VOLUME ONE

CLINICAL PEDIATRIC UROLOGY

Panayotis P. Kelalis, M.D.

Anson L. Clark Professor of Pediatric Urology
Mayo Medical School and Mayo Foundation
Rochester, Minnesota
and
Mayo Clinic Jacksonville
Jacksonville, Florida

Lowell R. King, M.D.

Professor of Surgery/Urology
Associate Professor of Pediatrics
Head, Section on Pediatric Urology
Department of Surgery
Duke University Medical Center
Duke University School of Medicine
Durham, North Carolina

A. Barry Belman, M.D.

Professor of Urology and Pediatrics
George Washington University School of Medicine
Chairman, Department of Pediatric Urology
Children's Hospital
Washington, D.C.

W.B. SAUNDERS COMPANY

Harcourt Brace Jovanovich, Inc.
Philadelphia   London   Toronto   Montreal   Sydney   Tokyo

THIRD EDITION

W. B. SAUNDERS COMPANY
Harcourt Brace Jovanovich, Inc.

The Curtis Center
Independence Square West
Philadelphia, Pennsylvania 19106

Library of Congress Cataloging-in-Publication Data

Clinical pediatric urology / Panayotis P. Kelalis, Lowell R. King,
A. Barry Belman.—3rd ed.
p. cm.

Includes bibliographical references and index.

ISBN 0–7216–3233–5

1. Pediatric urology. I. Kelalis, Panayotis P.
   (Panayotis Petrou). II. King, Lowell R.
   III. Belman, A. Barry.

[DNLM: 1. Urologic Diseases—in infancy & childhood.
WS 320 C643]

RJ466.C53 1992   618.92′6—dc20

DNLM/DLC   92–3593

Editor: W. B. Saunders Staff

Designer: Terri Siegel

Cover Designer: Megan Costello Connell

Production Manager: Peter Faber

Manuscript Editors: Carol Robins and Linda Weinerman

Illustration Specialist: Peg Shaw

Indexer: Mark Coyle

Clinical Pediatric Urology, 3rd edition   ISBN Volume I 0–7216–4449–X
                                                             Volume II 0–7216–4450–3
                                                          Two-Volume Set 0–7216–3233–5

Last digit is the print number: 9   8   7   6   5   4   3   2   1

☐ Contributors

IAN A. AARONSON, M.A., M.B., B.CHIR., F.R.C.S.

Professor of Urology and Pediatrics, Medical University of South Carolina. Chief of Pediatric Urology, Medical University Children's Hospital, Charleston, South Carolina.
Sexual Differentiation and Intersexuality

DAVID M. BARRETT, M.D.

Professor of Urology, Mayo Medical School. Chairman, Department of Urology, Mayo Clinic, Rochester, Minnesota.
Physiology of Micturition and Urodynamics

STUART B. BAUER, M.D.

Associate Professor of Surgery (Urology), Harvard Medical School. Associate in Surgery (Urology), Director of Neuro-urology, The Children's Hospital, Boston, Massachusetts.
Neuropathology of the Lower Urinary Tract

A. BARRY BELMAN, M.D.

Professor of Urology and Pediatrics, George Washington University School of Medicine. Chairman, Department of Pediatric Urology, Children's Hospital, Washington, DC.
Anomalies: Hypospadias and Other Urethral Abnormalities

DAVID A. BLOOM, M.D.

Associate Professor of Surgery, The University of Michigan Medical School. Chief, Pediatric Urology, Mott Children's Hospital, The University of Michigan, Ann Arbor, Michigan.
Disorders of the Male External Genitalia and Inguinal Canal

WILLIAM A. BROCK, M.D.

Professor of Urology, Albert Einstein School of Medicine, Bronx, New York. Chief, Division of Pediatric Urology, Schneider Children's Hospital, New Hyde Park, New York.
Cloacal Abnormalities and Imperforate Anus

MARK W. BURNS, M.D.

Assistant Professor of Urology, University of Washington School of Medicine. Staff Physician, Children's Hospital and Medical Center, Seattle, Washington.
Urinary Undiversion and Augmentation Cystoplasty

ROBERT L. CHEVALIER, M.D.

Professor and Vice-Chair, Department of Pediatrics, University of Virginia. Attending Pediatric Nephrologist and Director of Research and Development, Children's Medical Center, University of Virginia Health Sciences Center, Charlottesville, Virginia.
Renal Physiology and Function

BERNARD M. CHURCHILL, M.D.

Professor of Surgery, University of Toronto. Chief, Division of Urology, Hospital for Sick Children, Toronto, Ontario, Canada.
Pediatric Renal Transplantation

JACK S. ELDER, M.D.

Associate Professor of Urology, Case Western Reserve University School of Medicine. Director of Pediatric Urology, Rainbow Babies and Children's Hospital and Metro Health Hospital, Cleveland, Ohio.
Obstructive Uropathy: Obstruction: The Calyx

MAJID ESHGHI, M.D.

Associate Professor of Urology, Department of Urology, New York Medical College. Chief, Section of Endourology, Westchester County Medical Center, Valhalla, New York.
Obstructive Uropathy: Endoscopic Surgery of the Upper Tract in Children

R. BRUCE FILMER, M.B., B.S., F.R.A.C.S., F.R.C.S.

Associate Professor, Department of Urology, Thomas Jefferson University Medical School, Philadelphia, Pennsylvania. Chief, Division of Urology, Alfred I. duPont Institute, Wilmington, Delaware. Consultant, Pediatric Urologist, Thomas Jefferson University Hospital, Philadelphia; Medical Center of Delaware, Newark, Delaware; and St. Francis Hospital, Wilmington.
Renal Dysplasia, Renal Hypoplasia, and Cystic Disease of the Kidney

HOWARD C. FILSTON, M.D.

Professor of Pediatric Surgery and Pediatrics, University of Tennessee Graduate Medical Center. Chief, Division of Pediatric Surgery, Department of Surgery, University of Tennessee Memorial Medical Center. Active Staff, East Tennessee Children's Hospital, Knoxville, Tennessee.
Fluid and Electrolyte Management

STEVEN C. FLASHNER, M.D.
Associate, Pediatric Urology, Duke University Medical Center, Durham, North Carolina.
Obstructive Uropathy: Ureteropelvic Junction

ISRAEL FRANCO, M.D.
Assistant Professor of Urology, New York Medical College. Assistant Attending Physician, Westchester County Medical Center, Valhalla, New York.
Obstructive Uropathy: Endoscopic Surgery of the Upper Tract in Children

JOHN P. GEARHART, M.D.
Associate Professor of Pediatric Urology, Johns Hopkins University School of Medicine. Director of Pediatric Urology, James Buchanan Brady Urological Institute, Department of Urology, Johns Hopkins Hospital, Baltimore, Maryland.
Anomalies: Bladder and Urachal Abnormalities: The Exstrophy-Epispadias Complex

KENNETH I. GLASSBERG, M.D.
Professor of Urology, State University of New York, Brooklyn, New York. Director, Division of Pediatric Urology, State University Health Science Center, Kings County Hospital Center, and Long Island College Hospital, Brooklyn. Attending Physicians, Urology, Maimonides Medical Center, Brooklyn.
Renal Dysplasia, Renal Hypoplasia, and Cystic Disease of the Kidney

EDMOND T. GONZALES, JR., M.D.
Professor of Urology, Scott Department of Urology, Baylor College of Medicine. Head, Department of Surgery, and Chief, Urology Service, Texas Children's Hospital, Clinical Care Center, Houston, Texas.
Anomalies: Anomalies of the Renal Pelvis and Ureter

RICARDO GONZALEZ, M.D.
Professor, Department of Urologic Surgery, University of Minnesota. Director of Pediatric Urology, Variety Club Children's Hospital, University of Minnesota Hospital. Attending Urologist, Minneapolis Children's Medical Center, Minneapolis, Minnesota.
Urinary Incontinence

TERRY W. HENSLE, M.D.
Professor of Urology, Columbia University College of Physicians and Surgeons. Director, Pediatric Urology, Babies Hospital, and Columbia-Presbyterian Medical Center, New York, New York.
Urinary Diversion

DAVID E. HILL, M.D.
Clinical Assistant Professor of Urology and Pediatrics, Vanderbilt University School of Medicine. Active Staff, Baptist Hospital, Centennial Medical Center, and St. Thomas Medical Center, Nashville, Tennessee.
Genitourinary Infections: Specific Infections of the Genitourinary Tract

ALAN D. HOFFMAN, M.D.
Associate Professor of Radiology, Mayo Medical School. Staff Consultant, Saint Mary's Hospital and Rochester Methodist Hospital, Rochester, Minnesota.
Uroradiology: Procedures and Anatomy

WILLIAM C. HULBERT, JR., M.D.
Assistant Professor of Urology and Pediatrics, University of Rochester School of Medicine and Dentistry. Associate Chief of Urology, Rochester General Hospital; Attending Physician in Urology and Pediatrics, Strong Memorial Hospital and Rochester General Hospital. Attending Pediatric Urologist, University of Rochester Easter Seals Center, Rochester, New York.
Renal and Adrenal Vascular Thrombosis

GERALD R. JERKINS, M.D.
Assistant Professor of Urology, and Assistant Professor of Pediatrics, University of Tennessee. Active Staff, LeBonheur Children's Medical Center, and Consultant, St. Jude Children's Research Hospital, Memphis, Tennessee.
Genitourinary Trauma

GEORGE W. KAPLAN, M.D., M.S.
Clinical Professor of Surgery and Pediatrics, and Chief, Pediatric Urology, University of California at San Diego School of Medicine. Chief of Urology, Children's Hospital, San Diego, California.
Obstructive Uropathy: Infravesical Obstruction

EVAN J. KASS, M.D.
Chief, Division of Pediatric Urology, William Beaumont Hospital, Royal Oak, Michigan.
Obstructive Uropathy: Megaureter

ROBERT KAY, M.D.
Head, Section of Pediatric Urology, Cleveland Clinic Foundation, Cleveland, Ohio.
Genitourinary Tumors: Genital Tumors in Children

PANAYOTIS P. KELALIS, M.D.
Anson L. Clark Professor of Pediatric Urology, Mayo Medical School and Mayo Foundation, Rochester, Minnesota, and Mayo Clinic Jacksonville, Jacksonville, Florida.
Genitourinary Tumors: Upper Urinary Tract Tumors

DAVID W. KEY, M.D.
Staff Urologist, Miami Valley Hospital, Kettering Medical Center, and Dayton Children's Medical Center, Dayton, Ohio.
Disorders of the Male External Genitalia and Inguinal Canal

LOWELL R. KING, M.D.
Professor of Surgery/Urology; Associate Professor of Pediatrics; and Head, Section of Pediatric Urology, Department of Surgery, Duke University Medical Center, Durham, North Carolina.
Obstructive Uropathy: Ureteropelvic Junction

STANLEY J. KOGAN, M.D.
Clinical Professor of Urology, New York Medical College, Valhalla, New York. Adjunct Associate Professor of Pediatrics, Albert Einstein College of Medicine, Bronx, New York. Co-Director, Section of Pediatric Urology Westchester County Medical Center, Valhalla. Attending Pediatric Urologist, Montefiore Medical Center, Weiler Hospital of the Albert Einstein College of Medicine, and affiliated hospitals, Bronx.
Cryptorchidism

STEPHEN A. KRAMER, M.D.
Associate Professor of Urology, Mayo Medical School. Head, Section of Pediatric Urology, Mayo Clinic and Mayo Foundation, Rochester, Minnesota.
Genitourinary Infections: Specific Infections of the Genitourinary Tract; Vesicoureteral Reflux

R. LAWRENCE KROOVAND, M.D.
Professor of Surgery (Pediatric Urology) and Pediatrics, and Head, Section on Pediatric, Adolescent, and Reconstructive Urology, The Brenner Children's Hospital, Bowman Gray School of Medicine of Wake Forest University, Winston-Salem, North Carolina.
Endoscopy

ANDREW J. LeROY, M.D.
Associate Professor of Diagnostic Radiology, Mayo Medical School. Consultant in Diagnostic Radiology, Mayo Clinic, Rochester, Minnesota.
Uroradiology: Procedures and Anatomy

MASSOUD MAJD, M.D.
Professor of Radiology and Pediatrics, George Washington University School of Medicine, and Adjunct Professor of Radiology, Georgetown University School of Medicine. Director, Division of Nuclear Medicine, Department of Diagnostic Imaging and Radiology, Children's Hospital, Washington, D.C.
Nuclear Medicine in Pediatric Urology

JAMES MANDELL, M.D.
Associate Professor of Surgery, Harvard Medical School. Associate in Surgery, The Children's Hospital, Boston, Massachusetts.
Antenatal Diagnosis and Intervention in Urologic Diseases

PATRICK H. McKENNA, M.D.
Pediatric Urologist, Portsmouth Naval Hospital, Portsmouth, Virginia.
Pediatric Renal Transplantation

GORDON A. McLORIE, M.D., F.R.C.S.(C)
Associate Professor of Surgery, University of Toronto. Staff Urologist, Hospital for Sick Children, Toronto, Ontario, Canada.
Disorders of the Female Genitalia

PAUL A. MERGUERIAN, M.D.
Assistant Professor of Surgery (Urology) and Maternal and Child Health (Pediatrics), Dartmouth Hitchcock Medical Center and Dartmouth Medical School, Hanover, New Hampshire.
Disorders of the Female Genitalia

HRAIR-GEORGE J. MESROBIAN, M.D.
Associate Professor of Surgery and Pediatrics, University of North Carolina School of Medicine. Director of Pediatric Urology, University of North Carolina Hospitals, Chapel Hill, North Carolina.
Genitourinary Tumors: Upper Urinary Tract Tumors

DAWN S. MILLINER, M.D.
Assistant Professor of Pediatrics and Internal Medicine, Mayo Medical School. Staff Physician, St. Mary's Hospital and Methodist Hospital, Rochester, Minnesota.
Renal Parenchymal Disorders

MICHAEL E. MITCHELL, M.D.
Professor of Pediatric Urology, University of Washington School of Medicine. Chief, Division of Pediatric Urology, Children's Hospital and Medical Center, Seattle, Washington.
Urinary Undiversion and Augmentation Cystoplasty

BRUCE ZACHARY MORGENSTERN, M.D.
Assistant Professor of Pediatrics, Mayo Medical School. Pediatric Nephrologist, St. Mary's Hospital, Rochester Methodist Hospital, Rochester, Minnesota.
Renal Parenchymal Disorders

C. RICHARD MORRIS, M.D.
Associate Professor, University of North Carolina. Attending Physician in Pediatrics, University of North Carolina Hospitals, Chapel Hill, North Carolina.
Acute and Chronic Renal Failure in Children

H. NORMAN NOE, M.D.
Professor of Urology, Chief, Pediatric Urology, University of Tennessee. Chief of Urology, LeBonheur Children's Medical Center, and Consultant, St. Jude Children's Research Hospital, Memphis, Tennessee.
Genitourinary Trauma

ALBERTO PEÑA, M.D.
Professor of Surgery, Albert Einstein College of Medicine, New York, New York. Chief, Pediatric Surgery, Schneider Children's Hospital, Long Island Jewish Medical Center, New Hyde Park, New York.
Cloacal Abnormalities and Imperforate Anus

CRAIG A. PETERS, M.D.
Assistant Professor of Surgery, Harvard Medical School. Assistant in Surgery, The Children's Hospital, Boston, Massachusetts.
Antenatal Diagnosis and Intervention in Urologic Diseases

RONALD RABINOWITZ, M.D.
Professor of Urology and Pediatrics, University of Rochester School of Medicine. Attending Pediatric Urologist, Strong Memorial Hospital and Rochester General Hospital. Chief of Urology, Rochester General Hospital. Attending Pediatric Urologist, University of Rochester Children's Disability Center, Rochester, New York.
Renal and Adrenal Vascular Thrombosis

EDWARD F. REDA, M.D.
Assistant Professor of Urology at New York Medical College. Assistant Attending Physician, Westchester County Medical Center. Director of Pediatric Urology Lincoln Hospital, Valhalla, New York.
Obstructive Uropathy: Endoscopic Surgery of the Upper Tract in Children

KENNETH S. RING, M.D.
Clinical Instructor in Urology, College of Physicians and Surgeons of Columbia University, New York, New York. Attending Urologist, Overlook Hospital, Summit, New Jersey.
Urinary Diversion

MICHAEL RITCHEY, M.D.
Assistant Professor, Section of Urology, University of Michigan. Staff Physician, Mott Children's Hospital, Ann Arbor, Michigan.
Anomalies: Anomalies of the Kidney

KENNETH N. ROSENBAUM, M.D.
Associate Professor, Department of Pediatrics, George Washington University. Chairman, Medical Genetics, Children's Hospital, Washington, D.C.
Genetics and Dysmorphology

H. GIL RUSHTON, M.D.
Associate Professor Urology and Pediatrics, The George Washington University School of Medicine. Vice-Chairman, Department of Pediatric Urology, Children's Hospital, Washington, D.C.
Genitourinary Infections: Nonspecific Infections; Enuresis

HAL C. SCHERZ, M.D.
Assistant Clinical Professor Surgery/Urology, University of California, San Diego. Staff Physician, Children's Hospital Health Center, Pediatric Urology, and University of California San Diego Medical Center, San Diego, California.
Obstructive Uropathy: Infravesical Obstruction

JOSEPH W. SEGURA, M.D.
Carl Rosen, Professor of Urology, Mayo Medical School. Consultant in Urology, Mayo Clinic, St. Mary's Hospital, and Methodist Hospital, Rochester, Minnesota.
Urolithiasis

CURTIS A. SHELDON, M.D.
Associate Professor of Urology, University of Cincinnati. Director of Pediatric Urology, Children's Hospital Medical Center, Cincinnati, Ohio.
Obstructive Uropathy: Multicystic Kidney Disease; Pediatric Renal Transplantation

ARNOLD SHKOLNIK, M.D.
Professor of Clinical Radiology, Northwestern University Medical School. Attending Radiologist, Head, Division of Ultrasound, The Children's Memorial Hospital, Chicago, Illinois.
Ultrasonography of the Urogenital System

DANIEL SHOSKES, M.D.
Fellow, University of Oxford, Headington, Oxford, England.
Pediatric Renal Transplantation

STEVEN J. SKOOG, M.D.
Associate Professor of Urology, Uniformed Services University of the Health Sciences, Bethesda, Maryland. Director Pediatric Urology, Walter Reed Army Medical Center, Washington, D.C.
Prune-Belly Syndrome

LYNWOOD H. SMITH, M.D.
Professor of Medicine, Mayo Medical School. Consultant, Nephrology, Internal Medicine and Urol-

ogy, and Staff, St. Marys Hospital, and Methodist Hospital, Rochester, Minnesota.
Urolithiasis

BRENT W. SNOW, M.D.

Associate Professor of Surgery, University of Utah School of Medicine. Staff Physician, Primary Childrens Medical Center, Salt Lake City, Utah.
Genitourinary Tumors: Tumors of the Lower Urinary Tract

HOWARD McC. SNYDER III, M.D.

Associate Professor of Urology in Surgery, University of Pennsylvania School of Medicine. Associate Director, Division of Pediatric Urology, Children's Hospital of Philadelphia, Philadelphia, Pennsylvania.
Genitourinary Tumors: Adrenal Sympathetic Chain, and Retroperitoneal Tumors

JEFFREY WACKSMAN, M.D.

Assistant Professor of Urology, University of Cincinnati. Associate Director of Pediatric Urology, Children's Hospital Medical Center, Cincinnati, Ohio.
Obstructive Uropathy: Multicystic Kidney Disease

R. DIXON WALKER III, M.D.

Professor of Surgery and Pediatrics, University of Florida College of Medicine. Chief, Pediatric Urology, Shands Hospital, Gainesville, Florida.
Presentation of Genitourinary Disease and Abdominal Masses

JULIAN WAN, M.D.

Lecturer, University of Michigan Medical School. Fellow, University of Michigan Hospitals, Ann Arbor, Michigan.
Disorders of the Male External Genitalia and Inguinal Canal

ALAN J. WEIN, M.D.

Professor and Chairman, Division of Urology, University of Pennsylvania School of Medicine. Chief of Urology, Hospital of the University of Pennsylvania, Philadelphia, Pennsylvania.
Physiology of Micturition and Urodynamics

ROBERT M. WEISS, M.D.

Professor and Chief, Section of Urology, Yale University School of Medicine. Attending Physician in Urology, Yale–New Haven Hospital, New Haven, Connecticut.
Obstructive Uropathy: Pathophysiology and Diagnosis

DELBERT R. WIGFALL, M.D.

Assistant Professor of Pediatrics, Duke University. Acting Chief, Division of Pediatric Nephrology, Duke University Medical Center. Director of Pediatric Dialysis, Duke University Hospital, Durham, North Carolina.
Systemic Arterial Hypertension in Children and Adolescents

□ Preface

Sixteen years have passed since the first edition of *Clinical Pediatric Urology*. During this interval, epochal changes have occurred, the most significant of which, beyond any doubt, is the recognition of pediatric urology as the first true subspecialty of urology. Even though to this day pediatric urologists have not been duly recognized by certification, we are found in all major medical centers, devoting our time and effort almost exclusively to the practice of our subspecialty. This need for specialized training and development of expertise has been duly recognized by the Residency Review Committee in Urology in their publication *Special Requirements in Training for Pediatric Urology*.

All chapters in the third edition have been completely rewritten, in many instances by new authors, thus bringing the subject matter up to date, clearly reflecting the changes in the field, and adding a new perspective in the approach to the clinical problems.

We earnestly believe that the information in this edition is the "state of the art." At the same time we realize that, in a work of this magnitude, omissions may occur. This work is meant to be neither an encyclopedia nor, for that matter, a compendium of rare congenital anomalies. Rather, as in the previous editions, our overriding consideration has been to present material that lives up to the title of the book—clinical in orientation and, we hope, practical in presentation. We have made an effort to include detailed and comprehensive material seldom available in one place.

The multiauthor format in an area of constantly expanding knowledge permits the presentation of a complete and authoritative overview in each area; unavoidably, some areas overlap. We have generally viewed this as an advantage, realizing that this allows individual chapters to be developed in a coherent fashion. Therefore, any slight differences should serve to expand understanding rather than cause confusion.

The editors have not challenged statements, except for minor rewritings, that may conflict with the views of others, especially our own, since the contributors have tried not only to weigh the statements in their own experience but also to base these on scientific data when available.

Once again, we are deeply indebted to our contributors, past and present, for their sincere efforts and cooperation despite their ever-increasing professional commitments and other responsibilities. Without them, this work would have been impossible to complete. The truth is theirs; the mistakes are ours.

We also thank W. B. Saunders Company, our publisher, and Miss Carol Robins, manuscript editor, for their cooperation and understanding during the production of this work.

PANAYOTIS P. KELALIS
LOWELL R. KING
A. BARRY BELMAN

☐ Contents

VOLUME ONE

VOLUME TWO

1

☐ Antenatal Diagnosis and Intervention in Urologic Diseases

James Mandell and Craig A. Peters

DIAGNOSIS

Historical Perspectives

The development of fetal diagnosis has been closely linked with evolving aspirations of intervening on behalf of the fetus in order to prevent the progress of destructive processes. Although these goals remain somewhat elusive in the urologic realm, prenatal diagnostic capabilities are continuing to improve, thus providing the basis for possible effective prenatal therapy in the future. The early use of prenatal ultrasonography was similar to the use of plain film gestational radiography, in that it was used mainly for detecting fetal number, position, and size. This modality rapidly evolved through improvements both in imaging technology and observer experience to allow late first trimester diagnosis of gender, skeletal abnormalities, and parenchymal changes, especially the fluid-filled structures in the urinary tract. The ability to assess fetal digits, skin folds, and cardiac defects has led to earlier recognition of possible syndromic or chromosomal abnormalities (Benacerraf et al).

Prenatal Assessment

Ultrasonography

The fetal kidney and collecting systems are often detectable by ultrasound scanning as early as 15 weeks of gestation because of the acoustic characteristics of the tissue-fluid interface. Ultrasonography permits the early recognition of significant hydronephrosis and macrocystic dysplasias. Similarly, the amniotic fluid is readily visualized, and since this is composed mainly of fetal urine from 16 weeks of gestation onward, amniotic fluid volume serves as an additional reflection of urinary output (Seeds). Renal parenchymal dysplasia may be detectable as increased echogenicity. This is usually considered an irreversible condition, yet this finding is not uniformly detected when dysplasia is present. Real-time studies of the bladder permit an indirect assessment of urine production rates by way of bladder filling and emptying.

Anatomic resolution is usually precise enough to permit demonstration of renal duplications, a dilated ureter, a dilated posterior urethra, bladder wall thickness, and some penile abnormalities, all of which are important pieces of information in establishing the most accurate diagnosis. Maternal-fetal ultrasonography remains the cornerstone of prenatal urology, providing a highly sensitive, accurate, and noninvasive diagnostic tool, but it is not without its limitations.

Prenatal ultrasound scanning remains appreciably "operator-dependent," and variation in the reliability of examinations performed by different operators is a characteristic. Obstetric ultrasonography has been categorized into levels of thoroughness to attempt to reduce the impact of this feature. We recommend that any fetus with a suspected urinary tract abnormality should undergo a level 2 examination. We have found that although in a majority of the cases referred for further prenatal examination the suspected abnormality will be confirmed and evaluated in greater detail, a large number will be normal. In general, prenatal ultrasonography is a highly sensitive but less specific means of diagnosis, making it an ideal screening tool, for which it is being increasingly applied. When applicable, further diagnostic

1

options are specifically available for urologic anomalies.

Fetal Urine Electrolytes

Assessment of renal function in the postnatal period is most accurately accomplished with urinary electrolyte and clearance studies. These are available in the prenatal period to a limited extent. Urinary osmolarity and concentrations of sodium, chloride, and calcium have been studied and correlated to postnatal renal functional outcome (Grannum et al). Useful normal standards are just becoming available for comparison and may permit more precise interpretation of this information. At present, such tests are the best available and are reasonably safe, but remain nonspecific and subject to significant false-positive and false-negative interpretations. Prolonged in utero catheterizations of the urinary tract to permit measurements of urine flow rate and to obtain clearance data have been achieved but are subject to much higher risks of infection and amniotic fluid leakage. Interpretation is not straightforward, in that few normals have been studied and prenatal urinary clearances are much lower than postnatal clearances and evolve throughout gestation. Sensitive and specific markers of prenatal renal status remain to be identified.

Fetoscopy

Direct visualization of the fetus has been used in the identification of certain disorders with gross physical manifestations and has been applied on an experimental basis for intervention. As a method of placing shunting catheters under direct vision, this may permit prenatal therapy with significantly reduced morbidity. At present, its role remains speculative.

Chorionic Villus Sampling, Percutaneous Umbilical Blood Sampling, and Amniocentesis

Chorionic villus sampling (CVS) and percutaneous umbilical blood sampling (PUBS) have become, in recent years, key tools in the armamentarium of the obstetrician. Very early diagnosis of chromosomal abnormalities, at 8 to 10 weeks, is possible with CVS. New techniques also permit early diagnosis of various genetic diseases. PUBS has become a safe, accepted technique for fetal diagnosis and therapy, permitting direct access to the blood stream of the fetus. Amniocentesis remains the standard invasive fetal diagnostic tool and allows a wide variety of diagnoses to be made before 20 weeks' gestation. New experimental techniques that may enhance the ability to assess and treat the fetus include direct in utero tissue biopsy, amnioinfusion, and in utero cardiac catheterization and valvuloplasty.

Clinical Spectrum

Fetal diagnosis of ureteropelvic junction obstruction (Fig. 1–1), ureterovesical obstruction (Fig. 1–2), bladder outlet obstruction (Fig. 1–3), multicystic dysplasia (Fig. 1–4), autosomal recessive polycystic kidney disease (ARPD) (Fig. 1–5), duplex anomalies (Fig. 1–6), and urinoma (Fig. 1–7) is possible in most instances. Less common diagnoses include the prune-belly syndrome, megalourethra, bladder and cloacal exstrophy, virilizing adrenal hyperplasia, imperforate anus with urinary tract involvement, and retroperitoneal cystic neuroblastoma.

In any prenatal urologic assessment, certain features should always be sought and integrated into the final diagnosis. The gestational age, body size, sex, and movements of the fetus are important basic parameters. The presence of other major structural anomalies, including skeletal, cardiac, and neurologic defects, may be critical in the determination of management. The amount of amniotic fluid, particularly over time, is particularly important in the assessment of bladder outlet obstruction and major renal abnormalities. Renal size and echogenicity, the presence of two kidneys, hydronephrosis, hydroureter, and bladder size and wall thickness must be determined. A dilated posterior urethra should be sought and the external genitalia assessed. Although the presence of a phallus most likely means a male fetus, intrascrotal testes are diagnostic. These features permit as accurate a diagnosis as possible on a single examination. Serial examinations add valuable information regarding growth and the evolution of the findings, all of which may contribute to the management plan.

Accuracy

The prenatal assessment of genitourinary defects can be fairly complete yet remains

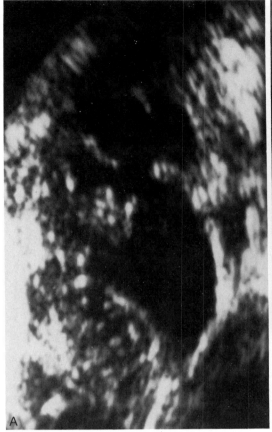

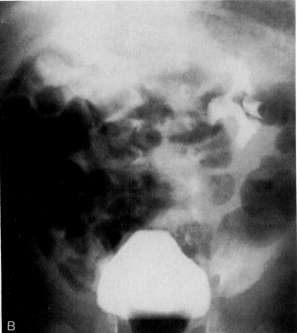

Figure 1–1 □ *A*, Maternal-fetal ultrasonogram at 36 weeks demonstrates dilated fetal renal pelvis and calyces on the right side. *B*, Postnatal excretory urogram shows similar anatomy with right ureteropelvic junction obstruction.

nonspecific in terms prediction of renal function. The condition of the renal parenchyma is often very difficult to determine with accuracy (Avni et al; Blane et al; Scott and Renwick), and although renal echogenicity in the setting of hydronephrosis is reasonably specific for dysplasia, it is not uniformly present. There is also a relatively large margin of error in defining the exact level of obstruction in many cases. Inability to visualize a dilated ureter resulting from positioning of the fetus, operator inexperience, or misinterpretation as bowel is a frequent cause for these misdiagnoses. Reflux may be difficult to diagnose prenatally with any degree of certainty (Scott). The late development of ARPKD can also lead to very difficult decisions for the family and physician (Townsend et al).

Natural History of Fetal Hydronephrosis

Much remains to be learned about the natural history of antenatally diagnosed genito-urinary defects. What we have seen is that the milder degrees of hydronephrosis occasionally worsen but most often remain stable or improve (Mandell et al). There is also a recognized overestimation of the degree of hydronephrosis compared with that seen on the postnatal examination (Kleiner et al). The more severe the degree of dilatation of the pelvis and calyces, the more likely the infant will need surgical correction (Arger et al; Mandell et al). The specific finding of caliectasis is an important indicator of the need for postnatal follow-up.

In view of the fact that no specific predictions regarding postnatal outcome may be made on the basis of prenatal ultrasonographic findings, postnatal follow-up evaluation is essential in all but the very mildest cases. As a result of physiologic neonatal oliguria during the first 2 days of life, the initial postnatal scan should be performed after that time and within 2 weeks. In cases of suspected total outlet obstruction, (i.e., males with a history of bilateral hydronephrosis and megacystis), prompt postnatal evaluation is appropriate.

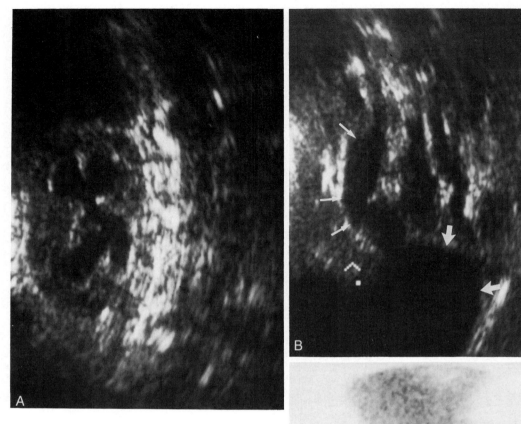

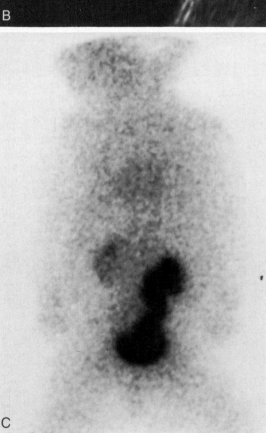

Figure 1–2 □ *A,* Maternal-fetal ultrasonogram at 32 weeks demonstrates dilated fetal pelvis and calyces on the right side. *B,* The dilated distal ureter (*small arrows*) can be seen entering the fetal bladder (*large arrows*). *C,* The postnatal renal scan shows the prolonged washout of radionuclide from the right pelvis and ureter after furosemide (Lasix) administration. (Used with permission from Mandell J, Peters CA, Retik AB: Current concepts in the perinatal diagnosis and management of hydronephrosis. Urol Clin North Am 17:247, 1990.)

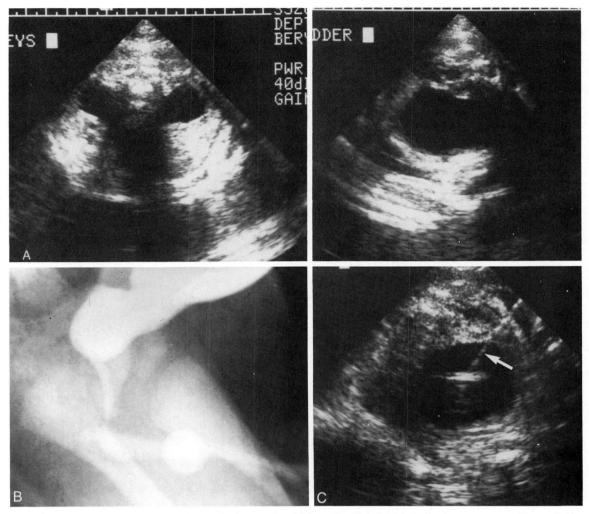

Figure 1–3 □ *A,* The composite maternal-fetal scan shows bilaterally dilated upper collecting systems and large, fluid-filled fetal bladder. *B,* The neonatal voiding cystourethrogram shows the dilated prostatic urethra characteristic of posterior urethral valves. (Used with permission from Mandell J, Peters CA, Retik AB: Current concepts in the perinatal diagnosis and management of hydronephrosis. Urol Clin North Am 17:247, 1990.) *C,* Ultrasound image of a fetal bladder tap at 22 weeks performed to obtain urinary indices. Arrow indicates the percutaneously introduced needle.

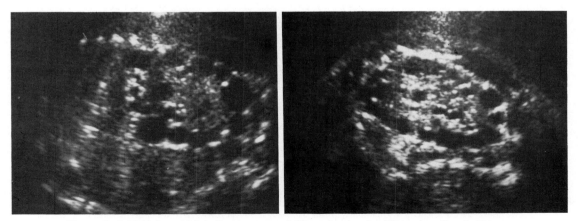

Figure 1–4 □ Maternal-fetal ultrasonogram at 28 weeks showing bilateral multicystic kidneys.

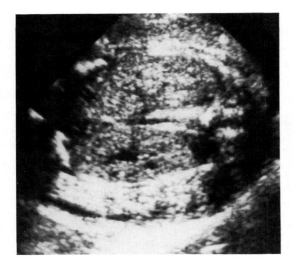

Figure 1–5 □ Maternal-fetal ultrasonogram at 24 weeks demonstrating bilaterally large, echogenic kidneys characteristic of autosomal recessive polycystic kidney disease.

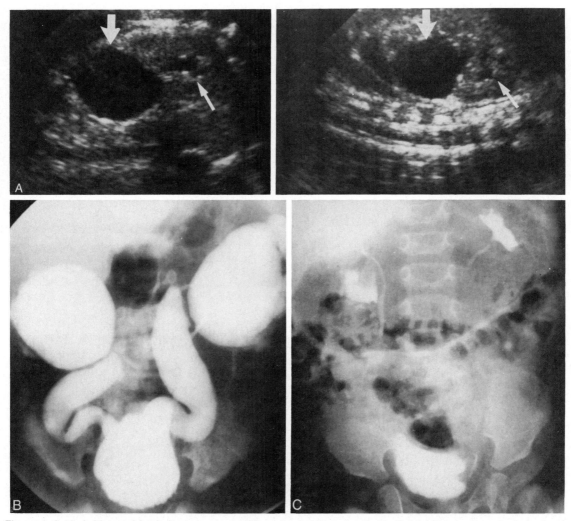

Figure 1–6 □ *A*, Maternal-fetal ultrasonogram at 36 weeks demonstrates that both fetal kidneys have hydronephrotic *lower* pole systems (*large arrows*) with delicate *upper* systems (*small arrows*). *B*, Postnatal voiding cystourethrogram shows massive bilateral lower pole reflux. *C*, Excretory urogram demonstrates both systems on the right and the upper pole on the left. The left lower pole did not function on radionuclide scans.

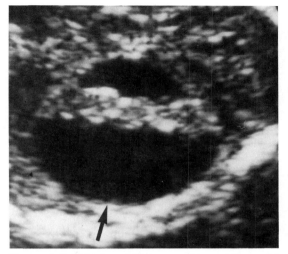

Figure 1–7 □ Maternal-fetal scan demonstrates mild fullness of the fetal renal pelvis with large perinephric urinoma (*arrow*).

PRENATAL INTERVENTION

Historical Aspects

Prenatal intervention for urologic diseases barely has a decade of history, yet the concept of treating the fetus and thereby necessarily exposing the mother to specific risks is certainly not new. Previous in utero medical therapies have included cardiotropic agents for fetal tachyarrhythmias (Harrigan et al; Newberger and Keane), exogenous thyroid hormone supplementation for hypothyroidism (Redding et al), medical treatment for Rh isoimmunization (Stenchever), treatment of congenital adrenal hyperplasia to prevent virilization in the affected female (Pang et al), and corticosteroid administration to hasten fetal lung maturity (Depp et al).

The historical aspects of a more invasive interventional approach also go back many years. Liley in 1963 reported intrauterine fetal transfusion in severe erythroblastosis (Liley). This was performed under fluoroscopy with about a 50 per cent accuracy in placement but allowed repeated transfusions until delivery was appropriate. Shortly thereafter, Freda and Adamsons, followed by Ascencio et al, reported the use of open hysterotomy with direct cannulation of the fetus as a method of permitting exchange transfusion with subsequent continuation of the pregnancy. Over time, the percutaneous method of transfusion became the standard method of treatment and further modifications have included direct fetal umbil-

ical vessel cannulation under ultrasound guidance (Seeds and Bowes). Fetal and maternal morbidity have been reduced to acceptably low levels.

Other types of direct intervention, including fetal ventricular shunting for hydrocephalus (Glick et al, 1984), have already fallen into disfavor, whereas experience with intrauterine open correction of congenital diaphragmatic hernia remains in its infancy (Harrison et al, 1990). The emerging field of ultrasonography in these instances, as in many others, has revolutionized the field of fetal diagnosis and has encouraged the possibility of altering the course of certain morbid fetal conditions.

In 1982, two important developments occurred that began the widespread scientific and public interest in the field of fetal urinary intervention. Golbus et al reported the percutaneous placement of a vesicoaminiotic shunt in one of twins at 32 weeks' gestation. This fetus, who was found to have severe hydronephrosis and megacystis presumed to be secondary to bladder outlet obstruction, was born 2 weeks later with the apparent diagnosis of prune-belly syndrome. The baby did well with subsequent postnatal therapy. The same group had previously reported an open hysterotomy with fetal urinary diversion for a 21-week gestational fetus presumed to have the same diagnosis (Harrison et al, 1981). That pregnancy continued to 35 weeks, but at birth the infant could not be ventilated and died. These cases as well as others created a media response that fueled the hope for in utero correction of congenital defects. Equally significant, perhaps, was the establishment in the same year of the International Registry of Fetal Surgery at the University of Manitoba, Canada. This represented the first attempt to gather and compile data on patients on whom interventions had been performed with an attempt at outcome analysis. The registry involved voluntary reporting of cases from several institutions with no specific prospective protocols for selection or treatment. Many individual reports continued to be published in the next few years involving acute and chronic drainage procedures for fetal hydronephrosis.

The indications for these procedures, the existing fetal conditions, and the maternal and fetal outcomes varied considerably between reports (Appleman and Golbus; Berkowitz et al; Bruno et al; Harrison et al, 1982a, 1982b; Kirkinen et al; Manning et al, 1983; McFadden et al; Shalev et al). The first survey from the fetal registry was published in 1986 (Manning et al, 1986) and provided further information as to the prenatal conditions affecting the patients in whom these procedures were performed. The wide variety of indications suggested a lack of consensus as to the role of these procedures. The perinatal mortality was 52 per cent, with a relatively high rate of complications. Multiple procedures (from two to seven per patient) were performed in more than 90 per cent of the patients. Poor documentation of postnatal diagnosis and renal function further clouded the reported success rate. Subsequent review articles questioned whether the overall benefit of prenatal intervention had been documented despite the large number of reports (Elder et al; Kramer; Sholder et al).

Some reports have demonstrated that technical innovations are still being made in this field. Changes in catheter configuration may have allowed longer-term diversion with less need for multiple procedures (Rodeck, personal communication). Open fetal vesicostomy has also been shown to be technically feasible with maintenance of pregnancy (Cromblehome et al, 1988). However, the reported details of prenatal and postnatal urologic parameters in these patients do not permit a definitive conclusion as to the actual benefit of the in utero intervention.

At present, the initial wave of enthusiasm for prenatal intervention for urologic diseases has ebbed. Few new cases are being reported to the Registry. This appears to be a product of the realization that although prenatal intervention is technically feasible and is sometimes clinically and experimentally justified, the risks and uncertainties must be well balanced by the anticipated benefits in the specific case. Concurrently, a strong interest in the natural history and pathophysiologic issues surrounding congenital obstructive uropathy is developing. This hiatus in clinical activity is also affording an opportunity for more careful development of the medical field of prenatal urology. This text reviews the major issues involved to provide a framework with which to evaluate the inevitable evolution of this field.

Aims of Intervention

The ultimate goal of a prenatal intervention for urologic conditions may not be as obvious as at first glance. Although decompression of the urinary tract is the clear initial aim, the ultimate goal may vary from saving the life of the newborn, to prolonging the interval until renal dialysis, to relieving maternal symptoms. Congenital hydronephrosis has been reported to induce maternal complications such as pain, hypertension, and toxemia (Seeds et al). Obstetric complications may also occur with an enlarged, obstructed urinary tract. Decompression in utero has a clear aim in those unusual cases.

At present the usual goal is to save the life of the newborn by preventing or reversing pulmonary hypoplasia, the usual cause of neonatal death in children with bladder obstruction and oligohydramnios. The clear-cut distinction between life or death provides a more acceptable justification for the maternal risks of the procedure. As those risks change and the ability to prognosticate with regard to renal outcomes improves, that goal may necessarily also evolve. Preventing significant renal damage alone may become similarly acceptable, even if the child's life is not immediately threatened. If in utero intervention would permit a child to live for 2 years without renal dialysis, in contrast to requiring it shortly after birth, the risks of prenatal intervention might be considered acceptable. Indeed, these risks will have probably been appreciably reduced by the time such determination is possible. The complications of neonatal renal dialysis or transplant are substantial in contrast to those in an older child. However, any consideration of expanding the aims of intervention in such a way is completely dependent upon an improved understanding of the natural history and pathophysiology of these diseases.

Indications for Therapy

At the current time, what are the indications for fetal intervention? Sonographic findings that indicate severe obstructive uropathy caused by bladder outlet obstruction include severe, persistent bilateral hydroureteronephrosis; cortical "thinning"; an enlarged, thick-walled bladder with impaired emptying; and reduced amniotic fluid. The degree of echogenicity of the renal parenchyma provides a rough estimate of the degree of maturational maldevelopment; we call this obstructive dysplasia (Mahony et al). This finding is not always present and is, in our experience, not uniformly predictive. If present and if accompanied by widespread microcystic changes, this finding suggests irreversible renal damage. Bladder refilling after aspiration provides some idea about urine flow rate, but not the quality of glomerular or tubular function. Many attempts have been made to provide a functional correlation with fetal urinary indices. Urine sodium, chloride, calcium, osmolality, and creatinine have been investigated (Cromblehome et al, 1990; Glick et al, 1985; Grannum et al, 1989). None of these, however, either singly or in combination, is uniformly predictive (Ruess et al; Wilkens et al). When taken together, all of these structural and biochemical findings may permit the categorization of renal outcome to a fairly good prognosis (with or without intervention) or to a very dismal one despite our best efforts. Fetuses with indeterminate findings are the ones we need to know more about, since they would be the ones most likely to benefit from timely intervention. It is in this group that further investigation into renal tubular enzymes and proteins, urinary metabolites, and other molecular markers may prove to be most helpful.

In addition to renal anatomic and functional indices, the fetal karyotype, general somatic survey, and indications of fetal maturity are important to determine. Unfortunately, no reproducible means of assessing lung maturation have been agreed upon (Nimrod et al). The ability to understand the interaction of fetal lung and kidney development may provide clues as to how to favorably influence this unique system.

In general, then, the situation in which we would consider intervening antenatally would be a male fetus younger than 30 weeks' gestation, with severe bilateral hydroureteronephrosis; an enlarged, thick-walled bladder; reduced amniotic fluid; "favorable" urine indices and renal parenchymal appearance; a normal karyotype; an otherwise normal fetal survey. Several options must be considered.

Management Options

Once a genitourinary defect has been noted, there are several potential options open for management.

Observation

The most obvious option is serial observation, not only to learn more about that particular patient's condition but also to gather information about the natural history of similar defects. One can determine serial measurements of renal pelvic diameter, notation of the renal parenchymal thickness and consistency, ureteral dilatation, bladder size, wall thickness and emptying, and amniotic fluid (Mandell et al, 1990). These findings all represent indirect assessment of fetal renal functional as well as structural status. How often to reassess these findings must be decided on the severity of the abnormality. We often recommend a second maternal-fetal ultrasonogram for what we consider moderate or severe dilatation, especially if the first study is performed before 30 weeks' gestation.

Termination

If the defect is felt to be incompatible with postnatal life, either with or without any type of fetal intervention, termination is currently a management option, in most states, before 24 weeks. For less severe defects, we simply inform the family of the range of expected outcomes based on the initial or subsequent findings.

Early Delivery

Early delivery becomes an option only if the continued maintenance of the pregnancy either offers no benefit or presents a threat to the health of the mother or fetus. One obvious example is premature rupture of the membranes, which is usually not specifically related to any urologic lesion. The mother is at risk for chorioamnionitis, and the child may not gain any further lung maturity. There are rare instances, however, in which either late occurrence or diagnosis of oligohydramnios is seen with obstructive uropathy or in which intervention has allowed continuation of the pregnancy for a limited time. In this situation, if the gestational age is 30 weeks or greater and the lecithin-to-sphingomyelin (L/S) ratio indicates lung maturity with or without steroid treatment (Depp et al), early delivery becomes a viable alternative. In most situations in which fetal genitourinary defects are diagnosed, we recommend routine obstetric care with full-term delivery at the primary care facility.

Percutaneous Shunting

The interventional technique of percutaneous drainage of the fetal urinary system has been performed in many centers. Very few have experience with more than a few cases, and often there is limited communication between obstetric and pediatric urologic consultants prior to these procedures. In the milieu of an experienced, multidisciplinary fetal research, diagnostic, and treatment center, fetal intervention can be performed with reasonable safeguards for technical considerations, coordination with postnatal caregivers, and adequate counseling for the mother. This technique, performed with the mother under local anesthesia and sedation, requires the creation of an artificial amniotic space by ultrasound-guided instillation of saline (Seeds and Mandell, 1988). The catheter is then placed into the fetal bladder, with one end left in the recreated amniotic space. Several catheters have been used for this. Earlier catheters (Glick et al, 1984; Seeds and Mandell, 1986) have been plagued by limited time of performance because of dislodgment or occlusion from debris. The Rodeck catheter (Rocket-London) appears to provide a longer period of time with adequate drainage, but this is a large catheter (13 Fr.), and several cases of iatrogenic bowel herniation through the abdominal wall have been seen (Robichaux et al, in press). The optimal catheter system, in terms of size, shape, and delivery, has yet to be devised.

Open Fetal Surgery

Direct fetal surgery through the open uterus has proved effective in providing adequate drainage and maintaining pregnancy (Cromblehome et al, 1988). Whether this technique, given the added risk to the mother for subsequent pregnancies, will prove to be beneficial enough remains to be seen. Certainly, a greater number of patients and better data will need to be collected. For example, two of the three survivors in the initial series of open fetal operations for urinary obstruction were females and without an identifiable cause for the presumed obstructive uropathy. Their natural outcome, if the patient is untreated, is very uncertain.

The future optimal management of those rare cases in which one sees severe obstructive uropathy with evidence of diminishing amniotic fluid remains a clear challenge. Certainly, if we are to prevent irreversible renal damage as well as pulmonary insufficiency, the criteria for treatment need to be more specific and sensitive. Perhaps fetoscopy with direct

placement of catheter drainage will become one technical option. Improved catheter configuration and placement techniques may allow safer, more permanent drainage. Open vesicostomy may yet prove to be the gold standard. An improved understanding of the natural history of prenatal urinary obstruction and the significance of available markers of renal function and irreversible fetal obstructive uropathy is essential in order to select and assess cases for fetal therapy. Combined clinical and laboratory initiatives offer the only solutions to these problems.

Ethics

Important ethical issues have been raised regarding the potential conflicting rights of the mother and fetus and the obligations of the involved physicians. There are necessary safeguards that need to be built into the process of decision making, including the participation of uninvolved physicians and nonphysicians; intra-institutional review boards; completely informed consent; and adequate levels of physician expertise. These interventions should be currently considered "experimental" and accepted as exposing the mother *and* fetus to specific risks. The issue of informed consent involves the understanding by the parents that treatment outcome may result in considerably less than normal renal and pulmonary function.

POSTNATAL CONSIDERATIONS

The principal advantages of prenatal diagnosis of congenital uropathies occur in the early postnatal period, permitting prompt protection of the newborn with prophylactic antibiotics and early definitive diagnostic evaluation. The prevention of sepsis and the early definitive treatment of severe obstruction are clearly the greatest present benefits of prenatal urologic diagnosis.

In most cases, evaluation may be deferred for several days to 2 weeks postnatally. Only in cases of possible bladder outlet or bilateral renal obstruction is immediate evaluation useful. In fact, renal ultrasonographic imaging in the first 2 days of life may be falsely normal because of the physiologic postnatal oliguria (Laing et al). Serum creatinine levels represent the mother's renal function, not the child's. Antibiotic administration to prevent infection in a possibly abnormal system, however, must be initiated immediately, with definitive diagnosis to follow. There is little risk to the newborn with the use of a penicillin-based agent. Sulfonamides should probably not be used within the first 1 to 2 months of life.

In cases of suspected bladder outlet obstruction, such as males with bilateral hydroureteronephrosis, immediate postnatal evaluation is appropriate. If decompression is indicated, it should be performed as soon as possible. Bilateral primary obstructive megaureters or bilateral vesicoureteral reflux may produce similar ultrasound findings. However, completely different management approaches are required.

The specifics of the postnatal management of congenital uropathies are dealt with elsewhere. The direction and pace of evaluation, rather than the particular diagnostic modalities, should be guided by the prenatal urologic findings.

Laboratory Research and Future Potential

The current status of assessment and treatment of fetal uropathies is that of a newly developing field of study (Peters and Mandell). Much remains to be learned, and careful clinical studies interrelated with investigation into the natural history and mechanisms of prenatal obstructive uropathy will be required. The tools of molecular and cellular biology are well suited and available to be applied in these investigations into the complex changes of obstruction imposed upon a dynamically growing and developing organ system with poorly defined interrelationships with other organ systems. The future for clinical intervention appears to be limited by the many ethical, legal, medical, and social factors one must deal with in such a field. The research potential, however, remains unlimited and must be the basis for subsequent clinical developments.

Bibliography

Acensio SH, Figueroa-Long JG, Pelegrina IA: Intrauterine exchange transfusion. Am J Obstet Gynecol 95:1129–1134, 1966.

Appelman Z, Golbus MS: The management of fetal urinary tract obstruction. Clin Obstet Gynecol 29:483–487, 1986.

Arger PH, Coleman BG, Mintz MC, et al: Routine fetal genitourinary screening. Radiology 156:485–489, 1985.

Avni EF, Rodeck F, Schulman CC: Fetal uropathies: diagnostic pitfalls and management. J Urol 134:921–925, 1985.

Benacerraf BR, Gelman R, Frigoletto FD Jr: Sonographic identification of second trimester fetuses with Down's syndrome. N Engl J Med 317:1371–1409, 1987.

Berkowitz RL, Glickman MG, Smith GJW, et al: Fetal urinary tract obstruction: what is the role of surgical intervention in utero? Am J Obstet Gynecol 144:367–375, 1982.

Blane CE, Koff SA, Bowerman RA, et al: Nonobstructive fetal hydronephrosis: sonographic recognition and therapeutic implications. Radiology 147:95–99, 1983.

Bruno AW, Lavin JP, Nasrallah PF: Ultrasound experience with prenatal genitourinary abnormalities. Urology 26:196–202, 1985.

Crombleholme TM, Harrison MR, Golbus MS, et al: Fetal intervention in obstructive uropathy: prognostic indicators and efficacy of intervention. Am J Obstet Gynecol 162:1239–1244, 1990.

Cromblehome TM, Harrison MR, Langer JC, et al: Early experience with open fetal surgery for congenital hydronephrosis. J Pediatr Surg 23:1114–1121, 1988.

Depp R, Boehm JJ, Nosek JA, et al: Antenatal corticosteroids to prevent neonatal respiratory distress syndrome: risk vs benefit benefit considerations. Am J Obstet Gynecol 137:338–350, 1980.

Elder JS, Duckett JW, Snyder HM: Intervention for fetal obstructive uropathy: has it been effective? Lancet 2:1007–1010, 1987.

Freda VJ, Adamsons K: Exchange transfusion in utero: report of a case. Am J Obstet Gynecol 89:817–821, 1964.

Glick PL, Harrison MR, Golbus MS, et al: Management of the fetus with congenital hydronephrosis. II. Prognostic criteria and selection for treatment. J Pediatr Surg 20:376–387, 1985.

Glick PL, Harrison MR, Nakayama DR: Management of ventriculomegaly in the fetus. J Pediatr 105:97–105, 1984.

Golus MS, Harrison MR, Filly RA, et al: In utero treatment of urinary tract obstruction. Am J Obstet Gynecol 142:383–388, 1982.

Grannum PA, Ghidini A, Scioscia A, et al: Assessment of fetal renal reserve in low level obstructive uropathy. Lancet 1:281–282, 1989.

Harrigan JT, Kangos JJ, Sikka A, et al: Successful treatment of fetal congestive heart failure secondary to tachycardia. N Engl J Med 304:1527–1529, 1981.

Harrison MR, Filly RA, Parer JJ, et al: Management of the fetus with a urinary tract malformation. JAMA 246:635–639, 1981.

Harrison, MR, Golbus, MS, Filly RA, et al: Fetal surgery for congenital hydronephrosis. N Engl J Med 306:591–593, 1982a.

Harrison MR, Golbus MS, Filly RA, et al: Management of the fetus with congenital hydronephrosis. J Pediatr Surg 17:728–742, 1982b.

Harrison MR, Langer JC, Adzick NS, et al: Correction of congenital diaphragmatic hernia in utero. V. Initial clinical experience. J Pediatr Surg 25:47–55, 1990.

Kirkinen P, Jouppila P, Tuononen S: Repeat transabdominal renocenteses in a case of fetal hydronephrotic kidney. Am J Obstet Gynecol 142:1049–1052, 1982.

Kleiner B, Callen PW, Filly RA: Sonographic analysis of the fetus with ureteropelvic junction obstruction. Am J Roentgenol 148:359–363, 1987.

Kramer, SA: Current status of fetal intervention for congenital hydronephrosis. J Urol 130:641–646, 1983.

Laing FC, Burke VD, Wing VW, et al: Postpartum evaluation of fetal hydronephrosis: optimal timing for follow-up sonography. Radiology 152:423–424, 1984.

Liley AW: Intrauterine transfusion of foetus in haemolytic disease. Br Med J 2:1107–1109, 1963.

Mahony BS, Filly FA, Callen PW, et al: Fetal renal dysplasia: sonographic evaluation. Radiology 152:143–146, 1984.

Mandell J: Prenatal diagnosis and treatment of obstructive uropathies. *In* Problems in Urology. Edited by SA Kramer. Philadelphia, JB Lippincott, in press.

Mandell J, Blyth B, Peters CA, et al: Structural genito-urinary defects detected in utero. Radiology 178:193, 1991.

Mandell J, Peters CA, Retik AB: Current concepts in the perinatal diagnosis and management of hydronephrosis. Urol Clin North Am 17:247–262, 1990.

Manning FA, Harman LR, Lange IR, et al: Antepartum chronic fetal vesicoamniotic shunts for obstructive uropathy: a report of two cases. Am J Obstet Gynecol 145:819–822, 1983.

Manning FA, Harrison MR, Rodeck C: Catheter shunts for fetal hydronephrosis: report of the International Fetal Surgery Registry. N Engl J Med 315:336–340, 1986.

McFadden IR: Obstruction of the fetal urinary tract: a role for surgical intervention in utero? Br Med J 288:459–462, 1984.

Newberger JW, Keane JF: Intrauterine supraventricular tachycardia. J Pediatr 95:780–786, 1979.

Nimrod C, Davies D, Stanislaw I, et al: Ultrasound prediction of pulmonary hypoplasia. Obstet Gynecol 68:495–498, 1986.

Pang S, Pollack MS, Marshall RN, Immken L: Prenatal treatment of congenital adrenal hyperplasia due to 21-hydroxylase deficiency. N Engl J Med 322:111–115, 1990.

Peters CA, Mandell J: Experimental congenital obstructive uropathy. Urol Clin North Am 17:437–447, 1990.

Redding RA, Douglas WHJ, Stern M: Thyroid hormone influence upon lung surfactant metabolism. Science 175:994, 1972.

Robichaux AG III, Mandell J, Greene MF, et al: Fetal abdominal wall defect: A new complication of vesicoamniotic shunting. Fetal Diagnosis and Therapy. In press.

Ruess A, Wladimiroff JW, Pijpers L, Provoost A: Fetal urinary electrolytes in bladder outlet obstruction. Fetal Ther 2:148–153, 1987.

Scott JES: Fetal ureteric reflux. Br J Urol 59:291–296, 1986.

Scott JES, Renwick M: Antenatal diagnosis of congenital abnormalities in the urinary tract. Br J Urol 62:295–300, 1987.

Seeds AE: Current concepts of amniotic fluid dynamics. Am J Obstet Gynecol 138:575–586, 1980.

Seeds JW, Bowes WA: Ultrasound guided fetal intravascular transfusions in severe rhesus immunization. Am J Obstet Gynecol 154:1105–1107, 1986.

Seeds JW, Cefalo RC, Herbert WN, et al: Hydramnios and maternal renal failure: relief with fetal therapy. Obstet Gynecol 64:26S, 1984.

Seeds JW, Mandell J: Congenital obstructive uropathies: pre- and postnatal treatment. Urol Clin North Am 13:155–165, 1986.

Seeds JW, Mandell J: Prenatal diagnosis and management of fetal obstructive uropathies. *In* Urologic Surgery in Neonates and Young Infants. Edited by LR King. Philadelphia, WB Saunders Co, 1988, pp 41–55.

Shalev E, Weiner E, Feldman E, et al: External bladder-amniotic fluid shunt for fetal urinary tract obstruction. Obstet Gynecol 63:315–345, 1984.

Sholder SJ, Maizels M, Depp R, et al: Caution in antenatal intervention. J Urol 139:1026–1029, 1988.

Stenchever MA: Promethazine hydrochloride: use in patients with isoimmunization. Am J Obstet Gynecol 130:665–668, 1978.

Townsend RR, Goldstein RB, Filly RA, et al: Sonographic identification of autosomal recessive polycystic kidney disease associated with increased maternal serum/amniotic fluid alpha-fetoprotein. Obstet Gynecol 71:1008–1012, 1988.

Wilkens IA, Chitkara V, Lynch L, et al: The nonpredictive value of fetal urinary electrolytes: preliminary report of outcome and correlations with pathologic diagnosis. Am J Obstet and Gynecol 157:694–698, 1987.

2

☐ Ultrasonography of the Urogenital System

Arnold Shkolnik

Since the 1985 edition of this text, the utilization of ultrasound scans for imaging the urogenital system of the pediatric patient has continued to increase at a rapid rate. This increase for diagnostic purposes, as well as for the guidance of interventive procedures, can be attributed to several factors.

Significant technologic advances have further broadened the clinical scope of ultrasound imaging. This is exemplified by the development of duplex and color-flow Doppler imaging. Increased use of prenatal ultrasound scanning has also resulted in the detection of a greater number of fetal urogenital abnormalities, which has further mandated greater utilization of ultrasonography for postnatal monitoring of these abnormalities. Additionally, larger numbers of requests for ultrasound examination continue to emanate from the referring pediatric physicians, who are continually updated regarding the state of the art by the ultrasound hospital staff; from local and national meetings; and from reports published in specialty journals.

THE ULTRASOUND EXAMINATION

The ultrasound examination is the most innocuous, and the most flexible, of the "special imaging" procedures. Its particular attributes are as follows:

1. The examination is essentially painless, and other than for the necessity or desirability of having the patient's bladder well distended during at least a part of the study, there is no special preparation required.

2. No significant biologic damage has been noted as a result of pulsed diagnostic ultrasonography (Baker and Dalrymple). Therefore, wherever applicable, this method of imaging is understandably highly desirable for primary investigations and for repetitive examinations when indicated (Slovis and Perlmutter).

3. The parents (or other family members or a favorite nurse) are encouraged to attend the study. In the vast majority of instances, this enhances patient reassurance, comfort, and cooperation. In my experience covering the past 15 years or more, the use of straps, tape, or other restraints for patient immobilization is seldom required and the need for patient sedation, other than for ultrasound-guided percutaneous procedures, has been exceedingly rare.

4. Scanning units are easily transportable, allowing examination of the compromised patient in the optimal life-support environment (Fig. 2–1). This capability has also resulted in further use of ultrasound guidance for a variety

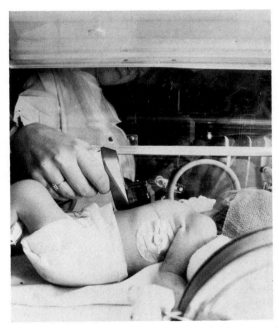

Figure 2–1 ☐ Real-time abdominal scanning in neonatal intensive care unit, performed through porthole of isolette.

13

of procedures undertaken in the operating room.

5. Imaging of each area examined is accomplished in at least two planes. To obtain comprehensive detail, however, additional imaging is frequently required in various obliquities, which can be readily accomplished. Also, the scanning can be performed with the patient in virtually any position.

6. There is very rapid accumulation of information. Since imaging is not dependent on organ function, instantaneous delineation of an abnormal kidney can be achieved (Shkolnik, 1977). To the deeply concerned parents of a child with a newly discovered flank mass, the relative benefit of promptly establishing the presence of hydronephrosis, as opposed to an intrarenal mass lesion, cannot be overlooked. Rapid recognition of a mass lesion is also associated with obvious benefits relative to decision making regarding further diagnostic procedures and treatment.

7. Real-time scanning, which has essentially supplanted articulated arm scanning, provides cross-sectional "echofluoroscopy," which can be directly viewed on the television monitor. Although diagnostic "freeze-frame" sector and linear sonograms, such as those displayed in the text, are routinely recorded on film, the examination can also be tape recorded, thereby allowing review of the dynamic as well as static aspects of the study. Although the majority of the sonograms presented in this chapter were achieved during real-time scanning, a number of the older, articulated arm images, which serve well to illustrate certain points, have been retained, allowing comparison of both methods.

THE UPPER URINARY TRACT

Kidney

Sonography enables kidney location and size to be determined. Linear measurements can be obtained in all three dimensions, thereby providing the means for calculating renal volume as well. A number of reports relative to renal measurements are listed in the bibliography.

Kidney configuration and morphology can also be delineated. Pelvocalyceal dilatation is quickly apparent. Variations from the normal echopattern of the renal parenchyma can aid in the recognition of parenchymal abnormalities and inflammatory processes as well as mass lesions and infiltrative disorders. Information in regard to renal vascular morphology and flow can be obtained.

Normal Kidney

The sonographic appearance of the normal kidney in the neonate is quite distinct (Fig. 2–2). The echogenicity of the relatively thin cortex (including the columns of Bertin), is essentially equal to that of normal liver parenchyma. In contrast, the *medullary pyramids* are prominent and hypoechoic; it is important that they not be mistaken for dilated calyces or cysts (Haller et al). Primarily as a result of paucity of fat, the renal sinus of the neonate is poorly echogenic and therefore at times quite indistinct. Conversely, the arcuate arteries are seen as strongly echogenic punctate foci (Cook et al), which provide a rough measure of peripheral cortical thickness.

The accentuated echogenicity of the neonatal renal cortex has been ascribed to an increased number of acoustic interfaces. This is a consequence of a greater percentage of glomeruli as well as greater cellularity of the glomerular tuft in the cortex of neonates. Additionally, 20 per cent of the loops of Henle are in the neonatal cortex rather than in the

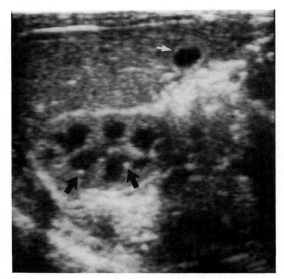

Figure 2–2 □ Normal kidney in neonate. Transverse linear sonogram demonstrates equal echogenicity of renal cortex and adjacent normal liver parenchyma. Arcuate arteries *(dark arrows)* are noted at base of hypoechoic medullary pyramids. Renal sinus echogenicity is vague. The gallbladder *(light arrow)* is mildly distended.

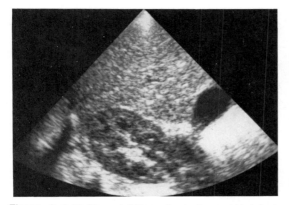

Figure 2–3 □ Normal kidney in a 1-year-old infant. Transverse sector sonogram demonstrates "adult" type parenchymal echogenicity, which is less intense than that of the normal liver parenchyma. Compared with neonatal kidney, there is increased thickness of the cortex with less pronounced corticomedullary demarcation. The renal sinus is more echogenic as a result of accumulation of fat. Several arcuate arteries can be seen. A distended gallbladder is noted.

medulla (Hricak et al). Progression to the "adult parenchymal pattern" (Fig. 2–3) occurs in 90 per cent of patients by 4 months of age (Hayden and Swischuk).

Prenatal Anomalies

The fetal kidneys can be identified initially by the 15th week of gestation. However, the definition of internal renal architecture is generally not feasible until after the 20th week (Hadlock et al), following which one or both kidneys can be identified approximately 95 per cent of the time (Lawson et al). The parameters of fetal kidney size and volume have been correlated with gestational age (Jeanty et al). The fetal bladder is also identifiable early in the second trimester, and changes in volume reflecting fetal urination can be noted with both static and real-time scanning. Oligohydramnios is a consistent manifestation of severe bilateral renal compromise in the fetus. Bilateral renal agenesis is additionally characterized by absence of bladder filling, even with the added stimulus of intravenous administration of furosemide to the mother.

The list of sonographically identifiable morphologic abnormalities of the fetal urogenital tract is extensive (Mahony). The most common abnormality noted during prenatal sonography is dilatation of the urinary tract. An example of ureteropelvic junction (UPJ) obstruction in a 35-week-old fetus is shown in Figure 2–4. In

Figure 2–5, the findings are demonstrated in a 26-week-old male fetus with subsequently documented posterior urethral valves.

The confirmation of posterior urethral valves has been achieved in utero by means of antegrade pyelography effected under ultrasonographic guidance (Gore et al). Intrauterine decompression of the kidneys, by means of ultrasonographically guided bladder drainage or nephrostomy, has been achieved in the presence of posterior urethral valves (Harrison et al) and bilateral UPJ stenosis (Vallancien et al). At the present time, however, the value and status of fetal urologic intervention are uncertain. Blane et al have pointed out that preservation of renal function in a fetus with severe obstructive hydronephrosis may necessitate very early intervention. However, an appreciable error rate in the diagnosis of certain fetal renal abnormalities can hinder the undertaking of interventive procedures. Avni et al reported that even with sequential fetal ultrasonography following previously detected abnormalities, a correct diagnosis was made in only 70 per cent of cases. The most common diagnostic problems were distinguishing be-

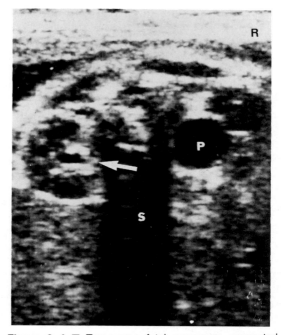

Figure 2–4 □ Transverse fetal sonogram, generated during real-time scanning, is displayed with white echoes on a black background. The right renal pelvis (P) is markedly dilated. Note mildly dilated appearance of left renal pelvis *(arrow)*, considered within normal limits, and the acoustic shadow (S) produced by the fetal spine. (Courtesy of Dr. Carlos Reynes, Loyola University Medical Center, Maywood, Illinois.)

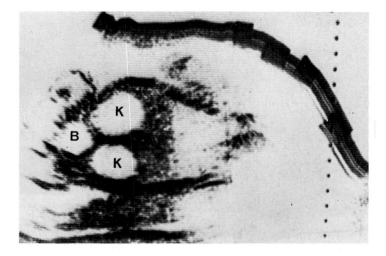

Figure 2–5 ☐ Articulated-arm antenatal sonogram demonstrates marked hydronephrosis of each kidney (K) and a prominently distended urinary bladder (B) in a 26-week fetus. (Courtesy of Dr. Carlos Reynes, Loyola University Medical Center, Maywood, Illinois.)

tween multicystic dysplastic kidney and ureteropelvic junction obstruction as well as differentiating dilatation as a result of severe reflux versus obstruction. Small, hypoplastic kidneys were infrequently visualized.

Findings in the Neonate

There are a number of clinical indications for renal assessment in the neonate, among which are a flank mass, urosepsis, evidence of renal failure, ascites, and abdominal distention of unknown etiology. In addition, a variety of physical findings and a number of syndromes are also known to be associated with an increased incidence of renal abnormalities (Dunbar and Nogrady). Some examples include malformed ears, abnormal external genitalia, imperforate anus, myelomeningocele, and the Eagle-Barrett syndrome.

Beyond the Neonate

All of the indications for renal assessment in the neonate may apply as well during infancy and beyond. However, as the patient grows older, the majority of requests for renal ultrasound assessment are for the purpose of investigating the cause for urinary tract infections and for patients requiring renal monitoring. This latter category includes patients with conditions predisposing to urinary tract infections, such as those with myelomeningocele as well as with those with a history of Wilms' tumor, and with conditions predisposing to the development of Wilms' tumor. Periodic evaluation

not infrequently is required for patients with renal transplant and other renal postoperative conditions.

Hydronephrosis

As mentioned, pelvicalyceal dilatation is readily identifiable. However, the cross-sectional appearance suggesting mild hydronephrosis may be normal, such as with a generous-sized extrarenal type pelvis. Additionally, a mild degree of true pelviectasia may also be clinically insignificant. This is exemplified by the transient dilatation of the renal pelvis during the phase of rapid diuresis following oral intake of a large volume of fluid (Fig. 2–6). A similar, but perhaps more persistent, distention may be present during the administration of parenteral fluids.

When observed during the real-time scanning procedure, the sudden appearance of or increase in pelvicalyceal dilatation (which may include evidence of turbulence) is consistent with high-grade vesicoureteral reflux (Kessler and Altman). This conclusion is also warranted when similar findings are noted either during or immediately following emptying of the bladder by the patient. Conversely, a post-voiding decrease in hydronephrosis can also be a valuable point of information.

In a large series of newborns with significant hydronephrosis, 75 per cent of which was discovered prenatally, Brown reported that no abnormality would have been suspected at birth in the majority, since the majority of the infants were asymptomatic. However, when an abdominal mass was noted in the newborn,

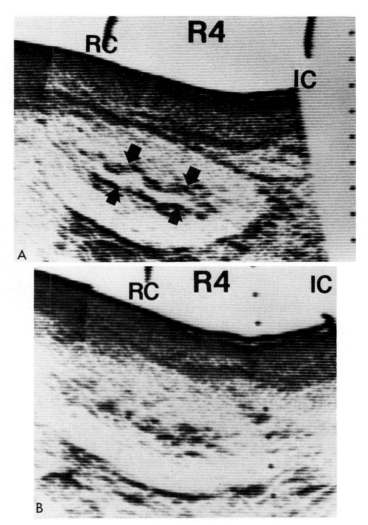

Figure 2–6 □ *A,* Longitudinal sonogram of a prone 6-year-old boy, 4 cm to right of midline, taken 15 minutes after copious oral fluid intake. There is mild separation of the walls of the renal pelvis *(arrows).* RC, base of rib cage; IC, posterior-superior iliac crest. *B,* On sonogram in same plane generated 15 minutes later, there is no evidence of pelvic dilatation.

obstructive uropathy accounted for the vast majority.

Ureteropelvic Junction Obstruction

The ureteropelvic junction represents the most common site of obstruction of the upper urinary tract and is one of two most common sources of a palpable flank mass in the neonate (the other being a cystic dysplastic kidney) (Lebowitz and Griscom). During the first year of life, there is a tendency toward bilaterality, particularly in boys. There is also an increased association of contralateral multicystic dysplastic kidney. Nearly all cases are congenital, as a result of intrinsic narrowing or extrinsic vascular compression at the UPJ.

Sonographically, pelvocalyceal dilatation without evidence of ureteral dilatation is noted. With more pronounced obstruction, the dilated pelvis extends downward and medially (Fig. 2–7) and, ultimately, pelvicalyceal differentiation becomes obliterated. The accompanying presence of a dilated ureter can reflect coexistent vesicoureteral reflux (Lebowitz and Blickman), or the underlying problem may be a primary megaureter.

Cystic Renal Disease

Cystic abnormalities affecting the kidneys range from diffuse involvement with profound renal impairment to focal asymptomatic lesions, some of which can be associated with a variety of congenital abnormalities.

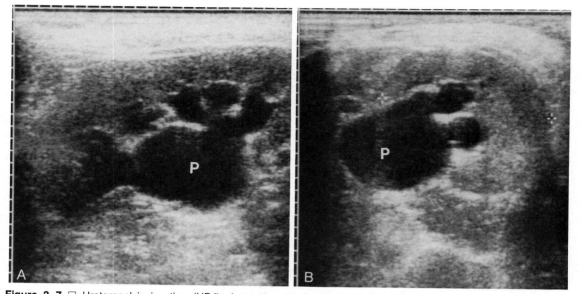

Figure 2–7 □ Ureteropelvic junction (UPJ) obstruction. *A,* On longitudinal linear sonogram, a moderately severe degree of pelvicalyceal dilatation is noted. There is no evidence of parenchymal loss, and cortical echogenicity appears normal. *B,* Corresponding appearance on transverse sonogram demonstrates prominent medial extension of the markedly dilated renal pelvis. Renal parenchyma, again visualized, is unremarkable in appearance. P, renal pelvis.

Multicystic Dysplastic Kidney

Multicystic dysplastic kidney (MDK) represents the most common cause of renal cystic disease presenting during infancy and, when hydronephrosis is excluded, the most common cause of an abdominal mass presenting in the neonate (Fernbach). There is a 20 to 25 per cent incidence of abnormality of the contralateral kidney, most commonly UPJ obstruction.

The appearance of the classic type of MDK is that of a cluster of discrete noncommunicating cysts ("bunch of grapes"). The largest cysts are peripheral (Stuck et al), and there is no evidence of a renal pelvis (Bearman et al) (Fig. 2–8). A less common hydronephrotic form of

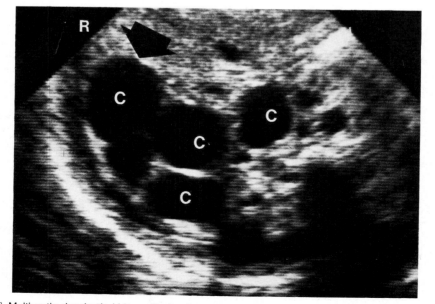

Figure 2–8 □ Multicystic dysplastic kidney. Supine transverse sector sonogram of a 6-day-old male with right flank mass, revealing multiple noncommunicating renal cysts (C), the largest of which is lateral *(arrow)*. A renal pelvis could not be identified.

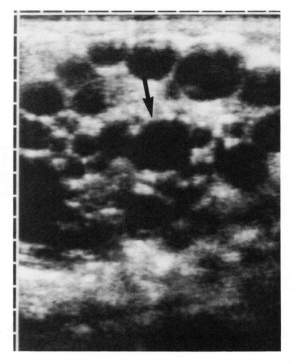

Figure 2–9 □ Multicystic dysplastic kidney. Linear longitudinal display of multicystic dysplastic kidney, with suggested presence of dilated renal pelvis *(arrow)*. A corresponding central appearance was also noted transversely.

MDK has been described (Felson and Cussen) in which a renal pelvis has been identified (as suggested in Fig. 2–9), and in which some degree of cyst communication has been documented.

At times, there may be difficulty in the sonographic differentiation of MDK from severe UPJ obstruction. In such instances, the radionuclide documentation of renal function is most often indicative of severe hydronephrosis. In rare instances, however, renal function has also been recorded in MDK. Thus, ultrasound-guided cyst puncture (with fluid analysis) and/or antegrade pyelography offers an additional or alternate means of diagnostic confirmation.

There has been a growing trend toward the nonsurgical approach to management of a patient with MDK (Gordon et al). Following serial sonography of 19 patients with MDK for a mean of 33.5 months, Vinocur et al reported that 9 per cent of the lesions disappeared within the first 3 years of follow-up and suggested that when the diagnosis of a classic MDK is made, the abnormal kidney may not have to be removed unless there is growth of the mass during the first year of life. Another form of cystic dysplasia exists in which large cysts form a less obvious component of this spectrum. The parenchyma appears dense, and normal architecture is absent (Fig. 2–10).

Autosomal Recessive Polycystic Kidney Disease (Infantile Polycystic Kidney Disease) (ARPKD)

Polycystic kidney disease presenting in the neonatal period is most often of the autosomal recessive type. The disease typically presents with poorly functioning, enlarged kidneys. There may be associated respiratory distress, as a result of pulmonary hypoplasia, and Potter's facies. The "cysts" represent ectatic renal tubules that provide innumerable acoustic interfaces, which are the source of the diffusely intense echogenicity characterizing these kidneys (Grossman et al). There is loss of corticomedullary differentiation, and unless there is dilatation of the pelvocalyceal system, loss of the renal sinus demarcation will also be evident.

A peripheral hypoechoic or sonolucent rim can be seen (Fig. 2–11). This was felt to represent the peripherally compressed renal cortex (Hayden and Swischuk). However, histologic examination of this area in one patient revealed replacement of the cortex by elongated, thin-walled cystic spaces (Currarino et al). Increased hepatic echogenicity is noted secondary to mild hepatic fibrosis and ductal hyperplasia.

In the spectrum of autosomal recessive polycystic kidneys, the degree of renal tubular

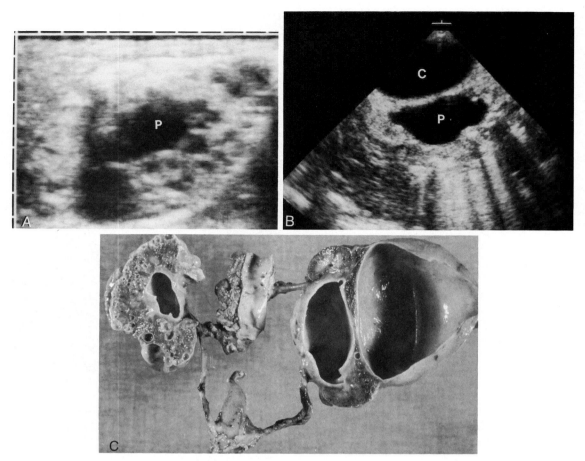

Figure 2–10 □ Severe bilateral obstructive dysplasia.

A, Longitudinal right linear sonogram in an anuric 3-day-old infant with bilateral flank masses demonstrates renal enlargement; configuration of the dilated renal pelvis suggests UPJ obstruction. There is blunting of the infundibulae, and multiple small cystic structures are noted throughout the parenchyma.

B, Coronal sector sonogram of the left kidney demonstrates appearance of renal pelvis (P) consistent with UPJ obstruction. A large noncommunicating peripheral ovoid cyst (C) is incorporated within the densely echogenic renal tissue.

C, Necropsy specimen with hemisection of each kidney. Obstruction of the proximal ureter was documented on each side by retrograde ureteral injection of methylene blue.

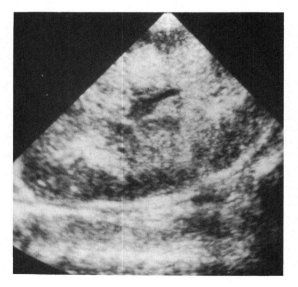

Figure 2–11 □ Autosomal recessive polycystic kidneys. Longitudinal presentation of markedly enlarged left kidney with intense somewhat heterogeneous echogenicity of the parenchyma. In the center of the parenchyma, a mildly dilated renal pelvis is visible. Peripheral echogenicity is diminished. The right kidney is essentially similar in appearance.

20

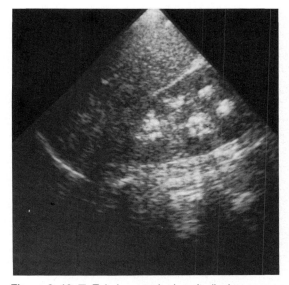

Figure 2–12 □ Tubular ectasia. Longitudinal sonogram of right kidney. Increased medullary echogenicity is apparent. The left kidney produced a similar appearance. On other views of the liver, some irregular increase in liver parenchymal echogenicity was identified, consistent with hepatic fibrosis.

ectasia and renal symptomatology may be minimal. The clinical picture then evolves later in childhood and is accompanied by portal hypertension and gastrointestinal bleeding resulting from hepatic fibrosis (Six et al). In this condition, the dilated collecting tubules can be seen during excretory urography, in the region of the renal pyramids. Sonographically, there is pronounced medullary echogenicity (Fig. 2–12).

Autosomal Dominant Polycystic Kidney Disease (Adult Polycystic Kidney Disease) (ADPKD)

This autosomal dominant abnormality has been identified prenatally and in infants and children, but it is much more frequently manifested in the adult. Typically, the well-defined cysts can be identified in the kidneys (Fig. 2–13). Cysts can also be found in the liver and, at times, in the spleen and pancreas as well. Berry aneurysms of the cerebral circulation occur in 10 to 15 per cent of patients. Ultrasonography is extremely sensitive for the detection of this condition, with a capability of identifying the cysts before they become large enough to produce their characteristic mass effect noted during excretory urography. For this reason, ultrasonography is useful for detecting the presence of this abnormality in family members of patients suspected of having ADPKD (Lufkin et al).

Parapelvic Cyst

Parapelvic cysts, rare in the pediatric age group, should not be mistaken for hydronephrosis (Cronan et al). As shown in Figure 2–14, a typical mass effect is seen on the excretory urogram. Ultrasonography confirms the presence of a cystic mass, displacing, rather than distending, the renal pelvis (Hidalgo et al).

Simple Cysts

Simple cysts are readily defined on ultrasound scans. These lesions are found in the variety of syndromes, including, among others, tuberous sclerosis, von Hippel–Lindau's disease, Zellweger's cerebrohepatorenal syndrome, and the Ehlers-Danlos syndrome. In normotensive, asymptomatic children, conservative management is suggested (Bartholomew et al) with or without cyst puncture (Kramer et al).

Uncomplicated Duplex Kidney

A fairly common abnormality, uncomplicated duplex kidney is characterized by a discontinuity in the renal sinus complex (Fig. 2–15).

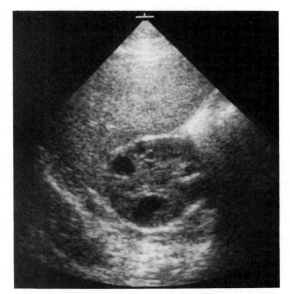

Figure 2–13 □ Autosomal dominant polycystic kidneys (ADPKD). Transverse sector sonogram demonstrates multiple cysts in the upper pole of an essentially normal-sized right kidney. Similar macrocysts are present in the left kidney. A maternal aunt had been known to have ADPKD.

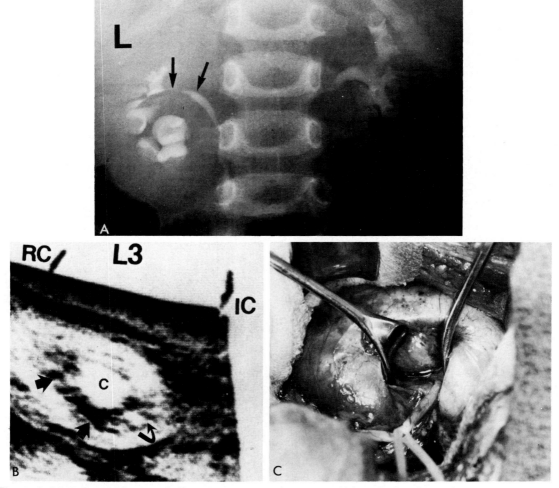

Figure 2–14 ☐ Parapelvic cyst. *A,* Excretory urogram of a 3-year-old boy displayed in posteroanterior projection reveals pressure effect on left ureter *(arrows).* The renal pelvis is not seen. Mild ectasia of lower pole calyces is evident. *B,* Longitudinal prone sonogram of left kidney demonstrates anterior displacement of renal pelvic echoes *(solid arrows)* by adjacent cystic mass (C). Lower pole calyectasis is demonstrated *(curved arrow).* RC, base of rib cage; IC, posterior-superior iliac crest. *C,* Intraoperative appearance of cyst.

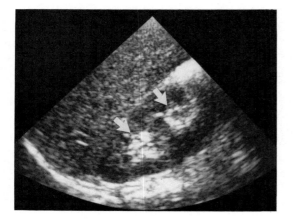

Figure 2–15 ☐ Uncomplicated duplex kidney. Longitudinal sector sonogram of right kidney demonstrates both components *(arrows)* of renal sinus.

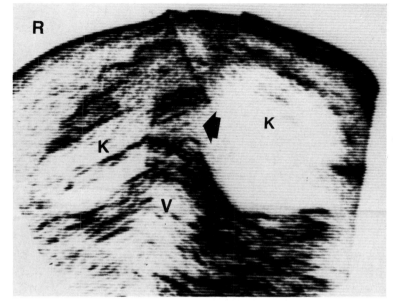

Figure 2–16 □ Horseshoe kidney. Supine transverse sonogram demonstrating isthmus *(arrow)* of horseshoe kidney. Note anterior position of both kidneys (K) relative to vertebra (V) and markedly hydronephrotic left kidney, the result of ureteropelvic junction obstruction.

Horseshoe Kidney

In the presence of a horseshoe kidney, renal malalignment is generally readily evident during the scanning procedure. To confirm this abnormality, however, delineation of the isthmus connecting the inferior renal poles is necessary (Mindell and Kupic). Although this can be accomplished sonographically, at times it may be quite difficult because of overlying gas-filled bowel. Documentation may be facilitated when there is an additional intrinsic morphologic abnormality of one of the kidneys (Fig. 2–16).

Renal Ectopia

The abnormally positioned kidney can result in radiographic or physical findings suggesting a pathologic mass. The presence of a thoracic kidney (Fig. 2–17) can be identified. A pelvic kidney (Fig. 2–18) as well as crossed renal ectopia (Fig. 2–19) can be verified.

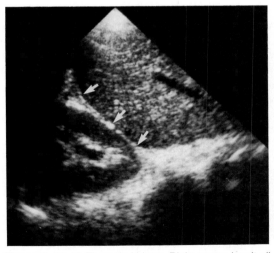

Figure 2–17 □ Thoracic kidney. Right sector longitudinal sonogram of a 4-year-old boy with radiographic evidence of a right-sided chest mass documented an intrathoracic kidney lying immediately above the right hemidiaphragm *(arrows)*. There is mild distention of the renal pelvis.

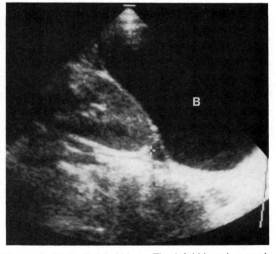

Figure 2–18 □ Pelvic kidney. The left kidney is seen in a longitudinal plane in the left upper pelvis, immediately adjacent to the distended urinary bladder (B).

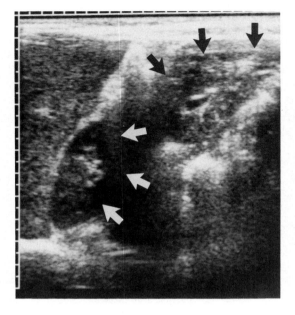

Figure 2–19 □ Crossed renal ectopia. Left linear longitudinal sonogram demonstrates both kidneys in essentially the same plane. The left kidney *(white arrows)* is in normal position and is unremarkable in appearance. The ectopic kidney *(black arrows)* is anterior and inferior in position, and there is slight fullness of the renal pelvis apparent. Kidney fusion, if present, could not be established in this case.

Renal Neoplasms

Other than for a possible radiograph of the abdomen, ultrasonography is generally the first diagnostic imaging modality in the assessment of a palpable abdominal mass. The consistency of the mass (solid, fluid, mixed) can be established. As stated by Markle and Potter, ultrasound imaging is "one part of a multimodal evaluation to (1) confirm the organ of origin and gross extent of the tumor, (2) identify large blood vessel involvement, (3) identify metastases, and (4) define the status of the opposite kidney."

Congenital Mesoblastic Nephroma

Congenital mesoblastic nephroma represents the most common renal tumor of the neonate. This lesion may be hyperechoic or hypoechoic (Fig. 2–20), or it may produce a mixed echo pattern (Hartman et al). This neoplasm is benign and thought to be a part of a spectrum of mesenchymal renal neoplasms of infancy, including some that are malignant (Gonzalez-Crussi et al, 1981). These mass lesions are sonographically indistinguishable from Wilms' tumor. As with any suspected primary renal neoplasm, nephrectomy is indicated. Additional treatment is rarely required.

Wilms' Tumor

Wilms' tumor represents the most common malignant abdominal tumor in children. One third of the cases are found in children under 1 year of age, and three fourths are found in children under 4 years of age (Markle and Potter). The tumor is usually large by the time of discovery, generally presenting as a palpable mass. In 10 to 15 per cent of cases, the tumor is bilateral (Fig. 2–21). The renal origin of a predominantly exophytic Wilms' tumor may be difficult to establish (Jaffe et al). Teele has stressed the importance of carefully imaging the entire outline of the kidney (Fig. 2–22). When the tumor has largely displaced the kidney, specific ultrasonographic documentation of its renal origin may be virtually impossible. The depiction of multiple fluid compartments within the mass, though suggestive of a retroperitoneal teratoma, is also compatible with Wilms' tumor, since areas of cystic necrosis are a common feature of this neoplasm and are reflected sonographically (Fig. 2–23). Conversely, a neuroblastoma most often appears entirely solid (Hartman and Sanders).

Vascular Extension. Real-time scanning has greatly facilitated the detection of Wilms' tumor growth into the renal vein, inferior vena cava (Fig. 2–24) (Slovis et al, 1981), and heart (Shkolnik). Such tumor extension, even when reaching the right atrium, can be totally asymptomatic (Slovis et al, 1978). Because the goal of surgery is total removal of the neoplasm, documentation of Wilms' tumor extension can have a significant bearing in determining the surgical approach (Fig. 2–25).

Monitoring the Patient at Risk. Sonography is now widely accepted as the means for peri-

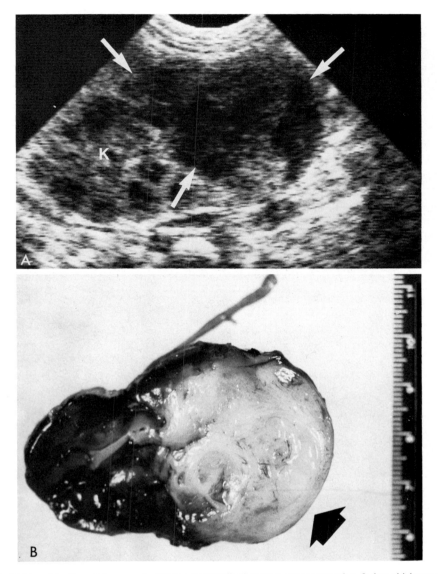

Figure 2–20 □ Mesoblastic nephroma. *A,* Supine longitudinal sector sonogram of a 2-day-old boy with right-sided abdominal mass displays focal hypoechoic mass *(arrows)* in the lower half of the right kidney. *B,* Excised hemisected specimen showing tumor in the lower pole *(arrow).* Histologic examination confirmed benign hamartoma.

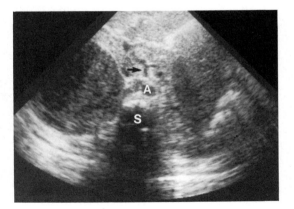

Figure 2–21 □ Bilateral Wilms' tumor. Transverse sector sonogram demonstrates bilateral renal mass. Detail on left is not as well delineated because of intervening bowel gas. The aorta (A) is seen immediately anterior to the left side of the spine (S). The celiac artery *(arrow)* is identified.

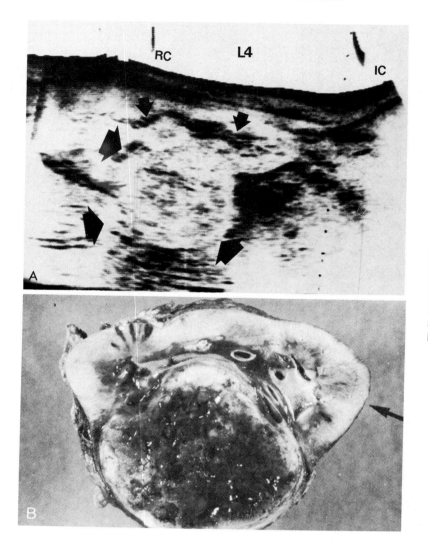

Figure 2–22 □ Wilms' tumor. *A,* Left longitudinal sonogram of a prone 3-year-old girl reveals echogenic mass *(large arrows)* extending from mid-anterior left kidney. Note displacement of superior aspect of renal sinus echoes *(small arrows). B,* Hemisected surgical specimen. Lower pole is indicated *(arrow).*

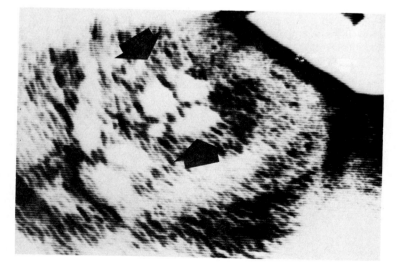

Figure 2–23 □ Wilms' tumor. Supine left longitudinal sonogram demonstrates multiple cystic compartments *(arrows)* within a large mass. No associated recognizable renal structure could be identified.

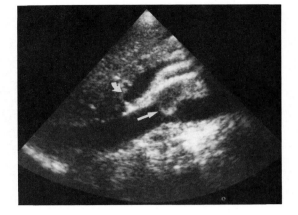

Figure 2–24 □ Wilms' tumor extension to the inferior vena cava (IVC) via the left renal vein. A longitudinal sector sonogram in the plane of the IVC documents intrusion of a solid mass *(straight arrow)* representing intravascular tumor extension from left-sided Wilms' tumor. Portal vein *(curved arrow)* is shown just prior to entering liver.

odic renal monitoring of individuals who are at risk for the development of Wilms' tumor. This includes patients with a previous Wilms' tumor or a family history of Wilms' tumor or sporadic aniridia (Friedman). Sonographic surveillance, similarly, is utilized for the detection of renal and extrarenal tumors in patients with Beckwith-Wiedemann syndrome or syndromes associated with hemihypertrophy (Tolchin et al).

Nephroblastomatosis

Nephroblastomatosis is an abnormality that is found in the kidneys of infants and children. It is characterized by the presence of persistent foci of immature renal blastema, which may be diffuse, focal, or multifocal. This lesion

may result in renal enlargement and gross alteration in the renal parenchyma pattern (Fig. 2–26). It can be found in up to one third of kidneys with Wilms' tumor and can also be found in the contralateral kidney (Fig. 2–27). There is also an increased incidence of nephroblastomatosis in patients with Beckwith-Wiedemann and hemihypertrophy syndromes and some major chromosomal abnormalities (Franken et al).

The management and prognosis of nephroblastomatosis is uncertain. A decrease in renal size has been noted in some patients with nephromegaly who are treated with vincristine and actinomycin D. All patients with this condition, regardless of type, remain at risk for the development of Wilms' tumor (Franken et al).

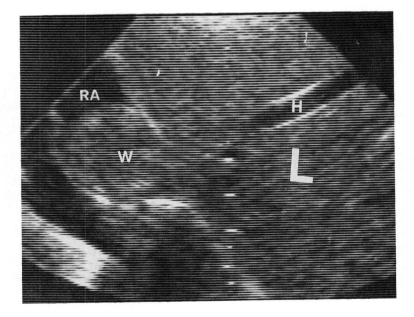

Figure 2–25 □ Wilms' tumor extension to the heart. Tumor mass (W) is seen in right atrium (RA) on longitudinal sector sonogram in an otherwise asymptomatic 2-year-old girl with a left-sided intrarenal mass. The inferior vena cava and left renal vein were virtually occluded by tumor growth. The neoplasm was totally excised by means of a combined abdominal-thoracic surgical approach. L, liver; H, hepatic vein.

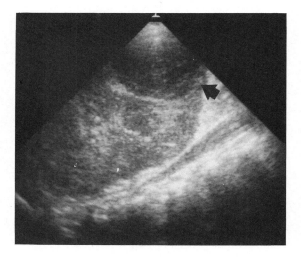

Figure 2–26 □ Nephroblastomatosis. Grossly abnormal and enlarged right kidney, as delineated on a sector longitudinal sonogram. A somewhat more discrete hypoechoic mass-like area *(arrow)* is seen in the lower pole. The left kidney was also grossly abnormal in appearance.

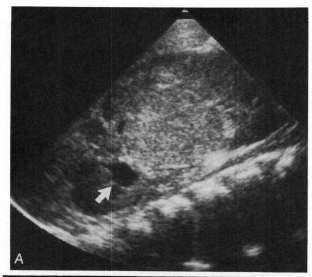

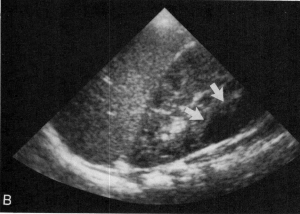

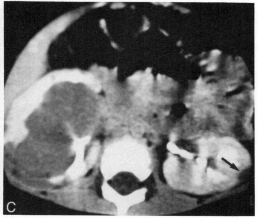

Figure 2–27 □ Wilms' tumor with contralateral nephroblastomatosis. *A,* Sector longitudinal sonogram of right kidney reveals large solid mass lesion. An ectatic portion of the upper collecting system is noted *(arrow). B,* Longitudinal view of left kidney reveals ovoid hypoechoic area posteriorly *(arrow). C,* CT study demonstrates large intrarenal mass on the right and the focus of subsequently confirmed nephroblastomatosis of left kidney *(arrow).*

Multilocular Cystic Nephroma

A relatively uncommon neoplasm, multilocular cystic nephroma is characterized by well-circumscribed, noncommunicating, fluid-filled loculi that ultrasonographically produce a whorled pattern (Madewell et al). An example of this neoplasm is demonstrated in Figure 2–28. The structural similarity of these lesions, compared with Wilms' tumor (Gonzalez-Crussi et al, 1982), supports the concept that nephrectomy is the treatment of choice. Indeed, both lesions have been found in the same kidney (Fig. 2–29).

Leukemia and Lymphoma

Leukemic deposits or lymphomatous infiltration of the kidneys results in nephromegaly and distortion of the collecting systems. Lymphomatous infiltrate is typically hypoechoic in appearance. Leukemic infiltrate can be either hypoechoic or hyperechoic. Gore and Shkolnik noted that renal enlargement, as an indicator of reactivated leukemia, can precede bone marrow changes by up to 12 days. Ultrasonography also provides the means for monitoring gross renal changes in response to therapy (Fig. 2–30).

Parenchymal Abnormalities

Renal parenchymal disease occurring in the glomerulus or in the interstitium results in recognizable, though nonspecific, changes in the internal echo pattern of the kidney. Cortical echogenicity becomes greater than that of

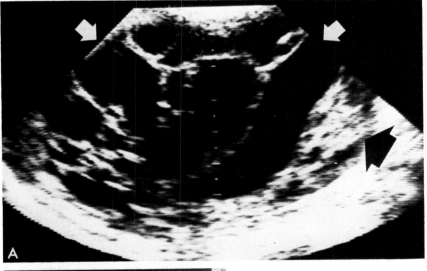

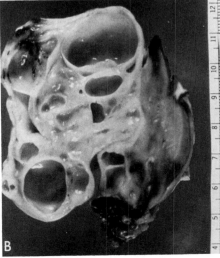

Figure 2–28 □ Multilocular cystic nephroma. *A,* Longitudinal supine sector sonogram of an 8-month-old girl demonstrates a large right renal mass, predominantly composed of multiple fluid compartments *(light arrows).* A solid portion is noted inferiorly *(dark arrow).* *B,* Corresponding cystic and solid components are seen in the surgical specimen.

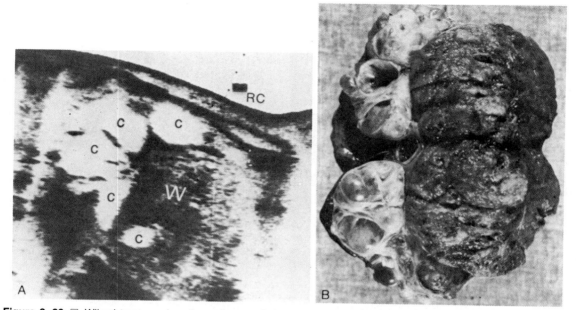

Figure 2–29 □ Wilms' tumor and cystic nephroma. *A*, Longitudinal sonogram of prone patient demonstrates a large renal mass. The central solid component (W) proved to be a Wilms' tumor. The cystic components (C) represent a multilocular cystic nephroma. *B*, Hemisected specimen (From Shkolnik A: The role of ultrasonography in the diagnosis and management of Wilms' tumor. *In* Wilms' Tumor: Clinical and Biological Manifestations. Edited by C Pochedly, ES Baum. New York, Elsevier, 1984.)

normal liver parenchyma, with or without disruption of the normal recognizable corticomedullary junction. Increased echogenicity may be the result of glomerular sclerosis or interstitial changes, such as fibrosis, tubular atrophy, interstitial infiltrate, or deposition of collagen or calcium. Examples of the renal appearance in the nephrotic syndrome (Fig. 2–31), acute tubular necrosis (Fig. 2–32), and the hemolytic uremic syndrome (Fig. 2–33) are shown.

Nephrocalcinosis and Urolithiasis

Nephrocalcinosis, with or without urolithiasis, can occur as a result of renal tubular syndromes, enzyme disorders, hypercalcemic states, parenchymal disease, or vascular phenomena; at times, the cause may be unknown (Foley et al). The sensitivity of ultrasound scanning in the detection of calcifications is well documented, and its application in this regard can be categorized as follows:

1. Confirming a renal or extrarenal location of calculi identified radiographically (Figs. 2–34 and 2–35).

2. Assessing the urinary tracts of patients who are at risk for nephrocalcinosis (Fig. 2–36) or urolithiasis (Hufnagle et al) or who present with suggestive clinical findings.

3. Monitoring for evidence of increase in size or number, or passage or resolution of renal calculi.

4. Intraoperative localization of renal stones. Such definition can expedite the optimal surgical removal of such calculi (Cook and Lytton). With the scan head encased in an appropriately sterile container, scanning is preferably initiated prior to nephrotomy via the surface of the intact kidney.

Inflammatory Disease

Hayden et al suggests that ultrasonography be used for initial imaging in screening children with suspected or confirmed urinary tract infections because (1) significant congenital urinary tract anomalies can be identified, (2) accurate kidney measurement is provided for assessment of present and future renal growth, (3) the presence of hydronephrosis can be confirmed, and (4) information can be provided regarding anatomy of the bladder, the ureterovesical junction, and the proximal ure-

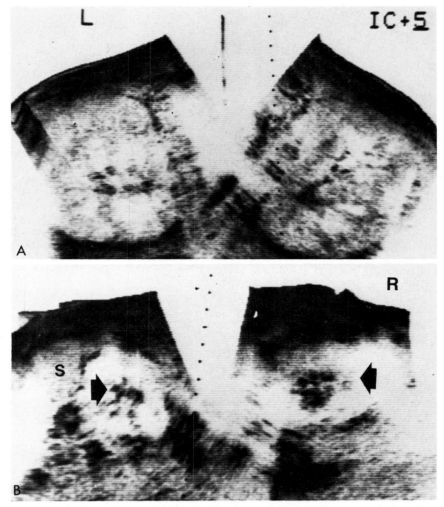

A

B

Figure 2–30 □ Renal leukemic infiltration. *A,* Transverse prone sonogram reveals symmetrically enlarged kidneys with disordered internal echogenicity in a 12-year-old boy with acute lymphoblastic leukemia. *B,* Post-therapy sonogram reveals marked decrease in renal size and essentially normal appearance of renal sinus echo complex bilaterally *(arrows).* S, spleen.

Figure 2–31 □ Nephrotic syndrome. Longitudinal sector sonogram demonstrates enlarged right kidney with marked increase in parenchymal echogenicity and loss of corticomedullary demarcation. Pleural effusion *(arrow)* is also noted at the right base. Left kidney was similar in appearance.

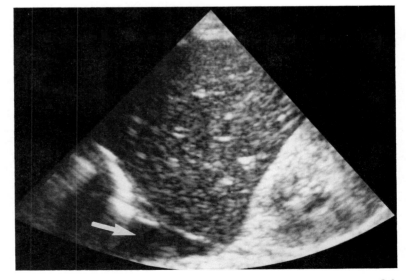

31

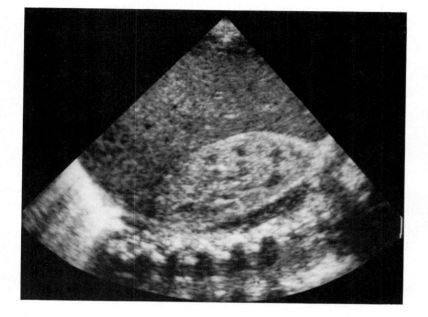

Figure 2–32 □ Acute tubular necrosis, confirmed at autopsy. Longitudinal sector sonogram of right kidney in a 3-day-old infant reveals increased echogenicity of the renal cortex with some degree of preservation of the corticomedullary demarcation. The left kidney was similar in appearance. When the infant was 1 day of age, the sonographic appearance of the kidneys had been unremarkable.

Figure 2–33 □ Hemolytic uremic syndrome. Sector longitudinal sonogram in a 7-year-old boy demonstrates enlargement of the right kidney with a marked increase in cortical echogenicity, accentuating the corticomedullary differentiation. The left kidney was essentially identical in appearance.

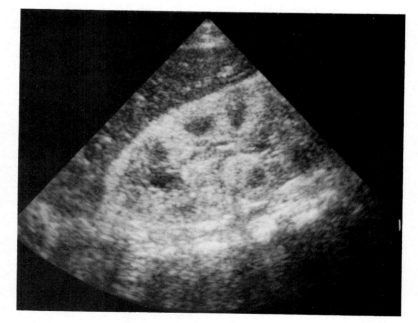

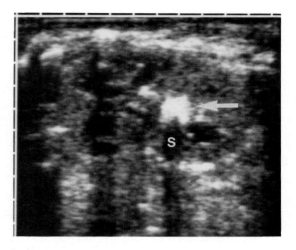

Figure 2–34 ☐ Renal calculus in an infant with severe cardiovascular disease. Supine left longitudinal renal sonogram confirms calculus *(arrow)* in lower pole, with characteristic acoustic shadow (S) deep to the calculus. This study was performed in the neonatal intensive care unit. Treatment included the long-term administration of furosemide.

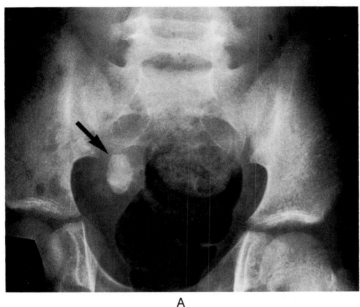

A

Figure 2–35 ☐ Distal left ureteral calculus. *A,* Large calculus *(arrow)* of unknown etiology in right lower quadrant of a 9-year-old boy. The cystogram was unremarkable. An excretory urogram revealed hydronephrosis of the right kidney. *B,* Longitudinal sector sonogram confirms impaction of stone *(dark arrows)* at ureterovesical junction; the obstructed, dilated, distal ureter is noted (U). Marked right-sided hydronephrosis was also documented on renal scans. An inflammatory polyp *(curved arrow),* noted only on the ultrasound study, was also removed at surgery. S, acoustic shadow.

B

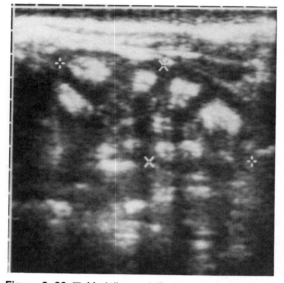

Figure 2–36 □ Medullary calcification. Linear longitudinal sonogram of the right kidney in an infant with clinical and laboratory findings consistent with those of distal renal tubular acidosis reveals densely echogenic medullary pyramids with associated acoustic shadowing. Left kidney was similar in appearance. (Markers outline renal contour.)

thra. Leonidas et al conclude that "in the absence of vesicoureteral reflux, children with urinary tract infection should be studied with sonography, and no further study is needed if a good quality sonogram is within normal limits."

Pyelonephritis

In the acute phase of pyelonephritis, ultrasonography can show swelling of the affected kidney and diminished echogenicity of the parenchyma as a result of edema (Fig. 2–37). Reflux nephropathy is characterized by shrunken kidneys that demonstrate loss of renal parenchyma, retraction of one or more calyces, and increased echogenicity resulting from interstitial fibrosis (Kay et al). At times, mild dilatation of the pelvocalyceal system can be observed. A similar appearance may be seen in virtually any chronic end-stage renal condition (Babcock).

Acute Focal Bacterial Nephritis (Acute Lobar Nephronia)

This abnormality is an acute, localized renal infection resulting in a mass without liquefaction (Rosenfield et al). Retrograde infection with gram-negative bacteria secondary to vesicoureteral reflux is felt to play a major etiologic role (Siegal and Glasier). Lobar nephronia can simulate a mass lesion on the excretory urogram.

Sonographically, a mass-like appearance is noted. Unlike Wilms' tumor, it is typically less echogenic than the surrounding renal tissue. A rapid change in the sonographic appearance typifies the response of this infectious process to antibiotic therapy (Fig. 2–38).

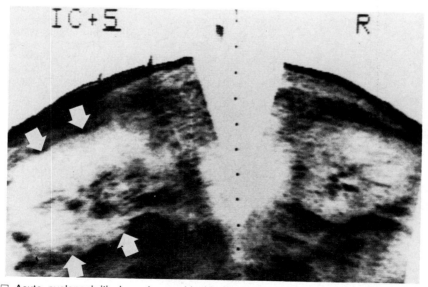

Figure 2–37 □ Acute pyelonephritis in a 4-year-old girl. Swollen left kidney *(arrows)* seen on transverse, prone sonogram. The edematous parenchyma is hypoechoic. Cortical-medullary distinction is obliterated.

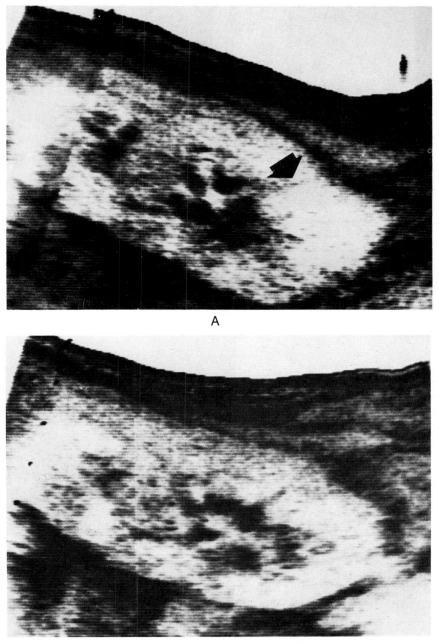

A

B

Figure 2–38 □ Lobar nephronia in a 5-year-old girl. *A*, Hypoechoic area noted in lower pole of the left kidney *(arrow)* on longitudinal prone sonogram. *B*, Sonogram following 7 days of antibiotic therapy reveals essentially normal appearance of lower pole.

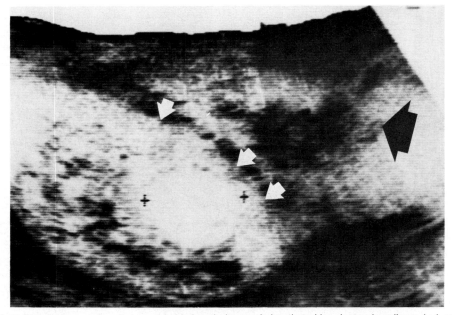

Figure 2–39 □ Renal abscess in a 2-year-old girl. Anechoic area is bracketed by electronic calipers (+), which yielded a measurement of 3 cm. Immediately adjacent to the posterior margin of the lower pole *(white arrows),* which is displaced anteriorly, lies a complex echogenic area *(dark areas).* The abscess and a posterior extrarenal extension *(dark arrow)* were surgically drained.

Renal Abscess

Sonographically, a walled-off mass, which may be anechoic or may contain echogenic inflammatory debris, is noted. An important aspect of ultrasonography is the ability to define an extrarenal extension of the process (Fig. 2–39).

Candidiasis

The occurrence of fungal balls in the renal pelvis secondary to *Candida albicans,* resulting in hydronephrosis, is well known in adults and children, particularly in those who are immunosuppressed or in those with diabetes mellitus. Similar findings (Fig. 2–40) secondary to systemic candidiasis have been reported in a low-birth-weight premature neonate (Kintanar et al).

Pyonephrosis

In the presence of obstruction, persistent, dependent echoes in the dilated pelvicalyceal system, producing a fluid-debris level (Fig. 2–41), has been described as one of the manifestations of pyonephrosis (Coleman et al). Thus, this appearance in the proper clinical setting is consistent with an inflammatory process. Ad-

ditional findings include a dependent shift of the debris as the patient changes to an upright, decubitus, or prone position. Other findings that were described include echoes with acoustic shadowing as a consequence of gas-forming

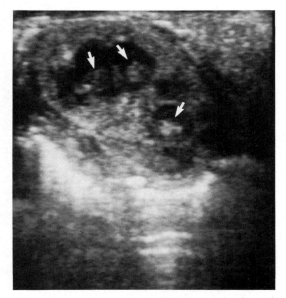

Figure 2–40 □ Fungal balls. Multiple round echogenic masses *(arrows)* are delineated within several dilated calyces on longitudinal renal sonogram of an infant with systemic candidiasis.

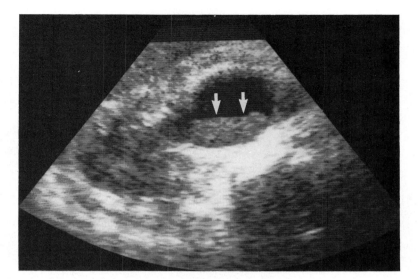

Figure 2–41 □ Pyonephrosis. Echogenic debris *(arrows)* layering dependently in dilated, obstructed renal pelvis. Movement of debris was apparent as the patient changed position. Surgical drainage followed.

pathogens or low-level echoes completely filling the distended collecting system without layering.

Imaging Following Renal Trauma

Determining the status of renal function is paramount in the presence of overt or suspected renal trauma. Therefore, contrast-enhanced computed tomography (CT), which reflects both renal morphology and function and provides an overview of the entire abdomen as well, is considered the initial imaging technique of choice. Ultrasonography can provide complementary information, and as in the case illustrated in Figure 2–42, it is particularly useful when follow-up renal monitoring is indicated.

Postsurgical Imaging

Following pyeloplasty, ureteral reimplantation or reconstruction, urinary diversion and undiversion procedures, and ureteral stent placement, ultrasound scanning is utilized to document changes in pelvocalyceal and/or ureteral dilatation. Postoperative fluid collections of blood, lymph, or urine (Fig. 2–43) can be identified. Follow-up scanning can be used to assess renal growth and to rule out late obstruction. As with all methods of diagnostic imaging, a totally unsuspected and valuable finding may be elicited (Fig. 2–44).

Complications of Renal Transplant Surgery

Prior to duplex and color-flow Doppler scanning, the following sonographic findings were associated with renal allograft rejection. These included transplant enlargement (Maklad) and/or enlarged and markedly hypoechoic medullary pyramids with coexistent diminution of renal sinus echogenicity (Fig. 2–45) (Hricak et al, 1982), or evidence of parenchymal infarction (Fig. 2–46). As mentioned above, hydronephrosis and perirenal fluid collections can be detected. A lymphocele in the renal transplant bed, which can at times produce symptomatology simulating renal allograft rejection, is typically well defined and septated (Fig. 2–47).

Text continued on page 42

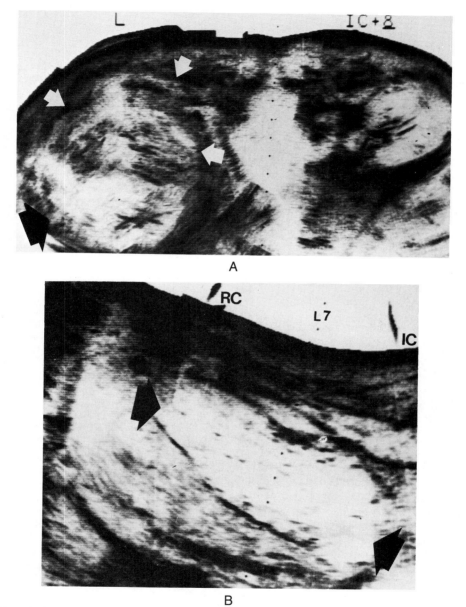

Figure 2–42 □ *A,* Subcapsular renal hematoma displaying heterogeneous echogenicity *(light arrows),* displacing left kidney *(dark arrow)* anteriorly, following left flank trauma to this 16-year-old boy. Renal function was not impaired. *B,* Hemolysis of clot, resulting in diminished echogenicity *(arrows),* is apparent on longitudinal sonogram performed 2 weeks later. The kidney remains displaced. Serial sonograms documented clot resorption and return of the left kidney to normal position.

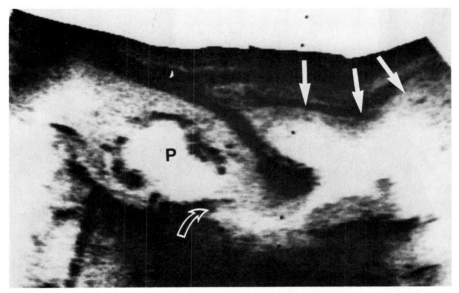

Figure 2–43 □ Post-pyeloplasty urinoma. Fluid mass *(solid arrows)* below left kidney, extending from the repair site *(open arrow)* of ureteropelvic obstruction in a 4-year-old boy. Lower pole of kidney is displaced anteriorly by the fluid mass.

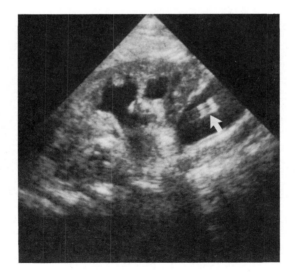

Figure 2–44 □ Ureteral stent *(arrow)* in a hydronephrotic patient with a history of "previous removal." Subsequent surgery documented retained fractured portion of stent.

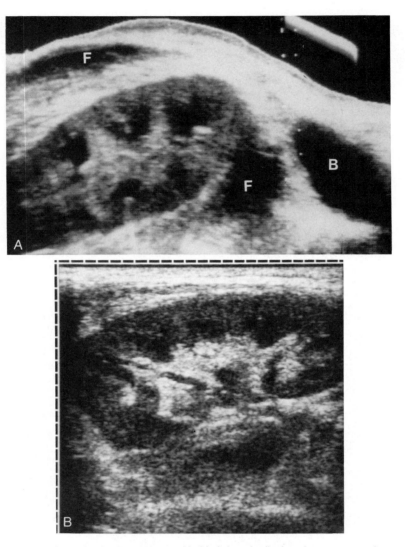

Figure 2–45 □ Renal transplant rejection in a 13-year-old girl. *A,* Longitudinal supine post-transplant sonogram reveals crescentic subcutaneous fluid collections beneath abdominal wall and adjacent to lower pole of the renal transplant (F). Clinical and laboratory findings suggesting allograft rejection were supported by rather prominent hypoechoic medullary pyramids and hypoechoic renal sinus complex. The patient responded to conservative management. *B,* A clinically normal renal transplant is shown for comparison.

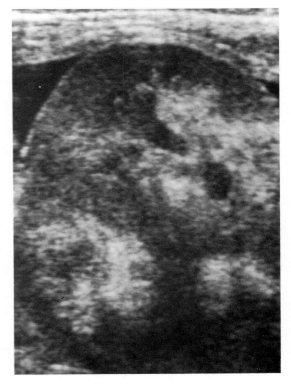

Figure 2–46 □ Renal transplant—parenchymal infarction. Post-transplant linear sonogram in a patient with evidence of renal failure reveals multiple irregular areas of increased echogenicity corresponding to areas of infarction and necrosis confirmed at subsequent surgery. Adjacent pararenal fluid collection is noted superiorly.

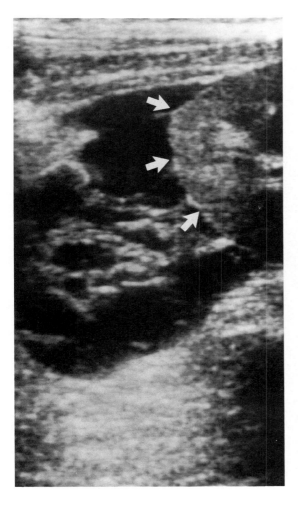

Figure 2–47 □ Post-transplant lymphocele. Longitudinal linear sonogram documents a septated fluid collection surrounding the upper pole *(arrows)* of a renal transplant.

Guidance for Percutaneous Renal Puncture

Renal biopsy remains the definitive method for establishing the etiology of parenchymal renal disease. Ultrasonography is widely utilized for guiding percutaneous renal biopsy, including renal transplants (Spigos et al), and for guidance of renal cyst puncture. Percutaneous needle renal penetration of the dilated renal pelvis for antegrade pyelography, nephrostomy drainage (Babcock et al), and Whitaker testing can likewise be facilitated.

Although transducer-affixed biopsy guides are available, the procedure can also be quite accurately accomplished in a "blind" manner after choosing an appropriate tissue plane by means of ultrasonography (Fig. 2–48). During the procedure, the position of the needle can also be monitored by scanning via the flank region. The presence of a post-biopsy hematoma can be documented (Nybonde and Mortensson).

The technique illustrated is also applicable for renal cyst puncture or nephrostomy tube placement. An example of the documentation of accurate nephrostomy tube placement and the rapid resolution of severe hydronephrosis is demonstrated in Figure 2–49. Similar monitoring has been utilized for diagnostic aspiration, drainage of inflammatory renal processes (Kuligowska et al), or drainage of post–renal transplant accumulations (Silver et al).

THE LOWER URINARY TRACT

Ureterovesical Junction Obstruction

Ureterovesical junction (UVJ) abnormalities reflect muscular dysfunction or narrowing of the distal ureter. Wood et al, reporting on a series of 40 asymptomatic patients, primarily detected during prenatal ultrasound studies, noted hyperperistalsis of the lower ureter and a sharply incurving adynamic segment ranging from 1 to 3 cm in length. Pronounced dilatation of the distal ureter may be quite disproportionate to that of the pelvocalyceal system (Fig. 2–50).

Ectopic Ureterocele

Ureteroceles, which occur more commonly in females, are often obstructions causing dilatation of the upper segment of a completely duplicated renal collecting system. Many of

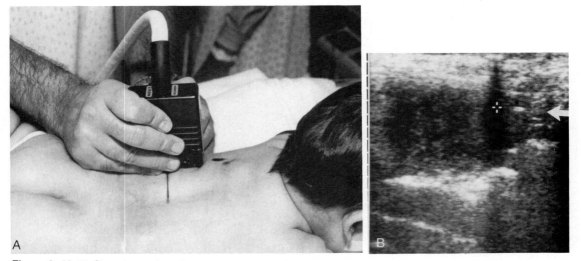

Figure 2–48 □ Choosing a plane for percutaneous renal puncture.

A, Linear longitudinal scan of the left kidney in an infant scheduled for diagnostic renal biopsy. A thin metallic needle has been placed between the face of the transducer and the skin and perpendicular to the plane of imaging. (A cotton-tipped swab can also be used.)

B, Corresponding sonogram, in plane, lateral to the renal sinus. An acceptable plane for biopsy crossing the lower pole of the kidney is indicated by the acoustic shadow produced by the needle. The lower tip of the kidney is indicated *(arrow).* Measurement by cursor (+) indicates depth necessary for posterior penetration of the kidney. The procedure was repeated to confirm biopsy plane in a transverse projection. Skin site was marked.

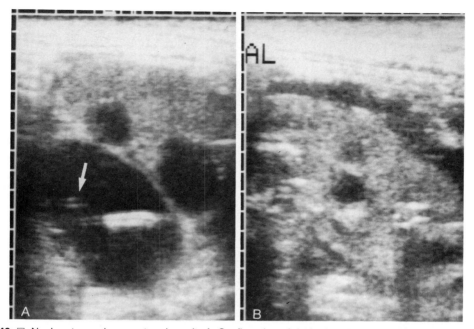

Figure 2–49 □ Nephrostomy placement and result. *A,* Confirmation of desired position of pigtail catheter, tip of which is indicated *(arrow),* in dilated left renal pelvis of 6-month-old boy with severe UPJ obstruction. The right kidney was absent. Pyuria was present, and the infant was in severe renal failure. *B,* Repeated scan minutes later documents marked decompression of the pelvocalyceal system. The catheter, not seen in this view, was well defined in other images. Following a course of nephrostomy drainage and administration of antibiotics, pyeloplasty was undertaken.

these defects are found initially on antenatal sonograms; however, infection of the obstructed unit is most often responsible for its clinical presentation postnatally.

The sonographic delineation of an upper pole fluid mass, in continuity with a dilated ureter, and an ipsilateral intravesical fluid mass (Fig. 2–51) is diagnostic of this entity (Mascatello et al). A large intravesical ureterocele (Fig. 2–52) can also obstruct the ipsilateral lower pole moiety as well as the collecting system of the contralateral kidney. Distention

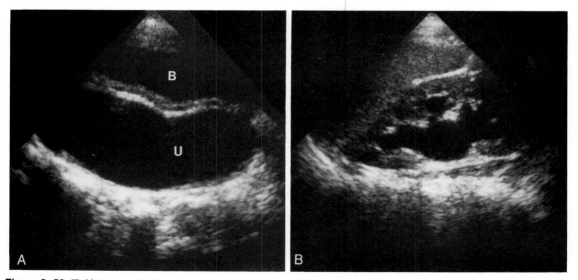

Figure 2–50 □ Ureterovesical junction obstruction. *A,* Longitudinal sector sonogram crossing left side of urinary bladder demonstrates a markedly dilated distal left ureter. *B,* Longitudinal sector sonogram of left kidney demonstrates moderate pelvocalyceal dilatation.

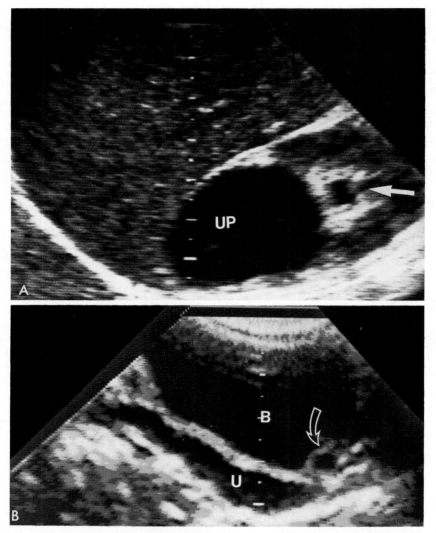

Figure 2–51 □ Ectopic ureterocele. *A,* Longitudinal sector sonogram defines upper pole (UP) fluid mass of right kidney in a supine infant. Mildly dilated pelvis of lower pole moiety is seen *(arrow). B,* Longitudinal, supine sonogram displays distal portion of dilated right upper pole ureter (U). Relatively small ureterocele *(arrow)* is seen protruding into the lumen of the distended bladder.

and contraction of the ureterocele may be evident during the real-time study.

The Urinary Bladder

The distended urinary bladder, ideally suited for ultrasonographic delineation, serves as an anatomic reference point. More importantly, it provides an optimal acoustic window for transmission of sound away from and back to the scanning transducer, thereby facilitating imaging of the surrounding pelvis and lower abdominal contents. Indeed, optimal assess-ment of the pelvis, in most instances, necessi-tates a well-distended bladder.

Urachal remnants, particularly when fluid-filled (Fig. 2–53), can be documented. Echo-genicity within a urachal cyst, as in other fluid compartments, may be a reflection of hemor-rhage or infection (Fig. 2–54). This is similarly true when this finding is noted within the distended urinary bladder (Fig. 2–55). An in-travesical calcification (Fig. 2–56) is readily apparent.

The forceful flow of fluid into fluid, as typi-fied by the ureteral jet phenomenon, can be observed (Fig. 2–57) during real-time scan-

Figure 2–52 □ Large ureterocele *(arrow)* within left posterior bladder lumen is seen on transverse articulated-arm sonogram. The ureterocele produced hydroureteronephrosis of each moiety of the duplicated left kidney and of the nonduplicated right kidney.

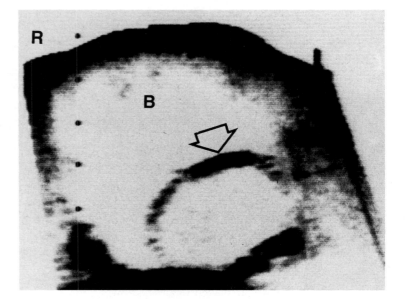

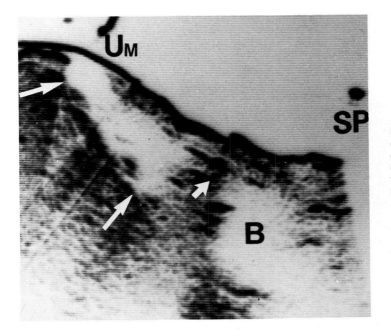

Figure 2–53 □ Urachal cyst. Surgically confirmed urachal cyst *(large arrows)* delineated on midline longitudinal sonogram in a 6-month-old girl with drainage from the umbilicus (UM). Connection with bladder (B) was suggested *(small arrow)*. SP, symphysis pubis.

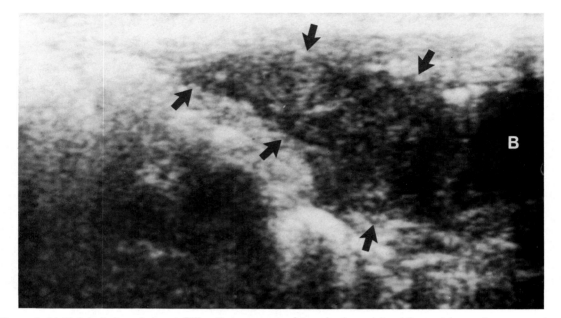

Figure 2–54 ☐ Infected urachal cyst. Diffuse heterogeneous internal echogenicity of the cyst *(arrows)* was secondary to a purulent process. Some movement of debris was evident during the scanning procedure.

ning. Three-dimensional measurements allow the assessment of bladder volume as well as the estimation of post-voiding residual (Erasmie and Lidefelt).

Bladder wall thickening (Fig. 2–58) can be documented. However, it must be remembered that a pseudothickened appearance may be simulated when the urinary bladder is inadequately distended. Conversely, hyperdis-tention of the urinary bladder may thin out a truly thickened bladder wall. As reported by Jequier and Rousseau, a measurement of the posterior bladder wall of 3 mm or greater with the urinary bladder well distended, or 5 mm or greater with the urinary bladder *incompletely* distended, is considered significant for bladder wall thickening. In patients with chronic bladder outlet obstruction or infection or with a neuropathic bladder, bladder wall trabeculation (Fig. 2–59) can also be apparent.

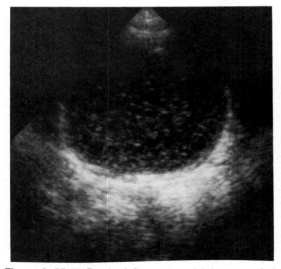

Figure 2–55 ☐ Pyuria. Inflammatory debris suspended in the bladder urine of a 4-year-old boy, as seen on transverse sonogram.

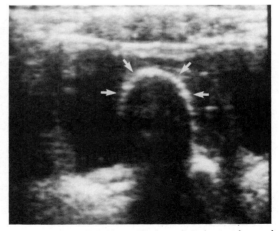

Figure 2–56 ☐ Bladder calculus. Anterior surface of large calculus *(arrows)* in the bladder of 6-year-old boy with myelomeningocele.

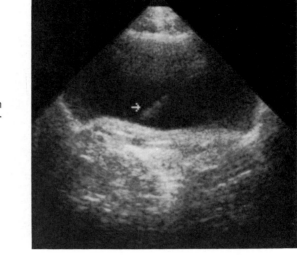

Figure 2–57 □ Ureteral jet. Transverse sector sonogram of bladder demonstrates oblique course *(arrow)* of intravesical flow of urine from right ureter.

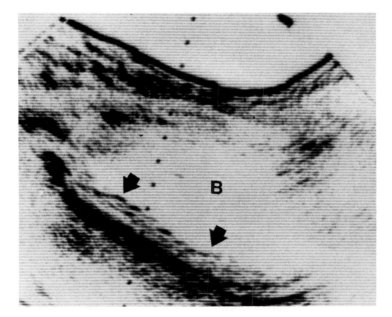

Figure 2–58 □ Bladder wall thickening. Midline longitudinal sonogram of bladder in an 8-year-old boy with cystitis demonstrates a thickened posterior bladder wall *(arrows)*. Edema of the bladder wall was confirmed cystoscopically.

Figure 2–59 □ Bladder wall trabeculation. Midline sector sonogram in a 3-year-old hydrocephalic girl with myelomeningocele displays coarse trabeculation of the posterior bladder wall. A small volume of shunted cerebrospinal fluid *(arrow)* is seen in the pouch of Douglas.

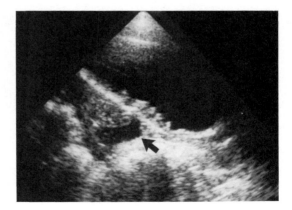

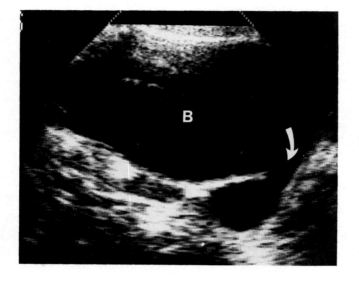

Figure 2–60 □ Bladder diverticulum. Diverticulum *(arrow)* at the left posterior aspect of bladder, as seen on transverse sector sonogram.

Also readily identified is a bladder diverticulum (Fig. 2–60) or polyp (Fig. 2–61).

Mass lesions arising from the bladder wall or protruding into the bladder lumen from the posterior urethra or prostate gland (Fig. 2–62A) can be identified (Bree and Silver). Monitoring the therapeutic response of a neoplasm (Fig. 2–62B) can be accomplished.

Posterior Urethral Valves

Posterior urethral valve (PUV) represents the most common cause of a bilateral flank mass in the male infant. The hydroureteronephrosis is not infrequently asymmetric. The simulta-

neous delineation of both distal dilated ureters can be achieved by scanning in a transverse plane across the distended urinary bladder (Fig. 2–63). Definitive confirmation of urethral obstruction is attained with a voiding cystourethrogram. Gilsanz et al, however, have described a classic sonographic combined appearance of bladder wall thickening and characteristic dilatation of the prostatic urethra (Fig. 2–64). A perirenal urinoma and/or urinary ascites can occur as a result of rupture of a calyceal fornix or a tear in the renal parenchyma, resulting from high-pressure vesicoureteral reflux. Characteristic septations of perirenal urinoma (Fig. 2–65) have been described (Feinstein and Fernbach).

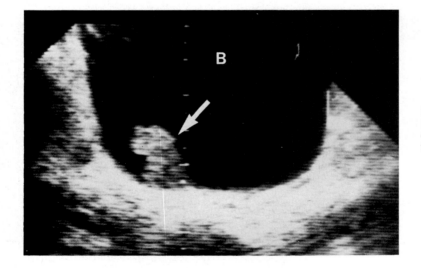

Figure 2–61 □ Bladder polyp. Myxomatous polyp *(arrow)* subsequently excised from the right posterior bladder wall.

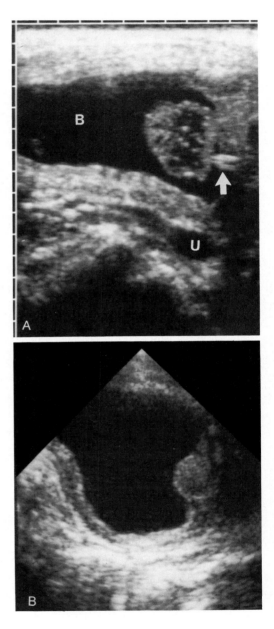

Figure 2–62 □ Rhabdomyosarcoma. *A,* Large, slightly lobulated, heterogeneous mass defined at the base of the bladder on a linear longitudinal sonogram in a 3-year-old boy. A catheter *(arrow)* is seen, with the proximal tip abutting the mass. Dilatation of the distal right ureter (U) is evident. *B,* Longitudinal sector sonogram following course of chemotherapy. Although the scale is smaller than in *A,* there is an obvious decrease in size of the mass, which also appears more homogeneous. Mild thickening of the bladder wall is noted.

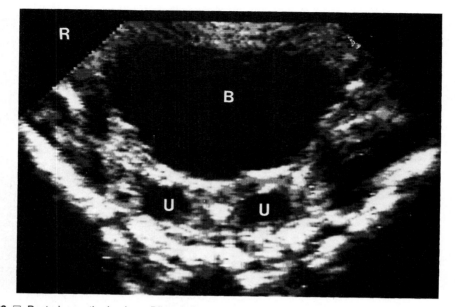

Figure 2–63 □ Posterior urethral valves. Dilated distal ureters (U) seen posterior to the bladder on transverse sector sonogram. Renal scanning documented moderately severe bilateral hydronephrosis.

Postoperative Imaging

Postoperative morphology of the bladder can be provided by ultrasonography following bladder augmentation (Fig. 2–66). Also, the site of subureteric polytef (Teflon) (Fig. 2–67), instilled as an antireflux measure, can be monitored (Gore et al, 1989).

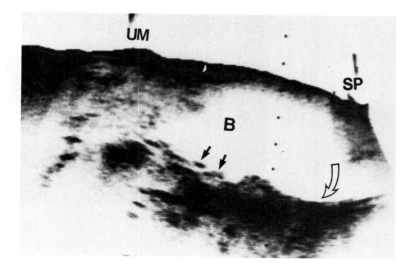

Figure 2–64 □ Posterior urethral valves. Longitudinal midline articulated-arm sonogram shows characteristic dilatation of prostatic urethra *(curved arrow)* in male infant. Bladder trabeculation is also noted *(arrows)*. SP, symphysis pubis; UM, umbilicus.

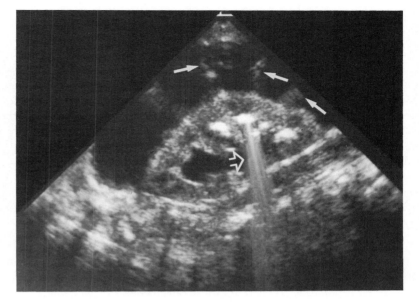

Figure 2–65 □ Perirenal urinoma secondary to posterior urethral valve. Large perirenal septated *(solid arrows)* fluid collection in left upper quadrant. Mild to moderate hydronephrosis. Intense intracalyceal echogenicity, including one example of classic reverberation artifacts *(open arrow)*, reflects presence of air, which was introduced into the bladder during catheterization, and ascended to the upper collecting system.

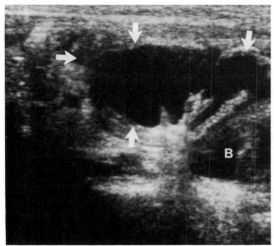

Figure 2–66 □ Bladder augmentation. Cecal component *(arrows)* of urinary bladder, defined on longitudinal scan slightly to right of midline.

Figure 2–67 □ Subureteric polytef (Teflon). Cursors (+) on right longitudinal sector sonogram, defining 8 mm length of subureteric Teflon, which produces a corresponding acoustic shadow.

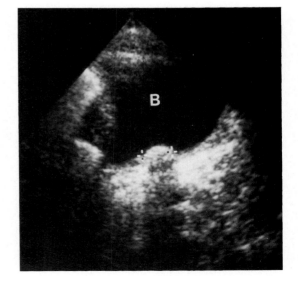

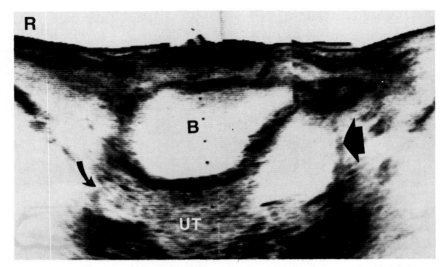

Figure 2–68 ☐ Ovarian cyst. Large left ovarian cyst *(large arrow)* in a 14-year-old girl with left lower quadrant pain. The right ovary *(curved arrow)* is normal. The patient was managed conservatively, and follow-up sonography documented involution of the cyst. UT, uterus; B, bladder.

GONADAL IMAGING

Uterus, Ovaries, Vagina

Ultrasonography serves as the primary imaging modality for the young girl presenting with lower abdominal pain and is likewise warranted when there is clinical suspicion or overt evidence of a pelvic mass. Pregnancy can be determined, the presence of hydrocolpos or hydrohematometrocolpos can be documented, and an ovarian cyst becomes quickly apparent (Fig. 2–68). Large ovarian cysts, capable of

reaching the upper abdomen, have been identified sonographically in the fetus and the neonate. Conversely, small transient ovarian cysts are also consistently seen in the neonate (Fig. 2–69) and young female (Nussbaum et al, 1988). Ovarian torsion produces an enlarged ovary that can appear as a hypoechoic mass. Engorged peripheral vessels may simulate cystic components. Free fluid in the cul-de-sac is not infrequently noted (Graif and Itzchak). The presence and consistency of an ovarian neoplasm may be confirmed (Fig. 2–70).

Ultrasonography of the pelvis can be of

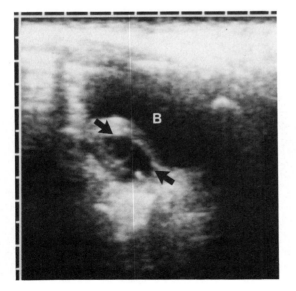

Figure 2–69 ☐ Linear longitudinal sonogram in a newborn girl demonstrates slightly enlarged ovary *(arrows)* containing a septated cyst or two immediately adjacent cysts. No evidence of abnormality was found on a follow-up study several months later.

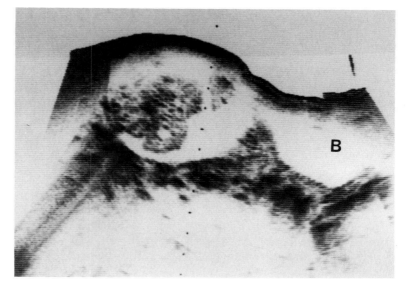

Figure 2–70 □ Ovarian teratoma. Longitudinal sonogram demonstrates anterior abdominal protuberance and a palpable mass in a female infant. A large complex mass is identified extending from just above the dome of the urinary bladder to the upper abdomen.

value in the presence of a purulent vaginal discharge. The appearance of pelvic inflammatory disease varies with the status of inflammation and abscess formation. Depending on its density, the presence of a foreign body may be detected (Fig. 2–71). Mass lesions of the vagina may also be identified.

Ambiguous Genitalia

Canty et al state:

The newborn with ambiguous genitalia must be regarded as a relative surgical emergency . . . parents should not be requested to take a newborn with ambiguous genitalia home before proper gender has been assigned and a carefully explained description given as to specific plans for surgical reconstruction and endocrinological management.

Ultrasonography provides a valuable addition to the multifaceted evaluation required in such newborns. The neonatal uterus, which is prominent as a result of maternal estrogen stimulation, can be consistently identified in the neonate (Nussbaum et al, 1986). Such delineation in a newborn with ambiguous external genitalia (Fig. 2–72) underscores the likelihood of a virilized female and, further, alerts the clinician to the risk of the salt-losing

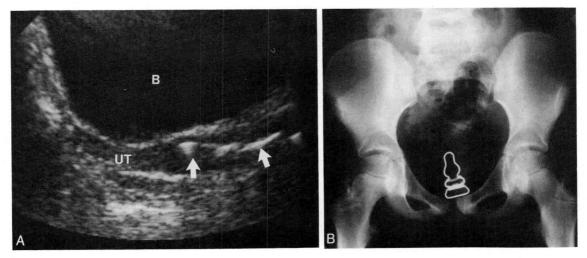

Figure 2–71 □ Vaginal foreign body. *A,* Linear echogenic structure *(arrows)* delineated in the vagina of 8-year-old girl with vaginal discharge. No palpable mass was found on rectal examination. *B,* Metallic foreign body identified on subsequent radiograph.

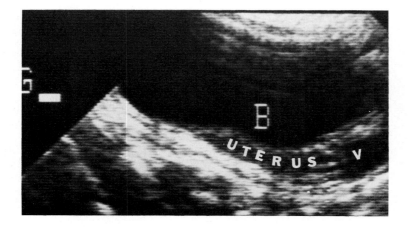

Figure 2–72 □ The infantile uterus is identified on a longitudinal sector sonogram of a neonate with ambiguous genitalia who proved to be a girl with virilizing adrenal hyperplasia. The fluid-distended vagina (V) was the result of labial fusion.

form of adrenal hyperplasia (Lippe and Sample). A müllerian duct remnant associated with abnormal external genitalia (Fig. 2–73), as well as one with which there is no gross evidence of external abnormality (Fig. 2–74) may otherwise escape detection unless discovered fortuitously or when becoming symptomatic.

prostate. A lesion arising in the prostate may extend into the bladder. These lesions often are not diagnosed until there is urinary obstruction requiring catheterization (Raffensperger), as was the case illustrated in Figure 2–62.

Prostate Gland

Approximately 50 per cent of rhabdomyosarcomas in childhood originate in the bladder or

Scrotum

The diagnosis of scrotal disease is highly dependent on clinical history and physical examination. Palpation can be severely compro-

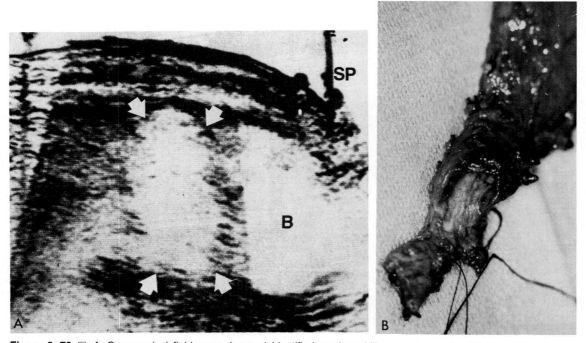

Figure 2–73 □ *A,* Supravesical fluid mass *(arrows)* identified on the midline sonogram of a 19-year-old male with dysuria. There had been a previous history of undescended testes and multiple surgical repairs for severe hypospadias. *B,* Müllerian duct remnant ("uterus masculinis") at surgery was fluid-filled. No adnexal structures were present.

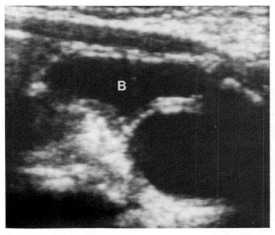

Figure 2–74 □ Midline linear sonogram demonstrates large fluid-filled utricle adjacent to the base of the bladder.

mised in the presence of marked tenderness of the scrotum or of the scrotal contents. Ultrasonography provides a complementary or alternative means of assessment. With the use of a stand-off pad placed on the scrotum, the scanning can be accomplished essentially without discomfort to the patient.

Hydrocele

The diagnosis of hydrocele is most often readily made by examination and transillumination of the scrotum. In questionable cases, verification can be made quickly and easily by ultrasonography. The testis and epididymis can be readily visualized with the hydrocele sac (Fig. 2–75).

Extratesticular Mass

The accuracy of ultrasonography in distinguishing between testicular and extratesticular masses has been stressed by a number of investigators (Carroll and Gross; Richie et al; Sample et al). An example is presented in Figure 2–76.

Neoplasms

The echogenicity of the cancerous testis reflects its tissue consistency, as displayed in Figure 2–77. In the leukemic patient who is in bone marrow remission, the ultrasonographic definition of a focal or diffuse hypoechoic region in an enlarged testicle has been documented as the initial site of an extramedullary relapse (Lupetin et al).

Torsion of the Spermatic Cord

Torsion of the spermatic cord, representing a surgical emergency, is usually accompanied by a history of sudden onset of scrotal pain and swelling. In a newborn, findings may be confined to swelling and redness of the scrotum (Hricak and Filly). Ultrasonographic changes following torsion occur rapidly and are characterized by an enlarged and hypoechoic testis.

Figure 2–75 □ Normal right testis (T) and epididymis (E) are surrounded by large hydrocele (H) on sector sonogram obtained during real-time scanning of the scrotum in a 2-month-old boy.

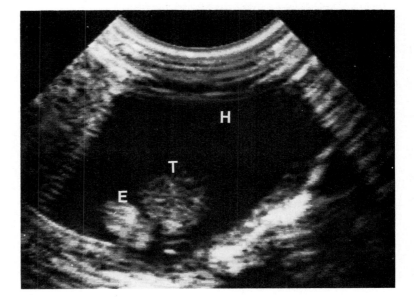

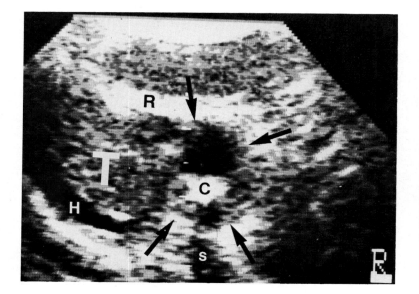

Figure 2–76 □ Palpable mass *(arrows)* at inferior aspect of right testicle in a 9-year-old boy with a previous episode of local pain. Strongly echogenic structure (C) with acoustic shadowing (S) is identified in the lower portion of otherwise predominantly fluid mass. Note reactive hydrocele (H) around the right testis (T). At surgery, the mass was found to be the result of torsion of a distal portion of the epididymis, resulting in a cystic mass, also containing a calcification in area of earlier tissue necrosis. R, median raphe of scrotum.

Radionuclide imaging with technetium 99m pertechnetate is widely accepted as the gold standard diagnostic imaging modality. However, ultrasonography can provide valuable complementary information (Mueller et al). Color-flow Doppler scanning (p. 60) offers significant potential as a primary imaging tool.

Epididymitis and Orchitis

Before a male is age 20, the ratio of epididymitis to testicular (spermatic cord) torsion is 3:2, with the ratio increasing to 9:1 after the age of 20 (Krone and Carroll). It is most often of unknown origin. The importance lies in distinguishing epididymitis from torsion of the spermatic cord in the patient presenting with an acute scrotum. In the acute stage, the involved epididymis appears enlarged and hypoechoic. In the chronic form, there may be a nodular hyperechoic painless mass within the epididymis.

Epididymitis may also accompany orchitis, which in young boys is usually the result of trauma. Orchitis can also occur in later years as a complication of mumps, epididymitis, or systemic disorders. The involved testicle ap-

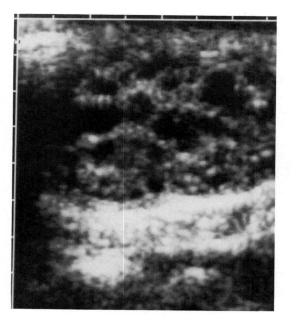

Figure 2–77 □ Enlarged, multicystic-appearing left testis proved to be a granulosa cell tumor in a 2-day-old infant.

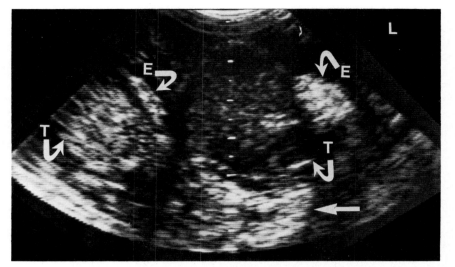

Figure 2–78 □ Orchitis and epididymitis in 13-year-old boy with parotitis and left-sided testicular and scrotal pain. Enlarged hypoechoic left testis (T) and prominent hyperechoic left epididymis (E) seen during sector real-time scanning. Accentuated echogenicity *(straight arrow)* was the result of scrotal inflammation.

pears enlarged and hypoechoic, while the involved epididymis may appear hypoechoic or hyperechoic (Figure 2–78).

Testicular Trauma

Sonographic abnormalities of testicular rupture include alterations of testicular echogenicity as a result of areas of infarction and/or hemorrhage; infrequently, there may be visualization of the fracture plane (Hricak and Jeffrey). In the presence of a traumatized scrotum, the sonographic detection of an intact testis may preclude unnecessary surgery. Acute scrotal hemorrhage may be similar in appearance to a hydrocele, whereas in a more chronic form varying degrees of septations are characteristic.

Cryptorchidism

In the great majority of instances, the undescended testis is located in the inguinal canal and may be palpable or identifiable sonographically (Madrazo et al). Limited success has been reported in the detection of intra-abdominal testes located on the surface of the iliac vessels (Wolverson et al).

Other Applications

The fluid nature of a spermatocele and varicoceles renders these abnormalities amenable

to ultrasonographic identification (Goodman and Haller). Color-flow Doppler imaging has particularly improved the ability to identify a varicocele rapidly. The diagnosis of scrotal hernia is most often achieved by physical examination. Ultrasonographically, this abnormality is supported by identification of loops of bowel within the scrotum, continuous with a hernia sac in the inguinal region (Subramanyam et al).

VASCULAR IMAGING

Starting with articulated arm scanning, cross-sectional imaging has been able to provide useful information relative to the cardiovascular system. Dramatic improvements have been afforded by real-time imaging and by the subsequent development of duplex and color-flow Doppler scanning.

Iatrogenic Vascular Thrombus Formation

In the care of the severely compromised premature neonate, central line placement is virtually a standard procedure that facilitates aspects of both diagnosis and therapy. Thrombus formation is a known complication of indwelling vascular catheters, and, depending upon site and extent, such thrombi have the potential for significant renal compromise. As with the detection of intravascular tumor extension previously described, ultrasonography offers a

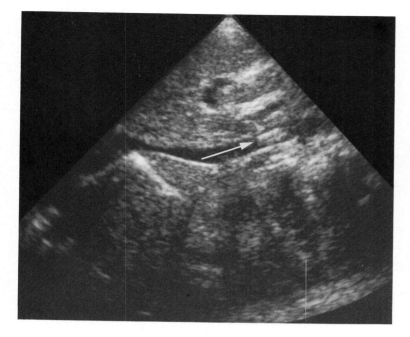

Figure 2–79 □ Thrombus *(arrow)* partially occluding the inferior vena cava in an infant in whom a central catheter had been placed previously.

ready means for thrombus identification (Figs. 2–79 and 2–80) (Oppenheimer et al). Monitoring of thrombus size and extent can be accomplished when treatment is deferred or when a thrombolytic agent is utilized. Likewise, following thrombectomy, the affected segment of the vessel can be assessed.

Renal Vein Thrombosis

Renal vein thrombosis is likely to occur in the dehydrated or septic neonate and is more prevalent in infants of diabetic mothers. One or both kidneys may be involved. Clinically, there is renal enlargement and hematuria. There may also be proteinuria and a low platelet count as a result of consumptive coagulopathy (Rosenberg et al). Azotemia may be noted, even when only one kidney is involved. If the thrombus reaches the renal vein or inferior vena cava, it may be directly visualized within these vessels. However, thrombosis occurs initially in the small intrarenal venous branches, extending toward the renal

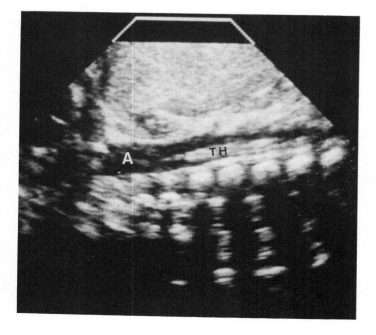

Figure 2–80 □ Large and extensive post-catheter intra-aortic (A) thrombus (TH). (From Shkolnik A: Applications of ultrasound in the neonatal abdomen. Radiol Clin North Am 23:141, 1985.)

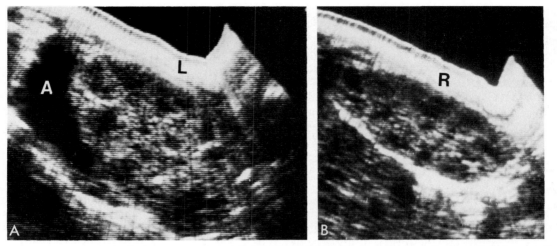

Figure 2–81 □ *A,* Longitudinal sonogram demonstrates large left kidney with a disordered echo pattern in a septic, dehydrated neonate. The presence of coexistent acute (liquid) adrenal hemorrhage is indicated by suprarenal anechoic structure (A). *B,* Normal right kidney. (Courtesy of Dr. Carol Rumack, Health Sciences Center, University of Colorado, Denver.)

hilum (Slovis et al, 1989). At this stage, the enlarged kidney presents a nonspecific and disordered heterogeneous internal echo pattern, reflecting the extent and severity of involvement. There may be coexistent adrenal hemorrhage, particularly on the left side where the adrenal vein drains directly into the renal vein (Fig. 2–81). In the majority of instances, significant function is regained. A reticulated pattern of calcification within the involved intrarenal veins may subsequently be seen.

Doppler Imaging

Doppler imaging is based on the change in frequency (Doppler shift) that occurs when insonated sound strikes a moving target, such as circulating red blood cells. The basic principles, instrumentation, and pitfalls of Doppler ultrasound scanning are well presented by Taylor and Holland, and the clinical applications are discussed by Scoutt et al. An excellent review of the basic principles and current applications of color Doppler imaging has been provided by Lewis et al. Additionally, Patriquin and Paltiel have authored an excellent overview of clinical applications of abdominal Doppler studies in children, and Keller has provided an insightful overview of the applications and potential applications of renal Doppler sonography in infants and children.

Renal Transplantation

The use of ultrasonography for assessment of post-transplant hydronephrosis and peri-

transplant fluid accumulations has been previously discussed. The Doppler examination, with calculation of

$$\text{resistive index} = \frac{A - B}{B}$$

(where A = peak systolic blood flow velocity and B = end systolic blood flow velocity) has been applied to the assessment of renal transplant dysfunction. A high resistive index has been reported as most often indicative of vascular transplant rejection (Buckley et al; Don et al; Fleischer et al; Rifkin et al; Townsend et al). However, a number of reports have questioned the value and reliability of this index (Allen et al; Drake et al; Genkins et al; Kelzc et al; Perrella, et al).

The detection of acute renal vein thrombosis in renal allografts by means of duplex Doppler ultrasonography (Reuther et al), as well as a post-biopsy arterial pseudoaneurysm (Weissman et al), has been reported. Stringer et al reported detection of renal artery stenosis in the transplanted kidney of a pediatric patient.

Other Applications

As Keller has further pointed out, Doppler sonography is capable of documenting causes of diminished urine output, such as renal arterial occlusion and renal vein thrombosis. The site of renal artery stenosis, likewise, may be detected in the hypertensive child.

Characterization of renal masses by means of Doppler ultrasound (Kuijpers and Jaspers) is a topic of great interest. In an important study by Patriquin et al, it was noted that during the oliguric or anuric phase of the hemolytic uremic syndrome, there was either absence of intrarenal arterial flow or absence, reversal, or marked reduction of diastolic flow. Diuresis was found to occur within 24 to 48 hours after diastolic Doppler shifts returned to normal. These findings enabled a prediction of recovery of renal function, thereby allowing the curtailment or avoidance of dialysis in some cases.

Duplex Doppler Scanning

In duplex Doppler scanning, real-time delineation of the blood vessel allows direct placement of a cursor within a portion of the vessel, providing for interrogation of a small volume within the Doppler beam. The rebounding sound waves from an artery produce the characteristic audible whooshing sound of systolic-diastolic blood flow. A lower-pitched, smoother sound characterizes venous flow. This information is also displayed simultaneously, with the real-time image on the television screen, as a spectral wave form that reflects the velocity of blood flow. An example of an arcuate artery inter-

rogation in a transplanted kidney is demonstrated (Fig. 2–82). Figure 2–83 displays the spectral tracing of the renal vein in a transplanted kidney.

Color-Flow Doppler Scanning

A color-flow renal sonogram is demonstrated in Color Figure 2–1 (see p. 62). The delineation of long segments of the renal artery and vein, including the smaller intrarenal branches, has greatly shortened the examination time, in that the sampling cursor is more readily placed in an appropriate position. An accompanying presentation of the spectral pattern can also be achieved as in Figures 2–82 and 2–83.

The sonogram in Figure 2–84 was instrumental in documenting torsion of the left spermatic cord in a neonate. There was no evidence of blood flow to the enlarged left testes during color-flow Doppler scanning. Similar findings in five adults have been documented in a report by Middleton and Melson. This use of color-flow Doppler scanning, as well as the overall clinical scope of color-flow imaging relative to the urogenital system of the pediatric patient, is sure to increase dramatically.

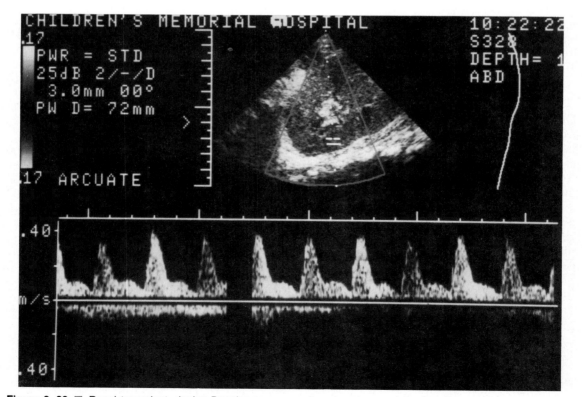

Figure 2–82 □ Renal transplant, duplex Doppler sonogram. Arcuate artery systolic-diastolic wave form. Blood flow, toward the transducer, is projected above the baseline.

Hricak H, Filly RA: Sonography of the scrotum. Invest Radiol 18:112, 1983.

Hricak H, Jeffrey RB: Sonography of acute scrotal abnormalities. Radiol Clin North Am 21:595, 1983.

Hricak H, Romanski RN, Eyler WR: The renal sinus during allograft rejection: Sonographic and histopathologic findings. Radiology 142:693, 1982.

Hufnagle KG, Khan SN, Penn D, et al: Renal calcifications: a complication of long-term furosemide therapy in preterm infants. Pediatrics 70:360, 1982.

Jaffe MH, White SJ, Silver TM, et al: Wilms' tumor: ultrasonic features, pathologic correlation and diagnostic pitfalls. Radiology 140:147, 1981.

Jeanty P, Dramaix-Wilmet M, Elkhazen N, et al: Measurement of fetal kidney growth on ultrasound. Radiology 144:159, 1982.

Jequier S, Paltiel H, LaFortune M: Ureterovesical jets in infants and children: duplex and color Doppler US studies. Radiology 175:349, 1990.

Jequier S, Rousseau O: Sonographic measurements of the normal bladder wall in children. AJR 149:563, 1987.

Kay CT, Rosenfield AT, Taylor KJW, et al: Ultrasonic characteristics of chronic atrophic pyelonephritis. AJR 132:47, 1979.

Kelcz F, Pozniak MA, Pirsch JD, Oberly TD: Pyramidal appearance and resistive index: insensitive and nonspecific sonographic indicators of renal transplant rejection. AJR 155:531, 1990.

Keller MS: Renal Doppler sonography in infants and children. Radiology 172:603, 1989.

Kessler RM, Altman DH: Real-time sonographic detection of vesicoureteral reflux in children. AJR 138:1033, 1982.

Kintanar C, Cramer BC, Reid WD, Andrews WL: Neonatal renal candidiasis: sonographic diagnosis. AJR 147:801, 1986.

Kramer SA, Hoffman AD, Aydin G, et al: Simple renal cysts in children. J Urol 128:1259, 1982.

Kremer H, Dobrinski W, Mikyska M, et al: Ultrasonic in vivo and in vitro studies on the nature of the ureteral jet phenomenon. Radiology 142:175, 1982.

Krone KD, Carroll BA: Scrotal ultrasound: symposium on ultrasonography of small parts. Radiol Clin North Am 23:121, 1985.

Kuijpers D, Jaspers R: Renal Masses: differential diagnosis with pulsed doppler US. Radiology 170:59, 1989.

Kuligowska E, Newman B, White SJ, et al: Interventional ultrasound in detection and treatment of renal inflammatory disease. Radiology 147:521, 1983.

Lawson TL, Foley WD, Berland LL, et al: Ultrasonic evaluation of fetal kidneys: analysis of normal size and frequency of visualization as related to stage of pregnancy. Radiology 138:153, 1981.

Lebowitz RL, Blickman JG: The coexistence of ureteropelvic junction obstruction and reflux. AJR 140:231, 1983.

Lebowitz RL, Griscom NT: Neonatal hydronephrosis: 146 cases. Radiol Clin North Am 15:49, 1977.

Leonidas JC, McCauley RGK, Klauber GC, Fretzayas AM: Sonography as a substitute for excretory urography in children with urinary tract infection. AJR 144:815, 1985.

Lewis BD, James EM, Charboneau JW, Reading CC, Welch TJ: Current applications of color Doppler imaging in the abdomen and extremities. RadioGraphics 9:599, 1989.

Lippe BM, Sample WF: Pelvic ultrasonography in pediatric and adolescent endocrine disorders. J Pediatr 92:897, 1978.

Lufkin EG, Alfrey AC, Trucksess ME, et al: Polycystic kidney disease: earlier diagnosis and using ultrasound. Urology 4:5, 1974.

Lupetin AR, King W, Rich P, et al: Ultrasound diagnosis of testicular leukemia. Radiology 146:171, 1983.

Madewell JE, Goldman SM, Davis CJ, et al: Multilocular cystic nephroma: a radiographic-pathologic correlation of 58 patients. Radiology 146:309, 1983.

Madrazo BL, Klugo RC, Parks JA, et al: Ultrasonographic demonstration of undescended testes. Radiology 133:181, 1979.

Mahony BS: The genitourinary system. *In* Ultrasonography in Obstetrics and Gynecology. Edited by PW Callen. Philadelphia, WB Saunders Co, 1988, pp 254–276.

Maklad NF, Wright CH, Rosenthal SJ: Gray scale ultrasonic appearance of renal transplant rejection. Radiology 131:711, 1979.

Markle BM, Potter BM: Surgical diseases of the urinary tract. *In* Ultrasound in Pediatrics. Edited by JO Haller, A Shkolnik. New York, Churchill Livingstone, 1981, pp 135–164.

Mascatello VJ, Smith EH, Carrera GF, et al: Ultrasonic evaluation of the obstructed duplex kidney. AJR 129:113, 1977.

Middleton WD, Melson GL: Testicular ischemia: color Doppler sonographic findings in five patients. AJR 152:1237, 1989.

Mindell HJ, Kupic EA: Horseshoe kidney: ultrasonic demonstration. AJR 129:526, 1977.

Mueller DL, Amundson GM, Rubin SZ, Wesenberg RL: Acute scrotal abnormalities in children: diagnosis by combined sonography and scintigraphy. AJR 150:643, 1988.

Nussbaum AR, Sanders RC, Hartman DS, Dudgeon DL, Parmley TH: Neonatal ovarian cysts: sonographic-pathologic correlation. Radiology 168:817, 1988.

Nussbaum AR, Sanders RC, Jones MD: Neonatal uterine morphology as seen on real-time US. Radiology 160:641, 1986.

Nybonde T, Mortensson W: Ultrasonography of the kidney following renal biopsy in children. Acta Radiol 29:151, 1988.

Oppenheimer DA, Carroll BA, Garth KE: Ultrasonic detection of complications following umbilical arterial catheterization in the neonate. Radiology 145:667, 1982.

Patriquin H, Palteil H: Abdominal doppler US in children: clinical applications. *In* Syllabus: A Categorical Course in Diagnostic Radiology, Pediatric Radiology. Edited by AK Poznanski, JA Kirkpatrick Jr. Presented at the 75th Scientific Assembly and Annual Meeting of the Radiological Society of North America. 1989, pp 185–196.

Platt JF, Ellis JH, Rubin JM, DiPietro MA, Sedman AB: Intrarenal arterial doppler sonography in patients with nonobstructive renal disease: correlation of resistive index with biopsy findings. AJR 154:1223, 1990.

Raffensperger JG: Soft tissue tumors. *In* Swenson's Pediatric Surgery, 4th ed. New York, Appleton-Century-Crofts, 1980, pp 405–414.

Reuther G, Wanjura D, Bauer H: Acute renal vein thrombosis in renal allografts: detection with duplex doppler US. Radiology 170:557, 1989.

Richie JP, Birnholz J, Garnick MB: Ultrasonography as a diagnostic adjunct for the evaluation of masses in the scrotum. Surg Gynecol Obstet 154:694, 1982.

Rifkin MD, Needleman L, Pasto ME, Kurtz AB, Foy PM, et al: Evaluation of renal transplant rejection by duplex Doppler examination: value of the resistive index. AJR 148:759, 1987.

Rosenberg ER, Trought WS, Kirks DR, et al: Ultrasonic

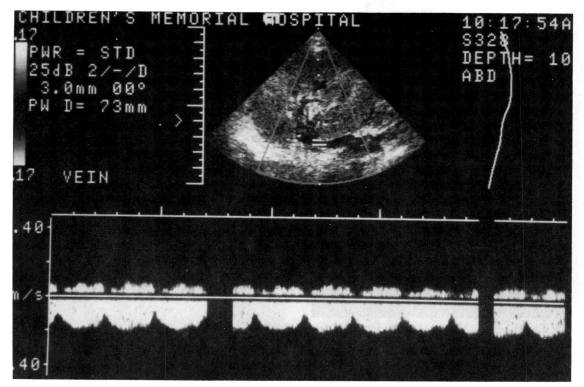

Figure 2–83 □ Renal transplant, duplex Doppler sonogram. Flow pattern of renal vein elicited during longitudinal scanning. Flow away from transducer projects below baseline.

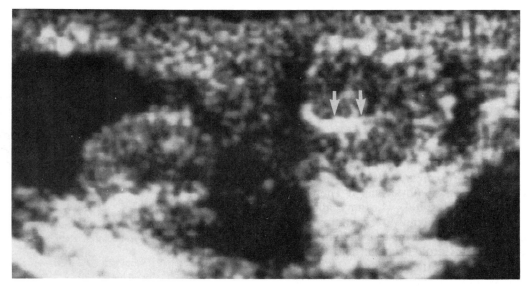

Figure 2–84 □ Transverse scan of swollen scrotum in a 1-day-old boy. There is a hydrocele around the normal-sized right testis. Testicular color flow appeared normal. The left testis is enlarged, and the mediastinum testis (arrows) is identified. No evidence of color flow to the left testis was observed during Doppler color flow imaging. At surgery, the left testicular torsion was confirmed and the testis removed.

diagnosis of renal vein thrombosis in neonates. AJR 134:35, 1980.

Rosenfield AT, Glickman MG, Taylor KJW, et al: Acute focal bacterial nephritis (acute lobar nephronia). Radiology 132:553, 1979.

Sample WF, Gottesman JE, Skinner DG, et al: Gray scale ultrasound of the scrotum. Radiology 127:225, 1978.

Sanders RC, Nussbaum AR, Soloz K: Renal dysplasia: sonographic findings. Radiology 167:623, 1988.

Scoutt LM, Zawin ML, Taylor KJW: Doppler US. Part II. Clinical applications. Radiology 174:309, 1990.

Shkolnik A: B-mode ultrasound and the nonvisualizing kidney in pediatrics. AJR 128:121, 1977.

Shkolnik A, Foley MJ, Riggs TW, et al: New application of real-time ultrasound in pediatrics. RadioGraphics 2:422, 1982.

Siegel MJ, Glasier CM: Acute focal bacterial nephritis in children: significance of ureteral reflux. AJR 127:257, 1981.

Silver TM, Campbell D, Wicks JD, et al: Peritransplant fluid collections: ultrasound evaluation and clinical significance. Radiology 138:145, 1981.

Six R, Oliphant M, Grossman H: A spectrum of renal tubular ectasia and hepatic fibrosis. Radiology 117:117, 1975.

Slovis TL, Cushing B, Reilly BJ, et al: Wilms' tumor to the heart: clinical and radiographic evaluation. AJR 131:263, 1978.

Slovis TL, Perlmutter AD: Recent advances in pediatric urological ultrasound. J Urol 123:613, 1980.

Slovis TL, Philippart AI, Cushing B, et al: Evaluation of the inferior vena cava by sonography and venography in children with renal and hepatic tumors. Radiology 140:767, 1981.

Slovis TL, Sty JR, Haller JO: *In* Imaging of the Pediatric Urinary Tract. Philadelphia, WB Saunders Co, 1989.

Spigos D, Capek V, Jonasson O: Percutaneous biopsy of renal transplants using ultrasonographic guidance. J Urol 117:699, 1977.

Stringer DA, O'Halpin D, Daneman A, Liu P, Geary DF: Duplex Doppler sonography for renal artery stenosis in the post-transplant pediatric patient. Pediatr Radiol 19:187, 1989.

Stuck KJ, Koff SA, Silver TM: Ultrasonic features of multicystic dysplastic kidney: expanded diagnostic criteria. Radiology 143:217, 1982.

Subramanyam BR, Balthazar EJ, Raghavendra BN, et al: Sonographic diagnosis of scrotal hernia. AJR 139:535, 1982.

Surratt JT, Siegel MJ, Middleton WD: Sonography of complications in pediatric renal allografts. RadioGraphics 10:687, 1990.

Taylor KJW, Holland S: Doppler US. Part I. Basic principles, instrumentation, and pitfalls. Radiology 174:297, 1990.

Teele RL: Ultrasonography of the genitourinary tract in children. Radiol Clin North Am 15:109, 1977.

Tolchin D, Koenigsberg M, Santorineou M: Early detection of Wilms' tumor in a child with hemihypertrophy and ovarian cysts. Pediatrics 70:135, 1982.

Townsend RR, Tomlanovich SJ, Goldstein RB, Filly RA: Combined Doppler and morphologic sonographic evaluation of renal transplant rejection. J Ultrasound Med 9:199, 1990.

Vallancien G, Dumez Y, Aubry MC, et al: Percutaneous nephrostomy in utero. Urology 20:647, 1982.

Vinocur L, Slovis TL, Perlmutter AD, Watts FB, Chang C-H: Follow-up studies of multicystic dysplastic kidneys. Radiology 167:311, 1988.

Weissman J, Giyanani VL, Landreneau MD, Kilpatrick JS: Postbiopsy arterial pseudoaneurysm in a renal allograft: detection by Duplex sonography. J Ultrasound Med 7:515, 1988.

Wladimiroff JW: Effect of furosemide on fetal urine production. Br J Obstet Gynaecol 82:221, 1975.

Wolverson MK, Houttuin E, et al: Comparison of computed tomography with high-resolution real-time ultrasound in the localization of the impalpable undescended testis. Radiology 146:133, 1983.

Wood BP, Ben-Ami T, Teele RL, Rabinowitz R: Ureterovesical obstruction and megaloureter: diagnosis by real-time US. Radiology 156:79, 1985.

3

☐ Uroradiology: Procedures and Anatomy

Alan D. Hoffman and Andrew J. LeRoy

Methods for imaging the urinary tract in children have proliferated significantly in recent years. Nuclear imaging, ultrasonography, computed tomography (CT), and magnetic resonance imaging (MRI) have been added to the more traditional armamentarium of radiographic examinations. In view of their impact on diagnosis and management, it is important that the indications, limitations, and complications of these procedures be familiar to urologists, pediatricians, and radiologists who deal with urinary tract disease in children. In various settings, the availability of the newer modalities as well as the experience and interest of the radiologists involved in the performance and interpretation of examinations will have an influence upon the method to be used. The radiologist should tailor the imaging workup of such patients. With this approach, the number of examinations, the expense, the irradiation, and patient discomfort are minimized, whereas the useful clinical information is maximized.

Ultrasonography and nuclear voiding cystography and renography are becoming increasingly more important as first-line examinations. However, excretory urography and image-intensified, fluoroscopically monitored voiding cystourethrography are still the most commonly employed procedures for the evaluation of the urinary tract in the practice of pediatric urology and nephrology (Figs. 3–1 and 3–2). This chapter emphasizes these latter examinations.

Ultrasonography and nuclear imaging are discussed in detail in Chapters 2 and 4. The diagnostic usefulness of the information about genitourinary anatomy and urinary tract disease that these techniques provide depends upon the manner in which the examinations are conducted. The high-quality excretory urogram or voiding cystourethrogram expected as a matter of course in adult urography certainly can be achieved in pediatric urography. However, unnecessarily sophisticated roentgenographic examinations with an excessive number of films are sometimes performed to diagnose problems that could have been evaluated adequately on a high-quality excretory urogram monitored by a physician experienced in solving problems encountered in pediatric uroradiology. With a knowledge of the usual pathologic processes, the physician can generally perform a fairly simple routine examination using only a few films. Appropriate tailoring of the examination by the radiologist is often necessary.

EXCRETORY UROGRAPHY

Intravenous urography is an important roentgenographic examination used to evaluate the urinary tract in infants and children. Although ultrasonography provides excellent anatomic detail and nuclear renography reveals detailed functional information, the excretory urogram is an examination that furnishes both anatomic and functional information.

An initial radiograph prior to the intravenous injection of contrast material is an important baseline for the evaluation of the urinary tract and the entire visualized abdomen. Following the injection of contrast material intravenously, the physician can evaluate sequentially the renal parenchyma, intrarenal collecting system, ureters, and bladder.

Many technical details of the procedure are variable, offering the examiner opportunities for critical choices. Peak kilovoltage and mil-

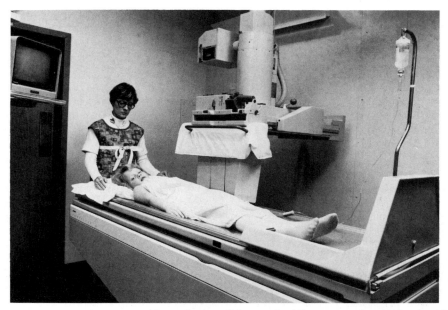

Figure 3–1 □ The fluoroscopic room used for pediatric radiology and voiding cystourethrography should be equipped with an image intensifier and spot film device capable of instantaneous recording of significant findings. In addition, television video recording can be useful for restudy and teaching.

liamperage; duration and timing of exposures; type and dosage of contrast medium; filming technique, including choice of x-ray film and screen combinations; positioning of the pa-

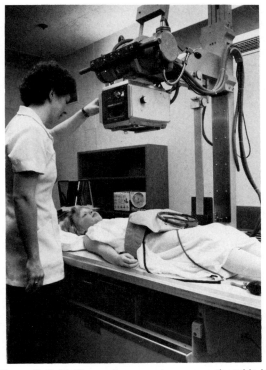

Figure 3–2 □ The modern excretory urography table is equipped for tomography; a ureteral compression device is shown in place.

tient; use or omission of tomography; and ureteral compression and catheter drainage of the bladder—all are crucial to achieving the desired accuracy of diagnosis. Careful selection among these technical variables is of utmost importance in excretory urography and voiding cystourethrography.

Indications

With the addition of new methods of imaging the urinary tract, the indications for an initial excretory urogram have undergone some change. Urinary tract infection remains the most common clinical indication for excretory urography in children. However, if a voiding cystourethrogram is normal, many physicians will perform ultrasonography rather than excretory urography (Lebowitz and Mandell; Leonidas et al). Other indications for excretory urography include hematuria or suspicious abdominal pain suggesting urinary calculus. Abnormal findings on a renal ultrasonogram often indicate the need for the performance of excretory urography. Patients with failure to thrive and moderately elevated serum creatinine levels may also be evaluated by a screening excretory urogram (Stannard and Lebowitz). Depending upon the availability of high-quality ultrasonography and isotopic scanning, these examinations may replace initial excretory urography in certain situations. Screening for associated congenital anomalies, abdominal mass, and abdominal pain, or searching for renal vascular causes for hypertension might best be initiated using these modalities. A considerable number of excretory urograms are taken as postoperative or follow-up examinations when the primary diagnosis is known. Not infrequently, the number of radiographs in such examinations might be reduced below the number routinely used.

Contraindications

A number of contraindications exist to the performance of excretory urography in children. Dehydration, particularly in a neonate, is a relative contraindication because of the hyperosmolarity of current contrast materials. Shock is an invariable contraindication. Hyperuricemia seen in children in a hypercatabolic state secondary to primary tumor breakdown or as a response to therapy of malignancy is also a contraindication. In such patients, uric acid may be precipitated in renal tubules as a result of a normal dose of contrast material (Kelly; Poslethwaithe and Kelly).

It has long been known that the glomerular filtration rate in neonates in the first days of life is low; as a result, excretory urography attempted on these infants often has limited usefulness because of poor visualization. If urography is performed, markedly delayed films may be useful. Generally, unless there are overwhelming clinical considerations, it is advantageous to delay excretory urography until at least the second week of life. This approach is particularly appropriate when high-quality ultrasonography and nuclear medicine are available.

Personnel and Equipment

More vital to successful diagnosis than any technical detail of equipment design is the participation of interested personnel—radiographers, nurses, and radiologists—involved in the performance of the examination. People choosing to work in the area where children are seen must be empathetic and skilled in the art of blending the proper degree of gentleness and occasional firmness required to achieve excellent technical results while keeping the patient reasonably happy. Technologists must be dedicated to the concept of high-quality

genitourinary radiography while keeping the radiation exposure to the patient to a minimum. Nurses must have an understanding of their role in the performance of examinations, and the radiologists involved must be knowledgeable and interested in the normal anatomy and pathology involved in urinary tract problems of children.

The roentgenographic systems intended for the evaluation of pediatric patients must have capability for fast exposure times inasmuch as patient motion is a prime cause of poor results in any roentgenographic procedure. Several acceptable systems exist that might be adaptable to the requirements of a given department or individual physician. Currently, radiographic systems for generating digital films allowing manipulation of images and reduction of radiation dose are being evaluated (Fajardo et al).

Gonadal Protection

It is the responsibility of the radiologic technologist and the physician to insist that gonadal shielding and the basic fundamental techniques of radiation protection be applied to all pediatric patients as well as to paramedical personnel and physicians involved in the use of ionizing radiation.

Gonadal protection should apply to all pediatric patients whenever it is feasible to do so without obscuring the part of the genitourinary system being evaluated. The male gonads can be shielded on all films taken for an excretory urogram, and the female gonads can be shielded on all films centered on and coned for the kidneys.

A simple and practical shielding method consists of using vinyl-covered lead sheeting (0.5 mm of lead) cut into various sizes to shield the male gonads without obscuring the pelvis. The female gonads can be protected with a vinyl-lead sheet placed over the pelvis, but the shield must be removed when films of the lower ureters and bladder are taken. Triangular pieces of vinyl-lead sheeting, cut into various sizes so that they do not obscure the bones of the pelvis or hips, also can be used to shield female gonads for other roentgenographic procedures (Fig. 3–3) (Godderidge). Alternatively, a lead "shadow shield" can be attached to the x-ray tube. With a full-field light localizing system, such a shield can be positioned to block radiation to either the male or female gonads (Fig. 3–4).

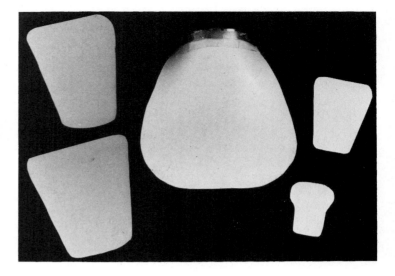

Figure 3–3 □ A variety of sizes of lead gonadal shields can be used for both males and females.

Preparation of Patient

Feeding

Food and fluids are not withheld from infants except for the feeding just prior to the excretory urogram. Preschoolers and older children usually have a liquid meal in the evening prior to the examination and are restricted from fluids on the morning of the examination to avoid aspiration of gastric contents in the occasional patient who vomits after the injection of contrast material. No attempt at dehydration should be made in pediatric patients; this is particularly important in infants or in any patient who may already be dehydrated. In the past, dehydration has been implicated in renal failure occurring after excretory urography. One possible explanation for renal failure following excretory urography is tubular obstruction by a "gel" formed by contrast medium in combination with the Tamm-Horsfall urinary mucoprotein (Fig. 3–5) (Berdon et al, 1969).

Bowel Preparation

Preparation of the gastrointestinal tract prior to excretory urography may be varied according to the patient's age. Infants do not require any type of bowel preparation. In preschoolers and older children, bisacodyl suppositories (Dulcolax) administered in the morning a few hours before the examination are often helpful in eliminating excess amounts of fecal material from the colon. Adolescents generally tolerate a normal adult preparation. Some radiologists, however, prefer to avoid bowel preparations altogether and rely upon tomography for proper visualization of the kidneys. Enemas are not usually used because they may actually interfere with the examination if air is introduced into the colon during administration of the enema.

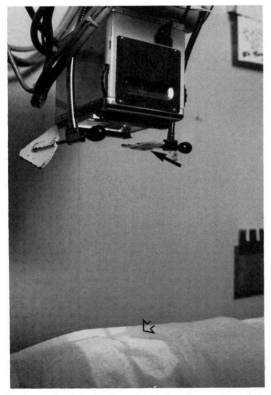

Figure 3–4 □ A shadow shield (solid arrow) casting a shadow over the gonad region (open arrow) is shown with the collimator light on.

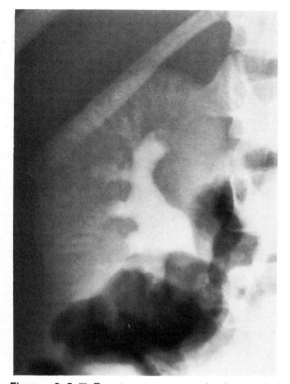

Figure 3–5 □ Excretory urogram showing typical striated nephrogram usually attributed to the interaction of contrast medium and Tamm-Horsfall mucoprotein.

Patient Education

An important consideration in the preparation of the child for a urographic or any radiographic examination that is frightening or uncomfortable is patient education. A successful method of educating young patients and also their parents about such examinations may be provided by using patient education materials that can be made available to the parent at the time that the examination is initially requested. If this occurs a day or more before the time the examination is actually performed, it is likely that both parent and child will have a reasonable idea of what to expect and overall anxiety will be reduced. These patient education materials can be written in simplified language with cartoon-like pictures that will appeal to young children. Frequently, children as young as 4 or 5 years will have reasonable understanding of these examinations and will be more fully cooperative during their performance. Figure 3–6 shows pamphlets based on those originally devised by Haas and Solomon.

Possibility of Pregnancy

Adolescent females should be asked for the time of their last menstrual period prior to a radiographic examination of the abdomen. If pregnancy is a likely consideration, such examinations should be delayed unless there is a major, acute clinical indication. Alternatively, ultrasonography might be performed.

Contrast Media

New low osmolar contrast materials (LOCMs) have become available to compete with the standard or high osmolar contrast materials (HOCMs) that had been utilized with a high degree of safety over the previous 30 years (Magill et al). Two large studies (Katayama and Tanaka; Palmer) show fewer side effects with the newer agents. Fatal outcome is rare with HOCMs (Hartman et al) but has not been sufficiently defined with LOCMs. However, the significantly higher cost of the LOCMs in the United States has prompted debate over which type of contrast material should be used in specific circumstances. Medical as well as ethical and economic considerations have been used to define under which circumstances LOCMs might be used instead of HOCMs (Bettmann; McClennan). There is, however, a lack of uniformity among radiologists over which patients should receive the LOCMs (Steinberg et al). As a result, some radiologists have switched over completely to the use of LOCMs, whereas many will use these contrast materials only in specific situations including previous contrast material reaction, debilitated or unstable patients, or a patient who is more likely to vomit after the administration of contrast material.

Dosage

The dosage of contrast medium to be used can be determined by several guidelines. At our institution, we utilize 1.0 ml/lb up to a dose of 50 ml, which is our standard adult dose. In children with renal failure or urinary tract obstruction and in newborn infants, the dosage of contrast medium may be increased up to a maximum of 1.5 to 2.0 ml/lb.

The dosages recommended by manufacturers of contrast media are usually considerably smaller than those suggested above. Nonetheless, increasing the dose of contrast material

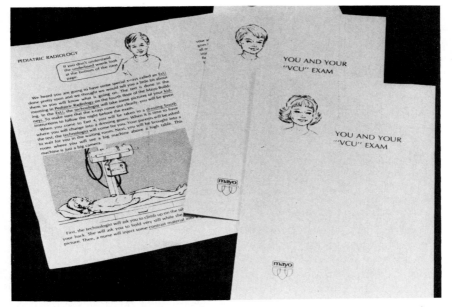

Figure 3–6 □ Educational pamphlets explain the excretory urogram *(left)* and voiding cystourethrogram *(right)* in language that is understandable for parents and children.

has substantially improved the quality of the urogram without increasing the incidence or severity of untoward reactions. For HOCMs, there is a dose beyond which improvement of the image does not occur, which is probably related to the diuretic effect of the contrast material itself (Fischer et al).

Administration

Contrast media should always be injected intravenously. Any one of a number of injection sites may be selected. Although an antecubital vein is most often used in adults and older children, it may be difficult to maintain a needle in this location in infants and young children. As a result, the most apparent superficial vein of any extremity may be utilized. Occasionally, an external jugular vein may be used by one experienced with the use of this route. In infants, scalp veins are occasionally used, but the femoral vein route is not appropriate because of the danger of a septic hip joint as a complication of a misdirected injection. Successful venipuncture requires careful immobilization, especially in the uncooperative patient. Butterfly needles or conventional needles may be used, depending upon the experience of the person performing the venipuncture.

The total amount of iodine injected is the important determinant in renal parenchyma and collecting system opacification. Inasmuch as maximal opacification is achieved by presenting to the renal filtration apparatus the highest concentration of contrast material, the injection is performed as a single bolus rather than a drip infusion (Dure-Smith et al). In patients who are thought to be predisposed to contrast medium reactions, access to an intravenous route is maintained by leaving the needle in the vein and keeping it open with a slow infusion of saline or a heparin-lock solution for the duration of the examination.

Reactions

Although Gooding and associates suggest that the incidence of hypersensitivity reactions to contrast media is lower in children than in adults, the full range of reactions does occur, including, rarely, death (Dunbar and Nogrady). Testing for hypersensitivity has been tried but does not seem to be predictive and could potentially give a false sense of security. A history of allergy to iodine and prior reactions to iodinated contrast material may be helpful in predicting an increased risk for subsequent examinations (Witten et al). There is renewed interest in the allergic, antibody-mediated hypothesis for contrast media reactions (Brasch). However, some of the most severe reactions reported have occurred in patients with no history of allergy or prior exposure to contrast media.

Fortunately, most reactions to contrast media are not serious. Although nausea and vomiting occur occasionally, they are not considered true hypersensitivity reactions. Erythema and urticaria are relatively common but, if mild, will usually disappear after a short period. When these cutaneous reactions are irritating to the patient, treatment with oral or parenteral antihistamines such as diphenhydramine hydrochloride (Benadryl), a histamine H_1-receptor antagonist, will usually provide relief. Recent work (Philbin et al) suggests that cimetidine, a histamine H_2-receptor antagonist, may supplement the action of a histamine H_1-receptor antagonist. Such cutaneous reactions may occur even after only the retrograde instillation of contrast material into the bladder for voiding cystourethrography (Currarino et al). A previous cutaneous reaction to contrast material generally is not a contraindication to a future examination utilizing contrast material. Pretreatment of high-risk patients with H_1-receptor and H_2-receptor blockades, as well as corticosteroids, has been suggested (Bielory and Kaliner). Such patients should receive low osmolar contrast material.

Serious reactions are uncommon, but an appropriately equipped emergency cart like that shown in Figure 3–7 and a physician who is trained in the treatment of hypotension, cardiovascular collapse, cardiac arrest, and bronchospasm or laryngospasm must be immediately available in the uroradiology area when such examinations are done. Medications that may be needed on such an emergency cart are listed in Table 3–1. Appropriate therapy depends upon the predominant symptoms. Because each serious reaction has its unique characteristics, the personnel and equipment must be available to respond to any of the above clinical situations. It should be noted that the medications listed include several appropriate in the resuscitation of adults. Certainly, an anxious parent or grandparent accompanying a pediatric patient might, in a rare instance, undergo a cardiorespiratory emergency, and it is for that possibility that a departmental emergency cart is so stocked.

General Technique

After arriving in the radiology department for excretory urography, the patient is asked to void prior to the examination. If the patient

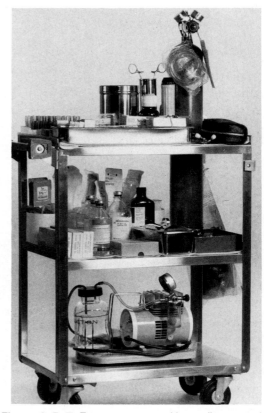

Figure 3–7 ☐ Emergency cart with ventilatory equipment, suction apparatus, sphygmomanometer, stethoscope, oxygen, fluids, and various medications.

generally empties his or her bladder by performance of the Credé maneuver or self-catheterization, these methods should be employed. Occasionally, a bladder catheter open to drainage is necessary during the examination.

In the routine excretory urogram, an abdominal film is obtained prior to the intravenous injection of contrast medium. This film, often referred to as a KUB (kidneys, ureter, and bladder), is taken with the patient in the supine

Table 3–1 ☐ Medications on Emergency Cart

Aminophylline	Hydrocortisone sodium succinate
Atropine	
Calcium gluconate	Intravenous fluids
Chlorpheniramine	Lidocaine
Diazepam	Mephentermine
Diphenhydramine	Metaraminol
Dopamine	Nitroglycerin
Ephedrine	Oxygen
Epinephrine, 1:1000	Sodium bicarbonate

position. It is coned to include the area between the diaphragm and symphysis pubis from flank to flank. Evaluation of this film before contrast medium is administered affords the radiologist and technologist the opportunity to check radiographic quality. Furthermore, the findings on this examination may suggest the need for a variety of actions other than the anticipated routine examination. Additional preparation of the patient, supplementary preliminary films, or performance of an examination other than an excretory urogram may be the result of careful evaluation of the KUB. This evaluation also affords an oppor-

tunity to evaluate the lumbosacral spine for abnormalities prior to its being obscured by contrast material.

If a significant amount of barium is in the bowel from a prior examination, a cleansing enema may be necessary or the excretory urogram may be postponed. Densities that might represent renal calculi might lead to further filming prior to injection of contrast material. Overlying bowel and its contents may make the precise definition of small renal stones difficult. Linear tomography frequently will overcome this difficulty (Fig. 3–8). Additionally, this technique helps significantly in the

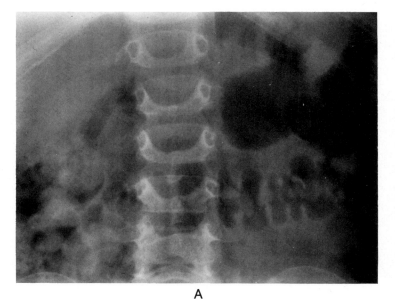

A

Figure 3–8 □ A, Both kidneys are largely obscured by overlying bowel content on the plain film. B, Tomogram obtained before injection of contrast medium clearly delineates dense calculus in lower pole of left kidney and poorly opacified calculus in upper pole of right kidney (arrows).

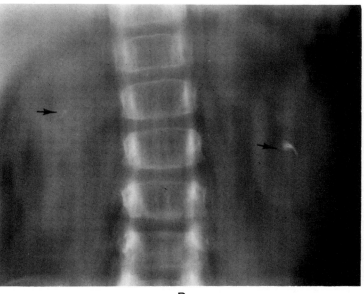

B

differentiation of intrarenal from extrarenal calcific densities. Tomographic evaluation generally obviates the necessity for oblique radiographs of this area. Other plain radiographs, including prone or cross-table lateral views, may be useful in the evaluation of poorly defined soft tissue densities.

In the case of a clinically palpable abdominal mass, a KUB is often taken prior to ultrasound, computed tomography, or even isotope scanning. In most instances, one of these examinations is appropriate rather than an excretory urogram.

When excretory urography is to be performed for other indications, the radiologist should review the KUB prior to the injection of contrast material. At this time, it should be determined whether it is appropriate to proceed with the excretory urogram and, if it is, what the initial sequence and timing of filming is to be. Monitoring should be performed from a problem-solving point of view, with several factors kept in mind. The number of films should be limited to those required to identify the clinical problem ˜and to visualize adequately the anatomy of the genitourinary system. Radiation exposure should be closely monitored and restricted to the minimum required to produce a high-quality examination.

Our routine urogram consists of only three films taken after the injection of contrast medium. The first film, properly coned and localized to the renal area, is taken 3 to 5 minutes after the injection. A single tomogram also coned to the renal area is taken immediately after the first film. At this early period, the density of the nephrogram is greatest and the collecting systems are most often adequately filled (Davidson). The use of tomography commonly overcomes the obscuring effect of the considerable amounts of overlying bowel and its contents common in infants and children. The third film, centered to include the entire urinary tract, is taken at 10 minutes after the injection, and the upper collecting systems, ureters, and bladder usually are adequately demonstrated (Fig. 3–9).

Although these routine films are sufficient in 80 to 90 per cent of our pediatric excretory urograms, careful on-line evaluation of films by the radiologist reveals the need for additional radiography in some patients. Further tomography, or prone, lateral, upright, or delayed filming may be indicated. A post-voiding film of the bladder is rarely useful inasmuch as the significance of "residual" urine (contrast material) after voiding is questionable unless the bladder empties completely. Actually, detailed analysis of the bladder is often impossible with excretory urography because of the variable amount and concentration of contrast material reaching the bladder at any given point during the procedure. On rare occasions, we will attempt to visualize the male urethra utilizing the contrast material that has reached the bladder. This extension of the excretory urogram is best made using fluoroscopically obtained spot films in a fashion similar to the voiding phase of a voiding cystourethrogram. The concentration, and consequently the density of the contrast medium, is generally only fair, but gross lesions such as partial obstruction of the urethra can often be excluded (Fig. 3–10). Improved visualization of the posterior urethra is often achieved by the use of a Zipser penile clamp (Fitts et al).

Ureteral compression is used routinely during excretory urography in adults. The procedure is extremely helpful in enhancing distention and adequate filling of the pelvicalyceal systems and upper ureters. This technique can also be used in children, resulting in improvement of the quality of urograms. There are, however, several situations in which ureteral compression is not used in children, either because it cannot be easily applied or because it may potentially obscure a diagnosis. In the former category, it is not used for infants or very young children up to about age 18 months, for patients with external urine collecting devices, or for those who have just had abdominal surgery. Patients in whom ureteral compression may be detrimental in diagnosis include those with an abdominal mass or possible obstructive uropathy.

When ureteral compression is not contraindicated, it is applied using a band with two inflatable bags. The band is placed around the upper pelvis, and the bags are positioned so that, when inflated, the ureters will be compressed between the device anteriorly and the upper pelvis posteriorly (Fig. 3–11). The compression is applied just after the contrast material has been injected so that its effect is seen on the early view of the renal area and on the tomogram. These films are evaluated immediately after they are developed, and if no further tomography is necessary, the compression is released immediately prior to exposure of the full-length film. In this way, the entire ureter may be shown on this film. If it is not appreciated that this is an immediate post-

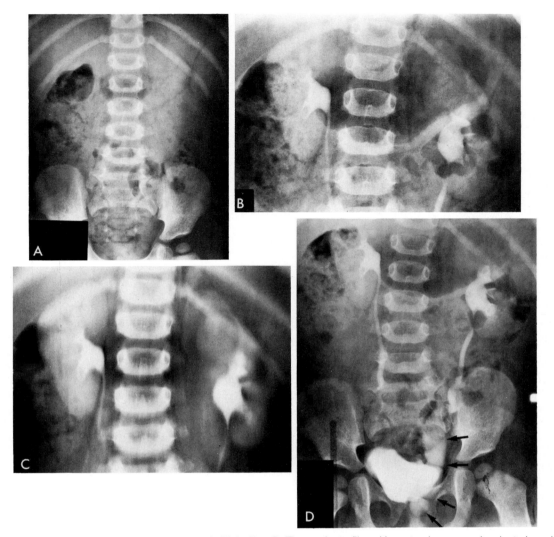

Figure 3–9 □ Four-film excretory urogram. *A*, Plain film. *B*, Three-minute film with ureteral compression (not shown). *C*, Three-minute thick-section tomogram of the renal area shows better definition of the renal outline and displays an obstructed upper pole collecting system on the left. *D*, Ten-minute film obtained shortly after the release of ureteral compression. The dilated ureter draining the upper pole of the left kidney is shown emptying below the bladder *(arrows)*.

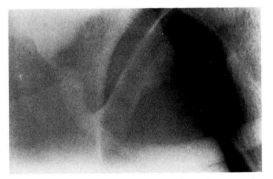

Figure 3–10 □ Antegrade (excretory) urethrogram done following excretory urogram in a 14-year-old male. This additional film was obtained to exclude posterior urethral valves.

decompression film, one might inadvertently assume that there is some degree of distal obstruction, reflux, or atony based upon the principle that a ureter fully outlined with contrast material on one film is usually abnormal.

The most common cause for inadequate visualization of the renal parenchyma and upper collecting system is overlying bowel content. Several techniques have been used to overcome this difficulty. Administration of a carbonated beverage distends the stomach with gas, displacing the overlying bowel away from the kidneys (Fig. 3–12). Distention of the stomach is especially helpful if the left kidney is obscured, but it can also be of help in

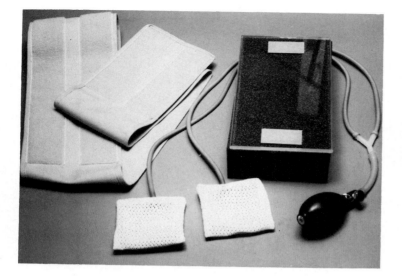

Figure 3–11 □ Compression device used temporarily to partially obstruct the ureters to better delineate the upper collecting system.

visualizing the right kidney, especially if a right posterior oblique film is obtained. However, if this gas passes through the pylorus and into the small bowel, it may obscure renal detail. Oblique films taken without administration of a carbonated beverage may help to visualize kidneys that are obscured by bowel content on conventional films.

These methods, however, suffer from a lack of reliability and reproducibility. In recent years, it has become increasingly apparent that tomography is technically feasible even in infants and young children and surpasses these other methods for defining renal outlines. Thin-section tomograms used for urography in adults require long tube travel distance and proportionately long exposure times. Such exposure times are unacceptable for infants and young children because respiratory motion would result in most cases. Consequently, decreased-amplitude (thick-section) tomography is used and generally exposure times are short enough to minimize patient motion and allow adequate visualization of renal parenchyma and renal outlines. Thick-section tomograms or zonograms have the additional advantage of permitting a reduction in the number of films exposed. Generally, a single properly executed tomogram is sufficient; with consideration of all three postinjection films routinely obtained, we find that adequate definition of both renal outlines can generally be satisfactorily accomplished (Fig. 3–13). In older children who can cooperate and hold their breath and in situations where finer detail is necessary, increased amplitude (thin-section) tomography can be done in the same manner as in adult urography.

Thick-section renal tomograms in young children are done using high milliamperage, low kilovoltage, and a short arc (20 degrees). The focus of the tomogram is at one third of the distance from the back of the patient to the front. Our routinely obtained tomogram is taken 3 to 5 minutes following injection of the contrast medium, when the nephrographic effect is greatest (Davidson). Additional tomograms are occasionally ordered after viewing the initial film.

The timing of filming is a critical factor in obtaining optimum urography. In the majority of patients, the schedule outlined above provides the appropriate diagnostic information with a minimum number of films.

In the neonate, however, delayed films are frequently required because of a combination of factors, including a lower glomerular filtration rate and a poorer concentrating ability. The excretion time for contrast medium is prolonged, and the concentration of contrast medium in the urinary tract is decreased. The peak excretion that occurs in older children and adults during the first 3 to 5 minutes may require from 30 minutes to as long as 3 hours in the neonate (Dunbar and Nogrady). Therefore, delayed films are advisable in infants when visualization of the kidneys and collecting systems is unsatisfactory on initial films. Ultrasonography, in conjunction with isotope scanning, has largely replaced excretory urography to define renal abnormalities in neonates.

In patients with obstruction of the urinary tract, delayed films also are essential in order to demonstrate the degree of hydronephrosis and to identify the site of obstruction. Rein-

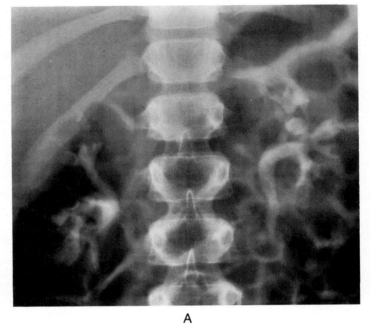

A

Figure 3–12 □ *A,* Kidneys are largely obscured by overlying gas in the small intestine. *B,* Immediately after administration of a carbonated beverage, the stomach is noticeably distended with gas, displacing loops of the small intestine inferiorly and allowing an unobstructed view of both kidneys.

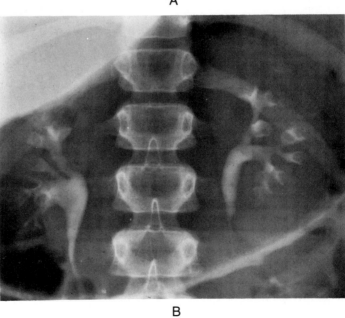

B

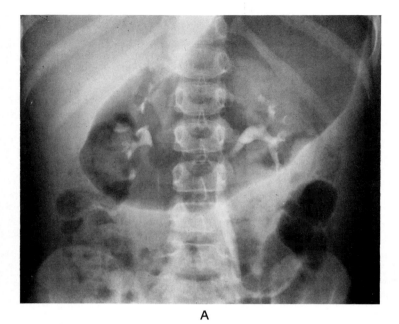

A

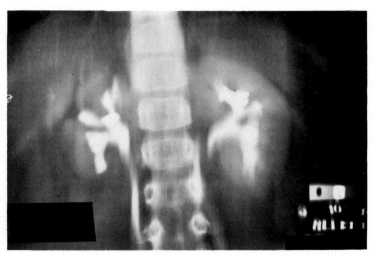

B

Figure 3–13 □ *A*, After administration of a carbonated beverage, both kidneys remain partially obscured by overlying bowel content. *B*, Linear tomography provides excellent visualization of both kidneys, revealing multiple areas of scarring of the right kidney and compensatory hypertrophy of the left kidney.

jection with an additional dose of contrast medium usually can be avoided by using ultrasonography in conjunction with excretory urography.

When a renal collecting system remains dilated following an operative procedure, it is often difficult subsequently to determine if obstruction is present on routine excretory urography. Augmentation of urinary flow can readily be accomplished by intravenous administration of a potent diuretic such as furosemide (Lasix). If this is injected at the end of a routine urogram, a radiograph of the abdomen exposed after an additional 20 or 30 minutes will show further dilatation if the renal collecting system is significantly obstructed. In such cases, the patient may experience colicky pain that simulates the symptoms that prompted the evaluation. The "Lasix test" can also be done in conjunction with an isotopic renal scan, described in Chapter 4.

Another technique for assessing possible partial obstruction of the urinary tract is the pressure-flow method of Whitaker. This requires placement of a percutaneous nephrostomy tube. If this test is done in the fluoroscopic suite, opaque contrast material is used so that a nephrostogram will show any areas of partial obstruction. This technique is described in detail in Chapter 16.

Anatomic Considerations

Accurate interpretation of the excretory urogram requires knowledge of the normal renal anatomy and experience in recognizing the many anatomic variations found in the normal individual. No attempt is made in this chapter to discuss all possible variations, but some that cause diagnostic difficulty have been singled out for emphasis.

Kidney Size

The size of the normal kidney in children varies according to age and to length and weight of the body. Renal lengths not only are easy to obtain from high-grade urograms but also have been shown to correlate well with actual renal size (Ludin). The pole-to-pole measurement of the left kidney of infants is usually a few millimeters longer than the right; in older children, the difference in measurement may be as much as 0.5 to 1.5 cm. Ultrasonography is also utilized to measure kidneys.

Just as pediatricians use growth charts to mark the progress of their patients, so is it important that those involved with renal disease in children be aware of renal growth over a period of time in their patients. The acceptance of this principle has resulted in the development of a number of renal growth charts. Although height correlates more consistently with renal size and growth than does age (Hodson et al), we utilize a renal growth chart that relates renal length to the patient's chronologic age, inasmuch as date of birth is readily obtained (Currarino). This chart has an additional tracing that represents the normal expected hypertrophy when only one kidney is present and functioning (Laufer and Griscom) (Fig. 3–14). In certain clinical circumstances, height or bone age may be the appropriate parameter to be related to renal length (Lebowitz et al).

Factors involved in the examination itself that might change the renal measurements include difference in centering, change in the axis of the kidneys with respiration, and swelling of the kidneys during the postinjection period as a result of the diuretic effect of the contrast medium. Hernandez and colleagues

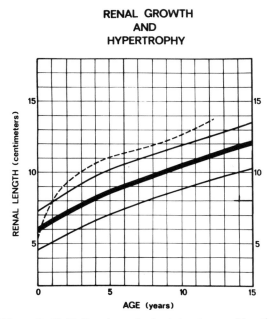

Figure 3–14 □ Renal growth chart showing renal length as a function of age. The bold line is the mean renal length; the thinner lines above and below show two standard deviations about the mean. The dotted line shows expected compensatory hypertrophy, which does not begin to deviate from the mean until birth. (From Lebowitz RL, Hopkins T, Colodny AH: Measuring the kidneys—practical applications using a growth hypertrophy chart. Pediatr Radiol 4:37, 1975. Courtesy of Springer-Verlag, Heidelberg.)

feel that the first two factors are the more significant ones. Partly to obviate some of these factors, the films taken at the same stage on each examination should be used for the measurement of renal size.

Certain anatomic factors that may affect pole-to-pole measurement of the kidneys include anomalies of position such as ectopy or malrotation. In addition, the normal kidney with a bifid collecting system has a pole-to-pole length longer than its nonduplicated mate. Bilateral duplication results in pole-to-pole measurements that appear as bilateral enlargements when compared with standard charts. Hydronephrosis or renal mass may also result in misleading renal measurements. Severe dehydration rarely may cause a decrease in overall renal size due to diminished blood flow.

Kidney Position

The right kidney is lower than the left kidney under normal conditions in more than 90 per cent of patients. Both kidneys tend to be mobile, and their positions relative to the spinal column will vary with different phases of respiration. The left kidney occasionally may be situated just beneath the diaphragm; the right kidney is seldom seen at this level because of the location of the liver in the right upper quadrant (Fig. 3–15). The lower pole of the right kidney commonly descends over the iliac crest in adults; this position is seen only occasionally in children (Figs. 3–16 and 3–17).

The upper poles of the kidneys are normally situated 1 to 2 cm closer to the midline than the lower poles, resulting in a characteristic angulation such that the axes of the kidneys parallel the psoas muscles. Variations in the degree of angulation are common, especially in infants and young children, in whom the axis normally parallels the longitudinal axis of the body. The lower pole of the kidney will, however, not normally be situated medial to the upper pole unless there is incomplete rotation or a horseshoe-shaped kidney (Fig. 3–18).

A mass in the suprarenal region or medial aspect of the upper pole of a kidney may result in a change in the axis of the kidney so that it is parallel to the spine or even reversed so that the upper pole lies lateral to the lower pole. When only the lower pole is being visualized, the abnormal axis may be the first indication of an obstructed, nonvisualized upper pole.

The location of the kidneys varies with changes in body position. By convention, the routine urogram is obtained with the patient in the supine position. If the patient is positioned on his or her right side, the anterior movement of the left kidney is greater than

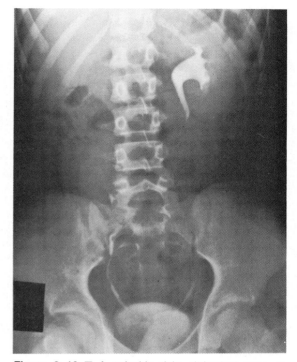

Figure 3–16 □ A palpable right abdominal mass is shown by excretory urography to be a low-lying, normal right kidney.

that of the right, and vice versa. Both kidneys normally may descend several centimeters when the patient is upright or prone. These factors must be kept in mind when interpreting films taken in positions other than the supine; otherwise, normal variations may be misinterpreted.

When the left kidney is not visualized on an excretory urogram, its presence or absence may be further ascertained by appreciation of the "splenic flexure" sign (Mascatello and Lebowitz; Meyers et al). When a left kidney is present in the left renal fossa, the splenic flexure of the colon is normally attached to the posterolateral abdominal wall by the phrenicocolic ligament. Absence or ectopia of the left kidney is associated with nondevelopment of the phrenicocolic ligament and resultant malposition of the anatomic splenic flexure of the colon so that it occupies the empty renal fossa (Fig. 3–19).

Renal Parenchyma

Since the mid 1960s, use of improved roentgenographic techniques and larger intravenous doses of contrast medium has made it possible

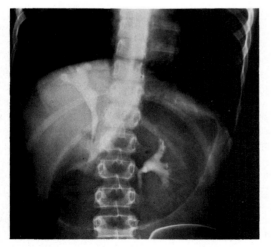

Figure 3–15 □ "Intrathoracic" right kidney demonstrated by excretory urography.

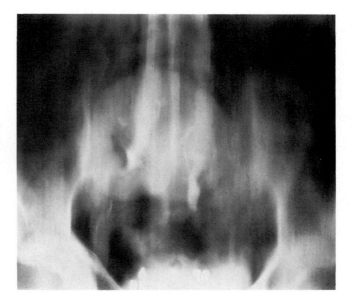

Figure 3–17 □ Fused pelvic kidney (pancake kidney) that was not visualized adequately on conventional films. Linear tomogram of the presacral region clearly demonstrates the anomalously fused pelvic kidney.

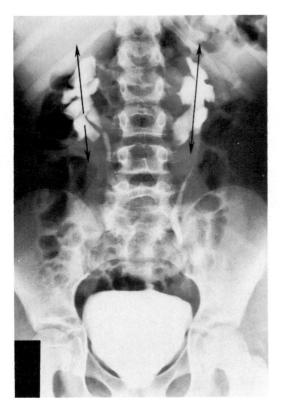

Figure 3–18 □ Horseshoe kidney in an 8-year-old girl. Arrows indicate the abnormal orientation of the renal axes.

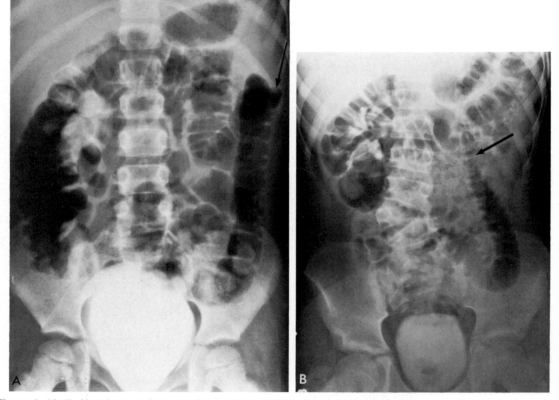

Figure 3–19 □ Air colograms in two patients whose left kidney had not been visualized by excretory urography. *A*, Arrow shows the normal position of the anatomic splenic flexure in this patient, who had a multicystic dysplastic kidney shown by ultrasonography and subsequently at operation. *B*, Abnormal position of the anatomic splenic flexure in a patient who was shown not to have any renal tissue in the renal fossa.

to visualize the renal parenchyma during the nephrographic phase of excretory urography. Previously, emphasis was placed on the pyelographic phase, and consequently on the secondary effects on the pelvicalyceal system produced by disease processes within the renal parenchyma. Other chapters in this book present detailed discussion of various disease processes whose parenchymal changes can be demonstrated on high-quality excretory urography.

It is the role of the radiology team to achieve the optimal demonstration of the renal parenchyma outline. However, as the clinical situation dictates, and in the interest of minimizing radiographic exposure, there are cases, especially in infants, in which less than complete visualization of the renal border is accepted. Nonetheless, it is generally readily possible to demonstrate the renal outline clearly on the nephrographic phase, permitting (1) accurate measurement of the pole-to-pole measurement of the kidneys, (2) determination of the rela-

tionship of the cortical margin to the calyceal tips, and (3) differentiation of anatomic variations that may mimic renal disease.

The simple technique of constructing the "interpapillary line" is often quite useful in establishing the relationship of the renal outline to the calyceal tips and in determining the thickness of the renal parenchyma (Fig. 3–20).

The relationship of abnormalities of the renal parenchyma to the calyces is often the key to the diagnosis. The thickness of the renal parenchyma at the upper and lower poles is usually symmetric and greater than the thickness of the parenchyma along the lateral margin of the kidney. The renal parenchyma is frequently prominent at the medial aspect of the upper pole of the kidney (Fig. 3–21).

The most common normal variation of renal parenchyma seen on an excretory urogram is persistent fetal lobulations. Fetal lobulations frequently persist during the first year of life and can be detected on high-quality urograms. In some persons, distinct indentations persist

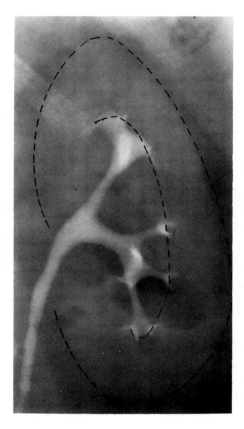

Figure 3–20 □ Localized view of left kidney with interpapillary line superimposed and renal margin outlined. Renal poles are equal in thickness, and there is slight thinning of upper lateral portion of kidney as a result of splenic impression.

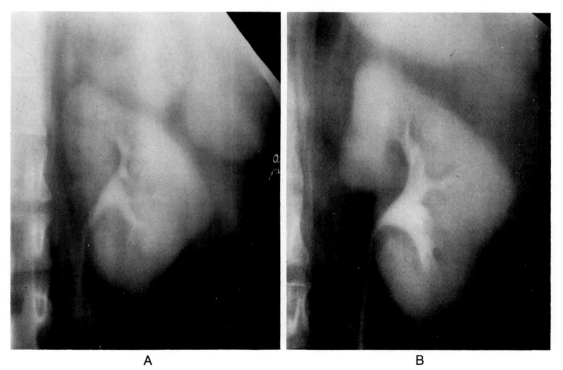

A   B

Figure 3–21 □ Tomograms of two kidneys with prominent areas of normal parenchyma that may be mistaken for renal tumor. *A,* Lower lateral aspect of left kidney (dromedary hump). *B,* Medial aspect of the upper pole of left kidney adjacent and superior to hilus (hilar lip) and at lateral margin of left kidney.

throughout life; these normal indentations should not be confused with scarring of the renal parenchyma or with a renal mass. Normal indentations are typically well demarcated and distinct and lie between calyces (Fig. 3–22).

Thin-section or thick-section tomograms taken during the nephrographic phase of the excretory urogram are often vitally important in demonstrating inflammatory scars, infarcts, renal masses, and perinephric abnormalities. Areas of persistent fetal lobulation, prominent but normal areas of renal parenchyma, localized areas of compensatory hypertrophy in a scarred kidney, and other "pseudotumors" that may be confused with a renal mass can usually be differentiated on good-quality excretory urograms (Fig. 3–23). Occasionally, isotopic scanning is required to differentiate the pseudotumor caused by septa of Bertin (Parker et al) from an intrarenal mass.

Prior to the widespread use of ultrasonography and other cross-sectional imaging, the technique of total body opacification during excretory urography was a method for evaluation of abdominal masses in infants and chil-

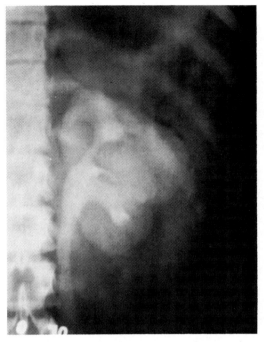

Figure 3–23 ☐ Localized compensatory hypertrophy resulting in pseudotumor in left kidney. Tomogram obtained during excretory urography reveals scarring of both poles. Localized compensatory hypertrophy on lateral aspect of the kidney simulates an intrarenal mass.

dren (Griscom and Neuhauser; O'Connor and Neuhauser). Cystic masses could be differentiated from solid ones. This technique depends upon administering the appropriate dose of contrast material intravenously as a bolus. A film of the renal area and the region of any known mass is obtained immediately. Total body opacification allows visualization of the contrast medium within the vascular compartment and the extracellular fluid compartment of the abdominal organs. A cystic avascular abnormality such as a multilocular cystic kidney, a multicystic dysplastic kidney, or hydronephrosis may be visualized as a radiolucent mass with walls that are enhanced by the contrast material (Fig. 3–24). Solid masses and other abdominal masses, on the other hand, may be visualized either as masses with a homogeneous increased density or as masses with a "mottled" opacity caused by alternating areas of increased and decreased density. Currently, high-quality ultrasonography or computed tomography (which, when performed with intravenous contrast material, utilizes the same principles as total body opacification) allows better definition of most abdominal masses, either cystic or solid, than does excre-

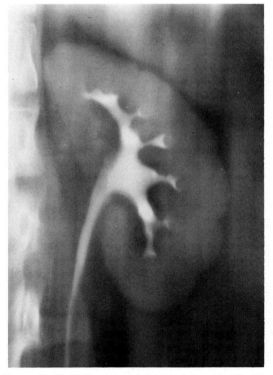

Figure 3–22 ☐ Persistent fetal lobulation identified by classic appearance of sharp indentations of renal cortex between underlying calyces.

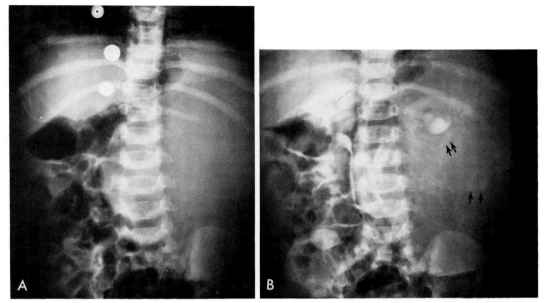

Figure 3–24 ☐ Total body opacification (TBO) effect. *A*, Preliminary film demonstrates left abdominal mass displacing bowel to the right. *B*, Radiograph of renal areas 2 minutes after an intravenous injection of contrast media. The right kidney is normal; the left kidney is markedly distorted. Arrows indicate enhancing septa in a multilocular cyst of the kidney.

tory urography with total body opacification (Fig. 3–25). Nonetheless, because of its ease, if excretory urography is being done, an early film is often obtained because of the additional information that might thus be obtained.

Pelvis and Calyces

The pelvicalyceal system of human kidneys is extremely variable in appearance. The usual number of calyces varies from 6 to 8, but as many as 12 are often found. The calyces usually are arranged in two distinct rows, one projecting anteriorly and the other projecting posteriorly (Fig. 3–26). The anterior calyces drain the anterior portion of the kidney and, when seen in profile, are situated closer to the lateral margin of the kidney than are the posterior calyces. The relative positions of the anterior and posterior rows of calyces result

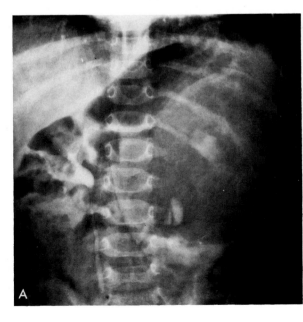

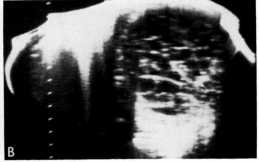

Figure 3–25 ☐ Multilocular cyst of the kidney presenting as a large left abdominal mass. *A*, Excretory urogram demonstrating a normal right kidney and a distorted left kidney largely replaced by a mass that appears relatively radiolucent. Distortion of the collecting system is noted. *B*, Transverse ultrasonogram graphically displays the cystic nature of the mass more readily than does the excretory urogram. (From Hoffman AD: Pediatric case of the day. Am J Roentgenol 142:1069, 1984; ©1984, American Roentgen Ray Society.)

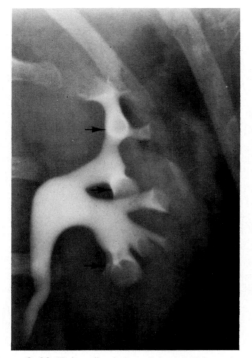

Figure 3–26 ☐ Localized view of the left kidney. Arrows indicate three posterior calyces. The remaining calyces make up the anterior row.

from the normal rotation of the kidney on its axis. As a result of this calyceal deployment, minor changes in the papilla, fornices, and renal parenchyma are more readily recognized anteriorly than posteriorly. Anatomically, the area of renal parenchyma drained by the posterior row of calyces is usually smaller than that drained by the anterior row.

"Papillary blush," a vague, cloud-like area of increased density, is frequently observed at the papillary tips. It represents concentration of contrast medium in the collecting ducts. This "blush," which is enhanced when larger doses of contrast medium, high-quality films, and ureteral compression are employed, is a normal phenomenon; it should not be confused with ectasia or cystic dilatation of the collecting ducts (medullary sponge kidney) (Figs. 3–27 and 3–28).

Renal papillae are usually funnel-shaped, but they may be rounded or elongated. Multiple papillae frequently drain into compound calyces, particularly at the polar regions of the kidney (Fig. 3–29). Such compound calyces are of considerable significance, inasmuch as it has now been shown that because of the anatomy of collecting tubule ostia of these papillae, the possibility of intrarenal reflux at

these sites is enhanced. The phenomenon of intrarenal reflux is occasionally demonstrated on voiding cystourethrography (Ransley).

Multiple variations in the size, shape, and location of renal papillae are common (Fig. 3–30). A papilla associated with an ectopic minor calyx that drains into an infundibulum may be confused with a filling defect. In cases of this normal anatomic variation, however, a dense rim of contrast medium within the fornix of the calyx usually can be seen around the papilla (Fig. 3–31).

The renal pelvis may be partially intrarenal and partially extrarenal in location, or it may be entirely intrarenal or extrarenal (Fig. 3–32). The renal pelvis commonly appears to vary in size and shape in response to changes in the position of the kidney. These variations may be observed fluoroscopically or on films made with the patient in various positions. Variations of this type do not indicate an abnormality and must not be mistaken for obstruction at the ureteral-pelvic junction.

The size of the renal pelvis is volume dependent; it can look normal on one examination but "ectatic" on an examination performed during diuresis or when filled with refluxed urine.

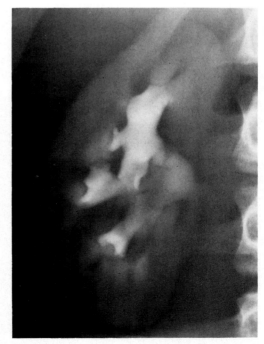

Figure 3–27 ☐ Papillary blush is present in all papillae of the right kidney. This finding should not be confused with pathologic conditions such as papillary necrosis or medullary sponge kidney.

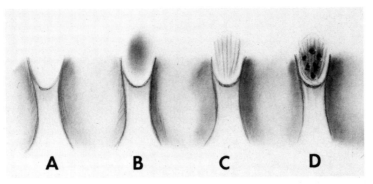

Figure 3–28 □ Drawings demonstrating possible appearances of the renal papilla during excretory urography. *A*, Usually, no contrast medium is identifiable within the renal papilla. *B*, Papillary blush, resulting in hazy, indistinct papillary opacification. *C*, Linear striations of the papilla, representing opacification of ectatic collecting tubules. *D*, Ectatic collecting tubules and tiny spherical collections of contrast medium as seen in medullary sponge kidney.

Ureters

In addition to urography, the methods available to image the ureters include ultrasonography, if the ureters are sufficiently dilated, and computed tomography. The anatomic course of the ureters is normally quite variable; therefore, any diagnosis of a retroperitoneal mass based only on an apparently unusual position of the ureter on the excretory urogram must be considered with caution. The ureters usually overlie the transverse processes of the lumbar vertebrae and, on rare occasions, may project as far medially as the pedicles in normal persons (Fig. 3–33).

A cross-table lateral view of the kidneys, ureters, and bladder can be especially helpful when one suspects a retroperitoneal mass. Because the position of the kidneys shifts when the patient is on his or her side or prone, supine cross-table lateral films should be obtained. Alterations in the anteroposterior axis shown on these films are not related to renal motion but reflect instead the actual anatomic relationship of the kidneys to the retroperitoneal structures. On cross-table lateral views, the kidneys normally are superimposed over the vertebral column and the ureters course along the anterior margin of the vertebral bodies to the level of the sacrum (Fig. 3–34).

Because of the para-aortic location of lymph nodes within the abdomen, enlarged nodes may be associated with lateral displacement of the upper ureters. The pelvic lymph nodes, on

Figure 3–29 □ Composite calyces, both poles of the kidneys. Numerous variations in appearance of calyces are possible. Composite (multipapillary) calyx, most commonly seen at poles of kidney, predisposes to intrarenal reflux and foci of reflux nephropathy.

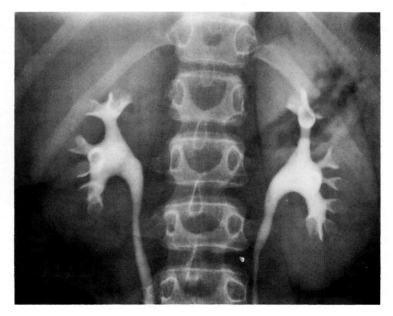

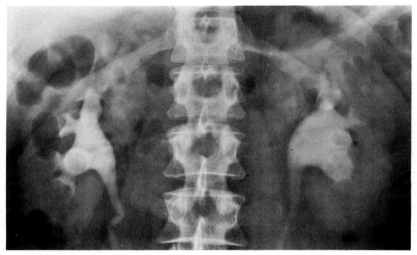

A

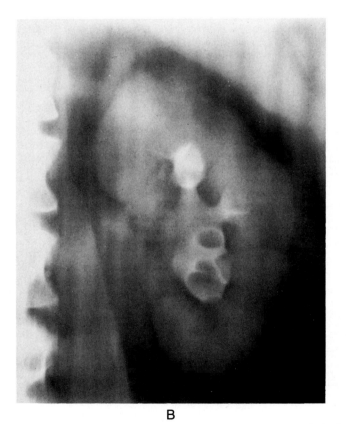

B

Figure 3–30 □ Variation of normal. *A*, Excretory urogram shows unusually large papillae in both kidneys. *B*, Tomogram of left kidney shows in detail persistent fetal lobulation and size of papillae of lower pole.

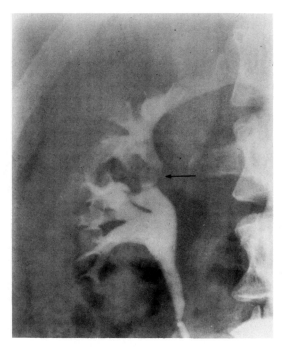

Figure 3–31 □ Localized view of right kidney reveals a radiolucent filling defect in infundibulum of upper pole *(arrow)* caused by an ectopically located papilla.

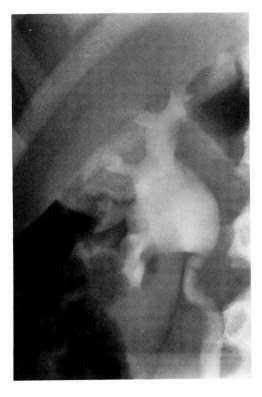

Figure 3–32 □ Right kidney showing a prominent extrarenal pelvis, which is a variation of normal and should not be mistaken for ureteropelvic junction obstruction.

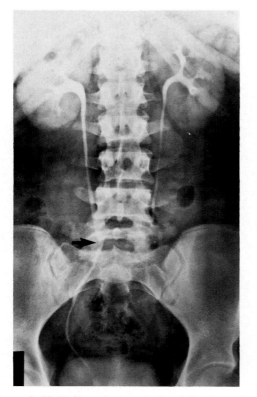

Figure 3–33 □ Normal amount of variation in ureteral course *(arrow)* on excretory urogram in a 16-year-old female.

diatric excretory urograms (Kaufman et al). This phenomenon was more commonly seen on the right than the left and is felt to be related to slight compression by the crossing iliac vessels. This dilatation was seen less frequently in infants than in older children.

A normal variant sometimes noted on the excretory urograms of infants is transverse folds in the proximal ureter. Histologically, folds of tissue are seen projecting into the ureteric lumen and are thought to represent persistence of normal fetal structures (Kirks et al).

On urographic studies, ureteric filling is quite variable because of normal active peristalsis. Successive films in the course of a single excretory urogram commonly show various parts of the ureters filled or empty. Generally, in a normal system, an entire ureter is not filled with contrast material on a single film unless a ureteral compression device has just been released. If this method is utilized, complete visualization of the ureter is frequently seen. A less commonly seen cause for dilatation of a ureter and even of the upper collecting system is a full bladder (Fig. 3–37). Because of this phenomenon, it is always appropriate to insist upon a film with an empty bladder before making the diagnosis of hydroureteronephrosis. If the patient is unable to void sufficiently, catheter drainage of the bladder should be employed.

Occasionally, reflux of contrast material into the ureter and upper collecting system of a nonfunctioning kidney may mimic excretion (Fig. 3–38), or reflux of nonopaque urine may make a well-functioning kidney appear to have diminished function. Errors may be avoided if such a situation is anticipated and if open catheter drainage of the bladder is maintained

the other hand, are lateral to the lower ureters, and enlarged nodes in this location produce medial displacement (Fig. 3–35).

The normal course of the ureters is oblique and anterior to the iliac vessels. Because of this relationship, extrinsic indentations and localized ureteral dilatation may be seen on excretory urograms (Fig. 3–36). Such ureteral dilatation has been found in one third of pe-

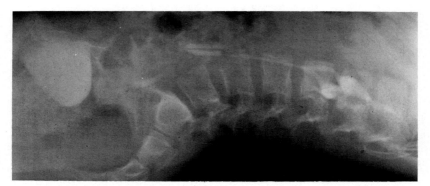

Figure 3–34 □ Cross-table lateral view demonstrates the normal relationship of kidneys and ureters to lumbar vertebrae.

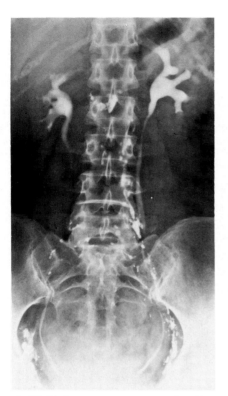

Figure 3–35 □ Excretory urogram made after a lymphangiogram, showing relationship between para-aortic and iliac lymph nodes and ureters.

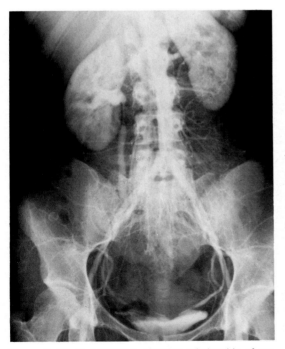

Figure 3–36 □ Aortogram showing relationship of ureters and iliac arteries.

while the excretory urogram is performed. Thus, contrast material or nonopaque urine is drained from the bladder instead of refluxing into the pelvicalyceal system.

Bladder

The ability to recognize anatomic abnormalities of the bladder must not be overestimated on the excretory urogram. Generally, on the pediatric exam, only a single view is available with the patient in a supine position, so that the amount of contrast medium seen in the bladder is variable. On the voiding cystourethrogram, on the other hand, there is the opportunity to visualize the bladder with various degrees of filling, and with the use of fluoroscopy, any degree of obliquity can be obtained.

On the single frontal view generally available on the excretory urogram, a common source of asymmetry is extrinsic compression by the feces-filled rectosigmoid (Fig. 3–39). The bichambered nature of the bladder may cause misinterpretation, particularly on prone films in which contrast material may be seen only in the superior portion of the bladder (Lebowitz and Avni). Significant pathologic lesions of the bladder, such as a mass, diverticula, or the vertically oriented, trabeculated bladder seen with neurogenic disorders, can generally be shown on excretory urography.

CYSTOURETHROGRAPHY

After excretory urography, the imaging examination most often performed to define the pediatric urinary tract is the voiding cystourethrogram (VCU, VCUG). This examination has appropriately supplanted examinations of the past, including static retrograde cystography, expression cystourethrography, and excretory cystourethrography. The VCU is superior because it provides better anatomic detail while recording normal physiologic events. The VCU is superior to excretory urography in the demonstration of bladder and urethral anatomy and abnormalities; additionally, vesicoureteral reflux and its precise extent are best defined with the VCU.

Voiding cystourethrography is most often performed after a child has had a urinary tract infection and it becomes important to find out if that patient also has vesicoureteral reflux. Often, excretory urography or ultrasonog-

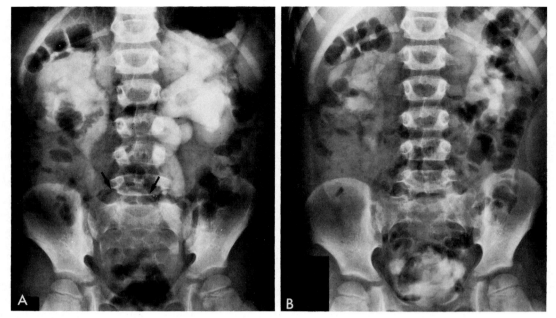

Figure 3–37 □ Transient dilatation of the upper collecting systems secondary to a full bladder. *A*, Prone film from an excretory urogram showing dilatation of the upper collecting systems. Arrows indicate dome of the bladder, which is filled with only slightly opacified urine. *B*, Prone post-voiding film shows a marked decrease of the apparent obstructive process, which was largely caused by a full bladder.

raphy is performed later on the same day to appraise renal integrity. Voiding cystourethrography should precede the other examinations inasmuch as the results of the VCU may determine which additional examination is to be done. Similarly, the sequence of VCU and diagnostic urologic examinations is important. Because the decision to proceed with cystoscopy often depends on the findings on a

VCU, it is appropriate to perform the radiographic examination. However, when a VCU and a cystometrogram are to be taken, the chemical irritation resulting from the contrast medium of the VCU may distort the findings on the latter exam. Consequently, the cystometrogram should precede the VCU or be performed a few days after it.

Voiding cystourethrography should not be

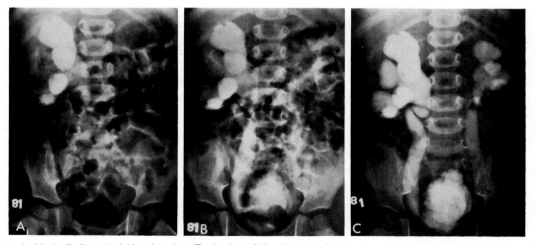

Figure 3–38 □ Reflux mimicking function. Evaluation of the changes during an excretory urogram *(A)* at 10 minutes, *(B)* at 40 minutes, and *(C)* at 2 hours shows progressively increasing opacification of the left collecting system after the bladder has filled from contrast material excreted on the right side. On an isotopic renal scan, there was essentially no function on the left.

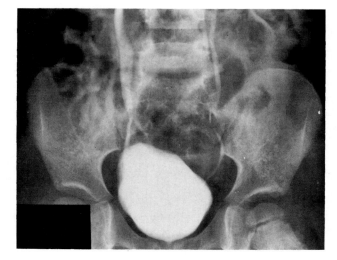

Figure 3–39 □ Impression on dome of bladder on the left is caused by a feces-filled sigmoid colon; this is a common appearance on pediatric excretory urograms.

performed routinely during an acute urinary tract infection, principally because bacteria in the lower urinary tract in the patient with vesicoureteral reflux may cause ureteral atony, which could exaggerate the grade of vesicoureteral reflux. It has not, however, been convincingly shown that urinary tract infection causes vesicoureteral reflux. The concern that bladder infection may result in reflux is not borne out by a study by Gross and Lebowitz, who showed an equal rate of vesicoureteral reflux in children with and without microscopic bacteria.

Contrast Media

The choice of contrast medium is of considerable importance. The medium must be nonirritating to the bladder in order to minimize spasm and edema of the vesicle wall, which some believe may lead to transient reflux (Shopfner, 1967). Large volumes of high-concentration contrast material result in inflammatory changes in the bladder wall of animals (McAlister et al). Currently, commercially available 17.2 per cent iothalamate meglumine (8.1 per cent iodine) (Cysto Conray II) is suitable for voiding cystourethrography. In addition to being less irritating than higher-concentration compounds, the decreased density allows visualization of filling defects in the bladder. The density of this contrast material is still great enough to adequately define subtle grades of vesicoureteral reflux and intrarenal reflux adequately and to show the detail necessary to define urethral lesions (Fig. 3–40).

Method of Exam

Voiding cystourethrography is performed as a dynamic examination; that is, the events occurring during micturition are seen as they occur (Colodny and Lebowitz, 1974a). Image-intensified fluoroscopy allows monitoring during the examination and spot films obtained in the course of the examination provide a permanent record. Another way to decrease the radiation dose during this examination is to use low fluoroscopic milliamperage (Sane and Worsing). This reduces the definition on the fluoroscopic examination; however, the definitive diagnosis is usually based on the spot films. A further adjunct is video taping of the television fluoroscopic image for review and teaching. The advantages of camera films obtained from the output phosphor of the image intensifier in a 70-, 90-, 100-, or 105-mm format include rapid filming sequence, good detail, and lower radiation than conventional films. In some radiology departments, digital radiography systems are now in use. These allow further reduction of radiation and manipulation of images to heighten diagnostic detail (Templeton et al).

Preparation of the patient for this examination is carried out in a fashion similar to that for excretory urography in that educational sheets explaining the voiding cystourethrogram are available for the parents and child at the time that the examination is scheduled (see Fig. 3–6). However, for voiding cystourethrography, no bowel preparation is required. Sedation should not be used because appropriate reassurance makes its use unnecessary; if it is

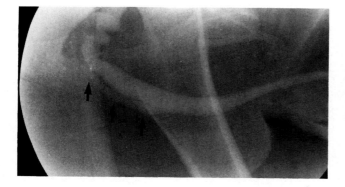

Figure 3–40 □ Spot film of the urethra from a voiding cystourethrogram using a 17.2 per cent concentration of contrast material. The detail of reflux into Cowper's duct is well demonstrated *(arrows)*.

used, it could impede normal voiding, which this examination is intended to simulate as closely as possible.

Using aseptic technique, the clinician gently catheterizes the child using a soft, straight catheter. Generally, an 8 Fr. infant feeding tube with an opaque line is best. Occasionally it is necessary to utilize a 5 Fr. feeding tube in premature infants, certain patients following urethral surgery, and those with urethral stricture. To minimize discomfort, lidocaine jelly may be introduced intraurethrally in older males prior to catheterization. Balloon catheters are not used. The urine obtained at the time of catheterization may be used for urinalysis, culture, sensitivity testing, and colony count.

After successful catheterization, the catheter tip is attached to conventional intravenous tubing, and the contrast material is instilled into the bladder by a gravity drip from a container suspended from an intravenous (IV) pole. The distance from the reservoir to the table top should not exceed 100 cm (Koff et al). In the rare instance when catheterization cannot be performed in infants, suprapubic needle insertion, a method frequently employed by pediatricians, may be used. A full bladder is necessary, and its presence can be ascertained by ultrasound (Fletcher et al).

In the performance of voiding cystourethrography, gross areas of pathology are defined on the fluoroscopic examination. More importantly, fluoroscopy allows appropriate position, timing, and collimation for spot films, which often define more subtle abnormalities. In this manner, a set of routine films is taken, utilizing only a minimal amount of fluoroscopy time.

Our routine films include (1) steep oblique views of each ureterovesical junction area toward the end of bladder filling, (2) urethral films during voiding; (3) a film of the bladder at the end of voiding, and (4) a film of each renal fossa at the end of voiding or, if vesicoureteral reflux is present, when it is maximal. Inasmuch as radiographically definable pathology of the female urethra is exceedingly rare, only a single anteroposterior urethral view is exposed during voiding (Fig. 3–41). For the male, a steep oblique position is best to see the urethra in profile. Two films of the posterior urethra and one of the anterior segment are routinely obtained (Fig. 3–42). Modification of this routine may be required as a result of clinical information, abnormalities on previous exams, or findings noted at fluoroscopy during the current examination (Fig. 3–43).

To gain the cooperation of a patient to initiate and continue the act of voiding under fluoroscopic visualization requires a carefully planned setting and what might be considered the "art" of radiology. A dimly lit room and a limited number of people in the fluoroscopic room are helpful. Adolescents, particularly females, have the greatest difficulty voiding during such examinations; the gender of the examiner does not seem to be as important as the experience and reassurance provided by the person performing the examination (Poznanski and Poznanski). Different positions, including supine, sitting, or standing, may be utilized. We find that most patients of any age are able to void in a recumbent position—females supine and males in a steep oblique so that the urethra is seen in profile. Others may find that specialized potty-chairs or a variety of urine receptacles are more efficacious. A variety of measures are used to help the patient initiate the urinary stream, including repeated assurance, warm water poured over the perineum, and suprapubic pressure, particularly for those with a neurogenic bladder. However, the primary method to ensure

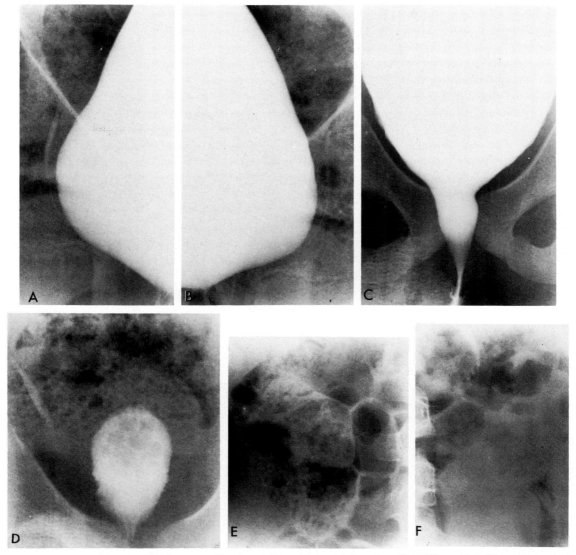

Figure 3–41 □ Voiding cystourethrogram. Usual spot films obtained in females. Right *(A)* and left *(B)* ureterovesical junctions at the end of filling. *C*, Anteroposterior view of urethra during voiding. *D*, Bladder at the end of voiding. Right *(E)* and left *(F)* renal fossae at the end of voiding. Bilateral grade I vesicoureteral reflux is faintly seen on *A* and *B*.

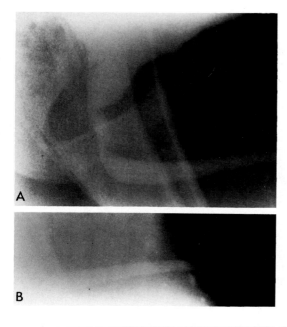

Figure 3–42 □ Male voiding cystourethrogram varies from the female voiding cystourethrogram in that oblique views of the urethra are obtained. *A*, Posterior urethra (usually two views are obtained). *B*, Anterior urethra.

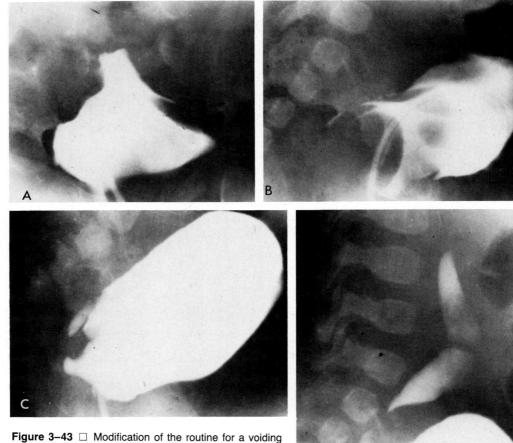

Figure 3–43 □ Modification of the routine for a voiding cystourethrogram in a child with bilateral duplication of renal collecting systems and bilateral ectopic ureteroceles.

A, Anteroposterior view; bilateral impressions on the bladder superiorly.

B, Lateral view during early filling demonstrates rounded negative defects caused by the ureteroceles, which are associated with the upper pole ureters.

C, Lateral view during the later filling phase shows beginning eversion of one of the ureteroceles.

D, Lateral view at the end of filling demonstrates complete intussusception of one of the ureteroceles into the ureter. Also noted is reflux into a lower pole ureter.

voiding is continued filling of the bladder until the contrast material stops dripping. Removal of the catheter should be avoided until the patient is producing a good urinary stream. This technique should be used particularly in infants, who often require refilling before adequate filming can be performed. There should be no concern that voiding is prevented by the presence of the catheter, inasmuch as even very young patients can readily void around the small catheters used. Spot films of the urethra are taken just after the catheter is slipped out. In a small minority of patients, voiding is not initiated even after the methods suggested above are employed. It may then become appropriate to allow the patient to void in a nearby bathroom and quickly return to the radiographic room for a post-voiding film. This maneuver compromises the examination, particularly in the male, in whom visualization of potential urethral pathology then is not obtained.

Anatomic Considerations

The definition of vesicoureteral reflux is the most common finding of the VCU. Many ob-servers have noted that the degree of vesico-ureteral reflux and, indeed, its absence or presence can vary from one examination to the next or from one day to another. Therefore, the technique used for voiding cystoure-thrography should be rigidly standardized in order to minimize error introduced by the examination itself. The significance of transitory reflux and the effects of medical and surgical management are discussed elsewhere in this book.

The degree of reflux has a significant bearing on the prognosis for the resolution of reflux as well as the development of complications, such as reflux nephropathy and, consequently, the therapy for each patient. As a result, a number of grading systems have been devised. One currently in use by the International Reflux Study Committee has five gradations (Fig. 3–44) (Levitt et al). Because of the significant implications regarding prognosis and treatment, this or one of the other systems of grading should be utilized.

Infrequently, when vesicoureteral reflux into the upper collecting system is seen, detection of further extension of contrast material into collecting tubules is also demonstrated. Such intrarenal reflux most often occurs when compound calyces, which are those draining more

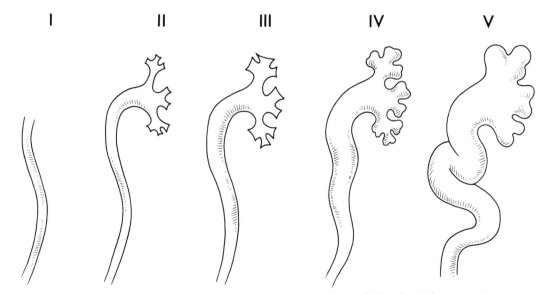

Figure 3–44 □ Radiographic grades of reflux (according to the International Reflux Study Committee).
Grade I, ureter only.
Grade II, ureter and upper collecting system without dilatation.
Grade III, mild or moderate dilatation of ureter and mild or moderate dilatation of renal pelvis, but no or slight blunting of fornices.
Grade IV, moderate dilatation and/or tortuosity of ureter with moderate dilatation of renal pelvis and calyces and complete obliteration of sharp angles of fornices, but maintenance of papillary impressions and the majority of calyces.
Grade V, gross dilatation and tortuosity of ureters, renal pelves, and calyces; papillary impressions are not visible in the majority of calyces.

than a single papilla, are present (Fig. 3–45); these are most common in the polar regions of the kidney.

The position of the ureterovesical junctions at the posterolateral aspects of the bladder determines the optimal patient position for filming to show vesicoureteral reflux and peri-ureteric bladder diverticula. With a straight anteroposterior position, reflux into the lower ureter may be obscured by contrast material in the bladder. The right ureterovesical junction is therefore best demonstrated with right anterior oblique position, and the left uretero-vesical junction is best seen in the left anterior oblique position. If the urethral catheter is shown on the oblique film and if the patient has vesicoureteral reflux, the relative position of the refluxing ureter to the urethra is established. Closer proximity than usual indicates ureteral ectopy (Fig. 3–46).

It is appropriate to perform radionuclide voiding cystography for (1) the follow-up of known vesicoureteral reflux, (2) determination of whether reflux has been corrected by reimplantation of the ureter, and (3) initial detection when a positive family history is the indication for investigation. Although anatomic detail is poorer, a significant reduction in radiation dose is achieved. This subject is more fully covered in a subsequent chapter.

To evaluate a voiding cystourethrogram properly, one must carefully assess patient position, filming sequence, variations in the appearance of the bladder and urethra, and changes in urethral caliber during voiding. Correct interpretation of bladder and urethral findings depends on a clear, thorough compre-

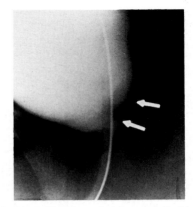

Figure 3–46 ☐ Ectopic ureter demonstrated by voiding cystourethrography during voiding. Arrows mark the left ureter, which drains into the urethra, marked by the opaque line of the bladder catheter.

hension of anatomic and physiologic variations that are normal in these organs (Fig. 3–47). For example, normal anatomic variations visualized in the region of the vesical neck and the prostatic urethra of males, and in the entire urethra of females, have been misinterpreted in the past as representations of lower urinary tract disease. Although unusual configurations of the vesical neck may sometimes suggest abnormalities when viewed on a single film, it has been clearly demonstrated that most such contours represent normal variations of the anatomy of the trigonal region or sphincteric mechanism reflecting the dynamics of micturition.

The normal anatomic relationships of the bladder base plate, the anterior and posterior trigonal plate, the trigonal canal, the bladder neck, the intermuscular incisura, and the urogenital diaphragm have been stressed by Shopfner and Hutch (Fig. 3–48). The roentgenographic appearances of these anatomic units of the bladder and urethra were elegantly illustrated by Shopfner (1971) in a monograph on cystourethrography.

Variations in the caliber and contour of the urethra are dependent on the volume and rate of flow during voiding; therefore, a roentgenographic diagnosis of an apparent stricture or other cause of urethral obstruction must be documented on more than one film during maximal distention of the urethra (Fig. 3–49). However, because of the extreme rarity of abnormalities in the female urethra, it is our policy routinely to obtain only a single spot film in the anteroposterior projection. A common finding is vaginal reflux (Kelalis et al)

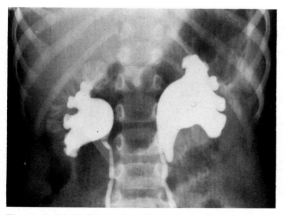

Figure 3–45 ☐ Bilateral vesicoureteral reflux resulting in complete filling of both collecting systems and associated with intrarenal reflux (IRR) on right.

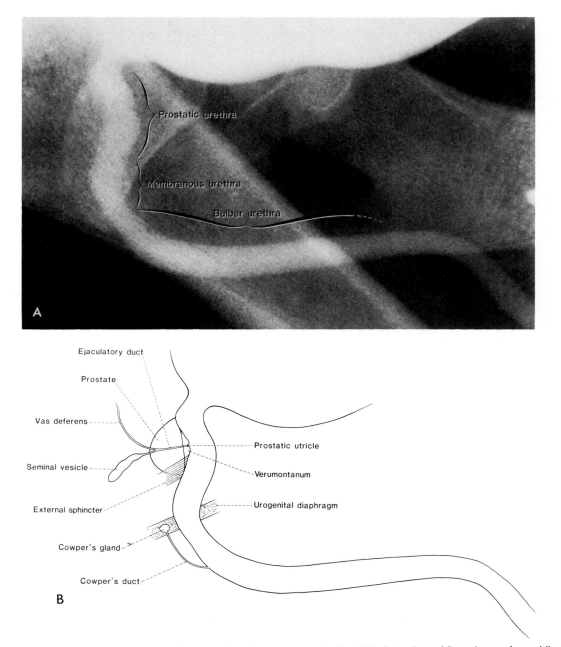

Figure 3–47 □ Posterior portions of a normal urethra in a boy. *A*, Spot film from the voiding phase of a voiding cystourethrogram. The segments of the posterior urethra are indicated. *B*, Diagram drawn from the spot film, indicating the various important structures immediately adjacent to the posterior urethra.

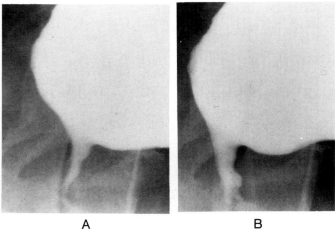

A

B

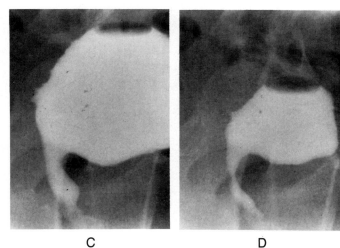

C

D

Figure 3–48 □ Sequence of spot films in steep oblique projection during voiding cystourethrography in a 5-year-old girl. The variation in appearance of the bladder base and urethra during voiding is shown. *A*, Early voiding. *B, C*, Mid voiding. *D*, Late voiding.

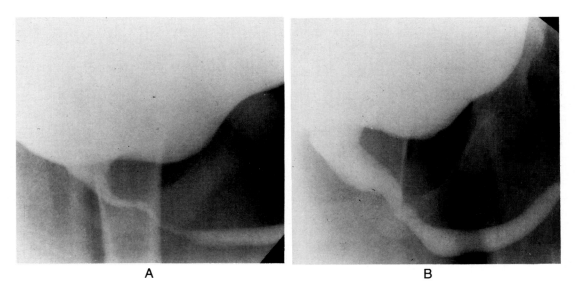

A

B

Figure 3–49 □ Voiding cystourethrogram spot films in an 8-year-old boy. *A*, Early voiding with urethra incompletely distended. *B*, A later stage demonstrates normal urethral appearance, with the urethra distended by a good urine flow.

(Fig. 3–50). Vaginal reflux is accentuated in the presence of female hypospadias or labial adhesions but usually results from voiding in the supine position. In males, variations such as prominent muscular incisura (Fig. 3–51) or narrowing caused by constriction of the bulbocavernosus muscle (Currarino) must be differentiated from true stricture. External sphincter spasm or fibrosis (Fig. 3–52) (Mandell et al) is a feature commonly seen in patients with a neuropathic bladder. In the absence of proximal dilatation, irregularity of the urethra does not generally indicate an obstructing lesion. Video tape recording of each examination permits restudy of changes in caliber and contour without repeat examination and further radiation exposure to the child. Evaluation by video tape is particularly important when a questionable abnormality

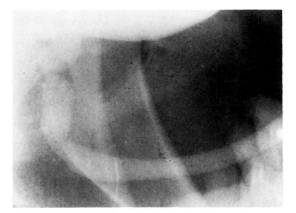

Figure 3–51 ☐ Voiding cystourethrogram spot film from a 4-year-old boy with a prominent intramuscular incisura that could be mistaken for a urethral lesion.

has been seen on the spot films taken during the procedure.

Adjunctive Examinations

Definition of abnormalities in the pelvis is often insufficiently accomplished by filling of the bladder alone. To define a tumor in this region adequately, it is often useful to obtain spot films or radiographs in the lateral projection after filling of the rectum and sigmoid with barium or air (Fig. 3–53). In this manner, a tumor is localized to a specific region in the pelvis (e.g., presacral, prerectal, or even prevesical), and depending upon the sex of the patient, the differential diagnostic possibilities are significantly reduced. Cross-sectional im-

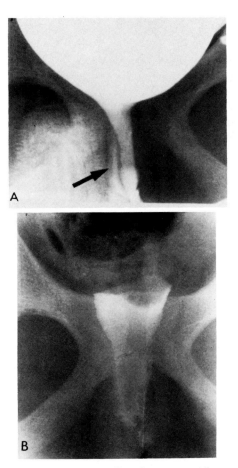

Figure 3–50 ☐ Vaginal reflux shown on voiding cystourethrogram in a 7-year-old girl with dribbling after voiding. *A,* Urethra during voiding, anteroposterior view; vagina *(arrow)* is shown. *B,* Post-voiding anteroposterior view; vagina clearly outlined by contrast material.

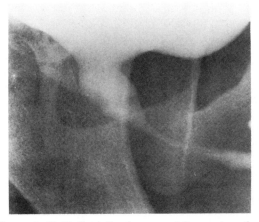

Figure 3–52 ☐ Spot film from a voiding cystourethrogram in a 14-year-old male with myelodysplasia. Narrowing of the posterior urethra at the level of the external sphincter persisted on this examination, suggesting sphincter dyssynergia.

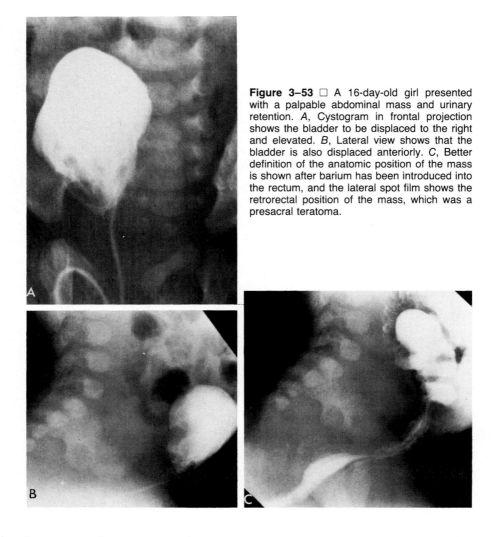

Figure 3–53 □ A 16-day-old girl presented with a palpable abdominal mass and urinary retention. *A*, Cystogram in frontal projection shows the bladder to be displaced to the right and elevated. *B*, Lateral view shows that the bladder is also displaced anteriorly. *C*, Better definition of the anatomic position of the mass is shown after barium has been introduced into the rectum, and the lateral spot film shows the retrorectal position of the mass, which was a presacral teratoma.

aging by ultrasonography or computed tomography will also contribute to anatomic definition in these cases.

For children and particularly infants with ambiguous genitalia or intersex, another adjunct to voiding cystourethrography is often helpful in the definition of anatomy. *Genitography* is the term used to describe the radiographic examination in which an attempt is made to fill all genital cavities with opaque contrast material (Shopfner, 1964). The method of examination is similar to that used in cystourethrography. After filling the bladder in the usual fashion, the physician advances a second catheter into any other genital orifice and again instills contrast material. Fluoroscopy and spot films in frontal, lateral, and occasionally oblique projections are used. An alternative means for filling these structures is the "flush method," in which a leak-proof seal is attempted by the use of a tapering connector or syringe tip. This tip is gently inserted into the visualized genital orifice, and contrast material is injected. Another method for performing genitography utilizes a feeding tube passed through a single-hole disposable nipple that is filled with cotton (Peck and Poznanski). The nipple acts as an obturator, and the tube can be passed the desired distance into the genital orifice. If the bladder cannot be catheterized, its position and anatomic connections can be determined after excretory urography (Fig. 3–54).

OTHER UROGRAPHIC EXAMS

Loopography

The kidneys and ureters draining into an ileal or sigmoid conduit should be evaluated periodically (yearly) by excretory urography,

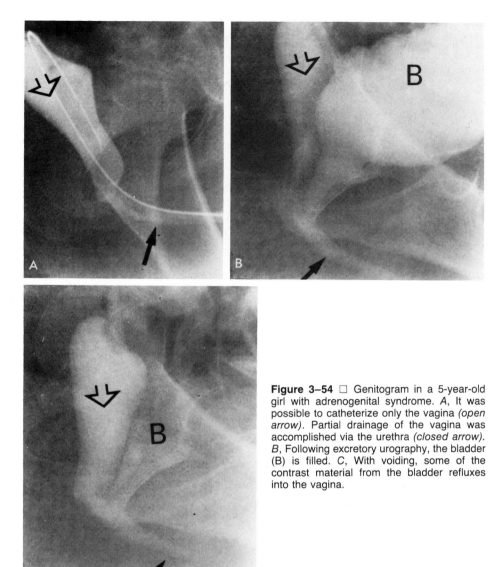

Figure 3–54 □ Genitogram in a 5-year-old girl with adrenogenital syndrome. *A,* It was possible to catheterize only the vagina *(open arrow).* Partial drainage of the vagina was accomplished via the urethra *(closed arrow). B,* Following excretory urography, the bladder (B) is filled. *C,* With voiding, some of the contrast material from the bladder refluxes into the vagina.

radionuclide studies, or ultrasonography as long as the conduit is present (Hardy et al; Lebowitz; Shapiro et al). The approximate length, width, and peristaltic activity of the conduit also can be evaluated fluoroscopically during the excretory urogram. If elongation or dilatation of the ureters or intestinal segment is noted on any of these examinations, a retrograde study of the ileal or sigmoid conduit should be done.

A retrograde loopogram can be obtained by introducing a catheter into the stoma, occluding the stoma around the catheter, and instilling contrast medium into the conduit by gravity drip under fluoroscopic guidance. Occlusion of the stomal lumen can be accomplished by inserting the tip of a Foley catheter into the stoma, with the balloon inflated outside the stoma. Alternatively, one end of a straight rubber catheter can be inserted through a predrilled hole into a small rubber ball, and the tip of the catheter can then be inserted into the stoma. The patient, if cooperative, presses the ball or balloon against the stoma with sufficient force to occlude the external opening. The examination should be combined with the use of fluoroscopy and spot filming so that proper positioning, sequential filming, adequate distention of the conduit, and the degree of reflux and peristalsis of the ureters and conduit can be observed and recorded.

Normal conduits are easily distended, and reflux is generally demonstrated during the examination of an ileal conduit with opacification of the ureters and pelvicalyceal system (Fig. 3–55) (Nogrady et al). Reflux should not occur with sigmoid conduits or ileal conduits in which an antireflux procedure has been performed.

Obstruction of the stoma may be evaluated by removing the catheter and fluoroscopically observing the peristaltic activity and emptying of the conduit. Vigorous peristaltic waves and ineffectual emptying of the ileal loop may indicate stomal obstruction. In unobstructed systems, a drainage film 20 minutes after an examination generally shows almost complete drainage of contrast material from the collecting systems and the conduit.

Loopography for sigmoid or other conduits that have had antirefluxing anastomoses need be performed initially only to exclude the presence of ureteral reflux. Periodic follow-up is accomplished by excretory urography, radionuclide studies, or ultrasonography. If hydronephrosis develops, cutaneous antegrade pyelography can be helpful in defining ureteral sites of obstruction; intrinsic sigmoid conduit strictures have not yet been reported (Lebowitz). Fluoroscopic evaluation of the sigmoid

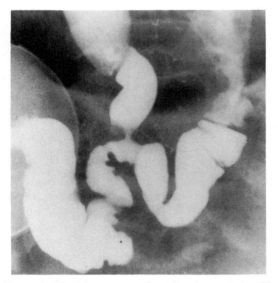

Figure 3–55 □ Loopogram. Spot film demonstrates filling and distention of the ileal conduit. A stricture is seen at the anastomosis between the right ureter and the ileal loop.

conduit is less informative because the colonic conduit behaves more like a conducting tube, with only minimal peristalsis, or even none at all.

Retrograde Urethrography in the Male

Visualization of the urethra is an integral part of voiding cystourethrography. Even though the entire urethral profile may be seen with the voiding method, the anatomy distal to a site of urethral obstruction often is not accurately depicted because urethral distention may be incomplete and significant lesions may be missed. Therefore, retrograde urethrography may be employed for the evaluation of the urethra distal to a site of urethral obstruction.

Water-soluble contrast medium in a concentration of 17 per cent may be used for retrograde injection. A syringe fitted with an adapter of appropriate size may be inserted into the urethral meatus to inject the medium. Alternatively, a small, 8 or 10 Fr. Foley catheter can be introduced into the urethra so that the balloon just passes through the meatus. If 0.5 to 1.0 ml of fluid is injected into the balloon, it will seat in the fossa navicularis. As a result, the catheter will be maintained in position and leakage of contrast material will not occur (McCallum and Colapinto). The contrast material is then gently injected through the catheter, and the urethra is viewed fluoroscopically in a lateral or steep oblique projection. Appropriate spot films are obtained.

Retrograde urethrography is particularly applicable in the evaluation of strictures, diverticula, and urethral trauma when rupture of the urethra is suspected. However, caution must be exercised in interpreting the films, inasmuch as the region of the membranous urethra is often incompletely distended because the external sphincter is not relaxed and apparent narrowing in this region could be falsely interpreted as stricture (Fig. 3–56).

Retrograde Pyelography

The need for retrograde pyelography was greatly reduced with the advent of modern excretory urography. The use of this examination has been reduced even further as other

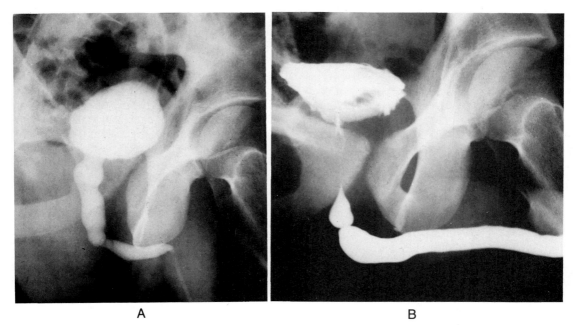

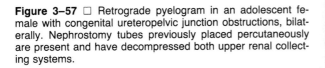

Figure 3–56 □ Lesions such as urethral strictures are well delineated with the complementary use of *(A)* a voiding cystourethrogram and *(B)* a retrograde urethrogram. The addition of the retrograde study shows the limited length of a bulbar urethral stricture *(arrows)*. Adequate filling of the area beyond the stricture frequently is not shown on the voiding examination alone.

modalities, such as isotopic studies, ultrasonography, and computed tomography have demonstrated renal anatomy when excretory urography is inadequate. Furthermore, percutaneous studies are increasingly employed in children with dilated collecting systems, and using catheters introduced in this manner, one can perform antegrade studies of the renal collecting systems. Therefore, retrograde pyelography is infrequently necessary. However, in a small percentage of cases in which these other examinations are not available or will not show the ureter beyond an obstruction, retrograde pyelography may be appropriate (Fig. 3–57).

Combining retrograde pyelography with

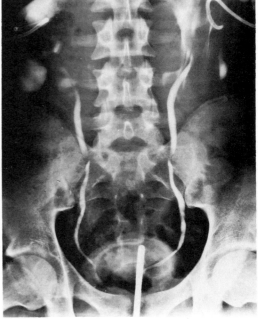

Figure 3–57 □ Retrograde pyelogram in an adolescent female with congenital ureteropelvic junction obstructions, bilaterally. Nephrostomy tubes previously placed percutaneously are present and have decompressed both upper renal collecting systems.

fluoroscopy in the cystoscopic suite eliminates the disadvantage of blind filling and filming technique and allows the ureteral catheter to be positioned optimally at the site of suspected lesion. With the use of fluoroscopy, overdistention of the renal pelvis and possible extravasation of contrast medium can be avoided. Also, questionable obstruction to the outflow of urine in the upper urinary tract is best evaluated with fluoroscopy.

ANTEGRADE PYELOGRAPHY AND INTERVENTIONAL PROCEDURES

Antegrade pyelography was initially introduced in the 1950s to facilitate further definition of the anatomy of the upper urinary tracts. Within the past decade, technical advances have greatly expanded the role of percutaneous antegrade procedures in children, providing access for complex endourologic diagnostic and therapeutic intervention (Towbin). The optimal clinical application of these procedures has resulted from continuing frequent consultation and interaction between radiologists and urologists.

The technique of antegrade pyelography is minimally invasive, requiring only mild sedation to limit anxiety. After injection of local anesthesia at the puncture site, the operator percutaneously advances a 21- or 22-gauge needle into the renal collecting systems. Real-time ultrasonic guidance of the needle tip limits renal trauma and facilitates rapid completion of the examination. With grossly dilated collecting systems, fluoroscopic needle guidance is equally effective. Following aspiration of urine for bacterial cultures, contrast medium injection under fluoroscopic observation provides the optimal anatomic information (Man and Ransley). Because small needles are used, minimal complications result, thus allowing outpatient evaluation (Riedy and Lebowitz).

Percutaneous nephrostomy placement is a direct extension of antegrade pyelography. Following percutaneous puncture of a renal calyx, a guide wire is placed through the needle and coiled in the renal pelvis. Infants are adequately drained by placement of a 5 to 6 Fr. pigtail catheter. For larger children, especially those with viscous, infected urine, better drainage is accomplished with 8 to 10 Fr. catheters. The use of self-retaining loop drainage catheters greatly reduces the incidence of

catheter dislodgment and requires considerably less external catheter fixation to the child's skin.

The complications of percutaneous nephrostomy placement are minimal (Ball et al). Postprocedural hematuria is universal, but clears within 24 hours. Rare (less than 1 per cent) arterial injuries may cause severe hemorrhage and are best treated with selective transcatheter angiographic embolization. Percutaneous catheter placement into an infected collecting system may induce clinical signs of sepsis; this complication is best limited by minimizing the tube manipulations required in the acute setting. Nephrostomy-related flank pain is usually minimal after 48 hours.

The establishment of external urinary drainage through a nephrostomy tube permits many diagnostic and therapeutic options. Temporary drainage allows healing of obstructive postoperative edema, direct assessment of renal function, or drainage of grossly purulent urine prior to definitive therapy. Although pyelography through small needles may be utilized, pressure-flow relationships (the Whitaker test) are most reliably defined through nephrostomy tubes. After infusion of fluid at a specified rate, elevated renal pelvic pressures relative to the bladder indicate ureteral obstruction in those complex cases with postoperative collecting system dilatation (Fig. 3–58). The pres-

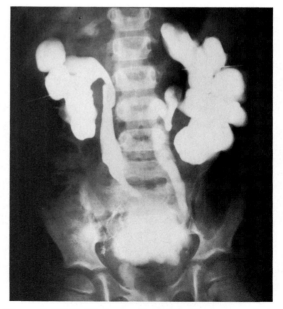

Figure 3–58 □ Bilateral antegrade pyelograms exclude ureteral obstruction in a patient with persistent dilatation after ureteroneocystostomies. Subsequent Whitaker tests were normal.

ence of the nephrostomy tract facilitates subsequent intervention including percutaneous removal of renal or ureteral calculi, antegrade ureteral stent placement, ureteral occlusion for malignant fistulas, or percutaneous intrarenal surgery such as endopyelotomy. The introduction of these techniques to the pediatric patient population with renal transplants has paralleled the adult experience (Bennett et al) (Fig. 3–59).

More complex endourologic procedures require additional equipment, expertise, and optimally the active cooperative efforts of both radiologists and urologists. General anesthesia is usually necessary for nephrostomy tract dilatation sufficient to allow percutaneous introduction of therapeutic endoscopic equipment for stone removal (Woodside et al), endopyelotomy, or foreign body removal (Douenias et al). Extensive antegrade manipulations within the ureter and bladder are often best managed with general anesthesia as well in pediatric patients.

Percutaneous drainage of renal, perinephric, and retroperitoneal abscesses has been shown to be an effective alternative to surgical intervention in selected cases. Technically, these drainage procedures are similar to the well-described activities in adults. External drainage and the use of appropriate antibiotics allow many abscesses to heal completely. In those patients with an underlying anatomic abnormality, preoperative percutaneous abscess drainage and patient defervescence often permit a single-stage surgical reconstruction rather than a staged surgical procedure.

Percutaneous biopsy of renal and abdominal masses in the pediatric population is a safe and effective procedure. Utilizing ultrasound, CT, or fluoroscopic guidance, one can approach nearly any lesion. Although the clinician need not perform a biopsy on obvious surgical lesions, the question of recurrent mass, new metastatic lesion, or parenchymal abnormality can be resolved without an open surgical procedure. The use of mild sedation, local anesthesia, and small biopsy needles facilitates outpatient evaluation.

VASCULAR STUDIES

Lymphangiography (Lymphography)

Newer imaging modalities such as CT and ultrasonography have reduced the need for lymphangiography in children. Generally, lymphangiography has been technically more difficult to do in children than in adults. However, with modern techniques and experienced radiologists, success in accomplishing lymphangiography and diagnostic accuracy and interpretation in pediatric patients can be expected to equal the rates achieved with adults (Dunnick et al).

A 30- or 31-gauge, rather than a 29-gauge needle, should be used, and sedation or anesthesia is almost always required in younger children. Evans blue dye is injected into the webbing between the great and second toe to opacify the lymph channels. After cannulation, iodized oil (Ethiodol) is slowly infused until the contrast material reaches the L4-5 interspace. The total average infusion is 0.2 ml of Ethiodol/kg of body weight. The relatively low

Figure 3–59 □ Percutaneous nephrostomy tube in the pelvis of a renal transplant in a 14-year-old male. After anastomotic edema resolved, no obstruction was present and the catheter was removed.

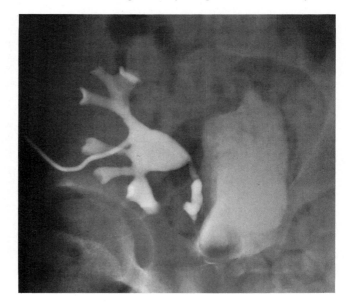

dose results in decreased adverse effects from pulmonary embolism. Films are obtained after contrast material has reached the lumbar level and at 24 hours (Fig. 3–60).

The procedure is most often performed in the evaluation of lymphoma or of gonadal or other pelvic malignancies that may also require staging lymphangiography. Demonstration of abnormal lymph nodes acts as a guide to the surgeon when biopsy or lymphadenectomy is to be done. In addition, because the contrast material stays in the nodes for weeks to months, progress of therapy and the extent of disease may often be followed simply with plain x-ray films of the abdomen. Inasmuch as not all lymph nodes are opacified with lymphangiographic contrast material, some metastases may be missed. However, the recognition of the entity of reactive hyperplasia and the ability to distinguish it from malignant involvement have reduced the rate of false-positive interpretations (Castellino).

Angiography

Inferior Venacavography

In the past, inferior venacavography in conjunction with excretory urography was the method most frequently used as the initial roentgenographic study in the evaluation of abdominal mass in infants and children. Currently, more reliable opacification of the inferior vena cava can be achieved by a formal inferior venacavogram using the Seldinger technique and a femoral vein route (Fig. 3–61). Even with good opacification of the inferior vena cava, extrinsic compression deformities may be confused with tumor invasion and interpretation is therefore often difficult.

Modern ultrasonography has largely supplanted contrast studies of the inferior vena cava in the pediatric patient with an abdominal mass. The sonogram not only gives information about the mass but also usually readily demonstrates the inferior vena cava (Slovis et al). Computed tomography and MRI also demonstrate the inferior vena cava.

One of the remaining roles for catheterization via the femoral vein is to gain access to the renal vein for sampling of renin levels in the evaluation of hypertension.

Arteriography

Arteriography may be helpful in evaluating certain abdominal masses in children, but it is not indicated in most instances. The majority of such masses are best evaluated by other less invasive imaging modalities, including excre-

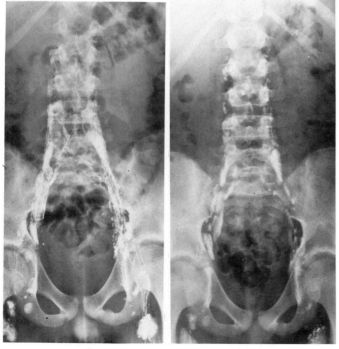

A   B

Figure 3–60 □ Selected films from a lymphangiogram. *A,* Anteroposterior film immediately after injection of contrast material demonstrating filling of lymph ducts and early filling of lymph nodes. *B,* Similar view 24 hours later shows lymph node architecture with some bilateral enlargement of femoral nodes and enlargement of left para-aortic node. Oblique projections are also routinely obtained.

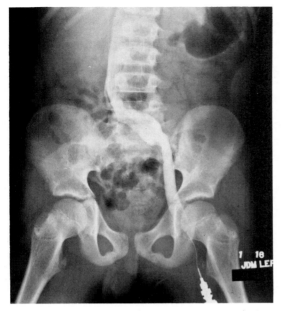

Figure 3–61 □ Normal inferior venacavagram (antero-posterior view) after left femoral vein injection.

tory urography, ultrasonography, radionuclide studies, CT, and MRI. Arteriography may have a role, however, in evaluation of certain tumors, for example, bilateral Wilms' tumor or a right-sided mass that may be hepatic in origin. Other indications for renal arteriography include childhood hypertension when renal vascular hypertension is suspected, renal trauma when vascular injury is suspected, and, rarely, inflammatory masses of the kidney. In the newborn with anuria, nonpalpable kidneys, or Potter facies, neonatal angiography by the transumbilical route may be indicated. Inasmuch as hydronephrotic kidneys are best shown by ultrasonography, this examination should usually be done first.

Transumbilical Neonatal Angiography

In infants during the first several days of life, the umbilical vessels provide an easily accessible site for performing rapid angiography. The lumen of the umbilical artery may be reopened and the recut ends expanded with forceps to allow the insertion of a catheter. A 5 Fr. infant feeding tube with an opaque line is frequently used. The catheter is advanced under fluoroscopy to the level of the renal arteries for the injection of radiopaque medium (Fig. 3–62).

Percutaneous Transfemoral Retrograde Aortography and Selective Renal Arteriography

Percutaneous transfemoral introduction of the catheter by the Seldinger technique can be performed safely, providing diagnostic accuracy by those skilled in this technique. Certain risks are inherent in the procedure, however, and the referring physician as well as the radiologist must be aware of these potential complications.

Bleeding may occur from the site of the arterial puncture after the catheter is removed. However, this may be avoided by applying continuous pressure over the arterial puncture site for a period of 10 minutes or more. Vascular occlusion in the legs due to clot formation on the catheter may occur, and arterial spasm can result in ischemia of the leg.

Arterial peak flow has been shown to be reduced in a percentage of children below the age of 8 years. For this reason, particularly in this age group, the smallest catheter that can deliver the necessary flow should be utilized (Kirks et al). Hypersensitivity reactions to the contrast material can occur, but the risk of

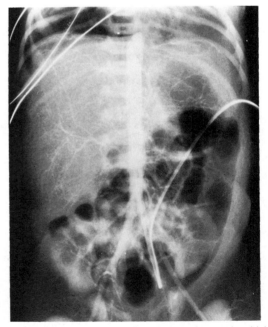

Figure 3–62 □ Single film from an arteriogram in which contrast material was injected through an indwelling umbilical artery catheter. The kidneys had not been identified on an ultrasound examination. This neonate with Potter's syndrome demonstrates no filling of renal arteries and was shown to have renal agenesis at postmortem examination.

such reactions is less than that incurred during intravenous excretory urography. With the advent of low osmolar contrast material, contrast reactions and discomfort during the examination should be reduced (Murphy et al). The heightened incidence of hypersensitivity reactions to venous, as opposed to arterial, injections is thought to be due to the release of histamine from the lungs when contrast material is injected intravenously.

Patient preparation in regard to hydration and bowel status should be similar to that used for excretory urography. Intramuscular sedation or a general anesthetic agent, such as ketamine, used without endotracheal intubation may be necessary to achieve the immobility necessary for optimal filming.

A detailed discussion of the technical aspects of angiography is not appropriate in this chapter. However, the physician in charge of pediatric angiography must become thoroughly familiar with the special considerations affecting examinations in infants and small children before attempting the procedure. Small catheters should be used to minimize intimal trauma, to prevent bleeding at the puncture site, and to increase the probability of successful arterial catheterization. In infants and children, the initial examination should be a midstream aortic injection (Fig. 3–63).

Several technical variations of the examination may be of significant value in children. Magnification arteriography has been utilized, and this may be especially helpful in visualizing tiny normal and pathologic vessels. Methods of radiographic subtraction and utilization of digitalized images have been introduced. The initial promise of the latter has not been ful-

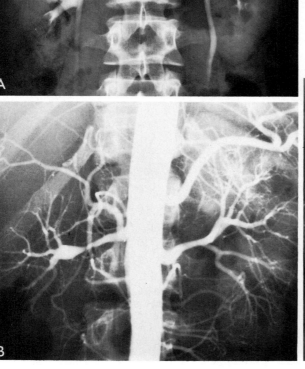

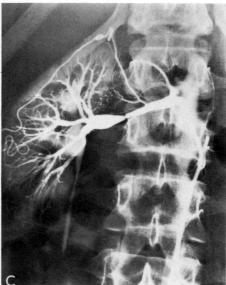

Figure 3–63 □ The patient is a 14-year-old female with renal vascular hypertension. *A,* Excretory urogram shows significant variation in renal size. Right renal length is 12.3 cm and left, 15.1 cm. Aortogram *(B)* and right selective renal arteriogram *(C)* show right renal artery stenosis.

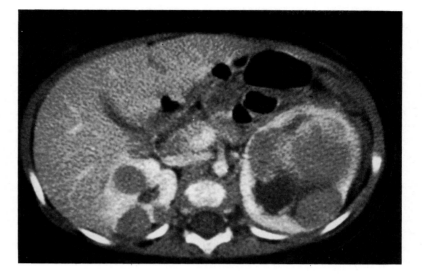

Figure 3–64 □ Ultrafast CT scan of the kidneys in a 1½-year-old. Intravenous contrast material has been given and the image is done early during the arterial and nephrographic phase. The image was exposed in 0.1 second, and no sedation was necessary. The vascular anatomy is sharply seen, and the multiple low-density masses within both kidneys can be appreciated in this patient with nephroblastomatosis.

filled because of resolution limitations. Percutaneous angioplasty has also been performed successfully in children (Korogi et al).

BODY COMPUTED TOMOGRAPHY

One of the most revolutionary changes in radiologic imaging has occurred with the advent and proliferation of computed tomography. This technique was first used for the evaluation of intracranial contents, but subsequently technology was quickly expanded to permit imaging of the entire body. Radiographic images are acquired from a number of angles in axial projection; slice thickness may be varied. Accurate measurement of attenuation coefficients (density) of each small volume (voxel) of tissue results in excellent anatomic detail. The large amount of data generated is collated by a computer, and the resultant images can be electronically manipulated to best define anatomy and pathology. Often intravenous or oral contrast materials are given to the patient to further define structures in the abdomen. However, scanning done before the administration of intravenous contrast material is helpful in the detection of renal calcifications.

The advantages of body CT are the remarkable image resolution displayed in full cross-sectional views and the relative noninvasiveness of the technique. Images obtained are not as dependent on function as in excretory urography, and they are not obscured by gas and bone as in ultrasonography. However, the cost and limited plane of view of the examination can be disadvantages. Radiation dose, particularly compared with that in ultrasonography, must be considered. In pediatric examinations of the renal area and retroperitoneum, additional problems of resolution occur because of respiratory motion and lack of retroperitoneal fat. Faster, newer generations of CT machines can partially obviate respiratory motion, but refinements in other imaging modalities—ultrasonography, radionuclide studies—have limited the use of CT as a primary imaging modality for urologic problems in children.

When body CT is to be used in young children, sedation is often required, particularly for children between the ages of 1 month and approximately 5 years. Immobilization may be necessary, and attention to maintenance of body temperature during the examinations in infants is particularly important. Ultrafast CT scanners are available in a limited number of institutions allowing subsecond imaging and obviating the need for sedation and possibly limiting the amount of contrast material necessary (Fig. 3–64) (Brasch).

A major role for body CT in pediatric patients is the demonstration of extension of renal, other retroperitoneal, and pelvic masses. This is particularly important when excretory urography and ultrasonography have failed to define these lesions adequately. Computed tomography has been shown to more accurately detect tumor extent and the relationship to surrounding structures; this information often has therapeutic and prognostic significance (Fig. 3–65).

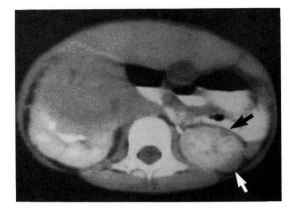

Figure 3–65 □ CT scan with oral and intravenous contrast material through the upper renal region in a 4-year-old patient. There is a large mass in the upper portion of the right kidney extending far anteriorly that was thought to be a Wilms' tumor. Two peripheral low-density nodules can be seen in the left kidney *(arrows)*. The lesion on the right was not thought to be initially operable and excisional biopsy specimens of the left renal lesions demonstrated renal blastema. Consequently, chemotherapy and radiotherapy could be given for the right renal lesion; subsequently, the kidney was resected with little difficulty.

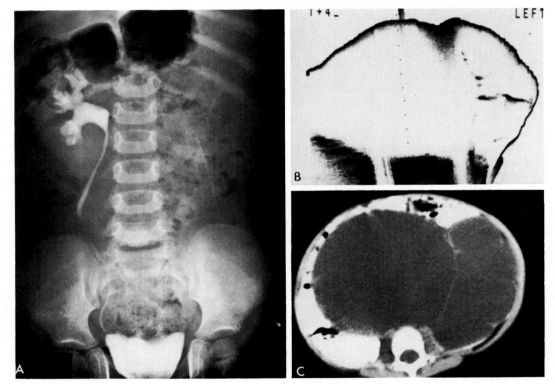

Figure 3–66 □ Hydronephrosis secondary to ureteropelvic junction obstruction in a 2-year-old girl who presented with abdominal prominence. *A,* Excretory urogram, 1-minute film showing a normal right kidney and nonopacification of the left kidney. *B,* Transverse ultrasonogram showing large cystic structures in the abdomen that are not as well defined as on CT. *C,* CT slice with oral contrast material in the markedly displaced bowel; the massively dilated renal pelvis is seen centrally and calyces are displayed to the right (patient's left).

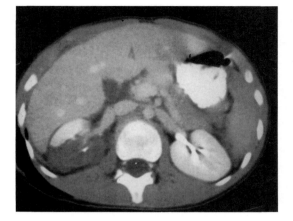

Figure 3–67 □ CT scan of the upper renal region with oral and intravenous contrast material in a 10-year-old who was being evaluated after a motor vehicle accident. Nonfunction of the upper 60 per cent of the right kidney was shown on this and other images. The renal veins can be well seen on this examination, and the renal arteries were seen on other images, excluding vascular lesions that would need repair. The patient also had a hepatic contusion (not shown) and was treated nonoperatively.

Recurrence of such tumors is often best shown on CT scans (Brasch et al). Computed tomography is occasionally used as a secondary examination in the evaluation of renal cystic disease, some inflammatory lesions, and severe hydronephrosis (Fig. 3–66). Body CT has become the primary examination in the evaluation of significant trauma involving the kidneys and other intra-abdominal structures (Fig. 3–67) (Yale-Loehr et al). Changes in renal transplants can also be shown well on computed tomography.

MAGNETIC RESONANCE IMAGING

The newest clinically applicable method of imaging is magnetic resonance imaging. This method is currently used to detect and define lesions of the urinary tract in infants and children (Boechat and Kangarloo; Harris and Cohen). The advantages of this method include excellent tissue-contrast differentiation, high resolution multiplanar capability, and a lack of ionizing radiation or any other known biologic risk.

For renal and perirenal masses, MRI appears to have advantages over other modalities in defining the origin of the mass, the evaluation of vascular patency, the detection of lymph node involvement, and the evaluation of direct invasion of the adjacent organs (Fig. 3–68) (Hricak et al).

To maximize diagnostic accuracy while minimizing excessive numbers of examinations and risk, it is critical to have an appreciation not only for which imaging modality is best for the

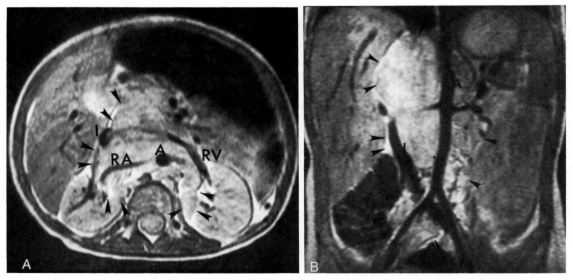

Figure 3–68 □ MRI of the abdomen in a 3-year-old with a large retroperitoneal neuroblastoma. Axial *(A)* and coronal *(B)* images (TE30 TR2000) demonstrate the extent of the mass *(arrowheads)* and the vascular anatomy, including aorta (A), inferior vena cava (I), renal artery (RA), and renal vein (RV). Marked anterior and lateral displacement of the inferior vena cava can be seen on the two images, and there is splaying of the renal veins with encasement of the other vascular structures. No invasion in the spinal canal was demonstrated on this examination.

presumptive diagnosis in the individual clinical situation but also for which examination is best performed in a particular setting or specific institution.

Acknowledgments

Drs. Glen W. Hartman and Robert R. Hattery were the authors of this chapter in the first edition of this book. Dr. Robert L. Lebowitz kindly reviewed the chapter for the second edition. Their contributions are gratefully acknowledged.

Bibliography

EXCRETORY UROGRAPHY

Berdon WE, Baker DH: The significance of a distended bladder on the interpretation of intravenous pyelograms obtained on patients with "hydronephrosis." Am J Roentgenol 120:402, 1974.

Berdon WE, Baker DH, Leonidas J: Advantages of prone positioning in gastrointestinal and genitourinary roentgenology studies in infants and children. Am J Roentgenol 103:444, 1968.

Berdon WE, Schwartz RH, Becker J, et al: Tamm-Horsfall proteinuria: its relationship to prolonged nephrogram in infants and children and to renal failure following intravenous urography in adults with multiple myeloma. Radiology 92:714, 1969.

Bettmann MA: Guidelines for use of low osmolality contrast agents. Radiology 172:901, 1989.

Bielory L, Kaliner MA: Anaphylactoid reactions to radiocontrast materials. Int Anesthesiol Clin 23:97, 1985.

Binder R, Korobkin M, Clark RE, Palubinskas AJ: Aberrant papillae and other filling defects of the renal pelvis. Am J Roentgenol 114:746, 1972.

Brasch RC: Allergic reactions to contrast media: accumulated evidence. Am J Roentgenol 134:797, 1980.

Cook IK, Keats TE, Seale DL: Determination of the normal position of the upper urinary tract on the lateral abdominal urogram. Radiology 99:499, 1971.

Currarino G: Roentgenographic estimation of kidney size in normal individuals with emphasis on children. Am J Roentgenol 93:464, 1965.

Currarino G, Weinberg A, Putnam R: Resorption of contrast material from the bladder during a cystourethrography causing an excretory urogram. Radiology 123:149, 1977.

Davidson AJ: Radiology of the Kidneys. Philadelphia, WB Saunders Co, 1985, pp 1–12.

Dunbar JS, Nogrady B: Excretory urography in the first year of life. Radiol Clin North Am 10:367, 1972.

Dure-Smith P, Simenhoff M, Zimsking PD, Kodroff M: The bolus effect of excretory urography. Radiology 101:24, 1971.

Fajardo LL, Hillman EJ, Hunter TB, et al: Excretory urography using computed radiography. Radiology 162:345, 1987.

Fischer HW, Rothfield NJH, Carr JD: Optimum dose in excretory urography. Am J Roentgenol 113:423, 1971.

Fitts FB Jr, Mascatello VG, Mellins HZ: The value of compression during excretion voiding urethrography. Radiology 125:53, 1977.

Gill WB, Curtis GA. The influence of bladder fullness on upper urinary tract dimensions and renal excretory function. J Urol 117:573, 1977.

Godderidge C: Female gonadal shielding. Appl Radiol 8:65, 1979.

Gooding CA, Berdon WE, Brodeur AE, Rowen M: Adverse reactions to intravenous pyelography in children. Am J Roentgenol 123:802, 1975.

Green WM, Pressman DB, McLennan BL, Casarella WJ: "Column of Bertin": diagnosis by nephrotomography. Am J Roentgenol 116:714, 1972.

Griscom NT, Neuhauser EBD: Total body opacification. J Pediatr Surg 1:76, 1966.

Haas EA, Solomon DJ: Telling children about diagnostic radiology procedures. Radiology 124:521, 1977.

Hartman GW, Hattery RR, Witten DM, et al: Mortality during excretory urography: Mayo Clinic experience. Am J Roentgenol 139:919, 1982.

Hernandez RJ, Poznanski AK, Kuhns RL, McCormick TL: Factors affecting the measurement of renal length. Radiology 130:653, 1979.

Hodson CJ, Davies Z, Prescod A: Renal parenchymal radiographic measurement in infants and children. Pediatr Radiol 3:16, 1975.

Kassner EG, Elguezabal A, Pochaczevsky R: Death during intravenous urography: overdosage syndrome in young infants. NY State J Med 73:1958, 1973.

Katayama H, Tanaka T: Clinical survey of adverse reactions to contrast media. Invest Radiol 23:S88, 1988.

Kaufman RA, Dunbar JS, Gob DE: Normal dilatation of the proximal ureter in children. Am J Roentgenol 137:945, 1981.

Kelly WM: Uricosuria and x-ray contrast agents. N Engl J Med 284:975, 1971.

Kirks DR, Currarino G, Weinburg AG: Transverse folds in the proximal ureter: a normal variant in infants. Am J Roentgenol 130:463, 1978.

Kumar D, Cigtay OS, Klein LH: Case reports: aberrant renal papilla. Br J Radiol 50:141, 1977.

Laufer I, Griscom NT: Compensatory renal hypertrophy: absence in utero and development in early life. Am J Roentgenol 113:646, 1971.

Lebowitz RL: Pediatric uroradiology. Annual Meeting American College of Radiology, Boston, 1982.

Lebowitz RL, Avni FE: Misleading appearances in pediatric uroradiology. Pediatr Radiol 10:15, 1980.

Lebowitz RL, Hopkins T, Colodny AH: Measuring the kidneys—practical applications using a growth hypertrophy chart. Pediatr Radiol 4:37, 1975.

Lebowitz RL, Mandell J: Urinary tract infection in children: putting radiology in its place. Radiology 165:1, 1987.

Leonidas JC, McCauley RGK, Klauber GC, Fretzayas AM: Sonography as a substitute for excretory urography in children with urinary tract infection. Am J Roentgenol 144:815, 1985.

Ludin H: Radiological estimation of kidney weight. Acta Radiol [Diagn] (Stockh) 6:651, 1967.

Lutzker LG, Goldman HS: A method for improved urographic visualization for children. Radiology 111:217, 1974.

Magill HL, Clarke EA, Fitch SJ, et al: Excretory urography with iohexol: evaluation in children. Radiology 161:625, 1986.

Mascatello V, Lebowitz RL: Malposition of the colon in left renal agenesis and ectopia. Radiology 123:371, 1976.

McClennan BL: Low-osmolality contrast media: premises and promises. Radiology 162:1, 1987.

Meyers MA, Whalen JP, Evans JA, et al: Malposition and displacement of the bowel in renal agenesis and ectopia: new observations. Am J Roentgenol 117:323, 1973.

Nogrady MB, Dunbar JS: The technique of roentgen investigation of the urinary tract in infants and children. Prog Pediatr Radiol 3:3, 1970.

O'Connor JF, Neuhauser EBD: Total body opacification in conventional and high dose intravenous urography in infancy. Am J Roentgenol 90:63, 1963.

Palmer FJ: The RACR survey of intravenous contrast media reactions: final report. Australas Radiol 32:426, 1988.

Parker JA, Lebowitz RL, Mascatello V, Treves S: Magnification renal scintigraphy in the differential diagnosis of septa of Bertin. Pediatr Radiol 4:157, 1976.

Philbin DM, Moss J, Akins CW, et al: The use of H_1 and H_2 histamine antagonists with morphine anesthesia: a double-blind study. Anesthesiology 55:292, 1981.

Poslethwaithe AE, Kelly WN: Uricosuria effects of radio-contrast agents: a study in man of more commonly used preparations. Ann Intern Med 74:845, 1971.

Ransley PG: Opacification of the renal parenchyma in obstruction reflux. Pediatr Radiol 4:226, 1976.

Stannard M, Lebowitz RL: Urography in the child who wets. Am J Roentgenol 130:959, 1978.

Steinberg EP, Anderson GF, Powe NR: Use of low osmolality contrast media in a price sensitive environment. Am J Roentgenol 151:271, 1988.

Whitaker RH: Methods of assessing obstruction in dilated ureters. Br J Urol 45:15, 1973.

Witten DM, Hirsch FD, Hartman GW: Acute reactions to urographic contrast medium: incidence, clinical characteristics and relationship to hypersensitivity states. Am J Roentgenol 119:832, 1973.

CYSTOURETHROGRAPHY

Colodny AH, Lebowitz RL: The importance of voiding during cystourethrogram. J Urol 111:838, 1974a.

Colodny AH, Lebowitz RL: A plea for grading vesicoureteral reflux. Urology 4:357, 1974b.

Currarino G: Narrowing of the male urethra caused by contractions or spasms of the bulbocavernosus muscle: cystourethrographic observations. Am J Roentgenol 108:641, 1970.

Fletcher EWL, Forbes WS, Gough MH: Superpubic micturating cystourethrography in infants. Clin Radiol 29:309, 1978.

Gross GW, Lebowitz RL: Infection does not cause reflux. Am J Roentgenol 137:929, 1981.

Kelalis PP, Burke EC, Stickler GB, et al: Urinary vaginal reflux in children. Pediatrics 51:941, 1973.

Koff SA, Fischer CP, Poznanski AK: Cystourethrography: the effect of reservoir height upon intravesical pressure. Pediatr Radiol 8:21, 1979.

Leibovic SJ, Lebowitz RL: Reducing patient dose in voiding cystourethrography. Urol Radiol 2:103, 1980.

Levitt SB, Duckett J, Spitzer A, Walker D: Medical versus surgical treatment of primary vesicoureteral reflux. Pediatrics 67:392, 1981.

Lucaya J: A simple technique of retrograde urethrography in male infants. Radiology 102:402, 1972.

Mandell J, Lebowitz RL, Hallett M, et al: Urethral narrowing in region of external sphincter: radiologic-urodynamic correlations in boys with myelodysplasia. Am J Roentgenol 134:731, 1980.

McAlister WH, Cacciarelli A, Shackelford GD: Complications associated with cystography in children. Radiology 111:167, 1974.

Peck AG, Poznanski AK: A simple device for genitography. Radiology 103:212, 1972.

Poznanski E, Poznanski AK: Psychogenic influences on voiding: Observations from cystourethrography. Psychosomatics 10:339, 1969.

Sane SM, Worsing A Jr: Voiding cystourethrography: recent advances. Minn Med 58:148, 1975.

Shopfner CE: Clinical evaluation of cystourethrographic contrast media. Radiology 88:491, 1967.

Shopfner CE: Cystourethrography. Med Radiogr Photogr 47:2, 1971.

Shopfner CE: Genitography in intersex states. Radiology 82:664, 1964.

Shopfner CE, Hutch JA: The trigonal canal. Radiology 88:209, 1967.

Templeton AW, Dwyer SJ III, Cox GG, et al: Digital radiography imaging system: description and clinical evaluation. Am J Roentgenol 149:847, 1987.

Vlahakis E, Hartman GW, Kelalis PP: Comparison of voiding cystourethrography and expression cystourethrography. J Urol 106:414, 1971.

OTHER UROGRAPHIC EXAMS

Hardy BE, Lebowitz RL, Baez A, Colodny AH: Strictures of the ileal loop. J Urol 117:358, 1977.

Hudson HC, Kramer SA, Anderson EE: Identification of uretero-ileal obstruction by retrograde loopography. Urology 17:147, 1981.

Lebowitz RL: Urinary diversion. *In*: Postoperative Pediatric Uroradiology. New York, Appleton-Century-Crofts, 1981, pp 103–130.

McCallum RW, Colapinto V: Urologic Radiology of the Adult Male Lower Urinary Tract. Springfield, Ill, Charles C Thomas, 1976, p 43.

Nogrady MB, Peticlerc R, Moir JD: The roentgenologic evaluation of supravesical permanent urinary diversion in childhood (ileal and colonic conduit). J Can Assoc Radiol 20:75, 1969.

Shapiro SR, Lebowitz R, Colodny AH: Fate of 90 children with ileal conduit urinary diversion a decade later: analysis of complications, pyelography, renal function and bacteriology. J Urol 114:289, 1975.

ANTEGRADE PYELOGRAPHY AND INTERVENTIONAL PROCEDURES

Ball WS Jr, Towbin R, Strife JL, Spencer R: Interventional genitourinary radiology in children: A review of 61 procedures. Am J Roentgenol 147:791, 1986.

Bennett LN, Voegeli DR, Crummy AB, et al: Urologic complications following renal transplantation: Role of interventional radiologic procedures. Radiology 160:531, 1986.

Douenias R, Smith AD, Brock WA: Advances in the percutaneous management of the ureteropelvic junction and other obstructions of the urinary tract in children. Urol Clin North Am 17:419, 1990.

Man DWK, Ransley PG: Percutaneous antegrade pyelography in children. Br J Urol 56:237, 1984.

Riedy MJ, Lebowitz RL: Percutaneous studies of the upper urinary tract in children, with special emphasis on infants. Radiology 160:231, 1986.

Towbin RB: Pediatric interventional procedures in the 1980's: a period of development, growth, and acceptance. Radiology 170:1081, 1989.

Woodside JR, Stevens GF, Stark GL, et al: Percutaneous stone removal in children. J Urol 134:1166, 1985.

VASCULAR STUDIES

Berdon WE, Baker DH, Santulli TV: Factors producing spurious obstruction of the inferior vena cava in infants and children with abdominal tumors. Radiology 88:111, 1967.

Berk RN, Wholey MH, Stodkcale R: Angiographic diagnosis of splenic and hepatic trauma. J Can Assoc Radiol 21:230, 1970.

Castellino RA: Observations in "reactive (follicular) hyperplasia" as encountered in repeat lymphography in the lymphomas. Cancer 34:2042, 1974.

Castellino RA, Bergeron C, Markovits P: Experience with 659 consecutive lymphograms in children. Cancer 40:1097, 1977.

Castellino RA, Markovits P, Musumeri R: Lymphography. *In* Pediatric Oncologic Radiology. Edited by BR Parker, RA Castellino. St Louis, CV Mosby, 1977, pp 58–84.

Dunnick NR, Parker BA, Castellino RA: Pediatric lymphography: Performance interpretation and accuracy in 193 consecutive children. Am J Roentgenol 129:639, 1977.

Fellows K: Angiography. *In* Pediatric Oncologic Radiology. Edited by BR Parker, RA Castellino. St Louis, CV Mosby, 1977, pp 11–39.

Fellows KE Jr, Nebesar RA: Abdominal, hepatic and visceral angiography. *In* Angiography in infants and children. Edited by MT Gyepes. New York, Grune and Stratton, 1974, pp 193–232.

Fitz CR, Harwood-Nash DC: Special procedures and techniques in infants. Radiol Clin North Am 13:191, 1975.

Harper AP, Yune HY, Franken EA Jr: Spectrum of angiographically demonstrable renal pathology in young hypertensive patients. Pediatr Radiol 123:141, 1977.

Kirks DR, Fitz CR, Harwood-Nash DC: Pediatric abdominal angiography: practical guide to catheter selection, flow rates and contrast dosage. Pediatr Radiol 5:19, 1976.

Korobkin M, Pick RA, Merten DF, et al: Etiologic radiographic findings in children and adolescents with nonuremic hypertension. Radiology 110:615, 1974.

Korogi Y, Takahashi M, Bussaka H, et al: Percutaneous transluminal angioplasty for renal branch stenosis—a report on a 6-year-old boy. Br J Radiol 58:77, 1985.

Mortensson W, Hallbook T, Lundstrom N-R: Percutaneous catheterization of the femoral vessels in children.
I. Influence on arterial peak flow and venous emptying rates in the calves. Pediatr Radiol 3:195, 1975.

Murphy G, Campbell DR, Fraser DB: Pain in peripheral arteriography: an assessment of conventional versus ionic and non-ionic low-osmolality contrast agents. J Can Assoc Radiol 39:104, 1988.

Nebesar RA, Fleischli DJ, Pollard JJ, Griscom NT: Arteriography in infants and children with emphasis on the Seldinger technique and abdominal diseases. Am J Roentgenol 106:81, 1969.

Slovis TL, Philippart AI, Cushing B, et al: Evaluation of the inferior vena cava by sonography and venography in children with renal and hepatic tumors. Radiology 140:767, 1981.

Tucker AS: The roentgen diagnosis of abdominal masses in children: intravenous urography vs inferior venacavography. Am J Roentgenol 95:76, 1965.

BODY COMPUTED TOMOGRAPHY

Berger PE, Kuhn JP, Brusehaber J: Techniques for computed tomography in infants and children. Radiol Clin North Am 19:399, 1981.

Brasch RC: Ultrafast computed tomography for infants and children. Radiol Clin North Am 26:277, 1988.

Brasch RC, Randel SB, Gould RG: Follow-up of Wilms' tumor: comparison of CT with other imaging modalities. Am J Roentgenol 137:1005, 1981.

Kuhn JP, Berger PE: Computed tomography of the kidney in infancy and childhood. Radiol Clin North Am 19:445, 1981.

Reiman TAH, Siegel MJ, Shackelford GD: Wilms tumor in children: abdominal CT and US evaluation. Radiology 160:501, 1986.

Yale-Loehr AJ, Kramer SS, Quinlan DM, et al: CT of severe renal trauma in children: evaluation and course of healing with conservative therapy. Am J Roentgenol 153:109, 1989.

MAGNETIC RESONANCE IMAGING

Boechat MI, Kangarloo H: MR imaging of the abdomen in children. Am J Roentgenol 152:1245, 1989.

Harris TM, Cohen MD: Abdominal magnetic resonance imaging. Pediatr Radiol 20:10, 1989.

Hricak H, Demas BE, Williams RD, et al: Magnetic resonance imaging in the diagnosis and staging of renal and perirenal neoplasms. Radiology 154:709, 1985.

4

☐ Nuclear Medicine in Pediatric Urology

Massoud Majd

The use of nuclear medicine in the diagnosis and management of urologic problems in infants and children has dramatically increased over the past several years. Major factors that have contributed to this rapid growth include the introduction of better radiopharmaceuticals, the improvement in imaging devices (gamma cameras), and the use of computers in analysis of the functional parameters of the genitourinary system. The introduction of the mobile gamma camera–computer system has expanded the use of nuclear medicine studies to the intensive care unit, the operating room, and the patient's bedside.

Nuclear medicine procedures are generally noninvasive, require neither fasting nor bowel preparation, are performed without anesthesia or sedation, and do not require hospitalization. Radiopharmaceuticals have no systemic pharmacologic effects and do not cause any allergic reaction. Absorbed radiation doses from the radionuclide studies do not reach a harmful range and, in some instances, are much lower than the doses from comparable radiographic tests. Most importantly, radionuclide studies offer quantitative functional information currently not available with other imaging modalities. Furthermore, they lend themselves to a variety of physiologic and pharmacologic interventions that can enhance their diagnostic accuracy. Notable examples of the use of pharmacologic intervention in renal studies are diuretic renography and captopril-enhanced renal scintigraphy. Many disorders of the genitourinary system in children are part of a dynamic process that necessitates serial assessment. Noninvasive radionuclide studies provide optimal means of evaluating and following the course of such disorders.

RENAL IMAGING AND FUNCTIONAL ANALYSIS

Radiopharmaceuticals

Radionuclide renal studies are used to assess renal perfusion and certain aspects of renal function and structure. The information gained depends upon which radiopharmaceutical is used. Currently, the following radiopharmaceuticals are used for the evaluation of the kidneys.

Technetium 99m DTPA

Technetium 99m diethylenetriaminepentaacetic acid (DTPA) is commonly used for renal studies. Renal clearance of DTPA is almost exclusively by glomerular filtration with no significant tubular secretion or cortical retention. Therefore, its rate of clearance provides an accurate measurement of the glomerular filtration rate (GFR). Its initial transit through the kidney reflects renal perfusion. Accumulation of the tracer in each kidney between 1 and 3 minutes after injection is proportional to its GFR. Because of rapid clearance, the high concentration of technetium 99m DTPA in the urine provides excellent visualization of the pelvicalyceal systems, ureter, and bladder. Because of its low retention in the renal cortex, however, this agent may fail to demonstrate small cortical lesions.

Technetium 99m GHA

Technetium 99m glucoheptonate (GHA) is cleared by a combination of glomerular filtra-

117

tion and tubular extraction. Most of the agent is rapidly excreted in the urine, allowing moderately good visualization of the pelvicalyceal systems, ureters, and bladder. Approximately 20 per cent of the administered dose of glucoheptonate, however, remains in the renal cortex, firmly bound to the tubular cells. Therefore, delayed imaging at 2 to 4 hours provides visualization of renal cortex. Glucoheptonate, owing to its complex mode of clearance, is not a suitable agent for measuring GFR. However, its accumulation in each kidney between 1 and 3 minutes after injection is a measure of relative renal function. Cortical uptake of glucoheptonate in each kidney on the delayed images can also be used for calculation of renal differential function, provided that there is no retention of the tracer in the pelvicalyceal system.

Technetium 99m DMSA

Technetium 99m dimercaptosuccinic acid (DMSA) is presently the best cortical imaging agent available. The majority is tightly bound to the renal tubular cells, and only a small amount is excreted in the urine. DMSA allows excellent visualization of the renal parenchyma without interference from pelvicalyceal activity and is therefore recommended for detection of cortical lesions such as acute pyelonephritis, cortical scars, or infarcts. The uptake of technetium 99m DMSA by each kidney is an accurate measure of relative functioning tubular mass and in most situations correlates well with the relative GFR and other parameters of renal function (Taylor, 1982).

Iodine 131 OIH

Iodine 131 orthoiodohippurate (OIH, Hippuran) is primarily a tubular agent. Approximately 80 per cent of OIH entering the kidney is extracted with each pass, of which 85 to 90 per cent is removed by tubular secretion and the remaining 10 to 15 per cent by passive glomerular filtration. Despite these excellent biologic properties and its early popularity, iodine 131 OIH currently has little place in pediatric nuclear medicine. The major disadvantages of this agent are poor characteristics of its radiation for imaging and high radiation dose resulting from the emission of beta particles. This necessitates the use of a low dose of the tracer, leading to a poor-resolution image.

Iodine 123 OIH

Iodine 123–labeled OIH, on the other hand, is an excellent renal imaging agent (Zielinski et al). Iodine 123 is a pure gamma emitter with an energy level suitable for imaging with the scintillation camera. It can be used in millicurie doses with a significantly lower radiation dose than would be received from microcuries of iodine 131 OIH. Radiochemically pure iodine 123 OIH, however, is not readily available.

Technetium 99m MAG 3

Technetium 99m mercaptoacetyltriglycine (MAG 3) is a new renal radiopharmaceutical that combines the desirable biologic properties of OIH and physical properties of technetium 99m. This agent is rapidly cleared by tubular secretion and is not retained in the parenchyma of normal kidneys. Although extraction of MAG 3 from blood in each passage through the kidney is less than that of OIH, the rate at which the two tracers appear in the urine are almost identical. This is primarily due to the fact that MAG 3 is more highly protein-bound than OIH and a greater percentage of the injected dose remains in the intravascular compartment. Furthermore, in contrast to OIH, very little, if any, MAG 3 enters the red blood cells. Therefore, a higher percentage of the injected dose of MAG 3 is available for renal clearance (Taylor et al, 1989).

Owing to its superior imaging qualities and lower radiation doses, technetium 99m MAG 3 is rapidly gaining acceptance as a replacement for iodine 131 OIH. The quality of MAG 3 images is also superior to the quality of DTPA images. This is due to a much smaller volume of distribution and a faster clearance, resulting in a higher target-to-background ratio. Therefore, MAG 3 appears to be a good replacement for DTPA in certain applications, such as diuretic renography. The favorable qualities of technetium 99m MAG 3 make it particularly appealing for use in the pediatric age group.

Procedures

Renal Scintigraphy

The conventional renal scan should consist of a radionuclide angiogram followed by sequential functional images of the kidneys, ureters, and bladder. The techniques used in different institutions vary greatly. The following technique is currently used in our laboratory.

After a rapid intravenous injection of an appropriate amount of the tracer (DTPA, GHA, or MAG 3), a series of 2-second dynamic posterior images of the kidneys is obtained during the first minute (angiographic phase) (Fig. 4–1A). This is followed by a series of 1-minute images of the kidneys, ureters, and bladder for 20 minutes for the evaluation of renal excretion and drainage of the tracer (Fig. 4–1B). Further delayed images are obtained if necessary.

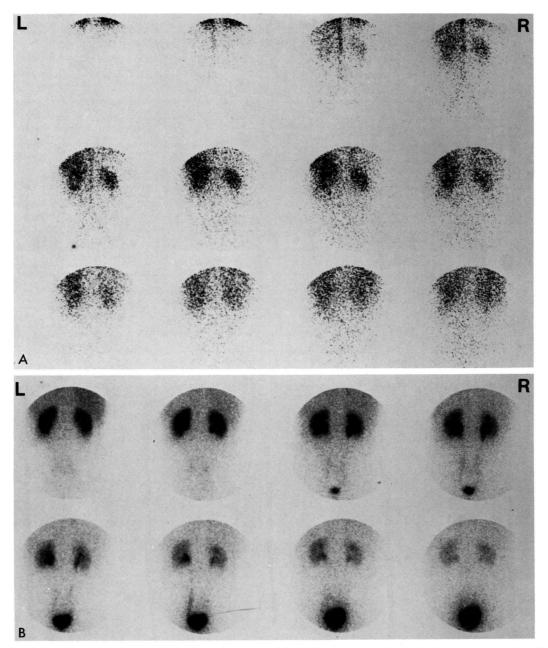

Figure 4–1 □ Normal technetium 99m DTPA dynamic renal function study. *A,* The perfusion phase or radionuclide renal angiogram demonstrates prompt and equal perfusion to both kidneys. *B,* The sequential static images show uniform distribution of the tracer in the cortex of both kidneys, early visualization of the collecting systems, and normal drainage.

Digital images are also acquired on a computer at the rate of one image per second for 60 seconds (angiographic phase) followed by a series of 15-second images for 20 minutes. The early digital images, after the angiographic phase and before accumulation of the tracer in the collecting systems, are used to calculate relative renal function.

Although analogue images allow for a rough visual assessment of renal vascular perfusion (Fig. 4–1*A*), computer analysis is essential for a precise assessment. Areas of interest are flagged over the abdominal aorta and the kidneys. Time-activity curves are generated from these areas of interest. The renal slopes are then compared with each other and with the aortic slope (Fig. 4–2).

Renal cortical imaging is accomplished by delayed imaging 2 to 3 hours after injection of either technetium 99m GHA or technetium 99m DMSA. Magnified, high-resolution images of each kidney, in posterior and posterior oblique projections, are obtained using a pinhole collimator. In addition, a posterior image of the kidneys using a parallel hole collimator is obtained for calculation of renal differential function (Fig. 4–3). Single photon emission computed tomography (SPECT) images of the kidneys are obtained in selected cases.

Relative Renal Function

The differential or relative function of each kidney can be calculated by determining the accumulation of the tracer in each kidney between 1 and 3 minutes after injection. During this period, all the radioactivity within the kidney is confined to the vessels and functioning renal parenchyma, as the tracer has not yet reached the collecting system. Regions of interest are selected for each kidney and its background. Background activity is then subtracted from corresponding renal activity. The net counts within each kidney are expressed as a percentage of the total renal counts (Fig. 4–4*A*). The same principle can be used in calculating the relative contribution of different segments of a kidney to its total function. The pitfalls of the differential function analysis, based on the 1 to 3 minutes' accumulation of the tracer in the kidneys, are as follows:

1. The technique is operator-dependent, and selection of the frames and the regions of interest affects the results. This is particularly critical for the background regions of interest, which may include a portion of the liver and spleen, which have a high concentration of the tracer.

2. The results may be invalid in the presence of extreme hydronephrosis. When the cortex is thin and poorly functioning, selecting an area of interest is difficult. Attenuation of the counts from the anterior parenchyma, which is widely displaced by the dilated, urine-filled pelvicalyceal system, results in inaccurate calculation of the total activity contained in the entire renal parenchyma.

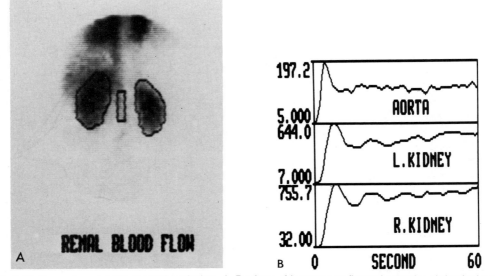

Figure 4–2 ☐ Computer analysis of renal perfusion. *A*, Regions of interest are flagged over the abdominal aorta and the kidneys. *B*, Time-activity curves of the first transit of the tracer through the abdominal aorta and the kidneys demonstrate similar slopes, indicating normal symmetric renal blood flow.

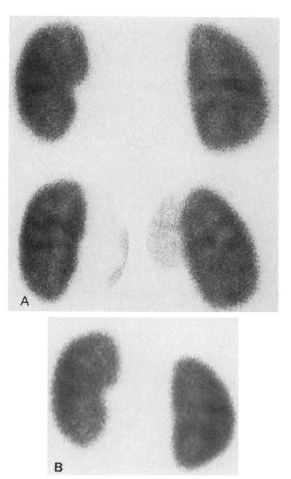

Figure 4–3 □ Normal DMSA scan. *A,* High-resolution magnified images of each kidney in posterior and posterior-oblique projections using a pinhole collimator. *B,* Posterior image of the kidneys obtained with a parallel hole collimator.

The relative renal function can also be calculated on delayed images (2 to 3 hours) using technetium 99m DMSA or technetium 99m glucoheptonate. There are advantages to this method:

1. The background activity is negligible by that time, and thus one source of potential error is eliminated.

2. Both anterior and posterior images can be obtained from which a geometric mean value can be calculated. The geometric mean may be more reliable than the count ratios from posterior images alone as routinely obtained when DTPA is used, particularly when the kidneys are at different depths.

Several investigations have confirmed the validity of these methods of calculating differential renal function by comparing results from DMSA, DTPA, and ureteral catheterization studies with split creatinine clearances (Powers; Price). The percentages calculated using DTPA and glucoheptonate are the same, in spite of their different modes of renal excretion. Furthermore, the glucoheptonate ratios calculated on the basis of early and delayed images are similar.

The differential renal functional analysis is an index only of relative function of the kidneys and does not provide information about absolute function of each kidney.

Total and Separate Glomerular Filtration Rates

Since technetium 99m DTPA is excreted almost exclusively by glomerular filtration, its rate of clearance from blood is an accurate measure of GFR. A variety of methods may be used to calculate GFR using technetium 99m DTPA (Dubovsky and Russell; Malligan et al). The simplest method, which employs three blood samples drawn between 2 and 3 hours after injection, is based on single compartmental analysis of the DTPA clearance (Fig. 4–4*B*). There is excellent correlation

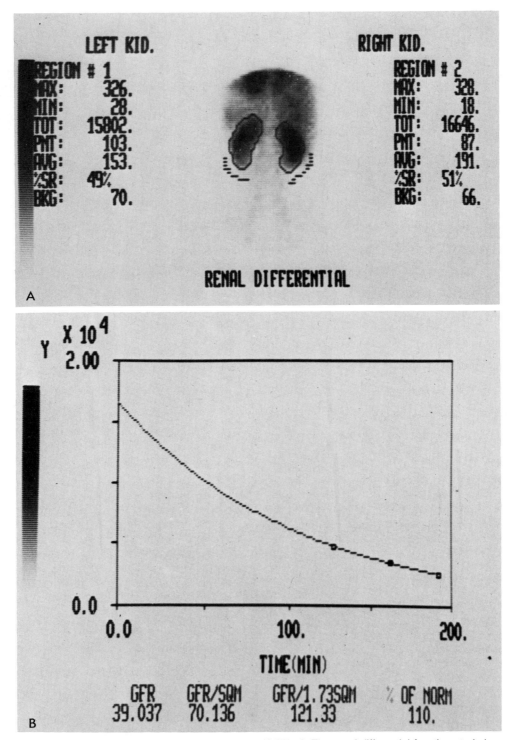

Figure 4–4 □ Total and separate glomerular filtration rate (GFR). *A,* The renal differential function study based upon the relative accumulation of the tracer in each kidney at the interval between 1 and 2 minutes after injection of technetium 99m DTPA shows that the kidneys function equally. *B,* The total GFR calculated on the basis of plasma clearance of technetium 99m DTPA is 121 ml/minute/1.73 M². The GFR from each kidney, therefore, is about 60.5 ml/minute/1.73 M².

between this technique and 24-hour urinary creatinine clearance (Braren et al). Absolute GFR of each kidney can then be calculated by multiplying the total calculated GFR in milliliters per minute by the percentages obtained from the renal differential function. This method of GFR calculation is relatively noninvasive and obviates the need for 24-hour urine collection. Because of the need for multiple venous punctures, however, the test is unpleasant for children and their parents. Because of uncertainty about the effect of diuretics on the GFR in different pathologic states, the test cannot be reliably performed in conjunction with diuretic renography.

Other methods of calculating GFR based on external counting without blood samples or with a single blood sample have been developed (Gates; Piepsz et al, 1978; Shore et al). These methods have become popular in adult nuclear medicine, but their reliability for use in children remains uncertain.

Radionuclide Renography

The radionuclide renogram is a time-activity curve of renal extraction and excretion of a radiopharmaceutical. Conventional iodine 131 Hippuran renography is seldom used in children. A modification of iodine 131 OIH or technetium 99m DTPA renography applying deconvolution analysis is used to measure renal parenchymal transit time of the tracer (Diffey et al; Whitfield et al, 1978, 1981). Parenchymal transit time is prolonged in patients with obstructive uropathy or renal ischemia. Diuretic radionuclide renography is another modification of conventional renography used in the evaluation of hydronephrosis. These procedures are explained in detail later in this chapter.

Clinical Applications

Although the renal scan lacks the anatomic resolution of the excretory urogram, it has several advantages, including quantitative assessment of renal function, independence of image quality from overlying bowel contents and bony structures, and ability to visualize renal tissue with a very low level of function. These advantages are particularly important in neonates. At birth, the GFR is about 21 per cent of the corrected adult value and reaches only 44 per cent by 2 weeks of age (McCrory). The low GFR, together with overlying bowel

gas, generally results in poor visualization of kidneys on the excretory urogram and often necessitates multiple radiographs and, occasionally, tomography for adequate visualization. This may expose the child to an unacceptably high radiation dose. In addition, the urographic contrast media, with the exception of newer non-ionic media, may produce osmotic side effects (Magill; Wood and Smith). Radionuclide scanning, which is limited only by renal function, is superior to excretory urography for localization and functional analysis of the kidneys in all ages, including the newborn.

Congenital Anomalies

Any functioning renal tissue, irrespective of its location, can be visualized on renal scan. Ectopic kidneys, which are often superimposed on bones and may remain obscure on an excretory urogram, can be easily demonstrated and differentiated from renal agenesis (Fig. 4–5). The horseshoe kidney and other variants of fused kidneys are also often better evaluated on a renal scan than on an excretory urogram (Figs. 4–6 and 4–7).

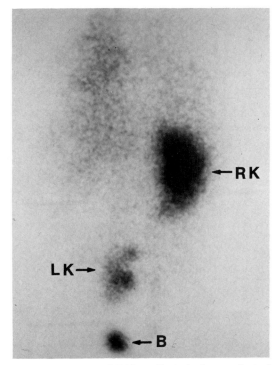

Figure 4–5 □ Ectopic kidney. Posterior image of a technetium 99m DTPA renal scan demonstrates ectopic (pelvic) left kidney. The right kidney is normal. RK, right kidney; LK, left kidney; B, bladder.

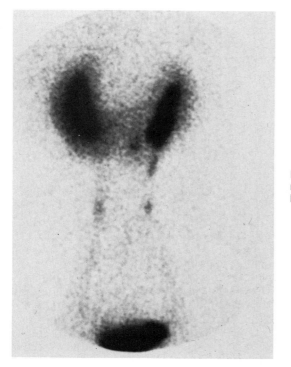

Figure 4–6 □ Horseshoe kidney. Anterior image of a technetium 99m DTPA renal scan demonstrates fusion of the lower poles of the kidneys.

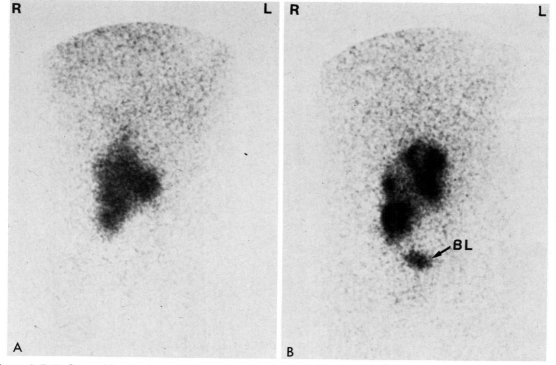

Figure 4–7 □ Crossed fused ectopia. *A,* The anterior image of a technetium 99m DTPA renal scan obtained 2 minutes after injection demonstrates a single irregular mass of functioning renal tissue located in the mid-lower abdomen. *B,* The image obtained at 10 minutes after injection shows two separate sets of pelvicalyceal systems. BL, bladder.

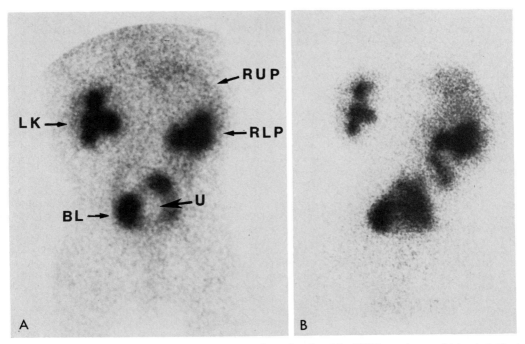

Figure 4–8 □ Ectopic ureterocele. The posterior images of a technetium 99m DTPA renal scan obtained at 10 minutes *(A)* and 30 minutes *(B)* after injection demonstrate duplication of the right renal collecting systems. The upper pole is hydronephrotic and shows delayed and decreased function. The collecting system of the lower pole of the right kidney is tilted. There is a filling defect in the bladder. This constellation is characteristic of ectopic ureterocele. The left kidney is normal. LK, left kidney; RUP, right upper pole; RLP, right lower pole; BL, bladder; U, ureterocele.

The renal scan is frequently useful to confirm renal duplication suspected on excretory urogram or sonogram or even to diagnose unsuspected cases. The function of each moiety of a duplicated kidney relative to the other and to the opposite kidney can be assessed. This may be important in deciding whether there is enough function to salvage the hydronephrotic, poorly functioning moiety (Fig. 4–8). Occasionally, a dysgenetic, nonfunctioning whole kidney or one moiety of a duplicated kidney is visualized on renal scan by reflux of the tracer from the bladder into the corresponding ureter and pelvicalyceal system (Fig. 4–9).

The multicystic dysplastic kidney and hydronephrosis caused by congenital ureteropelvic junction (UPJ) obstruction are the two most common flank masses in the neonatal period. The multicystic dysplastic kidney is caused by atresia of the ureter, renal pelvis, or both during the metanephric stage of renal development and is probably the end of the spectrum of ureteral obstruction (Felson and Cussen; Griscom et al). The continuing function of a few glomeruli and tubules creates hydronephrosis proximal to the obstruction. The altered excretory function inhibits cellular development, and the kidney becomes dysplastic. Depending on the number of functioning glomeruli remaining, the kidney may show minimal or no function. On the other hand, a kidney with congenital UPJ obstruction without dysplasia of the renal parenchyma usually retains significant function, unless prolonged obstruction has existed or infection has supervened. Therefore, management is dictated by the presence or absence of functioning renal tissue.

Sonography is the ideal initial imaging procedure in the evaluation of neonatal abdominal masses. It shows whether the mass is of renal or extrarenal origin and establishes the tissue character of the mass (solid, cystic, mixed). The next step should be renal scintigraphy to evaluate renal function. Both multicystic kidney and severe hydronephrosis appear as an avascular mass on the angiographic phase of the examination. The functional images in multicystic kidney show either no evidence of functioning renal tissue or only very minimal function on the delayed images (Fig. 4–10). On the other hand, the salvageable hydronephrotic kidney demonstrates a cap of function-

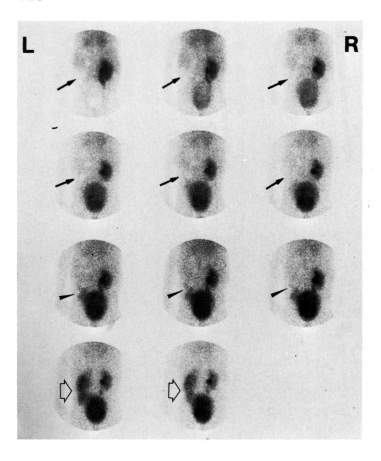

Figure 4–9 □ Dysgenetic nonfunctioning left kidney. Sequential 2-minute posterior images obtained from 2 to 14 minutes after injection of technetium 99m DTPA demonstrate a photon-deficient area in the left flank *(arrows)*. The 14- to 20-minute images show appearance of the tracer in the distal left ureter *(arrowheads)*. The 20- to 24-minute images show retrograde filling of a dilated left pelvicalyceal system and ureter *(open arrows)*. The left kidney is nonfunctioning, and the sudden appearance of the tracer in the left ureter on the delayed images is due to reflux. The right kidney is normal.

ing cortex of varying thickness at the periphery on the early static images while the delayed images show significant accumulation of the tracer in the dilated pelvicalyceal system (Fig. 4–11).

Hydronephrosis

Patients with hydronephrosis or hydroureteronephrosis may present with urinary tract infection (UTI) or an abdominal mass. With the increasing use of antenatal sonography, however, renal anomalies, including hydronephrosis, are being diagnosed much earlier and with greater frequency. Assessment of renal function and differentiation between obstructive and nonobstructive hydronephrosis are essential in the management of these patients. The diagnostic procedures used in the evaluation of hydronephrosis include cystography, excretory urography with or without diuretic enhancement, retrograde pyelography, renal scanning and renography with or without diuretic enhancement, renal parenchymal transit time, and pressure perfusion studies (the *Whitaker test*).

Vesicoureteral reflux as the cause of hydronephrosis is readily diagnosed by radiographic or radionuclide cystography. It should be noted, however, that reflux and obstruction may coexist (Lebowitz and Blickman). The conventional excretory urogram is occasionally diagnostic of obstruction but frequently does not differentiate between obstructive and nonobstructive hydronephrosis. A retrograde pyelogram may define the site of the change in ureteral caliber but does not provide any functional information. The conventional renal scan and renogram demonstrate the presence, extent, and severity of hydronephrosis and allow quantitative assessment of residual renal function. They do not, however, differentiate obstructive from nonobstructive hydronephrosis.

The pressure perfusion study (the Whitaker test) is based on the hypothesis that the dilated upper urinary tract can transport 10 ml/minute without an inordinate increase in pressure. The hydrostatic pressure in the system is then within physiologically normal levels and should not cause deterioration of renal function, and the degree of obstruction, if any, is insignifi-

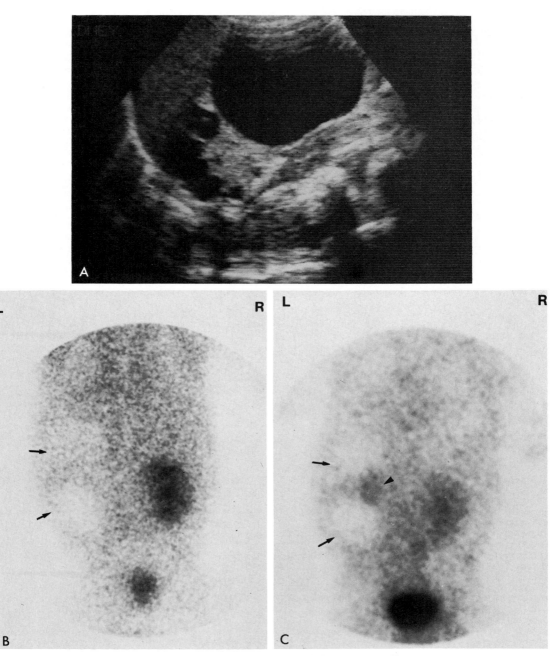

Figure 4–10 □ Multicystic dysplastic kidney in a newborn with a left flank mass. *A*, The renal sonogram demonstrates cystic lesions in the left kidney. *B*, The early image of a renal scan obtained at 4 minutes after injection of technetium 99m DTPA shows photon-deficient areas in the left flank *(arrows)* with no renal function on that side. *C*, The 3-hour delayed image shows persistence of the photon-deficient areas *(arrows)* and accumulation of a small amount of the tracer in the medial portion of the region between the photon-deficient areas *(arrowhead)*.

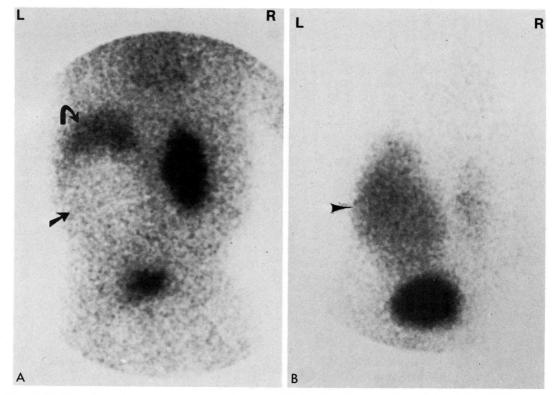

Figure 4–11 □ Hydronephrosis due to congenital ureteropelvic junction obstruction in a newborn with a left flank mass. *A,* The early image of the renal scan obtained at 10 minutes after injection of technetium 99m DTPA demonstrates a large photon-deficient area in the left flank *(straight arrow)* with a cap of renal tissue *(curved arrow). B,* The delayed 60-minute image shows filling of the photon-deficient area, which represents a massively dilated pelvicalyceal system *(arrowhead).*

cant. The Whitaker test is generally accepted as the standard for distinguishing obstructive from nonobstructive hydronephrosis. Its invasive nature, however, makes it undesirable for screening purposes and particularly for serial assessments. Furthermore, it does not provide any information about the renal function.

Diuretic excretory urography is based on the principle that, in the presence of significant obstruction, the urinary tract is unable to transport fluid over the physiologic range of flow rate and diuresis produces significant increase in the dimensions of the pelvicalyceal system. A 20 to 22 per cent increase in the area of the pelvicalyceal system after furosemide-induced diuresis has been reported to indicate significant obstruction (Nilson et al; Whitfield et al, 1977). Quantification by planimetry of the changes in the size of the pelvicalyceal system, however, is imprecise, and the test is not reliable. The following modifications of radionuclide renography offer more objective means of differentiating obstructed from nonobstructed dilatation.

Diuretic-Augmented Radionuclide Renography

This provocative test is based on the hypothesis that the prolonged retention of the tracer in the nonobstructed, dilated upper urinary tract is due to a reservoir effect and that increased urine flow following diuretic administration should result in prompt washout of the tracer, whereas in obstructive hydronephrosis there should not be any significant washout. The techniques and analytical methods used by different investigators vary widely. Diuretic renography is dependent upon several physiologic, mechanical, and technical factors. Understanding of the principles of the test, its limitations, and the sources of error is essential in the interpretation of the results and effective use of the test.

Factors Affecting the Renogram. The factors that affect the rate of the washout of the tracer and the shape of the renogram curve include the following.

Variable Degrees of Obstruction. Practically

all cases of obstruction are partial with varying degrees of severity. It is often difficult to predict what degree of obstruction will lead to deterioration of renal function. Some cases of obstruction are intermittent. Furthermore, the obstructive process, particularly in a young infant, may be progressive. Therefore, definition of significant obstruction remains imprecise.

Variable Impairment of Renal Function. The rate of accumulation of radionuclide in the dilated collecting system, as well as the response to diuretic, are dependent upon renal function. Therefore, in the presence of poor renal function the test is unreliable. Unfortunately, the level of renal function below which the diuretic renogram becomes unreliable is not clearly defined. Our experience suggests that when the collecting system does not completely fill within 1 hour after injection of the tracer, or if the affected kidney has less than 20 per cent of the total renal function, a prolonged washout may not be absolutely indicative of obstruction.

Capacity and Compliance of the Dilated System. In the presence of massive hydroureteronephrosis, even a very good response to furosemide may have little effect on the washout of tracer from the huge pool of retained tracer and may cause false-positive results. Distensibility or compliance of the dilated collecting system also plays a role.

State of Hydration. Adequate hydration is essential for diuresis. In addition to prescribing oral intake of fluid before the test, we routinely hydrate the patient with intravenous infusion of 5 per cent dextrose in one-third normal saline. This improves excretion of the tracer, enhances the response to furosemide, and prevents dehydration.

Fullness of the Bladder. Increased intravesical pressure associated with a full bladder may significantly affect the drainage from the upper urinary tract. We routinely insert an indwelling catheter for continuous drainage of urine from the bladder. This has the following advantages:

1. It eliminates the effect of a full bladder on the washout.
2. It allows measurement of the urine output at any chosen interval before and after injection of furosemide.
3. It eliminates the discomfort of a full bladder, which can cause the patient to move during acquisition of computer data.
4. It decreases radiation dose to the gonads by rapidly draining the radioactive urine.

5. It eliminates the effect of vesicoureteral reflux should reflux exist.

Dose of Diuretic. The response to furosemide is dose-dependent. We have found a dose of 1 mg/kg (maximum 40 mg) to be very effective and safe.

Time of Diuretic Injection. Some have advocated injection of the diuretic shortly (2 to 3 minutes) after injection of the tracer (Sfakianakis, 1988). This may not adversely affect the washout curves of the mildly dilated nonobstructed systems, but more severely dilated systems will probably remain incompletely filled during the acquisition of the computer data and the washout will appear falsely prolonged. Others have advocated injection of furosemide 15 minutes before injection of the tracer (English et al, 1987). This is based on the assumption that the peak effect of furosemide is at about 30 minutes after injection. In our experience, based on routine measurement of urine output at 10-minute intervals in more than 1000 patients, maximum diuresis usually occurs within a few minutes after injection of furosemide in the hydrated child. Therefore, it seems logical to administer furosemide after most of the injected tracer has cleared from the blood, at which time concentration of the tracer in the retained urine is at its maximum and in the incoming urine at its minimum. In well-hydrated patients with normal renal function, this occurs at about 20 to 30 minutes after injection of the tracer.

Patient Position. Washout of the retained tracer is occasionally affected by the position of the patient. The easiest and most practical position for immobilization and observation of the patient and for performance of diuretic renography in the pediatric age group is supine, with the camera positioned underneath the patient. We routinely perform the test using the supine position. However, if drainage is markedly delayed during the first 30 minutes after diuretic injection, the patient is placed in the prone position and additional images are obtained for 10 to 15 minutes. Markedly improved drainage with the patient in the prone position makes high-grade obstruction less likely and is usually associated with preservation of renal function.

Radiopharmaceutical. The ideal radiopharmaceutical for diuretic renography should have rapid blood clearance, a short physical half-life, and radiation characteristics suitable for imaging, and it should be readily available. At present, technetium 99m MAG 3 is clearly the radiopharmaceutical of choice for diuretic renography.

Region of Interest. Appropriate regions of interest should be chosen for generation of the curves. The changes in the amount of tracer in a portion of a dilated system may not be representative of the drainage from the entire system. In the presence of both pelvic and ureteral dilatation, the ureter can function as a reservoir for the tracer drained from the renal pelvis. Therefore, the region of interest should include the entire dilated collecting system.

Technique of Diuretic Renography. It is desirable to adopt a standard technique that eliminates or reduces the effect of as many of the aforementioned variables as possible. The following technique has evolved at our institution and has been used effectively since 1978.

The patient is positioned supine on the scanning table with the gamma camera underneath. A venous line is established, and an indwelling bladder catheter is inserted. The patient is hydrated by intravenous administration of 5 per cent dextrose in one-third normal saline during the test (total 15 ml/kg, starting before the injection of the tracer). A conventional renal scan using either technetium 99m DTPA (100 μCi/kg, minimum 1 mCi) or, more recently, technetium 99m MAG 3 (50 μCi/kg, minimum 500 μCi) is obtained. Accumulation of the tracer is continuously monitored, and when the dilated system is entirely filled with tracer, furosemide is injected intravenously in a dose of 1 mg/kg, up to 40 mg. Digital images are stored on a computer at the rate of four frames per minute from the time of injection of the tracer until 30 minutes after injection of furosemide. Simultaneously, sequential 1- to 2-minute images are obtained on the film. Urine output is measured during the period before injection of furosemide and afterward at 10-minute intervals. The computer data are then processed for generation of the renogram curve and calculation of the clearance half-time of the tracer from the dilated upper urinary tract (Fig. 4–12).

Analysis and Interpretation of Diuretic Renography. There are basically two methods for analyzing a diuretic renogram curve: (1) pattern recognition, and (2) quantitative analysis.

The *pattern recognition* method is based on the subjective analysis of the shape of the curve (O'Reily et al; Thrall et al). There is a spectrum of responses ranging from a very rapid drainage to no drainage at all (Fig. 4–13). Characteristic patterns are seen at the ends of the spectrum for nonobstructed hydro-

nephrosis and for high-grade obstruction that are easily recognizable. However, many curves demonstrate an intermediate response, which may indicate mild to moderate obstruction. Determination of the significance of obstruction, if any, based on the subjective interpretation of the shape of the intermediate curves is often impossible.

Quantitative analysis methods based on the washout half-time or some other measures of the washout rate help to reduce subjectivity in the interpretation of the curve and decrease the number of indeterminate results. This is particularly helpful when serial examinations are compared. Based on our extensive clinical experience, including surgical findings, comparative studies with Whitaker test, and long-term follow-up studies, we believe that a drainage half-time of ≥20 minutes is almost always associated with high-grade obstruction whereas a washout half-time of ≤10 minutes usually denotes no significant obstruction. The washout half-time of 10 to 20 minutes, particularly on a single study, is considered indeterminate and warrants close observation and a follow-up study. It should be remembered that in addition to the washout half-time, the shape of the curve should also be considered in the analysis of the diuretic renogram. The curve may show an initial rapid drop with a short calculated washout half-time, but instead of continuing to drop exponentially to a low level of residual activity, it may plateau at a high level of activity or it may even rise. These biphasic curves are almost always due to flow-dependent obstruction (Fig. 4–13F, G).

Improvement in the washout of the tracer after pyeloplasty varies greatly. In some, the half-time returns to the nonobstructed range in a short period of time (Fig. 4–14); in others, this may take significantly longer. In many instances, the washout half-time remains in the obstructed or equivocal range for at least 6 months. If function remains stable in that interval, there is no need for concern.

In summary, diuretic-augmented radionuclide renography appears to be a safe and valuable tool for the evaluation and management of hydronephrosis in infants and children. Its effectiveness is dependent upon the technique of the examination, meticulous analysis of the results, and recognition of its pitfalls and limitations.

Renal Parenchymal Transit Time

Parenchymal transit time of technetium 99m DTPA, based on deconvolution analysis of the

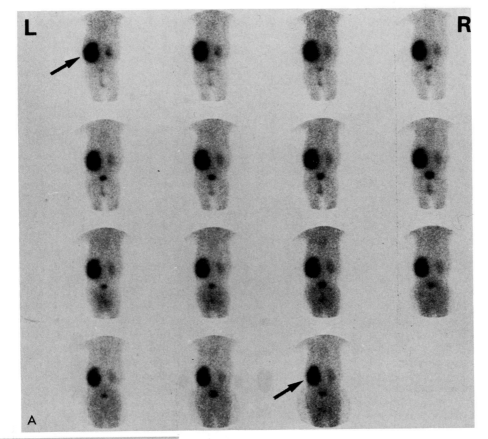

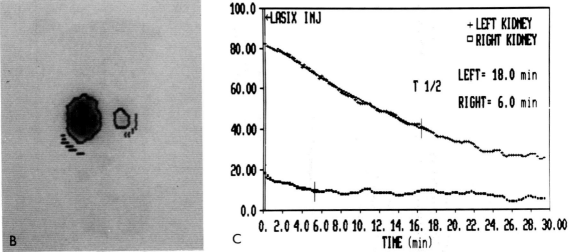

Figure 4–12 □ Diuretic-augmented renal scan and renogram in a child with left ureteropelvic junction obstruction. *A,* Sequential 2 minute images obtained after injection of furosemide show marked retention of the tracer in the dilated left pelvicalyceal system *(arrow).* The tracer from the normal right pelvicalyceal system washes out rapidly. For quantitative analysis of washout of the tracer, regions of interest for the pelvicalyceal systems and the corresponding backgrounds are selected *(B)* and the renogram curves are generated *(C).* The washout half-time is 18 minutes on the left and 6 minutes on the right. The relative flatness of the lower curve in *C* is due to the rapid washout from the nonobstructed right side of the tracer before the diuretic was injected.

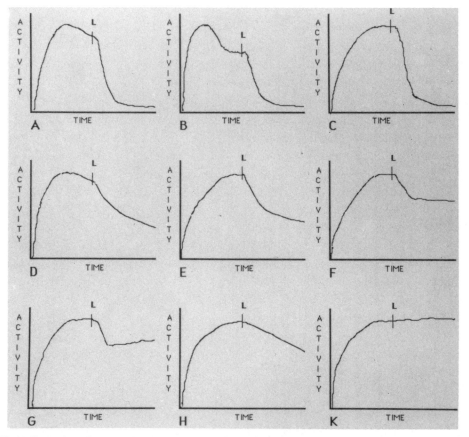

Figure 4–13 □ Examples of time-activity curves of hydronephrotic kidneys with diuretic injection (L) at the midpoint of a 60-minute acquisition. Patterns A, B, and C are seen with nonobstructed systems. Patterns F, G, H, and K indicate significant obstruction, patterns F and G being examples of a flow-dependent obstruction. Patterns D and E are equivocal.

cortical renogram curve, has been advocated as a sensitive indicator of obstructive nephropathy (Diffey et al; Nawaz et al; Whitfield et al, 1978, 1981). This test is based on the principle that, in the presence of renal outflow obstruction, the intratubular pressure is increased and reabsorption of salt and water is enhanced. The reabsorption of fluid from the tubular lumen leads to prolongation of the parenchymal transit time of nonreabsorbable tracers. Regions of interest are flagged over both the renal pelvis and the entire kidney, and time-activity curves are generated. The renal parenchymal time-activity curve is then derived by subtracting the pelvic curve from the whole kidney curve. Using the renal input function obtained by monitoring the cardiac blood pool activity, deconvolution analysis provides whole kidney and parenchymal curves corresponding to a theoretical instantaneous injection of the tracer into the renal artery.

Although deconvolution analysis appears promising, it is technically complex and there is some doubt about its efficacy in children (Piepsz et al, 1982).

Urinary Tract Infections

Urinary tract infection may be limited to the bladder (cystitis) or upper collecting systems (ureteritis, pyelitis), or it may involve the renal parenchyma (pyelonephritis). Acute pyelonephritis is a major cause of morbidity in children with UTI and can result in irreversible renal scarring. Well-recognized late sequelae of pyelonephritic scarring include hypertension and chronic renal failure. Clinical and experimental studies have demonstrated that renal scarring can be prevented or diminished by early diagnosis and aggressive treatment of acute pyelonephritis (Glauser et al, 1978; Ransley and Risdon, 1981; Winberg et al). Therefore, ac-

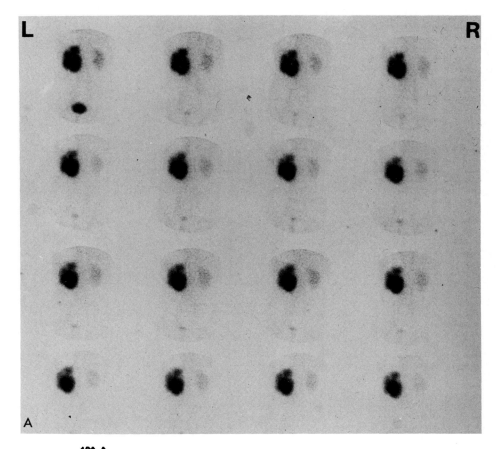

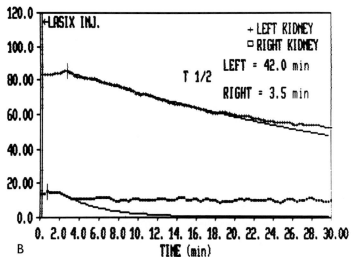

Figure 4–14 □ Diuretic-augmented renal scans and renograms in a patient with left ureteropelvic junction obstruction before and after pyeloplasty. The initial study demonstrates poor drainage from a markedly dilated left pelvicalyceal system *(A)* with a washout half-time of 42 minutes *(B)*.

Illustration continued on following page

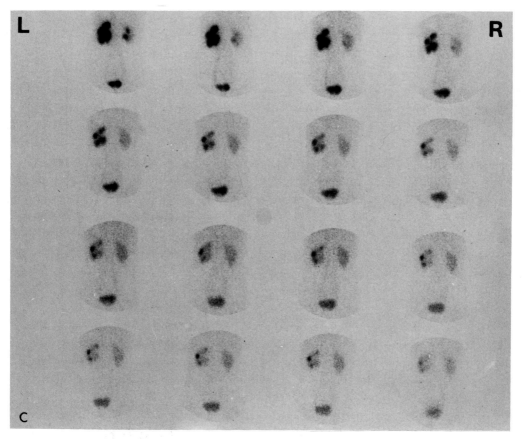

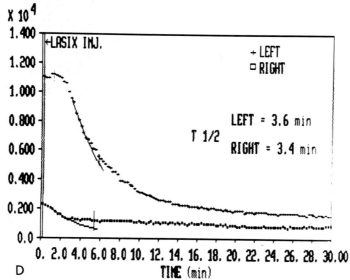

Figure 4–14 ☐ *Continued* The follow-up study 3 months after pyeloplasty *(C)* demonstrates residual mild dilatation of the left pelvicalyceal system and improved drainage with a washout half-time of 3.6 minutes *(D)*. In both *B* and *D*, the upper curve depicts the left kidney.

curate diagnosis of pyelonephritis has significant clinical relevance.

Acute pyelonephritis in adults is usually diagnosed on the basis of clinical signs and symptoms. In infants and children, however, differentiation of acute pyelonephritis from lower UTI based on clinical and laboratory findings is often difficult and the use of diagnostic imaging becomes necessary. Intravenous urography (IVP) has a very low sensitivity for the diagnosis of pyelonephritis (Silver et al). Computed tomography (CT) is probably a sensitive and effective technique, but its routine use in the evaluation of children with UTI is not practical (June et al; Montgomery et al). The role of magnetic resonance imaging (MRI) in the diagnosis of acute pyelonephritis is not clear (Raynaud et al). Radionuclide imaging procedures using gallium 67 citrate or indium 111–labeled leukocytes may be very reliable in the diagnosis of acute pyelonephritis (Fawcett et al; Mendez et al). These imaging procedures, however, result in high-radiation absorbed doses, require 24 to 48 hours to perform, and, more importantly, do not provide any information about the function or morphology of the kidneys. Renal sonography is useful in detection of renal or perirenal abscesses but is of little value in confirming acute pyelonephritis (Bjorgvinsson et al).

Clinical studies have shown renal cortical scintigraphy using technetium 99m–labeled DMSA or glucoheptonate to be significantly more sensitive than IVP and renal sonography in the detection of acute pyelonephritis (Handmaker, 1982; Traisman et al; Sty et al). Technetium 99m DMSA renal cortical scintigraphy has also been evaluated in experimentally induced acute pyelonephritis in piglets. In the study from our laboratory, unilateral vesicoureteral reflux of infected urine was surgically induced in 22 piglets. DMSA scans were obtained at 1 week (in nine piglets) or 2 weeks (13 piglets) after the introduction of bacteria into the bladder. Subsequently, the piglets were killed and the kidneys were examined for histopathologic evidence of acute pyelonephritis. The location and extent of pyelonephritic lesions found on histopathologic examination were compared with DMSA scan findings in a blinded fashion. Of the 22 kidneys subjected to vesicoureteral reflux of infected urine, 15 had histopathologic evidence of acute pyelonephritis. DMSA scans showed scintigraphic evidence of acute pyelonephritis in 13 of 15 kidneys (sensitivity = 87 per cent). The two

kidneys in which inflammation was not detected on the scans showed only minimal microscopic foci of inflammatory cells and were grossly normal. There were no false-positive scans in any of the 22 experimental kidneys (specificity = 100 per cent). There was an overall 94 per cent agreement between the DMSA scan and histopathologic findings for the detection of individual lesions (Rushton et al, 1988). Others have reported similar results (Parkhouse et al). Therefore, DMSA renal cortical scintigraphy is a highly sensitive and reliable technique for the detection and localization of acute pyelonephritis.

Renal cortical imaging has also proved to be more accurate than excretory urography in detection of pyelonephritic scarring. Merrick et al (1980) compared renal cortical imaging and excretory urography in 79 children with proven urinary tract infection followed for a period of 1 to 4 years. Both techniques were in agreement as to the presence or absence of scarring as well as to the extent of abnormality in 93.5 per cent of the kidneys studied. There was, however, discrepancy in ten kidneys. Excretory urography had a sensitivity of 86 per cent and a specificity of 92 per cent in the detection of pyelonephritic scarring, whereas renal cortical imaging had a sensitivity of 96 per cent and a specificity of 98 per cent.

The scintigraphic pattern of acute pyelonephritis is one of decreased cortical uptake of the tracer without any volume loss. This can be focal, multifocal, or diffuse (Fig. 4–15). Cortical scars are usually associated with loss of volume and present as a wedge-shaped defect or thinning and flattening of the cortex (Fig. 4–16) (Majd et al, 1991). Cortical imaging also offers the quantitative evaluation of relative renal function and a noninvasive method of assessing response to treatment.

The pathophysiologic mechanisms that account for the decreased uptake of DMSA in acute pyelonephritis are probably multifactorial. Cortical uptake of DMSA is determined primarily by intrarenal blood flow and proximal tubular cell membrane transport function. Any pathologic process that alters either or both of these parameters may result in focal or diffuse areas of decreased uptake. In an experimental study using sodium chromate (Cr 51) microspheres in the piglet model, we found that focal ischemia does occur in acute pyelonephritis and in some lesions the decrease in uptake of DMSA is proportional to focal de-

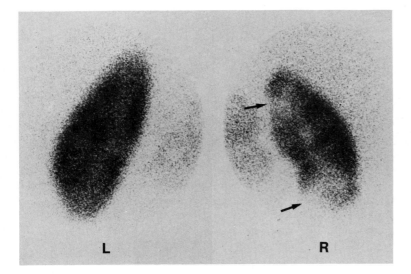

Figure 4–15 □ Acute pyelonephritis. The magnified posterior oblique views of the kidneys obtained 3 hours after injection of technetium 99m DMSA using a pinhole collimator demonstrate defects in the uptake of the tracer in the lower pole and the medial aspect of the upper pole of the right kidney *(arrows)*. The left kidney is normal.

creased blood flow; in other lesions, DMSA uptake is more severely decreased than focal blood flow. This suggests that focal ischemia is an early event that precedes tubular damage (Majd et al, 1990). Therefore, the DMSA scan may become positive in a very early stage of parenchymal inflammatory response to the invasion by bacteria. It is reasonable to assume that adequate treatment of acute pyelonephritis in this very early stage results in complete resolution without progression to scar formation.

Technetium 99m DMSA is an excellent renal cortical agent. About 60 per cent of the administered dose is tightly bound to the proximal tubular cells, and only a small amount is slowly excreted in the urine. DMSA allows visualization of renal parenchyma without in-

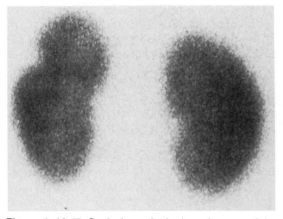

Figure 4–16 □ Cortical scar in the lateral aspect of the upper pole of the left kidney

terference from retained tracer in the collecting systems.

Concerns regarding higher radiation absorbed dose with DMSA have been expressed. It is true that radiation to the cortex of the kidneys per millicurie administered dose is about three times higher with DMSA as compared with glucoheptonate, but this is due to cortical fixation of a larger fraction of DMSA. Therefore, the administered dose of DMSA can be one third that of glucoheptonate. With this adjustment in the administered dose, total DMSA retained in the kidney and resultant renal radiation doses are equal to those of glucoheptonate; however, owing to the accumulation of a lesser amount of DMSA in the bladder, the gonadal radiation dose is significantly less. Therefore, DMSA is a preferred renal cortical imaging agent, particularly in infants.

Technetium 99m glucoheptonate is cleared by both glomerular filtration and cortical fixation. About 20 per cent of the administered dose is firmly bound to the tubular cells. Therefore, delayed imaging provides visualization of the cortex similar to DMSA images. Most of the administered dose is excreted in the urine, allowing moderately good visualization of the renal collecting systems. This additional information provided by glucoheptonate makes it the agent preferred by some. However, the status of the collecting systems is best evaluated on the renal sonogram, which is usually obtained in conjunction with the renal scan. There is often some hepatobiliary excretion of glucoheptonate, particularly in infants. Tracer in the gallbladder or small bowel may super-impose on the right kidney.

Trauma

Renal injuries are often due to blunt abdominal trauma or, less commonly, to penetration. Iatrogenic injuries may also occur as a result of surgical intervention, renal biopsy, retrograde pyelography, or interventional radiographic procedures. Diagnostic imaging procedures used in the evaluation of renal trauma include excretory urography with or without nephrotomography, sonography, CT, radionuclide studies, and arteriography. The position of these imaging modalities in the diagnostic algorithm depends on the patient's condition and associated injuries as well as the availability of equipment and expertise.

Excretory urography, the most readily available procedure, is sensitive in the detection of renal pedicle injuries but underestimates minor renal injuries. It has a low sensitivity for the detection of urinary leakage and does not provide information about injury to the other organs.

Renal sonography is useful in the detection of subcapsular and perirenal hematomas, lacerations, blood clots in the renal pelvis, and urinary tract obstruction. The use of Doppler studies allows evaluation of the renal blood flow. Renal sonography, however, does not provide any information about renal function, which may be a critical factor in the acute management of the patient. Nonvisualization of a kidney on an excretory urogram or renal scan may be due to renal agenesis, and unless a renal silhouette is observed on the plain abdominal radiograph, ultrasonography may be required to differentiate renal pedicle injury from renal agenesis.

Computed tomography of the abdomen with intravenous contrast enhancement provides superior anatomic detail, which allows accurate evaluation of the extent of renal trauma as well as simultaneous evaluation of other organs, the peritoneal cavity, and the retroperitoneum. It may be regarded as the single most informative imaging procedure in the evaluation of abdominal trauma. In a restless, injured child, however, motion artifacts may result in poor image quality.

Angiography is the best method for demonstrating vascular injury directly and also offers an opportunity to control active hemorrhage by selective arterial embolization

(Chuang et al). It is, however, invasive and not suitable for screening or serial evaluation. The role of digital subtraction angiography (DSA) is yet to be defined.

Radionuclide renal imaging provides information about overall and regional perfusion and function of the kidneys. It is extremely sensitive in detecting renal pedicle injuries (Fig. 4–17), segmental infarctions, contusions (Fig. 4–18), lacerations, and urine extravasation (Fig. 4–19). Pre-existing congenital anomalies, such as fusion, ectopia, and hydronephrosis, which make the kidneys more susceptible to trauma, are easily detected. Radionuclide renal studies, in conjunction with ultrasound scanning, are particularly useful in follow-up assessments of healing of traumatic injuries to the urinary tract and detection of secondary complications. The radiopharmaceutical of choice for the evaluation of renal trauma is technetium 99m glucoheptonate.

Renal Vascular Abnormalities

Renovascular Hypertension

Hypertension in children is often of renal origin. Therefore, radionuclide renal studies play an important role in the evaluation and management of hypertension in infants and children. Some of the renal causes of hypertension, such as infarction, post-pyelonephritic cortical scarring, and post-traumatic injuries, are easily diagnosed by conventional renal scanning. These methods, however, are less reliable in the diagnosis of renovascular hypertension. Renal artery stenosis is the cause of approximately 5 per cent of all cases of childhood hypertension (Hendren et al). The prevalence is considerably higher when the hypertension occurs in association with neurofibromatosis or aortic anomalies (Stanley and Frey). In half of all hypertensive children younger than 10 years of age, there is a vascular cause for the disease (Lawson).

Renal arteriography and renal vein renin measurements are needed for definitive diagnosis and management of the renal vascular causes of hypertension. Renal arteriography, however, is an invasive procedure and is not suitable for screening. The role of less invasive DSA for this purpose has yet to be defined. The so-called hypertensive excretory urogram is not sensitive enough to be used as a screening procedure. Lawson et al, reporting on a group of 107 hypertensive children, found ab-

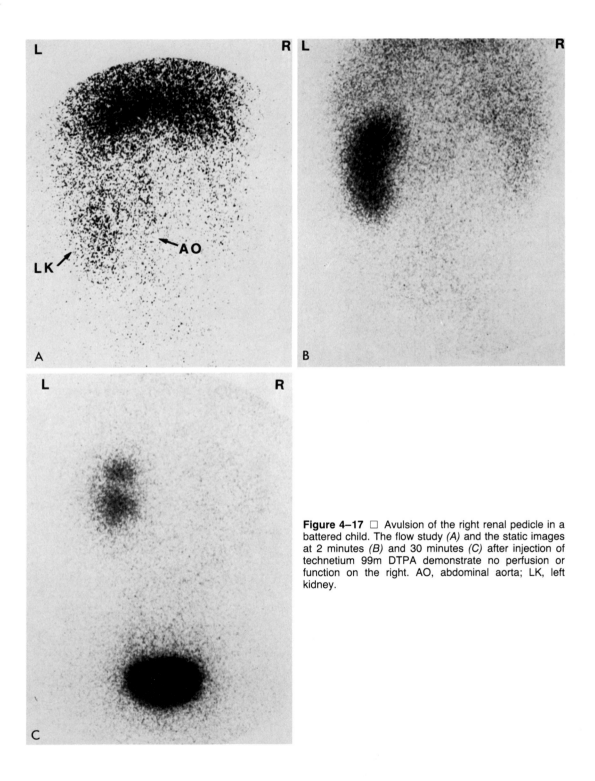

Figure 4–17 □ Avulsion of the right renal pedicle in a battered child. The flow study *(A)* and the static images at 2 minutes *(B)* and 30 minutes *(C)* after injection of technetium 99m DTPA demonstrate no perfusion or function on the right. AO, abdominal aorta; LK, left kidney.

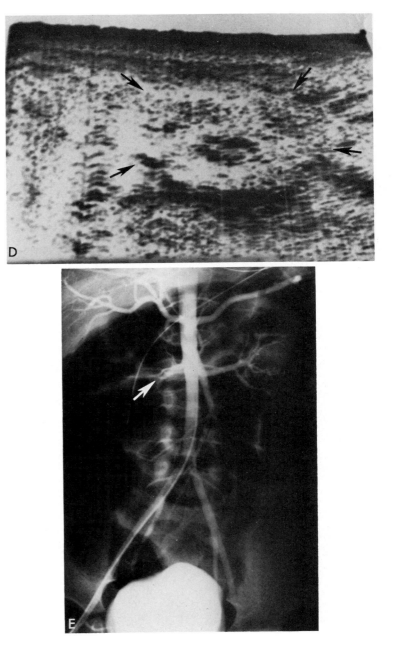

Figure 4–17 □ *Continued D*, The renal sonogram shows presence of the right kidney in its normal location *(arrows). E,* The abdominal aortogram demonstrates abrupt cut-off of the right renal artery *(arrow).* At surgery avulsion of the right renal pedicle was found and the nonviable kidney was removed.

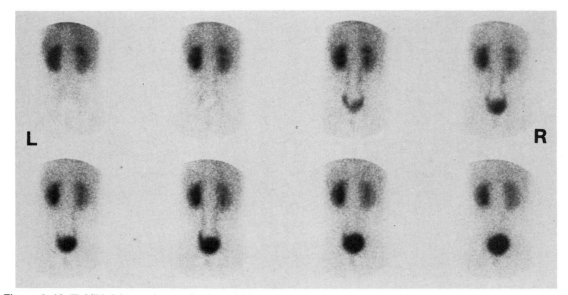

Figure 4–18 □ Mild right renal contusion in a child who presented with hematuria after trauma to the right flank. The posterior images obtained 2 to 30 minutes after injection of technetium 99m DTPA demonstrate minimal decrease in the right renal function with no evidence of laceration or extravasation.

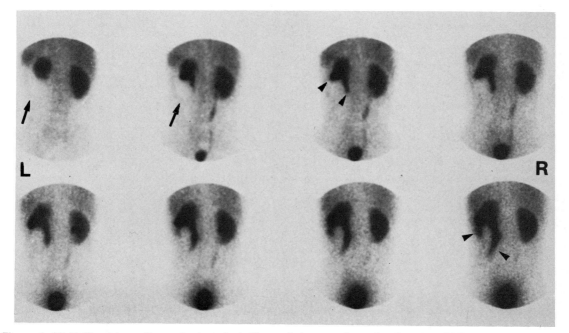

Figure 4–19 □ Renal laceration and urinary leak. The early images of a technetium 99m DTPA renal scan show a photon-deficient region below the functioning upper pole of the left kidney *(arrows)*. This area is occupied by the nonfunctioning lacerated lower pole of the kidney and surrounding fluid collection. The subsequent images show gradual accumulation of the tracer in this area and along the left paravertebral region as a result of urinary leak *(arrowheads)*.

normalities with rapid-sequence excretory urography in all patients with renal parenchymal disease but in only nine of 21 children (42 per cent) with renovascular disease. Stanley et al (1978) found abnormalities with rapid-sequence excretory urography in 11 of 17 children (65 per cent) with unilateral renovascular disease.

Conventional radionuclide imaging and renography in the presence of unilateral renal artery stenosis may show evidence of decreased renal perfusion and function on the affected side. In the presence of hypertension, however, the kidney with a stenotic artery may remain adequately perfused and, owing to the autoregulation mechanism, the renal scan and renogram may remain normal. Arlat et al, reporting on a group of 105 patients with angiographically proven unilateral renal artery stenosis and 45 patients with essential hypertension, found 18 per cent false-negative and 13 per cent false-positive renal scans for renal artery stenosis. The percentages for Hippuran renography were 17 and 26 per cent, respectively. Radionuclide studies are even less efficacious in the diagnosis of bilateral or segmental renal artery stenosis.

Captopril-Enhanced Scintigraphy

In 1982 we observed that captopril therapy in hypertensive children with renal artery stenosis caused dramatic but reversible deterioration of renal function that was easily detectable on renal scan. We proposed the use of captopril as a provocative test to increase the efficacy of renal scanning in the detection of renal artery stenosis (Majd et al, 1983). Subsequently, extensive experimental and clinical studies substantiated the usefulness of this pharmacologic intervention in the diagnosis of renovascular hypertension (Dondi et al; Hovinga et al; Sfakianakis et al, 1987).

In the presence of renal artery stenosis, the intrarenal perfusion pressure is decreased and there is a tendency for GFR to fall. However, within a wide range of perfusion pressure GFR is maintained at normal levels by an autoregulation mechanism mediated by the renin-angiotensin system. A major factor in maintaining GFR is the transcapillary pressure gradient across the glomerulus related to the difference in resistance at the level of the afferent and efferent arterioles. This is regulated by angiotensin II–induced selective constriction of the efferent arteriole of the glomerulus. Captopril,

an angiotensin-converting enzyme inhibitor, blocks the formation of angiotensin II, producing dilatation of the efferent arterioles and a decrease in the transcapillary pressure gradient. This leads to a significant, but reversible, decrease in renal function.

The choice of radiopharmaceutical, angiotensin-converting enzyme (ACE) inhibitor, and technique of examination varies among institutions (Dondi et al; Hovinga et al; Sfakianakis et al, 1987). Either glomerular or tubular agents can be used. The original work in pediatric patients was done with the use of DTPA and captopril (Majd et al, 1983). Subsequent experience has shown this to be a reliable method. Currently, MAG 3, which has replaced OIH for clinical use, is being evaluated for captopril renography and appears to be promising, particularly in cases of segmental renal artery stenosis. Either captopril or enalaprilat can be used as the choice of ACE inhibitor. Their mechanisms of action are similar, but the advantage of enalaprilat is that it is administered intravenously and, unlike oral captopril, its effect is not dependent on variable rate of absorption through the gastrointestinal tract. We routinely obtain a baseline renal scan, followed by a second study either 1 hour after oral administration of captopril or 10 minutes after intravenous administration of enalaprilat.

The scintigraphic manifestation of decreased renal function after administration of the ACE inhibitor depends on which radiopharmaceutical is used. With DTPA, there is decreased extraction and delayed appearance of the tracer in the collecting systems (Fig. 4–20); with MAG 3, there is prolonged parenchymal retention of the tracer.

Other Vascular Abnormalities

Other vascular abnormalities of the kidney, such as thrombosis of the main or segmental renal veins or arteries, can often be diagnosed on the radionuclide studies. Renal vein thrombosis occurs most often in neonates and is usually secondary to hemoconcentration. The renal scan generally shows both decreased perfusion and function in an enlarged kidney. Renal artery thrombosis in the neonate occurs most commonly as a complication of an indwelling aortic catheter. Renal artery thrombosis also causes decreased perfusion and function of the kidney but, unlike renal vein thrombosis, usually does not cause enlarge-

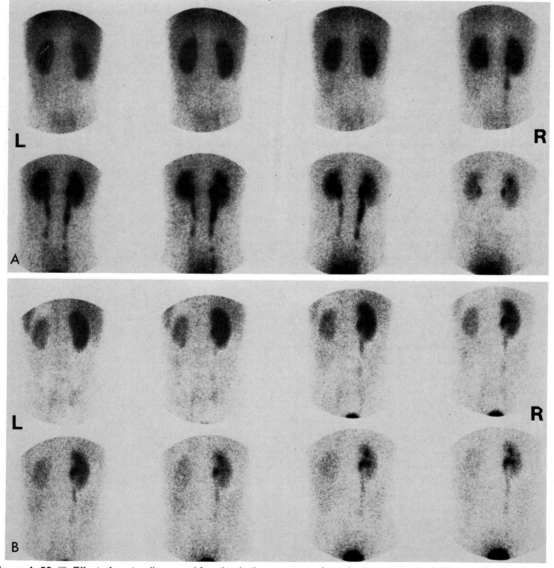

Figure 4–20 □ Effect of captopril on renal function in the presence of renal artery stenosis. *A,* The renal scan obtained as a part of the initial hypertensive workup was normal. *B,* The repeat study after 2 months of captopril therapy showed marked deterioration of the left renal function.

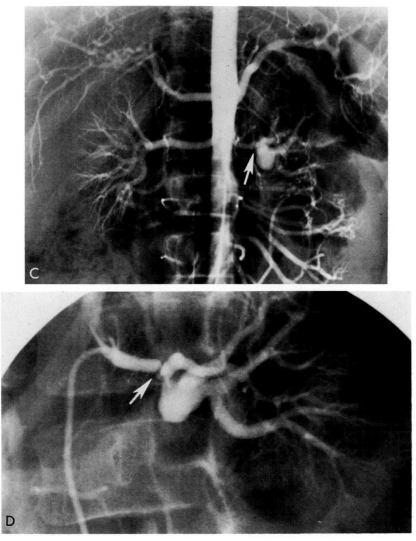

Figure 4–20 □ *Continued* Abdominal aortogram *(C)* and a selective left renal arteriogram *(D)* showed stenosis of the left renal artery *(arrow)* with poststenotic aneurysmal dilatation.

ment of the kidney. Scintigraphic findings of renal vascular occlusion are nonspecific and should be interpreted in the clinical context.

Renal Masses

Most renal masses are adequately localized and characterized by excretory urography, sonography, or CT. Radionuclide renal cortical imaging, however, may be of value in differentiating pseudotumors (such as prominent columns of Bertin [Fig. 4–21]), fetal lobulation, and dromedary humps from true pathology (such as tumor, infarct, or hemorrhage [Mazer and Quaife]).

The relative sensitivity of different diagnostic imaging modalities in early detection of

Wilms' tumor in children with aniridia or hemihypertrophy has not been defined. The combination of renal cortical imaging and sonography may be an effective approach to the periodic evaluation of these children during the risk period.

Renal Transplantation

Evaluation of Donor

Renal scanning (including total and separate GFR determination) is often used in the evaluation of the living-donor to ensure that he or she has two kidneys with normal function. This is usually followed by selective renal arteriography. When the use of the kidney from a

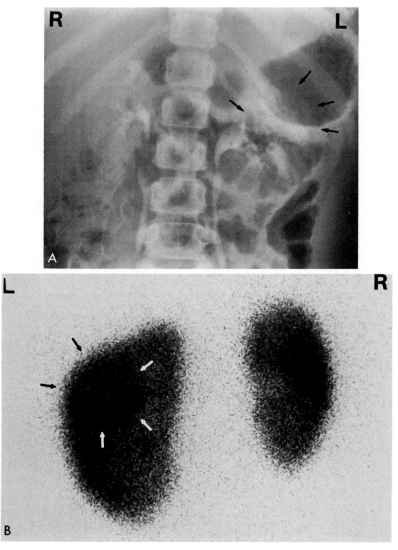

Figure 4–21 □ Column of Bertin. *A,* The excretory urogram shows a bump in the superior lateral aspect of the left kidney *(lateral arrows)* and an impression on the infundibulum of the upper calyx *(medial arrow)* suggestive of a space-occupying lesion. *B,* DMSA renal scan in posterior projection shows this area to be occupied by normal renal cortex *(arrows)*.

"brain-dead" patient is contemplated, a cerebral flow study may be performed as part of technetium 99m DTPA renal scan both to confirm brain death and to evaluate renal function.

Evaluation of the Transplanted Kidney

A variety of radionuclide studies have been used to evaluate perfusion and function of the transplanted kidney (George; Kirchner and Rosenthall). The most common procedure in children is technetium 99m DTPA renal scintigraphy, including evaluation of the first transit of tracer from the aorta and iliac artery to the transplanted kidney. The renal time-activity curve of the first transit is compared with that of the aorta or iliac artery. A normally perfused transplanted kidney shows a sharp rise and fall in the renal time-activity curve, which closely parallels the aortic curve (Fig. 4–22).

Complications

Possible complications following renal transplantation can be classified into two general categories: (1) those due to parenchymal failure, such as acute tubular necrosis (ATN),

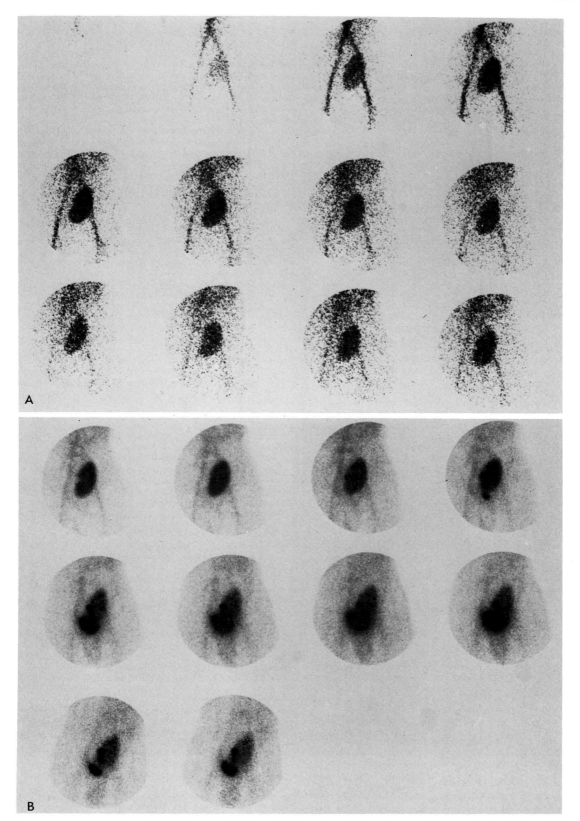

Figure 4–22 □ Renal transplant with normal function. *A,* The radionuclide angiogram shows prompt perfusion of the kidney. *B,* The static images from 2 to 35 minutes after injection of technetium 99m DTPA demonstrate prompt renal function and normal drainage.

Illustration continued on following page

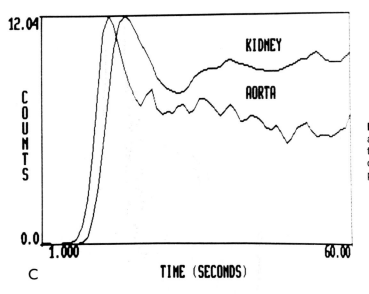

C

Figure 4–22 □ *Continued C,* The time-activity curves of first transit of the tracer through the kidney parallels that of the aorta, confirming normal blood flow to the transplant.

rejection, cyclosporine toxicity, and infection; and (2) those due to mechanical injuries, including complete or partial obstruction of blood vessels, ureteral obstruction, urinary leak, and lymphocele.

Certain complications occur at specific times after transplantation. Acute tubular necrosis secondary to ischemic damage prior to grafting is present in the majority of cadaveric transplants. It may rarely occur in a living related donor transplant as a result of technical problems at the time of surgery, severe hypotension, or reaction to radiographic contrast medium. Cyclosporine toxicity can occur at any time, but is less common during the first month of therapy. Hyperacute rejection occurs immediately or within the first 24 hours after transplantation. Acute rejection usually occurs 5 to 90 days after transplant. Chronic rejection is a slow process and is usually manifested months to years later.

Radionuclide studies are very useful in the diagnosis of acute renal vessel occlusion, poor parenchymal function, renal infarction, ureteral obstruction, and extravasation of urine. However, the scintigraphic patterns of parenchymal dysfunction are usually nonspecific and do not allow differentiation between ATN, rejection, and cyclosporine toxicity.

In ATN, renal function decreases whereas renal perfusion usually remains relatively normal (Fig. 4–23); in rejection, both perfusion and function decrease proportionally (Fig. 4–24). Differentiation of rejection from ATN on the basis of a single study, however, is often difficult, and serial studies over several days

or weeks may be necessary. A kidney injured by ATN generally displays its lowest level of perfusion and function by 24 to 48 hours after transplantation. Therefore, on serial examinations the perfusion and function should improve or remain unchanged. By contrast, deterioration of renal perfusion and function due to rejection, if untreated, is generally progressive.

It is important to obtain a baseline renal scan shortly after surgery, preferably within first 24 hours. The same protocol and technical parameters should be used in all follow-up examinations to facilitate comparison. The patient should be well hydrated and the bladder emptied before the examination.

Complete renal arterial or venous occlusion as well as hyperacute rejection results in nonperfusion of the transplant and cannot be differentiated by radionuclide angiography alone. The scintigraphic findings of a "photon-deficient" zone (renal activity distinctly less than surrounding background activity) indicates a nonsalvageable transplant (Fig. 4–25).

Hypertension may be due to stenosis of the vascular graft or vascular disease of the native kidney. Captopril-enhanced renal scintigraphy is helpful in the detection of renal artery stenosis.

Obstructive uropathy and urinary extravasation are readily detected on the renal scan, provided that renal function is adequate. A photon-deficient zone adjacent to the kidney on the early images may be due to urinary extravasation or lymphocele. In the case of urinary extravasation, delayed images demon-

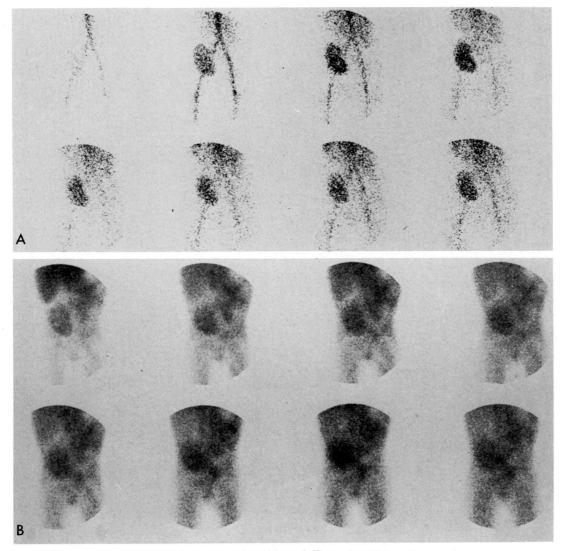

Figure 4–23 □ Acute tubular necrosis in a transplant kidney. *A,* The radionuclide angiogram shows normal blood flow to the kidney. *B,* The static images from 2 to 25 minutes after injection show decreased renal function.

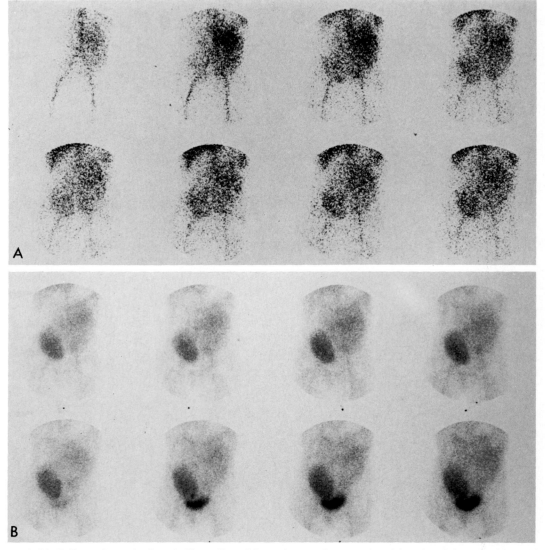

Figure 4–24 □ Transplant rejection. *A,* The radionuclide angiogram demonstrates delayed and decreased blood flow to the kidney. *B,* The static images from 2 to 35 minutes after injection show decreased renal function.

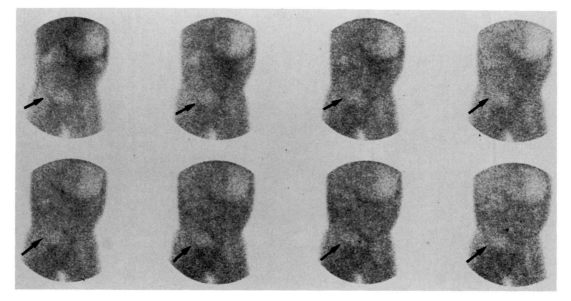

Figure 4–25 □ Nonsalvageable rejected transplant. Accumulation of the tracer in the region of the transplant *(arrows)* is less than in surrounding background.

strate accumulation of tracer in the area whereas a lymphocele remains photon-deficient. Sonography is complementary to scintigraphy in the detection of the urologic complications of renal transplantation.

RADIONUCLIDE CYSTOGRAPHY

The use of radionuclides for the detection of vesicoureteral reflux dates back to 1959, when Winter reported the appearance of radioactivity in the area of the kidneys after iodine 131 (iodopyracet [Diodrast]) or iodine 131 rose bengal had been instilled into the bladder. For these studies, scintillation probes were positioned over the kidneys. In 1964 Berne and Ekman reported the use of colloidal gold 198 for cystography and emphasized the advantage of its low radiation dose as compared with that of retrograde x-ray cystography. With the advent of the gamma camera and technetium 99m compounds, retrograde radionuclide cystography with isotope directly instilled in the bladder was modified by Corriere et al (1967, 1970) and by Blaufox et al and was popularized by Conway et al (1975). This technique is known as *direct radionuclide cystography*.

In 1963, Dodge reported his observation that a brisk rise in activity occurred in some patients with known reflux upon voiding at the end of a radionuclide renogram. This suggested a new technique for the detection of vesicoureteral reflux using intravenous injection of iodine 131 Hippuran and external scintillation counting over the renal area. This technique of *indirect (intravenous) cystography* was later modified by Handmaker and co-workers.

Direct (Retrograde) Radionuclide Cystography

No preparation or sedation is needed. The patient is supine with the gamma camera underneath. Following aseptic preparation, the urethra is catheterized with an 8 Fr. Foley catheter or an infant feeding tube. The bladder is emptied, and a urine sample is collected in a sterile bottle for culture. The catheter is connected to a bottle of normal saline by a regular intravenous infusion tubing set. The bottle of saline is placed 100 cm above the table top. After the flow of normal saline is established, 1 mCi of technetium 99m pertechnetate (0.5 mCi in neonates) is injected into the stream of saline through the rubber injection site of the infusion tube. The patient is positioned with the bladder on the lower edge of the field of view of the gamma camera.

While the bladder is filling, it is continuously monitored on the persistence scope of the gamma camera, and multiple analogue and digital posterior images of the bladder and upper abdomen are obtained. If bilateral reflux is observed, flow of normal saline is immediately discontinued. If no reflux is seen or only unilateral reflux occurs, the bladder is filled to capacity. The expected capacity of the bladder in children can be estimated from the following formula:

$$\text{bladder capacity} = (\text{age [years]} + 2) \times 30 \text{ ml}$$

The capacity of a hypertonic bladder, however, may be as low as 10 to 20 ml, whereas in those who void infrequently capacity may be greater than 500 ml. The signs of a full bladder include backup of saline in the tube, leakage around the catheter, upgoing toes, and crossing of the legs.

When reflux is seen, the volume of instilled saline is recorded. After adequate filling, the older patient is seated on a bedpan in front of the gamma camera, which has been placed in a vertical position. The catheter is removed, and the patient is encouraged to void. Analogue and digital images are obtained before, during, and after voiding (Fig. 4–26) (Majd and Belman). The number of counts on the pre-voiding and post-voiding images as well as total volume of instilled saline and the volume of the voided fluid are recorded. These values, together with the volume of instilled saline at the time of reflux, are used to calculate residual urine volume and bladder volume at the time of reflux (Weiss and Conway). The volume of reflux and the rate of its drainage back to the bladder can also be calculated. In infants, the voiding phase of the examination is carried on with the child in the supine position without measuring the voided urine volume. The volume of instilled saline at the time of reflux is accepted as the total bladder volume at that time.

Advantages

Low Radiation Dose. The most important advantage of direct radionuclide cystography is its extremely low radiation dose. With 1 mCi of technetium 99m pertechnetate in 200 ml of saline, the dose to the bladder wall during direct radionuclide cystography is about 1 mrad per minute of contact (Conway et al, 1972). In our experience, the average length of bladder exposure is only about 15 minutes, which results in a radiation dose of about 15 mrad to the bladder wall. The dose to the gonads, which in boys are at a considerable distance from the bladder wall, is probably less than 5 mrad. On the other hand, gonadal dose with standard x-ray voiding cystourethrography ranges from 75 mrad to several rads, depending on the fluoroscopy time and the number of films taken (Leibovic and Lebowitz). Therefore, on the average, the gonadal dose is about one one-hundredth (0.01) that of standard x-ray studies. The total body radiation that may result from possible absorption of a minimal amount of technetium 99m pertechnetate is negligible (Blaufox et al; Conway et al, 1972).

Sensitivity. Reflux is a dynamic, intermittent phenomenon. A considerable amount of reflux may vanish within a matter of seconds (Fig. 4–27). With standard x-ray voiding cystourethrography, continuous extended observation

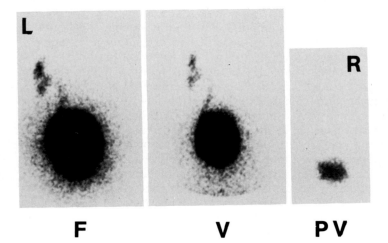

F   **V**   **P V**

Figure 4–26 □ Selected images from the filling (F), voiding (V), and post-voiding (PV) phases of a direct radionuclide cystogram. Left vesicoureteral reflux is seen during filling and voiding phases.

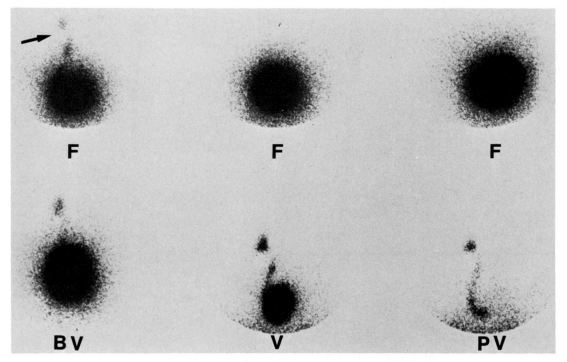

Figure 4–27 □ Intermittent reflux. Sequential images from a direct radionuclide cystogram show left vesicoureteral reflux in early filling phase *(arrow)*, which disappears on the subsequent images but reappears just before and during voiding. F, filling phase; BV, before voiding; V, during voiding; PV, post-voiding.

under fluoroscopy is unacceptable because of excessive radiation. With direct radionuclide cystography, the urinary tract is monitored continuously during filling, during voiding, and after voiding with no increase in the amount of radiation. In addition, reflux is more easily detected because overlying bowel contents and bones do not interfere with detection as they may during standard x-ray studies. The exception is minimal reflux to the distal ureter, which may be obscured by the isotope-filled bladder. Direct radionuclide cystography is more sensitive than x-ray cystography in detecting vesicoureteral reflux (Conway et al, 1972).

Quantitative Analyses. Parameters such as residual urine volume, bladder volume at the time of reflux, volume, and rate of clearance of reflux can be calculated. The clinical significance of these functional parameters is not clear. Bladder volume at the time of reflux appears to have a prognostic significance. If the bladder volume at the time of demonstration of reflux increases on annual serial examinations, it may indicate a better prognosis for spontaneous cessation of reflux (Nasrallah et al). Maizels et al recorded intravesical pressures during nuclear cystography and reported

that this combined information facilitates the management of children with vesicoureteral reflux and voiding abnormalities.

Disadvantages

The major disadvantage of direct radionuclide cystography is its unsuitability for evaluation of the male urethra. Therefore, its use for the initial study in boys with urinary tract infection is not advised unless the urethra is adequately evaluated on a voiding film obtained as part of an excretory urogram.

Because the anatomic resolution of direct radionuclide cystography is not as good as that of x-ray voiding cystourethrography, reflux cannot be graded accurately. The extremes of the spectrum (grades I, II, and V) can be differentiated, but grades III and IV cannot be accurately separated. Major abnormalities, such as large filling defects in the bladder (ureterocele), distortion and displacement of the bladder, and most duplications associated with reflux, can be appreciated (Fig. 4–28), but minor abnormalities of the bladder wall, such as diverticula, will be missed.

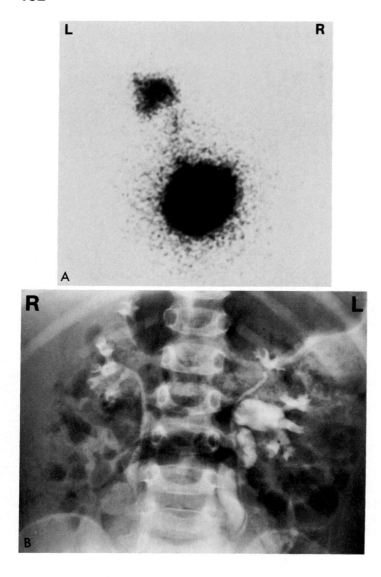

Figure 4–28 □ Reflux in a duplicated system. *A*, Posterior image of a direct radionuclide cystogram shows left vesico-ureteral reflux. The "drooping lily" appearance of the collecting system is suggestive of duplication. *B*, Excretory urogram shows bilateral duplication with dilatation of the pelvicalyceal system and ureter of the lower pole of the left kidney.

Indirect (Intravenous) Radionuclide Cystography

Indirect radionuclide cystography is a means of identifying reflux without urethral catheterization. It is based on the ideal condition of rapid and complete renal clearance of an intravenously injected radiopharmaceutical. The patient is normally hydrated (oral fluids). Following injection of 100 μCi/kg of technetium 99m DTPA or, preferably 50 μCi/kg of technetium 99m MAG 3, a conventional renal scan is obtained. The patient is instructed not to void and is monitored intermittently. When the upper urinary tract has drained and most of the tracer is contained in the bladder, the child is placed before the gamma camera in a sitting or standing position and analogue and digital images are obtained before, during, and after voiding. A sudden increase in radioactivity over a kidney or ureter indicates vesicoureteral reflux (Fig. 4–29).

Advantages

The theoretical advantages of indirect radionuclide cystography are that unpleasant catheterization is avoided, voiding may be more normal because the urethra is not irritated, and the study is performed without overdistending the bladder. A final advantage is that renal function and morphology as well as reflux may be evaluated simultaneously.

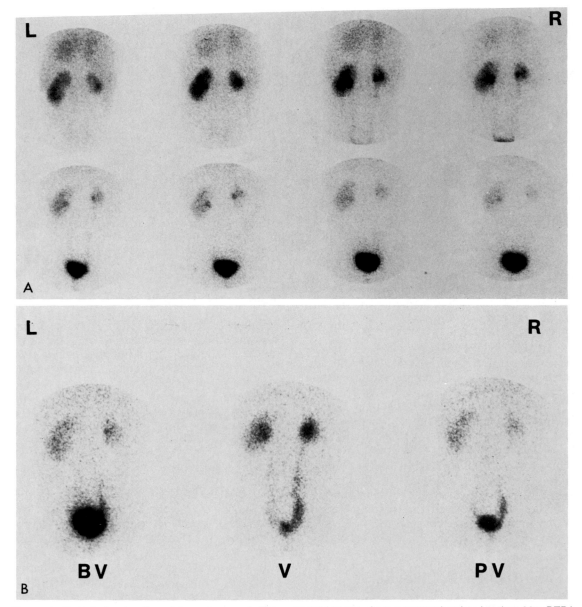

Figure 4–29 □ Indirect radionuclide cystogram. *A,* The sequential images from a conventional technetium 99m DTPA renal scan show prompt function and normal drainage bilaterally. The right kidney is small. *B,* The delayed images before (BV), during (V), and after (PV) voiding demonstrate bilateral vesicoureteral reflux, more severe on the right.

Illustration continued on following page

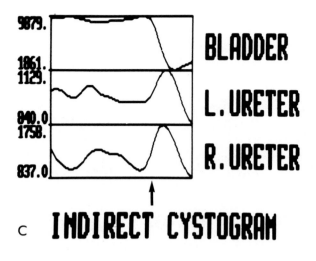

C **INDIRECT CYSTOGRAM**

Figure 4–29 □ *Continued C,* The time-activity curves of the regions of interest over the ureters and the bladder *(C)* demonstrate a rise in the activity over both ureters *(arrow)* as the bladder activity decreases during voiding. Slight terminal rise in the bladder activity curve is due to return of refluxed urine into the bladder during post-voiding phase.

Disadvantages

Although some reports indicate good correlation between indirect radionuclide cystography and x-ray voiding cystourethrography (Hedman et al; Merrick et al, 1977; Pollet et al), our study comparing the two radionuclide methods in 120 children with known reflux showed that the indirect technique using technetium 99m DTPA had a low sensitivity with an overall false-negative rate of 41 per cent (Fig. 4–30) (Majd et al, 1985). The use of technetium 99m MAG 3, which is cleared faster than technetium 99m DTPA, may improve the accuracy of indirect radionuclide cystography.

Other disadvantages of the indirect method include its dependence upon renal function and adequate drainage as well as cooperation by the patient, who must be able to void on request. The study is not practical in children who have a neuropathic bladder and in those who are not toilet-trained. The radiation dose is higher than that used for the direct cystogram and may become considerable if the child withholds urine for a protracted interval.

Clinical Applications

Direct Cystography

Direct radionuclide cystography, because of its superior sensitivity and minimal radiation dose, is the method of choice in the following situations:

1. All follow-up examinations in patients with known reflux who are on medical management or who have had antireflux surgery.
2. As a screening test to detect reflux in asymptomatic siblings of children with known reflux.
3. Serial evaluation of children with neuropathic bladder who are at risk for reflux to develop.
4. As the initial screening test for detection of reflux in girls with UTI.

Indirect Cystography

Indirect radionuclide cystography has a very low sensitivity for detection of reflux and should not be used as an initial screening test. In children with known reflux, if renal scanning with DTPA or MAG 3 is part of the follow-up evaluation, an indirect cystogram may be obtained. A positive study is reliable, but the negative studies should be confirmed by direct cystography.

SCROTAL SCINTIGRAPHY

Diagnostic testicular scanning was first proposed by Nadel et al in 1973. Since then, radionuclide scrotal imaging has been refined and has proved very useful in differentiating "surgical" from "nonsurgical" disorders of the scrotal contents. This study, if done properly in patients presenting with an acutely enlarged and painful hemiscrotum, may drastically decrease the number of unnecessary surgical explorations.

Technical Considerations

Thyroid uptake of technetium 99m pertechnetate is blocked by oral administration of

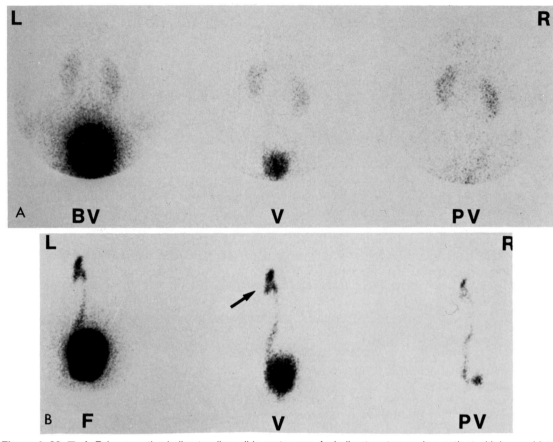

Figure 4–30 □ *A,* False-negative indirect radionuclide cystogram. An indirect cystogram in a patient with known history of left vesicoureteral reflux shows no evidence of reflux. *B,* A direct radionuclide cystogram obtained 7 days later demonstrates persistence of the left vesicoureteral reflux *(arrow).* BV, before voiding; V, during voiding; PV, post-voiding; F, filling.

potassium perchlorate in a dose of 5 mg/kg immediately prior to the test. The child is positioned supine on the imaging table. The penis is taped up over the pubis. The scrotum is supported by towels positioned between the thighs or by a tape sling. Lead shielding under the scrotum is not recommended for the angiographic phase of the examination (Holder et al), but is used for the static images, particularly in younger children. A lead shield under the scrotum facilitates detection of areas of decreased blood flow. The scrotum is positioned under the center of a gamma camera that is equipped with converging collimator or electronic magnification capability.

After rapid intravenous injection of technetium 99m pertechnetate in a dose of 200 μCi/kg, multiple 3-second dynamic images (radionuclide angiogram) are obtained. Immediately after the angiographic phase, early static images ("blood pool" or "tissue phase") are obtained. This is usually followed by the use

of a pinhole collimator to obtain high-resolution magnified static images.

Physical examination of the scrotum and accurate localization of the testicles by the nuclear physician are crucial in correct interpretation of the scintigraphic findings.

Scintigraphic Patterns

Basic knowledge of the vascular anatomy of the scrotum and its contents is essential for understanding the scintigraphic findings. A dual blood supply exists. The first pathway is composed of the vessels entering the spermatic cord: the testicular artery, which supplies the testicle, epididymis, and tunica vaginalis; the deferential artery; and the cremasteric artery. These three vessels enter at different levels and usually anastomose at the testicular mediastinum. The cremasteric artery forms a network over the tunica vaginalis and also participates in anastomoses with vessels supplying the scrotal wall. The second pathway is composed of the vessels that do not enter the spermatic cord. These include the internal pudendal artery and the superficial and deep external pudendal arteries. These arteries supply the scrotum and penis.

Normal Scrotal Scintigram

In a normal scrotal scintigram, the iliac arteries are well visualized. However, owing to their size and the relatively small amount of blood flow, the vessels supplying the scrotal contents are ill defined and the scrotum and its contents blur into a homogeneous area of tracer accumulation similar in intensity to that in the image of the thigh. Dartos activity cannot be separated from testicular or epididymal activity (Fig. 4–31).

Testicular Torsion

The scintigraphic pattern in testicular torsion depends on the duration of torsion.

Early Phase (Acute Torsion). In the early phase (probably within the first 6 hours), the radionuclide angiogram may show decreased blood flow to the hemiscrotum or may appear normal. Blood flow to the hemiscrotum is never increased at this stage. The static images ("tissue phase") show decreased accumulation of the tracer in the testicle without the reactive surrounding halo of increased activity seen in the later phases (Fig. 4–32).

Midphase. After a few hours, there is reactive hyperemia in the region supplied by the pudendal arteries. The radionuclide angiogram shows increased blood flow to the dartos, and the early static images show a halo of mildly increased activity around a cold center. The halo of increased activity gradually disappears on the subsequent images. This pattern is usually seen in patients who have been symptomatic for 6 to 18 hours.

Late Phase. If the patient with torsion does not seek immediate medical attention or is erroneously diagnosed, irreversible testicular infarction occurs. The pain and swelling resolve in a few days to weeks with subsequent atrophy of the testicle. It is important to diagnose late-phase testicular torsion in order to remove the necrotic testicle and to perform orchiopexy on the contralateral side.

Late-phase torsion reveals a characteristic scintigraphic pattern. The angiographic phase shows marked increased blood flow to the dartos, and static images reveal a complete rim or "halo" of increased activity around a cold center. The halo persists throughout the examination, which usually takes about 15 to 20 minutes (Fig. 4–33).

Spontaneous Detorsion. A spontaneously detorsed testicle may appear normal on the scans or may show slight, diffuse increased scrotal activity if the scan is obtained shortly after detorsion (Fig. 4–34). The diagnosis is best made on the basis of clinical history if examination has not been carried out prior to the detorsion. Demonstration of an intact blood supply to the testicle obviates only the need for emergency surgery. If the history is typical of intermittent torsion but physical examination shows the testis to be normally positioned and the scrotal scan shows intact perfusion and slightly increased activity, elective orchiopexy may be indicated (Lutzker).

Acute Epididymitis

In acute epididymitis, the radionuclide angiogram and the static images show markedly increased blood flow and blood pool activity to the area corresponding to the epididymis, or diffusely in the scrotum, if epididymoorchitis is present (Fig. 4–35). Intense, increased activity in the epididymis may occasionally resemble the halo of late-phase torsion. But, unlike the halo of late-phase torsion, the rim is incomplete and asymmetric (Fig. 4–36). Epididymitis in infants and young children may be secondary to an underlying anatomic abnormality, such as an ectopic ureter, and warrants complete investigation of the genitourinary system.

Torsion of the Testicular Appendages

Torsion of the appendix testis or epididymis may be visualized as a focal area of increased blood flow and blood pool activity, probably secondary to reactive hyperemia around the torsed appendix. The ischemic appendix itself is too small to be resolved on the images (Fig. 4–37). A more common scintigraphic pattern is that of mild generalized increased blood flow and "blood pool" activity indistinguishable

Text continued on page 161

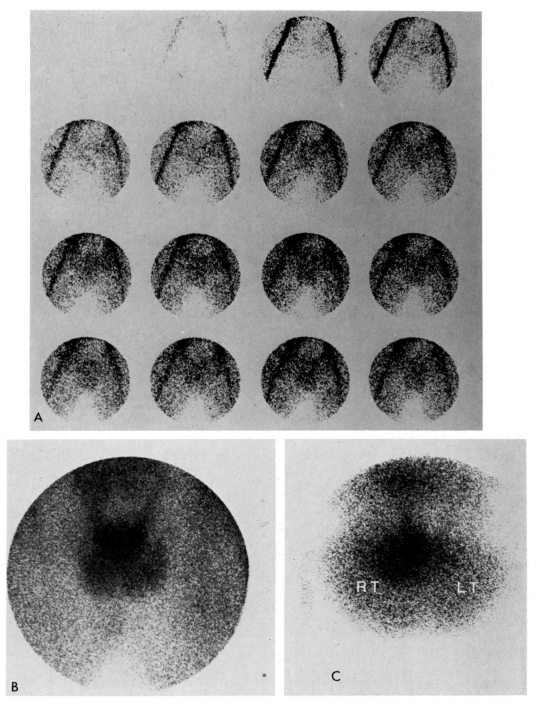

Figure 4–31 □ Normal scrotal scan. *A,* Sequential 3-second images of the radionuclide angiogram demonstrate excellent visualization of the iliac arteries. The vessels supplying the scrotum and its contents are not well defined. There is, however, homogeneous symmetrical accumulation of the tracer in the hemiscrotums. The unshielded static image *(B)* and the magnified image with the lead shield under the scrotum *(C)* also show symmetrical accumulation of the tracer in the testicles. RT, right testicle; LT, left testicle.

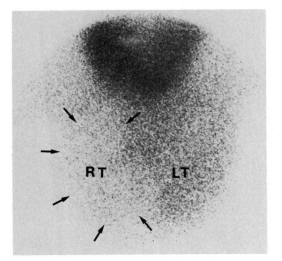

Figure 4–32 □ Acute testicular torsion in a 16-year-old boy with pain and swelling of the right testicle of 6 hours' duration. The static image using a pinhole collimator and lead shield under the scrotum shows decreased accumulation of the tracer in the right testicle *(arrows)*. RT, right testicle; LT, left testicle.

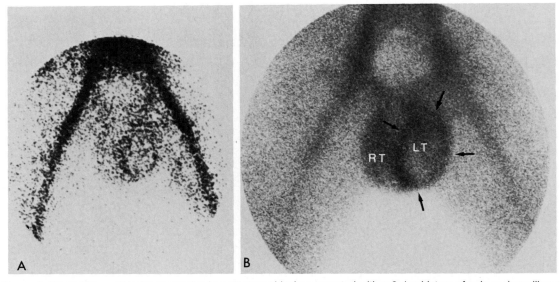

Figure 4–33 □ "Missed" testicular torsion in a 15-year-old who presented with a 2-day history of pain and swelling of the left hemiscrotum. *A,* A selected image of the radionuclide angiogram demonstrates increased blood flow *around* the left testicle. *B,* The static image shows decreased accumulation of the tracer in the left testicle associated with a surrounding rim or "halo" of increased accumulation of the tracer *(arrows)*. RT, right testicle; LT, left testicle.

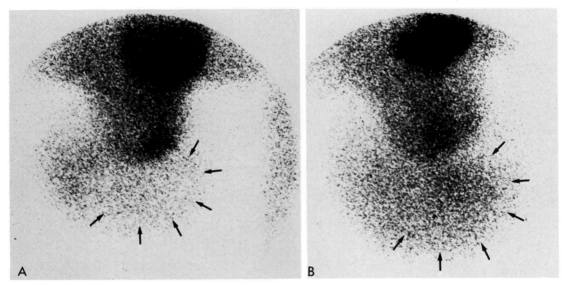

Figure 4–34 □ Spontaneous detorsion of the testicle in a 16-year-old boy who presented with a 4-hour history of pain and swelling of the left testicle. *A,* The magnified static image of the scrotum with a lead shield underneath shows decreased accumulation of the tracer in the left testicle *(arrows)* typical of an acute testicular torsion. Shortly after this image was obtained and while the patient was still on the scanning table, the pain abruptly subsided. *B,* Another image taken about 10 minutes after the image in *A* shows mild increased accumulation of the tracer in the left testicle *(arrows).* At surgery nonfixation of the testicle and evidence of spontaneous detorsion were found.

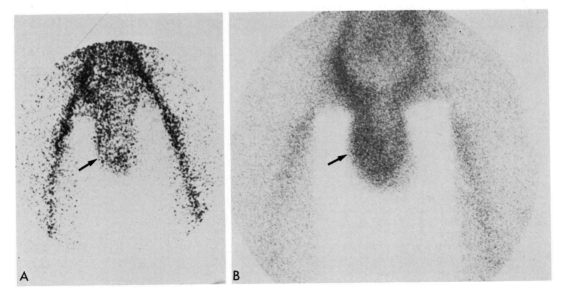

Figure 4–35 □ Acute epididymitis in a 15-year-old boy. The radionuclide angiogram *(A)* and the static image of the scrotum *(B)* show increased blood flow and accumulation of the tracer in the right hemiscrotum *(arrows).*

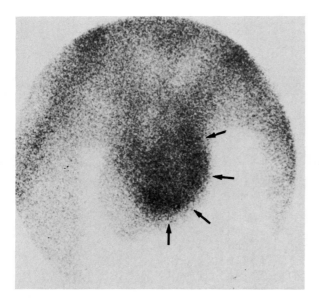

Figure 4–36 □ Acute epididymitis in a 17-year-old boy. The static image of the scrotum with a lead shield underneath demonstrates a semicircular area of increased accumulation of the tracer on the left corresponding to the epididymis *(arrows)*.

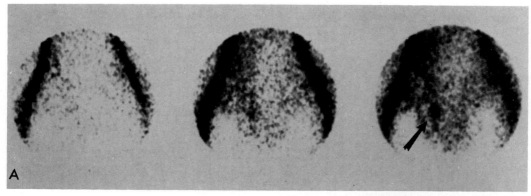

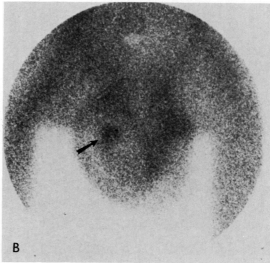

Figure 4–37 □ Torsion of the appendix testis in a 9-year-old boy who presented with a 2-day history of pain and swelling of the right hemiscrotum. The radionuclide angiogram *(A)* and the static image *(B)* of the scrotum demonstrate a small focal area of increased accumulation of the tracer on the right *(arrows)*.

from those seen with epididymitis (Fig. 4–38). This differentiation is of no surgical significance because both epididymitis and torsion of the appendix testis are generally considered to be nonsurgical problems. Radionuclide studies in the early phase of torsion of the appendix testis, prior to a significant inflammatory response, may be normal (Holder et al).

Scrotal Trauma

The scintigraphic pattern following scrotal trauma depends on the extent of injury as well as the time elapsed between the trauma and the scan. Mild, traumatic changes may appear as slightly to moderately diffuse increased tracer accumulation (Fig. 4–39). Intratesticular or intrascrotal hematoma may appear as a cold lesion with or without a surrounding halo of increased activity similar to testicular torsion (Fig. 4–40). Testicular rupture is also a surgical problem. Ultrasonography may be a useful adjunct in localizing a hematoma in relation to the testicle.

Hydrocele

The diagnosis of a simple hydrocele is made by physical examination and transillumination. In secondary hydrocele, which is seen in association with torsion, epididymitis, trauma,

or following herniorrhaphy, scintigraphic findings reflect the underlying condition. Hydroceles often appear as a horseshoe or a half-moon–shaped photon deficiency surrounding the testicle (Fig. 4–41).

Abscess

Scans of testicular or intrascrotal abscesses demonstrate a cold center surrounded by a rim of increased activity similar to that of late-phase torsion. The diagnosis is usually made in the context of the clinical history.

Clinical Applications

The scintigraphic patterns in the acute hemiscrotum can be divided into two groups.

1. Diffuse or focal increased blood flow and blood pool activity without any cold component. This pattern is seen in patients with epididymitis, torsion of the appendix testis, and minor post-traumatic abnormalities, all of which are nonsurgical conditions. The problem of differentiation between these conditions and spontaneous detorsion is usually solved on the basis of clinical history.

2. Cold lesions with or without a surrounding rim of increased activity (excluding typical hydrocele). This pattern is seen in patients

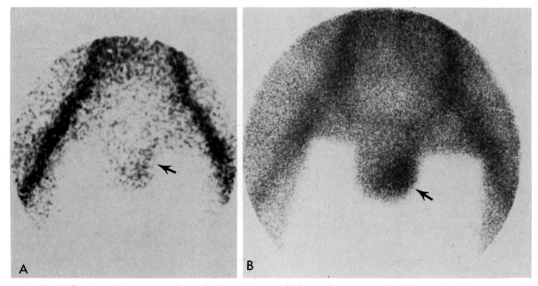

Figure 4–38 □ Torsion of the appendix testis in a 10-year-old boy who presented with a 3-day history of pain and swelling of the left hemiscrotum. The radionuclide angiogram *(A)* and the static image *(B)* demonstrate diffuse increased blood flow and accumulation of the tracer on the left *(arrows)* similar to the scintigraphic appearance of epididymitis.

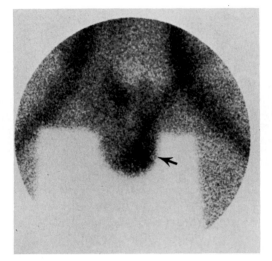

Figure 4–39 □ Scrotal trauma in a 16-year-old boy. He presented with a painful, swollen left testicle 2 days after direct trauma to his scrotum. The scan shows diffuse increased accumulation of the tracer on the left *(arrow)* similar to the scintigraphic pattern that may be seen in epididymitis or some cases of torsion of the appendix testis.

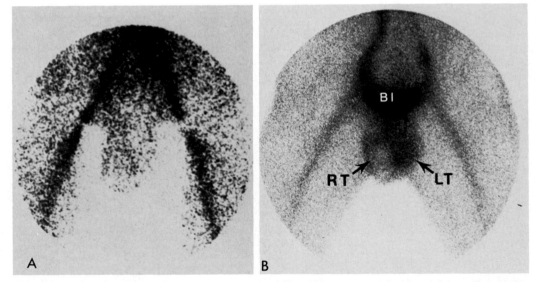

Figure 4–40 □ Testicular hematoma in a 12-year-old boy. The patient presented with painful swelling of the right testicle 14 hours after trauma to his scrotum. *A,* The radionuclide angiogram shows moderately increased blood flow around the right testicle. *B,* The static image shows decreased accumulation of the tracer in the right testicle with a "halo" of mildly increased activity. This scintigraphic pattern is similar to that of a missed torsion. Bl, bladder; RT, right testicle; LT, left testicle.

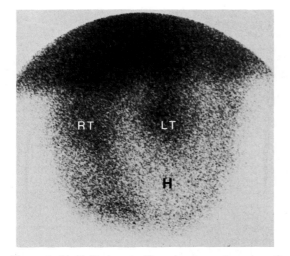

Figure 4–41 ☐ Hydrocele. There is a horseshoe-shaped area of decreased accumulation of the tracer surrounding the left testicle. RT, right testicle; LT, left testicle; H, hydrocele.

with testicular torsion, hematoma, and abscess, all of which are surgical conditions.

Acute Hemiscrotum

When the clinical presentation and physical findings are typical of the early phase of acute testicular torsion, surgery should be performed immediately without delaying for a testicular scan.

When the clinical presentation suggests inflammatory disease or conditions other than acute torsion, or when the patient cannot be properly examined because of extreme swelling and tenderness, testicular scanning is indicated and can reliably differentiate "surgical" from "nonsurgical" conditions.

Nonacute Indications

Testicular scanning may also be helpful (1) if there is any clinical doubt as to testicular viability after corrective detorsion and orchiopexy, and (2) in the occasional patient with suspected incompletely treated epididymoorchitis when the question of abscess arises.

Bibliography

Arlart I, Rosenthal J, Adam WE, et al: Predictive value of radionuclide methods in the diagnosis of unilateral renovascular hypertension. Cardiovascular Radiol 2:115, 1979.

Berne E, Ekman H: Method for clinical studies of vesi-coureteral reflux using colloidal 198 Au. Urol Int 18:335, 1964.

Bjorgvinsson E, Majd M, Eggli KD: Diagnosis of acute pyelonephritis in children: comparison of sonography and 99m Tc-DMSA scintigraphy. Am J Roentgenol 157:539, 1991.

Blaufox MD, Gruskin A, Sandler P, et al: Radionuclide cystography for detection of vesicoureteral reflux in children. J Pediatr 79:239, 1971.

Braren V, Versage PN, Touya JJ, et al: Radioisotopic determination of glomerular filtration rate. J Urol 121:145, 1979.

Chuang VP, Reuter SR, Schmidt RW: Control of experimental renal hemorrhage by embolization with autogenous blood clot. Radiology 117:55, 1975.

Conway JJ, Belman AB, King LR, et al: Direct and indirect radionuclide cystography. J Urol 113:689, 1975.

Conway JJ, King LR, Belman AB, et al: Detection of vesicoureteral reflux with radionuclide cystography: a comparison study with roentgenographic cystography. Am J Roentgenol Radium Ther Nucl Med 115:720, 1972.

Corriere JN Jr, Kuhl DE, Murphy JJ: The use of 99mTc labeled sulfur colloid to study particle dynamics in the urinary tract. Vesicoureteral reflux. Invest Urol 4:570, 1967.

Corriere JN Jr, Sanders TP, Kuhl DE, et al: Urinary particle dynamics and vesicoureteral reflux in humans. J Urol 103:599, 1970.

Diffey BL, Hall FM, Corfield JR: The 99mTc-DTPA dynamic renal scan with deconvolution analysis. J Nucl Med 17:352, 1976.

Dodge EA: Vesicoureteral reflux: diagnosis with iodine-131 sodium ortho-iodohippurate. Lancet 1:303, 1963.

Dondi M, Franchi R, Levorato M, et al: Evaluation of hypertensive patients by means of captopril enhanced renal scintigraphy with technetium-99m DTPA. J Nucl Med 30:615, 1989.

Dubovsky EV, Russell CD: Quantitation of renal function with glomerular and tubular agents. Semin Nucl Med 12:308, 1982.

English PJ, Testa HJ, Lawson RS, et al: Modified method of diuresis renography for the assessment of equivocal pelviureteric junction obstruction. Br J Urol 59:10, 1987.

Fawcett HD, Goodwin DA, Lantieri RL: In-111 leukocyte scanning in inflammatory renal disease. Clin Nucl Med 6:237, 1981.

Felson B, Cussen LJ: The hydronephrotic type of unilateral congenital multicystic disease of the kidney. Semin Roentgenol 10:113, 1975.

Gates GF: Glomerular filtration rate: estimation from fractional renal accumulation of 99mTc-DTPA (stannous). AJR 138:563, 1982.

George EA: Radionuclide diagnosis of allograft rejection. Semin Nucl Med 12:379, 1982.

Glauser MP, Lyons JM, Braude AL: Prevention of chronic experimental pyelonephritis by suppression of acute suppuration. J Clin Invest 61:403, 1978.

Griscom NT, Wawter GF, Fellers FX: Pelvoinfundibular atresia: the usual form of multicystic kidney: 44 unilateral and two bilateral cases. Semin Roentgenol 10:125, 1975.

Handmaker H: Nuclear renal imaging in acute pyelonephritis. Semin Nucl Med 12:246, 1982.

Handmaker H, McRae J, Buck EG: Intravenous radionuclide voiding cystography (IRVC): an atraumatic method of demonstrating vesicoureteral reflux. Radiology 108:703, 1973.

Hedman PJK, Kempi V, Voss H: Measurement of vesicoureteral reflux with intravenous 99mTc-DTPA compared to radiographic cystography. Radiology 126:205, 1978.

Hendren WH, Kim SH, Herrin JT, et al: Surgically correctable hypertension of renal origin in childhood. Am J Surg 143:432, 1982.

Holder LE, Melloul M, Chen D: Current status of radionuclide scrotal imaging. Semin Nucl Med 11:232, 1981.

Hovinga TKK, de Jong PE, Piers DA, et al: Diagnostic use of angiotensin-converting enzyme inhibitors in radioisotope evaluation of unilateral renal artery stenosis. J Nucl Med 30:605, 1989.

June CH, Browning MD, Smith LP, et al: Ultrasonography and computed tomography in severe urinary tract infection. Arch Intern Med 145:841, 1985.

Kirchner PT, Rosenthall L: Renal transplant evaluation. Semin Nucl Med 12:370, 1982.

Lawson JD, Boerth R, Foster JH, et al: Diagnosis and management of renovascular hypertension in children. Arch Surg 112:1307, 1977.

Lebowitz RL, Blickman JG: The coexistence of ureteropelvic junction obstruction and reflux. AJR 140:231, 1983.

Leibovic SJ, Lebowitz RL: Reducing patient dose in voiding cystourethrography. Urol Radiol 2:103, 1980.

Lutzker LG: The fine points of scrotal scintigraphy. Semin Nucl Med 12:387, 1982.

Magill HL, Clarke EA, Fitch SJ, et al: Excretory urography with Iohexol: evaluation in children. Radiology 161:625, 1986.

Maizels M, Weiss S, Conway JJ, et al: The cystometric nuclear cystogram. J Urol 121:203, 1979.

Majd M, Belman AB: Nuclear cystography in infants and children. Urol Clin North Am 6:395, 1979.

Majd M, Kass EJ, Belman AB: Radionuclide cystography in children: comparison of direct (retrograde) and indirect (intravenous) techniques. Ann Radiol 28:322, 1985.

Majd M, Potter BM, Guzzetta PC, et al: Effect of captopril on efficacy of renal scintigraphy in detection of renal artery stenosis. J Nucl Med 24:23, 1983.

Majd M, Rushton HG, Chandra R: Focal intrarenal blood flow changes in experimental acute pyelonephritis in piglets. Radiology 177(P)(Suppl):142, 1990.

Majd M, Rushton HG, Jantausch B, Wiedermann BL: Relationship among vesicoureteral reflux, P-fimbriated E. coli, and acute pyelonephritis in children with febrile urinary tract infection. J Pediatr 119:578, 1991.

Malligan JS, Blue PW, Hasbargen JA: Methods of measuring GFR with technetium 99m-DTPA: an analysis of several common methods. J Nucl Med 31:1211, 1990.

Mazer MJ, Quaife MA: Hypertrophied column of Bertin pseudotumors: radionuclide investigation (letter to the editor). Urology 14:210, 1979.

McCrory WW: Developmental Nephrology. Cambridge, Mass., Harvard University Press, 1972, p 96.

Mendez G Jr, Morillo G, Alonso M, et al: Gallium 67 radionuclide imaging in acute pyelonephritis. AJR 134:17, 1980.

Merrick MV, Uttley WS, Wild SR: A comparison of two techniques of detecting vesico-ureteric reflux. Br J Radiol 52:792, 1977.

Merrick MV, Uttley WS, Wild SR: The detection of pyelonephritic scarring in children by radioisotope imaging. Br J Radiol 53:544, 1980.

Montgomery P, Kuhn JP, Afshani E: CT evaluation of severe renal inflammatory disease in children. Pediatr Radiol 17:216, 1987.

Nadel NS, Gitter MH, Hahn LC, et al: Pre-operative diagnosis of testicular torsion. Urology 1:478, 1973.

Nasrallah PF, Conway JJ, King LR, et al: Quantitative nuclear cystogram: aid in determining spontaneous resolution of vesicoureteral reflux. Urology 12:654, 1978.

Nawaz MK, Nimmon CC, Britton KE, et al: Obstructive nephropathy: a comparison of the parenchymal transit time index and furosemide diuresis. J Nucl Med 24:16, 1983.

Nilson AE, Aurell M, Bratt CG, et al: Diuretic urography in the assessment of obstruction of the pelvi-ureteric junction. Acta Radiol (Diagn) (Stockh) 21:499, 1980.

O'Reily PH, Lawson RS, Shields RA, et al: Idiopathic hydronephrosis—the diuresis renogram: a new noninvasive method of assessing equivocal pelviureteral junction obstruction. J Urol 121:153, 1979.

Parkhouse HF, Godley ML, Cooper J, et al: Renal imaging with 99mTc-labelled DMSA in the detection of acute pyelonephritis: an experimental study in the pig. Nucl Med Commun 10:63, 1989.

Piepsz A, Denis R, Ham HR, et al: A simple method for measuring separate glomerular filtration rate using a single injection of 99mTc-DTPA and the scintillation camera. J Pediatr 93:769, 1978.

Piepsz A, Ham HR, Dobbeleir A, et al: How to exclude renal obstruction in children: comparison of intrarenal transit times, cortical times and furosemide test. In Radionuclides in Nephrology. Edited by AM Joekes, AR Constable, NJG Brown, et al. London, Academic Press, Inc, 1982, pp 199–204.

Pollet JE, Sharp PF, Smith FW: Radionuclide imaging for vesico-renal reflux using intravenous 99mTc-DTPA. Pediatr Radiol 8:165, 1979.

Powers TA, Stone WJ, Grove RB, et al: Radionuclide measurement of differential glomerular filtration rate. Invest Radiol 16:59, 1981.

Price RR, Torn ML, Jones JP, et al: Comparison of differential renal function determination by Tc-99m DMSA, Tc-99m DTPA, I-131 Hippuran and ureteral catheterization. J Nucl Med 20:631, 1979.

Ransley PG, Risdon PA: Reflux nephropathy: effect of antimicrobial therapy on the evolution of the early pyelonephritic scar. Kidney Int 20:733, 1981.

Raynaud C, Tran-Dinh S, Bourgugnan M, et al: Acute pyelonephritis in children: preliminary results obtained with NMR imaging. Contrib Nephrol 56:129, 1987.

Rushton HG, Majd M, Chandra R, Yim D: Evaluation of 99m technetium–dimercaptosuccinic acid renal scans in experimental acute pyelonephritis in piglets. J Urol 140:1169, 1988.

Sfakianakis GN, Bourgoignie JJ, Jaffe D, et al: Single-dose captopril scintigraphy in the diagnosis of renovascular hypertension. J Nucl Med 28:1383, 1987.

Sfakianakis GN, Sfakianakis ED: Nuclear medicine in pediatric urology and nephrology. J Nucl Med 29:1287, 1988.

Shore RM, Koff SA, Mentser M, et al: Glomerular filtration rate in children: determination from the Tc-99m DTPA renogram. Radiology 151:627, 1984.

Silver TM, Kass EJ, Thornbury JR, et al: The radiological spectrum of acute pyelonephritis in adults and adolescents. Radiology 118:65, 1976.

Stanley JC, Frey WJ: Pediatric renal artery occlusive disease and renovascular hypertension. Arch Surg 116:669, 1981.

Stanley P, Gyepes MT, Olson DL, et al: Renovascular hypertension in children and adolescents. Radiology 129:123, 1978.

Sty JR, Wells RG, Starshak RJ, Schroeder BA: Imaging in acute renal infection in children. AJR 148:471, 1987.

Taylor A Jr: Quantitation of renal function with static imaging agents. Semin Nucl Med 12:330, 1982.

Taylor A Jr, Ziffer JA, Steves A, et al: Clinical comparison of I-131 orthoiodohippurate and the Kit Formulation of Tc-99m mercaptoacetyltriglycine. Radiology 170:721, 1989.

Thrall JH, Koff SA, Keyes JW Jr: Diuretic radionuclide urography and scintigraphy in the differential diagnosis of hydronephrosis. Semin Nucl Med 11:89, 1981.

Traisman ES, Conway JJ, Traisman HS, et al: The localization of urinary tract infection with 99m Tc glucoheptonate scintigraphy. Pediatr Radiol 16:403, 1986.

Weiss S, Conway JJ: The technique of direct radionuclide cystography. Appl Radiol 4(3):133, 1975.

Whitfield HN, Britton KE, Fry IK, et al: The obstructed kidney: correlation between renal function and urodynamic assessment. Br J Urol 49:615, 1977.

Whitfield HN, Britton KE, Hendry WF, et al: The distinction between obstructive uropathy and nephropathy by radioisotope transit times. Br J Urology 50:433, 1978.

Whitfield HN, Britton KE, Nimmon CC, et al: Renal transit time measurements in the diagnosis of ureteric obstruction. Br J Urol 53:500, 1981.

Winberg J, Bollgren I, Kallenius G, et al: Clinical pyelonephritis and focal renal scarring: a selected review of pathogenesis, prevention and prognosis. Pediatr Clin North Am 29:801, 1982.

Winter CC: A new test for vesicoureteral reflux: an external technique using radioisotopes. J Urol 81:105, 1959.

Wood BP, Smith WL: Pulmonary edema in infants following injection of contrast media for urography. Radiology 139:377, 1981.

Zielinski FW, Holly FE, Robinson GD Jr, et al: Total and individual kidney function assessment with iodine-123 ortho-iodohippurate. Radiology 125:753, 1977.

5

□ Endoscopy

Lawrence Kroovand

In 1877 Max Nitze, with the help of instrument maker Wilhelm Deicke, invented and demonstrated the first practical light cystoscope in Dresden, Germany. Since then, progress in both technical innovation and clinical application has made possible the remarkably high quality of present-day urologic endoscopic equipment. Unfortunately, during this same time, the indications for pediatric cystoscopy have remained so poorly defined that some urologists believe that no pediatric urologic evaluation is complete without a cystoscopic examination, whereas others employ cystoscopy very sparingly. This chapter details rational indications and contraindications for pediatric cystoscopy, describes the endoscopic instruments currently available and the design of a pediatric cystoscopic suite, and discusses operative endoscopy. In addition, laparoscopy, percutaneous endourologic and ureteroscopic techniques, and their application to pediatric patients are reviewed.

CYSTOSCOPY: INDICATIONS AND CONTRAINDICATIONS

The Controversy

Cystourethroscopy is an established essential tool for adult urologic investigation. However, in view of the current sophistication of pediatric uroradiographic techniques and the types of common pediatric urologic problems, the role of cystoscopy in the evaluation and management of pediatric urologic problems appears limited. When recommending cystoscopy for the pediatric patient, one must consider the sometimes questionable diagnostic and therapeutic benefit to the child; this must be balanced against cost, the risk of anesthesia, and the potential for urethral trauma. Of course a cystoscopic examination should always be done when indicated.

Three publications (Dunn et al; Johnson et al; Walther and Kaplan) have systematically reviewed and analyzed large series of cystoscopic examinations in childhood. Each publication clarifies the indications for cystoscopic examination in childhood and reflects the declining indications for cystoscopy in childhood. The following section is intended to serve as an outline of the indications for diagnostic and operative pediatric cystoscopy.

Indications for Cystoscopy

Prior to any endoscopic evaluation of the urinary tract in a child, the basic anatomy of the upper and lower urinary tracts must be studied. Voiding cystourethrography defines the functional anatomy of the lower urinary tract and, if the voiding cystourethrogram is normal, renal ultrasonography provides appropriate upper tract evaluation. If the voiding cystourethrogram is abnormal, excretory urography is mandatory for upper tract evaluation, as this examination is more reliable than sonography in detecting parenchymal anomalies. Isotope renography may be substituted for excretory urography and is a more appropriate study in the neonate and young infant, where intestinal gas and renal functional immaturity may reduce the diagnostic yield of excretory urography. Voiding films during excretory urography are not as reliable as a voiding cystourethrogram. These uroradiographic studies will define the anatomic and functional status of the urinary tract and may suggest specific abnormalities to be evaluated at endoscopy. Because expression cystourethrography with the patient under general anesthesia may miss up to 50 per cent of known vesicoureteral reflux, its use for such purpose is discouraged (Timmons et al). Installation of methylene blue at the time of cystoscopy to detect vesicoureteral reflux is similarly inaccurate. Cystoscopy in children may be unwise or dangerous in the presence of active infection or blood dyscrasia.

Urinary Tract Infection

The most common indication for cystoscopic examination in childhood has been urinary tract infection. Many urologists, including this author, feel that the child with an uncomplicated urinary tract infection who has a normal uroradiographic evaluation does not have pyelonephritis and does not routinely require cystoscopy. The findings at cystoscopy in such children are almost invariably normal, or the abnormalities discovered at cystoscopy are incidental, not altering treatment or eventual outcome. However, cystoscopy certainly should be part of the evaluation of the child with persistent infection or multiple recurrent urinary infections. When a micturitional dysfunction is unexplained, cystoscopy may help to definitely exclude an anatomic obstruction. Children with such infections, usually girls over 5 with a history of urge incontinence, frequently have cystitis follicularis (cystitis cystica) and require long-term antibacterial treatment (6 to 12 months or more) combined with adjunctive anticholinergic medication to prevent recurrent infections and control associated voiding dysfunction. This regimen permits resolution of the inflammatory mucosal changes and secondary long-standing voiding dysfunction over time. In addition, documentation of chronic cystitis cystica may improve parental compliance with recommended long-term medication programs, although this has not been proved.

Children with urinary infection and abnormal x-rays will be discussed in more detail in the section specific to the disorder present.

Voiding Dysfunction without Urinary Infection

Children with voiding dysfunction (day wetting, frequency, urgency, or nocturnal enuresis) and without documented urinary infection usually have normal physical and neurologic findings, normal urinalyses, and normal uroradiographic evaluations. Because cystoscopy in this circumstance is generally normal or reveals only insignificant abnormalities not altering recommended therapy or ultimate outcome, cystoscopy is generally unnecessary. Even in those children with voiding dysfunction and abnormal uroradiographic studies, cystoscopic examination may only confirm or clarify the uroradiographic findings. These findings at cystoscopy are generally incidental and do not explain the child's symptoms, unless the identification of bladder trabeculation at cystoscopy makes the endoscopist consider the possibility of detrusor-sphincter-dyssynergia.

The value of urethral dilation in girls with urinary infection or voiding dysfunction, or both, remains controversial. Most pediatric urologists now believe that urethral manipulation (dilatation and/or urethrotomy) has little or no effect on the recurrence rate of infection or resolution of vesicoureteral reflux and only infrequently enhances resolution of symptoms. Routine urethral manipulation appears of little value in the treatment of children with urinary infection or voiding dysfunction, or with both (Kaplan et al, 1973).

Vesicoureteral Reflux

The role of cystoscopy as part of the evaluation and treatment of children with vesicoureteral reflux remains controversial. For older children with persistent vesicoureteral reflux, the decision to operate is most often based upon multiple factors, including the degree of reflux as judged from the voiding cystourethrogram, the presence or absence of recurrent infection while under prophylactic antibacterial management, renal growth arrest, or noncompliance with antibacterial therapy; less absolute indications include progression of renal scarring while under appropriate antibacterial prophylaxis and failure of reflux to resolve as anticipated.

Although cystoscopy at the time of initial evaluation may result in a recommendation for earlier ureteral reimplantation in some children, especially those with more severe grades of reflux (IV/V, V/V) and golf-hole orifices or large paraureteral diverticula, the majority of children with reflux and urinary infection are safely managed employing long-term prophylactic antibacterial coverage and careful periodic follow-up and re-evaluation. With cessation of recurrent urinary infection, renal growth usually resumes, renal scarring does not progress (although scars may mature), and the reflux may decrease in degree or completely resolve. Cystoscopy in children with reflux and infection appears to be of most value in assessing the prognosis of those with long-term persistent reflux by evaluating orifice configuration and permitting measurement of the length of the submucosal tunnel. A previously refluxing contralateral ureter may also be evaluated prior to ureteral reimplantation. Endoscopic evaluation in this context can generally be done at the time of the planned ureteral reimplantation, avoiding a separate anesthesia.

Hematuria

Some clinicians advocate routine cystoscopy for all children with hematuria. Such a reflex response appears unnecessary inasmuch as the most common causes of microscopic hematuria in childhood are infection and glomerulonephritis. Most causes of gross hematuria are not evident on uroradiographic studies, but some, such as tumors, stones, and cysts are more reliably detected on urographic studies than at cystoscopy (Chan; Khasidy et al).

All children with hematuria, gross or microscopic, should have excretory urography and voiding cystourethrography. When these studies are normal, cystoscopic evaluation invariably is normal and therefore appears unnecessary. As most significant bladder lesions in the pediatric age group are evident radiologically (Fig. 5–1); cystoscopy in this situation often serves only to confirm the uroradiographic findings. Persistent hematuria occasionally leads to cystoscopic examination (usually in desperation); causal lesions are seldom discovered.

A prolonged intensive course of antineoplastic chemotherapy (cyclophosphamide), especially when combined with concurrent pelvic radiation therapy, may result in an atrophic cystitis and profuse gross hematuria (Droller et al). Early cystoscopy in these children may confirm the diagnosis and alter the plan of chemotherapy.

In some boys anterior (bulbar) urethritis may present with a pathognomonic symptom complex of terminal hematuria and blood spotting on the under shorts, with or without dysuria but without pyuria, positive cultures, or abnormal uroradiographic study. A voiding cystogram is more reliable in detecting a valve of Guerin than ureteroscopy. Cystoscopy may suggest anterior urethritis as a cause (Color Plate 5–1 A) but the examination is rarely

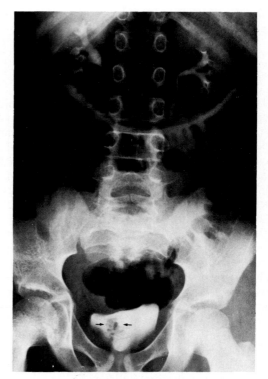

Figure 5–1 ☐ Inverted papilloma *(arrows)* in an 11-year-old girl with painless gross hematuria.

indicated because the symptoms and signs are so pathognomonic. Furthermore, cystoscopy in this condition has preceded stricture formation, giving rise to the clinical impression that the additional trauma of urethroscopy in this situation may contribute to later stricture formation (Kaplan and Brock).

Neoplasia

Urothelial malignancy involving the upper or lower urinary tract is infrequently encountered in the pediatric age group. When present, such lesions are usually visualized on uroradiographic study (see Fig. 5–1); cystoscopy then becomes confirmatory rather than diagnostic. Renal parenchymal tumors such as Wilms' tumor (more common) and renal cell carcinoma (less common) have such a characteristic appearance on intravenous urography that endoscopic evaluation and retrograde ureteropyelography are seldom necessary. Rhabdomyosarcoma of the bladder and prostate is usually very characteristic in appearance on uroradiographic evaluation; pretreatment endoscopy permits assessment of the extent of

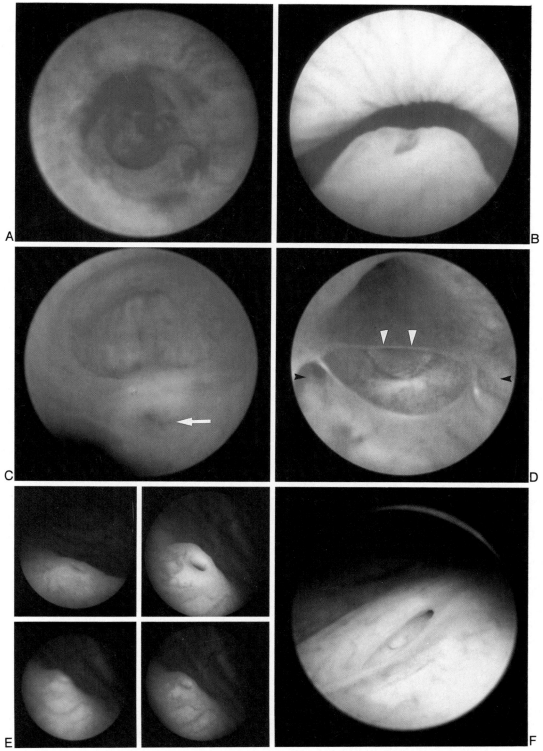

Plate 5–1 □ *A,* Anterior (bulbar) urethritis in a 10-year-old boy. *B,* Large prostatic utricle in a 4-year-old boy with penoscrotal hypospadias. *C,* Entrance of the vagina *(arrows)* into the urethra of a 3-year-old girl with congenital virilizing adrenogenital syndrome. *D,* Anomalous development of the Cowper's ducts with characteristic bulbar urethral diverticulum *(white arrows);* note the entrance of the Cowper's ducts into the urethra *(black arrows). E,* Cone- or volcano-shaped ureteral orifice. *F,* Stadium-shaped ureteral orifice.

the tumor and provides the opportunity to obtain a specimen for pathologic examination.

Malignant or benign lesions arising from other organ systems, such as the retroperitoneum, the internal genital ducts, or the intestinal tract, and appearing to impinge upon the urinary tract sometimes may be best defined by cystoscopy with retrograde ureteropyelography. The indications for endoscopic evaluation in this situation must be individualized.

Urinary Calculi and Foreign Bodies

Urinary calculi in childhood are relatively uncommon (Reiner et al). As in adults, up to 80 per cent pass spontaneously, whereas the remainder may require evaluation and manipulation by retrograde technique (Walther et al). For those ureteral or bladder calculi that do not pass spontaneously, the criteria for endoscopic retrieval (basket extraction, ureteroscopy) or open surgical removal are identical to those in the adult. Unfortunately, the small size of the prepubertal male urethra places constraints on instrument size for endoscopic manipulation of ureteral or vesical calculi. In girls the urethra is more distensible; gentle dilatation usually permits passage of adult-size instruments, thus increasing the options for endoscopic calculus manipulation. If the urethra will accommodate a 13 Fr. or large sheath, a 4 Fr. (13 Fr. sheath) Pfister-Schwartz, or 5 Fr. (14 Fr. sheath) Dormia stone retriever may facilitate ureteral calculus removal. Transurethral calculus manipulation in childhood carries the same risks as in the adult and should only be performed under fluoroscopic monitoring. When performing any transurethral procedure in childhood, the clinician must take particular care to avoid urethral injury; consistent gentleness of technique is mandatory. Bladder calculi and foreign bodies encountered in childhood usually require open surgical removal. Both are discussed later in the text. Percutaneous endourologic techniques are also discussed below. (See also Chapter 16, Endoscopic Surgery of the Upper Tract in Children.)

Retrograde Ureteral Catheterization

With the increasing sophistication in uroradiographic technique (conventional uroradiog-raphy, radionuclide imaging, and ultrasonography), the indications for retrograde ureteral catheterization have become relatively limited. Retrograde studies are only infrequently required to evaluate abnormalities of the upper urinary tract but may be useful whenever an obstructing process within the collecting system is incompletely visualized. Retrograde ureteropyelography should always be performed with appropriate fluoroscopic monitoring. A dilated megaureter that is incompletely visualized by intravenous urography or persistent ureterectasis following ureteral reimplantation or megaureter repair may be best defined by retrograde pyelography. In such instances fluoroscopy permits observation of ureteral peristalsis and drainage; manometric pressure perfusion recordings can be obtained if necessary.

In managing ureteropelvic junction obstruction, retrograde ureteropyelography, as a separate procedure, is generally not indicated unless another ureteral abnormality, not defined on excretory urography or during abdominal ultrasonography, is suspected. If indicated, retrograde ureteropyelography may be performed at the time of the definitive operative procedure, thereby avoiding a separate administration of anesthesia and reducing the potential complications for iatrogenic upper urinary infection.

Difficulties in obtaining adequate urine flow for split renal function studies through small caliber ureteral catheters plus the ill-defined effects of general anesthesia on renal function in the anesthetized child limit the success of this endeavor. Split renal function measurements or urine cultures, or both, may be obtained after copious bladder washing; percutaneous nephrostomy is now preferred for evaluation of renal function or severe upper urinary obstruction. When percutaneous drainage procedures fail, retrograde catheter placement can provide temporary upper tract decompression prior to definitive management. Retrograde manipulation of upper ureteral calculi into the renal pelvis prior to extracorporeal shock wave lithotripsy may facilitate calculus fragmentation.

For the child with ureteral obstruction after ureteral reimplantation or after endoscopic calculus manipulation or ureteroscopy, placement of a retrograde ureteral catheter or percutaneous decompression may be indicated. Unfortunately the smallest currently available double pigtail stent is 5 Fr. in size and therefore not usable with currently available pediatric panendoscopes. Such stents may sometimes be passed over a guide wire inserted through a suprapubic cystocath sheath with cystoscopic control.

Congenital Anomalies

Endoscopic evaluation may define developmental anatomic abnormalities associated with severe hypospadias, ambiguous genitalia, persistent urogenital sinus, and cloacal malformations not fully demonstrated uroradiographically. Although cystoscopy is not routinely performed in boys with hypospadias, those with severe hypospadias may have a large utriculus masculinus (müllerian duct remnant), not visualized on voiding cystourethrography, that may be easily identified endoscopically (see Color Plate 5–1*B*). Transurethral marsupialization of a particularly large utriculus with a narrow ostium may avoid urinary infection or calculus formation after hypospadias repair. The precise location of the narrow entrance of the distal vagina into the urogenital sinus may be identified at the time of genital reconstruction or vaginoplasty in girls with virilizing adrenogenital syndrome (see Color Plate 5–1*C*). When virilization is extreme, endoscopic placement of a Fogarty balloon catheter through the tiny connection of the urogenital sinus to the vaginal cavity aids in identifying the vagina and may reduce the extent of perineal dissection required during vaginoplasty and perineal reconstruction.

ENDOSCOPIC INSTRUMENTS

During the past 85 years, improvements in technique and instrumentation have made endoscopic evaluation of the lower urinary tract in infants and children a practical and safe procedure. Fiberoptic illumination and the Hopkins lens system now permit more reliable and intense illumination with increased perception and a clearer, less distorted visual field. One can visualize the lower urinary tract of infants and children accurately; transurethral manipulation and fulguration are easily accomplished. In addition, endoscopic photography and video recording are now routine at most pediatric urologic centers.

The essentials of a pediatric endoscopic unit include interchangeable telescopes (direct-vision and forward-oblique) and sheaths of assorted size to permit both observation (examination) and operative endoscopy. In addition, instruments to permit percutaneous endourology and ureteroscopic procedures in pediatric patients should be available. Several manufacturers (Storz, ACMI, Wolf, Olympus) produce a variety of pediatric endoscopic instruments. Most instruments are color-coded and engraved for easy identification of French size and retrograde capacity. The listed French (Fr.) sizes are approximate for sheaths with an oval cross section. Unfortunately, the true diameter of some of these instruments is sometimes greater than stated by the manufacturer; actual instrument size should be verified by the prospective buyer. Because these instruments are very delicate and are easily damaged, they should be handled with utmost care and gentleness. The quality and availability of instrument repair is variable from manufacturer to manufacturer and should be investigated by the prospective buyer prior to purchase. Even in careful use, these delicate instruments occasionally require repair.

Observation cystoscopes are available in 7 Fr. (Storz), 7.5 Fr. (Wolf), and 9 Fr. (Storz) sizes. Some have both observation (examination) and irrigating capability, whereas others permit observation only. This author has found neither type particularly useful because of the inability to fulgurate posterior urethral valves in small infants or to perform retrograde ureteropyelography. Urethroscopes of 7.5 Fr., 8.5 Fr., and 9.5 Fr. (Storz and Wolf) with a side channel that accommodates a 3 Fr. ureteral catheter are especially useful in small male infants for transurethral fulguration of posterior urethral valves (Fig. 5–2).

For larger infants and children, instruments of 10 to 14 Fr. sheath size are available; most accommodate one or two ureteral catheters.

Some instruments have an integrated (not interchangeable) sheath and telescope, while others have interchangeable direct-vision and forward-oblique telescopes. Integrated instruments may add unnecessary expense in equipping a pediatric endoscopic unit and therefore appear less desirable. However, such instruments may be more durable. For versatility, this author finds a 10 Fr. sheath with interchangeable direct-vision (0 degrees) and forward-oblique (30 degrees) telescopes most useful (Fig. 5–3).

Pediatric resectoscopes in sizes from 9.0 to 14 Fr. permit a wide variety of endoscopic

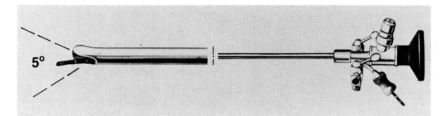

Figure 5–2 □ An 8 French infant cystoscope that will accommodate a 3 French ureteral catheter.

surgery (Fig. 5–4). Most instruments use an interchangeable direct-vision (0 degrees) or forward-oblique (30 degrees) telescope. Separate optical urethrotomes are also available in sizes starting at 8.5 Fr. (Wolf). Optical urethrotomes and infant resectoscopes appear to have interchangeable components; however, this may not necessarily be the case. Caution in application is encouraged. Endoscopic management of ureteral stricture is discussed later under Operative Endoscopy.

In addition, each manufacturer has available a variety of adjunctive endoscopic accessories, including operating bridges, grasping and foreign-body forceps, coagulating electrodes, and teaching attachments. Space limitations prevent a detailed review of these endoscopic accessories; the interested reader should consult the individual manufacturers' catalogues for additional information.

Light Sources

Fiberoptic light sources of variable intensity and flexible light-conducting systems are available from the various manufacturers. The Storz fluid light-conducting system greatly reduces the slight yellow hue that the fiber bundle imparts to the visual field, improving overall endoscopic visualization. Xenon light sources provide a brighter illumination than standard light sources and are useful when performing endophotography; caution must be

exercised to avoid thermal injury resulting from increased heat transfer when employing xenon light sources.

Teaching Attachments

Improved illumination and better visualization afforded by modern lens systems have revolutionized teaching attachments. It is now possible for both the endoscopist and the observer to have sufficient illumination for excellent endoscopic visualization. Both flexible and articulated attachments are available for teaching the student and house staff and for endophotography.

Retrograde Catheters

Sterile, disposable whistle-tip, pigtail, olivetip, and double pigtail ureteral catheters are available in 3 Fr. and larger sizes. The smallest cone-tip ureteral catheter available is an 8 Fr. tip on a 5 Fr. stem and is thus of limited application in pediatric patients.

Specialized ureteral stents, such as double pigtail catheters, are available in a 5 Fr. caliber and in 8-, 10-, and 12-cm lengths. Such indwelling catheters may be appropriate in selected situations when longer term ureteral intubation is necessary. Transurethral double pigtail catheter placement may not be possible in the small male as a result both of the small

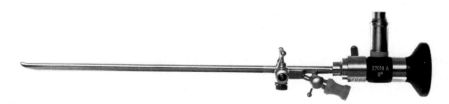

Figure 5–3 □ A 10 French sheath with interchangeable direct and forward-oblique lenses; the instrument will accommodate a 4 French ureteral catheter.

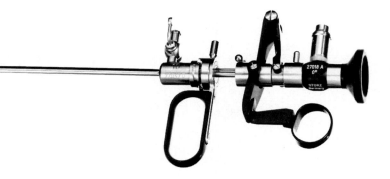

Figue 5–4 □ A 10 French pediatric resectoscope.

caliber of the male urethra and also of instrument limitations that do not permit passage of a 5 Fr. caliber catheter through the operating port. Transurethral catheter retrieval may be performed employing fine grasping forceps or by loop extraction employing a fine monofilament snare made with a shortened 3 or 4 Fr. ureteral catheter that can be passed through the operating port of a pediatric panendoscope.

Irrigating Solutions

Either sterile water or saline, warmed to body temperature, may be used as the irrigant for endoscopic examination. Because of the risk for hemolysis or electrolyte disturbance from intravascular absorption or intraperitoneal perforation during endoscopic surgery, sterile water is appropriate for endoscopic surgery only in brief procedures. Sterile water permits endoscopic fulguration and/or resection without changing irrigating solutions, but it is safer to use normal saline on a routine basis.

Hypothermia is a serious and potentially life-threatening complication of pediatric endoscopy. Utilization of warm irrigating solutions and monitoring of body temperature should prevent the development of systemic hypothermia and the associated acidosis (Meyers and Oh).

Bougies and Sounds

Otis bougies à boule and female urethral sounds are familiar and commonly available instruments requiring no special comment. The different curvature of the bulbous urethra and the rigidity of the urogenital diaphragm in the young male requires construction of infant male sounds with a shape and tip conforming to the shorter curvature of the urethra in the young boy, or unnecessary iatrogenic urethral injury may result.

ENDOSCOPIC SUITE

Because urologic endoscopic procedures in children necessitate some form of anesthesia, a fully equipped suite within an operating or anesthesia suite is safest. Cystoscopic examination under local anesthesia is not appropriate in childhood. Our cystoscopic table is hydraulically operated, including a movable table top. Customized clamps accommodate the smaller knee supports necessary for younger children (Fig. 5–5). An electrosurgical unit appropriately calibrated for pediatric endoscopic surgery should be a permanent part of any pediatric endoscopic unit. For convenience, there is a portable cabinet to organize and store endoscopic equipment. The top of this cabinet expands to provide a larger surface area for placement of the sterile endoscopic supplies (Fig. 5–6).

The importance of the dynamic factors in evaluating certain urologic disorders in childhood cannot be overemphasized; accordingly, an image intensifier is mounted on the endoscopic table in the unit. The size of the x-ray field is easily and accurately controlled by a variable collimator with separate vertical and lateral shutter adjustments as well as a swivel mount to rotate the axes of the field.

Video tape and 105-mm x-ray capability permit documentation of dynamic fluoroscopic studies for later review or for conversion to a video cassette for closed-circuit transmission to conferences or later review. In addition, there are 35-mm photographic and video cassette capabilities to record endoscopic observations.

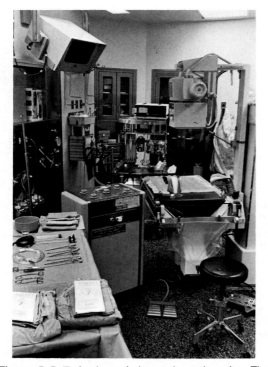

Figure 5–5 □ A view of the endoscopic suite. The power-operated table is as described. Custom clamps accommodate the smaller knee supports necessary for young children. Note the under table image-intensifier which includes a cine camera, variable collimator; the television monitor is conveniently located. The instrument storage cabinet, with side shelves elevated, serves as a surface for the sterile instrument table. A typical sterile setup is shown; less frequently used supplies are added as necessary. In actual use the electrosurgical unit and sterile table are positioned more conveniently for the endoscopist.

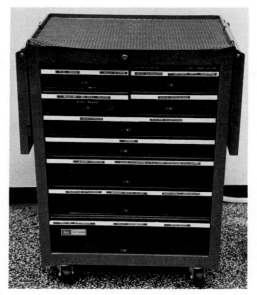

Figure 5–6 □ The author's portable instrument storage cabinet; the side shelves of the cabinet, when extended, serve as a surface for the sterile cystoscopic instrument table.

CYSTOSCOPIC TECHNIQUE

Cystoscopic technique in the infant and child is similar to that in the adult and therefore is not discussed in detail. However, certain precautions relevant to introducing the cystoscope into the urethra and a description of normal and abnormal endoscopic anatomy in childhood and adolescence are reviewed.

Cystoscopy is done with the child in the lithotomy position, although in small infants and young girls, an exaggerated frog-leg position is also acceptable. Appropriate sterile surgical preparation is done prior to cytoscopy; sterile technique is maintained throughout the procedure. The surgeon should scrub preoperatively and wear a mask (covering the nose), surgical cap, and sterile gown and gloves.

Particular care is required to avoid urethral

injury, and consistent gentleness of technique is mandatory. When the sheath is introduced, the obturator should be in place; a well-lubricated instrument must be guided, not forced, into the urethra. Forcing a sheath through a tight urethra may result in urethral laceration or false passage formation and later urethral stricture formation.

Although there is a normal range of urethral caliber for each sex and age group, this author uses the smallest caliber instrument that can be inserted without damaging the urethra. In the male child, the range of urethral size is limited (Allen et al). The narrowest portion of the male urethra is the external meatus. Meatotomy is infrequently required before cystourethroscopy; however, when necessary, a simple crush meatotomy permits easy passage of the instrument. Our experience demonstrates that most boys over 6 months of age will easily and atraumatically tolerate a 7.5 or 8.5 Fr. pediatric panendoscope, permitting retrograde ureteral catheterization or posterior urethral valve ablation using a 3 Fr. ureteral catheter passed through the operating port of the instrument. The male urethra of the toddler and older child usually accommodates a 10 or 13 Fr. sheath without difficulty.

Occasionally, the penile urethra is of insufficient size to permit passage of even the smallest infant cystoscope. In this situation, a perineal urethrostomy can be performed. Placing traction sutures in the urethral edges permits easy access to the larger caliber proximal bulbar urethra, thus allowing the endoscopic examination as well as fulguration of posterior urethral valves, retrograde ureteropyelography, or calculus manipulation. With the increased diagnostic yield of modern pediatric uroradiographic techniques, perineal urethrostomy solely for endoscopic observation appears unwarranted.

I do not advocate routine dilation of the urethra prior to cystourethroscopy, especially in the male child, as this may produce iatrogenic injury to the delicate urethral tissues and a potential for later stricture formation. Direct visual observation of the male urethra during passage of the instrument minimizes urethral trauma and permits observation of the entire urethra, preventing possible iatrogenic change. Prior to formal examination of the bladder, a urine specimen for urinalysis and culture and sensitivity testing should be obtained.

The elasticity and distensibility of the female urethra, even in the neonate, permits greater flexibility in the choice of instrument size and the type of operative endoscopic procedures applicable in little girls (Immergut and Wahman). In the female child, the sheath and obturator may be introduced directly into the bladder and the telescope then inserted.

The normal prepubertal male urethra is pale pink and of uniform caliber except at the penoscrotal angle and at the urogenital diaphragm, where physiologic narrowing or sphincter spasm may be misinterpreted as a urethral stricture. The entrances of Cowper's ducts are frequently visualized (see Color Plate 5–1D). In the deep bulbar urethra, the normal longitudinal vasculature of the urethra becomes more prominent at the urogenital diaphragm and should not be misinterpreted as anterior (bulbar) urethritis or some other inflammatory process. Similarly, the urothelium of the verumontanum, prostatic urethra, and bladder neck is usually more vascular than the urothelium of the penile urethra.

The bladder neck in both sexes is usually supple and not prominent. In boys with posterior urethral valves or long-standing voiding dysfunction, the bladder neck may be elevated and appear obstructive. Generally, this is not the case; treatment of the bladder neck itself is seldom, if ever, necessary inasmuch as the visual abnormalities of the bladder neck generally resolve after relief of the distal outlet obstruction or correction of the voiding dysfunction.

The trigone is normally pale and smooth. In the pubertal and adolescent girl, the trigone may become irregular or rugated, simulating cystitis cystica or chronic inflammation. This is generally not the case inasmuch as the observed changes are only seen to develop at puberty and most often in the absence of documented urinary tract infection, presumably the result of hormonal (estrogen) influence.

The ureteral orifices are located symmetrically within one or two visual fields (endoscopic) of the midline of the trigone. Orifice shape—cone, stadium, horseshoe, golf-hole (Fig. 5–7; Color Plate 5–2A and B; see Color Plate 5–1E and F)— and orifice position (Fig. 5–8) should be recorded with the bladder empty and after bladder filling. The visual appearance of the ureteral orifice varies, depending upon whether a direct vision (0 degrees) or forward-oblique (30 degrees) telescope is used. The endoscopist should develop a routine that permits consistent and reproducible observation.

The normal ureteral orifice is cone-shaped or volcano-shaped (see Color Plate 5–1E) and located at the "A" position on the trigone. The normal ureteral orifice retains its appearance and does not migrate laterally with bladder filling. The stadium orifice (see Color Plate 5–1F) is more laterally positioned ("B" position) on the trigone, is oval in shape, and may migrate laterally with bladder filling. The horseshoe orifice (see Color Plate 5–2A) has lost its medial rim and is usually in the "B" or "C" position on the trigone; lateral migration of the orifice usually occurs with bladder filling. The golf-hole orifice (see Color Plate 5–2B) has poor trigonal attachment and is usually found in the "C–D" position; there is little or no submucosal ureteral tunnel, producing the gaping golf-hole appearance of this orifice.

The length of the submucosal ureteral tunnel can be estimated or measured using a ureteral catheter. The length of the submucosal ureteral tunnel and the position of the ureteral orifice when the bladder is fully distended provide important guidelines in predicting spontaneous resolution of vesicoureteral reflux. The cystoscopy report should include the shape and position of the ureteral orifices and submucosal tunnel length, and the presence of ureteral duplication (see Color Plate 5–2C) or ectopia, trabeculation (see Color Plate 5–2D), diverticulum, tumor, stone, foreign body,

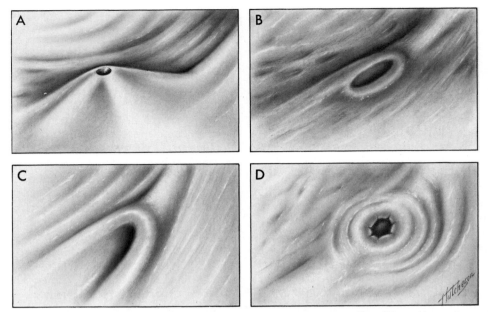

Figure 5–7 □ Appearances of ureteral orifice. Normal orifice *(A)*. Stadium-type orifice *(B)*, and horseshoe orifice *(C)* are variants of normal and generally do not reflux if a submucosal tunnel of adequate length is present. The "golf-hole" orifice *(D)* almost always refluxes. Generally, no submucosal tunnel is present.

bleeding points (see Color Plate 5–2E), or other abnormality, as well as bladder capacity. The cystoscopy report should become a permanent part of the medical record (see Fig. 5–8).

OPERATIVE ENDOSCOPY

Posterior Urethral Valves

Posterior urethral valves may be suspected after in utero fetal ultrasonography but may be confused with massive primary vesicoureteral reflux. A postnatal voiding cystourethrogram confirms the diagnosis of posterior urethral valves. Posterior urethral valves represent an obstructing diaphragm distal to the verumontanum with an eccentric annulus (see Color Plate 5–2F). Transurethral incision of the obstructing diaphragm (valves) can be done in the neonate and small infant through a 7.5 Fr. or larger infant panendoscope, or in the larger infant or young boy using a 13 or 14 Fr. sheath or 9.5, 10, or 13 Fr. pediatric resectoscope with a direct-vision or forward-oblique telescope. When a cystoscope sheath is used, a 3 or 4 Fr. ureteral catheter passed through the side channel may be converted into a satisfactory electrode using the catheter as the insulating sheath and advancing a wire

stylet 1 to 2 mm beyond the end of the catheter to serve as a straight electrode; alternately the wire may be fashioned into a small hook electrode. When employing an infant resectoscope, the clinician may use a loop electrode or right-angle resectoscope electrode to incise the valve leaflets. This author finds the right-angle electrode most useful and the safest for valve incision.

The electrosurgical unit should be calibrated before the valve leaflets are incised. This author uses a cutting current to insure a clean incision. It is not necessary to remove the entire valve leaflet, which is most commonly quite thin. Simple incision in several places—posterolaterally on each side, and distal to the verumontanum, taking care not to injure the verumontanum—usually provides satisfactory valve ablation and avoids accidental injury to the ejaculatory ducts or external sphincter. Residual obstruction is unusual and is easily managed at a later time. After incision of the valve leaflets, the clinician may instill contrast material into the bladder and perform an expression cystourethrogram to verify relief of the obstruction.

Anterior Urethral Valves and Urethral Diverticula

Anterior urethral valves and anterior urethral diverticula are rare causes of congenital uri-

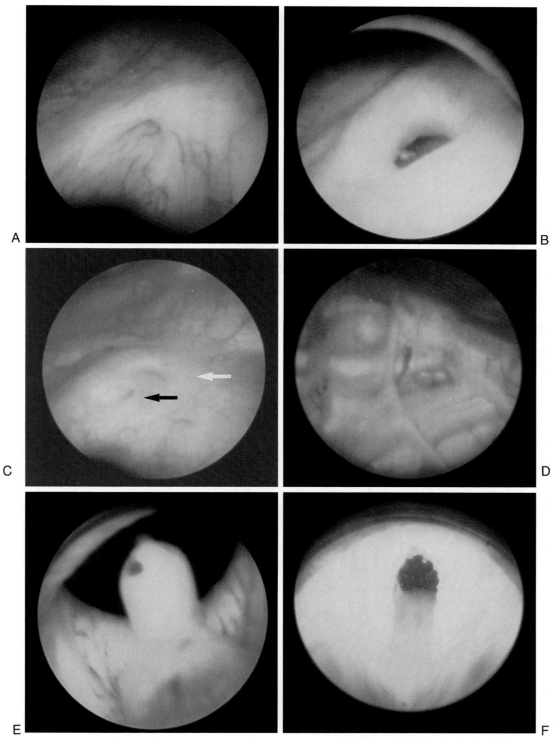

Plate 5–2 □ *A,* Horseshoe-shaped ureteral orifice; the orifice has lost its medial rim. *B,* Golf hole-shaped ureteral orifice; there is little or no submucosal ureteral tunnel. *C,* Duplicated ureteral orifices; the upper and more lateral orifice *(white arrow)* drains the lower renal segment; the lower and more medial orifice *(black arrow)* drains the upper renal segment. *D,* Bladder trabeculation in a boy with urinary outlet obstruction. *E,* A urethral polyp originating from the verumontanum in a boy with hematuria. *F,* Posterior urethral valves.

DO NOT WRITE IN THIS MARGIN

CYSTOSCOPIC EXAMINATION

DATE
PATIENT NO.
PATIENT NAME
MEDICAL RECORD NO.
BIRTH DATE SEX
PHYSICIAN

HISTORY ______________________________

PHYSICAL FINDINGS ______________________________

IVP ______________________________

CYSTOGRAM ______________________________

URINALYSIS
BLADDER ____________ (R) ____________ (L) ____________

URINE CULTURE
BLADDER ____________ (R) ____________ (L) ____________

INSTRUMENT SIZE ________ LENS ________ BLADDER RESIDUAL ________

URETHRA
MEATUS ________ LENGTH ________ MUCOSA ________

CALIBRATION FR. ____ DILATATION FR. ____ MEATOTOMY ____ URETHROTOMY ____ OTHER ____

BLADDER
BLADDER NECK ________ TRIGONE ________ CAPACITY ________

MUCOSA ________ TRABECULATION ________

URETERAL ORIFICES

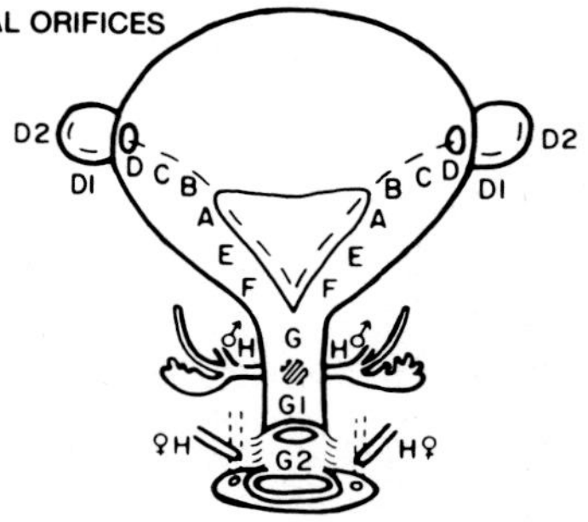

Rt. Orifice Posn								(✓)	Lt. Orifice Posn							
H	G	F	E	D	C	B	A	Shape	A	B	C	D	E	F	G	H
								✱ Golf Hole								
								Horseshoe								
								Stadium								
								Normal								
								Size								
								Small(S) Med.(M) Large(L)								
								Patulous(P) NonPat(NP)								
								Submucosal Tunnel m.m.								

RETROGRADE STUDIES (R) ________ (L) ________

PERISTALSIS (R) ________ (L) ________

OTHER OBSERVATIONS & CONCLUSIONS ______________________________

PLAN ______________________________

SURGEON ______________________________

FORM OR 3

▒ If ureteric orifice is duplicated, describe U.O. corresponding with cranial renal segment in shaded part of appropriate column.

✱ Paraureteral Diverticulum R. Present □ Not Present □ L. Present □ Not Present □

If present, denote site of U.O. in relation to diverticulum as shown on diagram D, D1, D2 when possible in D column/s.

White, MEDICAL RECORD — Canary, SURGEON — Pink, RESIDENT — Gold, DEPT.

Figure 5–8 □ Cystoscopy report. Endoscopic findings should be recorded on a cystoscopy record that becomes a permanent part of the patient record.

nary outlet obstruction. They appear to represent a similar entity, a fusion defect of the ventral urethral wall. The distal edge of the diverticulum may act as an obstructing flap during voiding, obstructing micturition. Anterior valves with limited urethral undermining are easily managed by transurethral incision or resection; larger diverticula or those with extensive urethral undermining necessitate open repair.

Ureterocele

The role of transurethral management of ureteroceles (Cendron et al; Monfort et al) is limited because transurethral incision or resection of an ectopic ureterocele usually trades obstruction for problematic reflux into a dilated, poorly functioning collecting system. Most authors agree that ectopic ureteroceles in infants and children are best treated by open surgery. However, large ectopic ureteroceles associated with severe urinary sepsis may be managed by transurethral incision on an emergency basis with planned delayed reconstruction. During endoscopic evaluation, an ectopic ureterocele may collapse with bladder filling or even evert through the ureteral hiatus and be mistaken for a bladder diverticulum (Color Plate 5–3A). Such endoscopic observations should not pose a diagnostic or therapeutic dilemma inasmuch as preoperative uroradiographic studies generally define the anatomy that will be encountered at endoscopic evaluation and/or management.

Simple ureteroceles are usually asymptomatic and are infrequently diagnosed in childhood. Occasionally, they may be associated with significant obstruction or stone formation, or both. Because incision of the ureterocele wall with a loop electrode usually permits postoperative vesicoureteral reflux, simple ureteroceles may be treated by careful medial incision of the stenotic meatus with a fine-tip flexible electrode or with endoscopic scissors avoiding the ureterocele wall. Significant post-incision vesicoureteral reflux is unusual but may be treated electively if it persists or becomes symptomatic. Similarly, a stenotic ureteral meatus may be minimally incised to relieve any obstruction present.

Occasionally, ureteral meatotomy is indicated for management of ureteral obstruction following ureteral reimplantation when the obstruction appears to be the result of distal ureteral fibrosis or an excessively long submucosal tunnel rather than the result of too tight a detrusor hiatus or extravesical ureteral kinking. Ureteral meatotomy may also be indicated when a calculus is lodged in the distal ureter. When carefully done, ureteral meatotomy may relieve the obstruction or allow calculus removal without producing postoperative vesicoureteral reflux.

Bladder Neck Obstruction

Bladder neck obstruction and bladder neck hypertrophy are uncommon diagnoses in childhood; bladder neck hypertrophy is usually secondary to distal obstruction (posterior urethral valves, urethral stricture, or detrusor-sphincter-dyssynergia) and will resolve after correction of the outlet obstruction. We have not had reason to perform transurethral surgery for management of bladder neck obstruction or hypertrophy. Retrograde ejaculation and vesicovaginal fistula are potential complications after bladder neck resection (or incision) in males and after deep resection of the bladder neck in females, respectively.

Urinary Calculi

Transurethral Calculus Management

The indications and techniques for transurethral management of urinary calculi in childhood are similar to those for adults. As noted previously, the small size of the male urethra in childhood may limit endoscopic manipulation of urinary calculi. The distensibility of the urethra in little girls permits use of adult-sized instruments and more latitude in transurethral management of urinary calculi. In either situation particular care is necessary to avoid urethral injury; consistent gentleness of technique is mandatory.

For manipulation of lower ureteral calculi, basket extractors are available in 4 and 5 Fr. sizes for use through a 13 or 14 Fr. pediatric panendoscope. Transurethral manipulation of lower ureteral calculi carries the same risks of complication as in the adult and always should be performed employing fluoroscopic monitoring.

Ureteroscopic management of urinary calculi in small children is now possible by using an 8.5 Fr. rigid ureteroscope or the newly

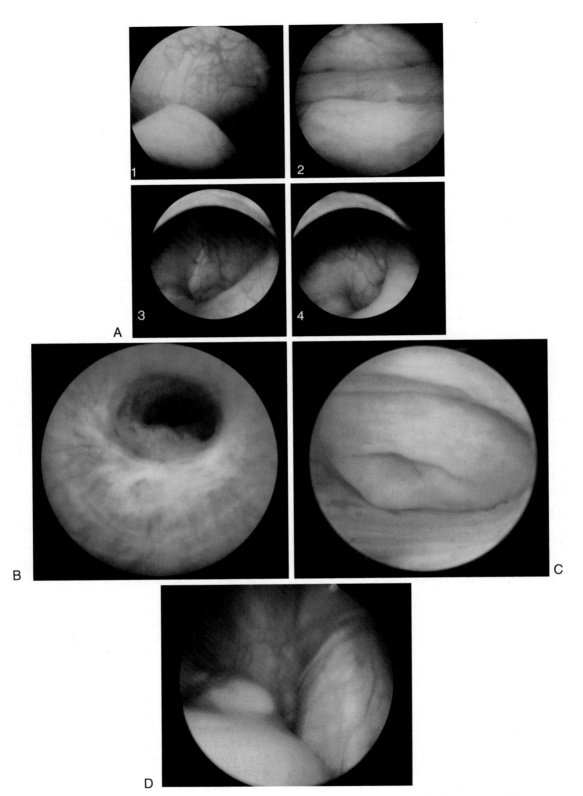

Plate 5–3 □ *A,* Ectopic ureterocele. The ureterocele bulges into the bladder (1), gradually flattens with increased bladder filling (2), and everts outside the bladder simulating a bladder diverticulum (3 and 4). *B,* Urethral stricture. *C,* Vaginoscopy; a normal prepubertal cervix. *D,* Laparoscopy; the lower pole of the testes and the gubernaculum *(black arrows)* at the internal ring *(open arrow)* in a boy with a nonpalpable undescended testicle. (Courtesy of M. Maizels and L. R. King.)

marketed 9.8 Fr. flexible or the 7.2 Fr. semi-rigid ureteroscope. Rigid or balloon ureteral dilators and double pigtail stents are now available in pediatric sizes. Once the calculus is visualized through the ureteroscope, calculus removal may be accomplished by employing a basket extractor or grasping forceps. Impacted calculi are manageable with either electrohydraulic, ultrasonographic, or pulsed dye laser lithotripsy under direct vision.

Electrohydraulic lithotripsy of ureteral calculi carries a risk of ureteral perforation and probably should be avoided if a laser or ultrasound unit is available. Decreased probe size (2.5 or 3 Fr.) and improved endoscopic equipment may eventually make electrohydraulic lithotripsy a less hazardous technique for management of ureteral calculi in childhood. Electrohydraulic lithotripsy usually results in calculus fragmentation, producing large fragments. Once the calculus has been electrohydraulically broken, the fragments must be additionally fragmented to a passable size or basket-extracted (Payne et al).

The most recent innovation for management of ureteral calculi is the pulsed dye laser (Ritchey et al; Dretler, 1987). The pulsed dye laser may be used within either a rigid or flexible ureteroscope. The laser fiber is quite small and may be used bare (without additional support), within a ureteral catheter, or in a laser stone-basket. The laser fiber must be in contact with the calculus (preferably perpendicular to it) for fragmentation to occur because calculus fragmentation results from direct light absorption by the calculus and the formation and expansion of a cloud of electrons called a "plasma" bubble. Laser fragmentation is precise, producing easily passable 2- to 3-mm calculus fragments. Gentle irrigation with saline disperses blood and laser heat during the procedure. Complications of laser ureteral lithotripsy are uncommon and most often related to the requisite ureteroscopy rather than to the laser action itself (Dretler, 1988). Laser lithotripsy has been applied only recently for management of ureteral calculi in childhood. Its use appears encouraging inasmuch as the morbidity is minimal. However, additional experience and long-term follow-up are necessary to establish the place for laser lithotripsy in management of ureteral calculi in childhood (Ritchey et al).

When considering ureteroscopic management of upper urinary calculi in childhood, one must recognize the risk of producing permanent damage to the ureterovesical junction as a consequence of dilating the small submucosal and intramural ureter of the child. Such iatrogenic injury may result in post-treatment vesicoureteral reflux or ureteral stricture, or both. Because of the infrequent reports of ureteroscopy in childhood, the actual incidence of postdilation vesicoureteral reflux and/or ureteral stricture is unknown. In adults the incidence of postdilation vesicoureteral reflux approaches 20 per cent when the distal ureter is dilated to 24 Fr. or greater (Segura). Distal ureteral stricture is uncommon. It appears prudent to dilate the distal ureter in children to a size only slightly larger than required to permit passage of the smallest useful ureteroscope. Reports of ureteroscopic calculus manipulation in young children are uncommon, and long-term follow-up is necessary to define the efficacy of ureteroscopy in childhood (Blute; Kostakopoulos).

Endoscopic Management of Vesicoureteral Reflux

Transurethral endoscopic management of vesicoureteral reflux by subureteric injection of polytetrafluoroethylene paste, "The Sting," was reported by Puri and O'Donnell in 1984. Their initial 2-year experience with more than 150 ureters resulted in an 85 per cent success rate (O'Donnell and Puri) without postoperative ureteral obstruction.

For subureteric polytef (Teflon) paste injection, a cystoscope with an offset lens (Wolf) is used combined with an "injection gun" with a specially designed 22-gauge needle (Storz) attached to the tip of the injection gun. The needle is slowly and accurately inserted at the 6 o'clock position beneath the mucosa of the ureteral orifice into the subureteric lamina propria of the distal ureter. Once the needle is in position, 0.3 to 0.8 ml of the polytetrafluoroethylene paste is slowly injected until a flattened crescentic ureteral orifice sits on a bead of the paste. Most procedures are performed on an outpatient basis.

Although the procedure is not as successful as an open surgical ureteral reimplantation, results after "The Sting" procedure improve with experience. Some question the efficacy and long-term wisdom of this procedure in childhood. Polytetrafluoroethylene particles have been injected for otolaryngologic procedures for many years; however, migration of polytetrafluoroethylene particles has been reported after urologic application (Malizia et al). Laboratory evaluation employing various collagen preparations is ongoing in an effort to eliminate the concerns related to polytetrafluoroethylene while maintaining a high success rate in correcting vesicoureteral reflux (Canning and Gearhart). In addition, it is unclear whether one might encounter late recurrence of the vesicoureteral reflux or ureteral obstruction. There is also uncertainty as to the long-term safety of polytetrafluoroethylene in infants and young children. Additional carefully monitored evaluation and follow-up of subureteric injection of polytetrafluoroethylene and collagen are mandatory to define their long-term efficacy in management of vesicoureteral reflux in childhood.

BLADDER CALCULI

Most bladder calculi encountered in childhood are endemic, formed around foreign bodies, or are the consequence of poor bladder drainage in children with a neurogenic bladder, bladder outlet obstruction, or intravesical foreign bodies (Griffith). Vesical calculi are most often large and may require open surgical removal, although some soft, infection-related calculi may be amenable to transurethral or suprapubic lithotripsy or litholapaxy. Electrohydraulic lithotripsy employing a 3.5 or 5 Fr. probe may permit transurethral fragmentation of bladder calculi using either rigid or flexible access to the bladder. The ultrasonographic lithotrite is of too large a diameter for routine transurethral use in childhood, especially in the male. When transurethral calculus removal is performed in males, the delicateness of the urethra in the young boy must be a primary consideration—precluding prolonged traumatic transurethral procedures and favoring open cystolithotomy.

Urethral Stricture and External Sphincter Spasm

Transurethral treatment of congenital or acquired urethral strictures (see Color Plate 5–3B) can be accomplished either by cold knife or by electroincision. A pediatric Otis urethrotome also may be used to incise strictures but is a blind instrument with a closed diameter of approximately 13 Fr. and therefore not appropriate for infants and young children. The cold knife or the Sachse urethrotome offers more versatility and permits direct-vision internal urethrotomy with inspection of the entire stricture and complete division of all scar under direct vision (Smith et al). Transcutaneous or transurethral injection of steroid into the stricture prior to incision may lessen postoperative reaction and stricture recurrence. Care must be exercised not to interchange the Storz pediatric urethrotome components with those of the infant or pediatric resectoscope. Even though they appear identical, the components are not interchangeable and may create a frustrating situation.

Urinary outlet obstruction as a result of narrowing of the urethra at the urogenital diaphragm may be the consequence of external sphincter spasm in some forms of neuropathic bladder dysfunction, in children with myelodysplasia, or in boys with prune-belly syndrome. Such inappropriate external sphincter contraction (narrowing) may interfere with bladder emptying and contribute to urinary infection or upper tract deterioration, or both. One form of treatment for such obstruction is anterior sphincterotomy at the 12 o'clock position; urethral incision at other locations may cause excessive bleeding. Overaggressive sphincter incision may result in intractable urinary incontinence and should be avoided.

Complications of Pediatric Endoscopy

Potential complications during or after pediatric endoscopy may be avoided or minimized by employing gentle technique and by keeping the endoscopic procedure as brief as possible. Adherence to meticulous sterile technique should make postinstrumentation urinary infection uncommon. Sepsis is more common after prolonged vigorous instrumentation or instrumentation of an anomalous or infected urinary tract with poor emptying characteristics. In such situations, maintenance of adequate post-instrumentation drainage or post-instrumentation administration of culture-specific antibiotics, or both, reduces or minimizes the possibility of urosepsis.

Mechanical injury to the urethra may occur with laceration, perforation, or false passage formation as the result of excessive trauma or the use of a tightly fitting sheath. Because stricture of the male urethra may follow instrumentation, even months or years later, a difficult or complicated endoscopic examination requires careful long-term follow-up.

Infants and small boys may experience temporary postoperative urinary retention because of dysuria or edema even after a gently performed cystoscopic examination. Temporary indwelling or clean intermittent catheterization may be necessary; trocar cystostomy is rarely necessary for management of postcystoscopy urinary retention.

Tearing of the bladder mucosa or rupture of the bladder may be the consequence of direct trauma from the cystoscope or overdistention of the bladder. Bladder capacity in childhood is estimated in ounces as age (years) plus or minus one, to about age 8.

Perforation of the ureter or renal parenchyma may occur during forceful ureteral catheterization, ureteroscopy, or percutaneous endoscopic manipulation of ureteral calculi. The potential for injury to the submucosal or intramuscular ureter after dilation prior to ureteroscopy has been previously discussed. Renal parenchymal injury may occur during establishment of percutaneous access, during percutaneous tract dilation or during definitive percutaneous endourologic procedures.

Deep resection of posterior urethral valves may result in injury to the ejaculatory ducts, urinary incontinence, or membranous urethral stricture. Transurethral resection of the female bladder neck or trigone may be complicated by postoperative urinary incontinence and/or vesicovaginal fistula and is not an appropriate maneuver.

An infrequent but potentially serious complication of cystoscopy is hypothermia from the use of cold or room temperature irrigating solutions. Every effort should be made to utilize body temperature irrigating solutions and to monitor body temperature carefully during cystoscopy to prevent systemic hypothermia and the associated metabolic acidosis (Meyers and Oh).

OTHER ENDOSCOPIC PROCEDURES

Vaginoscopy

The indications for vaginoscopy include vaginal discharge, genital malformation, vaginal tumor, and nonmenstrual vaginal bleeding. Vaginoscopy performed using a pediatric panendoscope with a direct-vision telescope (0 degrees) with the patient under general anesthesia provides a much clearer view of the vagina and cervix than can be obtained with a vaginal or nasal speculum. The childhood vagina is narrow and relatively long; the cervix is small, pale, and often hidden in mucosal folds of the vaginal fornix, where it may be difficult to visualize (see Color Plate 5–3C). A snug panendoscope and high water pressure should be avoided, as retrograde reflux of irrigating solution into the peritoneal cavity may cause peritonitis. Biopsy of vaginal or cervical lesions is rarely indicated but may be done with a biopsy forceps or a pediatric resectoscope.

Nephroscopy and Percutaneous Nephrostolithotomy

Percutaneous access to the pediatric kidney is an established technique. In pediatric urology, percutaneous endoscopy is useful to localize and manipulate intrarenal calculi and to identify the site of intrarenal bleeding. Pediatric nephroscopic techniques are analogous to those in the adult. Percutaneous management of surgically active upper urinary calculi in childhood may present problems because of the small size and mobility of the pediatric kidney, the small size of the collecting system, and the relatively large size of currently available percutaneous endourologic instruments (Krieger et al). Dilation of the percutaneous access tract to provide for percutaneous calculus manipulation and/or destruction has documented effectiveness in the adult. It has been demonstrated that the same endourologic techniques are applicable for management of upper urinary calculi in childhood (Payne et al). Some clinicians have concern about performing percutaneous procedures in infants or small children (younger than 5 years of age); improved (reduced) instrument size should facilitate percutaneous management of upper urinary calculi in small children (Boddy et al).

Percutaneous calculus management in childhood is conducted in a manner similar to that in the adult except in the very small child or infant, where instrument size may limit the applicability of percutaneous techniques (Papanicolaou et al). Percutaneous access is easily established under ultrasonographic or fluoroscopic monitoring using the Seldinger technique. A posterior or posterolateral subcostal approach is utilized to enter the collecting system. Pyelocalyceal anatomy is initially demonstrated by performing a thin needle (22 gauge) antegrade pyelogram or after excretory or retrograde ureteropyelography. This permits localization of the collecting system and planning the percutaneous access to facilitate calculus manipulation (Papanicolaou et al). Because most obstructing upper urinary calculi produce proximal urinary dilatation, antegrade percutaneous calculus manipulation may be facilitated (Marburger et al).

A variety of equipment is available to assist nephrostomy placement and tract dilation. Initial percutaneous tract dilation can be done after percutaneous puncture employing rigid dilators, progressively larger vascular dilators, or high-pressure balloon dilating catheters. Local bleeding may preclude calculus manipulation at the time of initial percutaneous access and tract dilatation. I usually perform percutaneous tract dilation and calculus manipulation in different sessions to lessen the risk for renal parenchymal laceration and hemorrhage during tract dilation and to facilitate calculus manipulation.

Rigid and flexible nephroscopes also may be used for calculus manipulation. Rigid nephroscopes are available in 24 to 26 Fr. size and easily accommodate either electrohydraulic or ultrasonographic lithotrites or percutaneous grasping forceps and stone basket extractors (Alken et al). Rigid nephroscopes may not permit location and management of multiple renal calculi without establishing multiple percutaneous tracts. The safety of establishing multiple percutaneous tracts in the pediatric kidney has not been established. Recently available flexible nephroscopes permit examination and calculus extraction from most areas of the collecting system and are usable in children.

Ultrasonographic lithotrites are preferable to electrohydraulic units for performing percutaneous lithotripsy because of a lesser risk for collecting system perforation and the greater efficiency of the ultrasonographic units. When the ultrasonographic lithotrite is used, the calculus is fragmented by sound waves generated and conducted down the lithotrite, the tip of which must be in contact with the calculus for fragmentation to occur. Calculus debris is extracted through the center of the

probe as lithotripsy is occurring. Completeness of calculus fragmentation and fragment removal is monitored by repeated fluoroscopy or ultrasonography.

For percutaneous electrohydraulic lithotripsy, a short-duration electrical discharge within a fluid medium creates a high-pressure bubble of steam (cavitation bubble), the expansion and contraction of which creates a shock wave in front of the calculus, fragmenting it. Percutaneous electrohydraulic lithotripsy carries a risk for injury to the collecting system wall. In addition, calculus fragments produced after electrohydraulic lithotripsy are large and require extraction or further electrohydraulic lithotripsy to reduce fragment size, further increasing the risk for collecting system injury. The choice of the type of percutaneous lithotripsy employed—laser, electrohydraulic, or ultrasound—is dependent upon the instrumentation available and the experience of the involved surgeon.

After completion of percutaneous calculus destruction, the clinician positions a nephrostomy catheter in the renal pelvis under uroradiographic monitoring. Plain and oblique x-rays taken a day or two postoperatively document complete calculus removal and fragment passage or indicate the necessity for additional calculus fragmentation or chemolysis. A nephrostogram documents distal ureteral patency. Overnight nephrostomy clamping ensures unobstructed drainage; the nephrostomy tube is then removed.

Current experience with percutaneous calculus removal in childhood is encouraging. Bleeding, urinary infection, and residual calculi are infrequent. Operative and postoperative morbidity are minimal, with hospital stay shorter and related medical expenses much lower than for open surgical procedures. It appears that long-term renal damage is minimal after percutaneous nephrostolithotomy in childhood despite establishing and dilating percutaneous tracts in the pediatric kidney (Hulbert et al; Mayo et al; Pfister et al).

Urinary calculus disease in childhood is often metabolic or infectious in origin with anticipated recurrences that may necessitate multiple additional procedures for future calculus management. Percutaneous nephrostolithotomy is a less invasive technique than open surgical lithotomy and appears to make additional procedures safer, especially when extracorporeal shock wave lithotripsy is not feasible or appropriate. If residual calculus remains after endoscopic nephrolithotomy, additional endourologic treatment is facilitated by the presence of an established percutaneous access to the kidney, or percutaneous irrigation with calculolytic solutions is possible. Additional experience and long-term follow-up should confirm the efficacy of percutaneous nephrostolithotomy for management of upper urinary calculi in childhood.

Laparoscopy

Laparoscopy using a pediatric laparoscope or panendoscope may permit identification of the nonpalpable undescended testis or an intraperitoneal anomaly such as an ovotestis, uterus, fallopian tube, or ovary. Identification of the internal spermatic vessels, vas deferens, or nonpalpable testicle (see Color Plate 5–3D) helps in the management of the nonpalpable testis (Bloom et al; Guiney et al; Joshi and Sotrel; Naslund et al). When the spermatic vessels and vas deferens end blindly in a scarlike area (vanishing testis syndrome), the child may be spared an operative exploration (Lowe et al).

Endophotography

Improved resolution and the wide viewing angle afforded by the newer lens systems, along with improvements in light sources and light transmission, have markedly improved the quality of endoscopic photographs and video recording for teaching and documentation of endoscopic findings. Any good single-lens reflex camera may be utilized for endophotography, although a special adaptor is necessary to secure the camera to the endoscopic eyepiece. Storz, Wolf, and Olympus offer excellent units with compatible light sources and flash generators. Additionally, motion picture and video technology has advanced to the point that endoscopic procedures may now be recorded with amazing accuracy in both detail and color. Such recordings subsequently become valuable teaching aids.

Bibliography

Alken P, Hutschenreeter R, Marburger M: Percutaneous stone manipulation. J Urol 125:463, 1981.

Allen JS, Summers JL, Wilkerson SE: Meatal calibration in newborn boys. J Urol 107:498, 1972.

Bloom DA, Ayers JWT, McGuire EJ: The role of laparoscopy in management of nonpalpable testes. Journal d'Urologie 94:465, 1988.

Blute ML, Segura JW, Patterson DE: Ureteroscopy. J Urol 139:510, 1988.

Boddy SAM, Kellett MJ, Fletcher MS, et al: Extracorporeal shock wave lithotripsy and percutaneous nephrolithotomy in children. J Pediatr Surg 221:223, 1987.

Canning DA, Gearhart JP: Limitations and alternatives to endoscopic correction of vesicoureteral reflux with polytef paste. Pediatr Surg Int 4:149, 1989.

Cendron J, Melin Y, Valayer J: Simplified treatment of ectopic ureterocele in 35 children. Eur Urol 7:321, 1981.

Chan JCM: Hematuria and proteinuria in the pediatric patient. Diagnostic approach. Urology 11:205, 1978.

Dretler SP: Laser photofragmentation of ureteral calculi: analysis of 75 cases. J Endourol 1:9–14, 1987.

Dretler SP: Techniques of laser lithotripsy. J Endourol 2:123, 1988.

Droller JM, Saral R, Santos G: Prevention of cyclophosphamide-induced hemorrhagic cystitis. Urology 20:256, 1982.

Dunn M, Smith JB, Abrams PH: Endoscopic examination in children. Br J Urol 50:586, 1978.

Griffith DP: Struvite stones. Kidney Int 13:372, 1978.

Guiney EJ, Corbally M, Malone PS: Laparoscopy and the management of the impalpable testis. Br J Urol 63:313, 1989.

Hulbert JC, Reddy PK, Gonzales R, et al: Percutaneous nephrostolithotomy: an alternative approach to the management of pediatric calculus diseases. Pediatrics 76:610, 1985.

Immergut MA, Wahman GE: The urethral caliber of female children with recurrent urinary tract infections. J Urol 99:189, 1968.

Johnson DK, Kroovand RL, Perlmutter AD: The changing role of cystoscopy in the pediatric patient. J Urol 123:232, 1980.

Joshi NP, Sotrel G: Diagnostic laparoscopy in apparent uterine agenesis. J Adolesc Health Care 9:403, 1988.

Kaplan GW, Brock WA: Idiopathic urethrorrhagia in boys. J Urol 128:1001, 1982.

Kaplan GW, Sammons TA, King LR: A blind comparison of dilation, urethrotomy and medication alone in treatment of urinary tract infections in girls. J Urol 109:917, 1973.

Kaplan WE, Dalton DP, Firlit CF: The endoscopic correction of reflux by polytetrafluoroethylene injection. J Urol 138:953, 1987.

Khasidy LR, Khashu B, Mallett B, et al: Transitional cell carcinoma of bladder in children. Urology 34:142, 1990.

Krieger JN, Rudd TG, Mayo ME: Infection stones in patients with myelomeningocele and ileal conduit urinary tract diversion.

Kostakopoulos A, Sofras F, Karayiannis A, et al: Ureterolithotripsy: report of 1000 cases. Br J Urol 63:243, 1989.

Lowe DH, Brock WA, Kaplan GW: Laparoscopy for localization of nonpalpable testes. J Urol 131:728, 1984.

Malizia AA, Reiman HM, Myers RP, et al: Migration and granulomatous reaction after periurethral injection of Polytef (Teflon). JAMA 251:3277, 1984.

Marburger M: Disintegration of renal and ureteral calculi with ultrasound. Urol Clin N Am 10:729, 1983.

Marburger M, Turk C, Steinkogler I: Piezoelectric extracorporeal shock wave lithotripsy in children. J Urol 142:349, 1989.

Mayo ME, Kreiger JN, Rudd TG: Effect of percutaneous nephrostolithotomy on renal function. J Urol 133:167, 1985.

Meyers MB, Oh TH: Prevention of hypothermia during cystoscopy in infants. Anesth Analg 55:592, 1976.

Monfort G, Morisson-Lacombe G, Coquet M: Endoscopic treatment of ureteroceles revisited. J Urol 133:1031, 1985.

Naslund MJ, Gearhart JP, Jeffs RD: Laparoscopy: its selected use in patients with unilateral nonpalpable testis after human chorionic gonadotropin stimulation. J Urol 142:108, 1989.

O'Donnell B, Puri P: Endoscopic correction of primary vesicoureteric reflux. Br J Urol 58:601, 1986.

Papanicolaou N, Pfister RC, Young HH, et al: Percutaneous ultrasonic lithotripsy of symptomatic renal calculi in children. Pediatr Radiol 16:13, 1986.

Payne SR, Ford TF, Wickham JEA: Endoscopic management of upper urinary tract stones. Br J Surg 72:822, 1985.

Pfister RC, Newhouse JH, Yoder IC, et al: Complications of percutaneous renal procedures: incidence and observations. Urol Clin North Am 10:563, 1983.

Puri P, O'Donnell B: Correction of experimentally produced vesicoureteric reflux in the piglet by intravesical injection of Teflon. Br Med J 289:5, 1984.

Reiner RJ, Kroovand RL, Perlmutter AD: Unusual aspects of urinary calculi in children. J Urol 121:480, 1979.

Ritchey M, Patterson DE, Kelalis PP, et al: A case of pediatric ureteroscopic lasertripsy. J Urol 139:1272, 1988.

Schulman CC, Simon J, Pamart D, et al: Endoscopic treatment of vesicoureteral reflux in children. J Urol 138 (Part 2):950, 1987.

Segura JW: Editorial comment. *In* Shepard P, Thomas R, Harmon EP: Urolithiasis in children: innovations in management. J Urol 140:790, 1988.

Smith PJB, Dunn M, Dounis A: The early results of treatment of stricture of the male urethra using the Sachse optical urethrotome. Br J Urol 51:224, 1979.

Timmons JW, Watts FB, Perlmutter AD: A comparison of awake and anesthesia cystography. Birth Defects 13:363, 1977.

Walther PC, Kaplan GW: Cystoscopy in children: indications for its use in common urologic problems. J Urol 122:717, 1979.

Walther PC, Lamm D, Kaplan GW: Pediatric urolithiasis: a ten year review. Pediatrics 65:1068, 1980.

6

☐ Physiology of Micturition and Urodynamics

Alan J. Wein and David M. Barrett

Neuromuscular disorders in children primarily affect the lower urinary tract by causing functional abnormalities of the bladder, the bladder outlet, or both. The upper urinary tract (ureter, renal collecting system, and renal parenchyma) is affected only secondarily, generally by the effects of distally generated backflow and back pressure. Normally, the upper tract manifests peristaltic activity, adapting its rate and rhythm to changes in diuresis and alterations in the state of bladder function. Peristaltic activity begins at pacemaker cells located at the junction of the renal parenchyma and the minor calyceal junctions (Weiss and Coolsaet). This pacemaker activity is propagated through the walls of the major calyces to the renal pelvis. The electrical activity is transmitted through the renal collecting system and across the renal pelvis and down the ureter by myogenic conduction. Whether an individual wave is transmitted from the renal pelvis to the ureter or not depends on the volume of urine in the renal pelvis.

Efficient propulsion of urine depends on the active and passive properties of the ureter and its ability to coapt its wall completely. Although contraction waves are subject to pharmacologic alteration in the laboratory, ureteral peristalsis in vivo seems to depend primarily on urine volume. Although autonomic nerve fibers exist in the muscularis of the renal collecting system and ureter, for the most part, they accompany small blood vessels and capillaries, and it is questionable whether, in vivo, they exercise any modulating effects on ureteral peristalsis (Wein et al; Weiss and Coolsaet). Urine passes into the lower urinary tract via the ureterovesical junction, which normally permits only antegrade transport. The lower urinary tract functions as a group of interrelated structures whose joint function is to bring about efficient bladder filling and urine storage and the voluntary expulsion of urine.

This chapter deals with the characteristics and manifestations of the primary effects of neuromuscular disease on the storage and emptying functions of the lower urinary tract. Generally, neuromuscular disorders do not affect the upper urinary tract primarily but only through infection, obstruction, or a sustained increase in intravesical pressure or vesicoureteral reflux. This section provides an overview of the anatomy, physiology, and pharmacology of lower urinary tract function in a framework of terms and concepts that is comprehensible and acceptable to practicing urologists and pediatricians.

RELEVANT ANATOMY AND TERMINOLOGY

The designation "lower urinary tract" includes the bladder, urethra, and periurethral striated muscle. Anatomically and embryologically, the bladder traditionally has been divided into detrusor and trigone regions. The terms "bladder body" and "bladder base" refer to a functional rather than anatomic division of bladder smooth muscle based on distinct differences in neuromorphology and neuropharmacology between the smooth muscle lying circumferentially above (body) and below (base) the level of the ureterovesical junction. The proximal urethra (i.e., extending to the urogenital diaphragm) in both sexes contains smooth muscle capable of affecting urethral resistance. The "smooth sphincter" refers to the smooth muscle of the bladder neck and proximal urethra. This sphincter is not anatomic but physiologic.

187

Some individuals refer to this area as the "internal sphincter," and some refer to it simply as the "bladder neck sphincter," emphasizing that virtually no physiologic or pathologic change affects the smooth muscle of the most proximal urethra without also affecting the smooth muscle of the bladder neck. Normally, resistance increases in the area of the smooth sphincter during bladder filling and urine storage and decreases during an emptying bladder contraction.

The classic view of the "external sphincter" is that of a striated muscle within the leaves of the urogenital diaphragm that, on contraction, is capable of stopping the urinary stream. This concept has been expanded to include intramural and extramural portions. The extramural portion corresponds roughly to the "classic" external urethral sphincter and the "urogenital diaphragm." The intramural portion denotes skeletal muscle in both sexes intimately associated with the urethra above the urogenital diaphragm, continuous from that level for a variable distance to the bladder neck, and forming an integral part of the outer muscular layer of the urethra. In males, although some striated muscle is seen in the prostatic capsule and parenchyma, the intramural striated sphincter is located primarily between the verumontanum and the urogenital diaphragm. Activity gradually increases in the striated sphincter during bladder filling and virtually disappears just prior to normal emptying.

Gosling's diagrams (Figs. 6–1 and 6–2) offer an excellent schematic representation of the muscular structures of the lower urinary tract necessary for radiographic interpretation. Not all of Gosling's terminology, however, is used in this chapter, and the differences are explained in the figure legends.

RECEPTOR FUNCTION AND INNERVATION OF THE LOWER URINARY TRACT

The physiology and pharmacology of the lower urinary tract cannot be separated from those of the autonomic nervous system. The terms "sympathetic" and "parasympathetic" refer simply to anatomic divisions of the autonomic

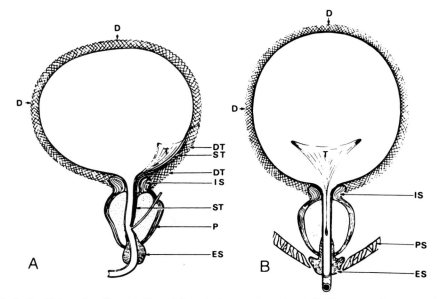

Figure 6–1 ☐ *A*, Sagittal section through the adult male lower urinary tract. *B*, Corresponding coronal section. The lumens of the bladder and urethra are dilated, and the right half of the trigone (T) in *A* and the entire trigone in *B* are shown as surface features. The detrusor muscle (D) is in direct continuity with the deep trigone (DT), with which it is morphologically and histochemically identical. The extension of the ureteric muscle formed by the trigonal muscle is represented as a thin layer (ST) extending inferiorly as far as the verumontanum. The smooth muscle of the bladder neck forms the internal urethral sphincter (IS), synonymous with the most proximal portion of the smooth sphincter mechanism, and is continuous with the prostatic capsule (P). ES represents the intrinsic (intramural) component of the striated sphincter, whereas PS represents the extrinsic or periurethral (extramural) component. (From Gosling J: The structure of the bladder and urethra in relation to function. Urol Clin North Am 6:31, 1979.)

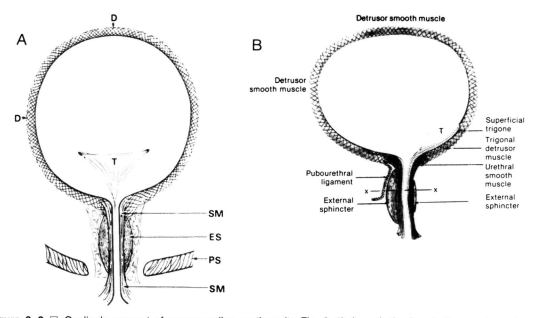

Figure 6–2 □ Gosling's concept of corresponding sections (to Fig. 6–1) through the female lower urinary tract. *A*, Sagittal view. *B*, Coronal view. The trigone (T) is represented as a surface feature. The detrusor smooth muscle (D) continues posterior to the superficial trigone and is replaced at the bladder neck region by a thin layer of smooth muscle (SM), which extends throughout the length of the urethra. The smooth muscle of the bladder neck constitutes the bulk of the smooth sphincter mechanism, but SM is also included in this designation. The intramural or intrinsic component of the striated sphincter is labeled external sphincter (ES); it is thickest along the middle third of the urethra and is relatively deficient posteriorly. This is separate from the extramural or extrinsic component, designated PS for periurethral striated muscle. The pubourethral ligament extends toward the pubis and lies anterior to the intramural component of the striated sphincter.

(*A*, From Gosling J: The structure of the bladder and urethra in relation to function. Urol Clin North Am 6:31, 1979. *B*, From Gosling JA: Anatomy. *In* Clinical Gynecologic Urology. Edited by SL Stanton. St. Louis, CV Mosby, 1984, pp 3–12. By permission of SL Stanton.)

nervous system. The sympathetic division consists of those fibers that originate in the thoracic and lumbar regions of the spinal cord, whereas the parasympathetic division refers to those fibers that originate in the cranial and sacral spinal nerves. The classic view of the peripheral autonomic nervous system involves a two-neuron system: preganglionic neurons emanating from the central nervous system and making synaptic contact with cells within ganglia, from which postganglionic neurons emerge to innervate peripheral organs. This relatively simple concept, however, although still useful for the purposes of discussion, has undergone much contemporary expansion and modification.

Most innervation of the lower urinary tract actually emanates from peripheral ganglia, which are at a short distance from, adjacent to, or within the organs they innervate (the urogenital short neuron system). Additionally, the efferent autonomic pathways do not necessarily conform to the classic two-neuron model: they are often interrupted by more than one synaptic relay. Furthermore, for many years the only autonomic neurotransmitters recognized were acetylcholine and norepinephrine. It has become obvious that additional transmitters are involved in various components of the autonomic nervous system. A once relatively simple concept of chemical neurotransmission has been expanded to include synaptic systems that involve modular transmitter mechanisms, prejunctional inhibition or enhancement of transmitter release, postjunctional modulation of transmitter action, cotransmitter release, and secondary involvement of locally synthesized hormones and other substances such as prostaglandins. All of these are subject to neuronal and hormonal regulation, desensitization, and hypersensitization. These relationships may be altered by changes that occur secondary to disease or destruction in the neuraxis, obstruction of the lower urinary tract, aging, and hormonal status. The interested reader is referred to more complete descriptions by Burnstock, Wein and Barrett (1988), and Elbadawi.

The classic model of smooth muscle involves synaptic release of a neurotransmitter in response to neural stimulation, with a subsequent combination of the transmitter agent with a recognition site, or receptor, on the postsynaptic smooth muscle cell membrane. The transmitter-receptor combination then initiates changes in the postsynaptic effector cell that ultimately result in the characteristic effect of that particular neurotransmitter on that particular smooth muscle. Clinicians are often confused because they assume that the terms sympathetic and parasympathetic imply particular neurotransmitters. These terms imply anatomic origin within the autonomic nervous system. Other adjectives are used to describe the nature of the neurotransmitter involved.

The term "cholinergic" refers to those receptor sites where acetylcholine is the neurotransmitter. All postganglionic parasympathetic fibers that terminate on lower urinary tract smooth muscle are cholinergic. Although other peripheral neurotransmitters in addition to acetylcholine may be released during parasympathetic nerve stimulation, acetylcholine is physiologically the most significant.

The term "adrenergic" is applied to those receptor sites where a catecholamine is the neurotransmitter. Adrenergic receptor sites include most postganglionic sympathetic fibers, including those to the lower urinary tract smooth muscle, where the catecholamine responsible for neurotransmission is norepinephrine. Adrenergic receptor sites are further classified as α or β on the basis of the differential effects elicited by a series of catecholamines and their antagonists. Classically, the term "α-adrenergic effect" designates vasoconstriction or contraction of smooth musculature, or both, in response to norepinephrine. The term "β-adrenergic effect" implies smooth muscle relaxation in response to catecholamine stimulation and also includes cardiac stimulation, vasodilatation, and bronchodilatation.

The pelvic and hypogastric nerves supply the bladder and urethra with efferent parasympathetic and sympathetic neurons, and both convey afferent (sensory) neurons from these organs to the spinal cord (Fig. 6–3). The parasympathetic efferent supply is classically described as originating in the gray matter of sacral spinal cord segments S-2 to S-4 and emerging as preganglionic fibers in the ventral nerve roots. This parasympathetic pregan-

glionic supply is ultimately conveyed by the pelvic nerve, which courses deep in the pelvis of humans on each side of the rectum as three or four trunks. Efferent sympathetic nerves to the bladder and urethra are thought to originate in spinal cord segments T-11 to L-2. These nerves traverse lumbar sympathetic (paravertebral) ganglia, and branches of these ganglia join the presacral nerve (superior hypogastric plexus), which is a plexiform nerve arrangement in the lumbosacral area anterior to the aorta. The presacral nerve divides into the right and left hypogastric nerves: Each of these is actually an elongated plexus. Bilaterally, at a variable distance from the bladder and urethra, the hypogastric and pelvic nerves meet and branch to form the pelvic plexus, sometimes known as the inferior hypogastric plexus or plexus of Frankenhäuser. This is a plexus of freely interconnected nerves in the pelvic fascia that is lateral to the rectum, internal genitalia, and lower urinary organs. Divergent branches of this plexus innervate these pelvic organs. Efferent innervation of the striated sphincter is generally thought to emanate from sacral spinal cord segments S-2 to S-4 via the pudendal nerve. Although this doubtless provides the primary basis for voluntary control of the external urethral sphincter, some authorities think that the striated sphincter is also innervated by somatic (voluntary) fibers within the pelvic nerve, whereas others think that the striated sphincter is innervated by branches of the autonomic nervous system as well.

All areas of the bladder of animals and humans receive abundant cholinergic innervation. There is general agreement that abundant cholinergic receptor sites exist throughout the bladder body and base of various animal species and humans. A sustained bladder contraction is produced by stimulation of the pelvic nerves, and it is generally agreed that reflex activation of this pelvic nerve excitatory tract is responsible for the emptying bladder contraction of normal micturition and the involuntary bladder contractions seen with various diseases of the neuraxis and in response to lower urinary tract obstruction. Whether acetylcholine is the sole neurotransmitter released during such stimulation is highly controversial.

Adrenergic innervation of the bladder and urethral smooth musculature has been demonstrated extensively in animals. These studies showed that the smooth musculature of the bladder base and proximal urethra possesses a rich adrenergic innervation, whereas the blad-

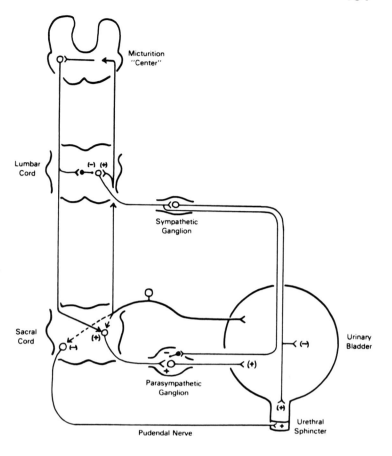

Figure 6–3 □ DeGroat's diagram of the reflex pathways involved in micturition. Plus and minus signs indicate excitatory and inhibitory synaptic actions, respectively. Voluntary control is accomplished by connection (not pictured) between the frontal cortex and pontine micturition center. Note the prominent role of the sympathetic nervous system and the synapse between the descending fibers from the micturition center (excitatory) and the preganglionic parasympathetic fibers in the sacral spinal cord. (From deGroat WC, Booth AM: Physiology of the urinary bladder and urethra. Ann Intern Med 92:312, 1980. By permission of the American College of Physicians.)

der body has a sparse (but definite) innervation of this type. The density of innervation seems in all areas to be less than that of the cholinergic systems. There is considerable disagreement as to a significant presence of postganglionic sympathetic innervation in the bladder and proximal urethra of humans, except for a consensus that the smooth muscle of the human male bladder neck possesses a dense adrenergic innervation. There is agreement that the smooth muscle of the bladder and proximal urethra in humans and various animals contains α- and β-adrenergic receptors. Alpha-adrenergic responses predominate in the bladder base and proximal urethra, whereas β-adrenergic responses predominate in the bladder body.

The postganglionic sympathetic fibers exert a significant inhibitory influence on parasympathetic ganglionic transmission. Those who advocate a major role for the sympathetic nervous system in the micturition cycle summarize the influences as follows. During bladder filling, a spinal sympathetic reflex is stimulated via sensory afferents to the thora-columbar area of the spinal cord. The efferent limb of this reflex acts, ultimately via postganglionic sympathetic fibers, (1) to increase outlet resistance by direct stimulation of the predominantly α-adrenergic receptors in the smooth muscle of the smooth sphincter area, (2) to inhibit bladder contraction by a blocking effect exerted on parasympathetic ganglion cell activity, and (3) to increase bladder accommodation through activation of the predominantly β-adrenergic receptors in the bladder body. Many authorities, however, believe that the sympathetic nervous system, although playing a major role in the micturition cycle of many animals, plays a minor role in humans, primarily having to do with function (2) above.

CENTRAL INFLUENCES ON LOWER URINARY TRACT FUNCTION

Micturition is basically a function of the peripheral autonomic nervous system. However, the ultimate control of lower urinary tract function resides at higher neurologic levels (Fig. 6–4). There is general consensus that the micturition "center" in the spinal cord is localized primarily to segments S-2 to S-4, with the major portion at S-3. However, there is little question that the brain stem, specifically the neurons of the pontine-mesencephalic gray matter, contains the nuclei that are the origin of the final common pathway to bladder motor neurons. Input to this area is derived from the cerebellum, basal ganglia, thalamus and hypothalamus, and cerebral cortex. Bladder contraction elicited by stimulation at or above this area seems to occur with a decrease in activity of the periurethral striated musculature, as in normal micturition. The region of the cerebral hemispheres primarily concerned with bladder function consists of the superomedial portion of the frontal lobes and the genu of the corpus callosum. Transection experiments indicate that the net effect of these areas is inhibitory.

IMPORTANT FUNCTIONAL QUESTIONS

What determines bladder response during filling? The normal bladder response to filling at a physiologic rate is an almost imperceptible change in intravesical pressure. There is little question that, during the initial stages of filling, this high compliance (compliance is defined as Δ volume/Δ pressure) is due primarily to purely passive properties of the bladder wall, summarized by the concepts of elasticity and viscoelasticity. At a certain level of bladder filling, a spinal sympathetic reflex is evoked in animals, and there is indirect evidence to support such a role in humans. The effects of this reflex are to facilitate the filling or storage phase of micturition. Endogenous opioids contribute a strong tonic inhibitory effect on bladder activity, at least at the level of the spinal cord and brain stem.

What determines outlet response during filling? Smooth and striated sphincteric elements contribute to a gradual increase in urethral pressure during bladder filling, attributable to different reflex mechanisms through their respective efferent innervations. The passive properties of the urethral wall also contribute to the maintenance of continence, because the tension that develops is a product of not only the active characteristics of smooth and striated muscle but also the passive characteristics of the elastic and collagenous tissue composition of the urethral wall. This tension must be exerted on a soft or plastic inner layer capable of being compressed to a closed configuration. Moreover, whatever the compressive forces, the lumen must be capable of being obliterated by a watertight seal (i.e., the "mucosal seal" mechanism).

Why does voiding ensue with a normal bladder contraction? During voluntarily initiated micturition, the bladder pressure becomes higher than the outlet pressure, certain adaptive changes occur in the shape of the bladder

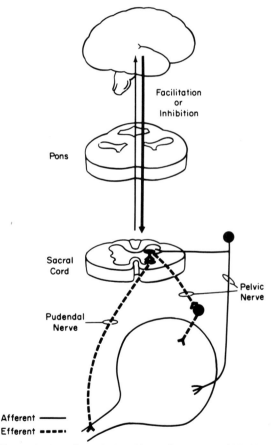

Figure 6–4 □ Sacral micturition reflex theory of bladder function. Bladder distention results in afferent pelvic nerve stimuli, which enter the sacral cord through the dorsal roots and synapse with pelvic and pudendal nerve nuclei, resulting in efferent discharges mediating bladder contraction and striated sphincter relaxation. Central nervous system pathways and local influences mediate facilitation and inhibition of this sacral reflex. (From Blaivas JG: The neurophysiology of micturition: A clinical study of 550 patients. J Urol 127:958, 1982. By permission of the Williams & Wilkins Company.)

outlet, and urine passes into and through the proximal urethra. There is a reflex coordination between a voluntarily induced bladder contraction of adequate magnitude and the active responses of the proximal urethra; that is, urethral pressure actually decreases prior to bladder contraction. Not only does intravesical pressure increase, but outlet resistance also decreases synergistically. The decrease in pelvic floor striated musculature electromyographic activity prior to voluntary bladder contraction strongly suggests that at least a portion of this decrease is secondary to a reflex mechanism involving the striated sphincter. It is tempting to speculate that a similar reflex coordination of smooth sphincter activity exists, mediated through a decrease in efferent hypogastric nerve activity. Additionally, there may be an active mechanism that decreases urethral smooth muscle activity and involves stimulation of β-adrenergic receptors or nonadrenergic noncholinergic receptors.

Why doesn't urinary leakage occur with abdominal straining? First of all, a coordinated bladder contraction does not occur in response to such stimuli. For urine to flow through a normal bladder neck and into a normal proximal urethra, an increase in intravesical pressure must occur and must be a product of a coordinated bladder contraction occurring through a neurally mediated reflex mechanism associated with characteristic changes in the bladder neck and proximal urethra. For the purposes of definition, the designation "detrusor pressure" indicates pressure produced by a bladder contraction, whereas the term "intravesical" or "vesical pressure" designates detrusor pressure plus any component contributed by intra-abdominal pressure (i.e., $P_{det} = P_{ves} - P_{abd}$). A major factor in the prevention of urinary leakage during increases in intra-abdominal pressure is the location of the bladder neck and proximal urethra (also called the sphincter unit). Normally, this unit is situated within the abdominal cavity to allow equal transmission of any increase in intra-abdominal pressure to the bladder neck and proximal urethra. Ligamentous and fascial structures normally support the sphincter area and prevent its descent into a position where intra-abdominal pressure increases are not transmitted at least equally. Alteration of these supportive structures allowing pathologic descent of the sphincteric unit with abdominal straining happens secondary to many etiologic factors,

predominantly in females; stress incontinence is the result.

EXTRAPOLATION

The following is a concise and simplified description of the normal processes involved in lower urinary tract function that seems consistent with existing data and opinions. The two functions of the lower urinary tract are the storage and active expulsion of urine. During bladder filling and urine storage at physiologic rates, intravesical pressure initially increases slowly despite large increases in volume. This phenomenon is due primarily to the passive properties of the smooth muscles and connective tissue of the bladder wall. There is little neural efferent activity until a certain critical intravesical pressure is reached. Whether this correlates with the first sensation or awareness of bladder filling is unknown. This is followed by an afferent pelvic nerve discharge, which results in a gradual reflex increase in somatic nerve efferent activity, primarily through the pudendal nerve, causing a gradual increase of contractile activity in the striated, or external urethral, sphincter. In animals, and perhaps in humans, an additional spinal sympathetic reflex also is initiated by pelvic nerve afferents. The efferent limb of this reflex is from the thoracolumbar segments through the hypogastric nerve and results in an inhibition of bladder contractile activity by means of an inhibitor effect on parasympathetic ganglionic transmission. It also produces an increase in bladder neck and proximal urethral tone because of active stimulation of the predominantly α-adrenergic receptors in that area. The net effect is that urethral pressure remains greater than detrusor pressure, and urine is stored rather than expelled. Normally, any increase in abdominal pressure (cough, strain) is reflected in an increase in vesical pressure and an equal or greater increase (due to an additional somatic reflex-involved striated sphincter contraction) in the bladder neck–proximal urethral area.

Although many factors are involved in the micturition reflex, it is increasing intravesical pressure producing a sensation of distention or the need to void that is primarily responsible for the initiation of voluntarily induced emptying of the lower urinary tract. The origin of the parasympathetic neural outflow to the bladder, the pelvic nerve, is in the sacral spinal cord. However, the actual organizational center for the micturition reflex in an individual with an intact neuraxis is in the brain stem, and the complete neural circuit for normal micturition includes the ascending and descending spinal cord pathways to and from this area and the facilitory and inhibitory influences from other parts of the brain.

Voluntary inhibition or cessation of the voiding reflex, as in the case of attempted inhibition of an involuntary bladder contraction, may be accomplished also through pudendal nerve–induced pelvic floor striated muscle contraction, which initiates a spinal reflex that inhibits further bladder contractile activity. The final step in voluntarily induced voiding involves inhibition of the pudendal nerve efferent activity to the striated sphincter and all aspects of the spinal sympathetic reflex evoked during filling. Immediately after the decrease in outlet resistance, efferent parasympathetic pelvic nerve activity is ultimately what is responsible for a highly coordinated contraction of the bulk of bladder smooth musculature. This occurs with adaptive shaping or funneling of the relaxed bladder outlet. These adaptive changes are due also to the anatomic interrelationships of the smooth muscle of the bladder base and proximal urethra. During voluntary interruption of the urinary stream, descending corticospinal pathways emanating from the motor cortex synapse in the pudendal nucleus, resulting in contraction of the striated sphincter. Urethral pressure increases above detrusor pressure, stopping urination directly and through an inhibitory reflex mechanism at the level of the sacral spinal cord.

OVERVIEW

Whatever disagreements exist, all investigators would agree on certain points. The micturition cycle involves two relatively discrete processes: (1) bladder filling and urine storage, and (2) bladder emptying. Whatever the neuromorphologic, neurophysiologic, neuropharmacologic, and mechanical details involved, one can summarize these processes from a conceptual point of view. Bladder filling and urine storage require (1) accommodation of increasing volumes of urine at low intravesical pressure and with appropriate sensation, (2) a closed bladder outlet at rest that remains so during increases in intra-abdominal pressure, and (3) absence of involuntary bladder contractions. Bladder emptying requires (1) a coordinated

contraction of adequate magnitude of the bladder smooth musculature, (2) a concomitant lowering of resistance at the level of the smooth and striated sphincters, and (3) absence of anatomic obstruction.

Any type of voiding dysfunction must result from an abnormality of one or more of the factors listed as involved in the two phases of the micturition cycle. This division, with its implied subdivision under each category into causes related to the bladder and causes related to the outlet, provides a logical rationale for the classification of all types of voiding dysfunction into disorders related to bladder filling or urine storage and disorders related to bladder emptying. There are indeed some types of voiding dysfunction that represent a combination of filling or storage and emptying disorders. Within this schema, these combined disorders become readily understandable. Furthermore, one may take all aspects of urodynamic, radiologic, and videourodynamic evaluation and classify the individual component studies in terms of either bladder or outlet activity during filling or storage or emptying. Finally, one can easily classify all known treatments for voiding dysfunction under the broad categories of an action primarily on the bladder or on the components of the bladder outlet.

CLASSIFICATION OF VOIDING DYSFUNCTION: ASSOCIATED DEFINITIONS

We have preferred to classify voiding dysfunction on a functional basis, describing the dysfunction simply in terms of whether the deficit produced is primarily in the filling or storage phase or in the emptying phase of micturition (Table 6–1) (Wein, 1986). This type of classification system is an excellent alternative when a particular dysfunction does not exactly lend itself to a generally agreed-on classification in one of the other systems, which in our expe-

Table 6–1 □ Functional Classification of Voiding Dysfunction

Failure to store
Because of the bladder
Because of the outlet
Failure to empty
Because of the bladder
Because of the outlet

From Wein AJ: Classification of voiding dysfunction: a simple approach. *In* Controversies in Neuro-Urology. Edited by DM Barrett, AJ Wein. New York, Churchill Livingstone, 1984, pp 239–250. By permission of the publisher.

rience occurs frequently. This simplified schema assumes only that, whatever their differences, authorities agree on certain general principles concerning the micturition cycle that have just been described. Such a system can be easily "expanded" to include etiologic or urodynamic connotations (Table 6–2). Proper use of this system for a given voiding dysfunction requires a reasonably accurate notion of what the urodynamic/radiologic/videourodynamic data show. However, an exact diagnosis is not required for treatment. Also, some patients do not have a single discrete storage or emptying failure; therefore, to properly utilize this system of classification, one must recognize the existence of combination deficits.

It is necessary to ensure a certain consistency in the use of terms that describe voiding dysfunction to be able to correlate the functional system of classification with the classification systems and (sometimes different) terms used by other authors to describe similar phenomena. Detrusor hyperactivity or overactivity may be secondary to either involuntary bladder contractions or decreased compliance. Involuntary contractions refer to phasic increases in detrusor pressure. When these occur in an individual with neurologic disease (and are presumed to be secondary to that disease), the term "detrusor hyperreflexia" is used. When these contractions are unrelated to neurologic disease, the term used to describe them is "detrusor instability."

Compliance refers to the ratio, change in volume over change in pressure ($\Delta V/\Delta P$). Decreased compliance refers to an inappropriate and steady increase in bladder pressure during filling ($\Delta V/\Delta P$) without phasic interruption. Involuntary bladder contraction may, however, be superimposed on decreased compliance. An involuntary bladder contraction or decreased compliance in an individual with normal sensation generally causes the symptom of urgency. If the abnormal pressure increase cannot be suppressed or controlled, then both urgency and incontinence will occur. Motor urgency refers to urgency that occurs in association with a demonstrable increase in detrusor pressure. Sensory urgency means that the sensation occurs in the absence of demonstrable involuntary contractions or decreased compliance.

Stress incontinence denotes involuntary loss of urine when the total intravesical pressure exceeds the maximal urethral pressure in the absence of detrusor activity. Urethral instability refers to episodic decreases in urethral pressure, causing either urgency or incontinence, in the absence of detrusor contraction. A synergic sphincter is one that exhibits appropriate relaxation during bladder contraction, enabling unobstructed micturition to occur. Striated sphincter dyssynergia, sometimes called external urethral sphincter dyssynergia or simply sphincter dyssynergia, refers to inappropriate contraction of the periurethral striated muscle during bladder contraction. This is fairly easy to detect radiographically and is generally distinguishable from a nonrelaxing striated sphincter, which also may cause functional obstruction but without active contraction. Smooth sphincter dyssynergia is sometimes called bladder neck or internal sphincter dyssynergia and, strictly speaking, refers to inappropriate contraction of the bladder neck or proximal urethral area during

---

Table 6–2 □ Expanded Functional Classification

Failure to Store
  Because of the bladder
    Detrusor hyperactivity
      Involuntary contractions
        Suprasacral neurologic disease
        Bladder outlet obstruction
        Idiopathic
      Decreased compliance
        Fibrosis
        Idiopathic
    Sensory urgency
      Inflammatory
      Infectious
      Neurologic
      Psychologic
      Idiopathic
  Because of the outlet
    Stress incontinence
    Nonfunctional bladder neck or proximal urethra
    Urethral instability
Failure to Empty
  Because of the bladder
    Neurologic
    Myogenic
    Psychogenic
    Idiopathic
  Because of the outlet
    Anatomic
      Prostatic obstruction
      Bladder neck contracture
      Urethral stricture
    Functional
      Smooth sphincter dyssynergia
      Striated sphincter dyssynergia

From Barrett DM, Wein AJ: Voiding dysfunction: diagnosis, classification, and management. *In* Adult and Pediatric Urology, Vol 1. Edited by JY Gillenwater, JT Grayhack, SS Howards, et al. Chicago, Year Book Medical Publishers, 1987, pp 863–962. By permission of the publisher.

bladder contraction. Because the normal bladder neck is radiographically closed during filling or storage, it is not possible to distinguish a bladder neck that is truly dyssynergic from one that simply fails to exhibit any adaptive changes or funneling. Failure of the bladder neck opening is normal during abdominal straining; during detrusor contraction, however, such failure is always abnormal.

The terms "upper motor neuron" and "lower motor neuron" are used primarily in conjunction with the Bors-Comarr classification (Table 6–3) of voiding dysfunction. This system applies only to patients with neuropathic dysfunction and assumes that the sacral spinal cord is the primary reflex center for micturition. Lower motor neuron describes collectively the preganglionic and postganglionic parasympathetic autonomic fibers that innervate the bladder and outlet and originate as preganglionic fibers in the sacral spinal cord. Upper motor neuron describes those descending autonomic pathways above the origin of the parasympathetic nerve supply to the lower urinary tract (above the sacral spinal cord). The terms "complete" and "incomplete" refer to the neurologic lesion, and this determination is made on the basis of a thorough neurologic evaluation. The terms "balanced" and "unbalanced" refer to the percentage of residual urine relative to bladder capacity. Unbalanced means the presence of more than 20 per cent residual urine in a patient with an upper motor neuron lesion and of 10 per cent in a patient with a lower motor neuron lesion. Some authors still use this terminology, and the use is best illustrated by example. An upper motor lesion, complete, imbalanced, is a neurologically complete lesion above the level of the sacral spinal cord that results in skeletal muscle spasticity below the level of the injury. Detrusor hyperreflexia exists, but with a residual urine volume greater than 20 per cent of bladder capacity, which implies that there is obstruction in the area of the bladder outlet (generally striated sphincter dyssynergia) during the hyperreflexic detrusor contraction. A lower motor neuron lesion, complete, imbalanced, is typified by a neurologically complete lesion at the level of the sacral spinal cord or the sacral roots that results in skeletal muscle flaccidity below that level. Detrusor areflexia results, and whatever maneuvers the patient may use to increase intravesical pressure are not sufficient to de-

Table 6–3 ☐ Bors-Comarr Classification

Sensory Neuron Lesion
  Incomplete, balanced
  Complete, imbalanced

Motor Neuron Lesion
  Balanced
  Imbalanced

Sensory Motor Neuron Lesion
  Upper motor neuron lesion
    Complete, balanced
    Complete, imbalanced
    Incomplete, balanced
    Incomplete, imbalanced
  Lower motor neuron lesion
    Complete, balanced
    Complete, imbalanced
    Incomplete, balanced
    Incomplete, imbalanced
  Mixed lesion
    Upper somatomotor neuron, lower visceromotor neuron
    Lower somatomotor neuron, upper visceromotor neuron
    Normal somatomotor neuron, lower visceromotor neuron

From Wein AJ: Classification of voiding dysfunction: a simple approach. *In* Controversies in Neuro-Urology. Edited by DM Barrett, AJ Wein. New York, Churchill Livingstone, 1984, pp 239–250. By permission of the publisher.

crease residual urine to less than 10 per cent of bladder capacity.

Lapides and associates contributed significantly to the care of the patient with neuropathic voiding dysfunction by popularizing a modification of a scheme originally proposed by McClellan (Table 6–4). The Lapides classification of neuropathic voiding dysfunction is the scheme most familiar to urologists; it describes in recognizable shorthand the clinical and cystometric condition in most types of dysfunction.

A sensory neuropathic bladder results from any disease that selectively interrupts the sensory fibers between the brain and spinal cord or the afferent tracts to the brain. Most commonly this is seen in patients with diabetes

Table 6–4 ☐ Lapides Classification

  Sensory neuropathic bladder
  Motor paralytic bladder
  Uninhibited neuropathic bladder
  Reflex neuropathic bladder
  Autonomous neuropathic bladder

Adapted from Wein AJ: Classification of voiding dysfunction: a simple approach. *In* Controversies in Neuro-Urology. Edited by DM Barrett, AJ Wein. New York, Churchill Livingstone, 1984, pp 239–250. By permission of the publisher.

mellitus, syphilis, and pernicious anemia. The first clinical changes consist only of impaired sensation. Unless voiding is initiated out of habit or on a timed basis, varying degrees of bladder overdistention often result, with resultant hypotonicity. Ultimately, with bladder decompensation, significant amounts of residual urine are found, and at this time the filling curve generally demonstrates a large bladder capacity with high compliance.

A motor paralytic bladder results from disease processes that destroy the parasympathetic motor innervation of the bladder. Extensive pelvic surgery or trauma or herpes zoster can produce a motor paralytic bladder. The early symptoms may vary from painful urinary retention to a relative inability to initiate and maintain normal micturition. In the early stages, compliance is normal, with normal sensation but without a voluntary contraction at bladder capacity. Later, chronic overdistention and bladder decompensation may occur and a large-capacity bladder with high compliance and a large residual urine volume results.

The uninhibited neuropathic bladder was originally described as resulting from injury or disease in what was called the "corticoregulatory tract." This concept presumed that the sacral spinal cord was the reflex center for micturition and that this corticoregulatory tract normally exerted an inhibitory influence on the primary micturition reflex. A destructive lesion in this tract would then result in overfacilitation of the micturition reflex. Cerebrovascular accident, brain or spinal cord tumor, and demyelinating disease are the most common causes of this type of lesion. This lesion generally results in a voiding dysfunction characterized clinically by frequency, urgency, and incontinence and cystometrically by normal sensation with detrusor hyperreflexia at low filling volumes. Residual urine volume is characteristically small or zero unless anatomic outlet obstruction or true involuntary smooth or striated sphincter dyssynergia occurs. The patient usually can initiate a bladder contraction voluntarily but is often unable to do so during cystometry because sufficient urine storage cannot occur before detrusor hyperreflexia is stimulated.

Reflex neuropathic bladder most commonly denotes the condition after spinal shock from complete interruption of the sensory and motor pathways between the sacral spinal cord and the brain stem. Typically, the patient has no bladder sensation and is unable to initiate micturition voluntarily. Incontinence results because of low volume detrusor hyperreflexia, which generally occurs with striated sphincter dyssynergia. This type of lesion is equivalent to a complete upper motor neuron lesion in the Bors-Comarr system.

An autonomous neuropathic bladder results from complete motor and sensory separation of the bladder from the sacral spinal cord. Any disease process that destroys the sacral cord or causes extensive damage to the sacral roots or pelvic nerves may result in this type of dysfunction. The patient is unable to initiate micturition voluntarily and has no bladder reflex activity and no specific sensation. This type of bladder is equivalent to the complete lower motor neuron lesion in the Bors-Comarr system. The characteristic cystometric pattern is initially similar to the late stages of the motor or sensory paralytic bladder, with a marked shift to the right of the filling curve and a large bladder capacity at low intravesical pressure. However, secondary changes in the filling limb may occur that cause decreased compliance. This may be secondary to chronic inflammatory change or the effects of the denervation itself. Emptying capacity may vary from essentially zero to a large percentage of bladder capacity, depending on the ability of the patient to increase intravesical pressure and the resistance offered during this increase by the smooth and striated muscle of the bladder outlet. It should be noted that "classic" cystometric patterns may be altered considerably or totally changed by infection, inflammation, or fibrosis.

With the development of more sophisticated urodynamic equipment and techniques to categorize bladder and outlet activity during filling or storage and emptying, systems of classification have been formulated based solely on objective urodynamic data (Table 6–5). When exact urodynamic classification is possible, this system provides a truly exact description of the particular voiding dysfunction under consideration. This system is easiest to use when detrusor hyperreflexia or normoreflexia is present, because sufficiently sophisticated and reproducible urodynamic techniques exist to describe the activity of the smooth and striated sphincters during bladder contraction. When a voluntary or hyperreflexic bladder contraction cannot be elicited, this system is more difficult to use because it is not appropriate to speak of true dyssynergia in the

Table 6–5 ☐ Krane-Siroky Urodynamic
Classification

Detrusor hyperreflexia (or normoreflexia)
Coordinated sphincters
Striated sphincter dyssynergia
Smooth sphincter dyssynergia
Nonrelaxing smooth sphincter
Detrusor areflexia
Coordinated sphincters
Nonrelaxing striated sphincter
Denervated striated sphincter
Nonrelaxing smooth sphincter

From Wein AJ: Classification of voiding dysfunction: a simple approach. *In* Controversies in Neuro-Urology. Edited by DM Barrett, AJ Wein. New York, Churchill Livingstone, 1984, pp 239–250. By permission of the publisher.

absence of an opposing bladder contraction. An additional problem with this type of system is that many times "experts" simply do not agree about the significance of certain data generated during a given urodynamic evaluation.

The International Continence Society (ICS) proposed a classification system based on the functional state of the bladder and urethra (Table 6–6). Overactive detrusor function is indicated when, during the filling phase, there are involuntary bladder contractions or decreased compliance that the patient cannot suppress. An overactive urethral closure mechanism contracts involuntarily against detrusor contraction (dyssynergia) or simply fails to relax during attempted micturition. An incompetent urethral closure mechanism implies urinary incontinence.

No single type of classification system for voiding dysfunction, regardless of cause, is ideal. Additionally, there are only a few terms that describe voiding function and dysfunction that are used in an entirely consistent fashion by all urologists and radiologists. Each of us must understand exactly what is meant when a problem is described in terms of its clinical

Table 6–6 ☐ International Continence
Society Classification

Detrusor	Urethra	Sensation
Normal	Normal	Normal
Overactive	Overactive	Hypersensitive
Underactive	Incompetent	Hyposensitive

From Barrett DM, Wein AJ: Voiding dysfunction: diagnosis, classification, and management. *In* Adult and Pediatric Urology, Vol 1. Edited by JY Gillenwater, JT Grayhack, SS Howards, et al. Chicago, Year Book Medical Publishers, 1987, pp 863–962. By permission of the publisher.

symptomatology and its urodynamic, radiologic, or videourodynamic findings; in addition, we must understand the nomenclature used within any given system of classification.

PEDIATRIC NEUROUROLOGIC EVALUATION

History and Physical Examination

For all purposes, neurourologic tests should not be conducted on a child with suspected vesicourethral dysfunction without first taking a complete history and doing a physical examination. A history suggestive of subtle central nervous system disease, such as a traumatic birth, neonatal anoxia, convulsive disorder, and head or back trauma, may explain many voiding abnormalities despite the absence of apparent neurologic disease.

During the initial interview with the child and parents, an assessment should be made of the fluid ingested in a 24-hour period. Historical approximations of this volume may be misleading, however, and when a voiding problem such as diabetes insipidus is being investigated, the child and parents should bring documentation of volumes ingested and voided.

The voiding history itself may hold the clue to which of the various available tests will offer the best opportunity for an accurate and cost-effective diagnosis. In the very young child, parents should be questioned about their observations of diaper wetness, number of diapers used, diaper rash, dripping loss of urine, leakage while crying, stream characteristics, straining during urination, and apparent pain or discomfort when voiding. The older child may be asked questions about painful urination, urgency, frequency, and unusual voiding positions, although corroboration from parents is often necessary for information related to enuresis, soiling, and malodor.

Aside from the potential damage to the bladder and upper tracts, vesicourethral dysfunction in children, especially when incontinence is involved, may have a dramatic impact on the psychologic and sociologic adjustment of the child or family as a unit. During the initial interview, an assessment should be made regarding the impact of the "voiding problem" on the child and parents. This information is important not only diagnostically, because psychogenic voiding dysfunction must be excluded, but also therapeutically, because eventual selection of therapeutic alternatives depends greatly on the psychosocial status of the patient and family.

The physical examination should be directed to those conditions that may foretell underlying neurologic diseases or suggest the more immediate problem of bladder overdistention and hydronephrosis. In the absence of overt neurologic problems, the examination should first be directed toward the integrity of the spinal column by looking for clues to vertebral dysraphism. Hairy patches, depressions, or dimples over the spine or sacral area may indicate underlying dysraphism or sacral agenesis. A rough estimate of intact reflex arc activity can be obtained by evoking deep tendon reflexes in the lower extremities, and also a rough estimate can be made of sensory neurologic integrity of the abdomen, perineum, and lower extremities. Further neurologic assessment should be left to a pediatric neurologist, and any clues that may be uncovered during the initial physical examination may lead to a consultation that would include more specificity.

After the initial history and physical examination have been completed and a urinalysis is performed, a determination must be made of the severity of the "voiding problem." Does it require further evaluation or can the child and parents be reassured that the symptoms are normal variants and there is no threat to the unseen portions of the urinary tract? Clinical judgment becomes the most important indicator at this time. Children with those conditions listed earlier will be evaluated further. However, in those children who cannot be placed in a particular category, one must weigh the relative costs and degree of invasiveness involved in additional tests against the risk of failing to diagnose a potentially serious vesicourethral abnormality.

Urodynamics

Urodynamics is a neurourologic diagnostic tool concerned with the identification and measurement of physiologic and pathologic factors involved in the storage, transportation, and evacuation of urine. The purpose of urodynamic testing is to identify and quantitate the causal factors that contribute to the voiding dysfunction, whether it is a problem of storage

or emptying. Because the bladder responds to various pathologic conditions with the same symptoms, the need for urodynamic testing becomes important before therapy is selected. Many studies have documented the poor correlation between the patient's symptoms and the findings of urodynamic testing. This is true for patients without (Farrar et al; Powell et al) and for patients with (Blaivas, 1980; Blaivas et al, 1979) neurologic disorders. In a study done in patients with multiple sclerosis, when treatment was based on symptoms and signs, it was effective in 27 per cent of patients. When treatment was based on urodynamic testing, it was effective in 83 per cent of patients (Blaivas, 1980; Blaivas et al, 1979).

Urodynamic tests are not without their limitations and potential for misinterpretation, especially in children. Ideally, the clinical symptom should be reproduced during the urodynamic testing sequence. If the symptom is not reproduced during routine testing, then the study must be repeated in as close an approximation as possible to the situation in which the patient's symptoms actually occur: rising, standing, coughing, laughing, or jogging. Older children should be asked to evaluate the similarity of their usual voiding to the voiding sequence evaluated urodynamically. This helps establish the credibility of the urodynamic data. On the other hand, there may be certain symptoms produced during the testing sequence that have urodynamic correlates but do not constitute a part of the patient's original complaints. These findings may represent artifact or may be early subclinical abnormalities not generally manifested during normal voiding.

Interpreting sensory data during urodynamic testing is subjective at best. This is unfortunate because many patients with voiding dysfunction have only sensation abnormalities and have no demonstrable urodynamic abnormalities. It is relatively easy to assess whether the sensation of bladder filling is normal, decreased, or absent. However, several sensations may occur during filling that are difficult to classify. The most troublesome of these is the symptom of urgency or the dire need to void. Although this can correlate with involuntary bladder contractions or detrusor hyperreflexia, it is not uncommon to reproduce this symptom during urodynamic testing and not be able to demonstrate a urodynamic abnormality. The test may not be sensitive enough to record the subtle changes that occur in the bladder or outlet, or the inhibitory factors that come into play in the laboratory setting may affect the test results.

Operator expertise in testing patients of all ages is essential for successful completion of most studies, and physician participation is recommended for the more complex tests.

There are four basic urodynamic modalities: (1) cystometry, (2) uroflowmetry (with residual volume determination), (3) urethral pressure profilometry, and (4) combined studies (with or without fluoroscopy, e.g., cystometrography-electromyography [CMG-EMG] or pressure-flow EMG). The exact sequence in which these tests are administered to the patient depends entirely on the presenting symptoms and the presumptive diagnosis based on other neurourologic tests. Table 6–7 lists the urodynamic modalities involved in evaluation of the bladder or the bladder outlet; in general, the simplest, least invasive test should be used.

The ability of the child to cooperate during testing may determine which tests are best, but general urologic practices will derive most benefit from simple uroflowmetry and cystometry. Sphincter EMG is important if patients with neuropathic bladder dysfunction make up a significant proportion of the study population. Complex cases that cannot be evaluated adequately in this manner are best referred to a urodynamic center capable of performing multifunction studies with the option of combined video cystourethrography; such a center should be staffed by a urodynamic technician with knowledge and expertise in this specialty.

Urodynamic testing is but one part of the overall evaluation of the child with voiding dysfunction. It is imperative that all portions of the neurourologic evaluation and the conclusions drawn from them be carefully reviewed and, when discrepancy exists between the symptoms and the urodynamic findings, that these studies should be questioned and repeated, especially before irreversible therapy is undertaken.

Cystometry

Cystometry is the method by which changes in bladder pressure are measured with progressive increase in bladder volume. The test is designed basically to evaluate the filling or storage phase of detrusor function. The presence or absence of a detrusor contraction, although an important observation, is not nec-

Table 6–7 ☐ Urodynamics Made Easy

	Bladder	**Outlet**
Filling or storage	$P_{det(FCMG)}$[1]	P_{ureth}[2] FLUORO[3]
Emptying	$P_{det(VCMG)}$[4]	P_{ureth}[2] FLUORO[3] EMG[5]
	FLOW[6] RU[7]	

Adapted from Barrett DM, Wein AJ: Voiding dysfunction: diagnosis, classification, and management. *In* Adult and Pediatric Urology, Vol 1. Edited by JY Gillenwater, JT Grayhack, SS Howards, et al. Chicago, Year Book Medical Publishers, 1987, pp 863–962. By permission of the publisher.
[1]Filling cystometrogram (recording of detrusor pressure during filling).
[2]Urethral pressure(s).
[3]Fluoroscopy.
[4]Voiding cystometry (recording of detrusor pressure during voluntary or involuntary emptying).
[5]Electromyography of periurethral striated muscle.
[6]Flowmetry.
[7]Residual urine determination.

essary to elicit important information from this test.

The normal bladder capacity varies with age: newborn, 50 to 100 ml, and adolescent, 300 to 600 ml. Within this capacity, bladder pressure should not increase above 15 cm H_2O before approaching capacity.

Schematically, the normal cystometrogram may be divided into four phases (Fig. 6–5). There is the initial increase in pressure to achieve resting bladder pressure. Then comes the second phase, the tonus limb, which reflects the vesicoelastic properties of the smooth muscle, collagen, and mucopolysaccharides of the bladder wall. During this filling or storage phase, bladder pressure should increase very

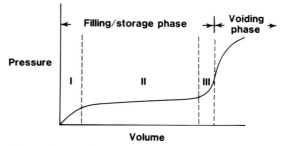

Figure 6–5 ☐ Characteristics of normal cystometrogram. (From Barrett DM, Wein AJ: Voiding dysfunction: diagnosis, classification, and management. *In* Adult and Pediatric Urology, Vol 1. Edited by JY Gillenwater, JT Grayhack, SS Howards, et al. Chicago, Year Book Medical Publishers, 1987, pp 863–962. By permission of the publisher.)

little because the normal bladder is able to accommodate to increasing urine volumes. Rapid filling rates may generate a steeper tonus limb. Bladder wall fibrosis from various causes (infection or radiation) and detrusor hypertrophy also may cause compromised accommodation, with a steeper tonus limb. At peak capacity, the detrusor muscle and other elastic tissue have stretched to their limit and any additional increase in volume will be accompanied by an increase in intravesical pressure. During this third stage, the patient still is able to suppress voluntary voiding contractions. Ruch and Tang demonstrated that the characteristic shape of the cystometry curve is independent of neural control and is an inherent property of the structural elements of the bladder wall.

The fourth phase of the normal cystometrogram is the generation of a voluntary voiding reflex that is dependent on intact neural pathways to the micturition center located in the brain stem. The untrained child lacks the maturation of this pathway, and detrusor contractility appears hyperreflexic. The older, toilet-trained child should be able to suppress voiding even when the bladder is at capacity.

It is not uncommon during a study to find that the patient is unable to generate a micturition reflex on command. This is more common in females and is related to psychologic inhibition resulting from the unnatural circumstances of the study. Performance of this phase of CMG with the male patient in an upright posture and the female on a commode may facilitate the generation of a micturition reflex. In the older child, voiding may be stimulated by administering 1.5 to 2.5 mg bethanechol subcutaneously. If voiding does not occur in response to bethanechol administration, the bladder should be emptied and filled again while the clinician measures bladder pressures to test for evidence of denervation supersensitivity (see Bethanechol Supersensitivity Test).

Either water or gas (carbon dioxide) can be used as the infusion medium during cystometry. Controversy exists as to the relative merits of each. From a practical point of view, there seems not to be a significant difference between the two. However, it is our preference to use water at 37° C to evaluate children. The advantage of gas (carbon dioxide) is that it is clean and efficient, allowing a rapid rate of bladder filling; thus, it takes little time to perform the test. On the other hand, when the

bladder is filled at a rapid rate, accommodation is impaired, with resultant erroneous values of total capacity and compliance. Carbon dioxide is irritating to the urothelium and some patients complain of discomfort and dysuria. Because gas is compressible, phasic bladder contractions of small amplitude may not be recorded, and significant high-pressure contractions may appear to be of low amplitude. Gas may also leak unobtrusively at instrument connections and also from the bladder around the catheter, particularly if outflow resistance is low.

The cystometric variables that may be observed during the study are those of compliance, contractility, sensation, capacity, and, if indicated, "leak-point pressure" (LPP). Although the stable bladder should remain so even at an unphysiologic rate of filling of 100 ml/minute, certain patients require a slower rate of bladder filling. These include patients with a known neurologic condition and suspected of having a hyperreflexic bladder, those with bladders with decreased compliance, and children. In these situations, the bladder should be filled at a rate of 25 to 50 ml/minute. During filling, a record is made of the bladder volumes at which first sensation of filling, sensation of urgency to void, and sensation of maximal capacity occur. During the filling phase, provocative measures such as coughing and the Valsalva maneuver should be used to look for increased detrusor contractility. The pressure measured within the bladder is composed of pressure induced by the detrusor itself and also by intra-abdominal pressure. Therefore, pressure increments recorded on a simple cystometrograph may at least partially reflect intra-abdominal pressure increases. To eliminate such artifactual interferences, it may be necessary to measure intra-abdominal pressure simultaneously by means of a rectal catheter. Cystometers are available that will electronically subtract the rectal pressure from the total bladder pressure, thus giving the subtracted bladder pressure or detrusor pressure. This measurement is important for provocative cystometry and for voiding studies to determine the efficiency of the voiding contraction.

Abnormal Cystometric Patterns

Abnormalities of bladder storage that may be detected by cystometry include decreased detrusor compliance, involuntary detrusor contractility or detrusor hyperreflexia, involuntary detrusor contraction, increased bladder compliance, and decreased detrusor contractility or detrusor areflexia.

Bladder compliance refers to the change in detrusor pressure that accompanies an increase in bladder volume during filling. Normally, this should not exceed 15 cm H_2O. A bladder with decreased compliance is one in which the pressure increases steeply with filling (Fig. 6–6). Decreased compliance may result from detrusor hypertrophy, fibrotic changes in the bladder wall, bladder wall inflammation, and possibly neurologic lesions.

Involuntary detrusor contraction refers to a phasic increase in bladder pressure. This may occur in response to provocation such as a cough, stress, or posture change, or it may occur spontaneously (Fig. 6–7). States of increased detrusor contractility have been referred to as "detrusor instability" or "detrusor hyperreflexia." In general, the term detrusor hyperreflexia refers to detrusor function that is a direct result of associated neurologic disease whereas detrusor instability is seen in the absence of neurologic disease (Hald). Detrusor hyperreflexia commonly occurs as a result of suprapontine cerebral disorders, such as cerebrovascular abnormalities or trauma. This condition also may occur in patients with suprasacral spinal cord disease processes, such as multiple sclerosis or trauma with or without concomitant detrusor-sphincter dyssynergia.

With marked detrusor instability (or hyperreflexia), the compliance may also be decreased, probably secondary to detrusor muscle hypertrophy (Fig. 6–8). At the most severe end of the spectrum of increased detrusor contractility is the bladder with decreased capacity, in which detrusor hyperreflexia occurs at a low volume (Fig. 6–9). Steepness of the curve is due to muscle contraction as well as to decreased compliance. This may have a neuropathic cause, although it may be seen in patients with severe outlet obstruction. Because both decreased compliance and detrusor hyperreflexia result in an increase in bladder

pressure, differentiation of the two can be difficult.

A large-capacity bladder with normal or increased compliance (Fig. 6–10) may result from decreased sensation; this is commonly seen in the diabetic patient or those with chronic outlet obstruction. Children with the non-neuropathic bladder syndrome will exhibit this type of detrusor function. It may also be a behavioral phenomenon in patients who learned to inhibit voiding voluntarily for long periods. Weir and Jaques found that 30 per cent of patients with bladder capacities in excess of 800 ml were urodynamically normal, so that increased bladder capacity in itself is not necessarily an indication of a pathologic condition, especially in patients who can generate a normal detrusor contraction and void to completeness.

Decreased bladder capacity may be purely sensory in origin (normal compliance and stability) and is commonly seen in females with idiopathic frequency syndrome and in those with an inflamed bladder. These patients usually are able to produce a voluntary detrusor contraction (Fig. 6–11).

Bethanechol Supersensitivity Test

Bethanechol chloride is an acetylcholine-like parasympathomimetic agent that exhibits a relatively selective action on the urinary bladder and gut, with little or no action at therapeutic dosages on ganglia or on the cardiovascular system (Koelle; Ursillo). It is cholinesterase-resistant and causes a contraction in vitro in smooth muscle from all areas of the bladder (Raezer et al). It has minimal effect on the normal bladder, decreasing the capacity slightly, increasing detrusor tone, and increasing the maximum voluntary micturition pressure. It does not cause the normal bladder to become unstable.

The bethanechol supersensitivity test is based on Cannon's law of denervation, which states that when an organ is deprived of its

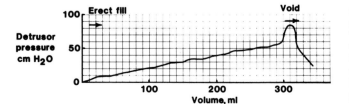

Figure 6–6 □ Cystometrogram depicting decreased detrusor compliance. (From Barrett DM, Wein AJ: Voiding dysfunction: diagnosis, classification, and management. *In* Adult and Pediatric Urology, Vol 1. Edited by JY Gillenwater, JT Grayhack, SS Howards, et al. Chicago, Year Book Medical Publishers, 1987, pp 863–962. By permission of the publisher.)

Figure 6-7 □ Cystometrogram depicting increased detrusor contractility. (From Barrett DM, Wein AJ: Voiding dysfunction: diagnosis, classification, and management. *In* Adult and Pediatric Urology, Vol 1. Edited by JY Gillenwater, JT Grayhack, SS Howards, et al. Chicago, Year Book Medical Publishers, 1987, pp 863–962. By permission of the publisher.)

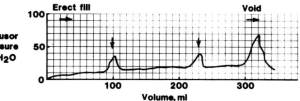

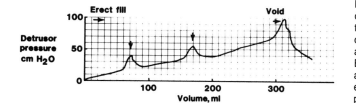

Figure 6-8 □ Cystometrogram showing decreased compliance and increased detrusor contractility. (From Barrett DM, Wein AJ: Voiding dysfunction: diagnosis, classification, and management. *In* Adult and Pediatric Urology, Vol 1. Edited by JY Gillenwater, JT Grayhack, SS Howards, et al. Chicago, Year Book Medical Publishers, 1987, pp 863–962. By permission of the publisher.)

Figure 6-9 □ Cystometrogram showing detrusor hyperreflexia. (From Barrett DM, Wein AJ: Voiding dysfunction: diagnosis, classification, and management. *In* Adult and Pediatric Urology, Vol 1. Edited by JY Gillenwater, JT Grayhack, SS Howards, et al. Chicago, Year Book Medical Publishers, 1987, pp 863–962. By permission of the publisher.)

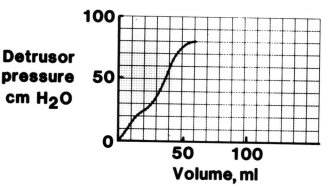

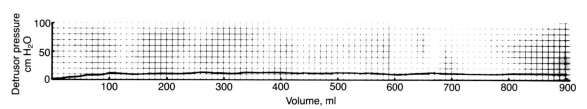

Figure 6-10 □ Cystometrogram demonstrating increased detrusor compliance. (From Barrett DM, Wein AJ: Voiding dysfunction: diagnosis, classification, and management. *In* Adult and Pediatric Urology, Vol 1. Edited by JY Gillenwater, JT Grayhack, SS Howards, et al. Chicago, Year Book Medical Publishers, 1987, pp 863–962. By permission of the publisher.)

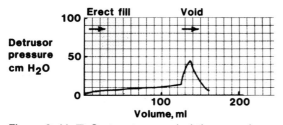

Figure 6–11 □ Cystometrogram depicting normal compliance and contractility but small capacity. (From Barrett DM, Wein AJ: Voiding dysfunction: diagnosis, classification, and management. *In* Adult and Pediatric Urology, Vol 1. Edited by JY Gillenwater, JT Grayhack, SS Howards, et al. Chicago, Year Book Medical Publishers, 1987, pp 863–962. By permission of the publisher.)

nerve supply, it will develop hypersensitivity to its own neurotransmitter substance. Lapides reported this to be quite accurate for patients with denervated bladder (Lapides et al). However, others (Blaivas et al, 1980) found significant rates of false-negative and false-positive responses.

A subcutaneous injection of 2.5 mg of bethanechol chloride is followed in 15 to 30 minutes by repeated cystometric examination. In patients with areflexic bladder of neuropathic origin, an increase in pressure results in at least 15 cm H_2O at 100 ml filling, in excess of the pretreated cystometric pressure (Fig. 6–12). This does not occur in normal patients and in those with myogenically decompensated bladders. A positive test result should not imply a potential benefit from the therapeutic use of bethanechol chloride given orally (Barrett, 1981).

The use of bethanechol chloride is contraindicated in patients with bronchial asthma, peptic ulcer, hyperthyroidism, enteritis, bowel obstruction, bladder outlet obstruction, cardiac

disease, or a history of recent gastrointestinal surgery (Wein, 1979, 1980).

Leak-Point Pressure Evaluation

In children who cannot speak, especially those with increased bladder contractility (instability or hyperreflexia) or decreased bladder compliance, the evaluation of LPP has significant prognostic implications. McGuire and colleagues emphasized, in evaluating children with myelodysplasia, that intravesical pressures exceeding 40 cm H_2O lead to insidious upper tract deterioration.

Leak-point pressure is determined during cystometry by using water in patients of all ages. Fluid is infused through a small-caliber catheter and intravesical pressure is recorded (CMG) simultaneously. The pressure at which fluid escapes through the urethra and around the catheter is the LPP. In the very young child with neurologic disease such as myelodysplasia, LPP determinations provide an excellent test to observe the internal bladder environment and its potential risk of upper tract disease (Fig. 6–13).

Uroflowmetry

Flow rate is defined as the volume of fluid expelled from the urethra per unit time and is expressed in ml/second. Modern instruments allow us to record not only the overall rate but also a flow trace (Fig. 6–14). The urine flow rate is an expression of the combined activity of the detrusor and urethra. A normal flow rate will usually indicate good function of both.

An obstruction in the urethra (e.g., urethral stricture) may be overcome by a more forceful detrusor contraction, which would bring higher

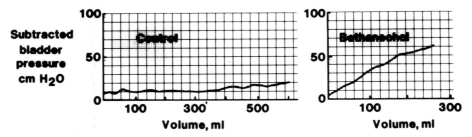

Figure 6–12 □ Cystometrogram showing positive response to bethanechol stimulation test. (From Barrett DM, Wein AJ: Voiding dysfunction: diagnosis, classification, and management. *In* Adult and Pediatric Urology, Vol 1. Edited by JY Gillenwater, JT Grayhack, SS Howards, et al. Chicago, Year Book Medical Publishers, 1987, pp 863–962. By permission of the publisher.)

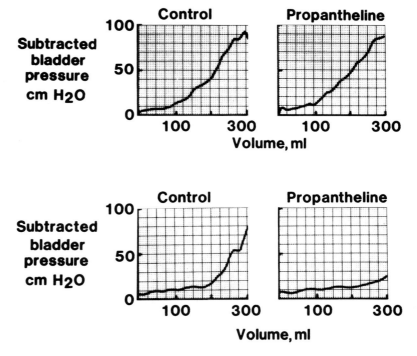

Figure 6–13 □ Cystometrogram before and after parenteral administration of 15 mg propantheline. A positive response is indicated by flattening of the tonus limb *(bottom panels)*. No change confirms inappropriate response *(top panels)*. (From Barrett DM, Wein AJ: Voiding dysfunction: diagnosis, classification, and management. *In* Adult and Pediatric Urology, Vol 1. Edited by JY Gillenwater, JT Grayhack, SS Howards, et al. Chicago, Year Book Medical Publishers, 1987, pp 863–962. By permission of the publisher.)

bladder pressures during the stage of micturition. This may result in an apparently normal peak flow rate—at least during the early stages of the obstruction—but a decreased average flow rate. Therefore, for a full definition of lower tract function, simultaneous pressure (cystometry) and flow studies during voiding may be indicated. However, a urine flow study alone has value as a screening test for lower urinary tract dysfunction, for preoperative and postoperative assessment of lower urinary tract surgery, and to study the effect of pharmacologic agents on urethral resistance and voiding efficiency.

Urine Flow Rate Variables

To the clinician, the urine flow rate variables (Table 6–8) of most importance are the maxi-

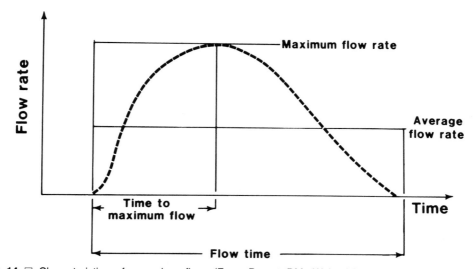

Figure 6–14 □ Characteristics of normal uroflow. (From Barrett DM, Wein AJ: Voiding dysfunction: diagnosis, classification, and management. *In* Adult and Pediatric Urology, Vol 1. Edited by JY Gillenwater, JT Grayhack, SS Howards, et al. Chicago, Year Book Medical Publishers, 1987, pp 863–962. By permission of the publisher.)

Table 6–8 □ Urine Flow Rate Variables

1. *Flow time*	Time during which measurable flow occurs
2. *Time to maximal flow*	Time from onset of flow to maximal rate
3. *Maximal flow rate*	Maximal rate of flow
4. *Voided volume*	Total volume expelled by way of the urethra
5. *Average flow rate*	Voided volume divided by flow time
6. *Voiding time*	Total duration of micturition, including interruptions
7. *Flow pattern*	May be continuous, interrupted, or specifically described

From Barrett DM, Wein AJ: Voiding dysfunction: diagnosis, classification, and management. *In* Adult and Pediatric Urology, Vol I. Edited by JY Gillenwater, JT Grayhack, SS Howards, et al. Chicago, Year Book Medical Publishers, 1987, pp 863–962. By permission of the publisher.

Table 6–9 □ Minimum Acceptable Urine Flow Rates

Age, Yr	Minimum Voided Volume (ml)	Male (ml/sec)	Female (ml/sec)
4–7	100	10	10
8–13	100	12	15
14–45	200	21	18
46–55	200	22	15
56–80	200	9	10

From Abrams P: The practice of urodynamics. *In* Urodynamics: Principles, Practice and Application. Edited by AR Mundy, TP Stephenson, AJ Wein. Edinburgh, Churchill Livingstone, 1984, pp 76–92. By permission of the publisher.

mal flow rate, voided volume, and flow pattern. Measurement of urine flow rate depends mostly on the patient's comfort with the environment in which the test is conducted and lack of intimidation in the urodynamics laboratory. Additionally, the patient must have an adequately full bladder because urine flow rate depends on voided volume. Ideally, interpretation of urine flow should be for volumes of at least 250 ml; flow rates with smaller voided volumes should be interpreted with caution. Large volumes may also be accompanied by decreased flow rates, perhaps due to decreased detrusor fibers stretching. However, flow rates are also related to the sex and age of the patient. Most data in the literature relate to measurements of flow in men younger than 55 years and cite norms of 15 ml/second and 25 ml/second for mean and maximal rates, respectively. Abrams (1984a, 1984b) stated correctly that normality should be defined in terms of age, and that the use of nomograms relating to young men for assessing the older male patient is a doubtful practice. Females have significantly higher flow rates than males matched for age and voided volumes. The values presented in Table 6–9 are from Abrams (1984a, 1984b) and represent the minimal flow rate for a given sex, age, and voided volume.

The normal flow pattern exhibits a rapid increase to maximal flow rate, attaining this level within one third of the ultimate voiding time, and in addition, at least 45 per cent of the total volume voided should be evacuated within this same period and before maximal flow rate is achieved. After achieving maximal

rate, flow decreases more slowly; hence, a true bell-shaped curve is not achieved. In normal patients, average flow rate should be approximately 50 per cent of the maximal urine flow rate.

If abdominal straining is used to augment voiding, the stream is interrupted (Fig. 6–15). Other causes of an interrupted stream may be voluntary sphincter contraction during voiding by the patient with detrusor sphincter dyssynergia or, more commonly, by an anxious patient, and artifactual recording, which most commonly occurs when a male patient directs his stream across the collecting funnel (Fig. 6–16).

In outlet obstruction, a flat, elongated curve with a low maximal flow rate is seen characteristically; maximal flow rate is reached in the initial part of the trace (Fig. 6–17). In the patient with detrusor underactivity, the flow pattern will be intermittent because abdominal muscles are used to augment voiding. The urine flow rate is decreased and the maximal flow rate is seen in the middle part of the tracing.

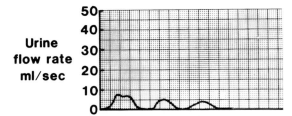

Figure 6–15 □ Uroflow with interrupted stream during straining to void. (From Barrett DM, Wein AJ: Voiding dysfunction: diagnosis, classification, and management. *In* Adult and Pediatric Urology, Vol 1. Edited by JY Gillenwater, JT Grayhack, SS Howards, et al. Chicago, Year Book Medical Publishers, 1987, pp 863–962. By permission of the publisher.)

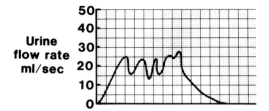

Figure 6–16 □ Uroflow with interrupted pattern as a result of intermittent sphincter activity. (From Barrett DM, Wein AJ: Voiding dysfunction: diagnosis, classification, and management. *In* Adult and Pediatric Urology, Vol 1. Edited by JY Gillenwater, JT Grayhack, SS Howards, et al. Chicago, Year Book Medical Publishers, 1987, pp 863–962. By permission of the publisher.)

Considerable care must be taken not to overinterpret flow study results, and considerable clinical judgment is necessary in their interpretation. Abnormal findings should be confirmed by the use of more elaborate urodynamic studies.

Residual Urine Volume

Residual urine volume is another variable that integrates the activity of the bladder and outlet during the emptying phase of micturition. A consistently increased residual urine volume generally indicates increased outlet resistance, decreased bladder contractility, or both. Absence of residual urine is compatible with normal lower urinary tract function during emptying but also may exist in the presence of significant disorders of filling or storage (incontinence) and disorders of emptying in which the intravesical pressure is sufficient to overcome increases in outlet resistance up to a certain point. A typical example of this is the patient with outlet obstruction as a result of urethral stricture. Initially, despite significant obstruction, the detrusor is capable of emptying the bladder by contracting with a greater force, leading to hypertrophy and increased

intravesical pressure. However, with time, the detrusor fails, leading to increased residual volumes and a decrease in intravesical pressures produced during voiding. This illustrates the fact that it is extremely rare to be able to make an adequate diagnosis on the basis of any single urodynamic study. All of the study results must fit together, and these must ultimately be compatible with the symptomatology and with the results of the rest of the neurologic evaluation.

Electromyography

EMG is the study of the bioelectric potentials generated by depolarization of skeletal muscle. Skeletal muscle is innervated by neurons whose cell bodies are in the anterior horn of the spinal cord. The anterior horn cell in the gray matter of the spinal cord, its axon, and all of the muscle fibers (the number may vary) innervated by it are called a motor unit. An excitatory impulse from an anterior horn cell causes contraction (by membrane depolarization) of all the muscle fibers in that motor unit. The electrical discharge produced on contraction of the muscle fibers of the motor unit is called a motor unit action potential. This may be detected by electrodes and displayed on an oscilloscope or strip chart, or it may be converted to an audible sound.

Individually recorded on an oscilloscope, the motor unit action potentials may take various configurations: biphasic, triphasic, or, rarely, polyphasic. In the relaxed state, the normal striated muscle is almost electrically quiescent and only infrequent action potentials are recorded. However, with progressive muscle contraction, increasing numbers of motor units are recruited and each motor unit fires at a more rapid rate. These firings can be individually recorded electromyographically, and the configuration of the action potentials is significant in diagnosis. At the point of maximal

Figure 6–17 □ Uroflow with abnormal flow rate characteristic of detrusor outlet obstruction. (From Barrett DM, Wein AJ: Voiding dysfunction: diagnosis, classification, and management. *In* Adult and Pediatric Urology, Vol 1. Edited by JY Gillenwater, JT Grayhack, SS Howards, et al. Chicago, Year Book Medical Publishers, 1987, pp 863–962. By permission of the publisher.)

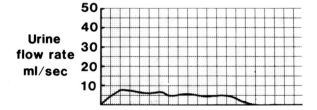

contraction, motor unit action potentials are so frequent that total overlap occurs and EMG separation cannot be achieved; an interference pattern results.

It takes considerable EMG experience to interpret the variables recorded on an oscilloscope during sphincter EMG. Identification of these variations is important in making an accurate neurologic diagnosis. Individual motor unit action potentials may be detected by needle electrodes placed directly into or near the muscle to be studied. When surface electrodes are used, individual motor unit action potentials are not visualized; instead, an overall gross recording of the activity of the muscle is detected (Barrett, 1980). If one is not interested in motor unit action potentials, surface electrodes are adequate. They can detect whether the pelvic floor muscles are contracting or relaxing at any given instant. However, because they are unable to detect individual motor unit action potentials, surface electrodes cannot help in assessing the integrity of these muscles and their nerve supply.

During cystometric bladder filling, there should be incremental increases in EMG activity as more motor units are recruited. This activity reaches a maximum when peak bladder capacity is reached, and at the command to void, there should be sudden cessation of sphincter activity, which should persist throughout voiding (Blaivas et al, 1977). On completion of bladder emptying, resumption of baseline sphincter activity occurs. In assessing external sphincter activity, the clinician asks the patient to interrupt voiding in the middle of the stream, at which point there should be an abrupt increase in sphincter activity, which should be sufficient to stop the flow. Resumption of voiding should occur thereafter; however, if the holding pattern is maintained, the detrusor reflex should ideally be lost in approximately 10 seconds (Webster).

Abnormal EMG patterns may be detected in a number of situations. Detrusor sphincter dyssynergia describes sphincter activity that is inappropriate to the activity of the detrusor. Three varieties of such discoordination (Fig. 6–18) were described (McGuire, 1979). One pattern involves an appropriate increase in EMG activity with bladder filling, which is followed by an inappropriate involuntary increase in activity at the onset of detrusor contraction. Thus, the detrusor contracts against a closed sphincter.

A second type of discoordination involves failure to develop a proper reflex detrusor contraction because of increased EMG activity during voiding, which causes inhibition of the detrusor motor nucleus in the sacral spinal cord with resultant inhibition of detrusor contraction. This type of discoordination may be seen in patients with suprasacral spinal cord injury.

The third type involves contraction and relaxation of the sphincter during bladder filling. This amounts to periods of uninhibited sphincter relaxation, which is associated with reflex detrusor contraction leading to urgency and urge incontinence.

Simultaneous EMG activity and an increase in intravesical pressure do not always indicate

DETRUSOR EXTERNAL SPHINCTER DYSSYNERGIA

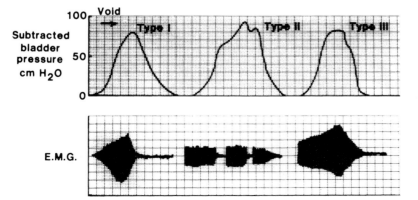

Figure 6–18 □ Varieties of external sphincter discoordination. (From Barrett DM, Wein AJ: Voiding dysfunction: diagnosis, classification, and management. *In* Adult and Pediatric Urology, Vol 1. Edited by JY Gillenwater, JT Grayhack, SS Howards, et al. Chicago, Year Book Medical Publishers, 1987, pp 863–962. Adapted from McGuire E: Electromyographic evaluation of sphincter function and dysfunction. Urol Clin North Am 6:121–124, 1979.)

sphincter dyssynergia. Detrusor striated sphincter dyssynergia is undoubtedly the most overdiagnosed entity in the field of voiding dysfunction. Patients suspected of having this diagnosis should always be further investigated urodynamically or radiologically, or both, in studies of the activity of the bladder and the outlet during the emptying phase of micturition. True detrusor striated sphincter dyssynergia is extremely uncommon (or does not exist) in patients without neurologic disease. This diagnosis in such a patient deserves exhaustive study before it is confirmed.

Sphincter EMG studies have gained popularity for the investigation of children with voiding dysfunction (Maizels and Firlit). It is suggested that learned dysfunctional sphincter habits may be responsible for voiding abnormalities and may result in recurrent urinary infections, reflux, and upper tract deterioration. An attempt has been made to retrain these sphincters by the use of biofeedback techniques utilizing sphincter EMG during voiding (Maizels et al). The patient can appreciate from an EMG audio monitor whether or not sphincter relaxation is being accomplished and, hence, by positive reinforcement may correct the problem.

Flow-EMG Evaluation

Because of the confusion relating to the diagnosis of detrusor–skeletal muscle sphincter dyssynergia in children without neurologic disease, we proposed a simple test using simultaneous flow and EMG in 1981 (Barrett and Wein). A cooperative child is required. Patch electrodes are placed on the perineum, and a uroflow-electromyogram is obtained. Children with complete absence of EMG activity noted throughout voiding do not have maturational dyssynergia. Interrupted stream or excessive bursts of EMG activity throughout voiding imply dyssynergia.

Evoked Responses

Evoked responses are potential changes in neural tissue that are recorded by using averaging techniques and result from distant stimulation, usually electrical stimulation (Sixth Report on the Standardization of Terminology of Lower Urinary Tract Function). Evoked responses may be used to test the integrity of peripheral, spinal, and central nervous pathways. As with nerve conduction studies, the conduction time (latency) may be measured. In addition, information may be gained from the amplitude and configuration of these responses.

For example, the sacral evoked response is measured by the latency of the bulbocavernosus reflex (Blaivas, 1984b; Blaivas et al, 1981b; Nordling and Meyhoff). The bulbocavernosus reflex arc is mediated by afferent and efferent pudendal nerve fibers. The reflex is seemingly polysynaptic, traversing at least several spinal cord segments. Clinically, the bulbocavernosus reflex is elicited by briskly squeezing the glans penis or clitoris and observing or feeling a reflex contractility response of the external anal sphincter or bulbocavernosus muscle. Alternately, the reflex may be stimulated by pulling the balloon of a Foley catheter against the bladder neck. The bulbocavernosus reflex is present in almost all normal men and in approximately 70 per cent of normal women. Absence of this reflex in a man strongly suggests a sacral neurologic lesion, but it is present in approximately 50 per cent of patients with an incomplete lower motor neuron lesion. Because it is difficult to grade the reflex clinically, measurement of the bulbocavernosus reflex latency offers a more quantitative means of evaluating the sacral reflex arcs. When one side of the penis is stimulated electrically, as by a surface stimulating electrode, there is a bilateral contractile response in the bulbocavernosus muscle that may be detected by needle electrodes placed bilaterally into this muscle (Blaivas et al, 1981b; Krane and Siroky). Considerable EMG expertise is required to determine the onset of the evoked response because of the possibility of interference from units that are firing either randomly or because of the patient's anxiety. Although some authors have recommended that evoked responses of 20 to 30 stimulations be electronically averaged to determine the latency, Blaivas (1984b) claimed that the shortest latency rather than the average is a more specific means of evaluating the sacral segments because the bulbocavernosus reflex is polysynaptic.

The bulbocavernosus reflex is a crossed response, and it is possible to stimulate on one side and record from the ipsilateral and the contralateral bulbocavernosus muscles. This is useful in detecting subtle abnormalities that affect only a single afferent or efferent pathway. Thus, when stimulating one side of the penis, the clinician may elicit recordings from both sides of the bulbocavernosus muscle. The other side of the penis is then stimulated, and the latencies from the bulbocavernosus muscle are again determined. In this fashion, it is possible to evaluate the right and left afferent and efferent pathways individually. The normal bulbocavernosus reflex latency varies from approximately 30 to 40 ms, but the exact values vary slightly from one laboratory to another. Any neurologic process that interferes with the integrity of the reflex arc will result in a prolonged latency. Common disorders that result in prolonged latencies include diabetes mellitus, alcoholic neuropathy, and prolapsed disks. Less commonly, a prolonged latency may be an early manifestation of a spinal cord tumor or of multiple sclerosis. Bulbocavernosus reflex latencies may also be obtained by stimulating the proximal urethra or bladder neck instead of the penis. However, limited experience has been gained with these techniques.

A word of caution is warranted in the interpretation of the result of sacral evoked responses. This test quantifies the integrity of innervation of the striated pelvic floor and perineal muscles and the supraspinal neurologic pathways involved in lower urinary tract function. It does not give information concerning the status of the smooth muscle of the detrusor, bladder neck, and proximal urethra. In general, it is reasonable to assume that when a neurologic lesion is found to affect the striated perineal floor muscles, it is likely that the same process also involves the detrusor because the pudendal and parasympathetic nuclei in the sacral spinal cord are practically adjacent to one another. Nevertheless, certain neurologic disorders may involve one portion of the nervous system and spare another.

Urethral Pressure Profile

The urethral pressure profile (UPP) is a graphic recording of the pressure within the urethra at each point along its length. In 1969, Brown and Wickham described a technique that is the basis for modern perfusion urethral profilometry. They utilized a specially designed catheter with multiple side holes and an occluded tip. Fluid infused along the catheter escaped through the side holes and the UPP measured the resistance of the urethral walls to distention by this escaping fluid. This resistance is expressed in terms of the pressure

necessary to maintain a steady flow of fluid through the catheter system. The UPP recording commences in the bladder, and constant withdrawal of the catheter is accomplished through the entire length of the urethra. Because the UPP measures the urethra's response to distention, various factors affecting urethral compliance alter the appearance of the profile curve. Contributing to the normal urethral compliance are smooth muscle activity, striated muscle activity, the fibroelastic component of the urethral wall, vascular tension resulting from the rich spongy network around the urethra, and an extrinsic compression component of varying degree. Alteration in any of these variables may significantly alter the appearance of the curve. However, the diagnostic value of the static UPP is limited because it is a study that is not done during filling or storage or emptying. It is a study done at rest, and it is difficult to prove that the events recorded bear any relationship to what goes on in the bladder or in the outlet during filling or storage or emptying.

Despite these shortcomings, static profilometry may help to evaluate artificial sphincter function, gel prosthesis function, and the success of medical or surgical therapy for sphincteric incontinence. Alterations in the static profile certainly correlate with some disease entities, such as stress incontinence, an enlarged prostate, and striated sphincter dyssynergia. However, the overlap is invariably large and, because of this, the utility of perfusion profilometry as a specific diagnostic study is limited. More recently, other methods of UPP measurement have been developed, including stress UPP and dynamic UPP. Before we elaborate on these more sophisticated techniques, we review some aspects of static UPP.

Static Urethral Pressure Profile. Although this technique may be modified by altering the position of the patient and the degree of bladder filling, the static UPP measures urethral pressure with the patient supine, the bladder at rest, and the urethra closed. Although perfusion profilometry may be the method most commonly used, the other two techniques used to measure static UPP are the balloon catheter technique and the catheter tip transducers.

Perfusion Urethral Pressure Profile. This technique uses a catheter with side holes through which saline is perfused with a motorized syringe pump. The pressure is measured via a side arm of the catheter. The pressure registered by the transducer represents the resistance to flow from the catheter side hole, as previously mentioned. Consequently, when the catheter is in the bladder, only bladder pressure opposes the outflow of saline, and the measured pressure is low. The catheter is then withdrawn at a constant rate through the entire length of the urethra. The initial pressure recorded is the intravesical pressure, followed by a positive deflection at the bladder neck and a progressive increase in urethral pressure to the midportion of the urethra in women (Fig. 6–19) and to the membranous urethra in men (Fig. 6–20). Beyond this point, pressure progressively decreases until the external meatus is reached.

Recommended nomenclature for UPP has been proposed by the International Continence Society. The most frequently measured variables are: (1) maximum urethral pressure, which is the maximum pressure of the profile; (2) maximum urethral closing pressure, which is the difference between the maximum urethral pressure and bladder pressure; and (3) functional profile length, which is the length of the urethra along which the pressure exceeds bladder pressure. Perfusion profilometry may be performed with gas instead of saline. However, it has been demonstrated that a CO_2 perfusion rate of 150 ml/minute is needed to achieve a satisfactory reading of urethral pressure. The use of such high flow rates makes

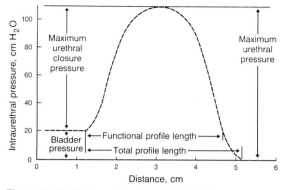

Figure 6–19 □ Normal perfusion urethral pressure profile for a woman. (From Barrett DM, Wein AJ: Voiding dysfunction: diagnosis, classification, and management. *In* Adult and Pediatric Urology, Vol 1. Edited by JY Gillenwater, JT Grayhack, SS Howards, et al. Chicago, Year Book Medical Publishers, 1987, pp 863–962. By permission of the publisher.)

the practical recording of urethral pressure very difficult because the bladder is filled rapidly and the investigator is measuring urethral pressure while the bladder is being distended swiftly. In addition, the speed of gas flow may theoretically lead to the recording of artificially high pressures as a result of the gas pushing the urethral walls apart. In this instance, the gas profile may be measuring urethral elasticity rather than urethral pressure.

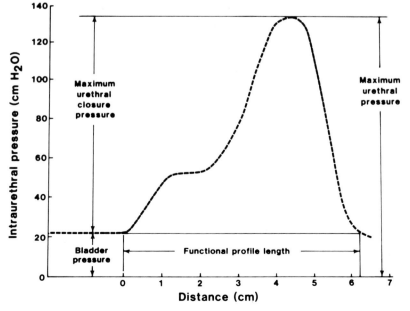

Figure 6–20 □ Normal perfusion urethral pressure profile for a man. (From Barrett DM, Wein AJ: Voiding dysfunction: diagnosis, classification, and management. *In* Adult and Pediatric Urology, Vol 1. Edited by JY Gillenwater, JT Grayhack, SS Howards, et al. Chicago, Year Book Medical Publishers, 1987, pp 863–962. By permission of the publisher.)

Balloon Catheter System. With this system, the eye holes of the catheter are covered by a fine plastic balloon. This technique relies on a closed system that must be free of all bubbles or leaks. Although this technique is accurate, frequent calibration and frequent replacement of balloon catheters is required owing to a gradual change in compliance of the thin-walled balloons.

Catheter Tip Transducer. This technique utilizes a catheter with either one or two transducers mounted on it. The transducer is at the site of recording and obviates the problems inherent in recording at a distance from the organ being monitored. It allows for urethral pressure measurement during voiding, and double transducer-tip catheters allow for the simultaneous measurement of intravesical and urethral pressure. The disadvantage of the Mickel transducer-catheter is its fragility and expense.

Whichever technique is used to measure UPP, it is probably essential to record external sphincter activity simultaneously. This ensures that unintentional external sphincter contraction does not cause an artifactual increase in maximal closing pressure. Many patients find it impossible to inhibit the external sphincter during the perfusion withdrawal process, and this is even more true of those with hypersensitive urethras and neuropathic bladder dysfunction. Simultaneous measurement of rectal pressure is advocated as a means of identifying unintentional abdominal straining, which might also alter the normal profile curve.

In normal female patients, there is a gradual tendency for the maximum urethral pressure to decrease with age. This occurs mainly after the menopause. The shape of the UPP curve is symmetric. In male patients, there is no decrease in maximum urethral pressure with age. However, there is a tendency for the length of the prostatic urethra to increase, particularly after age 45 years. The shape of the UPP curve in the male is asymmetric. In the proximal part of the profile, there is a variable plateau as a result of the bladder neck and prostatic tissues. In the distal part of the profile, the pressure recorded is higher than from the distal female urethra owing to the length and configuration of the male urethra. However, the distal urethra is rarely of clinical significance except on the unusual occasion when the profile is recorded in a patient with a urethral stricture.

Stress Urethral Pressure Profile. The stress UPP is measured best with a dual-sensor catheter tip transducer. The sensors should be separated by a 5- to 10-cm interval. The catheter is introduced into the bladder and then slowly withdrawn through the urethra while the patient is asked to cough at regular intervals. A slow withdrawal speed of 0.1 cm/second is used so that coughs may be recorded for each 0.2 cm of urethral length (Abrams, 1984a and 1984b).

In normal patients, the increased pressure seen on the intravesical pressure trace during coughing is also superimposed on the urethral pressure trace. Also in normal patients, the raised intra-abdominal pressure is transmitted to the proximal two thirds of the female urethra. In patients with genuine stress incontinence, there is a failure of pressure transmission. The findings on stress UPP have a far better correlation with the presence of genuine stress incontinence than do the findings on the static UPP. Stress urinary incontinence in women is the main indication for a stress UPP.

Dynamic Urethral Pressure Profile. Static perfusion profilometry is criticized mainly because it provides information on the pressure in the outlet only at rest. It supplies no information on the outlet's behavior during filling, storage, and voiding.

The dynamic urethral pressure profile is intended to show variation in sphincteric closure pressure under various physiologic events as well as under various stresses and commands. This dynamic pressure profile is obtained easily by the membrane catheter or microtransducer technique, but it is practically impossible to obtain by perfusion techniques (Tanagho, 1984). The pressure profile increases normally when the bladder is filled. In addition, postural change affects the urethral pressure. The lowest pressure is recorded when the patient is in the supine position. Sitting up causes an increase in pressure, and further increase in functional length and magnitude of closing pressure occurs when the upright position is assumed. A sharp increase in intra-abdominal pressure (by coughing) and a low sustained increase in intra-abdominal pressure (from bearing down) should result in a simultaneous increase of pressure in the urethra, which is normally much higher than the increase in intra-abdominal pressure.

A drop in urethral pressure just before normal voiding occurs has been reported (Tanagho, 1979). Whether meaningful information can be gleaned from urethral pressure measurement during voiding is debatable, and the technique is unlikely to replace the conventional ways of assessing dynamic urethral function by fluoroscopy. However, where fluoroscopic evaluation is unavailable, dynamic profilometry may be applied to diagnose such uncommon causes of obstruction as proximal sphincter dyssynergia. The establishment of a pressure gradient in an area of the urethra normally wide open with a detrusor contraction establishes the diagnosis of obstruction. An increased bladder pressure that decreases sharply at some point between the bladder neck and the bulbomembranous urethral junction is sufficient to diagnose proximal sphincter dyssynergia (McGuire, 1984). Dynamic UPP measurement may prove to be useful in the assessment of pharmacotherapy.

Multifunction Studies

As mentioned earlier in this chapter, the clinical applicability of urodynamics depends to a large extent on the re-enactment of the patient's symptom complex during the urodynamic assessment. Which urodynamic study to perform depends on the nature of the clinical problem, the available electronic equipment, the ease with which the study can be performed, and the interest and expertise of the urodynamicist. In most clinical settings, it is usually practical and cost-effective to screen patients by performing uroflowmetry, measurement of post-voiding residual volume, and cystometry (Blaivas, 1984a). These three simple tests help us to understand the patient's symptoms in the majority of cases. However, occasionally a more sophisticated study is needed. The indications include (Blaivas et al, 1981a): (1) the simple diagnostic procedures prove inconclusive, (2) the patient has persistent symptoms despite what appears to be appropriate treatment, (3) the patient has a pre-existing condition known to be associated with complex urodynamic abnormalities, and (4) the history and physical examination suggest a neuropathologic condition that requires more elaborate investigation before diagnosis.

Despite what has previously been stated, the patient with an overt neurologic disease, such as spinal cord injury or multiple sclerosis, in whom a urodynamic evaluation is required, should probably be routinely studied by a multifunction study, preferably with simultaneous cystourethrography. The reason for this

is that these conditions are often accompanied by unpredictable pathophysiologic conditions.

Ideally, abdominal pressure should be measured so that subtracted bladder pressure could be monitored during voiding studies because it is bladder pressure that alters in obstruction or detrusor dysfunction. This is particularly important when the detrusor contractions are of small magnitude and when voiding is accompanied by abdominal straining.

A poor urinary flow rate may be caused by outflow obstruction (Fig. 6–21), impaired detrusor contractility (Fig. 6–22), or a combination of both. From a practical standpoint, bladder outlet obstruction may be defined as a poor urinary flow rate in the presence of an "adequate" detrusor contraction (Blaivas, 1984a). For an individual patient, however, it may be difficult to determine whether or not the detrusor pressure is "adequate" with respect to the flow rate, and for this reason, many investigators have attempted to formulate a mathematical definition of bladder outlet obstruction by constructing a "resistance coefficient." The hydrodynamic principles from which these resistance coefficients are derived assume that the bladder behaves as a geometric sphere and that the urethra behaves as a rigid tube. This is clearly not the case, and this limits the usefulness of these formulas. If a bladder has normal contractility and the pressure generated during contraction is high with

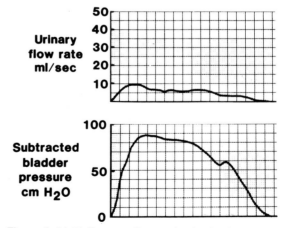

Figure 6–21 □ Pressure-flow study showing high bladder pressure and low flow rate. This is consistent with bladder outlet obstruction. (From Barrett DM, Wein AJ: Voiding dysfunction: diagnosis, classification, and management. *In* Adult and Pediatric Urology, Vol 1. Edited by JY Gillenwater, JT Grayhack, SS Howards, et al. Chicago, Year Book Medical Publishers, 1987, pp 863–962. By permission of the publisher.)

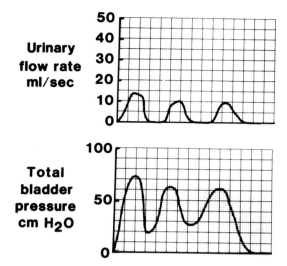

Figure 6–22 ☐ Variable flow rate and bladder pressure. Pattern may be seen in patients with detrusor-sphincter dyssynergia or abdominal straining. (From Barrett DM, Wein AJ: Voiding dysfunction: diagnosis, classification, and management. *In* Adult and Pediatric Urology, Vol 1. Edited by JY Gillenwater, JT Grayhack, SS Howards, et al. Chicago, Year Book Medical Publishers, 1987, pp 863–962. By permission of the publisher.)

a low flow rate produced (Fig. 6–21), a formula is not needed to tell us that obstruction exists. On the other hand, if the bladder is decompensated and incapable of producing a decent increase in intravesical pressure, there is no way that obstruction (or resistance) can be quantitated by these formulas. These formulas assume that if obstruction exists, the bladder is capable of producing a proportionate contraction in response, which is not always the case. If the bladder cannot contract, or contracts poorly, obstruction cannot be defined. Thus, it appears that when these formulas are most necessary, they are least accurate; therefore, they are of little clinical use at present.

Synchronous cystometry and sphincter EMG are useful urodynamic techniques for assessing neurologic function (Blaivas, 1984a; Blaivas et al, 1977). This examination helps to define the interrelationship between the striated external urethral sphincter and the detrusor during the storage and voiding phases of micturition.

The most important information to be gained from simultaneous cystometry and EMG relates to the presence or absence of detrusor external sphincter dyssynergia (DSD). In normal patients or those with detrusor instability or detrusor hyperreflexia due to neurologic lesions above the brain stem, the external urethral sphincter relaxes completely immediately prior to the onset of the increase in detrusor pressure. The relaxation continues throughout the detrusor contractions unless the patient voluntarily attempts to interrupt micturition. Detrusor external sphincter dyssynergia is characterized by an involuntary contraction of the external sphincter coincident with or immediately preceding the increase in detrusor pressure.

Blaivas and colleagues (1981a) classified DSD into three types (see Fig. 6–18). *Type I DSD* is characterized by an abrupt increase in EMG activity; the onset is approximately coincident with the onset of the measurable detrusor contraction. At the peak of the detrusor contraction, there is a sudden complete relaxation of the external sphincter, and widening ensues as the detrusor pressures decrease. In *type II DSD* there are sporadic sphincter contractions throughout the detrusor contraction. *Type III DSD* is characterized by a crescendo-decrescendo pattern of external sphincter contraction that parallels the detrusor contraction. Detrusor sphincter dyssynergia is an abnormal reflex that occurs only when the neurologic pathways between the pons and sacral micturition center are interrupted. In the absence of such a neurologic lesion, one should exercise extreme caution in diagnosing DSD.

Pseudodyssynergia is believed to be an abnormality of learned behavior in which the patient subconsciously attempts to inhibit micturition as it progresses (Wein and Barrett, 1982). This results in subconscious "voluntary" contraction of the external sphincter throughout micturition. Pseudodyssynergic syndromes are encountered most frequently in children with persistent voiding symptoms, in men with prostatitis, and in women with the urethral syndrome.

It is not possible to distinguish between true dyssynergia and pseudodyssynergia by simultaneous cystometry and EMG unless intra-abdominal pressure is measured concurrently. In pseudodyssynergia, there is usually some increase in intra-abdominal pressure as the patient tightens the abdominal and pelvic floor musculature.

Another, possibly more simple, way to screen for detrusor sphincter dyssynergia is by performing the combined test of uroflow and EMG (Barrett and Wein). When uroflow is accompanied by no external sphincter activity, dyssynergia may be excluded.

Stop Flow Test

This test is a combined measurement of uroflow and intravesical pressure; it is performed to evaluate the isometric detrusor pressure. The patient is asked to void. After the stream is initiated and intravesical pressure is recorded, the stream is abruptly stopped. In normal detrusor function, the detrusor pressure usually increases to a level well above voiding pressure. Theoretically, this test is a reflection of the integrity of detrusor tone and contractility.

Videourodynamics

Videourodynamics is a technique utilizing synchronously recorded urodynamic studies and cystourethrography for the evaluation of complex lower urinary tract problems. It comprises the performance of pressure-flow external sphincter EMG studies during filling, storage, and voiding phases of the micturition cycle, together with the periodic screening of the synchronous cystourethrographic appearance of the bladder and outflow tract.

Radiographic contrast material is infused for cystometry, permitting radiographic visualization of the lower urinary tract. Urodynamic variables are transduced and displayed on a storage oscilloscope. A television camera scans the oscilloscope screen, and the resulting image is displayed on a television monitor. The fluoroscopic image of the bladder and urethra is electronically mixed with that of the urodynamic data and displayed on the same monitor. The advantage of these studies is that they combine the objectivity of urodynamics with the visual radiographic image of the part being studied, allowing for far more logical interpretation of results. The financial investment required to establish such a study center limits its use to the medical center setting with a large enough patient population in whom such a study is indicated.

Videourodynamics has proved particularly valuable in the identification of complex bladder outlet obstruction problems. If bladder outlet obstruction has been diagnosed or is suspected but the site of obstruction is not clear, a micturitional static UPP determination usually provides definitive diagnostic data (Blaivas et al, 1981a). The demonstration of a decrease in pressure between the bladder and the membranous urethra during voiding, at which time the bladder and proximal urethra are normally isobaric, establishes the diagnosis of an obstruction between the bladder and the site of the decreased pressure. Fluoroscopy also allows visualization of the site of obstruction (Yalla et al).

Detrusor external sphincter dyssynergia is characterized by involuntary contraction of the external urethral sphincter during involuntary detrusor contractions (Fig. 6–23). This may be readily identified by fluoroscopy during voiding. If a patient was treated by external sphincterotomy and a question arises as to the efficacy of surgery, this may be evaluated best by a videourodynamic study.

Videourodynamics is also valuable in the evaluation of some women with stress incontinence. The symptoms of stress incontinence may be caused not only by urethral and bladder hypermobility but also by denervation of the smooth muscle of the proximal urethra (e.g., after radical pelvic surgery or in myelodysplasia). This latter condition may be diag-

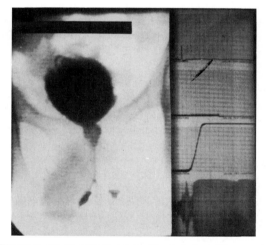

Figure 6–23 □ Videourodynamic study in a 15-year-old paraplegic (T-5) male who had high residual urine volumes and recurrent urinary infection. Intravesical pressure exceeded 100 cm H₂O (scale, 0 to 100 cm H₂O), and electromyographic activity was excessive during the detrusor contraction. Although the bladder neck opened, the prostatic urethra was dilated to a level of the external sphincter. There was no urinary flow *(top strip recording)* or increase in abdominal pressure *(second strip recording from top)*. This is classic detrusor–external sphincter dyssynergia. (From Barrett DM, Wein AJ: Voiding dysfunction: diagnosis, classification, and management. *In* Adult and Pediatric Urology, Vol 1. Edited by JY Gillenwater, JT Grayhack, SS Howards, et al. Chicago, Year Book Medical Publishers, 1987, pp 863–962. By permission of the publisher.)

nosed by demonstrating an open bladder neck during bladder filling and a proximal urethra that is isobaric with the bladder. The practical implication of this differentiation is the choice of surgical repair, which is quite different for the two conditions.

Bibliography

Abrams P: The practice of urodynamics. *In* Urodynamics: Principles, Practice and Application. Edited by AR Mundy, TP Stephenson, AJ Wein. Edinburgh, Churchill Livingstone, 1984a, pp 76–92.

Abrams P: The urethral pressure profile measurement. *In* Urodynamics: Principles, Practice and Application. Edited by AR Mundy, TP Stephenson, AJ Wein. Edinburgh, Churchill Livingstone, 1984b, pp 127–132.

Barrett DM: Disposable (infant) surface electrocardiogram electrodes in urodynamics: a simultaneous comparative study of electrodes. J Urol 124:663, 1980.

Barrett DM: The effect of oral bethanechol chloride on voiding in female patients with excessive residual urine: a randomized double-blind study. J Urol 126:640, 1981.

Barrett DM, Wein AJ: Flow evaluation and simultaneous external sphincter electromyography in clinical urodynamics. J Urol 125:538, 1981.

Blaivas J: Multichannel urodynamic studies. Urology 23:421, 1984a.

Blaivas JG: Electromyography and sacral evoked responses. *In* Urodynamics: Principles, Practice and Application. Edited by AR Mundy, TP Stephenson, AJ Wein. Edinburgh, Churchill Livingstone, 1984b, p 139.

Blaivas JG: Management of bladder dysfunction in multiple sclerosis. Neurology 30(part 2):12, 1980.

Blaivas JG, Bhimani G, Labib KB: Vesicourethral dysfunction in multiple sclerosis. J Urol 122:342, 1979.

Blaivas JG, Labib KL, Bauer SB, et al: A new approach to electromyography of the external urethral sphincter. J Urol 117:773, 1977.

Blaivas JG, Labib KB, Michalik SJ, et al: Failure of bethanechol denervation supersensitivity as a diagnostic aid. J Urol 123:199, 1980.

Blaivas JG, Sinha HP, Zayed AAH, et al: Detrusor-external sphincter dyssynergia: a detailed electromyographic study. J Urol 125:545, 1981a.

Blaivas JG, Zayed AAH, Labib KB: The bulbocavernosus reflex in urology: A prospective study of 299 patients. J Urol 126:197, 1981b.

Brown M, Wickham JEA: The urethral pressure profile. Br J Urol 41:211, 1969.

Burnstock G: The changing face of autonomic neurotransmission. Acta Physiol Scand 126:67, 1986.

Elbadawi A: Neuromuscular mechanisms of micturition. *In* Neurourology and Urodynamics: Principles and Practice. Edited by SV Yalla, EJ McGuire, A Elbadawi, et al. New York, Macmillan, 1988, pp 3–35.

Farrar DJ, Whiteside CG, Osborne JL, et al: A urodynamic evaluation of micturition symptoms in the female. Surg Gynecol Obstet 141:875, 1975.

Hald T: The Committee on Standardization of Terminology of Lower Urinary Tract Function. Copenhagen, International Continence Society, 1984.

Koelle GB: Parasympathomimetic agents. *In* The Pharmacological Basis of Therapeutics, 5th ed. Edited by LS Goodman, A Gilman. New York, Macmillan, 1975, pp 467–476.

Krane RJ, Siroky MB: Studies on sacral-evoked potentials. J Urol 124:872, 1980.

Lapides J, Friend CR, Ajemian EP, et al: Denervation supersensitivity as a test for neurogenic bladder. Surg Gynecol Obstet 114:241, 1962.

Maizels M, Firlit CF: Pediatric urodynamics: a clinical comparison of surface versus needle pelvic floor/external sphincter electromyography. J Urol 122:518, 1979.

Maizels M, King LR, Firlit CF: Urodynamic biofeedback: a new approach to treat vesical sphincter dyssynergia. J Urol 122:205, 1979.

McGuire E: Electromyographic evaluation of sphincter function and dysfunction. Urol Clin North Am 6:121, 1979.

McGuire EJ: Detrusor response to outlet obstruction. World J Urol 2:208, 1984.

McGuire EJ, Woodside JR, Borden TA, et al: Prognostic value of urodynamic testing in myelodysplastic patients. J Urol 126:205, 1981.

Nordling J, Meyhoff HH: Dissociation of urethral and anal sphincter activity in neurogenic bladder dysfunction. J Urol 122:352, 1979.

Powell PH, Shepherd AM, Lewis P, et al: The accuracy of clinical diagnoses assessed urodynamically. Prog Clin Biol Res 78:201, 1981.

Raezer D, Wein AJ, Jacobowitz D, et al: Autonomic innervation of canine urinary bladder: cholinergic and adrenergic contributions and interaction of sympathetic and parasympathetic nervous systems in bladder function. Urology 2:211, 1973.

Ruch TC, Tang PC: The higher control of the bladder. *In* Neurogenic Bladder. Edited by S Boyarsky. Baltimore, Williams & Wilkins, 1967, pp 34–45.

Sixth Report on the Standardization of Terminology of Lower Urinary Tract Function. The International Continence Society Committee on Standardization of Terminology, New York, May 1985.

Tanagho EA: Membrane and microtransducer catheters: their effectiveness for profilometry of the lower urinary tract. Urol Clin North Am 6:110, 1979.

Tanagho EA: Urethral pressure profile: membrane catheter. *In* Controversies in Neuro-Urology. Edited by DM Barrett, AJ Wein. New York, Churchill Livingstone, 1984, pp 55–65.

Ursillo RC: Rationale for drug therapy in bladder dysfunction. *In* Neurogenic Bladder. Edited by S Boyarsky. Baltimore, Williams & Wilkins, 1967, pp 187–190.

Webster GD: Urodynamic studies. *In* Diagnosis of Genitourinary Disease. Edited by MI Resnick, RA Older. New York, Thieme-Stratton, 1982, pp 173–204.

Wein AJ: Classification of voiding dysfunction. AUA Update Series 6:1, 1986.

Wein AJ: Pharmacologic approach to the management of neurogenic bladder dysfunction. J Cont Educ Urol 18:17, 1979.

Wein AJ: Pharmacology of the bladder and urethra. *In* Surgery of Female Incontinence. Edited by SL Stanton, EA Tanagho. Berlin, Springer-Verlag, 1980, pp 185–199.

Wein A, Barrett DM: Etiologic possibilities for increased pelvic floor electromyography activity during cystometry. J Urol 127:949, 1982.

Wein AJ, Barrett DM: Voiding Function and Dysfunction:

A Logical and Practical Approach. Chicago, Year Book Medical Publishers, 1988, pp 32–103.

Wein AJ, Leoni JV, Schoenberg HW, et al: A study of the adrenergic nerves in the dog ureter. J Urol 108:232, 1972.

Weir J, Jaques PF: Large-capacity bladder: a urodynamic survey. Urology 4:544, 1974.

Weiss RM, Coolsaet BLRA: The ureter. *In* Adult and Pediatric Urology, Vol 1. Edited by JY Gillenwater, JT Grayhack, SS Howards, et al. Chicago, Year Book Medical Publishers, 1987, pp 777–799.

Yalla SV, Sharma GVRK, Barsamian EM: Micturitional static urethral pressure profile: a method of recording urethral pressure profile during voiding and the implications. J Urol 124:649, 1980.

7

☐ Presentation of Genitourinary Disease and Abdominal Masses

R. Dixon Walker III

It has been more than 15 years since the first edition of *Clinical Pediatric Urology* was printed, and since that time, there has been a considerable change in the way children present with urologic disease. One can name many reasons why this is so, but clearly the most important one is the popularity of ultrasonography as a prenatal and postnatal screening tool. The result is that many diseases are diagnosed prior to the advent of signs or symptoms. Diseases for which this is commonly the case include vesicoureteral reflux, ureteropelvic junction (UPJ) obstruction, posterior urethral valves, megaureter, multicystic kidney, and duplex anomalies. This does not mean that the pediatric urologist does not need to be a sharp diagnostician: rather, the starting point is often different from that of previous years. Instead of an initiating sign or symptom, one now frequently starts with an ultrasound scan as the point from which diagnosis proceeds.

Moreover, the advent of sonography does not mean that the history and physical examination are not an integral part of the evaluation. Indeed, as the age of the patient has decreased, these have attained increased importance. Infants and small children are unable to communicate, and patience is required to obtain an adequate history from older children. Parents and grandparents who accompany the child can give meaningful histories, but they can also give misleading information; i.e., information received from family members may be colored by their own intellectual capacity and emotional response to the child's disease. Genetic history is more important than ever and may be more difficult to obtain than with diseases in other organ systems because of the secret nature of the abnormality,

particularly with genital abnormalities. Examination of the neonate necessitates a different set of skills than does examination of the older child and compels urologists to learn from neonatology colleagues. There is frequently more anxiety associated with disease in neonates and children than in adults, this anxiety often being transferred by the parents. Sometimes the anxiety is related to diseases that are associated with a poor prognosis; at other times it is related to abnormalities that are visible to the parents. Such is the case with genital surgery, in which the result is there for parents to clearly evaluate for themselves. Now, more than ever, the management of these serious problems should be in the hands of those who have had specialized training in pediatric urology.

SYMPTOMS OF GENITOURINARY DISORDERS

In the child who is old enough to complain, symptoms may be related directly to the urinary tract or to other organ systems. It is not uncommon for urologic disease to present with symptomatology that one may usually associate with the gastrointestinal tract. Nausea and vomiting may occur with uremia, acidosis, and acute pyelonephritis or in association with severe hydronephrosis. Weakness may be associated with metabolic acidosis, and bone pain may be related to disturbances of calcium or potassium metabolism. Uremia may be associated with nausea and vomiting, apathy, lethargy, coma, muscle twitching, headache, vertigo, anorexia, poor growth, melena, dyspnea,

218

or signs of congestive heart failure. Frequent headache is usually not related to renal disease but can be secondary to hypertension with hypertensive encephalopathy, with dismal results if it is not treated.

Abdominal Pain

Abdominal pain can be related to acute infection or distention of a hollow viscus. Patients with acute pyelonephritis may present with vague abdominal symptoms or with acute flank pain. Nausea and vomiting frequently precede the pain and sometimes are the only symptoms immediately apparent. Pain caused by distention of the renal pelvis or ureter can usually be distinguished by studying the history. Renal pelvic pain is most often localized in the flank with little radiation. Acute ureteral distention is characterized by sharp pain, which may radiate into the groin. Flank pain that is brought on by overhydration should always alert one to the possibility of an underlying obstruction of the ureteropelvic junction. There may be little correlation between the degree of hydronephrosis and the intensity of pain; indeed, patients with severe hydronephrosis may be asymptomatic.

Abnormalities of Voiding

Symptoms of voiding dysfunction include urinary retention, hematuria, dysuria, frequency and urgency, or straining to void. Each of these may indicate significant underlying urologic disease and thus must be taken seriously.

Urinary Retention

The neonate, infant, or child who exhibits symptoms of urinary retention or who has difficulty in initiating voiding may have a serious underlying disease. Urologic evaluation is always indicated in such children. Urine output in the first 2 days of life is normally low. If there is concern in this period about the volume of urine voided, a urinary collection bag may be applied so that accurate measures are taken. The average daily urine output for neonates, infants, and children is recorded in Table 7–1.

In the male neonate, *anuria* or urine retention should alert one to the possibility of

Table 7–1 □ Average 24-Hour Urine Output in Infants and Children

Age	Output in ml
Birth to 48 hours	15 to 60
3 to 10 days	100 to 300
10 days to 2 months	250 to 450
2 months to 1 year	400 to 500
1 to 3 years	500 to 600
3 to 5 years	600 to 700
5 to 8 years	650 to 1000
8 to 14 years	800 to 1400

From Campbell MF, Harrison JH: Urology, Vol 2, 3rd ed. Philadelphia, WB Saunders Co, 1970.

posterior urethral valves. This is virtually always associated with a large, palpable, distended bladder. Urine retention in the older child may be related to urethral stricture, urethral valves, urethral dyssynergia, or neuropathic bladder. Young male children can also have urinary retention secondary to severe pain associated with urethritis.

Hematuria

Hematuria is a common presenting symptom in neonates and children but has implications very different from its presentation in adults. In adults, hematuria is often associated with neoplasia; in children, neoplasia is a rare cause of hematuria. Most often, hematuria in children is medical in origin. Hematuria is discussed in greater detail in Chapter 27, but it is appropriate to mention one specific type of hematuria commonly seen by the pediatric urologist, *urethrorrhagia*. Kaplan and Brock have defined urethrorrhagia as urethral bleeding associated with dysuria occurring in boys. Urine culture is negative, and the characteristic symptom is "blood spotting on the undershorts." Dysuria and hematuria most often accompany this. The symptoms tend to occur at intervals several months apart and may persist for a decade. Cystoscopy does not show a treatable lesion; indeed, the procedure may be contraindicated because of the possibility of producing a stricture. An ultrasound scan of the abdomen and bladder most often suffices as far as radiologic screening is concerned. Treatment with low-dose, long-term antibacterials may be of help in some cases, but there is no scientific basis for this effect. Idiopathic urethrorrhagia is a benign lesion that appears to be self-limiting, and reassurance by the urologist is required as the principal mode of therapy.

A special situation that arises in adolescents is the presence of *stress hematuria*, particularly in association with sports. Most often seen in male patients, it can be seen in long-distance runners or in those who participate in contact sports. Figure 7–1 demonstrates an algorithm for evaluation and management of stress hematuria in adolescents.

Dysuria

Dysuria is another common voiding complaint of children and may or may not be associated with a urinary tract infection. As mentioned previously, dysuria may be associated with urethrorrhagia in males. It must be distinguished from the discomfort associated with uninhibited bladder contractions. Dysuria in the male may be specifically located to the urethra and may signal a nonspecific inflammatory process. Urine culture is indicated, and if results are positive, an appropriate radiologic evaluation should be performed. If specimens for urine culture are negative, the process is most often self-limited and no further evaluation is required. The patient should be managed by decreasing carbonated beverages, forcing fluids, and removing the presence of any chemical irritant such as soap. On occasion, alkalinizing the urine may be helpful.

Dysuria in girls may be related to inflammation outside the urinary tract, such as vaginitis. For this reason, it is important to ascertain whether the dysuria is occurring during the act of voiding or after the urine comes in contact with the vagina and paravaginal tissues.

Frequency and Urgency

Frequency and urgency are common complaints in young children and may be functional or may be associated with underlying disease. Urinalysis and culture may demonstrate associated infections. Patients who experience frequency as the sole symptom and who do not awaken at night virtually always have a functional problem that will resolve spontaneously

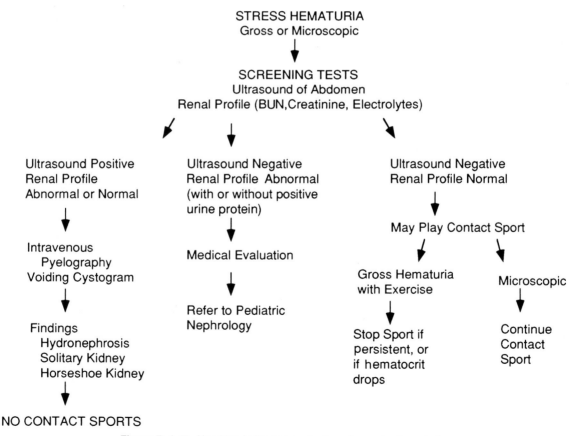

Figure 7–1 □ Algorithm indicating evaluation of exercise hematuria.

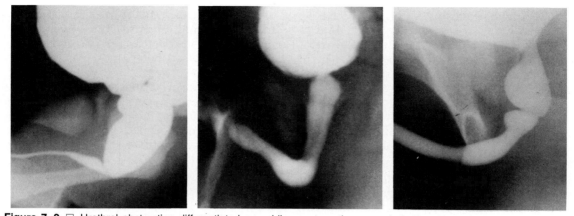

Figure 7–2 □ Urethral obstruction differentiated on voiding cystourethrogram. *Left,* Posterior urethral valve. *Middle,* Anterior urethral valve. *Right,* Urethral dyssynergia.

and that requires reassurance of the parents (Zoubek et al). Reassurance can be enhanced by screening with urine culture and ultrasonography of the kidneys and bladder. Severe cases of frequency may be treated with low doses of oxybutynin over a period of several months.

Frequency must be distinguished from *polyuria*. Polyuria is much less common, and if the parent gives a history of frequent voiding of large amounts of urine, a 24-hour urine volume should be established. Polyuria is seen in patients who have a severe concentration defect, such as with chronic pyelonephritis, hydronephrosis, renal cystic disease, and renal dysplasia. Polyuria is also seen in association with polydipsia and diabetes mellitus. Diabetes insipidus and Barter's syndrome are conditions also associated with polyuria and hydronephrosis.

Straining to Void

Straining to void almost always occurs in males and may be the only symptom of serious underlying disease. It is uncommon for females to strain with voiding, and anatomic urethral obstruction in the female is exceedingly rare. Straining to void in the male child may be either functional or anatomic. Functional obstruction, such as with sphincter dyssynergia, usually causes intermittency of flow and is diagnosed by urodynamic studies. Anatomic obstruction, such as a posterior or anterior urethral valves, is best diagnosed on voiding cystourethrography. The radiographic differences are depicted in Figure 7–2.

Dysfunctional voiding is a broad term that

encompasses a wide spectrum. At one end of the spectrum is *enuresis*, which may be physiologic in very young children but becomes dysfunctional as they get older. At the other end of the spectrum is the Hinman-Allen syndrome, in which patients have not only daytime and nighttime incontinence but also encopresis, hydronephrosis, and in some instances renal insufficiency or renal failure (Allen). Wetting problems are covered in Chapters 6 and 11 to 14. It is important to remember that enuresis is a normal phenomenon in infants and young children, characterized by a steady spontaneous resolution by age 6 (Table 7–2).

Other types of wetting problems may be associated with anatomic abnormalities of the ureter or urethra. Continuous dampness associated with normal voiding is strongly suggestive of ureteral ectopia. Continued leakage after voiding in females may be related to urethral diverticulum or retained urine in the vagina in obese patients; continued leakage after voiding in male patients may be related to scaphoid megalourethra or urethral diverticulum. Urine leakage is also commonly seen in

Table 7–2 □ Distribution of Enuresis by Age

Age	Percentage with Enuresis
1	92
2	40
3	13
4	10
5	6
6	4

Adapted from Klackenberg G: Primary enuresis: when is the child dry at night? Acta Paediatr Scand 44:513, 1955.

patients after extensive hypospadias surgery; in these situations, it is related to failure to empty the capacious penile urethra. Persistent incontinence is also a common problem in patients after exstrophy repair or bladder neck surgery.

GENITOURINARY AND OTHER ORGANIC ANOMALIES

The association of genitourinary anomalies with anomalies in other organ systems has been well established. Within the urinary tract two or more anomalies are frequently combined. Multiple defects may be coincidental or related. Abnormalities may be familial or genetic. These abnormalities may manifest themselves in one or more organ systems. Teratogenic agents may affect two organ systems at the same time during development. The maldevelopment of one organ system may so affect the fetal environment that abnormalities of other organ systems may appear. An understanding of these relationships is important in planning reparative procedures in children and in giving genetic counseling to parents.

Syndromes involving the genitourinary tract, to a major or minor extent, are legion, and no attempt is made to include all of them here. Rather, selected syndromes are employed as examples of problems involving an interrelationship between two organ systems. Many of these diseases are discussed in their respective chapters and are mentioned here only briefly.

It has been estimated that 20 to 25 per cent of all developmental anomalies are genetic, 10 per cent are environmental, and the remainder are of unknown etiology (Walker, 1987). Most familial anomalies are of genetic causation, some have both a genetic and environmental component, and a few are almost entirely environmental without any clear genetic determinants. The genetic aspects of genitourinary disease are described in Chapter 8. In broad terms, chromosomal abnormalities account for about 1 per cent of all congenital anomalies. These are not familial and are usually due to mutations of normal chromosomes. Single-gene defects are common and often related to abnormalities in other organ systems. Multifactorial disorders are the result of multiple genes acting in a given environment to produce a single abnormality. Examples of such abnormalities are vesicoureteral reflux, hypospadias,

and undescended testicle. It is less common for multifactorial abnormalities to have maldevelopment in other organ systems than for single-gene defects or chromosomal abnormalities.

Two multifactorial abnormalities that have been implicated as having associated anomalies are hypospadias and cryptorchidism. Concern is often raised about the need for excretory urography or ultrasonography to rule out abnormalities of the kidneys. Such studies are definitely indicated if the hypospadias or cryptorchid testicle is associated with a single-gene defect (Table 7–3) or a chromosomal abnormality (Table 7–4). If this is not the case, however, radiographic studies probably are not indicated. Radiologic studies with hypospadias are subject to interpretation as to whether the number of abnormalities is significant. Bauer et al investigated only those boys who had associated urinary tract infection and found that ten of 39 had abnormalities, two of which required surgery. Shima et al found six cases of ureteropelvic junction obstruction in 272 patients. All of the patients had proximal hypospadias, and none of 29 patients with glanular hypospadias had an upper tract anomaly. Vesicoureteral reflux was found in four of 272 patients, an occurrence probably similar to that in the normal population. Noble and Wacksman conducted a survey indicating that 50 per cent of pediatric urologists traditionally obtained an excretory urogram on boys with hypospadias. A reasonable compromise in suspected cases would be to perform abdominal ultrasound scanning, which is less invasive and expensive and probably screens adequately for significant anomalies.

Historically, Campbell and Harrison found 33 per cent of patients with undescended tes-

Table 7–3 □ Single-Gene Defects Associated with Genital Anomalies

Autosomal Dominant
Multiple lentigines syndrome; cryptorchidism, hypospadias
Noonan syndrome; hypogonadism, hypospadias
Opitz syndrome; hypospadias, cryptorchidism
Opitz-Frias (G) syndrome; cryptorchidism

Autosomal Recessive
Cryptophthalmos syndrome; hypospadias, cryptorchidism
Smith-Lemli-Opitz syndrome; cryptorchidism, hypospadias
Laurence-Moon-Biedl syndrome; genital hypoplasia
Adrenogenital syndrome
Pseudovaginal perineoscrotal hypospadias

Table 7–4 □ Chromosomal Syndromes Associated with Genitourinary Anomalies

Chromosome Number	Clinical Features	Renal Anomalies	Genital Anomalies
4 Autosome Wolf-Hirschhorn syndrome 4-P Trisomy 4-Q	Microcephaly Hemangiomas Hypertelorism Cleft lip/palate Low-set ears	Hydronephrosis	Hypospadias Undescended testicle
8 Autosome Trisomy 8	Large square head Prominent forehead Widely spaced eyes Slender body and limbs	Hydronephrosis Horseshoe kidney Reflux	Hypospadias Undescended testicle
9 Autosome 9-P Trisomy, 9-P Tetrasomy 9-P Monosomy	Small cranium Strabismus Large nose Webbed neck	Renal hypoplasia Pancake kidney	Hypospadias Undescended testicle Infantile male genitalia
10 Autosome 10-Q syndrome 10-P syndrome	Microcephaly Oval flat face Microphthalmia Short neck	Cystic kidney Hydronephrosis	Undescended testicle Small penis
11 Autosome 11-Q syndrome	High forehead Flat nose Wide glabella Cleft lip/palate		Micropenis
13 Autosome Patau syndrome Trisomy 13	Microcephaly Hypertelorism Polydactyly Congenital heart disease	Horseshoe kidney Hydronephrosis Cystic kidney	Undescended testicle
15 Autosome Monosomy 15-Q Prader-Willi syndrome	Obesity Hypotonia Retardation		Hypogonadism Cryptorchidism
18 Autosome Trisomy 18 Edwards syndrome	Micrognathia Hypertonia Congenital heart disease	Horseshoe kidney Hydronephrosis	Undescended testicle Small penis
20 Autosome 20 P syndrome	Round face Short nose Dental abnormalities Vertebral abnormalities	Hydronephrosis Polycystic kidney	Hypospadias
21 Autosome Trisomy 21 Down syndrome	Brachycephalic skull Congenital heart disease Nasal hypoplasia Broad, short hands		Undescended testicle Small penis
22 Autosome Trisomy 22	Microcephaly Pre-auricular skin tags Low-set ears Beaked nose Cleft palate		Undescended testicle Small penis
Sex chromosome-Y Klinefelter's syndrome XXY, XXXY XXXXY	Elongated legs Gynecomastia Eunuchoid body build Sparse body hair		Small penis Small testes
Sex chromosome X Turner's syndrome XO	Short stature Primary amenorrhea Webbed neck Broad chest Coarctation of aorta	Horseshoe kidney	Infantile genitalia

ticles had associated genitourinary abnormalities. Farrington and Kerr felt that cryptorchidism was associated with significant pathologic lesions of the urinary tract. Watson et al, however, found only 3 per cent displaying significant abnormalities on the excretory urogram. Donohue et al found only two major radiologic abnormalities in 100 cryptorchid patients. Noble and Wacksman, in their survey of pediatric urologists, found that 70 per cent did not routinely obtain an excretory urogram in patients with undescended testicle. One can conclude that the yield is quite low, probably not significantly different from what would be found in the normal population and that excretory urography is thus not routinely indicated. An exception is that the excretory urogram or ultrasonogram is desirable if, on exploration, no vas deferens or epididymis is identified.

Wilms' Tumor, Hemihypertrophy, and Aniridia

The incidence of hemihypertrophy is not known, but it is thought to be very low. It appears to be less common than aniridia, in which there is an incidence of 1 in 50,000 (Fontana et al). In patients with hemihypertrophy, there is an increased incidence of Wilms' tumor, adrenocortical tumors, hepatoblastoma, mental deficiency, club foot syndactyly, congenital heart disease, cryptorchidism, and hypospadias (Bjorklund). Wilms' tumor and hemihypertrophy may occur on opposite sides. The growth anomalies associated with Wilms' tumor may be divided into four categories: hemihypertrophy, hamartoma, visceral cytomegaly (Beckwith-Wiedemann syndrome), and malignant tumors of the adrenal and liver (Miller, 1981).

The incidence of congenital aniridia (1 in 50,000) is almost the same as that of exstrophy of the bladder. Aniridia is often associated with congenital glaucoma and cataracts (Miller et al), and there is usually a strong family history of 65 per cent of affected children having an affected parent. In children with both aniridia and Wilms' tumor, however, there is usually no family history (Mackintosh et al). Aniridia, in this instance, is due to a genetic mutation, and the absence of a family history has led to the use of the term congenital sporadic aniridia. Evidence has been presented that in children with sporadic aniridia, tumors may develop early; thus, close observation of these patients is recommended (Bracy et al).

Cardiovascular and Pulmonary Anomalies

The incidence of anomalies of the urinary tract is sufficiently high in patients with congenital cardiac defects to warrant evaluation. This can be done as part of cardiac angiography or as a separate screen with ultrasonography. Traditionally, a one-shot intravenous urogram was obtained as part of the cardiac catheterization, and when this was done, a significant number of urinary tract anomalies were discovered (Table 7–5). Most often, the present regimen is to obtain an ultrasound scan as part of the screening process in any child with congenital heart disease. The incidence of cardiovascular anomalies in association with horseshoe kidney is 11 per cent (Boatman et al). Of children with crossed or pelvic renal ectopia, 30 per cent had been found to have cardiovascular anomalies (Kelalis et al, 1973b). Engle found anomalies of the urinary tract in 7.7 per cent of children who had undergone intravenous urography as part of cardiac angiography. Many of the urologic abnormalities are ones that do not require surgical correction, and thus the incidence of surgically significant abnormalities may be much lower.

Urinary tract anomalies are also associated with pneumothorax and pneumomediastinum in the newborn. Bashour and Balfe found that 19 per cent of neonates with spontaneous pneumothorax or mediastinum had renal anomalies. All of the renal anomalies were significant and included posterior urethral

Table 7–5 ☐ Renal Anomalies Found on Intravenous Pyelogram after Cardiac Catheterization*

Type of Urinary Tract Abnormality	Number Found	Cardiac Patients Exhibiting Lesion (Per Cent)
Hydroureteronephrosis	18	4.06
Unilateral renal agenesis	4	0.90
Significant renal dysplasia	3	0.68
Fused kidney	2	0.45
Accessory renal mass	2	0.45
Ectopic kidney (in pelvis)	1	0.22
Large extrarenal pelvis without caliectasis	1	0.22
Duplication of collecting system	17	3.80
TOTAL	48	10.78

From King LR: Other congenital abnormalities. *In* Pediatric Surgery, Vol 2, 3rd ed. Edited by O Swenson. New York, Appleton-Century-Crofts, Inc, 1969.
*One film exposed after cardiac catheterization study performed because of congenital heart disease, 443 consecutive patients.

valves, infantile polycystic kidneys, renal agenesis, and multicystic renal dysplasia.

Neurologic and Musculoskeletal Anomalies

There is an obvious association of spina bifida with abnormalities of the urinary tract manifesting itself principally in the form of the accompanying neuropathic bladder with all of its sequelae. Neuropathic bladder can also occur with sacral lipoma, tethering, or absence of the sacral segments. Williams and Nixon have suggested that absence of as many as three sacral segments likely results in a neuropathic bladder.

Skeletal abnormalities may be associated with renal anomalies by themselves or as part of the VATER syndromes. (The VATER syndrome classically includes *v*ertebral defects, *a*nal atresia, esophageal atresia with *t*racheoesophageal fistula, *r*adial dysplasia renal anomalies, and cardiac defects. The presence of three anomalies qualifies a patient as having the VATER syndrome.) Vitko et al found that 30 per cent of children with kyphosis or scoliosis had a genitourinary anomaly. Avascular necrosis of the head of the femur is also associated with genitourinary anomalies in 4.3 per cent of patients. Curran and Curran reported renal and ureteral anomalies in children with oligodactyly, ectrodactyly, brachydactyly, and polydactyly.

Patients with the VATER syndrome may also have single umbilical artery, prenatal growth deficiency, large fontanelle, and minor defects of the external ear. Apold et al described abnormalities of the external genitalia in patients with VATER syndrome, including bifid scrotum, dysplastic penis, hypospadias, and testicular atrophy. Other authors have used the term VACTERL syndrome to add the *c*ardiovascular anomalies and *l*imb defects. Renal agenesis is the most common renal anomaly in the VACTERL syndrome (Khoury et al).

Gastrointestinal Anomalies

In addition to VATER and VACTERL syndrome, isolated gastrointestinal anomalies may be associated with anomalies of the genitourinary system. Atwell and Beard described abnormalities of the upper urinary tract in 50 per cent of patients with tracheoesophageal fistula, most of which were surgically significant. Weigel and Kaufmann reviewed urogenital abnormalities in patients with tracheoesophageal fistula and found a lesser incidence of genitourinary abnormalities (19 per cent). Reviewing six other series of patients, they found that the incidence of genitourinary anomalies ranged between 5 and 34 per cent.

Genitourinary anomalies are also common in patients with abnormalities of the lower intestinal tract. Constipation itself can be related to hydronephrosis and urinary tract infection in a significant number of children. Thompson and Grossman reviewed a series of female infants with low anorectal malformations, nine of whom had associated genitourinary abnormalities. The most severe anomaly seen with imperforate anus is the cloacal abnormality. Associated upper tract abnormalities may include pelvic kidney and crossed fused renal ectopia. In the most severe form of the anomaly, there is maldevelopment of the spine, with the resultant caudal regression leading to a neuropathic bladder. Williams and Grant have stated that the problems seen with imperforate anus are coexistent congenital disorders of the genitourinary tract, the result of associated anomalies of the spinal cord, complications of the accompanying fistula, or arising as complications from the definitive surgery. The level of rectal atresia correlates with genitourinary anomalies, with a greater number of anomalies existing in patients with high rectal atresia. Hoekstra et al evaluated 150 children with congenital anorectal malformations and found genitourinary abnormalities in 50 per cent. Vesicoureteral reflux was the most common finding.

Anomalies of Facial Development

In the mid 1940s, Potter described a case of abnormal facial development combined with renal agenesis and oligohydramnios. Numerous similar cases have been added to the literature, and the abnormality has come to be known as *Potter's syndrome*. Controversy still exists about the reason for the apparent association of abnormalities Potter described. Thomas and Smith felt that all of the nonrenal features of the syndrome could be caused by prolonged fetal compression secondary to oligohydramnios. Potter disagreed, however, stating that the prominent facial semicircular folds and the malposition of the ears cannot be explained on the basis of fetal compression.

Many patients have malformed ears but no other facial abnormalities. Reviewing a series of patients with malformed ears, Hilson found a wide range of genitourinary disorders besides renal agenesis, including duplication, cystic disease, hydronephrosis, and hypospadias. Taylor thought that renal abnormalities were much more likely to be found in children with underdeveloped facial bones and abnormal ears.

Renal-Genital and Multisystemic Anomalies

A large number of renal-genital anomalies are found in association with multisystemic defects, often with a lack of continuity between them. Some of the more common syndromes and their relationships are listed in Table 7–6.

Evaluation of the child with a non-urologic congenital abnormality and suspected abnormality in the genitourinary system should begin with urinalysis and an ultrasound scan. Patients who are suspected of having a neuropathic bladder, such as those with imperforate anus, should also undergo voiding cystourethrography. The finding of any degree of hydronephrosis, duplicated system, absence of a kidney, or displaced kidney should prompt the urologist to investigate further with voiding cystourethrography, intravenous urography, renal scan, and endoscopy.

EXAMINATION OF THE PATIENT

Examination of the pediatric patient with suspected genitourinary disease yields a quantity of useful data directly proportional to the diligence and thoroughness of the examiner. This is particularly so in pediatrics because, as mentioned, the history may be biased by the views of the parent or history giver and by the inability of the child to express the character of the symptoms. Thus, it is imperative that the scope of physical examination encompass more than just the abdomen and genitalia.

Neonatal Examination

Most often, the urologist examines the neonate only when called upon because of an obvious physical abnormality. The following text reviews the urologic examination performed by the pediatrician or neonatologist.

As part of the examination, one should evaluate the neonatal chart to look at the description of the umbilical cord. One per cent of newborns have only one umbilical artery with a frequent association with fetal anomalies. Originally, it was found that 27 per cent of neonates with a single umbilical artery had associated urogenital defects (Bourne and Benirschke) but that figure has been challenged by Froehlich and Fujikura. For that reason, contrast imaging of the kidneys is not necessary. Nonetheless, a strong index of suspicion is appropriate and ultrasonography can be used as a screen.

An obstetric history of polyhydramnios or oligohydramnios should draw attention to close scrutiny of the genitourinary tract. Conditions associated with polyhydramnios and oligohydramnios may include renal agenesis, posterior urethral valves, and prune-belly syndrome.

It is not uncommon for impaired respiration to be associated with congenital urogenital defects. Oligohydramnios is often associated with pulmonary hypoplasia. Impaired respiration may also occur secondary to a large intra-abdominal mass that is not allowing sufficient excursion of the diaphragm, thus compromising respiration. Abnormalities of the ears or other sequelae of intrauterine compression, such as flattened nose or recessed chin, should alert one to the possibility of Potter's syndrome, most often associated with renal agenesis. The presence of imperforate anus, spina bifida, a sacral dimple with hair, gluteal atrophy, or skeletal abnormalities should alert one to the possible presence of associated genitourinary abnormalities.

Findings consistent with aniridia, hemihypertrophy, or any growth abnormality may signify a risk of Wilms' tumor (see Chapter 34). Frequently, consultation may arise from the pediatric surgeon who has been called in because of a tracheoesophageal fistula or imperforate anus. Each of these entities warrants close physical examination by the urologist. Pyloric stenosis is a common entity in the newborn, and I have seen three cases of ureteral pelvic junction obstruction in association with this.

Indeed, the finding of any congenital anomaly is sufficient to alert one to the possibility of associated genitourinary disease. Appropriate screening can be most often accomplished by physical examination, determination of serum electrolyte and creatinine levels, and ultrasonography of the abdomen and pelvis. The finding of any significant abnormality on one of these studies would prompt further investigation.

Urologic examination of the neonate should begin with examination of the abdomen. One should evaluate the consistency of the abdominal musculature, palpating for any abdominal masses and determining whether the bladder is distended. It is appropriate to ask nursery personnel about urine output and whether anyone also has noted a distended bladder. A persistently distended bladder in a male patient, particularly if associated with the observance of a weak stream, signals the possibility of posterior urethral valves.

Examination of the genitalia of the neonate should include evaluation of the labia and clitoris in the female. Frequently, the urethra in the female neonate is difficult to visualize. Examination of the male neonatal genitalia should include evaluation of the penis and scrotal contents. The foreskin should be noted as to whether it is well formed; if it is not, the location of the urinary meatus should be ascertained. Frequently in hypospadias the meatus is quite small, and there is concern by the nursery personnel as to whether the meatus is large enough to allow voiding. Almost always, the meatus is adequate and it is extremely rare for a newborn male with hypospadias to require meatotomy. In patients with a normal foreskin, the corpora should be palpated. Any concern about penile size should result in comparison with nomograms so that if the penis is abnormally small (micropenis), appropriate management can be implemented. Examination of the scrotum and scrotal contents frequently shows a hydrocele. This is not uncommon in the newborn age group and resolves in the majority of cases. The presence of the testicles in the scrotum should be noted. Since the cremasteric muscle is not active in the newborn, retractile testes do not occur and thus an empty scrotum is representative of true nondescent, testicular ectopia, or anorchia. At least 6 months should be given to allow the testes to descend spontaneously in the neonate.

The finding of ambiguous genitalia is characterized by a phallus that is not distinctly male or female, a urethral meatus in an abnormal location, and the inability to palpate one or both gonads. There is a spectrum in ambiguity with variation in the size of the phallus, variation in the location of the meatus from the tip of the phallus to the perineum, and variation in the presence or absence of gonads. Sufficient variation to raise the question of ambiguity should immediately alert one to the possibility of an intersex problem. This should not be taken lightly, and adequate measures should be addressed to ensure that the sex assigned is in the best interest of the patient. In addition to obtaining consultation by an endocrinologist, appropriate studies include determination of serum and urine electrolyte levels, measurement of serum and urine adrenal steroid levels, ultrasound scan of the abdomen and pelvis, and a cystourethrogram/vaginogram/sinugram. Buccal smears allow early detection of chromatin material, and karyotype gives a definitive genetic diagnosis.

Examination of the Infant or Child

Both a general physical examination and a more extensive and sophisticated examination of the genitourinary tract are recommended.

Increased blood pressure is frequently associated with genitourinary pathology, and techniques of obtaining correct readings in the child are different from those used in the adult. Blood pressure cuffs should be of such size as to cover two thirds of the arm. If the blood pressure is difficult to auscultate, the Doppler ultrasound instrument may be used to considerable advantage.

Measurement of body length should be obtained at each clinic visit and growth plotted on a growth chart. Abnormalities in growth may be seen in patients with renal failure but are also common in diseases such as posterior urethral valves.

In addition to the routine vital signs of respiration and pulse, it is important that the temperature be taken at each clinic visit. The presence of fever should alert one to the possibility of urinary tract infection and is of particular importance when the infection is associated with obstruction or reflux.

The finding of any congenital abnormality on physical examination should alert one to the potential for associated genitourinary problems. This chapter indicates those associated anomalies for which further urologic evaluation is required.

Table 7-6 □ Multisystemic Anomalies with Genitourinary Pathology

Syndrome	Cardio-vascular	Gastro-intestinal	Neurologic	Musculo-skeletal	Integument	Facial	Genital	Urinary
Prune-Belly (Waldbaum and Marshall)		Occasional		Abdominal muscles absent			Undescended testicles	Hydronephrosis
Russell-Silver (Haslam et al)				Short stature Hemihypertrophy Short arms		Craniofacial dysostosis		Nonspecific renal anomalies
Curran				Acral anomalies				Renal agenesis Duplication
Turner Winter			Middle ear abnormalities				Vaginal atresia	Renal anomalies
Rüdiger			Motor instability	Short extremities Thick palms		Coarse facial features		Hydronephrosis
Goyer			Hearing loss		Ichthyosis			Renal disease
Von Hippel-Lindau (Malek and Green; Richards et al)		Pancreatic cysts	Cerebral medullary angioblastic tumor					Hypernephroid benign tumor
Holt-Oram (Silver et al)	Atrial septal defect			Defects of upper limb				Renal anomalies
Neonatal Ascites (Garrett et al; Lord)		Portohepatic obstruction Bowel perforation						Hydronephrosis
Turner's Female (XO) (Persky and Owens)				Wide chest Cubitus valgus		Webbed neck		Renal anomalies (70%)
Turner's Male (Noonan's) (Redman)				Wide chest Cubitus valgus		Webbed neck	Small testicles	Renal anomalies (50%)
Caudal Regression (Miller et al)		Imperforate anus		Inversion feet LS spine anomalies			Uterine and vaginal agenesis	Renal agenesis

VATER (Temtamy and Miller)	Ventricular septal defect	Imperforate anus Tracheoesophageal fistula		Vertebral defects Radial dysplasia Polydactyly Syndactyly				Renal dysplasia
Robinow's (Wadlington et al)				Hemihypertrophy			Small genitalia	
"G" (Opitz et al)		Neuromuscular defect of esophagus				Abnormal fascies Low-set ears	Hypospadias	
Smith-Lemli-Opitz (Ferrier)			Retardation	Syndactyly		Short upturned nose Microcephaly Epicanthal folds	Hypospadias Cryptorchidism	
Donohue's "Leprechaunism" (Gorlin and Sedano)					Hirsutism	Elfin face Prominent eyes Thick lips Low-set ears	Enlarged penis or clitoris	
Trisomy 13 (Hecht)	Ventricular and atrial septal defects	Omphalocele	Deafness Retardation	Polydactyly		Low-set ears	Cryptorchidism	Duplication Hydronephrosis
Trisomy 18 (Hecht)	Ventricular septal defect Patent ductus	Neonatal hepatitis TE fistula Malrotation	Retardation Hydrocephalus			Low-set ears Choanal atresia Cleft palate	Prominent clitoris Cryptorchidism	Horseshoe kidney Duplication Hydronephrosis
Trisomy 21 (Hecht)	Increased cardiac anomalies	Duodenal obstruction	Retardation	Muscle hypotonia		High arched palate	Small penis Cryptorchidism	Renal dysplasia

Examination of the Abdomen

Examination of a structure has traditionally included inspection, palpation, percussion, and auscultation.

Inspection of the abdomen includes not only an evaluation of abdominal size but also an inspection for abdominal masses. The presence of umbilical drainage should be noted, as should the condition of the skin. Anomalies such as gastroschisis, omphalocele, exstrophy of the bladder or cloaca, and prune-belly syndrome are readily apparent if present.

Palpation should be directed to the deep abdominal structures as well as to the superficial musculature and flank. If present, urachal cysts are superficial and situated in the midline. One should try to distinguish between ascitic fluid, bladder distention, the presence of intraabdominal or retroperitoneal masses, and hepatic or splenic enlargement. Ascites can be distinguished by its fluid wave. The presence of an abdominal mass should strongly alert one to the possibility of genitourinary disease because approximately 50 per cent of these masses are related to the urinary tract (Melicow and Uson).

Percussion and auscultation are perhaps of less importance in diagnosing genitourinary disease than are palpation, inspection, and transillumination, although percussion can give evidence of ascitic fluid or even of hydronephrotic fluid if the kidney is large.

Female Genitalia

Abnormalities related to the clitoris include complete absence as well as hypertrophy. Clitoral hypertrophy may be a manifestation—and perhaps the only physical sign—of adrenal genital syndrome and should be evaluated with appropriate hormonal and genetic studies. The labia in the female child should be well developed with an adequate introitus. Imperforate hymen may be associated with hydrocolpos or hematocolpos. The vagina should be inspected for the presence of foreign bodies. The urethral meatus should be just ventral to the vaginal introitus. Its absence from this location may signify that the patient has a urogenital sinus. In black pubescent or prepubescent girls, a circumferential prolapse of the urethral mucosa may present as a bleeding necrotic urethral mass. A prolapsed ureterocele also

appears as a perineal mass and may be difficult to distinguish from hydrocolpos.

The urologist should always be alert to the possibility of sexual abuse in children who present with genitourinary symptoms. Common symptoms may including wetting, recurring urinary tract infection, and urethral or vaginal discharge. Physical signs of abuse in the female may be tears at the vaginal fourchette, presence of condyloma, presence of a vaginal discharge, vaginal bleeding, or hypertrophy of the labial epithelium. On occasion, benign lesions, such as urethral prolapse, may be confused with the signs of sexual abuse. If there is any question in the mind of the examiner, the sexual abuse personnel in the local area should be contacted to resolve the issue.

Sarcomas are an uncommon malignancy in the pelvic area but, on occasion, may present as a polypoid pelvic mass extruding from the vagina.

Male Genitalia

Examination of the male genitalia should include evaluation of the urethral meatus, penis, and scrotal contents.

The male urethral meatus should be a cleft or slit at the tip or on the ventral surface of the glans penis. Meatal stenosis is characterized by a rounded non-elastic meatus; it may be associated with minimal urethral obstruction. The diagnosis should be confirmed with calibration of the meatus by bougie, observation of the urinary stream, and a urine flow rate. Table 7–7 indicates the average meatal size in the newborn. By age 18 months of age, 90 per cent of boys have a urethral meatus larger than 12 French (Fr.) units in size (Berry

Table 7–7 □ Meatal Calibration of Male Neonates

Calibration in French Units	Number of Cases
4	9
5	0
6	10
7	32
8	40
9	3
10	5
11	0
12	1

From Allen JS, Summers JL, Wilkerson JE: Meatal calibration of newborn boys. J Urol 107:498, 1972. © Williams & Wilkins, 1972 and Cross). The significance of the rounded, small meatus has not been definitely established, and its relationship to renal disease, urinary tract infection, and enuresis is incompletely understood. In asymptomatic patients, meatotomy should be reserved for those with objective evidence of a voiding disturbance.

Hypospadias is easily recognized by the triad of ventral urethral meatus, ventral chordee, and incomplete formation of the foreskin. The meatus is usually small. The most common hypospadias is glanular or coronal. *Epispadias* is characterized by a dorsal meatus, dorsal chordee, and incomplete formation of the foreskin. Epispadias is different than hypospadias, in that the most common presentation is in association with exstrophy and the least common presentation is a glanular epispadias. Other abnormalities of the penis may include chordee without hypospadias, penile torsion, webbed penis, and translocation of the penis and scrotum.

Microphallus is a diagnosis that should be restricted to boys who have a very small penis. Hinman's data indicate that the median length of the newborn penis, stretched or on erection, is 3.75 cm and by age 1 is 4.5 cm. In most cases of microphallus, the length at birth is less than 1 cm. In an obese youngster, a large mound of superficial fat may partially conceal the penis. The mons should be retracted, and stretched penile length and circumference should be measured. In most instances, an obese boy will have a penis of normal size. A prepubertal boy with a large phallus should be suspected of having male adrenogenital syndrome or congenital absence of erectile tissue. A large flaccid penis is characteristic of congenital absence of all corporal tissue (fusiform megalourethra). Fusiform megalourethra is a severe abnormality frequently associated with prune-belly syndrome. In these patients, there is no potential for erection. Serious consideration should be given to raising these patients as females. Patients with absence of only the corpus spongiosum (scaphoid megalourethra) frequently present with no functional defect. These patients may have a pseudodiverticulum of the penile urethra noticed with voiding and mild dorsal chordee. Except in extreme cases, they have adequate micturational and sexual function.

Parents are frequently concerned about the foreskin in uncircumcised males. Physiologic *phimosis* is normal in young children and may not resolve until puberty (Duckett). Forceful retraction of the foreskin is contraindicated. Mild penile glanular adhesions are common in the younger age group and break down spontaneously. Parents should be taught that active cleansing of the foreskin in the infant and young child is unnecessary. Between ages 3 and 5, the foreskin should retract spontaneously; if it does not, elective circumcision may be performed. Indications for circumcision in children would include those with severe phimosis who have difficulty in voiding, recurrent episodes of balanitis, or a history of paraphimosis.

The scrotum and its contents should be evaluated thoroughly. It must be established that the testes are present bilaterally as well as the vas deferens and epididymis. These structures may be difficult to palpate in children, but their absence may signal failure of the metanephric kidney to develop on the ipsilateral side.

Testes retract easily in infants and children because of activity of the cremasteric muscle. An overactive cremasteric muscle can be circumvented by trapping the testicle at the external ring or by examining the patient while he is in the squatting position. Hadziselimovic has described placing pressure on the ipsilateral femoral artery as a means of bringing a retractile testicle into the scrotum. Retractile testes are ones that come into the dependent scrotum and remain there after release. High scrotal testes or ones palpable in the groin are not retractile and should be appropriately managed. Acute scrotal swelling may be related to hydrocele or to torsion of the testicle or its appendages. Most often, a hydrocele is not associated with any inflammatory signs. Additionally, the swelling with hydrocele frequently incorporates part of the penile skin. A definitive diagnosis of hydrocele can be made by transillumination and by noting the testis within the hydrocele sac. Patients who present with torsion of the testis or its appendages have scrotal inflammation, scrotal pain, and swelling. The "blue dot sign" may indicate torsion of the appendix testis or appendix epididymis (Dresner). Doppler ultrasound scanning with pencil attachment can be used in evaluating blood flow in the acute scrotum. Epididymitis is almost unknown in boys and should be diagnosed only when there is associated pyuria, fever, and good blood flow on Doppler examination. Acute scrotal swelling associated with inflammation and pain should be assumed to be testicular torsion and should be surgically explored unless there is overwhelming evidence that the process is a torsion of an appendage or epididymitis.

Observation of Voiding

Observation can confirm likelihood of previously suspected obstructive lesions of the urethra. Male children should be able to generate a stream by some coaxing particularly after being given a fluid load. The stream should be forceful, continuous, not deviated, and not associated with pain. Parents may also observe for abnormalities in urine flow. Persistent abnormalities in urine flow warrant investigation.

Rectal Examination

Examination of the rectum can be invaluable in providing information about both the male and female patient: Suspected foreign bodies in the vagina can often be confirmed; abnormalities of the wolffian or müllerian duct structures, such as müllerian duct cyst and seminal vesicle cyst, can often be palpated; and the extent of pelvic tumors can be estimated. The rectal examination should be performed in a nonthreatening manner. Most often, the child should lie on the side with the knees to the chest. The well-lubricated, gloved index finger or little finger can be used, depending on the size of the child. Infants can be examined with the gloved, lubricated little finger while they are lying in the prone position.

Neurologic Evaluation

It is imperative that the urologist be capable of performing a limited neurologic evaluation because this is required in children presenting with enuresis, incontinence, and myelodysplasia. The limited neurologic examination begins with the general testing of sensation in the abdomen, perineum, buttock, and legs by means of a cotton applicator. A sharp instrument should not be used in small children. Knee-jerk reflexes should be examined with the hammer, and the feet are examined for the Babinski reflex and ankle clonus. Observation of walking may indicate abnormalities in gait. Examination of the buttock and lower spine for gluteal atrophy, hairy nevus, or spinal dimple is appropriate. Evaluation of the rec-

tum for sphincter tone and for the presence of the bulbocavernosus reflex completes the limited neurologic examination by the urologist.

ABDOMINAL MASSES

The presentation of an abdominal mass in an infant or child is a cause of immediate concern to parents and thus demands an urgent evaluation. Most abdominal masses are benign, and yet the chance of malignancy is real. Cancer rates are second to trauma as the cause of death in children, accounting for 10 per cent of all deaths in this age group (Public Health Service). Of malignant neoplasms, between 20 and 25 per cent may present as an abdominal mass. Most frequent is neuroblastoma, followed in decreasing order by Wilms' tumor, rhabdomyosarcoma, hepatoma, and Ewing's sarcoma (Morgan and Baum).

Each tumor is characterized by presenting signs and symptoms, some of which are similar and some quite different. Radiologic evaluation is required to establish the location and type of tumor. Although these topics are discussed in detail in Chapters 2, 3, 4, and 34, they are also briefly reviewed here. The focus of evaluation is the abdominal ultrasonogram. From this comes the lead into other radiologic studies. The algorithm in Figure 7–3 briefly outlines the radiologic evaluation of the abdominal mass.

Renal Masses

A renal tumor is suggested by palpating a flank mass. Definitive localization of the kidney can be done only with ultrasonography. The most common differential diagnosis of renal mass includes multicystic renal dysplasia, hydronephrosis, and Wilms' tumor (Fig. 7–4). Less common diagnoses are polycystic kidneys, multilocular cysts, simple cyst, and abscess.

Many cases of multicystic renal dysplasia and hydronephrosis are now discovered on fetal ultrasonograms. Multicystic kidneys are always present at birth and are easier to palpate at this time. They can be quite large, knobby to palpation, often crossing the midline. If very large, they may be associated with difficulty in urination because of bladder compression or with difficulty in breathing because of compromise of the diaphragm. The characteristic ultrasound appearance is of a kidney

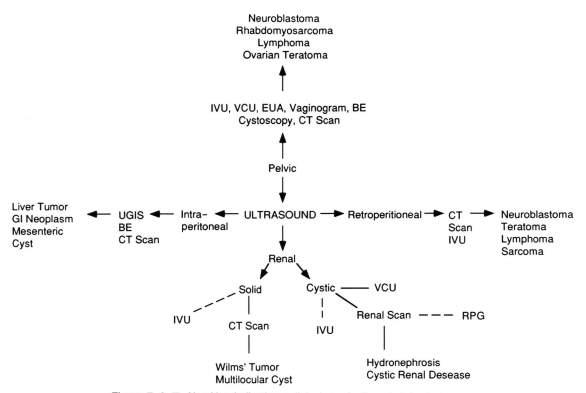

Figure 7–3 □ Algorithm indicating radiologic evaluation of abdominal mass.

without recognizable parenchyma and with multiple anechoic lesions of varying sizes representing the cysts. The other kidney should always be screened because about 40 per cent show pathology on the contralateral side (Greene et al).

Multicystic renal dysplasia occurs in a spectrum, and on occasion the cystic dysplasia may be segmental or may appear in a horseshoe kidney. Sometimes the cysts are large so as to resemble the renal pelvis, and there may also appear to be parenchyma present. Further differentiation of multicystic renal dysplasia can be obtained with a Tc-99m DTPA (diethylenetriamine pentaacetic acid) renal scan, which classically shows a cold nonperfused mass in the area of the kidney with less than background isotope present. Rarely, percutaneous nephrostomy or exploration is required to establish the diagnosis. Voiding cystourethrography frequently reveals mild reflux into the distal ureter.

Multicystic kidney persisting into childhood usually does not present as an abdominal mass but rather as an incidental finding. The reasons for this include the fact that multicystic kidney in the child is asymptomatic and the kidney is smaller in relationship to the child than it is to the neonate. Rarely, children with multicystic kidney may have hypertension, and recent reports of nephroblastoma cells in pathologic specimens has given rise to a concern about Wilms' tumor developing in nonoperated patients. To date, the number of such cases has been few (Peters and Mandell).

Hydronephrosis in the newborn is another common finding—usually suspected on prenatal ultrasonography and confirmed on postnatal studies. Hydronephrosis secondary to obstruction of the urethra (such as in posterior urethral valves) or ureteral vesicle junction obstruction usually does not present as an abdominal mass. Indeed, even ureteral pelvic junction obstruction with significant hydronephrosis may not result in a kidney that is easily palpable in the neonate. Those hydronephrotic kidneys that are palpable are smooth and mobile, rarely crossing the midline.

Ultrasound scanning confirms the large renal pelvis. The diagnosis of obstruction is best established with the furosemide (Lasix) infusion DTPA renal scan (Koff et al). The scan may give spurious results when performed in the first few days of life, and it is best per-

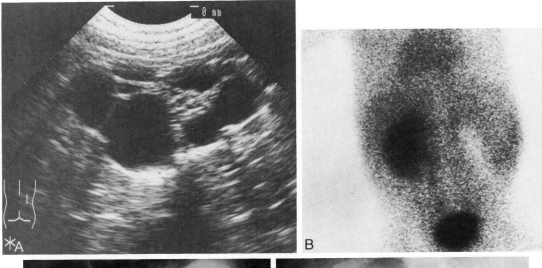

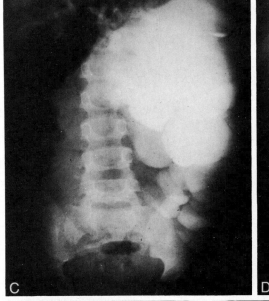

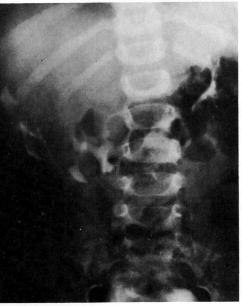

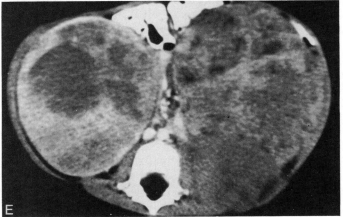

Figure 7–4 □ Radiologic differential diagnosis of abdominal mass of renal origin. *A*, Ultrasonogram, multicystic kidney. *B*, Renal scan, multicystic kidney. *C*, Intravenous urogram of hydronephrotic kidney. *D*, Intravenous urogram of Wilms' tumor. *E*, CT scan of bilateral Wilms' tumor.

formed after 1 to 2 weeks of age. The technique involves placing a catheter in the bladder and giving an intravenous injection of Tc-99m DTPA. Approximately 12 to 20 minutes after injection (ideally when renal perfusion is perceived on the gamma camera as maximum), the infant is given 0.3 mg/kg furosemide. Washout curves can be computer-generated and correlated with the degree of obstruction. Hydronephrosis in the child may also present as an abdominal mass; in active children, it is often associated with intermittent episodes of gross hematuria occurring after play. Hypertension is an uncommon associated finding. While the diagnosis may be suggested by physical examination, it is established with ultrasonography and renal scan. Obstructed kidneys in older children may be represented by shells of parenchyma and yet exhibit quite good recovery after repair.

Wilms' tumor is the most common solid renal mass in childhood (Walker, 1989). The presence of a solid mass in a neonate is suggestive of mesoblastic nephroma (a more benign variant) or a neuroblastoma. Whereas multicystic kidney and hydronephrosis uncommonly present as abdominal masses, Wilms' tumor commonly does. These masses may be discovered by the parent or the physician. The incidence is greatly increased with hemihypertrophy, Beckwith-Weidemann syndrome, and sporadic aniridia. There is a weaker association with anomalies of the external genitalia.

Most Wilms' tumors present as asymptomatic large abdominal masses. Pain may be associated with intratumor bleeding. Fever is common as is mild hypertension. On palpation, the tumor is large, firm to hard, and often immobile and may cross the midline slightly. The mass frequently can be seen on inspection of the abdomen. Ultrasonography confirms the solid nature of the tumor, the extent of which should be determined by computed tomographic (CT) scan. Bilateral Wilms' tumors occur in 10 per cent of cases. The diagnosis of Wilms' tumor is still occasionally made on excretory urography. The classic picture is that of the space-occupying lesion that displaces and distorts the intrarenal architecture.

Other renal masses that are less common may occur. Adult polycystic disease or autosomal dominant polycystic renal disease presents most often in adolescents or adults as bilateral palpable renal masses associated with hypertension and hematuria. Infantile polycystic disease or autosomal recessive polycystic disease usually does not present as an abdominal mass, but the large kidneys may be palpable. Multilocular cystic kidney is unilateral, may present as an abdominal mass, and requires full radiologic evaluation. The diagnosis is usually not established until the kidney is removed for pathologic examination.

Retroperitoneal Masses

An example of a retroperitoneal mass is depicted in Figure 7–5.

Lymphoma

Although lymphoma is one of the common solid tumors in childhood, most present with a cervical mass as the presenting sign. *Non-Hodgkin's lymphoma* may present as an abdominal mass often associated with ascites or bowel obstruction. *Burkitt's lymphoma* is particularly fast-growing and may be widespread at the time of diagnosis.

The diagnosis of lymphoma may be suggested on physical examination; however, the associated malaise of the child, cervical adenopathy, and abdominal pain point to the diagnosis. The diagnosis is further suggested by abdominal ultrasound and plain film to look for evidence of bowel obstruction or hydronephrosis. A CT scan delineates the extent of the disease, with the diagnosis established by biopsy of the abdominal mass or lymph nodes.

Neuroblastoma

Neuroblastoma is one of the more complex and difficult tumors to deal with in children (Walker, 1989). The presence of a solid mass in the neonate or young child is often suggestive of neuroblastoma. These aggressive tumors present as a large abdominal mass, accompanied by fever, malaise, and weight loss. In general, these children are more ill than children with Wilms' tumor, with the exception of the rhabdoid variant of Wilms' tumor, which may behave clinically like a neuroblastoma. Other symptoms associated with neuroblastoma may include diarrhea, paresthesia, or other neurologic symptoms.

On physical examination, the abdominal mass is hard, irregular, and fixed and frequently crosses the midline. It may sometimes

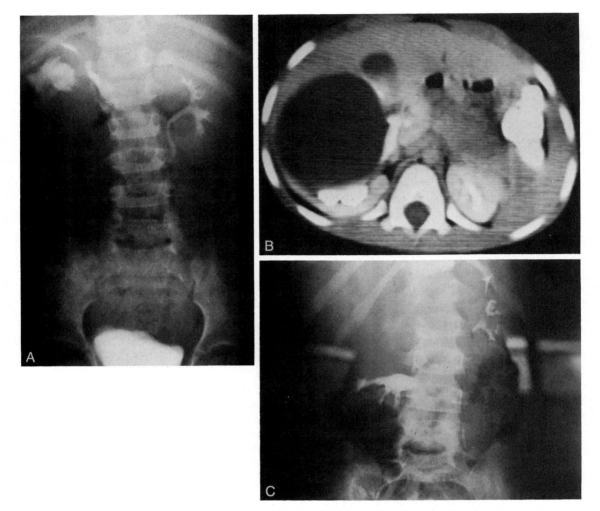

Figure 7–5 □ Radiologic differences in abdominal masses of nonrenal, retroperitoneal origin. *A*, Intravenous urogram, adrenal cyst. *B*, CT scan, adrenal cyst. *C*, Intravenous urogram, neuroblastoma.

present entirely as a midline or pelvic mass. Indeed, 30 per cent of neuroblastomas occur outside of the adrenal gland. Retro-orbital metastasis may cause proptosis, and subcutaneous metastatic nodules are occasionally seen. Radiologically, the disease is suggested by ultrasonography, although the extent of the tumor on physical examination occasionally prompts the physician to proceed directly to employing CT scan. The diagnosis is confirmed with 24-hour urine catacholemines, bone marrow aspiration, and tumor biopsy. The more mature form of neuroblastoma, *ganglioneu-*

roma, represents a more benign form of the disease. This tumor may be discovered incidentally, since size is not often sufficient to present as an abdominal mass.

Teratoma

Teratoma is an unusual retroperitoneal tumor (Raffensberger). The most malignant form is an *endodermal sinus tumor*, which can occur in the gonad or the retroperitoneum. More mature teratomas have also been found

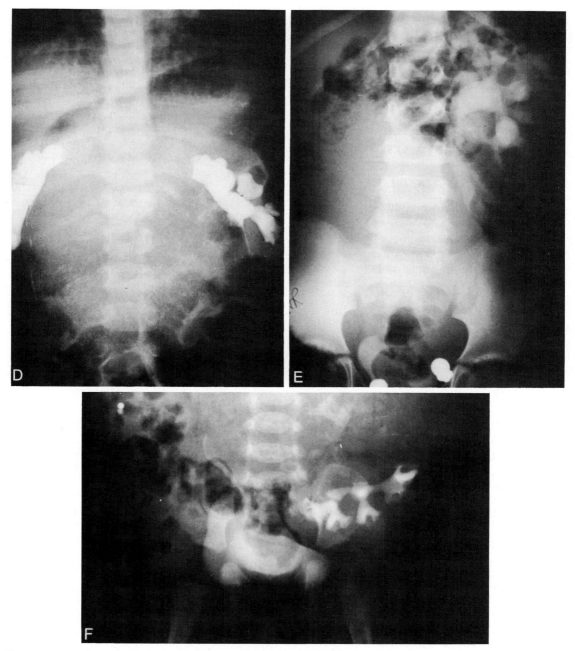

Figure 7–5 □ *Continued D*, Intravenous urogram, neuroblastoma. *E*, Intravenous urogram, lymphoma. *F*, Intravenous urogram, teratoma.

in the kidney, stomach, and other retroperitoneal areas.

The diagnosis of teratoma is usually not made until the mass is excised and sent for pathologic evaluation. Diagnosis may be suggested by a midline mass with radiologic evidence of calcification, such as bone or teeth. Teratomas may have elements from all three germ layers.

Sarcoma

Retroperitoneal sarcomas may arise from muscle, fat, connective tissue, or blood vessels and thus present as liposarcomas, fibrosarcomas, or rhabdomyosarcomas (Raffensberger). For all retroperitoneal tumors, there are no clearly identifiable presenting landmarks on physical examination. Those that present as abdominal masses are usually quite large when discovered. The extent of the tumor is determined by CT scan, and the diagnosis is established with biopsy.

Intra-abdominal Masses

An intraperitoneal mass may be in the abdomen or pelvis (Figs. 7–6 and 7–7). Those that are intra-abdominal are usually not urologic in origin, whereas those in the pelvis may be. A characteristic of the intra-abdominal mass is that it is usually easy to palpate. Those masses that involve mesentery, such as bowel tumors, mesenteric cysts, or ovarian tumors, are quite mobile on palpation. Liver tumors are rare and may be difficult to distinguish from retroperitoneal tumors on palpation. Ultrasonography can establish the difference between hepatosplenomegaly, liver tumors, or retroperitoneal tumors, with CT scan used in the latter two to further define the limits of the lesion. Malignant tumors of the liver may be associated with an abnormal liver profile, whereas benign tumors rarely are. The most common benign liver tumor is hemangioma, whereas both hepatoblastoma and liver carcinoma occur equally as the most common malignant liver tumor (Raffensberger).

Neoplasms and cysts of the gastrointestinal tract are also rare tumors in children. Most of these children present with symptoms of gastrointestinal bleeding rather than an abdominal mass. Those gastrointestinal tumors that are more likely to present as an abdominal mass include gastrointestinal lymphoma or carcinoid tumor. Tumors of the large bowel are more likely to present with obstructive symptoms.

Pelvic Tumors

Bladder Tumors

Bladder distention must be differentiated from an abdominal mass, and this can be easily accomplished with catheterization. Occasionally in females, a superpubic mass consistent with a distended bladder may represent hematocolpos or hydrocolpos. The diagnosis is further suggested by examination of the external genitalia and confirmed by abdominal ultrasonography.

Ovarian Tumors

Ovarian tumors are not uncommon. They may present as a cystic mass or as a benign or malignant tumor. They are mobile to palpation and may be associated with colicky abdominal pain, particularly if the weight is causing torsion of the ovarian pedicle. Cystic teratoma is the most common ovarian tumor in children. About 10 per cent of teratomas are malignant (Ehrin et al). Other germ cell tumors occur in lesser frequency. Ultrasound scanning is reliable in distinguishing a simple cyst of the ovary from a cystic teratoma or other solid ovarian neoplasm.

Rhabdomyosarcoma of the bladder, uterus, vagina, or prostate may present as a pelvic mass. These rapidly growing tumors cause symptoms because of their size. Most symptoms, therefore, are obstructive to either bowel or urine function. Hematuria is a late finding in genitourinary rhabdomyosarcoma. The tumors are frequently fixed in the pelvis and are easily palpable with bimanual examination. The diagnosis is suggested by ultrasonography. The limits of the tumor are defined with barium enema, cystourethrography, cystoscopy, and CT scan.

SPECIAL PROBLEMS OF CHILDREN WITH UROGENITAL DISEASE

Attitudinal Factors

Awareness of psychologic considerations specific to children is vitally important to successful medical management because all manifestations of disease in children must be taken into account in planning the treatment of the child's illness. Neither child nor parent is in a position to alter the course of management, and the urologist, in cooperative communication with the pediatrician, must assume that responsibility.

The attitude of the child toward the disease affects recovery and therefore must be evaluated carefully by the urologist. All sick children display anxiety, and the anxiety of the sick child is likely to differ both in origin and in effect from that of the sick adult. Children view their misfortune in terms of their immediate discomfort, and they lack the psychologic maturity and emotional control to cope with what is happening to themselves.

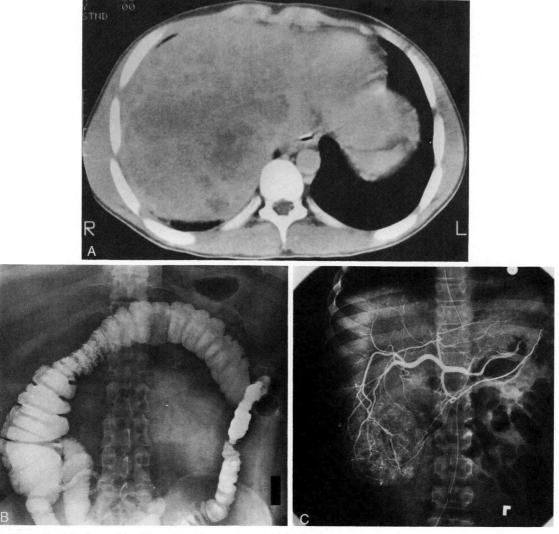

Figure 7–6 □ Radiographic differential of intraperitoneal abdominal mass. *A*, CT scan, hepatic carcinoma. *B*, Barium enema, descending colon adenocarcinoma. *C*, Arteriogram, hepatic carcinoma.

Separation Anxiety

Sick children are anxious because of their illness and pain, because they sense anxiety in the parents, and because the surroundings in the physician's office or the hospital are strange. The younger the child, the more he or she has relied upon the parents for control over the environment. Now, hospitalization has placed these children in an environment where they can make few decisions for themselves and where they are manipulated by a variety of people, many of them total strangers and all of them outside the immediate family. The child has no choice of bed, room, clothing, or food. Often these pediatric patients are placed in a bleak room, their bodies are routinely assaulted by repeated examination, painful venipuncture, and frightening machinery. The patient may be asked to inhale gases that have a peculiar smell and that induce a sleep from which one awakens, not rested and invigorated but suffering from sore throat and incisional pain, and unable to eat, void, defecate, or even talk. Moreover, these children may find themselves in yet more unusual and threatening surroundings, i.e., an intensive care unit.

The attitude and emotional responses of children to their illness and hospitalization do not remain static but change as they progress from the neonatal state to infancy, then through early childhood onward to adoles-

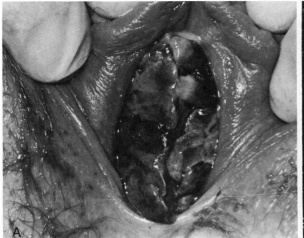

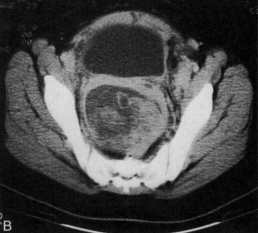

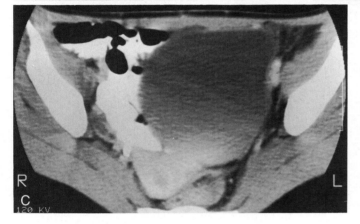

Figure 7–7 □ Radiographic differential of pelvic mass. *A*, Uterine rhabdomyosarcoma presenting at introitus. *B*, CT scan, uterine rhabdomyosarcoma. *C*, CT scan, ovarian teratoma.

cence. The neonate or infant has no comprehension of the disease process and is totally dependent on external forces. As children grow, they begin to identify with these surroundings and particularly with the mother. Thus, hospitalization during this early childhood period results primarily in separation anxiety (Edelston). Children are often able to comprehend the nature of this anxiety, even though they may not understand its origin. Separation anxiety can be relieved, at least in part, by allowing the parent to stay with the hospitalized child.

Emasculation Anxiety

Other anxieties have to do with the illness itself and vary with age. A child is not able to appreciate the nuances of a disease. A boy may be told that he will have an operation on his penis, but he does not have sufficient knowledge to interpret this information properly. Will he regard the procedure positively as one of reconstruction, or will he fear it as a process of emasculation? If his response is one of fear, will this fear be reinforced with each successive operation?

A 1973 study indicates that separation from the mother is most responsible for anxiety in the hypospadias patient aged 1½ to 3 years (Kelalis et al, 1973a). After age 3, the patient tends to develop anxiety about his genitalia; the anxiety progresses with increasing age and reaches a maximum at puberty. Robertson and Walker confirmed the existence of anxiety about genital abnormalities in older boys with hypospadias and demonstrated that this type of anxiety is quite different from that suffered by children with more obvious congenital abnormalities like cleft lip or palate.

Timing of Elective Genital Surgery

The best time to perform elective genital surgery remains controversial. The aforementioned data suggest that the problem with separation anxiety can largely be surmounted by having the mother stay with the child. Manley and Epstein have performed hypospadias repair successfully in 17 boys younger than 18 months of age. Belman and Kass reported similar results in 37 children under 1 year of age. In the hands of experienced pediatric anesthesiologists, the anesthetic risk in healthy infants is no different from that in older children. Penile size does not change significantly between 1 and 3 years of age. In boys with undescended testicles at age 6 months, it is extremely unlikely that the testes will descend spontaneously, at least until puberty. Histologic damage has been observed in the undescended testicle by 6 months of age. These data suggest that orchiopexy and hypospadias repair should be done when the child is at least 1 year of age or early in the second year of life.

Problems of Adolescence

Although the beginning and end of adolescence are not well defined, it is known that there are specific problems related to this period of intense physical and emotional growth. These are related to emancipation from dependency on parents, establishment of personal and sexual identity, development of personal moral and ethical codes, and the choosing of a career and lifestyle. Particular medical problems of adolescence are high suicide and accident rates, drug abuse, and increased incidence of venereal disease. The urologist must be aware that body image is extremely important to the adolescent and that such treatments as steroids, tumoricidal drugs, and urinary diversion procedures are likely to be met with great resistance.

Terminal Illness

Terminal disease and approaching death in the child present even more complex psychologic problems. It is probable that children with terminal disease have some foreknowledge of death. Experience indicates that children can be very perceptive of a terminal illness; such apprehension probably produces the ultimate separation anxiety.

Bibliography

BOOKS

Campbell MF, Harrison JH: Urology, Vol. 2, 3rd ed. Philadelphia, WB Saunders Co, 1970, pp 1629, 1730.

Duckett JW: The neonatal circumcision debate. *In* Urologic Surgery in Neonates and Young Infants. Edited by LR King. Philadelphia, WB Saunders Co, 1988, p 295.

Engle MA: Associated urologic anomalies in infants and children with congenital heart disease. *In* Associated Congenital Anomalies. Edited by M El-Shafie, CH Klippel. Baltimore, Williams & Wilkins, 1981, pp 137–142.

Ferrier PE: Disorders of sexual differentiation. *In* Metabolic, Endocrine, and Genetic Disorders of Children, Vol 2. Edited by VC Kelley. Hagerstown, Md, Harper & Row, 1974, pp 573–583.

Hadziselimovic F: Examinations and clinical findings in cryptorchid boys. *In* Cryptorchidism: Management and Implications. Edited by F Hadziselimovic. Berlin, Springer-Verlag, 1983, pp 95–98.

Hecht F: Autosomal chromosome abnormalities. *In* Metabolic, Endocrine, and Genetic Disorders of Children, Vol 1. Edited by VC Kelley. Hagerstown, Md, Harper & Row, 1974, pp 101–142.

King LR: Other congenital abnormalities. *In* Pediatric Surgery, Vol 2, 3rd ed. Edited by O Swenson. New York, Appleton-Century-Crofts, Inc, 1969, pp 1116–1127.

Miller RW: Relation between cancer and congenital malformations. *In* Associated Congenital Anomalies. Edited by M El-Shafie, CH Klippel. Baltimore, Williams & Wilkins, 1981, pp 67–70.

Morgan ER, Baum ES: Tumors. *In* Swenson's Pediatric Surgery. Edited by JG Raffensberger. Norwalk, Conn, Appleton & Lange, 1990.

Raffensberger JG: Teratomas, soft tissue tumors, liver tumors. *In* Swenson's Pediatric Surgery. Norwalk, Conn, Appleton & Lange, 1990.

REVIEW ARTICLES

Allen JS, Summers JL, Wilkerson JE: Meatal calibration of newborn boys. J Urol 107:498, 1972.

Allen TD: Voiding dysfunction in children. AUA Update Series, Vol VII, Lesson 22, 1988.

Apold J, Dahl E, Aarskoy D: The VATER association: malformations of the male external genitalia. Acta Paediatr Scand 65:150, 1976.

Atwell JD, Beard RC: Congenital anomalies of the upper urinary tract associated with esophageal atresia and tracheoesophageal fistula. J Pediatr Surg 9:825, 1974.

Bashour BN, Balfe JW: Urinary tract anomalies in neonates with spontaneous pneumothorax and/or pneumomediastinum. Pediatrics 59 (Suppl 6, pt 2):1048, 1977.

Bauer SB, Bull MJ, Retik AB: Hypospadias: a familial study. J Urol 121:474, 1979.

Belman AB, Kass EJ: Hypospadias repair in children under one year of age. J Urol 128:1273, 1982.

Berry CD Jr, Cross RR Jr: Urethral meatal caliber in circumcised and uncircumcised males. Am J Dis Child 92:152, 1956.

Bjorklund S-I: Hemihypertrophy and Wilms' tumour. Acta Paediatr Scand 44:287, 1955.

Boatman DL, Kolln CP, Flocks R II: Congenital anomalies associated with horseshoe kidney. J Urol 197:205, 1972.

Bourne GL, Benirschke K: Absent umbilical artery: a review of 113 cases. Arch Dis Child 35:534, 1960.

Bracy A, Randolph JG, Lilly JR: Children with congenital sporadic aniridia develop tumors early. Presented at the annual meeting of the American Pediatric Surgical Association, New Orleans, 1985.

Carlton CE Jr, Scott R Jr: Incidence of urological anomalies in association with major nonurological anomalies. J Urol 84:43, 1960.

Catteral A, Roberts GC, Wynne-Davies R: Association of Perthes' disease with congenital anomalies of genitourinary tract and inguinal region. Lancet 1:996, 1971.

Curran AS, Curran JP: Associated sacral and renal malformations: a new syndrome? Pediatrics 49:716, 1972.

Donohue RE, Utley WLF, Maling TM: Excretory urography in asymptomatic boys with cryptorchidism. J Urol 109:912, 1973.

Dresner ML: Torsed appendage: diagnosis and management; blue dot sign. Urology 1:63, 1973.

Edelston J: Separation anxiety in young children: a study of hospital cases. Genet Psychol Monogr 28:3, 1943.

Ehrin I, Mahove G, Isaacs H: Benign and malignant ovarian tumors in childhood and adolescence. Am J Surg 147:339, 1984.

Farrington GH, Kerr IH: Abnormalities of the upper urinary tract in cryptorchidism. Br J Urol 41:77, 1969.

Felton LM: Should intravenous pyelography be a routine procedure for children with cryptorchidism or hypospadias? J Urol 81:335, 1959.

Fontana VJ, Ferrera A, Perciaccante R: Wilms' tumor and associated anomalies. Am J Dis Child 109:459, 1965.

Froehlich LA, Fujikura T: Follow-up of infants with single umbilical artery. Pediatrics 52:6, 1973.

Gorlin RJ, Sedano H: Leprechaunism—Donohue's syndrome. Mod Med 48:86, 1972.

Goyer RA, Reynolds J Jr, Burke J, et al: Hereditary renal disease with neurosensory hearing loss, proteinuria and ichthyosis. Am J Med Sci 256:166, 1968.

Greene LF, Feinzaig W, Dahlin DC: Multicystic dysplasia of the kidney: with special reference to the contralateral kidney. J Urol 105:482, 1971.

Haslam RHA, Berman W, Heller RM: Renal abnormalities in the Russell-Silver syndrome. Pediatrics 51:216, 1973.

Hilson D: Malformation of ears as sign of malformation of genitourinary tract. Br Med J 2:785, 1957.

Hinman F Jr: Microphallus: characteristics and choice of treatment from a study of 20 cases. J Urol 107:499, 1972.

Hoekstra WJ, Scholtmeijer RJ, Molenaar JC, Schreeve RH, Schroeder FH: Urogenital tract abnormalities associated with congenital anorectal anomalies. J Urol 130:962, 1983.

Humphrey A, Munn HD: Abnormalities of the urinary tract in association with congenital cardiovascular disease. Can Med Assoc J 95:143, 1966.

Kaplan GW, Brock WA: Idiopathic urethrorrhagia in boys. J Urol 128:1001, 1982.

Kelalis PP, Bunge R, Barkin M: The timing of elective surgery on the genitalia of male children with particular reference to undescended testes and hypospadias. (Report by the Action Committee on surgery on the genitalia of male children.) American Academy of Pediatrics, Section on Urology, Chicago, October, 1973a.

Kelalis PP, Malek RS, Segura JW: Observations on renal ectopia and fusion in children. J Urol 110:588, 1973b.

Khoury MJ, Cordero JF, Greenberg F, James LM, Erickson JD: A population study of the VACTERL association: evidence of its etiologic heterogeneity. Pediatrics 71:815, 1983.

Klackenberg G: Primary enuresis: when is a child dry at night? Acta Paediatr 44:513, 1955.

Koff SA, Thrall JH, Keys JW: Diuretic radionuclide urography: a noninvasive method for evaluating nephroureteral dilation. J Urol 122:451, 1979.

Mackintosh TF, Girdwood TG, Parker DJ, et al: Aniridia and Wilms's tumour (nephroblastoma). Br J Ophthalmol 52:846, 1968.

Malek RS, Greene LF: Urologic aspects of Hippel-Lindau syndrome. J Urol 106:800, 1971.

Manley CB, Epstein ES: Early hypospadias repair. J Urol 126:698, 1981.

Melicow MM, Uson AC: Palpable abdominal masses in infants and children: a report based on a review of 653 cases. J Urol 81:705, 1959.

Miller RW, Fraumeni JF Jr, Manning MD: Association of Wilms's tumor with aniridia, hemihypertrophy and other congenital malformations. N Engl J Med 270:922, 1964.

Newman H, Molthan ME, Osborn WF: Urinary tract anomalies in children with congenital heart disease. Am J Roentgenol Radium Ther Nucl Med 106:52, 1969.

Noble MJ, Wacksman J: Screening excretory urography in patients with cryptorchidism or hypospadias: a survey and review of the literature. J Urol 124:98, 1980.

Opitz JM, Frias JL, Gutenberger JE, et al: The G syndrome of multiple congenital anomalies. Birth Defects 5 (part II):95, 1969.

Persky L, Owens R: Genitourinary tract abnormalities in Turner's syndrome (gonadal dysgenesis). J Urol 105:309, 1971.

Peters CA, Mandell J: The multicystic dysplastic kidney. AUA Update Series, Lesson 7, Vol VIII, 1989.

Potter EL: Facial characteristics of infants with bilateral renal agenesis. Am J Obstet Gynecol 51:885, 1946.

Potter EL: Oligohydramnios: further comment. J Pediatr 84:931, 1971.

Public Health Service: Vital statistics of the United States: 1973. Rockville, Md, HEW, 1975, Vol 2, Part B.

Redman JF: Noonan's syndrome and cryptorchidism. J Urol 109:909, 1973.

Richards RD, Mebust WK, Schimke RN: A prospective study on Von Hippel–Lindau disease. J Urol 110:27, 1973.

Robertson M, Walker D: Psychological factors in hypospadias repair. J Urol 113:698, 1975.

Rudger RA, Schmidt W, Loose DA, et al: Severe developmental failure with coarse facial features, distal limb hypoplasia, thickened palmar creases, bifid uvula, and ureteral stenosis: a previously unidentified familial disorder with lethal outcome. J Pediatr 79:977, 1971.

Shima H, Ikoma F, Terakawa T, et al: Developmental anomalies associated with hypospadias. J Urol 122:619, 1979.

Silver W, Steier M, Schwartz O, et al: The Holt-Oram syndrome with previously undescribed associated anomalies. Am J Dis Child 124:911, 1972.

Taylor WC: Deformity of ears and kidneys. Can Med Assoc J, 93:107, 1965.

Temtamy SA, Miller JD: Extending the scope of the VATER association: definition of the VATER syndrome. J Pediatr 85:345, 1974.

Thomas IT, Smith DW: Oligohydramnios: cause of the nonrenal features of Potter's syndrome, including pulmonary hypoplasia. J Pediatr 84:811, 1974.

Thompson W, Grossman H: The association of spinal and genitourinary abnormalities with low anorectal anomalies (imperforate anus) in female infants. Radiology 113:693, 1974.

Turner G: A second family with renal, vaginal, and middle ear anomalies (letter). J Pediatr 76:641, 1970.

Vitko RJ, Cass AS, Winter RB: Anomalies of the genitourinary tract associated with congenital scoliosis and congenital kyphosis. J Urol 108:655, 1972.

Wadlington WB, Tucker VL, Schimke RN: Mesomelic dwarfism with hemivertebrae and small genitalia (the Robinow syndrome). Am J Dis Child 126:202, 1973.

Waldbaum RS, Marshall VF: The prune belly syndrome: a diagnostic therapeutic plan. J Urol 103:668, 1970.

Walker RD: Familial and genetic urologic disorders in childhood. AUA Update Series, Vol VI, Lesson 30, 1987.

Walker RD: New concepts in the treatment of genitourinary cancer in children. Semin Surg Oncol 5:227, 1989.

Watson RA, Lennox KW, Gangai MP: Simple cryptorchidism: the value of the excretory urogram as a screening method. J Urol 111:789, 1974.

Weigel W, Kaufmann JH: The frequency and types of other congenital anomalies in association with tracheoesophageal malformations. Clin Pediatr 15:819, 1976.

Williams DI, Grant J: Urological complications of imperforate anus. Br J Urol 41:660, 1969.

Williams DI, Nixon HH: Agenesis of the sacrum. Surg Gynecol Obstet 105:84, 1957.

Winter JSD, John G, Mellman WJ, et al: A familial syndrome of renal, genital, and middle ear anomalies. J Pediatr 72:88, 1968.

Zoubek J, Bloom DA, Sedman AB: Extraordinary urinary frequency. Pediatrics 85:1112, 1990.

8

☐ Genetics and Dysmorphology

Kenneth N. Rosenbaum

In the last few years, the field of genetics, much like other specialties, has undergone a period of extremely rapid growth with development of clinical subspecialties, such as dysmorphology, along with dramatic advances in laboratory techniques. The urologist and geneticist share important roles in the management of the pediatric patient with a urologic abnormality. Both are frequently consulted shortly after delivery to define structural abnormalities of the genitalia; both are often placed in the position of coordinator of care for the infant with multiple malformations; yet each brings a unique but complementary approach to the clinical problem.

This chapter establishes a framework of basic principles in genetics and dysmorphology that the urologist may use when assessing the malformed or dysmorphic child. An understanding of these principles may aid the urologist in establishing etiology and answering questions related to prognosis, the need for investigation of other possible systemic malformations, and the risk of recurrence. More pressing, however, is the fact that the patient with a genetic disorder, especially the infant with a serious malformation, may require rapid decision making in the form of delivery room or nursery intervention. It is for this reason that all physicians dealing with infants should have an awareness of some of the conditions detailed later in the chapter. Areas covered include the process of genetic counseling, determination of risk figures for specific isolated urologic conditions, laboratory techniques, and prenatal diagnosis.

SIGNIFICANCE OF GENETIC DISORDERS IN THE PEDIATRIC POPULATION

Numerous studies detailing the significance of genetic disorders in the population have been published. Hall and associates reviewed admission data from a large pediatric center over a 12-month period and classified patients into five categories by diagnosis: (1) single gene or chromosomal disorder, (2) multifactorial/polygenic disorders, (3) developmental anomalies of unknown etiology and without figures for recurrence, (4) familial disorders without an otherwise well-known genetic basis, and (5) nongenetic disorders. The frequency of admission in the various categories was 26.6 per cent for single-gene, chromosomal, or multifactorial conditions, 13.6 per cent with a developmental anomaly, and an additional 13.2 per cent with a familial disorder. The authors demonstrated that the group of patients with genetic disorders were admitted more frequently, remained in the hospital for longer periods of time, and were less likely to have third-party coverage for their expenses. Comparable figures exist from other studies in the United States, Canada, and Europe (Day and Holmes; Scriver et al).

PRINCIPLES OF GENETICS

Consideration of a possible genetic basis for many urologic disorders dates back at least to the mid 1800s, when Virchow described three siblings with hydronephrosis (Raffle). Reports of familial clustering in other types of urologic abnormalities exist in the early to mid 1900s as well (Raffle). These observations, paralleling the growth of mendelian genetics, were initially explainable on the basis of single-gene inheritance. As new chromosomal abnormalities were identified and better understanding of multifactorial traits developed, the genetics of many malformations became less clear. The contribution of single-gene disorders in the production of human disease should not be underestimated, however; McKusick, in his most recent catalogue (Table 8–1), lists 4937 single-gene entries, with over 3000 autosomal dominant disorders alone. This represents an increase of more than 1500 disorders in 7 years, a number that will certainly rise in the next edition as new single-gene disorders continue to be recognized. It is also worth noting that this compilation does not include cytogenetic abnormalities or a number of dysmorphic syndromes of unknown etiology.

Dysmorphology

Fascination with malformations and genetic disorders is not a modern phenomenon. Ancient civilizations, even prior to recorded history, fashioned idols of their malformed offspring to protect the population from recurrence of the problem, which was thought to be supernatural in origin (Warkany). Many of the examples that remain represent varying types of conjoined twins, but other well-categorized conditions such as achondroplasia and other skeletal dysplasias have been found. The Egyptians, and later the Greeks, appreciated the "natural" origin of malformations. In the Middle Ages, scholars still viewed the birth of a malformed infant as an omen or the result of maternal impression, a concept that persists to the present.

Credit for the foundation of modern human genetics is usually given to Gregor Mendel, an Austrian monk, whose experiments with garden peas in the mid 1800s demonstrated that genetic characteristics were inherited independently rather than as a result of blending of traits as previously thought. Unfortunately, his work was poorly understood, at best, by his colleagues and its accuracy and impact remained unknown until 1900, when three other Europeans arrived at the same conclusion (Dewald). It is not practical to list the innumerable landmarks of human genetics since that time,

except to emphasize the foresight Mendel had in his observations more than 100 years ago.

The recognition of patterns of abnormal development, termed *dysmorphology* by Smith in 1966, led to more objectivity in the evaluation of the malformed child. Acronyms such as "FLK (funny-looking kid) syndrome" have given way to the term "dysmorphic child," which is more palatable to families and professionals. Numerous clinical centers now exist to provide for diagnosis and management of such children, and many excellent texts and journals on dysmorphology and syndromes are available (Buyse; Gorlin et al, 1990; Jones; McKusick). Classification continues to be a problem. Because the field is advancing so rapidly, the dysmorphologist is faced with the unusual scenario of having to decide (often daily) whether a given patient has a previously seen syndrome or a unique complex, a situation that is infrequent in other specialties (Cohen).

Classification

A report from an international group on errors of morphogenesis lists four categories of abnormal development with the following definitions (Spranger et al):

1. *Malformation.* A morphologic defect of an organ, part of an organ, or larger region of the body resulting from an intrinsically abnormal developmental process.

2. *Disruption.* A morphologic defect of an organ, part of an organ, or larger region of the body resulting from extrinsic breakdown of, or interference with, an originally normal developmental process.

3. *Deformation.* An abnormal form, shape, or position of part of the body caused by mechanical forces.

4. *Dysplasia.* Abnormal organization of cells into tissue(s) and its morphologic result(s).

Examples of these categories are shown in Table 8–2.

Table 8–1 □ Single-Gene Disorders

Autosomal Dominant	Autosomal Recessive	X-Linked	Total
1864*	631*	161*	2656*
(1183)†	(923)†	(175)†	(2281)†
3047	1554	336	4937

Adapted from McKusick VA: Mendelian Inheritance in Man: Catalogs of Autosomal Dominant, Autosomal Recessive and X-Linked Phenotypes, 9th ed. Baltimore, Johns Hopkins University Press, 1990.
*Denotes inheritance proved.
†Parentheses denote inheritance not proved, but suspected.

Table 8–2 □ Errors in Morphogenesis

Type of Error	Example	Urogenital Abnormality
Malformation (syndrome)	BBB syndrome	Hypospadias
Disruption	Fetal alcohol syndrome	Renal hypoplasia
Deformation	Oligohydramnios (Potter sequence)	Renal agenesis
Dysplasia	Neurofibromatosis	Urogenital neurofibromatosis

In this system, the term *syndrome* is used for a recurrent pattern of multiple malformations that are pathogenetically related. *Association* refers to a nonrandom occurrence of multiple anomalies, not part of a syndrome. Two additional concepts relating to morphogenesis are that of a field defect and sequence. A *field defect* is a pattern of anomalies derived from the disturbance of a single developmental field (functional embryologic unit). Examples of field defects are numerous and are seen in the facial variations of the child with a cleft lip or those frequently seen in children with underlying structural malformations of the brain. A *sequence* is a pattern of multiple anomalies derived from a single known anomaly or mechanical factor. Obvious clinical examples include the infant with myelomeningocele who develops limb wasting, clubfoot, and secondary renal disease.

The prevalence of minor and major anomalies varies greatly between populations and from examiner to examiner. Holmes (1976) studied 7742 infants, looking for the presence of specific minor anomalies and normal variations. He defined *major malformations* as those that were of medical, surgical, or cosmetic

significance; 2 to 3 per cent of patients in the sample had such a malformation. *Minor malformations* were unusual morphologic features of no significance and were seen in less than 4 per cent of patients. *Normal variations,* much like minor malformations, were of little significance but were found with a frequency of greater than 4 per cent. As seen in Table 8–3, wide differences in frequency were observed between race and sex. In an update of the study, he found that 6.8 to 10.3 per cent of infants had three or more minor anomalies, with 39 to 47 per cent having one or more (Holmes, 1982).

A final group of definitions concerning the results of gene action are in order before moving on to a discussion of principles:

1. *Heterogeneity.* This term describes situations in which a similar clinical picture is produced by different genetic mechanisms. Many examples of genetic heterogeneity are encountered. Excellent examples can be found among the mucopolysaccharidoses, with seven distinct types producing similar phenotypes, all the result of different enzymatic deficiencies.

2. *Variable expressivity.* Differences in clin-

Table 8–3 □ Prevalence of Minor Malformations and Normal Variations

Feature	White (%)		Black (%)	
	Male	*Female*	*Male*	*Female*
Epicanthal folds	1.2	1.6	0.7	1.2
Brushfield spots	7.4	7.0	0.0	0.3
Preauricular sinus (unilateral)	0.4	1.3	4.5	6.1
Diastasis recti	32.3	32.9	41.4	40.1
Umbilical hernia	0.4	1.0	3.6	8.6
Clinodactyly (fifth finger), both	5.8	4.5	5.2	8.7
Simian crease				
Unilateral	2.5	1.1	1.7	1.1
Bilateral	1.0	0.3	0.5	0.5

Adapted from Holmes LB: The malformed newborn: practical perspectives. Unpublished, 1976.

ical severity within the same condition. This term is not synonymous with "penetrance," (discussed next). This term does not apply if the observed clinical differences are the result of heterogeneity.

3. *Penetrance.* A population figure stating that a given gene manifests itself in a given percentage of individuals. Penetrance is an all-or-none phenomenon, *is never variable,* but is either incomplete or reduced.

4. *Pleiotropy.* Multiple phenotypic effects from a single mutant gene.

Chromosomal Disorders

Following confirmation of the chromosome number in humans as 46 and description of Down syndrome as the first clinically identified cytogenetic syndrome in 1959, there has been a proliferation of information on many new cytogenetic abnormalities. This is related primarily to the development of chromosomal banding techniques that allow for the identification of small aberrations along the length of the chromosome.

Prevalence studies performed on newborns prior to the availability of banding consistently demonstrated that 0.5 to 0.6 per cent of live births are associated with a significant chromosomal abnormality. Although this number is slightly greater when newer techniques are considered, the impact of this group, as shown by Hall and colleagues, is great.

Chromosome Nomenclature and Techniques

It is estimated that there are on the order of 50,000 structural genes in the human genome, with at least one gene mapped to each chromosome. Of the approximate 1800 loci that have been definitely mapped, more than 300 are on the X chromosome alone (McKusick). Recombinant DNA techniques should now allow for more rapid assignment of gene loci.

Chromosomes consist of two chromatids joined together at the centromere. With standard nomenclature used, the portion of the chromosome above the centromere is designated as the *p* or *short arm* and the portion below, the *q* or *long arm*. Proper notation for a normal male chromosome complement is 46,XY. If a + sign *precedes* a chromosome number, an entire additional chromosome is present as in Down syndrome (trisomy 21): 47,XY,+21. A chromosome number *followed* by a + or − sign denotes presence or absence of material on that particular chromosome: for example, 46,XY,6p+ or 46,XY,6p−. These patients are said to have a partial trisomy or partial monosomy state. Last, with banding techniques, chromosomes can be seen to be a series of light-staining and dark-staining bands (Fig. 8–1). The dark-staining bands tend to be rich in adenine-thymine base pairs and generally contain heterochromatin, or nonstructural genetic material. Lighter-staining areas are rich in guanine-cytosine base pairs and are thought to represent areas of euchromatin, or structural gene areas. The chromosome is subdivided into *regions* that are numbered and then further divided into *bands and subbands* within regions so that the example used above with deleted material on chromosome 6 may further be designated: 46,XY,del(6)(p23) to indicate the point at which chromosomal breakage and loss of material occurred. More sophisticated nomenclature systems have been developed to allow further subdivision of chromosomes as techniques progress.

Clinical Cytogenetic Syndromes

Urologic abnormalities are frequently seen in many classic cytogenetic syndromes (Table 8–4). Additions to the list include some patients who have aniridia associated with Wilms' tumor, primarily those with the aniridia–genital abnormality–retardation (WAGR) trait, who have been shown to have a small deletion of 11p13 (Riccardi et al, 1978, 1980; Turleau et al). It is worth noting that this deletion has not been detected in patients with aniridia and Wilms' tumor only, without other somatic abnormalities. An increased risk for gonadoblastoma has also been noted (Turleau et al).

An interstitial deletion of proximal chromosome 15q (band q11–q12) has been seen in a number of patients with the Prader-Willi syndrome (Butler, 1990; Butler et al; 1986; Kousseff; Ledbetter et al, 1981, 1982). As determined by sophisticated techniques, the frequency of this chromosomal abnormality in Prader-Willi children is approximately 50 per cent. Other abnormalities (partial trisomy, tetrasomy 15p) have also been seen, and the remaining cases may represent genetic heterogeneity or an as yet undetectable deletion at the same point. The origin of the deleted 15 chromosome has been found to be paternal in

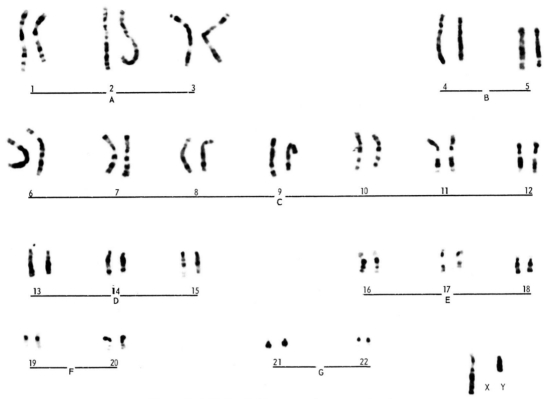

Figure 8–1 ☐ Banded karyotype from normal male.

virtually all cases studied. A lengthier discussion of the Prader-Willi syndrome appears later in the chapter.

Single-Gene Disorders

The category of single-gene disorders includes those conditions that follow simple mendelian patterns of inheritance and are not secondary to an observable cytogenetic alteration.

Autosomal Dominant Traits

In this form of inheritance, a mutation at a single locus on a given pair of chromosomes is sufficient to allow for expression (Table 8–5). An affected individual is *heterozygous* for the trait, meaning that only one gene is abnormal. Autosomal dominant traits may be said to demonstrate the following characteristics:

1. Vertical transmission; the disorder may be seen in more than one generation.
2. Males and females are affected equally.
3. In a large population, 50 per cent of offspring born to affected individuals would have the condition.
4. Spontaneous mutation; most dominant traits have a rate of spontaneous mutation in which the condition originates in a single ovum or sperm at or near the time of conception. Once established, a spontaneous mutation for a dominant trait will behave as expected.
5. The term *sporadic* is not synonymous with spontaneous mutation. It usually refers to the first affected individual within a family.
6. The risk of recurrence for an *affected* individual with a known dominant trait is, of course, 1 in 2 (1/2) or 50 per cent with every pregnancy. For *unaffected* parents of a child with a dominant trait, the risk of recurrence is extremely small and approaches the risk for the rest of the population. This assumes that the parents have been examined and are found to be unaffected, that pedigree data are negative, and that reduced penetrance is not a factor.

Autosomal Recessive Inheritance

In this form of inheritance, an affected individual has received two mutant genes (one

Table 8–4 □ Genitourinary Anomalies in Selected Chromosomal Syndromes

Chromosomal Syndrome	Malformations
Autosomes	
Trisomies (duplication)	
3q	B, E
4p	A, B, C, E
8 (mosaic)	A
9p	A, B, C, E
9 (mosaic)	A, C, E
10q	A, B, E
13	A, B, E
18	A, B, D, E
20p	A, C, E
21	A, C, E
22 (cat-eye syndrome)	E
Triploidy	A, C, E
Monosomies (deficiency)	
4p	A, B, E
5p	A, E
9p	A, C, D, E
11p	A, B, C, D
13q	A, B, E
15q (Prader-Willi syndrome)	A, C
18p	E
18q	A, C, D, E
Sex Chromosomes	
XXY	A, B, C
XXXXY	A, B, C
XYY	A, B, C
X (Turner syndrome)	E

Adapted from Jones KL: Smith's Recognizable Patterns of Human Malformation, 4th ed. Philadelphia, WB Saunders Co, 1988; and Barakat AY, Butler MG: Renal and urinary tract abnormalities associated with chromosome aberrations. Int J Pediatr Nephrol 8:215, 1987. Courtesy of Karger, Basel.

Abbreviations: A, cryptorchidism; B, hypospadias; C, microphallus; D, ambiguous genitalia; E, renal abnormalities (including agenesis, dysplasia, horseshoe kidney, hydronephrosis, other).

Table 8–5 □ Single-Gene Inheritance

Autosomal Dominant
Aa = affected heterozygote
aa = normal
Parental genotypes Aa × aa
Offspring genotypes Aa(1/2) or aa(1/2)

Autosomal Recessive
AA = normal
Aa = heterozygote (carrier)
aa = homozygote (affected)
Parental genotypes Aa × Aa
Offspring genotypes AA(1/4); Aa(1/2); aa(1/4)

X-Linked Recessive
XY = normal male
$X'Y$ = affected male (hemizygote)
XX = normal female
$X'X$ = carrier female
Parental genotypes X'X × XY
Offspring genotypes X'X(1/4); X'Y(1/4); XX(1/4); XY(1/4)

Parental genotypes XX × X'Y
Offspring genotypes X'X(1/2); XY(1/2)

from each parent) at corresponding points on a pair of chromosomes (Table 8–5). This individual is said to be *homozygous* for the trait. Here, spontaneous mutation is not a significant factor, and both parents are *obligate carriers* for the mutant gene, despite a lack of findings either clinically or often biochemically. Characteristics that may be demonstrated with autosomal recessive inheritance are:

1. Horizontal transmission; multiple siblings may be affected with unaffected parents. Because as humans have small families, affected sibs are frequently lacking even with well-known recessive disorders, such as Tay-Sachs disease, sickle cell anemia, and cystic fibrosis.

2. Males and females are equally affected.

3. Consanguinity increases the risk of having an affected child because first cousins share one in every eight genes.

4. Biochemical confirmation may be possible for certain recessive disorders, especially enzymopathies.

5. The risk of recurrence for two obligate carriers is 1 in 4, or 25 per cent with every pregnancy.

6. The offspring of an affected individual are *usually* unaffected, especially for rare recessive disorders, because the probability of meeting a carrier in the general population is low.

It is often necessary to calculate carrier frequencies for recessive disorders. Using the Hardy-Weinberg equilibrium

$$p^2 + 2pq + q^2 = 1,$$

where *p* represents the frequency of normal genes and *q* represents the frequency of mutant genes in the general population, the heterozygote frequency (*2pq*) is approximately equal to $2\sqrt{q^2}$ if *p* approaches 1. Thus, for example, if the frequency of cystic fibrosis in the population is 1 in 1600 births, then 1 in 20 individuals is a carrier for the gene ($2\sqrt{1/1600}$ = 1/20).

A second important calculation relates to the risk of an *unaffected* child born to a family with a recessive disorder having a child with the same condition. This can be determined by the following:

risk of carrying mutant gene
× risk of transmitting gene
× risk of mate's having gene

or $2/3 \times 1/4 \times 1/20 = 1/120$ for cystic fibrosis, using a carrier frequency of 1/20.

X-Linked (Sex-Linked) Inheritance

Geneticists spent years debating the mechanism of X chromosome gene action (dosage compensation) because males have only one X chromosome whereas females have two. The Lyon hypothesis accounts for this paradox by stating that shortly after conception, one X chromosome is inactivated in all cells with two X chromosomes (Vogel and Motulsky). This process is theoretically random, with 50 per cent of cells having the paternal X chromosome as the active one and 50 per cent the maternal, and is usually irreversible. The inactivated X is identifiable as the Barr body in interphase cells near the nuclear membrane. Females, therefore, are functional mosaics for genes located on the X chromosome.

X-linked inheritance may be either recessive or, in some instances, dominant. In X-linked recessive inheritance, the following may be observed (Table 8–5):

1. In a large pedigree, males are affected more frequently than females.
2. There is a lack of male-to-male transmission.
3. Detection of carrier females is often difficult.
4. For carrier females, the risk of having an *affected male* is 50 per cent with every pregnancy and 50 per cent for having a *carrier female* who will be clinically well. Spontaneous mutation does occur for X-linked traits. Although it has been suggested that one third of "lethal" X-linked traits arise as the result of spontaneous mutation, experience with conditions such as hemophilia and the fragile X syndrome show a lower rate of mutation, possibly 10 to 15 per cent of cases.
5. All daughters of an affected male are obligate carriers, as are sisters with more than one affected brother.

Calculation of probabilities for X-linked traits is based on Bayes' theorem, which takes into account the presence of additional historical information (such as numbers of male births) to develop a joint probability.

In X-linked dominant inheritance, females that have the mutant gene are more likely to express the trait than with X-linked recessive disorders but are more mildly affected than males. Numerous dysmorphic syndromes (hy-pohydrotic ectodermal dysplasia, incontinentia pigmenti, Goltz syndrome) feature this mode of inheritance. The risk of recurrence in the male and female offspring of an *affected* woman with an X-linked dominant trait is 50 per cent with each pregnancy. For an *affected* male, all daughters and none of the sons will be affected.

Multifactorial Disorders

Multifactorial disorders are the result of the action of multiple genes with small additive effects in combination with environmental influences. Although often used interchangeably with the term *polygenic inheritance,* the term *multifactorial* allows for the role of environmental factors in the production of such traits. Multifactorial disorders are characterized by the following features:

1. Increased frequency is observed in close relatives. Twin studies on clefting, for example, have shown greater concordance for the defect than would be expected by chance but less than for a single gene disorder.
2. Consanguinity increases the risk of multifactorial disorders, since relatives will have a greater share of common genes.
3. Most regional malformations and other ill-defined familial disorders are thought to have a multifactorial basis.

Multifactorial Model

Many measurable traits in the population, such as height, intelligence, blood pressure, and even serum cholesterol levels, reflect hereditary factors that are multifactorial and define a normal distribution or bell-shaped curve. These traits are said to be *continuous,* with no interruptions in the curve. At first glance, malformations appear to be *discontinuous* (either unaffected or affected), although it has been proposed that they also follow a gaussian curve representing liability or likelihood of developing a given condition (Fig. 8–2). When the liability (genetic component) reaches a certain point (the threshold), the disorder becomes manifest. Environmental components, either extrauterine or intrauterine factors, theoretically may function by altering the position of the threshold, thereby increasing liability. Affected individuals have a mean liability near the tail of the curve, and first-degree relatives

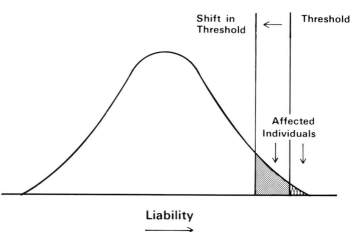

Figure 8–2 □ Liability curve representing model of multifactorial inheritance. (From Rosenbaum KN: The genetics of congenital heart disease. Clinical Proceedings of the Children's Hospital National Medical Center, 34:255–269, 1978.)

(siblings, parents, offspring) have a mean liability midway between the mean of the population and that of the affected group.

Calculation of Recurrence Risks

The multifactorial model has become the basis for the calculation of recurrence for most isolated regional malformations, including urologic abnormalities, congenital heart disease, and neural tube defects. After exclusion of chromosomal and single-gene disorders, the theoretical risk of recurrence for a presumed multifactorial trait, as Falconer has suggested, can be expressed as:

$$\text{risk} = \sqrt{\text{frequency for specific lesion}}$$

Observed risks in populations of at-risk individuals confirm the reliability of such calculations. Large amounts of data exist especially for congenital heart disease (Nora and Nora), but information is being accumulated for multifactorial urologic abnormalities and is discussed under the heading Counseling for Selected Isolated Urologic Conditions.

Caution must be exercised in the use of theoretical figures for counseling, however, since certain assumptions are made. The first is that a given family is of *average* liability and presents with a *single* affected individual. Although figures are sparse for families with two affected children or an affected parent and child, the risk of recurrence appears to increase sharply and may approach mendelian risks. It has also been observed that the more severe the defect, as in perineoscrotal versus glanular hypospadias, the greater the risk.

EVALUATION OF THE DYSMORPHIC CHILD WITH UROGENITAL ABNORMALITIES

The process of evaluation for the malformed child must often, of necessity, be performed rapidly and under stressful conditions. For some isolated urologic abnormalities, such as penile agenesis or severe degrees of genital ambiguity, response in terms of gender identification is required in the delivery room. The same is true for the dysmorphic child who presents with a urologic abnormality as part of a more generalized disorder. Steps that should be performed in the evaluation process are:

1. *In-depth antenatal history, family history, and physical examination.* Even in the delivery room, it may be possible to elicit important information related to prenatal drug exposure, fetal activity, maternal illness, and the presence or absence of urogenital or other malformations. A rapid physical examination should then be performed, with the urologist looking for nonurologic abnormalities and variations.
2. *Measurements.* Objective data on facial characteristics such as interpupillary distance (to determine whether the infant has hypertelorism), ear length, and philtrum length (midline depression on upper lip) among others are available to assist in assessment (Holmes, 1976; Jones). Visual cues are often misleading; therefore, it is ideal to obtain objective measurement, if possible.

3. *Knowledge of what is normal.* As detailed in Table 8–3, many facial variations are seen so frequently in the general population that they are of little significance. Conversely, many dysmorphic syndromes are characterized by a grouping of minor variations with few, if any, major malformations. The appearance of the child with Down syndrome is an excellent example of a situation in which there are multiple minor malformations and variations that individually are of little significance but that together allow for diagnosis.

4. *Interpretation of anomalies from the viewpoint of developmental anatomy.* A good knowledge of fetal development is essential in understanding which anomaly came first and whether it was primary or secondary. Does the patient have a true malformation, or is it explainable as a deformation or disruption?

5. *Laboratory evaluation.*
   a. Appropriate laboratory studies should be obtained early in the evaluation. For the child with an isolated urologic abnormality such as cryptorchidism or hypospadias, cytogenetic studies are not usually recommended because their yield is low. In cases of genital ambiguity, chromosomal analysis is mandatory. The buccal smear may still have a role in the laboratory armamentarium, but its limitations should be recognized. Buccal smears are *screening tests only,* and decisions should not be made based on buccal smear results. Falsely low percentages of Barr bodies are frequently seen in the normal newborn female, and some laboratories report low rates of false-positive Barr bodies in males. More specific is Y fluorescence, which stains the heterochromatic area of the Y chromosome intensely. Normal newborn males are 60 to 70 per cent Y-chromatin positive in the author's laboratory; again, however, this procedure remains a screening test.
   b. Preliminary chromosomal results can be obtained routinely in 72 hours; some laboratories harvest the sample as early as 48 hours if sex determination is the primary concern. High-resolution banding techniques to look for small additions or deletions usually take an additional 3 to 4 days. *It should be stressed that the majority of children with a rec-*

ognizable dysmorphic syndrome have normal chromosomes. Thus, a negative result may be falsely reassuring to physicians and parents. The greatest diagnostic yield can be anticipated from examination by an experienced clinical geneticist or dysmorphologist.
   c. Other laboratory studies should be obtained, depending on the specific abnormality. For the genetic female with genital ambiguity, levels of serum 17α-hydroxyprogesterone, renin, and urinary 17α-hydroxysteroids and 17-ketosteroids are necessary. The approach to the intersex child is detailed in Chapter 21.

6. *Radiographic studies.* Specific views of the urogenital system for the child with genital abnormalities are warranted. Depending on the clinical situation, ultrasonography, genitography, renal scanning, or voiding cystourethrography may be required.

7. *Photographs.* Documentation of physical differences is best performed with medical photographs. This is especially true of the child with life-threatening malformations or the stillborn infant, since efforts to make diagnoses often cease after death and are anticlimactic. Many geneticists routinely provide consultation through the mail on malformed infants that were not able to be seen, although this is often suboptimal. Photographs also serve the purpose of reducing the "mystique" and fears that parents often develop about their infant's malformations.

8. *Overall diagnosis for appropriate counseling.* Without a proper diagnosis, the clinician can give little correct information about prognosis and the presence of related abnormalities. Two of the primary considerations are whether the family is at risk for recurrence of the disorder and whether prenatal diagnosis is available.

SINGLE-GENE DISORDERS AND DYSMORPHIC SYNDROMES WITH UROLOGIC ANOMALIES

Autosomal Dominant Disorders

BOR Syndrome (Branchio-Oto-Renal Syndrome, Melnick-Fraser Syndrome)

Branchial arch anomalies are associated with hearing loss and structural renal disease

(Fraser et al, 1978; Melnick et al). As expected, marked variability of expressivity is noted in most affected patients. Auricular and branchial abnormalities include cupped ears with unusual helices, preauricular sinuses, branchial cleft sinuses, and ossicular abnormalities. Similarly, the renal anomalies have included renal agenesis, hypoplasia, polycystic disease, and calyceal dysplasia. The BOR syndrome is inherited as an autosomal dominant trait, with an estimated prevalence at 1 in 40,000 births (Jones). Prenatal diagnosis of an affected fetus with bilateral renal agenesis has been reported by Greenberg and colleagues.

Hypertelorism-Hypospadias Syndromes (BBB and G Syndromes, Opitz and Opitz-Frias Syndromes)

These two conditions are discussed together, since recent data raise the question as to whether they represent variable manifestations of the same syndrome. The genetics of this group of syndromes is also uncertain, with many investigators believing that the entities are autosomal dominant with sex-limited inheritance and others suggesting that this is an X-linked dominant trait (Cordero and Holmes; Funderburk and Stewart; Gonzalez et al; Opitz). Because of the ascertainment bias (finding that leads to investigation) with hypospadias, females may be underdiagnosed. Some instances of male-to-male transmission have been reported as well (Cordero and Holmes; Rosenbaum: unpublished observations, 1979).

BBB Syndrome (Opitz Syndrome)

Clinical findings seen most frequently in BBB syndrome include telecanthus, hypertelorism, and coarse facial features with a widow's peak, a large tongue, and clefting of the lip and palate (Fig. 8–3A). Eighty-six per cent of affected males in a recent report had hypospadias, with mental retardation and central nervous system abnormalities in approximately half (Funderburk and Stewart). Cryptorchidism has also been described in approximately 33 per cent of patients. In a review of 21 patients by Noe and coworkers, all had hypospadias (this was necessary for diagnosis), with 6 of 21 demonstrating cryptorchidism. Six of 18 patients had upper tract anomalies. A variety of other malformations, including congenital heart disease, imperforate anus, and ocular abnormalities, can be seen.

G Syndrome (Opitz-Frias Syndrome)

As noted, because of phenotypic similarities, some investigators have questioned whether this entity is distinct from the BBB syndrome. Patients with G syndrome were originally described because of swallowing dysfunction leading to recurrent aspiration. The clinical findings in the two syndromes are quite similar, with a decreased frequency of clefting in the G syndrome as compared with the BBB syndrome.

Nail-Patella Syndrome (Hereditary Osteo-Onychodysplasia [HOOD] Syndrome)

This autosomal dominant disorder may represent a connective tissue disorder, with patients manifesting a variety of skeletal and renal abnormalities. Linkage to the ABO blood group on chromosome 9 has been demonstrated in a number of pedigrees (Bennett et al; Jones; Silverman et al). Clinical findings seen with high frequency include nail hypoplasia (especially of the thumb), hypoplasia of the patellae, radial head abnormalities, unusual iliac bones, and a number of eye findings such as unusual iris pigmentation, microcornea, and keratoconus. In addition, approximately 30 per cent of patients have a glomerulonephropathy with proteinuria and, at times, hematuria. A characteristic microscopic appearance has been suggested (Bennett et al; Silverman et al).

Noonan Syndrome

One of the more common dysmorphic syndromes featuring autosomal dominant inheritance, Noonan syndrome has an estimated incidence of 1 in 3000 to 5000 live births (Nora et al). Previously, this condition had been mistakenly called the Turner-like syndrome with normal chromosomes and, on occasion, the male Turner syndrome despite the fact that males and females are affected with equal frequency. Clinical findings include craniofacial dysmorphism with frequent ptosis and epicanthal folds (see Fig. 8–3B), a low hairline with webbed neck, broad chest, and congenital heart disease (pulmonary stenosis in 40 to 50 per cent of patients) (Nora et al). Cryptorchidism is common in affected males.

Polycystic Kidney Disease

Much has been written in the urologic, nephrologic, and genetic literature about polycystic

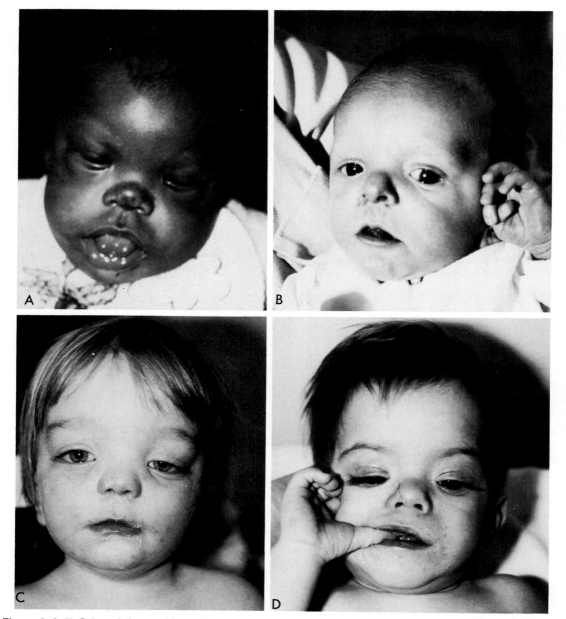

Figure 8–3 □ Selected dysmorphic syndromes. *A,* Hypertelorism-hypospadias syndrome. *B,* Noonan syndrome. *C,* Aarskog-Scott syndrome. *D,* Russell-Silver syndrome.

kidney disease. Classification on the basis of age of onset is fraught with difficulties because infants may have "adult type" disease (Anton and Abramowsky; Bear et al; Cole et al; Gal et al; Kaplan et al; Shokeir; Strand et al) and adults may have the "infantile" type (Piering et al). Distinction, however, on a genetic basis is still warranted, because most previously classified infantile forms are autosomal recessive and most adult forms are autosomal dominant.

Variability even within specific genetic forms of polycystic kidney disease is to be expected. These considerations are also important in regard to prenatal diagnosis of polycystic kidney disease.

"Adult" or Autosomal Dominant Polycystic Kidney Disease (ADPKD)

Linkage analysis has mapped the adult polycystic kidney disease gene (PKD1) to the distal short arm of chromosome 16 (16p) (Reeders et al). The PKD1 gene is closely linked to the alpha globin complex. A report by Kimberling and associates, however, describes a large family in which linkage could not be demonstrated. Although it is estimated that 90 per cent of autosomal dominant polycystic kidney disease is due to the 16p mutation, caution in interpreting DNA studies must be exercised until more information about heterogeneity is available.

The penetrance of this common gene is higher with increasing age of the patient and allows for determination of probability based on sonographic findings. The majority of patients come to attention because of renal failure or hypertension in their fourth decade. Cysts in a number of other organs are well described, and cerebral aneurysms have been found in 20 per cent of patients (Anton and Abramowsky; Milutinovic et al; Rosenfield et al; Sahney et al).

The reliability of ultrasonography alone in screening at-risk individuals is now well documented (Bear et al; Gabow et al; Rosenfield et al). The probability of detection by ultrasonography of an affected individual at 5, 15, and 25 years is 22.2, 65.7, and 85.5 per cent, respectively. Conversely, the chance of a normal result in affected individuals is 46, 28, and 14 per cent, respectively, in the first, second, and third decades (Bear et al).

Robinow Syndrome (Fetal Face Syndrome)

This disorder produces a wide spectrum of malformations, including mild shortness of stature, relative macrocephaly with a large anterior fontanelle, hypertelorism with unusual palpebral fissures, and, frequently, short forearms and other extremity variations (Jones). Genital abnormalities include microphallus and cryptorchidism, and often, hypoplasia of the clitoris and labia majora in affected females (Jones). Lee and colleagues have shown evidence for partial primary hypogonadism as evidenced by elevated serum follicle-stimulating hormone levels in men with the Robinow syndrome.

Autosomal Recessive Disorders

Asphyxiating Thoracic Dystrophy (Jeune Syndrome)

This infrequent disorder produces short stature and often leads to death in the perinatal period because of a constricted chest. Renal abnormalities include dysplasia and, in survivors, chronic nephritis leading to renal failure (Jones; Shah).

Bardet-Biedl Syndrome (Laurence-Moon-Biedl Syndrome)

This syndrome features some combination of obesity, mental retardation, and polydactyly of the hands, along with retinitis pigmentosa and genital hypoplasia or hypogonadism (Schachat and Maumenee). The hypogonadism is usually hypogonadotropic. Testicular failure has also been described (Jones). Renal involvement typically includes small kidneys, with histologic findings of glomerulosclerosis, interstitial fibrosis, and dysplasia (Linne et al). In the author's experience, patients with renal findings have progressive loss of function, often leading to end-stage renal failure.

Cryptophthalmos Syndrome (Fraser Syndrome)

This uncommon disorder features cryptophthalmos (eyes covered with skin) in association with an unusual facial appearance involving hypoplastic nares and auricular abnormalities. Affected males have been described with hypospadias and cryptorchidism, whereas affected females have hypoplastic external genitalia and may have müllerian abnormalities (Fraser; Jones).

Meckel-Gruber Syndrome

This well-known disorder involves neural tube formation presenting primarily with encephalocele in association with cleft lip and palate and polydactyly. Survival is unlikely in this condition. A variety of visceral anomalies have been seen, including hepatic cysts and renal dysplasia (Fraser and Lytwyn; Hsia et al; Seller). Cryptorchidism and ambiguity of external genitalia have been encountered as well.

"Infantile" or Autosomal Recessive Polycystic Kidney Disease (ARPKD)

Presentation within this subgroup is also variable, with some patients manifesting oligohydramnios and pulmonary hypoplasia and death in the perinatal period, and other patients surviving only to develop significant infantile hypertension, leading to dialysis and transplantation (Lieberman et al). In survivors, hepatic fibrosis, cirrhosis, and portal hypertension may become manifest (Lieberman et al).

Second-trimester prenatal diagnosis of polycystic kidney disease using a combination of restriction fragment length polymorphism (RFLP) analysis and ultrasonography (Ceccherini et al; Hadlock et al; Kaffe et al; Novelli et al; Shenker and Anderson) has been successfully performed. Caution, however should be exercised, especially when trying to exclude autosomal recessive polycystic kidney disease, because of the small cyst size and natural history of the disease.

Smith-Lemli-Opitz Syndrome

This is an infrequent disorder with characteristic facies secondary to scaphocephaly, ptosis of the eyelids with epicanthal folds, and a number of extremity variations. Affected individuals are profoundly mentally retarded, and survival is poor. Genital abnormalities reported in males include cryptorchidism, hypospadias, genital ambiguity, and recently, focal renal hypoplasia. Females have been noted to have fewer genital abnormalities (Akl et al; Jones). Genetic females with apparent sex reversal secondary to the Smith-Lemli-Opitz syndrome have been seen (Patterson et al).

Cerebrohepatorenal Syndrome (Zellweger Syndrome)

This is another uncommon syndrome that is frequently lethal in early infancy. Craniofacial findings include a flat face with sloping forehead, upslanting palpebral fissures, and a large anterior fontanelle. Affected infants usually have hepatomegaly and, on autopsy, have renal dysplasia and microcysts (Danks et al, 1975; Jones). Resemblance of patients to those with other dysmorphic and chromosomal syndromes such as Down syndrome is well established. The Zellweger syndrome is the prototype of peroxisomal disorders in man, a group of unusual metabolic conditions that includes adrenoleukodystrophy, infantile Refsum disease, and chondrodysplasia punctata (Moser et al).

X-Linked Disorders

Aarskog-Scott Syndrome

Affected individuals demonstrate some degree of short stature with a broad, relatively large cranium, downslanting palpebral fissures, and, often, ptosis (see Fig. 8–3C). Other craniofacial findings include a long philtrum. The genital abnormalities typically are that of a "shawl scrotum," representing a mild degree of penoscrotal transposition and cryptorchidism (Bawle et al; Escobar and Weaver; Fryns et al; Jones). In addition, in the author's own series and in the literature, absence or atrophy of a testis has been seen (Fryns et al).

The inheritance of the Aarskog-Scott syndrome is uncertain at this time. In a few of the families studied by the author, the mother of the affected child demonstrates mild manifestations of the Aarskog-Scott syndrome. This would be suggestive of X-linked dominant or possibly X-linked recessive inheritance. Escobar and Weaver, in a review of 10 pedigrees, felt that X-linked recessive inheritance was more likely because they found a paucity of affected daughters from affected men. Other investigators have suggested an autosomal dominant sex-limited mode of inheritance (Escobar and Weaver). The syndrome resembles in some ways the Noonan syndrome and Robinow syndrome.

Alport Syndrome (Hereditary Nephritis)

A number of single-gene disorders and dysmorphic syndromes feature the association of auditory, ocular, and renal abnormalities, either functional or structural. One of the best known in pediatric populations is the association of nephritis with hearing loss. Although the condition is named after Alport's description of the entity in 1927, investigators prior to this time were aware of the association (Gubler et al; Kenya et al; O'Neill et al). Significant debate has gone on regarding the genetics of this condition, with X-linked dominant inheritance now accepted as the most likely means of transmission for this gene given the increased severity and progression in males and a lack of male-to-male transmission in a number of pedigrees (Gubler et al; Tishler).

O'Neill and co-workers, in looking at 150 patients with hereditary nephritis in two large pedigrees, found no examples of male-to-male transmission. In addition, there was almost a 2:1 female-male ratio, and the risk of affected offspring born to affected females was approximately 50 per cent. O'Neill and colleagues felt that these findings were more compatible with X-linked dominant inheritance in their pedigrees. Diagnosis rested on the demonstration of microscopic hematuria. Gubler and associates reviewed the clinical experience in 58 pediatric patients with Alport syndrome. The most common presentations were microscopic hematuria and proteinuria. In regard to the auditory deficit in patients, 37 of 58 tested (63.8 per cent) had hearing loss, with males affected more than females, and a variety of ocular abnormalities were also seen, including anterior lenticonus and macular abnormalities. Heterogeneity of Alport syndrome, however, is still possible.

Histologic abnormalities of the glomerular basement membrane have led to a search for an abnormal collagen gene. An X-linked collagen gene, COL4A5, that codes for the 5 (IV) chain, maps to the same X chromosomal region as does Alport syndrome, Xq22. Barker and co-workers and Hostikka and colleagues have shown three distinct mutations of the COL4A5 gene that may account for the majority of X-linked Alport families.

Oculocerebrorenal Syndrome (Lowe Syndrome)

This uncommon disorder features renal tubular acidosis leading to progressive dysfunction in association with mental retardation and severe ocular handicap, usually caused by cataracts or glaucoma, or both (Abbassi et al; Jones). Affected infants at birth may appear relatively normal until the generalized aminoaciduria is detected. Carrier females may be discovered occasionally on the basis of their ocular abnormalities.

Menkes Syndrome (Kinky Hair Syndrome)

This is also an uncommon disorder characterized by sparse, kinky hair along with severe central nervous system abnormalities (primarily mental retardation and seizures) usually progressing to death (Danks et al, 1972). It appears that Menkes syndrome is a disorder of elastogenesis secondary to copper deficiency. A number of urinary tract findings have been described in patients with Menkes syndrome, including hydronephrosis, ureteropelvic junction obstruction, vesicoureteral reflux, and cryptorchidism. Daly and Rabinovitch described bladder diverticula in three of four patients studied. One of these patients was managed with intravenous copper infusions and was alive at age 7. His bladder diverticula on radiologic examination showed progressive enlargement, although the upper tracts were normal. The patient was also placed on intermittent catheterization. During therapy, calculi developed and a vesicostomy was then performed.

DYSMORPHIC SYNDROMES OF UNCERTAIN OR UNKNOWN CAUSE

CHARGE Association

CHARGE association is a recently described entity that is likely to be heterogeneous in etiology. The acronym CHARGE stands for *c*oloboma of the iris and/or retina, *h*eart lesions, *a*tresia choanae, *r*etardation of growth and/or development, *g*enital abnormalities, and *e*ar abnormalities and/or deafness. Pagon and associates (1981) reviewed a number of patients with the CHARGE association. The majority of patients were ascertained on the basis of their ocular and choanal abnormalities. However, a high frequency of genital abnormalities was noted in these patients. The CHARGE association is one of the more frequent colobomatous syndromes.

Facioauriculovertebral Dysplasia (Goldenhar Syndrome, Hemifacial Microsomia)

This disorder of unknown etiology is a relatively prevalent malformation syndrome with an estimated frequency of 1 in 5000 births (Gorlin et al, 1990; Jones). Although this syndrome is classically described in patients with ocular dermoids, many patients have much milder manifestations of the syndrome. Overall, 50 per cent of affected patients have vertebral anomalies, with 30 per cent of patients exhibiting cardiac malformations and a similar percentage having urogenital abnormalities. The structural abnormalities are varied and may include unilateral renal agenesis, hypoplasia, or dysplasia. The management of patients with the facioauriculovertebral syndrome depends on the spectrum of abnormalities. Patients with sufficient craniofacial abnormalities to confirm the diagnosis should at least undergo renal ultrasonography.

MURCS Association

The MURCS association was described by Duncan and colleagues in their review of 28 patients with vaginal atresia. In their study, they found a high frequency of cervicothoracic vertebral anomalies and renal abnormalities. They therefore coined the acronym MURCS (*mü*llerian duct aplasia, *r*enal aplasia, *c*ervicothoracic *s*omite dysplasia) for this group of patients. They proposed that the etiology of the MURCS association was an early embryologic event that involved the developing renal blastema and cervical somites.

The clinical findings in these patients are quite similar to those of the VATER association (*v*ertebral defects, *a*nal atresia, *t*racheoesophageal fistula, *r*enal and radial abnormalities) and may indicate that the MURCS association is a subgroup. Within the VATER association, which is a form of caudal regression, patients may have vaginal atresia and lower müllerian agenesis. The VATER association is discussed in more detail below. The major reason for identifying patients with the MURCS and VATER associations is to determine the need to search for renal anomalies in these patients.

Prader-Willi Syndrome

This disorder was first described in 1956 by Prader in patients with short stature, obesity, and mental retardation. More males than females are recognized with the disorder because of the overt hypogonadism and hypogenitalism in boys. Typically, at birth a male presents with a small phallus and cryptorchidism (Hall and Smith). Despite a few reports of apparent autosomal recessive inheritance, the etiology of the Prader-Willi syndrome has been unknown until recently.

As discussed earlier in this chapter under Clinical Cytogenetic Syndromes, Ledbetter and colleagues (1981, 1982) and Butler and associates have described a number of patients with an interstitial deletion of proximal 15q in the Prader-Willi syndrome. It would appear that this deletion is a cause of the condition in at least 50 per cent of patients, although heterogeneity cannot be excluded because some

patients with definite Prader-Willi syndrome have had normal chromosomes even on prometaphase banding (Butler; Butler et al; Kousseff; Ledbetter et al, 1982).

The urogenital abnormalities seen in patients with the Prader-Willi syndrome have been discussed by a number of authors. In their review of 32 cases, Hall and Smith found cryptorchidism in 84 per cent of males. In studying 30 affected males with the Prader-Willi syndrome, Uehling found cryptorchidism in 21 of 30 patients (70 per cent), with 14 of 30 patients (47 per cent) having both testes maldescended. Testicular biopsies were performed on four patients ranging in age from 4 to 21 years of age. It was found that all of the testes histologically had a Sertoli-cell–only appearance. Some of these obese children may have retractile rather than undescended testicles. Uehling used trials of gonadotropin therapy in an attempt to produce descent and was successful in two patients at 4 and 8 years of age and in a 5-year-old with unilateral cryptorchidism. Uehling recommended gonadotropin administration instead of immediate orchiopexy in patients with Prader-Willi syndrome.

Prune-Belly Syndrome (Sequence)

A review of the prune-belly syndrome (triad syndrome, Eagle-Barrett syndrome) is included in Chapter 20. It has been estimated that approximately 200 to 300 reports of this entity exist, with the overwhelming majority being affected infant males. Rabinowitz and Schillinger reported their experience and reviewed the literature on 17 affected females and concluded that most were incomplete examples of the syndrome.

There has been significant debate in the urologic and pediatric literature concerning the etiology of this syndrome. The prune-belly anomaly has been seen in association with fetal ascites, the Beckwith-Wiedemann syndrome, monosomy X (Turner syndrome), polycystic kidney disease, renal dysplasia, and anencephaly (Hodes et al; Lubinsky and Rapoport; Monie and Monie; Pagon et al, 1979; Pramanik et al). The perspective of the pediatric geneticist, who frequently deals with nonviable infants that have a prune belly, is often different from that of the urologist who sees a more homogeneous population (Woodhouse et al). Two cases of twins concordant for the prune-belly anomaly have been described (Garlinger and Ott), although there are a number of discordant presumed monozygotic twin pairs (Garlinger and Ott; Ives; Lubinsky and Rapoport). Garlinger and Ott reported a case with affected male siblings and male half–first cousins. Adeyokunnu and Familusi reported on the prune-belly syndrome in two male siblings and a male first cousin. One of the sisters had Turner syndrome.

The hypotheses that have been put forth to explain the prune-belly syndrome fall into two major categories: mesodermal dysgenesis and urethral dysgenesis (King and Prescott; Kroovand et al, 1982; Moerman et al; Nakayama et al; Pagon et al, 1979). Pagon and associates (1979) reviewed the sequence of events leading to the prune-belly syndrome, ostensibly from urethral obstruction. It was their feeling that the developmental complexity of the prostatic urethra in males increased the risk of an abnormality and accounted for the large predominance of affected males. Moerman and colleagues reviewed the histologic findings in seven males with prune-belly syndrome and observed severe prostatic hypoplasia in all. This would also account for the manifestations of the prune-belly syndrome in the other conditions noted above.

A genetic basis has been postulated by many authors as well (Adeyokunnu and Familusi; Garlinger and Ott; Ives; Riccardi and Grum). Riccardi and Grum suggested that the clinical data supported an unusual two-step autosomal dominant mutation with sex-limited expression partially mimicking X-linkage. Single-gene inheritance of a more conventional nature can be ruled out on the basis of the lack of affected monozygotic twins. It is likely that the prune-belly syndrome is multifactorially determined, as are most of the other regional urogenital malformations. The other manifestations (musculoskeletal) of the prune-belly syndrome are probably secondary to the initiating factor and not additional primary malformations. Counseling should be directed toward identification of the *specific* urologic lesion. Reports of a lethal recessive condition, the megacystis–microcolon–intestinal hypoperistalsis syndrome (Penman and Lilford), may mimic the manifestations of the prune-belly syndrome and account for some of the observed recurrences.

Prenatal diagnosis of the prune-belly syndrome is also possible (Bovicelli et al; Christopher et al). Pescia and coauthors (1982) reported on a case in which elevations of maternal serum alpha-fetoprotein levels were present at 15 weeks' gestation and the fetus showed abnormalities at 17 weeks' gestation on sonography. Other investigators have made a sonographic diagnosis of the prune-belly syndrome in the third trimester (Bovicelli et al; Christopher et al).

Russell-Silver Syndrome

Russell-Silver syndrome is associated with low birth weight and dwarfism along with asymmetry of body parts in 75 per cent of patients, minor craniofacial dysmorphism with triangular facies, down-turned corners of the mouth (Fig. 8–3D), extremity variations including clinodactyly and syndactyly of the toes, and developmental delay and/or mental retardation in approximately 20 per cent of patients (Escobar et al; Jones; Marks and Bergeson). Marks and Bergeson reported on a case of Russell-Silver syndrome with ambiguous genitalia and reviewed 148 cases reported in the literature. They found three other examples of ambiguous genitalia, cryptorchidism in 22 patients, and hypospadias in 12 others. In addition, precocious sexual development was seen in eight girls.

The etiology of the Russell-Silver syndrome is unknown. The majority of affected patients have had normal chromosomes. Escobar and associates reviewed the familial cases of Russell-Silver syndrome from a total sample of the 150 patients reported to date. Their findings were not conclusive for single-gene inheritance. There were a number of familial cases that did at least suggest the possibility of autosomal dominant inheritance. One problem in dealing with the Russell-Silver syndrome relates to the marked heterogeneity, with a number of disorders potentially resembling the Russell-Silver syndrome. With otherwise unaffected family members, the risk of recurrence for the Russell-Silver syndrome is low.

VATER Association

As noted earlier in the discussion of the MURCS association, the VATER association, which was first formally described in 1973 (Quan and Smith), represents a defect in mesodermal development at the primitive streak level. The acronym VATER (*v*ertebral defects, *a*nal atresia, *t*racheoesophageal fistula, *r*enal and radial anomalies) reflects the physical manifestations, with most affected patients having three VATER components. Additional features frequently include congenital heart disease and a single umbilical artery. Other authors have suggested extending the acronym to include other limb abnormalities as well (Temtamy and Miller). Renal anomalies are seen in approximately 50 per cent of patients and include renal agenesis, dysplasia, or hypoplasia (Jones; Temtamy and Miller). Abnormalities of the external genitalia have also been described. Uehling and colleagues reviewed the data on 23 VATER patients and found 21 with significant genitourinary involvement. Seven patients had renal agenesis, five had ureteropelvic junction obstruction, five had crossed fused ectopia, and an additional nine patients exhibited severe reflux. Hoekstra and associates documented that 50 per cent of patients in a large study of congenital anorectal malformations had urogenital anomalies. Complete evaluation of the urogenital system, including both cystography and visualization of the upper tracts, in patients who present with other components of the VATER association, especially imperforate anus and tracheoesophageal fistula, is likely to result in a high yield.

GENETIC COUNSELING

The process of genetic counseling is one that should be implicit in all discussions with families that include a malformed child or one with a genetic disorder. The purpose of such counseling is threefold: to provide useful information in an understandable fashion, to reduce the often overwhelming stresses on the family, and to develop reproductive alternatives related to the risk of recurrence. Counseling is more art than science. Most genetic counselors provide nondirective counseling without making an actual decision for the family. The steps in counseling a family include:

1. *Rapid diagnosis.* As noted above, everything hinges on a rapid, accurate diagnosis after consideration of syndromic etiologies.
2. *Counseling parents together.* The reasons for this are obvious. During counseling, individuals hear selectively and are often unable to relay information correctly to one another. Also, feelings of guilt are more equally divided when both members of a couple are present.

3. *Explanation of problems in biologic terms.* This step aids in reducing guilt by demonstrating that there is a scientific basis for the occurrence of a malformation or genetic disorder. Terms used should be understandable, but complex concepts (such as chromosomes and genes) should not be avoided.
4. *Discussion of recurrence risk.* Parents should be told what the theoretical risk of recurrence is, and it should be placed in a real-life situation. A demonstration of the mechanical basis of inheritance is reasonable at this point.
5. *Discussion of burden.* As important as risk figures may be to a family, the burden or impact of a condition on a family emotionally, financially, and medically may be what makes the decision for them. Each family views burden differently, and the counselor should not bias the information with his or her own view of burden.
6. *Consideration of reproductive options.* The availability of prenatal diagnosis and other options, including donor insemination and adoption, should be introduced in an objective fashion.
7. *Written summary.* Throughout the counseling session, both visual and auditory cues are used. The pace of the session should be leisurely, with periodic pauses where questions would be appropriate. If possible, some written material, either informal notes of the session highlighting key points or a more formal follow-up letter, should be provided.
8. *Repetition.* Much has been written on the imperfections of counseling. Although many families may retain risk figure information, the subtleties of what occurs in a counseling session are often lost. Repetition on the part of the urologist, geneticist, and other care providers is frequently necessary to ensure a clear perception of transmitted information. Excellent reviews on the counseling process demonstrate well the inherent difficulties in transmitting information to families (Leonard et al; Targum).

COUNSELING FOR SELECTED ISOLATED UROLOGIC CONDITIONS

The situation that the urologist most often faces is the child with an isolated urogenital malformation and parents who desire information on the risk of recurrence. As indicated throughout much of this chapter, it is currently thought that most regional malformations are multifactorially determined, with both environmental and genetic components. Excellent reviews are available detailing the genetic basis of isolated urologic malformations (Barakat et al, 1986; Burger and Burger; Klass; Mininberg).

Cryptorchidism

It has been estimated that 4 per cent of term infants have cryptorchidism (Bartone and Schmidt). A number of factors need to be considered in counseling families with cryptorchid children, most importantly, exclusion of other genitourinary external anomalies or evidence of a generalized dysmorphic syndrome that would influence the risk of recurrence. Jones and Young, in looking at 51 males with cryptorchidism, found that 9.75 per cent of their male siblings were affected. In addition, 3.9 per cent of their fathers had cryptorchidism as well. In second-degree relatives, the risk fell to 5 per cent overall.

A second important consideration in cryptorchidism is the frequency of associated chromosomal abnormalities. An early report by Mininberg and Bingol indicated that there was a high frequency of chromosomal abnormalities in cryptorchid patients. However, their data included syndromic causes and were obtained prior to the advent of advanced banding techniques. In addition, a number of what appear to be laboratory artifacts, such as random loss of chromosomes, were included as abnormalities. More recent studies, including those of Bartone and Schmidt, Dewald and associates, and Waaler, have shown no increase in the frequency of chromosomal abnormalities in *isolated* cryptorchidism. It is the author's recommendation that patients who have hypospadias or other genitourinary anomalies in addition to cryptorchidism should have a banded chromosomal analysis prior to gender assignment and naming.

Exstrophy-Epispadias

Bladder exstrophy is an uncommon malformation with an estimated frequency of 1 in 30,000 live births. Shapiro and co-workers, in a retrospective study of personal experiences from 53 pediatric urologists worldwide, iden-

tified approximately 2500 index patients. Recurrence of bladder exstrophy was seen in nine of the families (1 in 275). Exact risks of recurrence could not be calculated from the study because the precise number of siblings born to these families was unknown. Five sets of monozygotic male twins were concordant for exstrophy. No female twins were concordant. Their review of the literature included two women with epispadias and one woman with exstrophy who produced children with bladder exstrophy. The authors suggested that although the risk for recurrence of this complex was low (less than 1 per cent), the risk to offspring was greater than expected.

Hypospadias

The largest body of data in regard to recurrence is found in the hypospadias literature (Bauer et al; Burger and Burger; Czeizel et al; Editorial; Klass; Mininberg; Page). Bauer and associates reported their findings in 177 boys presenting with hypospadias. Forty-four of the 177 families (25 per cent) had a second affected family member in addition to the index case. Twelve families (7 per cent) had three affected members. When looking at the risk of recurrence, Bauer and associates found that among the families of 150 patients, 14 recurrences occurred in 125 additional male children (Table 8–6). The overall risk factor was therefore 11 per cent. As expected, the risk of recurrence was proportionate to the severity of the hypospadias, with no recurrences among patients with a coronal meatus, a 12 per cent risk in the penile hypospadias group, and a 19 per cent risk in the penoscrotal group.

Table 8–6 □ Risk of Recurrence of Hypospadias

Severity/Affected Individuals	% Recurrence
Index case only affected	
Severity	
Coronal	0
Penile	12
Penoscrotal	19
Index case + second affected family member (excluding father)	15
Index case + father affected	27

Adapted from Bauer SB, Bull MJ, Retik AB: Hypospadias: a familial study. J Urol 121:474, 1979. © by Williams & Wilkins, 1979.

Bauer and associates also investigated the probabilities of recurrence when another family member was affected in addition to the index case. The risk was 15 per cent if an index child and another family member exclusive of the father were affected and 27 per cent if the father and the index child were the affected members. A large study conducted by Czeizel and coworkers in Hungary demonstrated similar findings with 28 twin pairs that were affected among 907 patients with simple hypospadias. Four per cent of the first-degree relatives of the index patients were affected with forms of hypospadias. Interestingly, there was a significant difference between sex hormone therapy in the mothers of index cases compared with controls ($P < .01$). A follow-up study did not support this trend, however (Czeizel and Toth). Page reported evidence of presumed single-gene inheritance of hypospadias. Two families were presented with multigenerational involvement. This, however, does not preclude multifactorial inheritance.

Posterior Urethral Valves

As with other malformations, posterior urethral valves have been observed on occasion to be more frequent among siblings of affected children than in the general population. Hasen and Song described brothers with urethral valves, and Davidsohn and Newberger reported similar findings in twins. Kroovand and colleagues (1977) documented the presence of valves in confirmed monozygotic twins as did Livne and associates. Data for risk of recurrence are sparse but should be calculable using the equation given on page 251; the risk would be expected to be quite low.

Renal Agenesis

The infant or fetus with bilateral renal agenesis (BRA) is a frequent clinical problem. The incidence of BRA is estimated to be approximately 1 in 3000 live births, with 1 in 1000 infants exhibiting unilateral agenesis (Burger and Burger; Schinzel et al). Holmes (1989) found a prevalence of 0.3 per 1000 for bilateral renal agenesis/dysgenesis among 85,800 infants examined as part of a large malformation surveillance program. A number of reports exist of siblings with bilateral renal agenesis as do instances of a parent with unilateral agenesis.

Mauer and associates first described renal agenesis in twins, and Schinzel and co-workers found 14 families that had more than one affected child in a review of the literature. Pescia and colleagues (1976) presented data to suggest a multifactorial cause in two of 91 siblings of female index cases, and they established an empiric recurrence risk of 2 to 5 per cent. Carter and associates estimated the risk for recurrence at 3.5 per cent for bilateral renal agenesis; however, others have suggested this number is higher than expected for a multifactorial condition.

It has become apparent that BRA represents part of a spectrum of renal malformation that includes unilateral renal agenesis as well as renal dysgenesis. The term hereditary renal adysplasia (HRA) has been suggested as an appropriate one for this group of conditions, which also features an increased frequency of müllerian anomalies and other non-urologic malformations (Biedel et al). Reviews by Roodhooft et al, McPherson et al, and others (Biedel et al; Curry et al; Schimke and King) demonstrate that a significant portion of recurrences among families with BRA is due to the effect of an autosomal dominant gene with reduced penetrance. Using these data, McPherson et al estimate that the empiric risk for bilateral severe renal adysplasia is 15 to 20 per cent, with an additional risk for less severe abnormalities in families with hereditary renal adysplasia. Following the birth of a child with renal agenesis or dysgenesis, the clinician should perform sonography on the parents, looking for unilateral or bilateral abnormalities. Prenatal diagnosis should also be offered for future pregnancies even in the absence of parental pathology.

Vesicoureteral Reflux and Other Uropathology

Numerous examples of familial reflux and other forms of uropathology have been described (Burger and Burger; Burger and Smith; Dwoskin; Jerkins and Noe; Kerr and Pillai; Middleton et al; Miller and Caspari; Mobley; Mulcahy et al; Raffle; Sengar et al; Simpson and German; Zel and Retik). Raffle described four cases of hydronephrosis in two generations of a family. All affected patients were females. The etiology of the apparent ureteropelvic junction obstruction was not identified in his cases except for one individual with aberrant vessels.

Mulcahy and associates reviewed 211 Mayo Clinic patients with reflux and found a positive family history of urinary tract symptomatology (dysuria) or proven infection in 13.2 per cent of parents and siblings. The frequency of finding affected relatives with reflux has ranged from approximately 2 per cent to as much as 60 per cent (Burger and Smith; Mobley; Zel and Retik). Burger and Burger found that in screening the siblings of patients with reflux, 60 per cent were also found to have reflux. After two affected members, 33 per cent of the remaining asymptomatic sibs had reflux. Dwoskin found that 47.6 per cent of sibships had uropathology when reflux was the primary problem in the proband, and that 26.5 per cent of these patients also had reflux. When the uropathology was other than reflux, the number decreased to 13.2 per cent. Jerkins and Noe looked at the problem prospectively and found an incidence of reflux of 32 per cent in the siblings of index cases; 73 per cent of the siblings with reflux were asymptomatic. Aggarwal and Jones studied 33 first-degree relatives of affected individuals (mothers and siblings). Fifteen of 33 (52 per cent) had either upper tract anomalies or reflux. Lewy and Belman reported father-to-son transmission of reflux, suggesting autosomal dominant inheritance.

The genetic basis of reflux would seem to be multifactorial, although sex-linked sibships have been described (Middleton et al). One group of investigators has also looked at human leukocyte antigen (HLA) linkage and association (Sengar et al). In four families at risk for reflux and one with ureteropelvic junction obstruction, the urogenital abnormalities segregated with a particular HLA haplotype, suggesting linkage of reflux to the HLA complex. This finding is currently unconfirmed by other investigators.

TERATOGENIC INFLUENCES

Available literature on the effect of teratogens on the male genital system is concentrated in two areas: the effects of diethylstilbestrol (DES) and other estrogens on male genitalia, and the relationship of progestin exposure to the production of hypospadias. The latter question may be easier to answer than the former. Reports noting an increased associa-

tion between fetuses exposed to progestins during pregnancy and hypospadias have existed for a number of years (Aarskog; Czeizel et al; Kallen and Winberg; Mau; Schardein; Svensson). Aarskog, in reviewing the problem, found that of 130 patients with hypospadias, 11 had early progestin exposure. However, this report does not include an estimate of the population at risk, and the significance of his findings is unknown. He also referred to the United States Collaborative Perinatal Project, which examined 50,282 mother-child pairs. Here again there was a greater than expected rate of hypospadias among progestin-exposed infants, but no significant statistical differences existed between the exposed and unexposed groups. Other negative studies include that of Mau in West Germany and Kallen and Winberg's report from Sweden, which showed no statistical increase in the risk of hypospadias following progestin exposure. If there is any statistical association between progestin exposure and hypospadias, it is likely to be small.

Stillman has reviewed nicely the effects of in utero DES exposure on male offspring. Most of his discussion is based on the data of Gill and colleagues. These authors found a 31.5 per cent incidence of epididymal cysts and/or hypoplastic testes in men exposed to DES in utero compared with 7.8 per cent in placebo-exposed controls. There were also a large number of patients with abnormalities of spermatozoa function and formation. Sixty-five per cent of exposed men with testicular hypoplasia had a history of cryptorchidism. Because DES is no longer used to any great extent, continued problems related to this drug should decrease.

The teratogenic influences of both estrogens and progestins in male fetuses are, therefore, unresolved. It is possible that the action of these agents is to increase the genetic susceptibility in at-risk families through a multifactorial means.

Additionally, urogenital abnormalities have been described following exposure to cocaine and, frequently, alcohol. Chavez and colleagues have demonstrated a substantial increase in the risk for urinary tract defects with maternal cocaine use. The crude odds ratio for all urinary tract anomalies in their study was 4.39 and for genital organ abnormalities, 2.26. The possibility of a chance association, however, could not be excluded in the second group. The particular malformations seen in the study included an infant with bilateral congenital hydronephrosis leading to prune-belly syndrome, a second infant with unilateral congenital hydronephrosis, and a third with unilateral renal and ureteral agenesis, ambiguous genitalia, unilateral ectopia of a fallopian tube, gastroschisis, and additional anomalies. Three of four infants in the second group had hypospadias. Postulated mechanisms that would explain the occurrence of genitourinary malformations in these infants relate primarily to the vasoconstrictive effects of cocaine as well as its action on calcium availability. Chavez and colleagues suggest that the slower metabolism of cocaine in the fetus would allow for prolonged exposure of the fetal genitourinary tract to cocaine and its metabolites. Additionally, local ischemia and interference with peristalsis may contribute to the risk.

Renal anomalies in the fetal alcohol syndrome are well described (DeBeukelaer et al; Havers et al; Qazi et al). The fetal alcohol syndrome is one of the more common causes of preventable mental retardation, with a frequency of 1 to 3/1000 births. Systematic evaluation for renal anomalies in fetal alcohol syndrome has not been performed but may be reasonable. The spectrum of observed malformations is broad but primarily features hypoplasia. Renal agenesis, hydronephrosis, and ureteral duplication have been seen. The teratogenic mechanism of alcohol embryopathy, although not understood completely, may be similar to that described for cocaine because alcohol is a potent vasoconstrictor. Animal studies have also demonstrated that alcohol directly interferes with protein synthesis and cell growth.

PRENATAL DIAGNOSIS

Over the last 20 years, a number of tools have been developed that allow for assessment of the genetic make-up of the fetus. Although prenatal diagnosis of urologic abnormalities has been discussed in Chapter 1 and reviewed elsewhere (Barakat et al, 1989), a broad view of the issue is included here.

Indications

The leading indication for prenatal diagnosis is advanced maternal age, generally accepted as 35 years or older at the time of delivery. With increasing age of the mother, there is a corresponding increase in the risk of having a child with a chromosomal abnormality, primarily related to nondisjunctional events such as trisomy 21 (Down syndrome), trisomy 13, trisomy 18, and the Klinefelter syndrome. The risk for structural chromosomal abnormalities such as unbalanced translocations and for conditions such as the Turner syndrome is not increased. The risk for Down syndrome at selected maternal ages is shown in Table 8–7 (Hook and Lindsje).

Other indications for seeking prenatal diagnosis include:

1. *Positive family history.* The presence of a genetic disorder or birth defect in a close relative may warrant prenatal diagnosis. For families that have had a child with a single-gene disorder (dominant, recessive, or X-linked), prenatal diagnosis may exist for the condition. For certain X-linked traits, sex determination may be offered if a more exact diagnosis cannot be obtained.

2. *Previously affected child with chromosomal abnormality.* The risk of having a second live-born child with a chromosomal abnormality (e.g., Down syndrome) increases to approximately 1 per cent plus the age-related risk. This is equally true for less common conditions (trisomy 13, trisomy 18) where the risk seems related more to chromosomal nondisjunction in general. For families in which a parent has been identified as having a balanced translocation, with no net loss or gain of genetic material, the risk for unbalanced offspring may rise dramatically.

3. *Recurrent miscarriages or infant loss.* Approximately 5 per cent of couples experiencing more than two unexplained spontaneous abortions carry a balanced translocation in one member of the couple.

4. *Abnormal alpha-fetoprotein result.*

Table 8–7 ☐ Risk for Giving Birth to a Child with Down Syndrome at Selected Maternal Ages

Maternal Age	Risk at Birth
30	1/885
33	1/592
35	1/365
37	1/225
40	1/109
45	1/32

Adapted from Hook EJ, Lindsje A: Down syndrome in live births by single year maternal age interval in a Swedish study: comparison with results from a New York State study. Am J Hum Genet 30:19, 1978. Courtesy of the University of Chicago Press.

Screening for malformations of the neural tube in "low-risk" families has been accomplished by measurement of maternal serum alpha-fetoprotein (MSAFP) levels (Burton, 1986, 1988; Main and Mennuti). Elevations of this protein correlate well with an increased risk for myelomeningocele and anencephaly as well as other neural tube defects. Awareness of low MSAFP levels in fetuses with Down syndrome may allow for more accurate determination of risk. Using a cutoff value of 1/270 (comparable with the risk of having a child with Down syndrome at age 35), DiMaio and associates found that one quarter to one third of pregnancies in which the fetus had Down syndrome could be detected using alpha-fetoprotein screening. Most centers would view an MSAFP level below 0.5 multiples of the median as significant. Tables exist from a variety of sources to allow for more accurate calculations of exact risk in such a family (DiMaio et al).

5. *Abnormal fetal ultrasound scan.* This subject was discussed fully in Chapter 1.

6. *Drug exposure.* The exposure of the fetus to certain substances during pregnancy can substantially increase the risk for birth defects. Level II ultrasonography should be offered to these families for reassurance and management.

7. *Maternal illness.* The risk for malformations is increased for specific maternal illnesses, with diabetes the most prevalent (Mills et al). In this situation, the risk for malformation is at least 2 to 3 times greater than the general population. In a large collaborative study, Mills and co-workers have demonstrated that improved diabetic control can reduce, but not eliminate, the risk for malformation.

Methods and Techniques

Amniocentesis

Amniocentesis has been performed routinely since the late 1960s and has been clearly demonstrated to have high levels of accuracy and safety. Amniocentesis is generally performed at 16 to 18 weeks of gestation, after localization of the placenta. A small sample of amniotic fluid is removed and analyzed after culture for appropriate studies. The risk for procedure-related fetal loss in most centers is approximately 1 in 500 to 1 in 800.

Chorionic Villus Sampling

A newer technique that differs from amniocentesis in a few respects, chronic villus sampling (CVS), is performed at an earlier point in pregnancy than amniocentesis (10 to 11 weeks versus 16 to 18 weeks) and is usually conducted transcervically and not transabdominally. A small amount of placental material is removed and can be analyzed directly or placed in short-term culture. Chromosome results are usually available in less than 7 days. Fetal loss is on the order of 1 in 100.

Percutaneous Umbilical Blood Sampling

Direct sampling of fetal blood can be performed by means of percutaneous umbilical blood sampling (PUBS). This technique involves aspiration of umbilical cord blood near the placental insertion of the cord. A relatively pure sample of blood can be obtained at low risk to the fetus. The benefit of this technique is primarily to allow for rapid karyotyping of the fetus following identification of a sonographic abnormality.

Maternal Serum Alpha-Fetoprotein Screening

In 1972, Brock and Sutcliffe retrospectively demonstrated a correlation between high levels of alpha-fetoprotein (AFP) and infants who were born with neural tube defects. Alpha-fetoprotein is a prevalent albumin-like protein that is elaborated by the fetus as early as 6 to 7 weeks' gestation and that peaks in fetal serum at 13 to 14 weeks' gestation. AFP is detectable in amniotic fluid and in maternal serum as well through placental absorption. Alterations in AFP levels occur in many situations, but especially when there is leakage or transudation of fetal serum, for example, myelomeningocele, anencephaly, gastroschisis, omphalocele, and cystic hygroma.

A large United Kingdom collaborative study in the mid 1970s demonstrated the efficacy of maternal screening for neural tube defects with acceptable specificity and sensitivity. This study led to a number of similar projects in this country (Burton, 1986 and 1988; Main and Mennuti). Awareness of a trend toward low maternal serum AFP (MSAFP) levels in fetuses with Down syndrome and trisomy 18 has broadened the utilization of MSAFP testing to low-risk groups (DiMaio et al). Tables have been developed that allow for calculation of exact risks for having a child with Down syndrome based on a single AFP determination expressed as a multiple of the median (DiMaio et al).

Ultrasonography

Ultrasound diagnosis of urogenital abnormalities was comprehensively reviewed in Chapter 2. Two related areas deserve mention here.

The presence of an apparently isolated malformation on ultrasonography should routinely raise the question as to whether the malformation is truly isolated or is part of a broader malformation syndrome. Similarly, the frequency of chromosomal syndromes in this "isolated" group is significant. In the author's center, families are routinely offered amniocentesis or rapid fetal karyotyping in this situation. An abnormal karyotype has the potential for making profound changes in prenatal and postnatal management even if the abnormality is detected beyond 25 weeks' gestation. The frequency of chromosomal abnormalities in fetuses with ultrasonographically detected malformations ranges from 13 per cent to 35 per cent in selected reports (Donnenfeld and Mennuti; Eydoux et al; Hentemann et al; Nicolaides et al; Palmer et al; Platt et al; Williamson et al; Wladimiroff et al).

For genitourinary anomalies, four large series demonstrated an 11 to 30 per cent risk for chromosomal abnormalities, with trisomies 13, 18, and 21 the predominant syndromes (Eydoux et al; Hentemann et al; Nicolaides et al; Nyberg et al). The management strategy after detection of a sonographic abnormality, therefore, should include a comprehensive level II sonogram to look for additional malformations; consideration of a fetal echocardiogram, if not included in the original sonogram; a rapid karyotype, through amniocentesis, placental biopsy, or umbilical blood sampling; genetic counseling; and appropriate subspecialty visits as indicated.

Molecular Diagnosis

Revolutionary advances in the understanding of gene structure and function have provided a powerful tool useful in prenatal diagnosis (Boehm; Ostrer and Hejtmancik; Steel; Williamson and Murray). Until the molecular basis of most human genetic diseases is known, diagnosis generally rests upon linkage analysis using RFLPs. These are minor variations of the human genome upstream or downstream from the gene in question. "Linkage" refers to a situation in which genes on the same chromosome are located extremely close together. Information concerning one gene may, therefore, give information about the second gene. RFLP diagnosis also requires DNA from an affected individual before it can be determined that a family will be *informative*.

The process of DNA analysis using RFLPs is as follows: Genomic DNA is collected from an appropriate source (white blood cells, fibroblasts, amniotic fluid cells). The DNA is exposed to restriction endonucleases, enzymes that recognize only specific *sequences* of DNA and cleave DNA at these restriction sites. The DNA then undergoes gel electrophoresis and hybridization to a complementary DNA (cDNA). Finally, a radioactive label is added to the gel so that the cleaved fragments of interest can be identified. The final product using this method is called a *Southern blot*. Use of polymerase chain reaction (PCR) methods has added greatly to this field of DNA analysis by allowing for the use of small amounts of material for diagnosis. PCR methods make use of the complementary nature of DNA by generating additional copies of a gene from the "template." In a short period of time, multiple copies of the gene of interest can be amplified, allowing for more rapid diagnosis. This method has been used successfully to predict fetal sex by detecting Y-specific sequences in maternal blood (Adinolfi et al).

CONCLUSION

We have reached a point where technologic advances are occurring so rapidly that they frequently outstrip one's ability to incorporate advances into a reasonable plan of management. Prenatal sonographic recognition of urinary tract abnormalities in the second trimester is now routine, and a number of centers are experimenting with the possibilities of prenatal intervention for fetal urologic abnormalities (Berkowitz et al; Duckett; Harrison et al). This topic has been reviewed by a panel of pediatric urologists, and it appears that there are no *firm* indications for fetal urologic intervention. Still, in the early 1950s, the actual chromosomal number in humans was unknown, and in the mid 1960s amniocentesis was regarded as a research technique with little idea of its practical applications.

The desire to learn more about the fetus has heightened complex ethical issues that are also difficult to resolve. Fletcher defines four areas that are at the center of the problem: (1) possible conflicts of interest between fetus, parents, and physicians; (2) the inconsistency of fetal intervention on one hand and termination of pregnancy on the other; (3) the development of research guidelines for fetal therapy; and (4) the social and economic priorities that should be given to fetal therapy. These and other factors will demand that the urologist become a better geneticist.

Bibliography

Aarskog D: Maternal progestins as a possible cause of hypospadias. N Engl J Med 300:75, 1979.

Abbassi V, Lowe CU, Calcagno PL: Oculo-cerebral-renal syndrome—a review. Am J Dis Child 115:145, 1968.

Adeyokunnu AA, Familusi JB: Prune belly syndrome in two siblings and a first cousin—possible genetic implications. Am J Dis Child 136:23, 1982.

Adinolfi M, Camporese C, Carr T: Gene amplification to detect fetal nucleated cells in pregnant women. Lancet 2:328, 1989.

Aggarwal VK, Jones KV: Vesicoureteric reflux: screening of first degree relatives. Arch Dis Child 64:1538, 1989.

Akl KF, Khud GS, Der Kaloustian VM, et al: The Smith-Lemli-Opitz syndrome—report of a consanguineous Arab infant with bilateral focal renal dysplasia. Clin Pediatr 16:665, 1977.

Anton PA, Abramowsky CR: Adult polycystic renal disease presenting in infancy: a report emphasizing the bilateral involvement. J Urol 128:1290, 1982.

Barakat AY, Awazu M, Fleischer AC: Antenatal diagnosis of renal abnormalities: a review of the state of the art. South Med J 82:229, 1989.

Barakat AY, Butler MG: Renal and urinary tract abnormalities associated with chromosome aberrations. Int J Pediatr Nephrol 8:215, 1987.

Barakat AY, Seikaly MG, Der Kaloustian VM: Urogenital abnormalities in genetic disease. J Urol 136:778, 1986.

Barker DF, Hostikka SL, Zhou J, et al: Identification of mutations in the COL4A5 collagen gene in Alport syndrome. Science 248:1224, 1990.

Bartone FF, Schmidt MA: Cryptorchidism: incidence of chromosomal anomalies in 50 cases. J Urol 127:1105, 1982.

Bauer SB, Bull MJ, Retik AB: Hypospadias: a familial study. J Urol 121:474, 1979.

Bawle E, Tyrkus M, Lipman S, et al: Aarskog syndrome: full male and female expression associated with an X-autosome translocation. Am J Med Genet 17:595, 1984.

Bear JC, McManamon P, Morgan J, et al: Age at clinical onset and at ultrasonographic detection of adult polycystic kidney disease: data for genetic counselling. Am J Med Genet 18:45, 1984.

Bennett WM, Musgrave JE, Campbell RA, et al: The nephropathy of the nail-patella syndrome—a clinico-pathologic analysis of 11 kindred. Am J Med 54:304, 1973.

Berkowitz RL, Glickman MG, Smith GJ, et al: Fetal urinary tract obstruction: what is the role of surgical intervention in utero? Am J Obstet Gynecol 144:367, 1982.

Biedel CW, Pagon RA, Zapata JO: Müllerian anomalies and renal agenesis: autosomal dominant urogenital adysplasia. J Pediatr 104:861, 1984.

Boehm CD: Prenatal diagnosis and carrier detection by DNA analysis. Prog Med Genet 7:143, 1988.

Bovicelli L, Rizzo N, Orsini LF, et al: Prenatal diagnosis of the prune belly syndrome. Clin Genet 18:79, 1980.

Brock DJ, Sutcliffe RG: Alpha-fetoprotein in the antenatal diagnosis of anencephaly and spina bifida. Lancet 2:197, 1972.

Burger RH, Burger SE: Genetic determinants of urologic disease. Urol Clin North Am 1:419, 1974.

Burger RH, Smith C: Hereditary and familial vesicoureteral reflux. J Urol 106:845, 1971.

Burton BK: Alpha-fetoprotein screening. Adv Pediatr 33:181, 1986.

Burton BK: Elevated maternal serum alpha-fetoprotein (MSAFP): interpretation and follow-up. Clin Obstet Gynecol 31:293, 1988.

Butler MG: Prader-Willi syndrome: current understanding of cause and diagnosis. Am J Med Genet 35:319, 1990.

Butler MG, Meaney FJ, Palmer CG: Clinical and cytogenetic survey of 39 individuals with Prader-Labhart-Willi syndrome. Am J Med Genet 23:793, 1986.

Buyse ML (ed): Birth Defects Encyclopedia. Cambridge, Mass, Blackwell Scientific Publications, 1990.

Carter CO, Evans K, Pescia G: A family study of renal agenesis. J Med Genet 16:176, 1979.

Ceccherini I, Lituania M, Cordone MS, et al: Autosomal dominant polycystic kidney disease: prenatal diagnosis by DNA analysis and sonography at 14 weeks. Prenat Diagn 9:751, 1989.

Chavez GF, Mulinare J, Cordero JF: Maternal cocaine use during early pregnancy as a risk factor for congenital urogenital anomalies. JAMA 262:795, 1989.

Christopher CR, Spinelli A, Severt D: Ultrasonic diagnosis of prune belly syndrome. Obstet Gynecol 59:391, 1982.

Cohen MM: The Child with Multiple Birth Defects. New York, Raven Press, 1982.

Cole BR, Conley SB, Stapleton FB: Polycystic kidney disease in the first year of life. J Pediatr 111:693, 1987.

Cordero JF, Holmes LB: Phenotypic overlap of the BBB and G syndromes. Am J Med Genet 2:145, 1978.

Curry CJ, Jensen K, Holland J, et al: The Potter sequence: a clinical analysis of 80 cases. Am J Med Genet 19:679, 1984.

Czeizel A, Toth J: Correlation between the birth prevalence of isolated hypospadias and parental subfertility. Teratology 41:167, 1990.

Czeizel A, Toth J, Erodi E: Aetiological studies of hypospadias in Hungary. Hum Hered 29:166, 1979.

Daly WJ, Rabinovitch HH: Urologic abnormalities in Menkes' syndrome. J Urol 126:262, 1981.

Danks DM, Campbell PE, Stevens BJ, et al: Menkes' kinky hair syndrome. An inherited defect in copper absorption with widespread effects. Pediatrics 50:188, 1972.

Danks DM, Tippett P, Adams C, et al: Cerebro-hepatorenal syndrome of Zellweger—a report of eight cases with comments upon the incidence, the liver lesion, and a fault in pipecolic acid metabolism. J Pediatr 86:382, 1975.

Davidsohn I, Newberger C: Congenital valves of the posterior urethra in twins. Arch Pathol 16:57, 1933.

Day N, Holmes LB: The incidence of genetic disease in a university hospital population. Am J Hum Genet 25:237, 1973.

DeBeukelaer MM, Randall CL, Stroud DR: Renal anomalies in the fetal alcohol syndrome. J Pediatr 91:759, 1977.

Dewald GW: Gregor Johann Mendel and the beginning of genetics. Mayo Clin Proc 52:513, 1977.

Dewald GW, Kelalis PP, Gordon H: Chromosomal studies in cryptorchidism. J Urol 117:110, 1977.

DiMaio MS, Baumgarten A, Greenstein RM, et al: Screening for fetal Down's syndrome in pregnancy by measuring maternal serum alpha-fetoprotein levels. N Engl J Med 317:342, 1987.

Donnenfeld AE, Mennuti MT: Sonographic findings in fetuses with common chromosome abnormalities. Clin Obstet Gynecol 31:80, 1988.

Duckett JW (ed): Fetal intervention for obstructive uropathy. Dialog Pediatr Urol 5:1, 1982.

Duncan PA, Shapiro LR, Stangel JJ, et al: The MURCS association: müllerian duct aplasia, renal aplasia and cervicothoracic somite dysplasia. J Pediatr 95:399, 1979.

Dwoskin JY: Sibling uropathology. J Urol 115:726, 1976.

Editorial: Genetics of hypospadias. Br Med J 2:189, 1972.

Escobar V, Gleiser S, Weaver DD: Phenotype and genetic analysis of the Silver-Russell syndrome. Clin Genet 13:278, 1978.

Escobar V, Weaver DD: Aarskog syndrome—new findings and genetic analysis. JAMA 240:2638, 1978.

Eydoux P, Choiset A, Le Porrier N, et al: Chromosomal prenatal diagnosis: study of 936 cases of intrauterine abnormalities after ultrasound assessment. Prenat Diagn 9:255, 1989.

Falconer DS: The inheritance of liability to certain diseases, estimated from the incidence among relatives. Ann Hum Genet 25:51, 1965.

Fletcher JC: The fetus as patient: ethical issues. JAMA 246:772, 1981.

Fraser FC, Ling D, Clogg D, et al: Genetic aspects of the BOR syndrome—branchial fistulas, ear pits, hearing loss, and renal anomalies. Am J Med Genet 2:241, 1978.

Fraser FC, Lytwyn A: Spectrum of anomalies in the Meckel syndrome or: "Maybe there is a malformation syndrome with at least one constant anomaly." Am J Med Genet 9:67, 1981.

Fraser GR: Our genetical "load." A review of some aspects of genetical variation. Ann Hum Genet 25:387, 1962.

Fryns JP, Macken J, Vinken L, et al: The Aarskog syndrome. Hum Genet 42:129, 1978.

Funderburk SJ, Stewart R: The G and BBB syndromes: case presentations, genetics and nosology. Am J Med Genet 2:131, 1978.

Gabow PA, Ikle DW, Holmes JH: Polycystic kidney disease: prospective analysis of nonazotemic patients and family members. Ann Intern Med 101:238, 1984.

Gal A, Wirth B, Kaariainen H, et al: Childhood manifestation of autosomal dominant polycystic kidney disease: no evidence for genetic heterogeneity. Clin Genet 35:13, 1989.

Garlinger P, Ott J: Prune belly syndrome—possible genetic implications. Birth Defects 10:173, 1974.

Gill WB, Schumacher GF, Bibbo M, et al: Association of diethylstilbestrol exposure in utero with cryptorchidism, testicular hypoplasia and semen abnormalities. J Urol 122:36, 1979.

Gonzalez CH, Herrmann J, Opitz JM: Studies of malformation syndromes of man VB: The hypertelorism-hypospadias (BBB) syndrome. Eur J Pediatr 125:1, 1977.

Gorlin RJ, Cohen MM, Levin LS: Syndromes of the Head and Neck, 3rd ed. New York, Oxford University Press, 1990.

Gorlin RJ, Jue KL, Jacobsen U, et al: Oculoauriculovertebral dysplasia. J Pediatr 63:991, 1963.

Greenberg CR, Trevenen CL, Evans JA: The BOR syndrome and renal agenesis—prenatal diagnosis and further clinical delineation. Prenat Diagn 8:103, 1988.

Gubler M, Levy M, Broyer M, et al: Alport's syndrome—a report of 58 cases and a review of the literature. Am J Med 70:493, 1981.

Hadlock FP, Deter RL, Carpenter R, et al: Sonography of fetal urinary tract anomalies. Am J Roentgenol 137:261, 1981.

Hall BD, Smith DW: Prader-Willi syndrome—a resume of 32 cases including an instance of affected first cousins, one of whom is of normal stature and intelligence. J Pediatr 81:286, 1972.

Hall JG, Powers EK, McIlvaine RT, et al: The frequency and financial burden of genetic disease in a pediatric hospital. Am J Med Genet 1:417, 1978.

Harrison MR, Golbus MS, Filly RA, et al: Fetal surgery for congenital hydronephrosis. N Engl J Med 306:591, 1982.

Hasen HB, Song YS: Congenital valvular obstruction of the posterior urethra in two brothers. J Pediatr 47:207, 1955.

Havers W, Majewski F, Olbing H, et al: Anomalies of the kidneys and genitourinary tract in alcohol embryopathy. J Urol 124:108, 1980.

Hentemann M, Rauskolb R, Ulbrich R, et al: Abnormal pregnancy sonogram and chromosomal anomalies: four years experience with rapid karyotyping. Prenat Diagn 9:605, 1989.

Hodes ME, Butler MG, Keitges EA, et al: Prune belly syndrome in an anencephalic male. Am J Med Genet 14:37, 1983.

Hoekstra WJ, Scholtmeijer RJ, Molenaar JC, et al: Urogenital tract abnormalities associated with congenital anorectal anomalies. J Urol 130:962, 1983.

Holmes LB: Minor anomalies in newborn infants (abstr). Am J Hum Genet 34:94A, 1982.

Holmes LB: Prevalence, phenotypic heterogeneity and familial aspects of bilateral renal agenesis/dysgenesis. Prog Clin Biol Res 305:1, 1989.

Holmes LB: The Malformed Newborn: Practical Perspectives. Boston, Genetics Unit, Children's Service, Massachusetts General Hospital, 1976.

Hook EJ, Lindsje A: Down syndrome in live births by single year maternal age interval in a Swedish study: comparison with results from a New York State study. Am J Hum Genet 30:19, 1978.

Hostikka SL, Eddy RL, Byers MG: Identification of a distinct type IV collagen chain with restricted kidney distribution and assignment of its gene to the locus of X chromosome-linked Alport syndrome. Proc Natl Acad Sci USA 87:1606, 1990.

Hsia YE, Bratu M, Herbordt A: Genetics of the Meckel syndrome (dysencephalia splanchnocystica). Pediatrics 48:237, 1971.

Ives EJ: The abdominal muscle deficiency triad syndrome—experience with 10 cases. Birth Defects 10:127, 1974.

Jerkins GR, Noe HN: Familial vesicoureteral reflux: a prospective study. J Urol 128:774, 1982.

Jones IR, Young ID: Familial incidence of cryptorchidism. J Urol 127:508, 1982.

Jones KL: Smith's Recognizable Patterns of Human Malformation, 4th ed. Philadelphia, WB Saunders Co, 1988.

Kaffe S, Rose JS, Godmilow L, et al: Prenatal diagnosis of renal anomalies. Am J Med Genet 1:241, 1977.

Kallen B, Winberg J: An epidemiological study of hypospadias in Sweden. Acta Paediatr Scand [Suppl] 293:1, 1982.

Kaplan BS, Kaplan P, Rosenberg HK, et al: Polycystic kidney diseases in childhood. J Pediatr 115:867, 1989.

Kenya PR, Asal NR, Pederson JA, et al: Hereditary (familial) renal disease: clinical and genetic studies. South Med J 70:1049, 1977.

Kerr DN, Pillai PM: Identical twins with identical vesicoureteric reflux: chronic pyelonephritis in one. Br Med J 286:1245, 1983.

Kimberling WJ, Fain PR, Kenyon JB, et al: Linkage heterogeneity of autosomal dominant polycystic kidney disease. N Engl J Med 319:913, 1988.

King CR, Prescott G: Pathogenesis of the prune belly anomalad. J Pediatr 93:273, 1978.

Klass P: Hereditary factors in urogenital disease. Pediatr Ann 4:87, 1975.

Kousseff BG: The cytogenetic controversy in the Prader-Labhart-Willi syndrome. Am J Med Genet 13:431, 1982.

Kroovand RL, Al-Ansari RM, Perlmutter AD: Urethral and genital malformations in prune belly syndrome. J Urol 127:94, 1982.

Kroovand RL, Weinberg N, Emami A: Posterior urethral valves in identical twins. Pediatrics 60:748, 1977.

Ledbetter DH, Mascarello JT, Riccardi VM, et al: Chromosome 15 abnormalities and the Prader-Willi syndrome: a follow-up report of 40 cases. Am J Hum Genet 34:278, 1982.

Ledbetter DH, Riccardi VM, Airhart SD, et al: Deletions of chromosome 15 as a cause of the Prader-Willi syndrome. N Engl J Med 304:325, 1981.

Lee PA, Migeon CJ, Brown TR, et al: Robinow's syndrome—partial primary hypogonadism in pubertal boys, with persistence of micropenis. Am J Dis Child 136:327, 1982.

Leonard CO, Chase GA, Childs B: Genetic counseling: a consumer's view. N Engl J Med 287:433, 1972.

Lewy PR, Belman AB: Familial occurrence of nonobstructive, noninfectious vesicoureteral reflux with renal scarring. J Pediatr 86:851, 1975.

Lieberman E, Salinas-Madrigal L, Gwinn JL, et al: Infantile polycystic disease of the kidneys and liver: clinical, pathological and radiological correlations and comparison with congenital hepatic fibrosis. Medicine 50:277, 1971.

Linne T, Wikstad I, Zetterstrom R: Renal involvement in the Laurence-Moon-Biedl syndrome: functional and radiological studies. Acta Paediatr Scand 75:240, 1986.

Livne DM, Delaune J, Gonzales EJ: Genetic etiology of posterior urethral valves. J Urol 130:178, 1983.

Lubinsky M, Rapoport P: Transient fetal hydrops and "prune belly" in one identical female twin. N Engl J Med 308:256, 1983.

Main DM, Mennuti MT: Neural tube defects: issues in prenatal diagnosis and counselling. Obstet Gynecol 67:1, 1986.

Marks LJ, Bergeson PS: The Silver-Russell syndrome—a

case with sexual ambiguity, and a review of the literature. Am J Dis Child 131:447, 1977.

Mau G: Progestins during pregnancy and hypospadias. Teratology 24:285, 1981.

Mauer SM, Dobrin RS, Vermier RL: Unilateral and bilateral renal agenesis in monoamniotic twins. J Pediatr 84:236, 1974.

McKusick VA: Mendelian Inheritance in Man: Catalogs of Autosomal Dominant, Autosomal Recessive and X-Linked Phenotypes, 9th ed. Baltimore, Johns Hopkins University Press, 1990.

McPherson E, Carey J, Kramer A, et al: Dominantly inherited renal adysplasia. Am J Med Genet 26:863, 1987.

Melnick M, Bixler D, Nance WE, et al: Familial branchio-oto-renal dysplasia: a new addition to the branchial arch syndromes. Clin Genet 9:25, 1976.

Middleton GW, Howards SS, Gillenwater JY: Sex-linked familial reflux. J Urol 114:36, 1975.

Miller HC, Caspari EW: Ureteral reflux as genetic trait. JAMA 220:842, 1972.

Mills JL, Knopp RH, Simpson JL, et al: Lack of relation of increased malformation rates in infants of diabetic mothers to glycemic control during organogenesis. N Engl J Med 318:671, 1988.

Milutinovic J, Fialkow PJ, Rudd TG, et al: Liver cysts in patients with autosomal dominant polycystic kidney disease. Am J Med 68:741, 1980.

Mininberg DT (ed): Genetics in urology. Dialog Pediatr Urol 2:1, 1979.

Mininberg DT, Bingol N: Chromosomal abnormalities in undescended testes. Urology 1:98, 1973.

Mobley DF: Familial vesicoureteral reflux. Urology 2:514, 1973.

Moerman P, Fryns JP, Goddeeris P, et al: Pathogenesis of the prune belly syndrome: a functional urethral obstruction caused by prostatic hypoplasia. Pediatrics 73:470, 1984.

Monie IW, Monie BJ: Prune belly syndrome and fetal ascites. Teratology 19:111, 1979.

Moser AE, Singh I, Brown FR, et al: The cerebrohepatorenal (Zellweger) syndrome—increased levels and impaired degradation of very-long-chain fatty acids and their use in prenatal diagnosis. N Engl J Med 310:1141, 1984.

Mulcahy JJ, Kelalis PP, Stickler GB, et al: Familial vesicoureteral reflux. J Urol 104:762, 1970.

Nakayama DK, Harrison MR, Chinn DH, et al: The pathogenesis of prune belly. Am J Dis Child 138:834, 1984.

Nicolaides KH, Rodeck CH, Gosden CM: Rapid karyotyping in nonlethal fetal malformations. Lancet 1:283, 1986.

Noe HN, Peeden JN, Jerkins GR, et al: Hypertelorism-hypospadias syndrome. J Urol 132:951, 1984.

Nora JJ, Nora AH: The evolution of specific genetic and environmental counseling in congenital heart diseases. Circulation 57:205, 1978.

Nora JJ, Nora AH, Sinha AK, et al: The Ullrich-Noonan syndrome (Turner phenotype). Am J Dis Child 127:48, 1974.

Novelli G, Frontali M, Baldini D, et al: Prenatal diagnosis of adult polycystic kidney disease with DNA markers on chromosome 16 and the genetic heterogeneity problem. Prenat Diagn 9:759, 1989.

Nyberg D, Fitzsimmons J, Mack L, et al: Chromosomal abnormalities in fetuses with omphalocele: significance of omphalocele contents. J Ultrasound Med 8:299, 1989.

O'Neill WM, Atkin CL, Bloomer HA: Hereditary nephritis: a re-examination of its clinical and genetic features. Ann Intern Med 88:176, 1978.

Opitz JM: G syndrome (hypertelorism with esophageal abnormality and hypospadias, or hypospadias-dysphagia, or "Opitz-Frias" or "Opitz-G" syndrome)—perspective in 1987 and bibliography. Am J Med Genet 28:275, 1987.

Ostrer H, Hejtmancik JF: Prenatal diagnosis and carrier detection of genetic diseases by analysis of deoxyribonucleic acid. J Pediatr 112:679, 1988.

Page LA: Inheritance of uncomplicated hypospadias. Pediatrics 63:788, 1979.

Pagon RA, Graham JM, Zonana J, et al: Coloboma, congenital heart disease, and choanal atresia with multiple anomalies: CHARGE association. J Pediatr 99:223, 1981.

Pagon RA, Smith DW, Shepard TH: Urethral obstruction malformation complex: a cause of abdominal muscle deficiency and the "prune belly." J Pediatr 96:900, 1979.

Palmer CG, Miles JH, Howard-Peebles PN, et al: Fetal karyotype following ascertainment of fetal anomalies by ultrasound. Prenat Diag 7:551, 1987.

Patterson K, Toomey KE, Chandra RF: Hirschsprung disease in an 46,XY phenotypic female with Smith-Lemli-Opitz syndrome. J Pediatr 103:425, 1983.

Penman DG, Lilford RJ: The megacystis-microcolon-intestinal hypoperistalsis syndrome: a fatal autosomal recessive condition. J Med Genet 26:66, 1989.

Pescia G, Cruz JM, Weihs D: Prenatal diagnosis of prune belly syndrome by means of raised maternal AFP levels. J Genet Hum 30:271, 1982.

Pescia G, Evans KA, Carter CO: The risk of recurrence for renal agenesis (abstr). Fifth International Congress on Human Genetics, Mexico City, 1976.

Piering WF, Hebert LA, Lemann J: Infantile polycystic kidney disease in the adult. Arch Intern Med 137:1625, 1977.

Platt LD, DeVore GR, Lopez E, et al: Role of amniocentesis in ultrasound-detected fetal malformations. Obstet Gynecol 68:153, 1986.

Pramanik AK, Altshuler G, Light IJ, et al: Prune-belly syndrome associated with Potter (renal nonfunction) syndrome. Am J Dis Child 131:672, 1977.

Qazi Q, Masakawa A, Milman D, et al: Renal anomalies in fetal alcohol syndrome. Pediatrics 63:886, 1979.

Quan L, Smith DW: The VATER association—vertebral defects, anal atresia, TE fistula with esophageal atresia, radial and renal dysplasia: a spectrum of associated defects. J Pediatr 82:104, 1973.

Rabinowitz R, Schillinger JF: Prune belly syndrome in the female subject. J Urol 118:454, 1977.

Raffle RB: Familial hydronephrosis. Br Med J 1:580, 1955.

Reeders ST, Breuning MH, Davies KE, et al: A highly polymorphic DNA marker linked to adult polycystic kidney disease on chromosome 16. Nature 317:542, 1985.

Riccardi VM, Grum CM: The prune belly anomaly: heterogeneity and superficial X-linkage mimicry. J Med Genet 14:266, 1977.

Riccardi VM, Hittner HM, Francke U, et al: The aniridia-Wilms' tumor association: the critical role of chromosome band 11p13. Cancer Genet Cytogenet 2:131, 1980.

Riccardi VM, Sujansky E, Smith AC, et al: Chromosomal imbalance in the aniridia-Wilms' tumor association: 11p interstitial deletion. Pediatrics 61:604, 1978.

Roodhooft AM, Birnholz JC, Holmes LB: Familial nature of congenital absence and severe dysgenesis of both kidneys. N Engl J Med 310:1341, 1984.

Rosenbaum KN: The genetics of congenital heart disease. Clinical Proceedings of the Children's Hospital National Medical Center 34:255, 1978.

Rosenfield AT, Lipson MH, Wolf B, et al: Ultrasonography and nephrotomography in the presymptomatic diagnosis of dominantly inherited (adult-onset) polycystic kidney disease. Radiology 135:423, 1980.

Sahney S, Weiss L, Levin NW: Genetic counseling in adult polycystic kidney disease. Am J Med Genet 11:461, 1982.

Schachat AP, Maumenee IH: The Bardet-Biedl syndrome and related disorders. Arch Ophthalmol 100:285, 1982.

Schardein JL: Congenital abnormalities and hormones during pregnancy: a clinical review. Teratology 22:251, 1980.

Schimke RN, King CR: Hereditary urogenital adysplasia. Clin Genet 18:417, 1980.

Schinzel A, Homberger C, Sigrist T: Case report: bilateral renal agenesis in male sibs born to consanguineous parents. J Med Genet 15:314, 1978.

Scriver CR, Neal JL, Saginur R, et al: The frequency of genetic disease and congenital malformation among patients in a pediatric hospital. Can Med Assoc J 108:1111, 1973.

Seller MJ: Phenotypic variation in Meckel syndrome. Clin Genet 20:74, 1981.

Sengar DP, Rashid A, Wolfish NM: Familial urinary tract anomalies: association with the major histocompatibility complex in man. J Urol 121:194, 1979.

Shah KJ: Renal lesion in Jeune's syndrome. Br J Radiol 53:432, 1980.

Shapiro E, Lepor H, Jeffs RD: The inheritance of the exstrophy-epispadias complex. J Urol 132:308, 1984.

Shenker L, Anderson G: Intrauterine diagnosis and management of fetal polycystic kidney disease. Obstet Gynecol 59:385, 1982.

Shokier MH: Expression of "adult" polycystic renal disease in the fetus and newborn. Clin Genet 14:61, 1978.

Silverman ME, Goodman RM, Cuppage FE: The nail-patella syndrome—clinical findings and ultrastructural observations in the kidney. Arch Intern Med 120:68, 1967.

Simpson JL, German J: Familial urinary tract anomalies. JAMA 212:2264, 1970.

Smith DW: Dysmorphology (teratology). J Pediatr 69:1150, 1966.

Spranger J, Benirschke K, Hall JG, et al: Errors of morphogenesis: concepts and terms. J Pediatr 100:160, 1982.

Steel CM: DNA in medicine: The tools: Part I. Lancet 2:908, 1984.

Stillman RJ: In utero exposure to diethylstilbestrol: adverse effects on the reproductive tract and reproductive performance in male and female offspring. Am J Obstet Gynecol 142:905, 1982.

Strand WR, Rushton HG, Markle BM, et al: Autosomal dominant polycystic kidney disease in infants: asymmetric disease mimicking a unilateral renal mass. J Urol 141:1151, 1989.

Svensson J: Male hypospadias, 625 cases, associated malformations and possible etiologic factors. Acta Paediatr Scand 68:587, 1979.

Targum SD: Psychotherapeutic considerations in genetic counseling. Am J Med Genet 8:281, 1981.

Temtamy SA, Miller JD: Extending the scope of the

VATER association: definition of the VATER syndrome. J Pediatr 85:345, 1974.

Tishler PV: Healthy female carriers of a gene for the Alport syndrome: importance for genetic counseling. Clin Genet 16:291, 1979.

Turleau C, de Grouchy J, Dufier JL, et al: Aniridia, male pseudo-hermaphroditism, gonadoblastoma, mental retardation, and del 11p13. Hum Genet 57:300, 1981.

Uehling D: Cryptorchidism in the Prader-Willi syndrome. J Urol 124:103, 1980.

Uehling DT, Gilbert E, Chesney R: Urologic implications of the VATER association. J Urol 129:352, 1983.

UK collaborative study on alpha-fetoprotein in relation to neural-tube defects: Maternal-serum alpha-fetoprotein measurement in antenatal screening for anencephaly and spina bifida in early pregnancy. Lancet 1:1323, 1977.

Vogel F, Motulsky AG: Human Genetics: Problems and Approaches, 2nd ed. Berlin, Springer-Verlag, 1986.

Waaler PE: Clinical and cytogenetic studies in undescended testes. Acta Paediatr Scand 65:553, 1976.

Warkany J: Congenital Malformations: Notes and Comments. Chicago, Year Book Medical Publishers, 1971.

Williamson RA, Murray JC: Molecular analysis of genetic disorders. Clin Obstet Gynecol 31:270, 1988.

Williamson RA, Weiner CP, Patil S, et al: Abnormal pregnancy sonogram: selective indication for fetal karyotype. Obstet Gynecol 59:15, 1987.

Wladimiroff JW, Sachs ES, Reuss A, et al: Prenatal diagnosis of chromosome abnormalities in the presence of fetal structural defects. Am J Med Genet 29:289, 1988.

Woodhouse CR, Ransley PG, Innes-Williams D: Prune belly syndrome—report of 47 cases. Arch Dis Child 57:856, 1982.

Zel G, Retik AB: Familial vesicoureteral reflux. Urology 2:249, 1973.

9

☐ Fluid and Electrolyte Management

Howard C. Filston

One would think that the management of fluid and electrolytes in the human body would have been settled by the ancient Greek physicians; perhaps they had settled it for their time. However, the modern era of fluid and electrolyte management dates only to the 1960s, at which time better understanding of shock as a consequence of hypovolemia, of sequestration of fluids in spaces outside the vascular space, of the concept of perfusion, and of the role of aldosterone and antidiuretic hormone led to improved management of volume restoration.

In 1946, Wiggers created a laboratory shock model in dogs by shedding blood, dropping their systolic pressures to a third of normal, and maintaining this level of shock for 2 hours and 15 minutes. Despite complete restoration of the shed blood, the majority of the dogs (more than 80 per cent) died. From this came the idea of the irreversibility of shock. However, only in more recent times has understanding of the sequence of vasoconstriction, reduced flow, ischemic damage to the capillaries, and fluid shifts into the extravascular "third space" led to an appreciation of the need to restore sometimes massive volumes of fluid for internal shifts either accompanying blood loss or as an independent pathophysiologic event.

In the mid 1960s, Shires tied a great many evolving concepts together when he repeated Wiggers' shock model experiment, but in addition to restoring the shed blood, he restored variable volumes of balanced salt solution and found that he could, in fact, resuscitate the dogs from what had been thought to be an irreversible state of shock. The years since his findings have seen some fine-tuning of the concept of third space and the fluid requirements generated by these fluid shifts, but no major additional breakthroughs have occurred.

In the management of fluid and electrolytes in neonates and infants, the pendulum has swung back from the attitudes of Rickham and of Wilkerson, who, from the 1940s to the late 1960s, advocated considerable reduction in the volume of fluid administered to the neonate and young infant, especially to the neonate, whom they saw as a volume-overloaded individual. Wilkerson actually advocated early oral liquid feedings and early discontinuation (often on the operating table) of the intravenous line.

This chapter describes the pathophysiologic basis of hypovolemia and attempts to develop a logical and practical method of management of fluids and electrolytes in the surgical patient based on a thorough understanding of the circulatory responses to shock.

PATHOPHYSIOLOGY OF HYPOVOLEMIA

Were the circulatory system of the human animal made up of a series of rigid plastic tubes with no adaptive responses, blood pressure would be an excellent measure of the state of the vascular volume. Reductions of intravascular blood volume or fluid volume would result in a direct fall in pressure. However, the human vascular system is made up of a series of living, responsive vessels, and in response to a falling intravascular volume, vasoconstriction of the arterioles takes place, shutting down flow to large amounts of tissue to protect the perfusion of more vital organs. This maintains full volume in the vessels still being perfused and, therefore, maintains normal blood pressure until a very late and severe stage of hypovolemia makes such compensation no longer possible. Thus, blood pressure is a poor and delayed guide to hypovolemia.

By the time blood pressure falls from hypovolemia, one can be assured that ischemic damage has occurred to the endothelium of the capillaries in those tissues that have been hypoperfused as a result of the body's attempts to divert blood flow to more vital tissues. It is vitally important that this compensating mechanism be well understood and that the consequences to these tissues during this period of hypoperfusion be well recognized.

With the shutdown of flow to tissues to preserve flow to other more vital structures, the tissues involved in the reduced flow are forced to undergo an anaerobic type of metabolism, with build-up of two-carbon ketone fragments and disabling enzyme systems due to oxygen deprivation. As a result of this ischemic damage, the capillary endothelium, which is exquisitely sensitive to deprivation of oxygen and nutrients, becomes damaged and no longer acts as the semipermeable membrane essential to the life of all those animals that have a circulatory system. The result of this ischemic damage is a shift of fluid through the damaged capillary into the extravascular tissue, creating a "third-space" sequestration of fluid.

If the vascular space is understood as being the "first space," and the interstitial extracellular fluid and intracellular fluid are understood as the "second space," the second space is a space that will deliver fluid back to the intravascular volume should the intravascular volume become depleted. However, once the endothelial lining of the capillary is damaged, albumin and sometimes other protein molecules "leak" through the damaged membrane into the extravascular interstitial space and create a *reverse osmotic gradient* that prevents the return of fluid to the vascular space despite a depletion in volume and of hydrostatic pressure that would otherwise favor return of fluid from the extravascular tissues. The "third space" is a type of second space that is either opposite a damaged capillary so that fluid cannot return despite the need for fluid in the intravascular compartment, or a space in which some derangement such as a breaking-down hematoma creates a large "reverse" osmotic force, pulling fluid out of the vascular space and preventing restoration of the vascular space from this sequestered pool of fluid.

It is important to recognize that this whole matter is a dynamic one, and at any given time fluid may be re-entering the capillary from some areas and leaving the capillary from others. Any sequestration of fluid based on abnormal hydrostatic pressures or osmotic forces can create a third space. Other examples of third-spacing of fluid include the intestinal lumen under conditions of obstruction, ileus, or inflammation; the peritoneal cavity under conditions of massive peritonitis, pancreatitis, or increased portal pressure resulting in portal hypertension and loss of fluid from the mesenteric-portal capillaries with creation of ascites; and any area of edema formation.

Before the understanding of these concepts was well ingrained in clinical thinking, the role of aldosterone and antidiuretic hormone (ADH) was somewhat confusing. In the 1950s, the control of volume in the body was thought to be totally based on control of electrolyte balance, with water going everywhere passively to maintain electrolyte and osmolar normal tension. Thus, in the 1950s when Dr. Francis Moore and his colleagues at the Peter Bent Brigham Hospital in Boston looked at the postoperative, postanesthetic, or post-trauma patient and found high levels of circulating aldosterone as well as significant levels of ADH, they concluded that the body, under these stressful conditions, tended to hold onto salt and water. At that time, ADH was believed to be a minor modulator of electrolyte and osmolar balance that was normally secreted only under conditions of increased electrolyte concentration, whereupon it acted to hold onto water to restore electrolyte concentration to normal. Therefore, the finding of ADH in the postoperative, postanesthetic, post-trauma patient who exhibited a normal or slightly hypotonic electrolyte state was considered "inappropriate." These investigators recommended marked fluid restriction and almost total salt restriction in the postoperative patient.

With the evolution of work in the 1960s that delineated ADH as part of the major volume protective mechanism responding to monitors in the great venous system that signaled reductions in circulatory volume, it was demonstrated by several investigators that rapid volume restoration under the conditions of the postoperative, postanesthetic, post-trauma state, would in fact, "shut off" ADH and result in urine output (Shires et al; Wright and Gann). It is essential, therefore, to recognize that ADH is likely to be present in the postoperative patient who has sustained any volume depletion, and that until adequate volume restoration has been accomplished to "shut off'' ADH, an adequate urine output cannot be achieved.

CHOICE OF FLUIDS FOR VOLUME RESTORATION

Once the need for volume restoration in the intraoperative and postoperative periods has been recognized, the choice of fluid becomes extremely important. If one thinks about the vascular system as a "tank" containing electrolytes, proteins, and water, and registering a certain intravascular hydrostatic pressure, and then thinks about the surrounding milieu as being an equivalent one with a hydrostatic pressure and oncotic pressures due to crystalloids and colloids, the depletion of the "tank" initially produces a fall in hydrostatic pressure but no change in either protein or crystalloid oncotic pressure. This fall in hydrostatic pressure would ordinarily, under normal circumstances, lead to some shift of fluid from the extravascular back into the vascular compartment. Before this occurs, however, the depleted vascular compartment contains fluids and electrolytes and proteins in the same concentration as before the loss. This is the simple concept that drinking half the bottle of "Coke" leaves half a bottle of "Coke."

If one then attempts to restore vascular volume exogenously, one must look at the effect of various solutions upon the efficiency of this restoration. If one attempts to refill the depleted volume with water, one will begin to restore hydrostatic pressure to the intravascular space but will dilute out the concentrations of the electrolytes and the proteins, resulting in an excess of water relative to electrolyte in the vascular space. This will result in an attempt of electrolytes and proteins to shift inward from the extravascular space. However, proteins cannot shift because they will not pass through the semipermeable membrane, and although a small amount of electrolyte will shift into the vascular space, there is such an excess of water molecules that the net effect of this will be a loss of a significant amount of the water to the extravascular space, resulting in inefficient restoration of vascular volume.

If one were to refill the depleted volume with blood, this would be highly efficient except that if the loss were a noncellular one, one would gradually increase the concentration of cells to the point that flow in the microcirculation would be impeded by rouleaux formation.

Other fluids for restoration, therefore, fall on a scale between the very inefficient water and the highly efficient blood. Table 9–1 lists these fluids along with their relative contraindications. Essentially, blood has all of the relative contraindications, but is clearly indicated for the patient who needs oxygen-carrying capacity in the form of additional red blood cells. Plasma retains many of the contraindications, and is indicated for the patient who has a deficiency of clotting factors.

Albumin in balanced salt solution (lactated Ringer's solution) provides a highly efficient form of restoration of the vascular deficit and retains only those relative contraindications of availability and cost. The exception to this statement is that the individual whose capillary endothelium may be damaged, particularly when the pulmonary capillary endothelium is involved in the damage, may do poorly with initial volume restoration with albumin-containing fluids. The most common situation in which this exists is the patient in endotoxic shock with massive ischemic damage to the capillaries throughout the entire body. It does not apply to the average postoperative patient, even one who has had some mild hypovolemia during the operative experience.

Experimental and clinical studies related to the use of albumin are still somewhat equivocal. Experiments in which standard doses of endotoxin are given to primates followed by randomized restoration of volume losses with solutions of balanced salt solution compared with solutions of albumin in balanced salt solution suggest that the lungs are heavier in the animals restored with albumin-containing solutions (Holcroft and Trunkey; Moss et al). It has been suggested that there is an excellent clearing mechanism for interstitial fluid in the lung, and that this clearing mechanism becomes occluded when albumin shifts from the

Table 9–1 ☐ Fluids for Volume Restoration: Relative Contraindications

Fluid	Relative Contraindications*
Blood	V, T, H, I, A, $
Plasma	T, H, I, A, $
Albumin/lactated Ringer's	A, $
Lactated Ringer's/normal saline	
Hypotonic electrolyte solutions	
Water	

Abbreviations: *V, hyperviscosity; T, transfusion reactions; H, hepatitis; I, infection; A, availability; $, cost.

vascular to the interstitial space through the damaged pulmonary capillary, retarding clearing of the interstitial fluid (edema). On the other hand, similar experiments have shown that it takes three to eight times as much balanced salt solution to restore the volume deficit as it does albumin in balanced salt solution (Cervera and Moss), so that this inefficiency of the non–protein-containing solution should be kept in mind when restoring volume in those patients for whom the risk of albumin shifting into the pulmonary interstitial space is insignificant.

Although this concern for sequestration of fluid in the interstitial space of the pulmonary parenchyma occasionally limits the use of albumin-containing solutions in patients for whom this may be a concern, there is no contraindication to the use of the balanced salt solution. Therefore, a solution approximating the crystalloid concentration of plasma should be the solution of choice for restoration of volume in most instances. Remembering that the elimination of albumin from the solution creates an inefficiency resulting in the shift of two to seven volumes of fluid into the extravascular space for every volume that remains to provide restoration, one must rigorously avoid the introduction of a greater "coefficient of inefficiency" by using dilute electrolyte solutions and dextrose in water. Therefore, when planning volume restoration for a patient, one must ask the question whether the "tank" is depleted. *If the answer is yes, no solution less concentrated than a full balanced salt solution should be chosen for restoration, and other solutions that may be indicated for the patient such as those that provide maintenance water and electrolytes should be held back until full restoration of volume is accomplished, as indicated by the achievement of an acceptable urine output.*

A PRACTICAL GUIDELINE TO PARENTERAL FLUID AND ELECTROLYTE MANAGEMENT IN THE POSTOPERATIVE PEDIATRIC PATIENT

Losses of fluid—insensibly, measurably, or transcompartmentally—create the need for fluid and electrolyte administration and restoration in the intraoperative and postoperative patient. Every patient requires maintenance fluid and electrolytes to replace the normal physiologic losses of daily living.

Maintenance Fluid and Electrolytes

Insensible losses create the need for maintenance water administration. These occur from the loss of the water of hydration of the inhaled gasses, from simple evaporation from the body surface, and from the need for a "solvent" in which to dissolve the day's "solutes," the breakdown products of metabolism, and thus provide an adequate urine volume for excretion of these waste products. All of these insensible losses are in the form of free water, and water is the "solvent" necessary to dissolve the metabolic "solutes." However, a small amount of electrolyte is also lost insensibly in the stool and the urine and from the body surface, and so these electrolytes can be administered by dissolving them in the maintenance water.

An adult needs approximately 1 liter of water per square meter of body surface area per day, thus amounting to 1730 ml of water for the "average" adult with a body surface area of 1.73 meters square. This is approximately 25 ml/kg. The adult also requires 45 to 60 mEq of sodium and chloride and approximately 40 mEq of potassium for daily maintenance. This is equivalent to approximately 0.65 to 0.85 mEq of sodium and chloride per kilogram per day.

On the other hand, the child's requirements for maintenance water and electrolytes vary with body surface area and weight. Formulas have been developed which are essentially reduction formulas that describe the fact that the newborn infant with a massive surface area compared with weight has a much greater requirement for fluids and electrolytes than does the older child or adult. The most common formula in use is that which defines the child's needs as:

- 100 ml of water per kilogram for the first 10 kg.
- 50 ml for the next 10 kg (11 to 20 kg).
- 20 ml/kg above 20 kg.

A one-step simplified formula (Wallace) is:

$$(100 - 3 \times \text{the age in years})$$
$$\times \text{the weight in kilograms} = \text{maintenance}$$

By the time the child is large enough so that the calculations equal 1730 ml, the child is equal to an "average" adult and requires no more than the adult volume. This author arbitrarily holds maintenance volume to 1500 ml in the postoperative patient because of concern over shifts of dilute fluid out of the vascular space if a depletion exists.

Electrolyte requirements for the child are based on the newborn's need for 3 mEq of sodium, chloride, and potassium per kilogram per 24 hours. Because the newborn child and infant require 100 ml of water per kilogram and 3 mEq of sodium, chloride, and potassium per kilogram, a solution of water that contains 3 mEq of sodium and chloride per 100 ml would satisfy the salt requirement.

Normal saline contains 154 mEq of sodium chloride per liter or 15.4 mEq of sodium chloride per 100 ml (or per deciliter). One-fifth normal saline would contain 3.1 mEq of sodium chloride per 100 ml, and thus, a solution of one-fifth normal saline would act as an appropriate maintenance solution for the newborn infant. Reduction formulas appropriately reduce the volume of water administered to the child as he or she grows older and bigger and approaches adult body habitus. Similarly, the use of the reduction formulas in calculating the amount of one-fifth normal saline will provide a similar appropriate reduction of sodium chloride. The administration of 1500 ml of one-fifth normal saline to the adult will provide the adult with 45 mEq of sodium chloride, within the minimum requirement of 45 to 60 mEq per day. On the other hand, the use of the formula of 3 mEq/kg in the older individual would result in a 70-kg adult receiving 210 mEq of sodium chloride a day, a vast excess over requirements.

It is important to keep in mind, however, that this choice of solutions, that is, one-fifth normal saline, is appropriate only for the patient who is initially in electrolyte balance. This individual with normal electrolytes requires a maintenance electrolyte amount that is satisfied by the administration of one-fifth normal saline.

For the patient who is in electrolyte depletion, the amount of electrolyte that should be administered with the maintenance water is increased. For example, a 4-kg infant whose serum sodium is 120 mEq/L and whose serum chloride is 85 mEq/L lacks 20 mEq of sodium per liter from his sodium space, which is primarily extracellular fluid or 21 per cent of the body weight. Moreover, the infant lacks 20 mEq of chloride per liter from the chloride space, which is his total body water or 60 per cent of body weight.

It is essential to correct the electrolyte that is most deficient; therefore, this individual requires 20 mEq of sodium chloride × 60 per cent of his or her body weight. Because the infant weighs 4 kg, the requirement is 20 mEq × 4 × 0.6 or 48 mEq of sodium chloride. In addition, 3 mEq/kg of sodium chloride is required in the next 24 hours to restore insensible losses. Thus, the total requirement for the day is not 3 mEq/kg, which would be 12 mEq, but 48 mEq plus 12 mEq, or 60 mEq. The free water requirement is 100 ml/kg, or 400 ml. If one gave this water as one-fifth normal saline, one would leave out the 48 mEq required to restore the electrolyte deficit. This would then require that the child receive an additional 300 ml of normal saline (15.4 mEq of sodium chloride per 100 ml) to restore the electrolyte deficiency. If, on the other hand, maintenance fluid is given as normal saline rather than one-fifth normal saline, the infant would receive 60 mEq of sodium chloride in 400 ml of normal saline, thus providing the 400 ml of water, the 48 mEq of sodium chloride to restore the deficit, and the 12 mEq of sodium chloride to provide the anticipated maintenance requirement.

For patients who are in a *hypertonic state* of electrolytes, there is, in fact, no electrolyte requirement for the day. Their maintenance solution should be given as dextrose and water, which will allow them to excrete electrolyte through insensible losses and thereby bring the electrolyte concentration back to normal tonicity.

A good rule states that when fluids are being given at significantly greater than maintenance rates, the correction of the hypertonic electrolyte state should be done gradually to avoid running large amounts of free water into the hyperconcentrated fluids, which might result in the rapid dilution of the vascular concentrations relative to the intracellular concentrations, producing massive fluid shifts into the cells. Such shifting into the cerebral cells can result in brain edema and damage. Thus, no solution less concentrated than half normal saline should be utilized for correction of the hypertonic state when dehydration accompanies the hypertonic state and rapid fluid administration is required. However, when the patient is normovolemic and hypertonic, the use of electrolyte-containing solutions will result in failure to correct the hypertonic state. Thus, in the normovolemic patient, dextrose and water should be used as the maintenance solution for the patient with a hypertonic electrolyte state.

In this connection, it is important to understand that the original concept of the action of ADH as a modulator of electrolytes in the state of hypertonicity was not wrong but simply focused on a minor role of ADH rather than the major role of volume maintenance. When the patient is in a state of hypertonic electrolytes, ADH is, in fact, secreted. It is secreted in order to hold onto water to dilute the patient out of the hypertonic state. This situation commonly occurs in the postoperative period when balanced salt solution is administered to the patient long beyond the time when an adequate urine volume has been re-established, indicating the restoration of vascular volume. This prolonged administration of a balanced salt solution results in failure to restore adequate volumes of free water to replace the insensible losses and results in increased concentration of electrolytes. If the patient is normovolemic and hypertonic, the secretion of ADH under these circumstances will result in a reduced urine volume, giving the impression of hypovolemia. The response to such a state is often one of giving "pushes" of balanced salt solution because of fear of hypovolemia. Recognition of the role of ADH under these circumstances will result in appropriate administration of free water to correct the hypertonicity and to allow the ADH to be "shut off," with the resultant appropriate diuresis.

Measured Losses

Measured losses make up the simplest category to understand and correct. These are losses of fluid and electrolytes outside the body, and therefore they can be collected and measured. The electrolyte composition of the fluids can be analyzed in the laboratory, but generally the sources are gastric juice resulting from drainage of a nasogastric tube or gastrointestinal losses beyond the pylorus through such means as choledochostomy tubes, pancreaticocutaneous fistulas, ileostomies, or simply massive diarrhea. All of these entities represent some variation of an ultrafiltrate of the

plasma and can best be restored by the use of balanced salt solutions.

Gastric juice is essentially a combination of sodium, potassium, chloride, and acid. Its sodium concentration ranges between 60 and 75 mEq/L, its chloride concentration between 100 and 150 mEq/L, and its potassium concentration between 5 and 30 mEq/L; the acid concentration is variable. Gastric juice can be replaced by a solution of one-half normal saline, which would have 77 mEq of sodium and chloride per liter to which are added 30 mEq of potassium chloride per liter, producing a final solution having a sodium concentration of 77 mEq, with potassium concentration of 30 mEq and a chloride concentration of 107 mEq (Table 9–2).

Third-Space Volume Repletion

The earlier discussion of the need for replacement of fluids that shift into a third space and are thus temporarily unavailable to restore a vascular volume deficit included a description of the types of fluids that should be utilized. These ranged from blood for the patient who needed oxygen-carrying capacity through plasma to the patient who needed restoration of clotting factors to balanced salt solution (lactated Ringer's solution). Most patients having significant intra-abdominal procedures, all patients who sustain severe blood loss and hypovolemic hypotension, and patients in states of septic shock will require third-space fluid restoration.

Whereas the volume of fluid required for maintenance fluid and electrolyte restoration was calculated from formulas based on experimental analyses and measured losses were replaced by direct replacement of known volumes, the volume required for third-space shifts is variable, dynamic, and uncertain. There is no way to measure directly the vol-

Table 9–2 □ Solution for Replacing Losses of Gastric Secretions

Electrolyte	Gastric Juice (in mEq/L)	Replacement Fluid D5%/0.5 Normal Saline + 30 mEq/ KCl/L
Sodium	60–75	77
Chloride	105–130	107
Potassium	5–30	30
H+	0–65	0

umes of fluid shifting out of the vascular volume. However, the only important consideration is that the intravascular volume be restored. Therefore, again returning to the concept of a "tank," the tank will contain a certain residual volume to which one will mentally add the measured losses and the maintenance requirements and conclude that everything more that is needed to restore the volume of the tank is the third-space requirement.

The restoration of an adequate urine output signals adequate restoration of the intravascular volume. Such a urine output indicates that there is adequate renal blood flow and glomerular filtrate and that ADH is not being secreted, thus indicating that at least the physiologic monitor of the vascular space feels that adequate intravascular volume exists.

However, as one starts out, one has no idea what the state of that vascular volume is, nor does one know whether any urine will be forthcoming. Thus, one can only "guess" at the volumes of fluid required to restore this third-space depletion. *One knows that the correct volume of third-space repletion fluid when added to measured losses and maintenance and administered over a 24-hour period would result in a urine output that is adequate.* An adequate urine output for an infant is 40 ml/kg/day, or approximately 1.5 to 2 ml/kg/hour. Thus, one must initially "guess" at the volume required for third-space repletion, add it to the maintenance and measured-loss volumes, divide by 24 hours, and begin administering the third-space repletion solution at the rate determined by this calculation. Urine output is then monitored, and if the urine output falls within the range of 1.5 to 2 ml/kg/hour, the appropriate amount of fluid is being given. If the urine output is inadequate, the rate of administration must be increased. This effectively creates a requirement for additional amounts of third-space volume repletion fluids inasmuch as the originally calculated fluids will run out before the end of the 24 hours. On the other hand, if the amount of urine output is greater than 2 ml/kg/hour, the rate of administration must be slowed down, and if an adequate urine output is maintained, once the rate is down to that which would administer only maintenance fluid, the solution should be changed to the more hypotonic maintenance solution (assuming that the patient is not receiving an isotonic maintenance solution to correct for pre-existing electrolyte deficiencies).

Once a child reaches 30 kg, urine output would be 30 kg × 40 ml/kg/day or 1200 ml/day. Inasmuch as this is a perfectly adequate urine output for an adult, one does not ask a child to excrete more than this.

In utilizing urine output as a guide for fluid administration, it is essential to keep checking that the underlying assumptions enabling use of urine output as a guide to vascular volume restoration continue to hold true. These assumptions include:

- A normal cardiac output
- Normal kidney function with an intact drainage system and no obstruction to outflow of urine
- No inappropriate ADH, such as might be found in the patient receiving vasopressin for pulmonary hypertension with esophageal variceal hemorrhage
- No septic state, particularly that of endotoxemia, which might be causing inappropriate responses and damage to additional capillary systems
- A normally functioning liver with appropriate secretion of enzymes and hormones.

When the patient is "anuric" following surgery or trauma, it is essential to differentiate between the patient who is actually in renal shutdown from some renal dysfunction or injury and the patient who is still hypovolemic. For the patient for whom the evaluation of other organ systems reveals normal function, a volume "push" should be the initial response to an anuric situation.

The patient can tolerate a push of one fourth of the blood volume. The infant or young child has a blood volume equal to 8 per cent of body weight or 80 ml/kg. It has been shown that a healthy individual can tolerate a volume expansion of 25 per cent without any signs of overload. Thus, one fourth of 80, or 20 ml/kg, is a standard push.

Cardiac output is at least 2 times the blood volume. In a 20-kg individual with a blood volume of 1600 ml, the cardiac output per minute is at least 3200 ml. For a needle in a peripheral or central vein dripping in a volume push that is supposedly equal to one fourth of blood volume, or 400 ml, the volume going past the needle over time is going to determine whether or not the vascular volume sees a 25 per cent expansion push that will "shut off" ADH if it is being secreted in response to hypovolemia. If the push is given in 1 to 2 minutes, the expansion will, in fact, be rapid enough to create a one-fourth expansion of the vascular volume. However, if the push is given over 30 minutes, the volume going by the needle is equal to 30 × 3200, or 96,000 ml. Thus, the dripping of 400 ml into a volume equivalent to 96,000 ml would not be seen by the body as a push. The problem is that this "test" is based on the plan that if the urine output fails to materialize after the push, the patient would be treated as though he or she was in renal failure. This, of course, would require reduction and restriction of fluid and electrolytes when, in fact, hypovolemia requires the rapid administration of restorative volumes. Thus, the inappropriately slow administration of the push can mislead one into the wrong conclusion.

Whenever lack of response to a push is observed, or one is unable to confirm that other organ systems are functioning normally so that proper response to a volume push can be anticipated, better monitoring in the form of a central venous catheter must be instituted to enable the physician to look directly at the state of repletion of the vascular volume. Usually in children with any kind of normal cardiac function, a simple central venous line is all that is needed for such monitoring. A Swan-Ganz pulmonary wedge pressure catheter is reserved for those patients whose cardiac malfunction makes such a more sophisticated monitoring device essential.

Definition of "Correct" Volume for Repletion of Hypovolemic States Caused by Third-Space Shifts or Pre-existing Volume Deficits

If the circulatory system is understood to be a dynamic volume system, conceptualizing it as a "tank" that has an immeasurable leak together with several sources of ingress for fluids such that the only way to know when the tank is full is when it overflows, then a definition of the appropriate amount of third-space replacement can be constructed. *The correct volume for repletion of hypovolemic states due to third-space shifts is that volume of fluid containing appropriate amounts of crystalloid and colloid which when added to calculated maintenance volumes and measured losses and administered over a 24-hour period will achieve a urine output in a child of 1.5 to 2 ml/kg/per hour. Thus, at the end of 24 hours, if the patient has* *achieved an appropriate urine output, one has given the right amount of third-space repletion fluid.*

Prospectively, adequate amounts of repletion fluid each hour can be administered to achieve the desired urine output. If one works at this diligently on an hour-to-hour basis, it should be possible, by appropriate increases and/or decreases of the rate of administration, to come close to the ideal or "correct" volume of repletion fluid.

PRACTICAL APPLICATION OF PRINCIPLES

Case Example

A 7-kg 10-month-old infant has had recurrent urinary tract infections, and renal sonography shows a right dysplastic kidney and a left kidney with moderate hydronephrosis and hydroureter. On further evaluation, a moderately severe ureterovesical obstruction is demonstrated in the child, and he undergoes right nephroureterectomy and a left ureteroneocystostomy. During the operative procedure 100 ml of gastric drainage is noted from the nasogastric tube. What would be this infant's 24-hour postoperative fluid regimen?

Although the child will need maintenance fluid, replacement of the measured loss, and repletion fluid for third-space shifts, one's initial concern is to ensure that the vascular volume is rapidly restored. It is hoped that the anesthesiologist has provided adequate fluid to maintain vascular volume during the procedure, but one must assure this by providing appropriate amounts of repletion fluid, that is, fluid containing a minimum oncotic concentration equivalent to balanced salt solution, with appropriate adjustments upward in oncotic value as needed for the individual patient. This would be accomplished by adding 25 per cent albumin to the balanced salt solution to make 5 per cent albumin in D5%/lactated Ringer's (LR) or, in the case of a patient who needs either clotting factors or oxygen carrying capacity, the choice of plasma or blood for the repletion fluid. For this particular patient, assume that only balanced salt solution is necessary.

One's initial concern is to run in adequate amounts of the more concentrated repletion solution until an adequate urine output is demonstrated. However, one must initially calculate the child's maintenance, measured losses, and third-space fluid requirements.

Maintenance. Using the formula of 100 ml/kg for the first 10 kg, the 7-kg child would require 700 ml, which one would give in the form of 5 per cent dextrose/0.2 per cent normal saline (D5%/0.2% NS), to which we would add 3 mEq of potassium chloride per kilogram or 21 mEq of potassium chloride in 700 ml of D5%/0.2% NS.

Measured Loss. This amounts to 100 ml of nasogastric tube loss during the operation, which would be replaced by 100 ml of a solution of D5%/0.5% NS to which one would add 30 mEq/L or 3 mEq/dl of potassium chloride. Therefore, the measured loss solution would be 100 ml D5%/0.5 NS + 3 mEq KCl.

Third-Space Repletion Solution. Recognizing that this volume is a "guess," suppose one takes a really *wild* guess—4000 ml! . . . which one will give as D5%/ LR.

The total fluid regimen, therefore, looks like this:

Fluid Requirement	Fluid Regimen
Maintenance	700 ml D5%/0.2 NS + 21 mEq KCl
Measured loss	100 ml D5%/0.5 NS + 3 mEq KCl
Third space	4000 ml D5%/LR
Total	4800 ml

This amount is then divided by 24 to give a rate of 200 ml/hour, and one would start administering D5%/LR at 200 ml/hour and monitor urine output. This is, of course, a very excessive volume for this 7-kg infant.

Correcting "Wrong" Guesses

Since a major portion of the above fluid regimen is a guess, urine output must be monitored very carefully. Desirable urine output for this 7-kg infant would be 1.5 to 2 ml/kg/hour or a maximum of 14 ml/hour. As fluids are run at 200 ml/hour, urine output will be monitored and in all probability the urine output will *rapidly* exceed 14 ml.

As soon as one recognizes this *excessive* urine output, one *must* slow down the rate of administration and continue to slow it until the urine output comes down to 14 ml/hour. This effectively eliminates some of the fluid that would otherwise have been administered in the 24 hours and corrects the overly generous guess.

On the other hand, if in a different patient one guesses too little volume for the third-space requirement and the urine output fails to come up to 1.5 to 2 ml/kg/hour, the rate of hourly administration *must* be increased. This effectively causes the fluid regimen to be used up in less than 24 hours, and more fluid must be added. The most likely additional fluid needed would be the repletion fluid for the third space (assuming that the maintenance and the measured loss are calculated correctly). Thus, hourly monitoring of urine out-

put should allow one to come within a reasonable approximation of the child's actual requirements for the 24 hours.

If the child produces no urine output, one must assess the functioning of the various organ systems such as cardiovascular, respiratory, endocrine, and so forth, to be certain that the assumption of normalcy for these organs is correct. The urinary drainage system, including any catheter system, must also be patent. Once it is certain that these systems are working appropriately, one resorts to a volume push, as defined earlier, to "test" whether the child is hypovolemic or in renal or cardiac failure.

Improving the Guess after Abdominal Surgery

Many years of experience in clinical observation prompted the realization that there was a relationship between the extent of abdominal surgery and the requirement for third-space repletion (Filston et al). Thus, the extent of abdominal surgery can be related to the child's maintenance (and therefore size) by the observation that one quarter of the maintenance volume will be needed in the form of repletion solution (D5%/LR, etc.) for each quadrant of the abdomen that either an inflammatory or obstructive disease entity involves or that is operatively explored. This schema brings the "guess" to a level of an "educated guess" based on the extent of involvement of the abdominal cavity, a source of considerable third-space shifting. Application of this schema to the earlier case example would result in the same maintenance formula calculation and measured losses, but the third-space guess would be based on the evaluation of the extent of the operative procedure in the abdominal cavity. The obstructive uropathy was a chronic state, so that unless the child had ascites, no factor would be included for the disease entity's effect on the abdominal cavity. However, the surgical exploration might exteriorize the bowel for a considerable period of time with nephrectomy on one side and operative manipulations on the other. Therefore, a guess of two to four quadrants, depending on the extent of dissection and the facts regarding the exteriorization of the bowel, would be in order. Using a guess of three quadrants, the urologist calculates that the child would require three quarters of the maintenance level, or approximately 525 ml of D5%/LR for third-space repletion. This quantity, when added to 700 ml maintenance and 100 ml measured loss, would total 1325 ml for the 24 hours, or 55 ml/hour.

Once again, one would begin running the D5%/LR at 55 ml/hour and monitor the child's urine output, adjusting the rate of administration upward or downward appropriately to maintain hourly urine output between 1.5 and 2 ml/kg/hour.

The state of the child's preoperative hydration, the amount of fluid administered during the operative procedure, and the considerable variability in the "guess" as to the extent of involvement of the peritoneal cavity by the operative procedure and the disease will still leave a considerable possibility of error in this "educated guess." However, this additional calculation will help to avoid such blatant errors as that in the case illustration. The results of applying this schema to 50 consecutive infants undergoing abdominal surgery by six consecutive senior surgical house officers rotating through the pediatric surgical service at Duke University Medical Center are shown in Figure 9–1. The four patients who failed to come up to the ideal level were the sickest patients, all of them in endotoxic shock, and they actually received the most fluid administration and the most attention by the house officers of the 50 patients represented.

The 40 patients who are significantly above the ideal range all did well, but their urine outputs could have been kept closer to the ideal range by more diligent attention to the rate of fluid administration postoperatively. Realistically, the house officers tended to work hard to achieve a urine output in each of the postoperative patients, but because they had a multitude of other tasks and patients to care for, they failed to monitor the urine output carefully and make appropriate reductions in the rate of fluid administration when the urine output exceeded 2 ml/kg/hour. This only confirms that all systems of postoperative fluid management can only be estimates because of the extensive variability of the individual patient and his or her disease state and, therefore, can only serve as guidelines to be augmented by careful monitoring of the state of the vascular volume until its appropriate repletion is assured.

DIFFICULTIES IN RENAL INSUFFICIENCY AND URINARY TRACT OBSTRUCTIVE STATES

The above schema depends upon a urinary system in which the renal function is normal and the urinary drainage system is patent. Because a patent urinary system can become "obstructed" by a plugged drainage catheter, the patency of the drainage system must always be assured. However, often after urinary tract surgery, leakage from reconstructed urinary drainage tracts results in difficulty in effectively

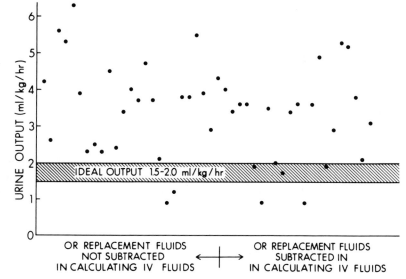

Figure 9–1 □ Distribution of average hourly urine outputs during first 24 hours after surgery for 50 infants undergoing abdominal surgery, with fluid estimates based on a "quadrant scheme" relating extent of disease and surgical trauma to maintenance fluid volumes. (OR, operating room; IV, intravenous.) (From Filston HC, Edwards CH III, Chitwood WR Jr, et al: Estimation of postoperative fluid requirements in infants and children. Ann Surg 196:76–81, 1982.)

monitoring the volume of urine output. More significantly, when it is known that renal function is impaired, this fluid administration system, based on the reliability of renal function, becomes relatively undependable.

When the operative procedure or the disease entity is likely to produce relatively little in the way of third-space volume shifts, the patient can be managed in a fairly straightforward manner by providing maintenance fluid and electrolytes, replacing measured losses, and perhaps administering a minimal amount of additional repletion solution. However, when hypovolemia, hypoxia, endotoxemia, or an extensive surgical procedure make the need for significant repletion volumes likely, it is essential then to monitor the vascular volume by providing central venous pressure measurements. These measurements cannot tell the exact amount of fluid to administer, but they can provide evidence of adequate volume repletion. Children with normal cardiovascular and respiratory function generally have low central venous pressures (CVPs), with newborns and young infants often having CVPs of 0 with adequate vascular volume. Thus, if the urine output cannot be relied upon as a measure of volume repletion, maintaining a central venous pressure in the range of 0 to 5 cm of water ensures adequate volume repletion. Generally, a range of 5 to 10 cm of water suggests adequate to excessive volume repletion and pressures above 10 cm of water would suggest overload. These numbers are in no way absolutes, however, and they must be adjusted for the overall clinical state of the patient. Not infrequently, patients who are in severe septic shock with multisystem failure, requiring intubated ventilation and inotropic cardiovascular support, will demonstrate CVPs well above the 8 to 10 cm of water range and still require additional fluids. Evaluation of tissue perfusion based on capillary refill and evaluation of arterial blood gases with particular attention to acid-base balance will help in the overall assessment of the patient's ongoing fluid needs.

GUIDELINES FOR ENTERAL FEEDING OF INFANTS AND CHILDREN

In an ideal world, it would be nice to demand that anyone who presumed to operate on infants or children first be able to feed them appropriately, maintain volume status enterally or parenterally, and demonstrate the ability to gain vascular access both peripherally and centrally. Although this may be unrealistic, it is important that a pediatric surgical specialist have some knowledge of these requirements.

Peripheral Versus Central Access

Peripheral access can usually be achieved by cannulating the veins of the forearm, wrist, or hand, or, in the lower extremities, the saphenous vein at the ankle or the veins of the foot (Filston and Johnson). Additional peripheral access can be obtained in newborns and young infants utilizing the prominent scalp veins. Success at cannulation of these tiny veins can be enhanced by immobilizing the extremity well, placing the bevel of the needle down so that the needle travels parallel to the lumen of the vein rather than coursing quickly through it as it does when the bevel is held in the upright position, utilizing a plastic cannula with inner needle stylet and attached syringe, which allows aspiration of blood with reinjection. This "balloons up" the vein, allowing the needle stylet to be advanced a millimeter or two further into the vein, assuring that the following cannula enters the vein before the needle stylet is removed. Additionally, one should never withdraw the needle while aspirating the syringe hoping to re-enter a pierced vein because the needle stylet may become plugged with tissue, preventing aspiration of blood. Greater success will be achieved by removing the needle stylet once the cannula is advanced to the depth that seems appropriate and then very slowly and carefully backing the cannula outward, hoping in this fashion to re-enter the lumen and gain flow. A slight twist will frequently seat the cannula well into the lumen of the vessel once backflow of blood is noted.

Central cannulation can be achieved either by means of a percutaneous subclavian approach or by incisional access to the external or internal jugular system in the neck. Both techniques are well established and well described in the literature (Filler et al; Filston and Grant).

Caloric Differences

Peripheral veins will tolerate little more than a concentration of dextrose equal to 12.5 per

Fluid Quantity	Nutrient	Grams per Kilogram	Kilocalories per Kilogram
50 ml	5 per cent protein hydrolysate	= 2.5 g/kg =	10 kcal/kg
30 ml	50 per cent dextrose	= 15 g/kg =	51 kcal/kg
33 ml	10 per cent intralipid	= 3.3 g/kg =	30 kcal/kg
113 ml	+ 7 ml water	= 120 ml/kg =	91 kcal/kg

cent. Maintenance fluid requirement for the child is equal to 100 ml/kg, but the child will easily tolerate 120 ml/kg. This can be made up as a solution of 50 ml of 5 per cent protein hydrolysate, which provides 2.5 g/kg of protein, or 10 kcal. Adding to this 30 ml of 50 per cent dextrose would provide 15 g of dextrose, which at 3.4 kcal/g would provide 51 kcal. One third of the total calories can be in fats, so 33 ml of 10 per cent intralipid would provide 30 kcal of a total of 91 kcal. This is a volume of 113 ml, and, in order to hold it to 12.5 per cent dextrose concentration, it would have to be diluted with water to a total volume of 120 ml as shown above.

However, 10 of these calories are protein calories, which are usually not counted as these should be used as "building blocks" for body protein, so that the actual nonprotein calories equal 81 kcal/kg.

By contrast, 120 ml/kg of total parenteral nutrition fluid delivered centrally could provide 132 kcal/kg in 120 ml by the following formula:

50 ml of 5 per cent protein	= 2.5 g/kg	= 10 kcal/kg
50 ml of 50 per cent dextrose	= 25 g/kg	= 85 kcal/kg
15 ml of 20 per cent lipid	= 3 g/kg	= 27 kcal/kg

115 ml provides 122 kcal/kg, or 112 nonprotein kcal/kg

Additionally, using 50 ml of 5 per cent protein hydrolysate and 72 ml of 50 per cent dextrose for a total volume of 122 ml/kg would provide 122 carbohydrate kcal/kg and 10 protein kcal/kg in 120 ml fluid/kg. If, in addition, one third of total calories were provided by fat, 36 ml of intralipid could be provided, giving a total fluid volume of 158 ml/kg and providing 188 nonprotein kcal/kg by this central route. Thus, it is clear that the central access route provides much greater flexibility and the possibility of giving a much greater caloric load. Nevertheless, most infants will grow well on 120 kcal/kg.

NUTRITIONAL REQUIREMENTS

Caloric requirements for an infant or young child are defined by the following formula (Wallace):

$$(100 - 3 \times \text{the age in years})$$
$$\times \text{ the weight in kilograms}$$
$$= \text{kilocalories per kilogram}$$

In actuality, the newborn and young infant require approximately 120 kcal/kg for adequate growth. As the child ages, this reduction formula provides a rough estimate of the number of kilocalories per kilogram provided. Thus, a 2-year-old child would require 100 − 6 = 94 kcal/kg.

When protein is being provided parenterally, the child tolerates best a solution of approximately 2.5 g/kg. By the enteral route, a bit more protein can be tolerated. It is recommended that the fat calories be limited to one third of the total calories and 3 g/kg. With the limitations described for protein and fat, the additional caloric requirement is then made up by carbohydrates.

Enteral feedings of infant formulas generally supply the minerals, vitamins, and trace elements needed for normal growth, development, and enzyme system functioning. During parenteral feedings, the 3 mEq/kg requirement for sodium, potassium, and chloride must be provided as well as calcium, phosphate, and magnesium.

Trace elements known to be required during long-term total parenteral nutrition include iron, manganese, selenium, copper, zinc, and molybdenum. All multivitamin preparations will provide adequate amounts of all but vitamin K. One must be careful with premature newborns to utilize vitamin preparations that appropriately limit vitamin A in this age group.

GUIDELINES FOR ENTERAL FEEDINGS OF INFANTS AND CHILDREN

Although "regular diet" and "diet for age" may be adequate orders for the older child and teenager, for the newborn and young infant, some understanding of infant formulas is essential.

All standard infant formulas are made up to approximate breast milk. The caloric level is 20 kcal/ounce which is the caloric level of normal breast milk. Most standard formulas have a protein content based on casein hydrolysate (cow's milk) to which sugars, starches, and fats are added proportionally along with minerals and vitamins. These formulas contain lactose and sucrose and require the digestive enzymes lactase and disaccharidase for digestion and absorption. Most standard infant formulas such as Similac,* Enfamil,† and SMA‡ are nearly isosmotic.

Various modified formulas can be utilized when a child has difficulty with digestion. The most common formula intolerance is intolerance to cow's milk protein, and for this, the substitution of soy-based protein in formulas such as ProSobee† and Nursoy‡ may be helpful. However, some children are even more violently allergic to soy protein than they are to cow's milk protein and may have a quite bloody diarrhea as a result of soy intolerance.

For those patients with an inability to tolerate fats, the substitution of medium-chain triglycerides as the fat source in formulas such as Portagen† will provide a fat source that is more easily tolerated inasmuch as the medium-chain triglycerides do not need to be emulsified and do not require the active cellular process of chylomicron formation and active transport. Instead, they are absorbed directly into the lymphatics and transported to the liver.

For the infant who has serious problems with digestive enzyme deficiencies, such as those with short-gut syndrome or those having had an hypoxic or septic injury to the mucosal enzyme systems, a "predigested" formula providing fats in the form of medium-chain triglycerides, a simplified protein base, and simple carbohydrates such as glucose and fructose will allow absorption of formula while mini-mizing the amount of digestion the child needs to provide by his or her own intestinal function. However, often these formulas are hyperosmolar and, therefore, need to be "titrated" until tolerance is gradually achieved.

Inasmuch as the standard formulas provide 20 kcal/kg, the child needs 150 ml of formula per kilogram to provide 100 kcal/kg and 180 ml/kg to provide 120 kcal/kg, the amount usually required for the newborn.

Individual feeding volume can then be determined by calculating the total required volume for the day and dividing it by the number of feedings. Premature infants usually have a small gastric capacity and need to eat every 2 hours in order to consume adequate calories at small-volume feedings. Normal full-term newborns will feed approximately every 3 hours around the clock and thus would require eight feedings per day. As the child reaches 2 to 3 months of age, he or she gradually moves to a 4-hour schedule and often drops a nighttime feeding, resulting in five feedings into which the total volume must be divided. Pediatricians vary considerably in their views as to when foods other than formula should be added to the diet. Some years ago, the child who was fed breast milk or formula well into the first year of life became an anemic "milk baby." Today, virtually all standard formulas have iron supplements, but the breast-fed baby will still require exogenous iron supplementation.

SUMMARY

Although many procedures in pediatric urology are straightforward technical operations that produce little alteration in the child's overall functional state, situations do arise in which sepsis, blood loss, or an internal fluid shift results in depletion of vascular volume with a consequent reduction in tissue perfusion and potential damage to the capillary endothelium. Many pediatric urologic procedures require complex reconstructive techniques often utilizing parts of the intestine for conduits or to augment a deficient bladder. Intraoperative fluid losses may be substantial during such procedures, and, perhaps of even more significance, these children may present subsequently with complications such as bowel obstructions that produce massive intraluminal fluid losses, creating marked hypovolemia. Recognition of these deficiencies and some

---

*Ross Laboratories, Columbus, Ohio.
†Mead Johnson Laboratories, Evansville, Indiana.
‡Wyeth-Ayerst Laboratories, Philadelphia, Pennsylvania.

facility with gauging the volumes and types of fluids needed for correcting this hypovolemic state are as essential to the successful management of these patients as is the skill to perform the technical maneuvers required for the reconstruction of the deficient urinary tract.

Bibliography

Cervera AL, Moss G: Progressive hypovolemia leading to shock after continuous hemorrhage and 3:1 crystalloid replacement. Am J Surg 129:670, 1975.

Filler RM, Eraklis AJ, Rubin VG, et al: Long-term total parenteral nutrition in infants. N Engl J Med 281:589, 1969.

Filston HC, Edwards CH III, Chitwood WR Jr, et al: Estimation of postoperative fluid requirements in infants and children. Ann Surg 196:76, 1982.

Filston HC, Grant JP: A safer system for percutaneous subclavian venous catheterization in newborn infants. J Pediatr Surg 14:564, 1979.

Filston HC, Johnson DG: Percutaneous venous cannulation in neonates and infants: a method for catheter insertion without "cut-down." Pediatrics 48:896, 1971.

Holcroft JW, Trunkey DD: Pulmonary extravasation of albumin during and after hemorrhagic shock in baboons. J Surg Res 18:91, 1975.

Moore FD: Metabolic Care of the Surgical Patient. Philadelphia, WB Saunders Co, 1959, p 292.

Moss GS, Siegel DC, Cockin MS, et al: Effects of saline and colloid solutions on pulmonary function in hemorrhagic shock. Surg Gynecol Obstet 133:53, 1971.

Rickham PP: The Metabolic Response to Neonatal Surgery. Cambridge, Harvard University Press, 1957.

Rickham PP: Preoperative and postoperative care: neonates. In Pediatric Surgery. Edited by WJ Mustard, MM Ravitch, WH Snyder Jr, et al. Chicago, Year Book Medical Publishers, 1969, p 38.

Shires T: Fluid therapy in hemorrhagic shock. Arch Surg 88:688, 1964.

Shires T: The role of sodium-containing solutions in the treatment of oligemic shock. Surg Clin North Am 45:365, 1965.

Shires T, Williams J, Brown F: Acute change in ECF associated with major surgical procedures. Ann Surg 154:803, 1961.

Wallace WM: Quantitative requirements of the infant and child for water and electrolyte under varying conditions. Am J Clin Path 23:1133, 1953.

Wiggers CJ: Physiology of Shock. New York, The Commonwealth Fund, 1950, p 137.

Wilkerson AW, Nagy G, Billing BH, et al: Excretion of chloride and sodium after operation. Lancet 1:640, 1949.

Wright HK, Gann DS: Correction of defect in free water excretion in postoperative patients by extracellular fluid volume expansion. Ann Surg 158:70, 1963.

10

☐ Genitourinary Infections

☐ NONSPECIFIC INFECTIONS

H. Gil Rushton

The last decade has been marked by many fascinating advances in the study of childhood urinary tract infection (UTI). Recent prospective epidemiologic studies in Swedish infants and children have reported a prevalence of urinary infection approximately twice as high as in previous studies. Extensive investigation of the complex host-parasite interaction in urinary infection has identified a number of genetically coded bacterial virulence factors, particularly adherence, which enhance the uropathogenicity of a limited number of bacterial clones. Bacterial virulence is relative and must be considered in relation to a number of host factors, ranging from vesicoureteral reflux to the secretor phenotype, that also influence an individual's susceptibility to urinary infection.

Animal model studies have led to a greater understanding of the pathogenetic chain of the events in acute pyelonephritis at a cellular level. These experimental studies, when combined with clinical reports, clearly demonstrate the critical role that infection plays in producing irreversible renal scarring. This recognition has led to greater emphasis on the nonsurgical management of conditions such as vesicoureteral reflux and nonobstructive hydronephrosis. Some animal studies also have demonstrated the effectiveness of vaccines against specific bacterial virulence factors in the prevention of ascending pyelonephritis. The next decade will undoubtedly witness their clinical application.

Urinary tract imaging in children with urinary infection, likewise, has changed with gradual replacement of intravenous pyelography by ultrasonography and/or renal scintigraphy. With renal cortical scintigraphy, accurate identification of upper UTI and documentation of the extent and progression of renal parenchymal damage, especially in young children, will allow for further refinement of therapeutic regimens. Already these localization studies have confirmed a higher than previously recognized incidence of nonreflux pyelonephritis in children. This chapter highlights the advances in childhood UTIs over the last several years, relating these to the existing fund of knowledge. The author acknowledges the scholarly contribution from the last edition of this text, which served as the foundation for the current chapter (Belman, 1985).

PREVALENCE OF BACTERIURIA

The prevalence of symptomatic and asymptomatic bacteriuria in childhood is influenced by the age and sex of the patient as well as the method of diagnosis. The overall incidence of neonatal bacteriuria has been reported as 1 to 1.4 per cent (Abbott; Littlewood et al; O'Doherty). The male-to-female ratio in neonates is reversed from that seen in older children (Table 10–1). From a compilation of screening studies of healthy newborns reviewed by Stamey, 1.5 per cent of boys versus only 0.13 per cent of girls had bacteriuria (Stamey, 1980). The reported incidence of *symptomatic* urinary infections in neonates ranges from 0.14 to 0.5 per cent, with a male-to-female ratio ranging from 2.8:1 to 5.4:1 (Bergström et al, 1972; Drew and Acton).

The actual incidence of UTI during infancy has probably been underestimated in the past, partly because of the nonspecificity of symptoms and the inability to verbalize in this age group. In a 3-year prospective screening study of 3581 infants (0 to 1 year) in Goteborg, Sweden, screening bacteriuria confirmed by

Table 10–1 □ Sex Ratio of Urinary
Tract Infections

	Females	Males
Neonate	0.4	1
1–6 mos.	1.5	1
6–12 mos.	4.0	1
1–3 yrs.	10.0	1
3–11 yrs.	9.0	1
11–16 yrs.	2.0	1

From Belman AB, Kaplan GW: Genitourinary Problems in
Pediatrics. Philadelphia, WB Saunders Co, 1981. Modified from
Winberg J, Andersen HJ, Bergström L, et al: Epidemiology of
symptomatic urinary tract infection in childhood. Acta Paediatr
Scand (Suppl) 252:1, 1974.

Table 10–2 □ History and Symptoms of 109
Children with "Screening" Bacteriuria

History/Symptoms	Per Cent
Previous urinary tract infection	20
Nocturnal enuresis	51
Diurnal enuresis	47
Urgency	54
Frequency	53
Dysuria	13
Unexplained fever	7
Flank pain	4
Nocturia	4
All symptoms (excluding nocturnal enuresis)	70

Modified from Savage DCL, Wilson MI, McHardy M, et al:
Covert bacteria of childhood. Arch Dis Child 48:8, 1973.

suprapubic aspiration of urine was found in 2.5 per cent of boys and in 0.9 per cent of girls (Jodal, 1987). Symptomatic bacteriuria occurred equally often in both sexes (1.2 per cent of boys versus 1.1 per cent of girls). Overall, 3.7 per cent of boys and 2 per cent of girls had bacteriuria during the first year of life. This is a much higher frequency of bacteriuria during the first year of life compared with the frequency noted in previous studies. The male dominance noted in the Goteborg study occurred during the first few months of life, confirming similar findings of others (Fig. 10–1) (Ginsburg and McCracken; Majd et al).

During preschool and school age, the sex

ratio for screening bacteriuria is reversed from that seen in infancy. Several large screening studies have shown that 0.7 to 1.9 per cent of girls and 0.04 to 0.2 per cent of boys have bacteriuria (Kunin et al; Lindberg et al, 1975b; Newcastle Group; Savage et al; Saxena et al). In these studies, as many as one third of the children had a prior history of urinary infection and many also had a history of voiding symptoms (Table 10–2). Based on an average annual incidence figure of 0.4 per cent, Kunin (1964) estimated that bacteriuria will develop in approximately 5 per cent of girls prior to graduation from high school. Other authors have reported a higher annual incidence rate of infection during childhood, suggesting that the risk for developing bacteriuria may even be greater (Savage et al). Additional data collected by Kunin (1970) revealed that infection will recur in 80 per cent of all white girls and 60 per cent of black girls within 5 years.

In a classic prospective epidemiologic study of symptomatic urinary tract infections in children living in Goteborg, Sweden, Winberg et al (1974) estimated that the aggregate risk for *symptomatic* urinary infection up to age 11 was at least 3 per cent for girls and at least 1.1 per cent for boys. However, in a more recent study of 7-year-old school entrants from the same city, 7.8 per cent of girls and 1.7 per cent of boys were found to have had a previous symptomatic UTI verified by urine culture (Jodal, 1990). These figures suggest that the true frequency of symptomatic urinary infection in children has been underestimated.

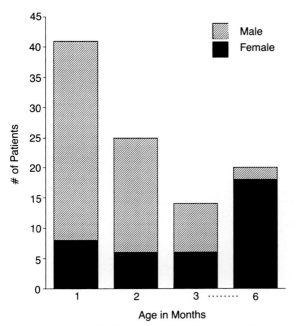

Figure 10–1 □ Distribution by sex and age of 100 infants with urinary tract infection. Dark squares represent females; diagonal squares represent males. (Modified from Ginsburg CM, McCracken GH: Urinary tract infections in young infants. Reproduced by permission of Pediatrics, Vol 69, p 409, © 1982.)

BACTERIOLOGY

The majority of uncomplicated UTIs are caused by a large family of gram-negative, aerobic bacilli known as Enterobacteriaceae. Included in this family are the species *Escherichia, Klebsiella, Enterobacter, Citrobacter, Proteus, Providencia, Morganella, Serratia,* and *Salmonella.* Of these, *Escherichia coli* is the most frequently isolated organism, being responsible for approximately 80 per cent of UTIs. This family of bacteria is generally characterized by a negative reaction to the oxidase test and the capacity to ferment glucose and reduce nitrates to nitrite. Identification of all of these organisms by standard culture techniques is routine and available in all laboratories and many office practices. *Pseudomonas* is also a gram-negative, aerobic bacillus but is distinct and unrelated to Enterobactericeae. Most of the *Pseudomonas* organisms that are recovered from the urine are of relatively low virulence and do not tend to invade tissue unless the host defense mechanisms are compromised. *Pseudomonas aeruginosa* is the most common uropathogenic strain in this family. The most common gram-positive organisms found in UTIs are *Staphylococcus* and enterococcus.

Although *E. coli* is the most common single organism, other organisms are frequently isolated from certain age-related and/or sex-related groups. For example, *Proteus* infections have been reported to be common in boys older than 1 year of age, staphylococcal infections are common at puberty, and *Klebsiella* is more often isolated from newborns than from older children (Table 10–3) (Hermansson et al; Winberg et al, 1974). The majority of uncomplicated infections are caused by a single organism. Patients with complicated infections, particularly those who have been managed with long-term catheterization, may have multiple organisms.

Anaerobic fecal flora rarely produce urinary tract infections despite being 100 to 1000 times more abundant than *E. coli* in stool (Brook; Ribot et al; Segura et al). Occasionally, unusual or fastidious organisms may produce infections that may be difficult to detect because they often do not grow well in commonly used culture media. *Haemophilus influenza* has been reported to cause urinary infections (Granoff and Roskes), and *H. influenza* epididymo-orchitis in infant males has been recognized (Thomas et al, 1981). Other unusual organisms include *Salmonella* and *Shigella.* Although *Lactobacilli, Corynebacteria,* and alpha-*Streptococcus* may rarely cause UTI, they probably should be considered contaminants unless they are found in culture of specimens obtained by suprapubic aspiration or by catheterization.

Serology

E. coli, the most common species of uropathogens, can be typed serologically by three major groups of antigenic structures capable of producing specific antibodies (Fig. 10–2). There are more than 150 O (cell wall) antigens, more than 50 H (flagellar) antigens, and approximately 100 K (capsular) antigens. Not all strains are typable. Serologic classification of *E. coli* in UTI is restricted mainly to O antigens. Early studies have attempted to correlate serologic markers with increased virulence or tissue invasiveness. Most of these were epidemiologic studies that were conducted prior to

Table 10–3 □ Infecting Bacteriuria (%) Isolated from "First-Time" Urinary Infection in Children Categorized by Age and Sex

Infecting Organism	All Neonates (%) (n = 73)	Females (%)		Males§ (%)	
		1 mo–10 yr‡ *(n = 389)*	*10–16 yr* *(n = 30)*	*1 mo–1 yr* *(n = 62)*	*1–16 yr* *(n = 42)*
Escherichia coli	57 (females) 83 (males)	83%	60%	85%	33%
Klebsiella	11%	4	0	2	2
Proteus	0	3	0	5	33
Enterococcus	3	2	0	0	2
*Staphylococcus**	1	4	30	0	12†
Other, mixed, or unknown	9%	11%	10%	8%	17%

Modified from Winberg J, Andersen HJ, Bergström T, et al: Epidemiology of symptomatic urinary tract infection in childhood. Acta Paediatr Scand (Suppl) 252:1, 1, 1974.

*No difference between boys 1 to 10 years and 10 to 16 years old, except for *Staphylococcus.* (Species of *Staphylococcus,* i.e., *epidermidis* versus *saprophyticus,* not analyzed.)

†Four of five patients older than 11 years of age.

‡No difference between girls 1 month to 1 year old and 1 to 10 years old.

§Males not routinely circumcised in Scandinavia.

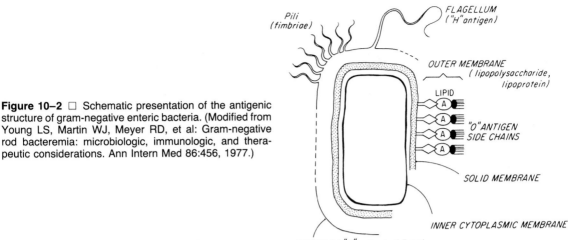

Figure 10–2 ☐ Schematic presentation of the antigenic structure of gram-negative enteric bacteria. (Modified from Young LS, Martin WJ, Meyer RD, et al: Gram-negative rod bacteremia: microbiologic, immunologic, and therapeutic considerations. Ann Intern Med 86:456, 1977.)

discovery of the special role of specific virulence factors, such as attachment factors. In contrast to patients with cystitis or asymptomatic bacteriuria, patients with pyelonephritis have been found to be more frequently infected with certain O typable strains and strains having certain K antigens. Eight O antigen types (O1, O2, O4, O6, O7, O18, O25, O75) were the cause of 80 per cent of cases of pyelonephritis in one report (Lindberg et al, 1975c). Another study reported that 70 per cent of isolates from patients with pyelonephritis were accounted for by *E. coli* possessing five K antigens (K1, K2, K3, K12, K13) (Kaijser et al, 1977). These earlier serologic studies have been extended to identify more specific O:K:H combination serotypes characteristic of pyelonephritogenic strains (Orskov et al; 1982, Orskov and Orskov, 1983).

Virulence Factors

Additional studies of pyelonephritogenic strains of *E. coli* reveal the presence of a limited number of bacterial clones that possess specific virulence factors that are expressed only in certain O groups (Orskov et al, 1982; Vaisanen-Rhen et al). The term virulence describes the ability of microorganisms to cause disease. The concept of uropathogenic bacteria refers to certain strains that are selected from the fecal flora, not by chance or based on prevalence but because of the presence of specific virulence factors that enhance colonization of the uroepithelium. Other virulence factors aid in persistence of bacteria in the

urinary tract and provide these organisms with the capacity to induce inflammation of the urethra, bladder, or renal parenchyma. Specific, recognized *E. coli* virulence factors include (1) adherence to uroepithelial cells, (2) high quantity of K antigen, (3) resistance to serum bactericidal activity, (4) hemolysin production, and (5) the ability of bacteria to acquire iron.

Adherence

Bacterial adherence is the initiating step in all infections, whereas tissue invasion, inflammation, and damage are secondary events. Bacteria are capable of adhering in a specific manner as the result of surface adhesins that bind to specific host cell receptors. The bacterial adhesins can be localized either in an outer coat or capsule or on specialized pili (also known as fimbriae) (Fig. 10–2). The extent of tissue binding can be determined by incubation of uroepithelial cells with bacteria. Alternatively, bacteria-host binding interaction can be studied based on the ability of bacteria to agglutinate red blood cells that possess similar surface receptors.

Considerable experimental and clinical evidence suggests that at least two distinct forms of pili or fimbriae exist that are important to bacterial adherence in the urinary tract. Type I fimbriae are found on most strains of *E. coli*. The specific receptor for this fimbria is D-mannosyl (Ofek and Beachey). Since either attachment to target cells or agglutination of red blood cells by type I fimbriated *E. coli* can be blocked by D-mannose, these fimbriae are referred to as "mannose-sensitive." In contrast, attachment or agglutination by type II pili is not inhibited by mannose; these fimbriae are therefore "mannose-resistant." Both types of fimbriae can coexist on the same bacterial strain.

Data regarding the role of type I fimbriae in the pathogenesis of urinary tract infection is contradictory. Some investigators have reported poor attachment of type I fimbriae to uroepithelial cells, although they adhere well to buccal epithelial cells (Hagberg et al, 1981). Other evidence suggests that type I fimbriae may play a role in the initiation of colonization of the lower urinary tract and/or vagina (Marre and Hacker; Ofek et al; Schaeffer et al, 1984). Experimental colonization of the urinary tract of mice with E. coli can be prevented by blocking adherence using mannose analogues (Aronson et al, 1979). Immunization with type I fimbriae prevents ascending infection in rats following bladder inoculation (Silverblatt and Cohen; Silverblatt et al). In one clinical study, a high prevalence of type I fimbriated E. coli strains was recovered from the bladder of patients with cystitis (88.9 per cent) compared with the prevalence found in fecal strains (44.1 per cent) (Nasu). Type I fimbriae are also recognized by phagocytes. Following tissue invasion, type I fimbriae may promote attachment to the phagocytes, resulting in greater killing of bacteria (Bar-Sharit et al; Blumenstock and Jann; Silverblatt and Ofek).

In contrast to type I fimbriae, type II or mannose-resistant fimbriae are expressed by only certain strains of E. coli. The receptor for type II fimbriae is a glycosphingolipid that is present on both the uroepithelial cell membrane and red blood cells (Kallenius et al, 1980; Leffler and Svanborg Edén). An oligosaccharide fraction of this glycosphingolipid, α-D-galactose-1-4-β-D-galactose (Gal 1-4 Gal), has been shown to be the specific receptor. Evidence includes competitive inhibition, induced by bacterial exposure to an isolated fraction of this purified oligosaccharide, of both attachment of type II fimbriated E. coli to uroepithelial cells and agglutination by type II fimbriated E. coli of P blood group erythrocytes. Furthermore, agglutination of previously nonagglutinable p red blood cells (which lack the P blood group antigen) occurs following coating of the red blood cells with a synthetic Gal 1-4 Gal analogue (Kallenius et al, 1982). Because the Gal 1-4 Gal receptor is part of the P blood group antigen, type II pili are commonly referred to as P-fimbriae. In addition to its role in colonization of the urinary tract, adherence mediated by P-fimbria may also provide more efficient delivery of endotoxin, present in the capsule of all E. coli, to the uroepithelial tissue (Mårild et al, 1988). Endotoxin is a lipopolysaccharide moiety that is thought to be an important mediator of both the local and systemic inflammatory response to infection.

Epidemiologic studies in adults and children have provided considerable evidence that the presence of P-fimbriae on E. coli organisms is a significant virulence factor, particularly in upper urinary tract infections. These studies have shown that 76 to 94 per cent of pyelonephritogenic strains of E. coli are P-fimbriated compared with 19 to 23 per cent of cystitis strains, 14 to 18 per cent of strains isolated from patients with asymptomatic bacteriuria and 7 to 16 per cent of fecal isolate strains. No such correlation was found with type I fimbriae (Kallenius et al, 1981; Vaisanen-Rhen et al). As shown in experimental and clinical studies, however, this does not necessarily negate a role for type I fimbriae in colonization of the bladder (Hagberg et al, 1983; Iwahi et al; Marre and Hacker; Nasu; Schaeffer et al, 1979).

Other evidence supporting the importance of P-fimbriae in causing upper urinary tract infections comes from animal model studies. Inoculation of the bladders of non-refluxing primates with P-fimbriated E. coli resulted in pyelonephritis in 66 per cent of animals. In contrast, pyelonephritis was not seen in any other monkeys inoculated with non–P-fimbriated E. coli (Roberts et al, 1985). Furthermore, immunization of primates with antifimbrial antibody affords protection against pyelonephritis following renal inoculation with P-fimbriated E. coli (Roberts et al, 1984).

Rapid-phase variation, whereby E. coli can alternate between nonfimbriated and fimbriated phases, has been demonstrated both in vitro and in vivo (Eisenstein; Kisielius et al; Nowicki et al, 1984; Pere et al). Consequently, strains of bacteria from different sites in the urinary tract can show phenotypic variation in the state of piliation (Kisielius et al). This variation creates a number of ways for bacteria to increase their pathogenic potential by enabling them to adapt to different microenvironments in the host. For example, it may be beneficial for E. coli strains that reach the kidney to "turn off" production of type I fimbriae in order to inhibit recognition and attachment by phagocytes. In vitro, several antibiotics can cause phase variation of P-fimbriated *E. coli* to a nonfimbriated state. Trimethoprim is particularly effective. This may explain, in part, the effectiveness of this antibiotic in low-dose prophylaxis for recurrent urinary infection (Vaisanen et al, 1982). Because of the variability in the phenotypic expression of fimbriae, more recent studies of bacterial virulence have emphasized evaluation of the specific genes that encode for the phenotypic expression of individual virulence factors (Hull et al; Normark et al; O'Hanley et al).

Additional adherence factors have been described. One group, known as X-fimbriae, are also mannose-resistant, but they attach to a completely different human epithelial receptor than P-fimbriae (Labigne-Roussel et al; Vaisanen et al, 1981). Its clinical significance has not been well studied. Another adhesion, Dr hemagglutin, recognizes a receptor on the Dr blood group antigen and has been shown to be a possible virulence factor for cystitis (Nowicki et al, 1989).

Bacterial adherence is only one of several factors believed to have a role in infection. Other bacterial virulence factors and host defense factors may play even a greater role in tissue invasion and inflammation. In an experimental study in mice, the presence of P-fimbriae was found to be necessary for colonization of the upper urinary tract but did not produce tissue invasion unless combined with other virulence factors (O'Hanley et al). Similarly, in a clinical study of children with febrile UTI, there was no difference in the incidence of P-fimbriated *E. coli* in those who had acute inflammatory parenchymal damage documented by DMSA renal scans versus those whose scans were normal, suggesting a role for other virulence factors in producing tissue invasion and damage (Majd et al).

Other Virulence Factors

K Antigen. Capsular polysaccharides afford K antigen specificity to *E. coli*. The quantity of K antigen has been found to be greater in strains recovered from children with pyelonephritis than in those from children with cystitis or healthy controls (Kaijser et al, 1977). K antigen has been shown to shield bacteria from complement lysis and phagocytosis and to enhance persistence of bacteria in the kidneys of experimental mice (Horwitz and Silverstein; Svanborg Edén et al, 1987).

Serum Resistance. In the presence of fresh human serum, many strains of *E. coli* are killed following activation of complement. Complement activation renders bacteria more sensitive to the toxic effects of lysozyme and phagocytosis by leukocytes (Taylor). Serum resistance has been related to virulence of gram-negative bacteria both in UTIs and gram-negative bacteremia (McCabe et al; Olling et al).

Hemolysin. Hemolysins are cytotoxic proteins produced by some strains of *E. coli*. These strains are isolated with greater frequency from patients with bacteremia and urinary infections than from feces of healthy controls (Fried and Wong; Hughes et al). The gene clusters controlling hemolysin production have been identified and are closely linked with mannose-resistance binding, supporting the clonal concept that a few virulent clones of bacteria possess a genetically determined "uropathogenic package" (Low et al). Hemolysin is capable of damaging renal tubular cells in vitro, and hemolytic strains of *E. coli* produce more severe experimental pyelonephritis in mice (Waalwijk et al). However, in one study of children with febrile UTI, there was no difference in hemolysin production between those who had parenchymal inflammatory changes documented by DMSA renal scan compared with those whose scans were normal (Jantausch et al).

Iron-Binding Capacity. Most bacteria require iron for optimal growth and metabolism and have developed mechanisms to acquire iron when there is limited supply. Aerobactin is an iron-binding protein, produced by certain strains of *E. coli*. The ability to manufacture aerobactin has been shown to be associated with increased virulence in epidemiologic studies (Carbonetti et al; Jacobson et al; Orskov et al, 1988). However, it is not known at which stage of the infectious process these strains have an advantage.

Although these virulence factors have been considered separately, the effect of virulence properties appears to be additive. The majority of isolates in patients with nonreflux acute pyelonephritis express three or four virulence properties in contrast to those with cystitis or asymptomatic bacteriuria (Table 10–4) (Lomberg et al, 1984). Interestingly, in this same study, the frequency of P-fimbriae and other virulence factors was significantly diminished

Table 10–4 □ Virulence Factors* in *Escherichia coli* Strains Causing Acute Pyelonephritis (Pyelo), Acute Cystitis, or Asymptomatic Bacteriuria (ABU) and Relationship to Vesicoureteral Reflux

No. of Virulence Factors	Without Reflux (%)			With Reflux (%)		
	Pyelo (*n = 105*)	*Cystitis* (*n = 46*)	*ABU* (*n = 219*)	*Pyelo* (*n = 77*)	*Cystitis* (*n = 10*)	*ABU* (*n = 54*)
0	0%	20%	24%	8%	10%	30%
1	12	24	36	31	20	39
2	13	37	26	26	40	20
3	36	13	10	22	20	7
4	38%	6%	4%	13%	10%	4%

Modified from Lomberg H, Hellström M, Jodal U, et al: Virulence-associated traits in *Escherichia coli* causing first and recurrent episodes of urinary tract infection in children with or without vesicoureteral reflux. J Infect Dis 150:561, 1984.

*Four virulence factors analyzed included one of O antigen groups (O1,O2,O4,O6,O7,O8,O16,O18,O25,O75) commonly associated with pyelonephritis, presence of P-fimbriae, resistance to serum killing, and production of hemolysin.

in patients who had vesicoureteral reflux, implying reduced host resistance. It was suggested that efforts aimed at preventing or treating urinary infection by interfering with "virulent" bacteria, such as by vaccination, may be of less value in patients with recurrent pyelonephritis and reflux, the group in whom renal scars are most likely to develop (Smellie et al, 1981). However, others have not demonstrated a significant difference in virulence traits among pyelonephritogenic strains in patients with and without reflux (Arthur et al).

Renal Scarring

Regardless of the role of virulence factors in the etiology of urinary tract infection, some studies suggest that there may be a paradoxical inverse relationship of bacterial virulence, defined by P-fimbriated binding, and renal scarring. Virulent clones occurred significantly less often in patients with recurrent pyelonephritis who developed renal scarring (22 per cent) than in patients who did not develop renal scars (62 per cent) (Lomberg et al, 1989a). Although the frequency of scarring among girls with vesicoureteral reflux was 57 per cent in contrast to 8 per cent of those without, this alone did not explain the selection of bacteria of low virulence in those patients with scar development. Lomberg et al concluded that reduced host resistance was essential for the tendency to renal scarring after acute pyelonephritis. These studies underscore the complexity of the host-parasite interaction in the etiology of UTIs and renal scarring. The definition of bacterial virulence for acute urinary infection may not necessarily equate with that for renal scarring (Svanborg Edén and de Man). Future studies are needed in order to

further clarify the specific roles of bacterial virulence factors.

HOST DEFENSE FACTORS

Interacting with bacterial virulence properties are an equally complex number of mechanical, hydrodynamic, anti-adherence, receptor-dependent, and immunologic host factors that affect an individual's susceptibility to UTI. These factors are, by necessity, closely interrelated to the pathogenesis of UTIs, beginning with the route of entry of bacteria into the urinary tract.

Route of Entry

Considerable clinical and experimental evidence has clearly established an ascending or retrograde route of entry of bacteria in the majority of UTIs. Ascent of bacteria into the urinary tract begins in the urethra, and the usual organisms are fecal flora that contaminate the perineum (Gruneberg). Stamey (1973) demonstrated that the same bacterial strains causing bladder infections in women with recurrent infections could be found on perineal cultures prior to bladder invasion, in contrast to negative cultures in healthy controls. Similar observations have been reported in children (Bollgren and Winberg, 1976b; Leadbetter and Slavins; Stamey, 1980). The predisposition to perineal colonization in girls and women prone to recurrent infection appears to be related in part to increased bacterial adherence to vaginal and periurethral cells (Fowler and Stamey; Kallenius and Winberg; Schaeffer et al, 1981). It has been postulated that an increased density or expression of receptor sites for attaching bacteria accounts for increased bacterial adherence in patients with recurrent urinary infections (Svanborg Edén and Jodal). Because increased adherence of bacteria to vaginal cells is associated with increased adherence to buccal cells from the same patients, genetic factors may be involved that influence the receptivity of vaginal, buccal, and uroepithelial cells to adhering bacteria (Schaeffer et al, 1981). Furthermore, in the absence of urologic abnormalities, a generalized epithelial defect characterized by diminished antibacterial activity of buccal and uroepithelial cells has been reported in children with recurrent urinary tract infection (Schofer et al).

The exception to the hypothesis of an ascending route of infection may be the newborn, in whom a hematogenous route has been suggested based on the more frequent association of urinary infection with bacteremia in this age group (Ginsburg and McCracken). However, this assumption has been questioned, as other studies have not demonstrated a significantly higher incidence of bacteremia in infants with urinary infections compared with older children (Hellström et al, 1989; Majd et al). Evidence supporting an ascending route of infection in infancy is the recently recognized increased risk for urinary infection in uncircumcised male infants compared with both females and circumcised males. Ginsburg and McCracken first noted that a high percentage (95 per cent) of male infants with UTIs were uncircumcised. Interestingly, prior epidemiologic studies reporting a male predominance in urinary infection in early infancy were from countries where boys were not routinely circumcised (Abbott; Drew and Acton; Winberg et al, 1974). Wiswell et al (1985, 1986) subsequently demonstrated a ten-fold to twenty-fold increase in the incidence of UTIs in uncircumcised male infants compared with males who had been circumcised (Table 10–5). This increased risk appears to extend up until 1 year of age (Herzog), corresponding to the time period when heavier colonization of the prepuce by gram-negative bacteria had been previously noted by others (Bollgren and Winberg, 1976a, 1976b). In vitro studies reveal that pathogenic fimbriated *E. coli* adhere well to the mucosal surface of the prepuce whereas nonpathogenic *E. coli* do not (Fussell et al). Colonization of the prepuce in infant boys as a risk factor for urinary infection suggests an

Table 10–5 □ Incidence of Urinary Tract Infection (UTI) in Female and Circumcised and Uncircumcised Male Infants (0–1 Yr) Born in U.S. Army Hospitals (1974–1983)

	Total No.	No. with UTI	Rate per 1000
All Males	217,116	661	3.0
Circumcised	175,317	193	1.1
Uncircumcised	41,799	468	11.2
Females	205,212	1164	5.7

Modified from Wiswell TE, Roscelli JD: Corroborative evidence for the decreased incidence of urinary tract infections in circumcised male infants. Reproduced with permission of Pediatrics, Vol 78, p 96, © 1986.

ascending route of infection similar to that described in girls. Circumcision may help to prevent urinary infection in male infants by removal of the mucosal surface necessary for bacterial adherence to occur.

The mere presence of bacteria in the periurethral region is not, by itself, sufficient to cause infection. Heavy periurethral colonization with gram-negative bacteria has been reported in 75 to 80 per cent of healthy infants and toddlers of both sexes (Bollgren and Winberg, 1976a), whereas only 1 to 3 per cent became infected (Winberg et al, 1974). The presence of bacteria decreases during the first year of life, becoming rare after 5 years of age. It has been postulated that other host factors are involved that mature during the first year of life, resulting in a decrease of both periurethral colonization and frequency of UTI. The normal bacterial flora of the periurethral area even may be protective against urinary infection by competitive interference with attachment of uropathogenic bacteria (Chan et al, 1984, 1985). This potential protective effect can be altered by the administration of antimicrobial agents, given for any reason. In a study of children with first-time acute pyelonephritis, significantly more children had been recently treated with antibiotics, usually for non–UTIs, compared with controls (Mårild et al, 1989). Other perineal factors that may enhance an individual's propensity to recurrent infection include vaginal pH greater than 4.4 (Stamey and Timothy) and decreased levels of vaginal secretory IgA (Tuttle et al).

Urethra

The short urethra in female infants relative to males appears to be the most ready explanation for the increased incidence of UTIs in girls past the first 6 months of life. Urethral caliber, historically blamed as the pre-eminent factor influencing susceptibility to lower urinary infections in girls, does not play a role. It has long been recognized that intrinsic urethral luminal size is not significantly different in those girls who are bacteriuric and in those who are never infected (Graham et al; Immergut and Wahman). In fact, both of these studies demonstrated that urethral diameter was slightly larger in infected groups than in those never infected.

In the past, passage of bacteria into the bladder has been attributed to turbulent flow during voiding or reflux into the bladder from retrograde closure of the proximal urethra at the completion of voiding (Caine and Edwards; Corriere et al; Hinman, 1966). However, probably more important for urethral ascent of bacteria into the bladder is the ability of uropathogenic bacteria to attach to uroepithelial cells. Similar to the findings with periurethral cells (Kallenius and Winberg), increased adherence of bacteria to uroepithelial cells has been demonstrated in children prone to urinary infections (Svanborg Edén and Jodal). This implies a difference in host receptor density or affinity that influences an individual's susceptibility to infection.

Bladder

Anti-adherence

Once bacteria have reached the bladder, adherence in animals has been shown to be partially inhibited by a thin layer of an acid-sensitive mucopolysaccharide that is thought to be produced locally by transitional epithelium lining the bladder (Parsons et al, 1975, 1977, 1978). Chemical analysis of this mucopolysaccharide has revealed a glycosaminoglycan that is hydrophilic and attracts an aqueous film of water or urine onto its surface (Parsons et al, 1979). Bacteria must penetrate this area in order to attach to specific uroepithelial cell receptors. Using in vivo saline bladder extracts and an in vitro anion exchange resin model, defective anti-adherence activity of the surface mucin layer against invading bacteria has been demonstrated in women and children with recurrent UTIs compared with healthy controls (Ruggieri et al).

Recently recognized is the association of the non-secretor phenotype for blood group antigens and proneness to UTI. As discussed earlier, blood group antigens are a group of carbohydrate determinants found on erythrocytes and certain epithelial tissues, including urothelium. The secretor gene is a regulatory gene that controls the ability to excrete the water-soluble glycoprotein form of the ABO blood group and Lewis antigens into body fluids and determines the terminal oligosaccharide structure in epithelial tissues (Cordon-Cardo et al). In non-secretors, who lack both of these functions, an increased attachment of bacteria to uroepithelial cells and overrepresentation among patients with recurrent UTIs has been noted (Kinane et al; Sheinfeld et al, 1989). The protective effect against adherence in secretors may be due to competive inhibition by free oligosaccharides secreted into the urine that bind to bacteria, thereby preventing their attachment to uroepithelium. Alternatively, the terminal oligosaccharide structure on the uroepithelial cells of secretors may shield uroepithelial receptors from bacteria and thereby inhibit bacterial binding (Lomberg et al, 1989b).

Recently, Sheinfield and associates (1990) reported an increased frequency of UTIs in children with genitourinary structural anomalies whose urothelium reflected the non-secretor phenotype. They suggested that the antigen profile of urothelium influences susceptibility to UTI and that it may prove to be important in identifying patients who would benefit from prophylactic antibiotics or earlier surgical intervention.

Urinary Inhibitory Factors

The urine itself from normal individuals may be inhibitory to bacterial growth and may actually be capable of killing bacteria when the inoculum is small. The most important inhibitory factors of urine are the osmolality, pH, and urea concentration, the latter being the most significant (Kaye). Tamm-Horsfall protein, a glycoprotein secreted by the ascending loop of Henle, may also be protective. This glycoprotein has been shown to be identical to uromucoid or urinary slime (Orskov et al, 1980). It contains abundant mannose residues. In vitro studies have shown adherence of large numbers of *E. coli* with type I (mannose-sensitive) fimbriae to uroepithelial cells coated with uromucoid in contrast to poor adherence to uroepithelial cells devoid of uromucoid (Chick et al). It has been postulated that free Tamm-Horsfall protein in the urine may trap

E. coli possessing type I fimbriae, thereby inhibiting attachment to uroepithelium. A study of UTIs in infants revealed a significantly lower mean concentration of Tamm-Horsfall protein in those with documented *E. coli* infections compared with healthy controls (Israele et al). Further investigation is needed to clarify this hypothetical role for Tamm-Horsfall protein as a host defense factor.

Voiding Dysfunction

The elimination of bacteria from the bladder by frequent and complete bladder emptying plays a significant role in preventing infection (Cox and Hinman). In a group of girls followed with asymptomatic bacteriuria (ABU), the incidence of recurrent bacteria correlated directly to bladder emptying. Average residual volumes in those with ABU was 23.7 ml, whereas the mean residual volume in normal controls was 1.1 ml. On follow-up, recurrences were present in 75 per cent of those with more than 5 ml of residual urine whereas only 17 per cent of those with less than 5 ml of residual urine had recurrences (Lindberg et al, 1975a). Various types of voiding dysfunction have been described in children ranging from the unstable bladder characterized by frequency, urgency, enuresis, and posturing to the infrequent voider who has associated constipation and/or encopresis. Numerous reports have linked dysfunctional voiding and recurrent UTIs (Allen; Hinman, 1974). More recently, attention has also focused on the association between dysfunctional voiding and vesicoureteral reflux in children with recurrent UTI (Koff and Murtagh). The predisposition to recurrent UTIs and vesicoureteral reflux in children with dysfunctional voiding is related to the presence of residual volume resulting from inadequate emptying of the bladder, increased intravesical pressure created by uninhibited bladder contractions, and bladder overdistention from infrequent voiding habits. The establishment of normal voiding habits in these children has been shown to reduce the incidence of recurrent UTIs.

Constipation

Similarly, there is a definite correlation between constipation and recurrent UTIs in children (Neumann et al; O'Regan et al). Although this may occasionally be the result of mechanical factors related to compression of the bladder and bladder neck by a hard mass of stool, it is more likely due to a relationship between constipation and dysfunctional voiding with incomplete bladder emptying. Improvement in bowel habits generally results in a decrease in the incidence of recurrent UTIs in some patients, particularly when coupled with a more normal voiding pattern.

Upper Urinary Tract

Receptors

Bacterial adherence mediated by the presence of P-fimbriae on certain strains of *E. coli* appears to be particularly significant in the pathogenesis of upper tract infections. As discussed earlier, a special class of glycosphingolipids, possessing the Gal 1-4 Gal oligosaccharide, act as receptors for P-fimbriated *E. coli.* (Kallenius et al, 1980; Leffler and Svanborg Edén). These receptors are antigens in the P blood group system. Since the P1 blood group phenotype is overrepresented in children with recurrent pyelonephritis in contrast to normal controls, this suggests that this phenotype increases host susceptibility to pyelonephritis by enhancing bacterial adherence (Lomberg et al, 1983; Tomisawa et al). However, this overrepresentation of the P1 blood group is seen only in patients with pyelonephritis who do not have associated vesicoureteral reflux (Lomberg et al, 1983).

Vesicoureteral Reflux

Vesicoureteral reflux, when present, continues to be the most significant single host risk factor in the etiology of pyelonephritis. In a prospective study of children hospitalized with febrile UTIs, 80 per cent of children with vesicoureteral reflux were found to have acute inflammatory changes on DMSA renal scans, including all with moderate or severe vesicoureteral reflux. In contrast, only 58 per cent of children without vesicoureteral reflux showed acute inflammatory changes (Majd et al).

The presence of vesicoureteral reflux appears to compensate for virulence of *E. coli* in patients with recurrent pyelonephritis (Lomberg et al, 1984). When there is reflux, bacteria do not need special properties, such as attaching ability, to ascend from the bladder to the kidney. In girls with recurrent pyelonephritis, infections were caused by P-fimbriated *E. coli* in only 38 per cent of those with reflux compared with 76 per cent of those without reflux (Lomberg, 1984). The presence of severe vesicoureteral reflux may also result in significant post-voiding residuals, another recognized risk factor in the etiology of infection (Linberg et al, 1975a). Despite the important role the vesicoureteral reflux plays when it is present, some studies have reported that as many as two thirds of children with pyelonephritis do not demonstrate vesicoureteral reflux (Hellström et al, 1989; Majd et al). This underscores the importance of bacterial virulence and other host defense factors in the pathogenesis of acute pyelonephritis in children.

Obstruction

Obstruction and other severe malformations of the upper urinary tract often present with infection and are obvious predisposing factors to renal damage. However, such anomalies are present in only a small minority of children with UTIs. The increased predisposition to infection results from impairment of urinary flow with resultant stasis that compromises bladder and renal defense mechanisms. Obstruction results in an increase in the residual volume of urine in the bladder or dilated urinary tract, permitting the multiplication of bacteria in the urine (Cox and Hinman). It also inhibits the mechanical washout or flushing effect associated with effective micturition or ureteral peristalsis and may alter other local defense factors. All of this results in increased susceptibility of the parenchyma to infection and damage.

Heredity

Evidence that heredity plays a role in determining individual susceptibility to UTI is accumulating. The daughters of mothers who had been bacteriuric in childhood show a higher incidence of UTI, and female siblings tend also to show a higher incidence of bacteriuria (Fennell et al; Gillenwater et al, 1979). In a more recent study of children with first-time pyelonephritis the patients significantly more often had relatives with a history of UTI than did controls (Mårild et al, 1989). Racially dependent differences in the prevalence of UTIs and in the rate of recurrent bacteriuria have also been reported. Kunin et al (1964)

reported a 1.2 per cent bacteriuria prevalence rate in white girls versus a rate of 0.5 per cent in black girls in the same age group. In a retrospective review, the number of black girls evaluated following UTI who were found to have vesicoureteral reflux was one-third that of white girls at an institution where equal numbers of black and white girls were hospitalized (Askari and Belman). This observation was confirmed by a prospective study of patients admitted to this same institution with febrile UTIs (Majd et al).

Immunology

The immunologic response to urinary infection has been studied at both the kidney and bladder level. Understanding the immune response to infection of the urinary tract is particularly important because immunization is currently being explored as a possible means of prevention of recurrent UTIs. The antibody response to infection also has been used diagnostically to localize the level of urinary infection to the upper or lower urinary tract (Hellerstein et al, 1978; Thomas et al, 1974).

Antibody Response

The focus of most of the clinical and experimental immunologic studies of urinary infection has been the immune response to pyelonephritis. During acute pyelonephritis, a systemic antibody response occurs, with antibody production primarily against the O antigen of the infecting bacteria. A lesser response is seen toward the K antigen (Ehrenkranz and Carter, Hanson et al, Kaijser; Kaijser et al, 1973; Winberg et al, 1963). Antibodies of the IgM, IgG, IgA, and secretory IgA type have all been demonstrated in the serum of children and experimental animals with acute pyelonephritis (Mattsby-Baltzer et al; Sohl-Akerlund et al). High IgG, IgA, and secretory IgA antibody levels have also been found in the urine of girls with pyelonephritis (Sohl-Akerlund et al).

Antibody response to pili also has been seen following pyelonephritis (Rene and Silverblatt). Antibody to pili of the secretory IgA and IgG type recovered from the urine of patients with acute pyelonephritis has been shown to prevent in vitro adherence of *E. coli* to human uroepithelial cells (Svanborg Edén and Svennerholm). Mannose-specific interactions between *E. coli* and the carbohydrate moiety of secretory IgA have been reported (Wold et al). Secretory IgA, when bound to the uroepithelium, may thus offer a receptor site for bacteria; when excreted, it may result in competitive inhibition of binding.

The presence of antibodies within the renal parenchyma enhances bacterial opsonization, the process by which bacteria are coated by substances that lead to further phagocytosis. The immune response may also confer immunity against reinfection by the same strain of bacteria. At this time, there is no convincing evidence that an abnormal immune response occurs in patients with pyelonephritis, except possibly in infants under 2 months of age (Winberg et al, 1963).

With regard to the immune response of the bladder to urinary infection, a systemic circulating antibody response to cystitis has not been demonstrated (Clark et al; Sohl-Akerlund et al). However, an elevation of secretory IgA antibody in the urine has been observed in children with UTI, suggesting local antibody production (Sohl-Akerlund et al; Uehling and Stiehm). A more recent study reported a decreased excretion rate of secretory IgA in uninfected children with a history of symptomatic infections compared with healthy controls. However, when these girls were subsequently studied at the time of symptomatic urinary infection, secretory IgA excretion rates were significantly higher than in controls (Fleidner et al). Other evidence supporting a role for secretory IgA as a host defense factor comes from animal studies. Attempts at local immunization of the urinary tract have shown that intravesical immunization is effective against experimentally induced ascending UTI in rats (Kaijser et al, 1978). The presence of secretory IgA in the urine following local bladder or vaginal immunization in rats has been shown to decrease adherence to uroepithelial cells (Uehling et al, 1978, 1982).

Cell-Mediated Immunity

The protective role, if any, of cell-mediated immunity in UTI is controversial (Hahn and Kaufmann). T and B cell lymphocytic response is seen in the kidney during experimental pyelonephritis (Hjelm). However, others have shown a depressed cell-mediated immune response during the early phase of renal infection when bacterial replication is maximal (Miller et al). Although such studies have documented cell-mediated host responsiveness to bacterial infection, they have not defined the role of this process in the pathogenesis of UTI. There is no strong clinical evidence to support an abnormality of cell-mediated immunity in patients prone to UTI. Similarly, in patients with compromised immune systems, an increased susceptibility to UTIs has not been reported. Studies to better define the role of the immune response in UTI are obviously needed.

Vaccine

Much of the significance of clarifying the immune response to UTI relates to the possibility of developing an effective vaccine to prevent urinary infections. Experimental evidence has accumulated to suggest that this may be possible in the future. Protection against experimental ascending pyelonephritis in rats has been demonstrated using isolated capsular antigen to stimulate antibody production directed at K antigen (Kaijser et al, 1983). Similarly, immunization with *E. coli* P-fimbriae in both mice and primates confers protection against ascending pyelonephritis, presumably by interfering with adherence of the organism to the uroepithelium (Pecha et al; Roberts et al, 1984). Immunization of rats with purified *E. coli* type I fimbriae also affords substantial protection against experimental ascending pyelonephritis in rats. (Silverblatt et al, 1982). A potential protective role against renal invasion and damage from immunization with hemolysin has been suggested (O'Hanley et al, 1985). The value of such vaccines to prevent pyelonephritis will be critically assessed only by appropriately controlled clinical trials. The next decade should provide an opportunity to assess this clinical potential.

DIAGNOSIS OF URINARY TRACT INFECTION

Urinary tract infection can be reliably diagnosed only by culture. Symptoms of dysuria, urgency, frequency, and enuresis are nonspecific and may be the result of vulvitis, urethritis, dysfunctional voiding, or nonspecific causes, such as dehydration associated with a febrile illness. In 34 children with lower urinary symptoms alone, urine culture demonstrated significant bacilluria in only 18 per cent; 40 per cent of those with sterile urine had upper respiratory infection (Dickinson). Similarly, Heale et al found that of 378 children with specific urinary complaints, only 14.3 per cent had urinary infection. Thirty-three per cent with flank pain, frequency, and/or dysuria and 31.5 per cent with the recent onset of wetting had UTI, whereas only 4.2 per cent with chronic nocturnal enuresis were infected. Of those without specific complaints, 4.4 per cent had UTI infection (there was little difference from those who were wet only at night).

Urinalysis

Although urinalysis can be helpful in calling attention to those who might be infected, the association of inflammatory cells in the urine by itself is at best only 70 per cent reliable (Ginsburg and McCracken; Kass, 1956) and is oftentimes less reliable (Corman et al; Pryles and Eliot). The finding of significant pyuria on routine urinalysis varies with the volume of urine centrifuged and examined, the force and duration of centrifugation, volume in which cells are resuspended, and observer error (Stamm). Pyuria in the absence of UTI may be found in children following viral immunization (Hart and Cherry) and in association with gastroenteritis (Pryles and Luders).

Microscopy

Urine microscopy for bacteria significantly improves the reliability of urinalysis for the detection of urinary infection, particularly when one combines this with examination of the urinary sediment for pyuria (Robins et al). Jenkins et al reviewed approximately 40 publications reporting urine microscopy for bacteria and found a wide variation in methodology and diagnostic criteria. They concluded that the least reliable method was examination of unstained uncentrifuged urine. When stained centrifuged urine was examined, the sensitivity using the criterion of one or more organisms per oil immersion field was greater than 95 per cent when compared with urine culture growing $\geq 10^5$ colony-forming units (CFUs) per ml. The specificity was at least 95 per cent when more than five organisms per oil immersion field were viewed.

Enzyme Tests

Partly as a result of the technique and operator-dependent variability with urine micros-

copy, a number of rapid enzymatic methods for detection of pyuria or bacteriuria have been developed over the last decade. The two most popular are leukocyte esterase test and the nitrate reductase (Greiss test). These studies are inexpensive, rapid, and easy to perform.

Leukocyte Esterase Test

The leukocyte esterase dipstick test demonstrates the presence of pyuria by histochemical methods that specifically detect esterases in the neutrophils. When compared with chamber count methods, studies have revealed a sensitivity of 88 to 95 per cent for detection of pyuria using a cutoff of 10 or more leukocytes/mm^2 (Gillenwater; Kusumi et al). Similar good results have been obtained in comparisons with less quantitative examinations of urinary sediment (Gelbart et al; Loo et al). The test is not interpretable when the dipstick is discolored by blood, bilirubin, rifampin, or nitrofurantoin. This test is probably no more reliable for the diagnosis of UTI than the finding of pyuria on urinalysis.

Nitrite Test

The nitrite method employs reagent paper impregnated with sulfanilic acid and alpha-naphthylamine. Nitrite diazotizes the sulfanilic acid, which then reacts with the alpha-naphthylamine to form a red azo dye. Given adequate contact, bacteria convert nitrate, normally present in the urine, to nitrite. Thus, a positive colorimetric reaction implies the presence of bacteria in the bladder. However, a relatively long incubation period (4 hours) is required for conversion of nitrate to nitrite. For this reason, the first morning urine sample is really the best specimen for this test. A single test done on randomly collected urine specimens was reported to have a sensitivity of only 29.2 to 44.9 per cent on 790 urine specimens using dipsticks from two manufacturers; however, the specificity was 98 per cent when the test was positive (James et al). This test has not proved to be a reliable office screening method when used alone (Marr and Traisman).

Combined Nitrite–Leukocyte Esterase Test

Combining the leukocyte esterase test and the nitrite test on a single dipstick* has im-

---

*Chemstrip LN, Bio-Dynamics Division of Boehringer Mannheim Diagnostics, Indianapolis.

proved the ability to detect or exclude UTI. In a review of rapid methods to detect urinary tract infections, Pezzlo reported a sensitivity for the combined nitrate-leukocyte esterase strips of 78 to 92 per cent and a specificity of 60 to 98 per cent. The accuracy of the test is affected by the probability that an individual is infected based on clinical symptoms (Bolann et al). According to these studies, it may be reasonable to eliminate urine culture when the dipstick test is negative and when the index of suspicion based on clinical symptoms is low. However, specimens for urine culture should be obtained in all patients with positive test findings or in any patient when the clinical index of suspicion is high, regardless of the dipstick results.

Filtration Test

Recent use of a filtration system in conjunction with a colorimetric test for bacteria has been used with both a semi-automated* and a simpler manual method† for rapid screening of urine specimens. A sample of urine is passed through an electronegatively charged filter pad that traps bacteria and white blood cells. Safranin O dye is then used to strain the trapped cells. Both tests can be performed in approximately 1 minute with a cost of $1.00 to $1.25 per test. The average sensitivity reported from seven studies evaluating the semi-automated Bac-T-Screen was 93.8 per cent (range 88.2 to 98 per cent) compared with urine cultures growing $\geq 10^5$ CFU/ml. The average negative predictive value was 97.5 per cent (range 94 to 97 per cent). False-positive rates often exceeded 25 per cent (Pezzlo).

In a report of 1198 randomly collected specimens, the simpler manual FiltraCheck–UTI system had a sensitivity of 96.5 per cent and a negative predictive value of 99.1 per cent when compared with urine cultures yielding $\geq 10^5$ CFU/ml (Longoria and Gonzalez). Both of these tests are uninterpretable in a small percentage of patients because of clogging of the filter. Although these easily performed and inexpensive tests may be useful in excluding the need for urine cultures in patients with negative results, the high false-positive rate mandates that a urine specimen for culture be obtained whenever a test is positive or when the results are uninterpretable as a result of clogging of the filter.

*Bac-T-Screen, Vitek Systems, Inc., Hazelwood, Mo.
†FiltraCheck–UTI, Vitek Systems, Inc.

Urine Culture

Specimen Collection

In the pre–toilet-trained group, the urine specimen is often initially obtained by applying a collection bag (U-Bag) to the perineum. Although this method has been justifiably criticized as producing a high rate of contamination, the technique is reliable when the specimen for culture is negative. Contamination is directly related to the length of time the collection device remains applied to the child. If a specimen has not been obtained within 30 minutes of application, reliability begins to fall. Removing the appliance and plating or refrigerating the urine immediately after the child voids is paramount. Having the parent apply the bag before leaving for the physician's office in an effort to shorten the wait is acceptable only when the specimen for culture is negative. Confirmation of all positive urine specimens for culture collected by the external appliance technique is advisable prior to treatment. Invasive means (catheterization or suprapubic aspiration) should be employed when the clinical situation dictates the necessity for immediate treatment.

When a clean specimen is difficult or impossible to obtain or the institution of therapy is urgent, urine should be collected by catheterization or direct bladder (suprapubic) aspiration (SPA). A feeding tube (8 to 10 Fr.) is ideal for catheterizations (Fig. 10–3). SPA has

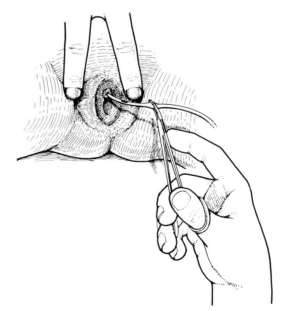

Figure 10–3 □ Sterile urethral catheterization for collection of a urine specimen for culture.

achieved great popularity in pediatric circles. This is most likely a response to the negative reputation urethral catheterization has gained through the years. Young children are particularly favorable candidates for SPA because of the abdominal location of their urinary bladders. However, the procedure cannot be expected to be successful when the bladder is empty. Therefore, a requirement for attempting aspiration is a palpable bladder. This requirement is the major drawback of SPA. If urine is not obtained initially, repeated attempts at aspiration should be delayed until such time as the bladder has filled.

SPA is performed after first cleaning the suprapubic area with an antiseptic solution. A 21- to 25-gauge needle is inserted perpendicular to the patient in the midline one fingerbreadth above the symphysis (Fig. 10–4). Although a local anesthetic can first be infiltrated, this appears not to be necessary and may actually cause more pain than a quick in-and-out aspiration. It is practical to apply a U-Bag to the perineum prior to cleansing the abdomen. Many times the child voids during preparation for aspiration, obviating the necessity for that procedure if the voided urine is immediately plated or refrigerated.

It has been stated that "any number of bacteria" obtained by suprapubic bladder puncture are significant (Kunin, 1987). Since the bladder is a reservoir and this method of

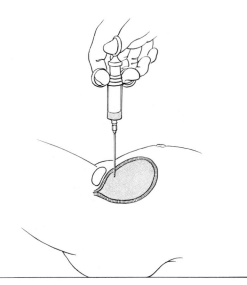

Figure 10–4 □ Suprapublic aspiration for collection of bladder urine with a full bladder. The needle is inserted 2 cm cephalad to the symphysis perpendicular to the axis of the child.

collection depicts the number of bacteria in that reservoir, one should not anticipate colony counts significantly different from those properly collected by other means and then handled in a similar manner. Ginsburg and McCracken demonstrated greater than 100,000 CFU/ml in 96 per cent and 40,000 to 80,000 colonies in the remaining 4 per cent of 100 infants, 5 days to 8 months of age, with bacilluria demonstrated on SPA. None showed fewer than 40,000 colonies. Nelson and Peters had previously reported similar results in a study of premature and term infants. Colony counts from the bladder of less than 10,000 are suspect regardless of the manner in which that urine was collected.

Reported complications resulting from SPA are few, although transient hematuria is common. Pelvic hematomas requiring transfusion have been noted (Morrell et al). Additionally, a report of two cases of abdominal wall abscesses following aspiration of intestinal contents reinforces the conclusion that a palpable bladder is an absolute prerequisite (Polnay et al).

Culture Techniques

The calibrated loop culture techniques of the bacteriology laboratory are supplemented by less complicated and less expensive methods applicable to standard office use. No matter the method of culture, the most significant determinant of the interpretive value of the findings on that culture is the time between collection of the specimen and inoculation into the culture medium (Fig. 10–5). If it is anticipated that inoculation is to be delayed for more than 10 minutes, the specimen should be immediately refrigerated or placed in an ice bath. Urine transported from the patient's home to the office or from the office to the laboratory should be kept in a cold environment.

Two commonly used office culture methods are the dipstick pad culture and the dip-slide method.

Dipstick Pad. This test employs a clear plastic strip with one chemical reagent pad impregnated with nitrite-sensitive dye and two pads impregnated with culture media. One of these two media supports only the growth of gram-negative organisms, making it possible to recognize false positive findings based on gram-positive contaminants. A semiquantitative colony count is achieved by comparison at

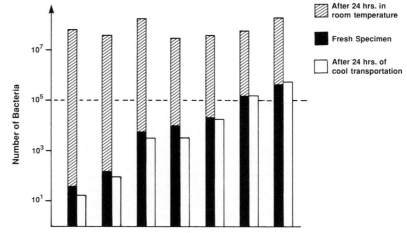

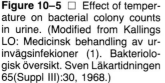

Figure 10–5 □ Effect of temperature on bacterial colony counts in urine. (Modified from Kallings LO: Medicinsk behandling av urinvägsinfekioner (1). Bakteriologisk översikt. Sven Läkartidningen 65(Suppl III):30, 1968.)

24 to 48 hours with a set of standards. This method correlates fairly accurately in the presence of infection (80 to 90 per cent) and is associated with a low incidence of false-negative results (Craig et al; Gillenwater et al, 1976; Winter).

Dip-Slide. Slides are coated with culture media. Numerous methods are available that also allow for subculturing if antibiotic sensitivities are indicated. A distinction can be made between gram-negative and gram-positive organisms with the different medium on each side of the slide. The accuracy of the slide method is comparable to that of the standard loop technique routinely used for quantitative cultures (Arneil et al). As in all culture techniques, accuracy depends on the rapidity of inoculation and experience in interpretation.

"Significant" Bacteriuria

The definition of significant bacteriuria, using the criteria established by Kass in 1957 of $\geq 100,000$ CFU/ml, has continued to be the most practical cutoff point for establishing the diagnosis of urinary tract infection in children. More than 95 per cent of children with UTI show culture yields greater than 100,000 CFU/ml (Ginsburg and McCracken), and most show colony counts exceeding 10^6 (Kunin, 1987). In almost all of the remainder, colony counts are greater than 10^4. Recent evidence in young adult women suggest that symptomatic lower UTIs (acute urethral syndrome) are often associated with lower "significant" counts of 10^2 to 10^3, confirmed by suprapubic aspiration or catheterization. More than 90 per cent of these

young women had pyuria, and repeated cultures revealed persistent bacteriuria (Stamm et al). Similar findings have not been reported in other age groups but might be expected in sexually active adolescents. In one study of screening bacteriuria in preadolescent girls, borderline bacterial counts between 10,000 and 50,000 CFU/ml were no more predictive of the subsequent development of new cases of urinary infection (defined by $\geq 10^6$ CFU/ml) than were bacterial counts $< 10,000$ CFU/ml (Walten and Kunin).

CLINICAL PRESENTATION AND LOCALIZATION

As one would anticipate, the classic signs and symptoms for UTI do not present themselves in the very young. Instead, nonspecific symptoms, such as irritability, poor feeding, failure to gain weight, vomiting, and diarrhea, may be the only signs suggestive of an underlying problem (Table 10–6). In one study of children with symptomatic urinary infections, only 9 per cent of 78 infants were initially referred with a suspected diagnosis of UTI (Smellie et al, 1964). Often absent in neonates, fever is present in most infants between 1 and 12 months (Winberg et al, 1974). A screening urine specimen for culture should be obtained whenever a nonverbal, non–toilet-trained child presents with unexplained fever.

As the child becomes verbal and is toilet-trained, urinary tract symptomatology is more easily detected. Fever continues to be relatively common in toddlers with first-time symptomatic infections. However, fever is not as

Table 10–6 □ Prominent Symptoms in Neonatal*
Nonobstructive Urinary Tract Infection (n = 75)

Symptom	Per Cent
Weight loss†	76
Fever	49
Cyanosis or gray color	40
Distended abdomen	16
CNS symptoms (purulent meningitis not included)	23
Generalized convulsions	7
Purulent meningitis	8
Jaundice (conjugated bilirubin increased)	7
Other	16

From Harrison JH, Gittes RF, Perlmutter AD, et al: Campbell's
Urology, 4th ed. Vol. 1. Philadelphia, WB Saunders Co, 1978.
*Zero to 30 days old.
†Registered for only 46 patients falling ill on days 0 to 10.
Weight loss was not explained by vomiting, diarrhea, or refusal to
eat.
Abbreviation: CNS, central nervous system.

frequently associated with recurrent and/or
long-standing infection. In older children, urgency, frequency, enuresis, and dysuria are
common presenting symptoms. Failure to become toilet-trained at the proper age may
occasionally herald underlying chronic lower
urinary infection. It is clear, however, that
these lower tract symptoms do not always
represent bacterial infection and may be the
result of vulvitis, urethritis, or dysfunctional
voiding. For example, the daytime urinary
frequency syndrome of childhood is characterized by severe daytime urgency and frequency
associated with voiding of small amounts of
urine. This syndrome is not associated with
infection, pyuria, or increased incidence of
underlying uropathology (Koff and Byard). It
is a self-limiting condition and is presumed to
be stress-related. Consequently, antibiotics
and anticholinergics are usually not beneficial.

There are few population-based studies of
symptomatic UTIs in childhood. The classic
epidemiologic study by Winberg et al (1974)
was carried out between 1960 and 1966 in
Goteborg, Sweden. The special organizational
structure of that city's pediatric medical care
has afforded unique opportunities to perform
ongoing epidemiologic studies of UTIs in children. Jodal (1987) reported a similar prospective epidemiologic study conducted in Goteborg from 1970 to 1979. There were 952
females and 225 male (4.2:1) below age 10
years of age who were treated for a first-time
symptomatic urinary infection (Fig. 10–6). Of
the 225 boys, 59 per cent presented during the
first year of life. The number of boys diagnosed

in the higher age groups was low, especially
over age 5. The number of first infections in
girls was also highest in the first year of life
(19 per cent). A gradual decrease in number
of girls with first-time infections was associated
with increasing age. In both girls and boys,
febrile infections, presumed to be pyelonephritis, predominated during the first year of
life. Acute cystitis was most commonly seen
between 2 and 5 years of age in both sexes,
with a marked peak frequency in girls during
the third year of life. As expected, infections
during infancy were the most difficult to characterize as pyelonephritis or cystitis.

Cystitis

Acute cystitis in children is rarely associated
with significant long-term morbidity. Typical
symptoms that accompany acute cystitis in
toilet-trained children include dysuria, frequency, urgency, and/or secondary-onset enuresis. Fever and systemic complaints are generally not a feature of the clinical picture. As
previously mentioned, however, these same
irritative lower tract symptoms are often seen
in the absence of bacterial cystitis, mandating
that a specimen for urine culture be obtained
prior to institution of therapy. Although the
recurrence rate of lower UTIs is high, most
cases can be considered little more than a
nuisance and recurrences tend to disappear by
adolescence. It is worth noting that many children prone to recurrent lower UTIs have voiding dysfunction, particularly infrequent voiding. Typically, these children do not void for
1 or 2 hours after awakening in the morning
and then may void only two or three times
throughout the day. Consequently, bladder
capacity is abnormally large and bladder emptying is often incomplete. Often these children
also have a history of chronic constipation.

Slightly fewer than 10 per cent of girls susceptible to urinary infection go on to have
recurrences virtually at the completion of each
course of antibiotic therapy. These children
have chronic symptoms of bladder instability
characterized by severe frequency, urgency,
and urge incontinence. Squatting or posturing
in response to unstable bladder contractions is
common in this group (Fig. 10–7). Many of
these children have chronic inflammatory
changes of the bladder. Endoscopically, multiple raised "cysts" are seen in the area of the
bladder neck and trigone. Histologically, sub-

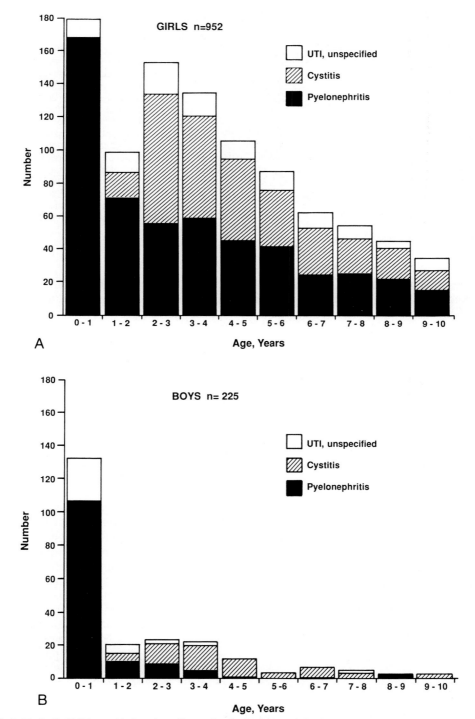

Figure 10–6 □ *A, B,* Children with first-time diagnosis of urinary tract infection at the Children's Hospital in Goteborg, Sweden, from 1970 to 1979 according to age and clinical diagnosis. (From Jodal U: Host risk factors in pyelonephritis. *In* Pyelonephritis: Pathogenesis and Management Update. Edited by HG Rushton, Dialogues in Pediatric Urology (Ehrlich RM, ed). Pearl River, NY, William J Miller Associates, 13:4, 1990.)

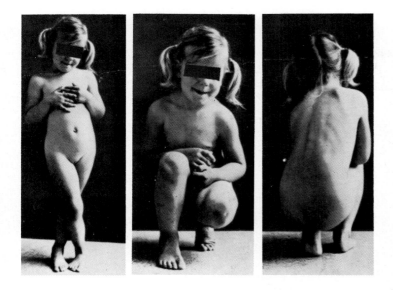

Figure 10–7 □ Typical posturing of child with the *urge syndrome,* characterized by an unpredictable urge to void, often associated with urge incontinence. To avoid wetting, the child assumes a posture that provides for external urethral compression, usually by squatting onto one heel until the urgency disappears. The urge incontinence is often associated with diurnal or nocturnal enuresis and may be associated with infection in some cases, although for many children the syndrome appears to be an abnormality of micturition. (From DeJonge GA: The urge syndrome. *In* Bladder Control and Enuresis. Edited by I Kolvin, RC MacKeith, SR Meadow. London, W. Heinemann Medical Books, Ltd. 1973.)

mucosal lymphoid follicles are present (Fig. 10–8). Clinically, this entity has been termed cystitis cystica, although the histologic appearance suggests it would be more accurately referred to as cystitis follicularis. The presence of these follicles suggests an immunologic response to chronic infection (Uehling and King).

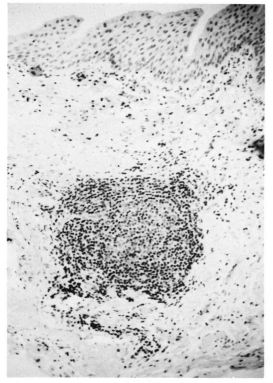

Figure 10–8 □ "Cystitis cystica." Submucosal lymphoid follicle (cystitis follicularis) is typical of the histologic changes seen in children with long-standing cystitis. (From Belman AB, Kaplan GW: Genitourinary Problems in Pediatrics. Philadelphia, WB Saunders Co, 1981.)

Asymptomatic Bacteriuria

The natural history and uroradiographic findings in patients with asymptomatic or covert bacteriuria vary according to the age of the patient and prior episodes of symptomatic infections. Screening bacteriuria does not necessarily represent asymptomatic bacteriuria, as approximately one third of school-aged girls with screening bacteriuria have a prior history of UTIs. It is unclear whether the prognosis is any different for children who have primary asymptomatic bacteriuria compared with those in whom asymptomatic bacteriuria develops after treatment of a symptomatic infection.

A study of asymptomatic and symptomatic bacteriuria in infants under 1 year of age reveals interesting differences in the two populations (Jodal, 1987). Among those with symptomatic infections, one patient had a significant ureteropelvic junction obstruction and 14 of 39 (36 per cent) had vesicoureteral reflux, including three with grade III or greater. In patients with asymptomatic bacteriuria, only mild reflux (grades I to II) was found, occurring in five of 46 (11 per cent). In two of 50 patients with asymptomatic bacteriuria, clinical acute pyelonephritis developed within 2 weeks of detection. In 37 of 45 left untreated, the bacteriuria cleared spontaneously and seven others became abacteriuric following antibiotic treatment for other reasons. Although asymptomatic recurrences developed later in six (13 per cent) no pyelonephritic recurrences occurred in this group during follow-up of at least 1 year and follow-up urography, done in 36, did not reveal any evidence of renal scarring. In contrast, in the symptomatic group, 14 of 40 (35 per cent) experienced recurrences, including six with acute pyelonephritis and three with cystitis, whereas asymptomatic bacteriuria was noted in five. It was concluded that infants with asymptomatic bacteriuria represent a low-risk group with a tendency to spontaneously become abacteriuric, usually within a few months.

Considerable variation in uroradiographic findings has been reported in school-aged children found to have bacteriuria on screening. These studies have reported vesicoureteral reflux in 19 to 35 per cent and renal scarring in 10 to 26 per cent (Kunin et al, 1964; Lindberg et al, 1975b; McLachlan et al; Newcastle Group; Savage et al). However, many of these children have a prior history of symptomatic UTIs and others undoubtedly had infections during infancy that were overlooked or misdiagnosed. The risk for development of acute pyelonephritis in a girl older than 4 years of age with untreated asymptomatic bacteriuria is small and seems to be associated with a change in bacterial strain, perhaps as a result of antibiotic treatment (Lindberg et al, 1978). Follow-up by the Cardiff-Oxford Bacteriuria Study Group revealed that those schoolchildren who presented initially with a radiographically normal urinary tract remained normal in spite of persistent asymptomatic bacteriuria. Only in those children who had previous renal scarring did new scars or progression of scarring develop, and all of these children had vesicoureteral reflux. Other studies have shown that asymptomatic bacteriuria is associated with low-virulence bacterial strains lacking the ability to adhere and cause symptoms (Kallenius et al, 1981; Svanborg Edén et al, 1976, 1978). These organisms may be commensal with the host and may even protect against infection by more virulent strains. Based on this information, it is reasonable that asymptomatic bacteriuria, particularly in older girls, be left untreated (Hannsson et al; Svanborg Edén et al, 1978).

Pyelonephritis

Over the last decade, experimental and clinical observations have provided us with consider-able insight into the pathogenesis of pyelonephritis and renal scarring. The potential morbidity of urinary infection in children has led to our current recognition of the importance of early diagnosis, appropriate antibiotic management, and complete evaluation of the urinary tract of children with documented infections. A brief review of the pathogenesis of pyelonephritis and renal scarring is fundamental to the rationale for evaluation and management of children with UTI.

Pathogenesis

Experimental studies by Roberts (1983) and others clearly suggest that the same acute inflammatory response that is responsible for the eradication of bacteria is also responsible for the damage to renal tissue and subsequent renal scarring. Through a series of experimental studies using the primate model, Roberts has developed a unified theory of the chain of events involved in the process that ultimately leads to renal scarring (Fig. 10–9). The initiating event is bacterial inoculation of the renal parenchyma, which elicits both an immune and inflammatory response. Whereas the immune response can be elicited by either live or heat-killed bacteria, the acute inflammatory response occurs only following inoculation by live bacteria (Roberts et al, 1981). Since heat-killed bacteria do not cause renal scarring, it appears that it is the acute inflammatory response that is more important in the subsequent development of permanent renal damage.

The inflammatory response of pyelonephritis

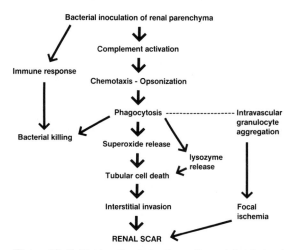

Figure 10–9 □ Hypothesis for the pathogenetic chain of events in acute pyelonephritis. (Modified from Roberts JA: Pathogenesis of pyelonephritis. J Urol 129:1102, 1983. © by Williams & Wilkins, 1983.)

is triggered by complement activation from bacterial lipopolysaccharides. This leads to chemotactic migration of granulocytes to the site of infection. Intravascular granulocyte aggregation occurs that, along with edema, creates focal ischemia (Kaack et al, 1986). The offending bacteria are phagocytized by the granulocyte, initiating a sequence of events. Direct bacterial killing by the granulocytes occurs. Simultaneously, toxic enzymes, such as lysozymes, are released both within the granulocyte and into the lumen of the renal tubules, causing damage to tubular epithelium. At the same time, the respiratory burst occurs, a phenomenon universal to acute inflammatory responses. This releases superoxide, which generates oxygen radicals that are toxic not only to the bacteria but also to the granulocytes and surrounding tubular cells (Roberts et al, 1982). Tubular cell death results, releasing the inflammatory response into the interstitium, causing even further damage. It is this interstitial damage from both toxic enzymes and ischemia that ultimately leads to renal scarring.

Renal Scarring

Most of our clinical knowledge regarding renal scarring is derived from studies of patients with vesicoureteral reflux. Older reports have shown that as many as 30 to 60 per cent of children with reflux and a history of symptomatic UTIs have scarring at the time of their initial evaluation (Smellie et al, 1975). Investigations conducted over a more recent time period suggest that the incidence of scarring may not be as high, perhaps reflecting the current trend toward more aggressive diagnosis and antibiotic management (Skoog et al).

The onset of renal scarring is usually an event that occurs early in life, usually before age 5 and most frequently under 3 years of age (McLachlan et al; Pylkkanen et al; Winberg et al, 1982). However, renal scarring is rarely demonstrated in neonates with symptomatic infections, even in the presence of vesicoureteral reflux (Table 10–7) (Abbott;

Table 10–7 □ Renal Scarring in Males at Time of "First" Urinary Tract Infection (UTI)

Age at First UTI	No.	No. with Scarring
1–30 days	54	0
2–12 mo	62	1
1–16 yr	44	11 (25%)

Modified from Winberg J, Bollgren I, Kallenius G, et al: Clinical pyelonephritis and focal renal scarring. Pediatr Clin North Am 29:801, 1982.

Table 10–8 □ Renal Scarring Compared with Grade of Reflux*

Grade of Reflux	Per Cent with Scarring†
1	5
2	6
3	17
4	25
5	50

Modified from Skoog SJ, Belman AB, Majd M: A nonsurgical approach to the management of primary vesicoureteral reflux. J Urol 138:441, 1987. © by Williams & Wilkins, 1987.
*Total number of kidneys evaluated = 804.
†Total number of kidneys with scarring = 97 (12%).

Drew and Acton; Winberg et al, 1982). Although rare, scarring may be acquired in older children (Smellie et al, 1985). New or progressive scarring is almost always associated with a history of UTI. The correlation between the severity of vesicoureteral reflux and renal scarring is also well established (Table 10–8) (Bisset et al; Jodal, 1987; Skoog et al). Scarring has even been reported in 3.5 to 5 per cent of children without vesicoureteral reflux who have had symptomatic urinary infection (Hellström et al, 1989; Jodal, 1987). The critical role that infection plays in the pathogenesis of renal scarring associated with reflux was clarified in Ransley and Risdon's classic experimental studies of vesicoureteral reflux in piglets (Ransley and Risdon, 1978). They demonstrated that in the face of vesicoureteral reflux and normal voiding pressures, renal scarring occurs only when urinary infection is present. Reflux in the absence of infection caused renal changes *only* when bladder outlet resistance was increased, so that obstruction, not reflux, was the pathophysiologic explanation for renal damage. It was suggested that the portions of the kidney at risk for scarring are those susceptible to pyelotubular backflow (intrarenal reflux) based on papillary morphology and configuration (Fig. 10–10).

Experimental studies and clinical experience have shown that a single episode of pyelonephritis can lead to significant renal damage (Fig. 10–11) (Ransley and Risdon, 1981; Smellie et al, 1985). Furthermore, a clear association between the number of pyelonephritic attacks and incidence of renal scarring has been reported (Fig. 10–12) (Jodal, 1987; Smellie et al, 1985). Both experimental and clinical studies have also shown that some renal scarring can be prevented or diminished by early antibiotic treatment of acute pyelonephritis (Figs. 10–13 and 10–14) (Glauser et al; Ransley and Risdon, 1981; Winberg et al, 1982; Winter et al). Furthermore, when reflux is

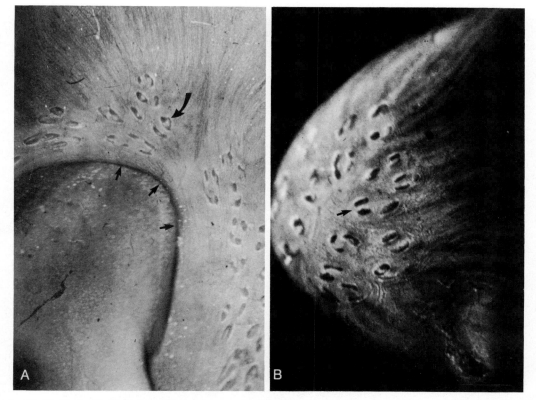

Figure 10–10 □ *A,* "Refluxing" papilla is compound with concave area cribosa *(arrows)* and gaping oval to round orifices of collecting ducts *(curved arrows). B,* "Nonrefluxing" simple papilla has conical configuration and slit-like orifices of collecting ducts *(arrow).* (From Rushton HG, Majd M, Chandra R, Yim D: Evaluation of 99m technetium-dimercaptosuccinic acid renal scans in experimental acute pyelonephritis in piglets. J Urol 140:1169, 1988. © by Williams & Wilkins, 1988.)

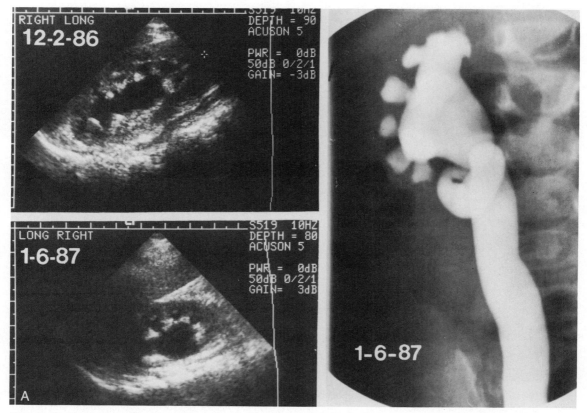

Figure 10–11 □ The patient is a 9-month-old girl who was admitted with an acute "first-time" febrile urinary tract infection (UTI).

A, Initial sonogram shows mild hydronephrosis of right kidney. Renal length measures 7.2 cm. Voiding cystourethrogram demonstrates right grade IV vesicoureteral reflux. Follow-up sonogram 5 weeks later reveals generalized scarring and contraction of right kidney, which now measures only 4.9 cm in length.

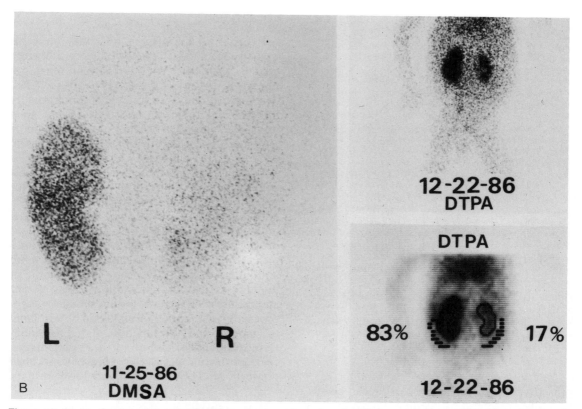

Figure 10–11 □ *Continued B,* Initial DMSA renal scan at time of acute UTI demonstrates marked diffuse decrease in uptake by right kidney consistent with generalized acute pyelonephritis. Three weeks later, a DTPA renal scan shows a small right kidney, which contributes only 17 per cent of total renal function.

Figure 10–12 □ Relationship of renal scarring to number of episodes of acute pyelonephritis. (Modified from Jodal U: The natural history of bacteriuria in childhood. Infect Dis Clin North Am 1:713, 1987.)

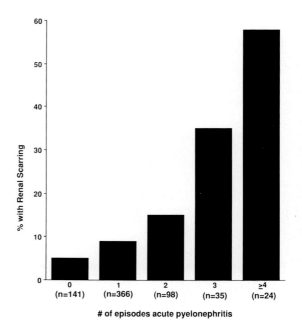

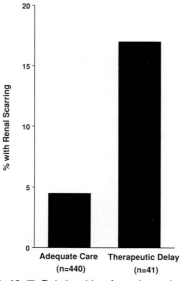

Figure 10–13 □ Relationship of renal scarring to adequate care in contrast to therapeutic delay at "first" infection. (Modified from Winberg J, Boillgren I, Kallenius G, et al: Clinical pyelonephritis and focal renal scarring. Pediatr Clin North Am 29:801, 1982.)

present, progressive renal scarring can be successfully prevented by keeping the patient free of infection (Bellinger and Duckett; Edwards et al; Skoog et al). Based on all of the above, it is clear that infection, not reflux alone, is a prerequisite for acquired renal scarring.

Localization

Infection of the urinary tract may be localized to the bladder (cystitis), upper collecting system (ureteritis, pyelitis), and/or renal parenchyma (pyelonephritis) (Fig. 10–15). The diagnosis of acute pyelonephritis traditionally has been made on the basis of classic clinical signs and symptoms of fever and flank pain or tenderness associated with pyuria and positive urine culture. However, accurate diagnosis using these clinical parameters often is difficult, especially in children (Busch and Huland). Neonates and infants in particular frequently present with nonspecific clinical findings (Winberg et al, 1974), and all too often the diagnosis is obscured by improper urine collection techniques or prior empiric antibiotic therapy. Accurate identification of upper UTI and documentation of the extent and progression of renal parenchymal damage, especially in young children, aid in determining the appropriate therapeutic regimens, long-term risks, and follow-up of these patients.

Direct techniques have been used to localize the level of UTI to the upper or lower urinary tract. These include split-urine cultures collected by ureteral catheterization (Stamey et al, 1965), the bladder washout test (Fairley et al), or thin-needle aspiration of renal pelvic urine under ultrasonic guidance. Although these efforts may accurately localize infection

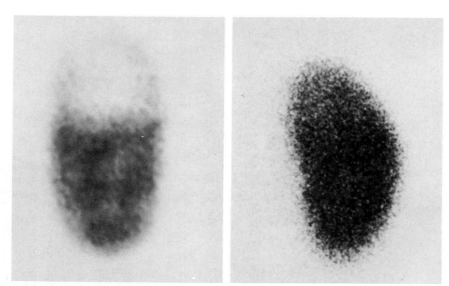

Figure 10–14 □ An 11-month-old boy presented with an acute febrile urinary tract infection.
Left, DMSA renal scan at the time of acute infection reveals severe acute pyelonephritis of the right upper pole. Typical findings of acute pyelonephritis are a decrease in uptake of DMSA with preservation of normal renal contour.
Right, Seven months later, a follow-up DMSA renal scan reveals resolution of pyelonephritis without residual scarring.

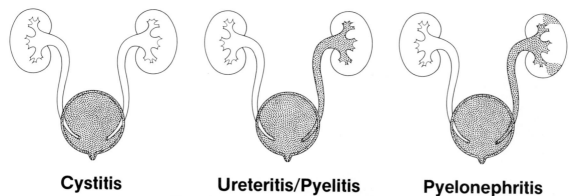

Cystitis   **Ureteritis/Pyelitis**   **Pyelonephritis**

Figure 10–15 □ Sites of acute urinary infection.

to the upper or lower urinary tract, they are obviously invasive and do not offer direct evidence of the presence or extent of parenchymal involvement. In other words, these tests cannot differentiate infection of the upper collecting systems (ureteritis, pyelitis) from pyelonephritis.

Numerous studies using various laboratory techniques for localization of urinary infection to the upper or lower urinary tract, such as elevated serum C-reactive protein and erythrocyte sedimentation rate (ESR) (Hellerstein et al, 1982; Jodal et al; Wientzen et al), increased urinary excretion of beta-2 microglobulin (Schardijn et al), presence of antibody-coated bacteria in the urine sediment (Hellerstein et al, 1978; Thomas et al, 1974), and elevated urinary lactic dehydrogenase isoenzymes (Lorentz and Resnick) have been reported. For a variety of reasons, including lack of specificity, impracticality, unreliability, and/or nonavailability, these have not gained widespread acceptance for the evaluation of children with acute UTIs (Durbin and Peter; Hellerstein et al, 1982, 1988; Lorentz and Resnick). Furthermore, none of these techniques provides any information regarding renal function or the extent of parenchymal involvement during acute pyelonephritis.

Several imaging modalities have been used for localization of acute infections of the lower or upper tract. Excretory urography (IVP) has been of limited value in establishing the diagnosis of acute pyelonephritis (Silver et al). Two clinical studies comparing ultrasonography, IVP, and technetium-99m glucoheptonate scintigraphy to detect renal parenchymal involvement in acute UTIs in children found IVP and ultrasonography to be far less sensitive than renal cortical scintigraphy with Tc-

99m glucoheptonate (Sty et al; Traisman et al). Computed tomography (CT) has also been used to establish the diagnosis of acute pyelonephritis in children (Greenfield and Montgomery). In these clinical reports, the various imaging modalities have been compared retrospectively with signs and symptoms such as fever, flank pain, and routine laboratory studies. However, these same clinical signs and symptoms have been shown to correlate poorly with direct localization studies (Busch and Huland).

Gallium-67 imaging has also been used to localize the site of urinary infection. One study that compared gallium scans with split ureteral catheterization and bladder washout studies report an accuracy rate of 85 per cent (Hurwitz et al). Gallium scintigraphy, however, does not provide any information regarding renal function or the extent of parenchymal damage; it exposes the metaphyseal growth complex to higher doses of radiation compared with cortical scintigraphy, and the study takes at least 6 to 24 hours to complete (Conway; Thomas et al, 1983).

An experimental study in piglets compared renal cortical imaging using Tc-99m DMSA (dimercaptosuccinic acid) directly with histopathologic findings of acute pyelonephritis. Typical pyelonephritic lesions were characterized by a focal decrease in uptake of isotope with preservation of the renal contour (Fig. 10–16). The DMSA renal scan was found to be a highly sensitive and reliable imaging modality for detection and localization of experimental acute pyelonephritis, with a sensitivity of 87 per cent and overall agreement rate of 94 per cent (Rushton et al, 1988). The only lesions that were not detected were microscopic foci of inflammation not associated with

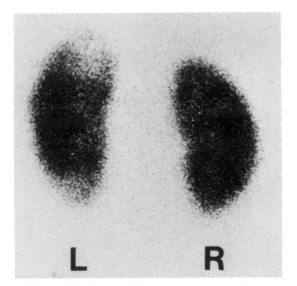

Figure 10–16 □ Posterior view of DMSA renal scan in piglet with acute pyelonephritis demonstrates upper and lower pole acute pyelonephritis characterized by focal decreased uptake of DMSA with preservation of normal renal contour.

significant parenchymal damage and not evident on gross inspection. DMSA renal cortical scintigraphy also provides reliable information regarding renal function and has been shown to be superior to IVP for the detection of chronic pyelonephritic scarring (Goldraich et al; Merrick et al), thus making it an ideal study for monitoring both the extent and progression of renal damage resulting from the acute pyelonephritic episode.

Renal Abscess

Renal abscesses, a rare form of renal infection, in the past were generally not thought to be caused by ascending infection. *Staphylococcus aureus,* historically, has been the offending organism, and in many cases a peripheral cutaneous site of origin could be localized (Rote et al). Diagnosis is often delayed in these patients because urine cultures are negative in most. With the advent of effective antistaphylococcal therapy, this complication of staphylococcal bacteremia has decreased. More cases of gram-negative infections in the presence of vesicoureteral reflux or other anatomic abnormalities of the urinary tract are now being seen (Timmons and Perlmutter).

Most patients with a renal abscess present with high fever, leukocytosis, and an elevated ESR, often accompanied by flank pain. A variety of imaging techniques have been used to diagnose renal abscesses, including IVP and angiography (Koehler), gallium-67 scintigraphy (Hopkins et al; Kumar et al), sonography and CT (Gerzof and Gale) (Fig. 10–17). The classic treatment of renal abscesses has been surgical drainage in addition to appropriate antibiotic therapy. However, improved antibiotics and diagnostic techniques, together with the ability to obtain a culture by percutaneous aspiration or drainage under ultrasonic control, have often obviated the necessity for surgery (Fig. 10–18) (Gerzof and Gale; Pederson et al). In seven patients reported by Schiff et al, 10 days of parenteral antibiotic treatment alone followed by an additional 2 weeks of appropriate oral therapy was successful.

Xanthogranulomatous Pyelonephritis

Xanthogranulomatous pyelonephritis is an atypical form of severe chronic renal parenchymal infection characterized by unilateral destruction of parenchyma and accumulation of lipid-laden foamy macrophages (xanthoma cells) either surrounding abscess cavities or as discrete yellow nodules. More than 50 cases of xanthogranulomatous pyelonephritis have been reported in children (Schulman and Denis; Watson et al; Yazaki et al). Age of presentation has ranged from infancy to 16 years. Most patients present with nonspecific symptoms of chronic infection, including weight loss, recurrent fever, failure to thrive,

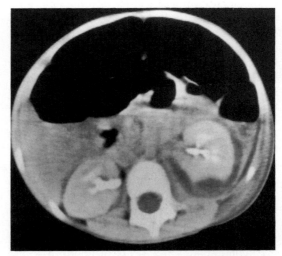

Figure 10–17 □ CT scan reveals a filling defect in upper pole of left kidney consistent with a renal abscess in a child with flank pain and fever.

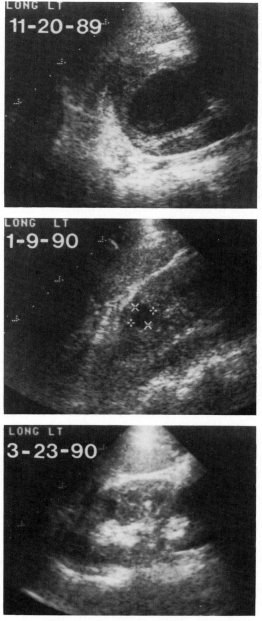

Figure 10–18 □ Sonogram in a 16-year-old girl who presented with fever and flank pain. *Top,* Sonolucent mass in the left upper pole consistent with a renal abscess. Needle aspiration under sonographic guidance yielded purulent material that grew *Escherichia coli.* Following 2 weeks of parenteral and 4 weeks of oral antibiotic therapy, sonograms 7 weeks later *(middle)* and 17 weeks later *(bottom)* show progressive resolution of abscess cavity.

pallor, and lethargy (Watson et al), although those with the focal form are often in good medical condition (Yazaki et al). A palpable abdominal mass is present in approximately one third of patients. Bacterial specimens for culture can be obtained from the urine or renal abscess in the majority of cases, with *Proteus* being the most common organism isolated.

Both diffuse and focal forms of the disease have been reported, with the focal form being more common in children than in adults (Schulman et al; Watson et al). The pathologic and radiologic differences between focal and diffuse xanthogranulomatous pyelonephritis have been described (Bagley et al). Radiographic evaluation in the diffuse form of the disease often reveals nonfunction of the involved kidney. Calcification or stones may be present, although this is less common in the focal form of the disease. Characteristic sonographic or CT appearances of xanthogranulomatous pyelonephritis also have been reported (Subramanyam et al). However, these features are nonspecific and often mimic neoplasia or other forms of chronic inflammatory renal parenchymal disease. Consequently, the correct diagnosis is seldom made preoperatively (Malek and Elder). Nephrectomy is curative, although partial nephrectomy may be adequate in focal disease, assuming that the diagnosis can be established. No incidence of recurrence in the contralateral kidney has been reported.

EVALUATION

Recommendations for evaluation of UTIs in children vary. The current trend toward early evaluation of young children following their first documented UTI is based on both experimental and clinical studies. Epidemiologic data collected by Kunin (1970) in school-aged girls revealed that reinfection occurs within 18 months in as many as 80 per cent of all white girls and in 60 per cent of black girls. Radiographic studies of girls with symptomatic urinary infection have revealed the presence of vesicoureteral reflux in approximately 35 per cent of cases (Smellie et al, 1975). The relative incidence of vesicoureteral reflux in black girls with UTI is about one-third that of whites (Askari and Belman, 1982). Unfortunately, other clinical parameters have proved unreliable in distinguishing those children with UTIs who also have reflux (Smellie et al, 1981).

Both clinical and experimental studies have proved that significant renal scarring can occur after a single UTI (Ransley and Risdon, 1981; Smellie et al, 1985). A higher incidence of renal scarring has been reported in children with vesicoureteral reflux and recurrent UTIs than in those with reflux who have had only a single infection (Jodal, 1987; Smellie et al, 1981; Winberg et al, 1975). Furthermore, the nonspecificity of signs and symptoms that typically accompany urinary infection in infants and toddlers often makes it impossible to determine whether an infection actually represents the first episode (Winberg et al, 1974). All of the aforementioned factors offer abundant reasons to pursue early evaluation of young children following their first documented UTI. Waiting until the child has had two or more urinary infections before proceeding with evaluation clearly increases the risk that permanent scarring (which might otherwise have been prevented) may occur.

Radiographic evaluation should be pursued after the first culture documented UTI in all boys and all white girls younger than 6 years of age. Furthermore, all girls with febrile or recurrent infections should be evaluated, regardless of age. In view of the decreased incidence of vesicoureteral reflux in the black population, evaluation of black girls might well be reserved for infants and those with febrile infection or uncontrollable recurrences.

Imaging

Recommended imaging studies for a child with a history of a culture-documented UTI are based, to some extent, on the experience of the radiologist and the availability of imaging modalities. However, evaluation should always include a cystogram to detect the presence of vesicoureteral reflux, ureteroceles, posterior urethral valves in boys, or bladder wall thickening and an examination of the upper tracts to look for obstruction, hydronephrosis, or other congenital malformations (Blickman et al).

Timing of Evaluation

The timing of evaluation is often a concern of the urologist, radiologist, and pediatrician. Children requiring hospitalization should at least be screened for obstruction with an ultrasound scan prior to discharge. It has been suggested that cystography be delayed 4 to 6 weeks following the acute infection to avoid demonstrating transient mild reflux secondary to inflammatory changes of the ureterovesical junction. However, it is rare for reflux to be detected during infection and then to disappear after treatment (Gross and Lebowitz). Furthermore, since the significance of reflux is greatest at the time of bacterial infection, demonstration of even transient reflux may be very meaningful. One potential disadvantage of obtaining a cystogram early in the course of a febrile infection is that ureteral dilatation secondary to the effect of endotoxins may result in overestimation of the grade of reflux (Hellström et al, 1987; Roberts, 1975). Nevertheless, a prolonged "waiting period" is not necessary. The cystogram can be performed whenever the patient is no longer symptomatic and when the urine is sterile (Lebowitz and Mandell, 1987). Regardless of when studies are performed, antibiotic prophylaxis should be maintained until that time, particularly in infants or in children with a previous febrile UTI, in order to prevent reinfection (Lebowitz and Mandell, 1987; Smellie et al, 1985).

Cystography

A contrast voiding cystourethrogram (as opposed to an isotope cystogram) with a preliminary radiograph (plain film) is indicated in all boys to exclude urethral pathology as well as vesicoureteral reflux. The spine should also be carefully inspected, and one should note the amount of stool present in the colon. Although visualization of the urethra in females is rarely helpful except in the unusual case of a refluxing ectopic ureter, a contrast cystogram may also be preferred for the initial evaluation in order to allow for grading of vesicoureteral reflux, if present. Several classifications have been used to grade vesicoureteral reflux. The scheme shown in Fig. 10–19 is widely accepted and has been endorsed by the International Reflux Study (1981). Isotope cystography, with its reduced radiation exposure and high sensitivity, is the best choice for a follow-up evaluation of children with known reflux and in documenting the results of antireflux surgery (Willi and Treves). It is also recommended in screening for sibling reflux (Lebowitz and Mandell, 1987). Regardless of one's preference, cystography should not be performed with the child under anesthesia because the information derived from the static cystogram is vastly inferior to that obtained with a dynamic voiding study (Lebowitz).

Upper Tract Imaging

Recommendations for evaluating the upper urinary tract in children presenting with UTI also vary from institution to institution. The

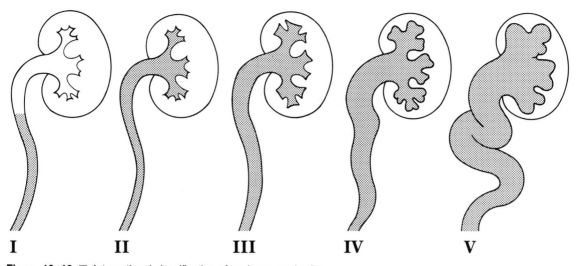

Figure 10–19 □ International classification of vesicoureteral reflux.
Grade I, Ureter only.
Grade II, Ureter, pelvis, calyces; no dilatation, normal calyceal fornices.
Grade III, mild or moderate dilatation and/or tortuosity of the ureter, and mild or moderate dilatation of the pelvis, but *no* or *slight* blunting of the fornices.
Grade IV, Moderate dilatation and/or tortuosity of ureter and mild dilatation of renal pelvis and calyces; complete obliteration of sharp angle of fornices but maintenance of papillary impressions in majority of calyces.
Grade V, Gross dilatation and tortuosity of ureter; gross dilatation of renal pelvis and calyces; papillary impressions are no longer visible in majority of calyces.
(Modified from International Reflux Committee: Medical versus surgical treatment of primary vesicoureteral reflux. Reproduced with permission from Pediatrics, Vol 67, p 392, © 1981.)

ideal study should be painless, safe, cost-effective, and associated with minimal or no radiation and yet should be capable of detecting clinically significant structural malformations as well as renal scarring. Unfortunately, such an all-encompassing study does not exist.

One approach is initial screening of all patients being evaluated for a history of UTI with a renal-bladder sonogram (Kangarloo et al). In children, sonography has been found to be as sensitive as IVP for the detection of any significant renal abnormality except for uncomplicated duplication anomalies and focal renal scarring (Horgan et al; Jequier et al; Kangarloo et al; Leonidas et al). Sonography is painless, noninvasive, simple to perform, radiation-free, and independent of renal function. It is critical that appropriate images of the ureters, bladder, and true pelvis be *routinely* obtained in order to detect the presence of ureteroceles or dilated ureters secondary to ureteral ectopia, ureterovesical junction obstruction, or severe vesicoureteral reflux. To do so, the bladder should be full during the examination. A post-voiding residual also can be demonstrated at the completion of the study. No further imaging of the urinary tract is required if both the cystogram and renal-bladder sonogram are normal.

In the absence of reflux, hydronephrosis revealed by sonography is best evaluated with diuretic renography using Tc-99m DTPA (diethylenetriaminepentaacetic acid) or Tc-99m MAG-3 (mercaptoacetyltriglycine) (Majd). Although the renal scan lacks the anatomic resolution of IVP, it has several advantages. The furosemide-enhanced renal scan, combined with computer analysis, can provide quantitative assessment of both renal function and drainage of the dilated collecting system (Kass et al). Evaluation of these two parameters more objectively differentiates nonobstructive dilatation from true obstruction compared with IVP. When combined with the findings of the renal-bladder sonogram, the site of obstruction can be reliably determined in almost all cases. When needed, further evaluation is best accomplished with percutaneous antegrade pyelography and pressure-perfusion studies (Whitaker test). The choice between diuretic renography or IVP in the evaluation of nonrefluxing hydronephrosis is determined in part by the availability of and experience with these imaging modalities (see Chapter 4).

Those children who are found to have vesicoureteral reflux are further evaluated with a cortical renal scan, using either Tc-99m labeled

DMSA or glucoheptonate, or with IVP to detect focal or generalized renal scarring. Merrick et al compared DMSA and glucoheptonate renal scans with IVP in 79 children who had proven urinary tract infection and who had been observed for a period of 1 to 4 years. The sensitivity of IVP for detection of pyelonephritic scarring in this group of patients was 86 per cent and specificity was 92 per cent, whereas renal cortical scintigraphy demonstrated a sensitivity of 96 per cent and a specificity of 98 per cent. Similar findings were reported by Goldraich et al in a more recent study of 202 children with documented UTI and vesicoureteral reflux. In addition to greater sensitivity and specificity for detection of renal scarring, cortical scintigraphy also provides quantitative assessment of differential renal function (Bingham and Maisey, Gordon; Handmaker; Majd). Since DMSA is a radionuclide agent that is fixed by renal tubules with only minimal excretion, it is optimal for morphologic visualization of functioning renal parenchyma and is considered the cortical scanning agent of choice for demonstrating postinflammatory renal scars (Fig. 10–20) (Goldraich et al; Gordon; Merrick et al).

Some authors have recommended a more tailored approach to the evaluation of children with UTI, beginning with a voiding cystogram (Ben-Ami et al; Blickman et al). If no reflux is present, a renal ultrasound scan is done to exclude hydronephrosis or other upper tract malformations. Otherwise, if reflux is demon-

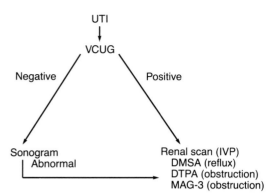

Figure 10–21 □ Algorithm for evaluation of children with urinary tract infection (UTI).

strated, the next study would be a renal cortical scan or IVP to detect renal scarring. This approach seems reasonable for the majority of cases (Fig. 10–21).

In the febrile child, renal cortical scanning, using either Tc-99m-labeled DMSA or glucoheptonate, has been recommended as a means to evaluate those suspected of having acute pyelonephritis. Both clinical and experimental studies have shown that cortical scintigraphy is highly reliable for detection of acute inflammatory changes of pyelonephritis (Handmaker; Rushton et al, 1988; Sty et al; Traisman et al). Cortical scintigraphy not only confirms the diagnosis of pyelonephritis, particularly in those children who are otherwise difficult to diagnose, but also identifies those patients who are at risk for subsequent renal scarring (Fig. 10–22) (Rushton et al, 1990). Generally, screening sonography should precede cortical scintigraphy in the acutely ill child (Reid et al).

TREATMENT

The obvious goals of treatment of UTI are symptomatic relief and prevention of new or progressive renal damage, especially in infants and young children who are at greatest risk for renal scarring. Initial treatment, ideally, should be based on in vitro sensitivity studies. Frequently, such testing is not done or treatment is instituted before the results are available. Fortunately, because the common uropathogens are susceptible to multiple antibiotics and the response to antibiotics correlates best with urine levels that are usually more highly concentrated than serum levels (Stamey et al, 1974), high cure rates have been reported in most therapeutic trials.

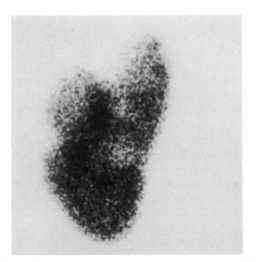

Figure 10–20 □ Left posterior oblique view of DMSA renal scan reveals renal scarring, characterized by loss of functioning cortex, involving the upper pole and mid zone of the left kidney.

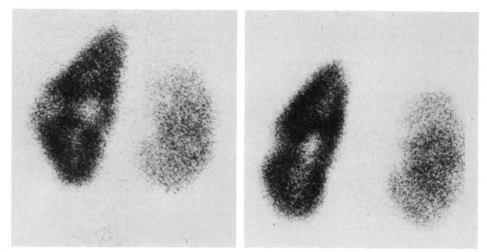

Figure 10–22 □ DMSA renal scan in a 13-month-old girl who presented with an acute febrile urinary tract infection.
Left, Left posterior oblique view on initial DMSA scan demonstrates acute pyelonephritis involving the mid zone of the left kidney with typical findings of a focal decrease in uptake of DMSA with preservation of the normal renal contour.
Right, Follow-up DMSA scan reveals progression to renal scar characterized by contraction and loss of functioning renal cortex.
(From Rushton HG, Majd M, Jantausch B, et al: Renal scarring following reflux and nonreflux pyelonephritis. J Urol, in press).

Uncomplicated Lower Urinary Tract Infection

Agents that have been used successfully for acute, uncomplicated lower urinary infections include sulfonamides, trimethoprim-sulfamethoxazole (TMP-SMX), nitrofurantoin, trimethoprim, and oral cephalosporins (see Appendix). Unfortunately, ampicillin and amoxicillin are used commonly by primary health care physicians. High intestinal levels of these two antibiotics often result in rapid development of resistant enteric organisms, which then become the reinfecting bacteria.

The emergence of resistant strains to ampicillin or amoxicillin has also limited its initial efficacy in treating urinary infections compared with other antibiotics (Rajkumar et al). This drawback of the synthetic penicillins has been diminished by the relatively recent combination of clavulanic acid with amoxicillin (Augmentin). Clavulanic acid inhibits the bacterial beta-lactamase enzymes, which render the beta-lactamic antibiotics ineffective. This combination has proved effective in eradication of UTIs in children, even when in vitro susceptibility testing demonstrates resistance to amoxicillin alone (Roomi et al; Ruberto et al, 1989). However, ampicillin-clavulanic acid is associated with a high incidence of side effects, is expensive, and is no more effective than the usual drugs.

A new class of oral antibacterials, the fluoroquinolones, have been shown to have a wide spectrum of activity that includes most grampositive and gram-negative organisms, including *Pseudomonas aeruginosa* and *Proteus* (Barry et al). These are bactericidal agents and are believed to work by inhibiting the essential bacterial enzyme deoxyribonucleic acid (DNA) gyrase, which is essential for DNA replication in bacterial cells (Hooper et al). Concern regarding adverse arthropathic effects, based on animal studies showing cartilage toxicity, has prevented its approval for use in children (Schluter). However, the same experimental toxic effects have been reported with all quinolones, including nalidixic acid, which is licensed for use and has been widely used in children (Bouissou et al). A retrospective match-controlled study of nalidixic acid in 11 children treated for 10 to 600 days with follow-up examination 3 to 12 years later did not reveal any differences in arthropathic adverse effects compared with controls (Schaad and Wedgwood-Krucko). Furthermore, clinical evidence of cartilage toxicity has not been reported in more than 100 children with cystic fibrosis treated with varying courses of high-dose ciprofloxacin (Ball). Despite the lack of clinical evidence demonstrating cartilage toxicity in children, the use of fluoroquinolones in growing children generally should be avoided until definitive studies have been performed.

Duration of Treatment

The optimal duration of treatment of acute uncomplicated lower UTIs in children is controversial. Several randomized, controlled studies have been published reporting the use of single-dose or short-course antimicrobial therapy in children. The potential advantages of short-course therapy include decreased costs, improved compliance, decreased antibiotic-related side effects, and decreased effect on the fecal flora. In 1982, Shapiro reviewed eight published studies of short-course therapy for urinary infection in children. It was concluded that although many children with uncomplicated lower UTIs would respond favorably to abbreviated regimens, the inability to distinguish easily those with cystitis from those with pyelonephritis and the relatively small number of children evaluated with short-course therapy precluded its routine use in children.

In 1988, Moffatt and associates reported a methodologic analysis by four independent reviewers of the eight reports reviewed by Shapiro and six subsequent randomized, controlled trials of short-course antimicrobial therapy for uncomplicated lower UTIs in children. Short-course therapy varied in these 14 studies, with nine using single-dose, one using 1-day, three using 3-day, and one using 4-day treatment. Conventional therapy ranged from 7 to 10 days. In two, short-course therapy was less effective. One study compared single-dose versus 10-day amoxicillin therapy (Avner et al), and one compared 1-day versus 10-day cefadroxil therapy (McCracken et al). The other 12 studies showed no difference in outcome. Interestingly, inadequate sample size was the major methodologic flaw in all except the two that reported a decreased efficacy in short-course treatment. The authors concluded that there is still insufficient evidence to recommend short-course therapy for UTIs in children.

A subsequent large clinical study reported 132 children with culture-documented "first-time" acute UTI who were randomly assigned to receive TMP-SMX in one dose, two doses daily for 3 days, or two doses daily for 7 days. There was no difference in bacteriologic cure rate for single-dose (93 per cent) versus multidose regimens (96 per cent). However, significantly higher recurrence rates at 10 to 12 or 28 to 37 days after treatment were found in the single-dose group (20.5 per cent) compared

with the 3-day (5.6 per cent) and 7-day (8 per cent) groups (Madrigal et al).

Another large study of 110 children with UTIs revealed no difference in initial cure or subsequent relapse rates in children treated with relatively short-course (3-day) therapy versus conventional therapy (10 days) using either cotrimoxazole or nitrofurantoin (Ruberto et al, 1984). At this time, the author considers it reasonable to treat acute *lower uncomplicated* infections in children with a "relatively" short 3- to 5-day course of antibiotics. However, young children with first-time infection should then continue to receive low-dose antimicrobial prophylaxis until radiographic evaluation is completed.

Asymptomatic Bacteriuria

Treatment of asymptomatic bacteriuria does not appear to be necessary if the urinary tract is otherwise normal (Eichenwald; Hannson et al; White). The risk for pyelonephritis in infants and young girls with untreated asymptomatic bacteriuria is small, and many demonstrate spontaneous remission. (Jodal, 1987; Winberg et al, 1974). A 4-year follow-up by the Cardiff-Oxford Bacteriuria Study Group did not reveal any new or progressive renal scarring in children 5 to 12 years of age with untreated covert bacteriuria except when vesicoureteral reflux was present. Furthermore, treatment of patients with asymptomatic bacteriuria is followed by a high recurrence rate up to 80 per cent (Kunin, 1970). Most are caused by new strains, which may carry the risk of being more virulent (Bergström et al, 1967; McGeachie). In contrast, studies have shown that asymptomatic bacteriuria is generally associated with low-virulence bacterial strains lacking the ability to adhere and cause symptoms (Kallenius et al, 1981; Svanborg Edén et al, 1976, 1978).

Pyelonephritis

The child with suspected pyelonephritis requires a greater degree of assurance of immediate therapeutic success, since the degree of scarring and renal damage resulting from an infection may be influenced by the rapidity of effective therapy (Glauser et al; Ransley and Risdon, 1981; Winberg et al, 1982; Winter et al). Oral medication can be initiated in older children who are not septic or vomiting as long as good compliance is ensured. Trimethoprim-sulfamethoxazole can be anticipated to be effective in most cases. Cephalosporins are also a good choice for initial therapy in the febrile child who does not require parenteral therapy. Treatment can be changed to include less expensive agents when the antibiotic sensitivities become available.

The toxic child and infants under 2 years of age with suspected pyelonephritis are candidates for immediate parenteral therapy. Also, young children with acute parenchymal damage documented by DMSA cortical scintigraphy should be considered for parenteral therapy to reduce the likelihood of subsequent irreversible renal scarring. After appropriate specimens for cultures have been obtained, combination therapy, including an aminoglycoside and synthetic penicillin, is initiated until culture and sensitivity results are known. Alternatively, one of the new third-generation cephalosporins may be used (see Appendix), but these are more expensive and do not provide comprehensive coverage of gram-positive organisms, including enterococcus. Antibiotic therapy should be continued for 10 to 14 days, although oral therapy can be substituted for parenteral treatment of sensitive organisms after the patient has been afebrile for 48 to 72 hours. Follow-up specimens for urine culture should be obtained at the completion of therapy, and prophylaxis should be instituted until evaluation of the urinary tract is completed.

Prophylaxis

Long-term, continuous antibiotic prophylaxis is recommended in children with vesicoureteral reflux (particularly under 8 years of age), those with frequent symptomatic recurrences, or those with endoscopically demonstrated cystitis cystica (cystitis follicularis). Antibiotic prophylaxis should also be considered in young children (under age 3) with non-reflux acute pyelonephritis when acute or chronic renal damage is documented by cortical scintigraphy. These children, in particular, appear to have bacterial virulence-host defense factors that place them at significant risk for pyelonephritic damage.

In children with vesicoureteral reflux, prophylaxis is usually continued until the reflux spontaneously resolves or is surgically corrected. Some advocate stopping prophylaxis in children older than 8 years of age who have low-grade vesicoureteral reflux. Girls with a history of UTI should be advised of the importance of surveillance urine cultures during pregnancy because they are at risk for pyelonephritis, which may be associated with increased rates of low-birth-weight infants and perinatal mortality (Norden and Kass). This is true regardless of whether or not reflux is present (Gillenwater et al, 1979). Even those who underwent successful surgical correction of reflux during childhood have been reported to be at increased risk for pyelonephritis during pregnancy (Austenfeld and Snow).

Children with recurrent symptomatic infections (three in 6 months, four in a year) or cystitis cystica should remain on prophylaxis for a minimum of 6 to 12 months. Periodic urine specimens for culture should be obtained every 3 to 6 months to monitor the success of prophylaxis. Medication should then be reinstituted for an additional 12 months if infection recurs within 3 months of discontinuation. It is not necessary to discontinue treatment to obtain urine specimens for culture. When breakthrough infection occurs, the offending organism will be resistant to the current agent; therefore, the culture media will not be sterilized by the excreted drug.

Although prophylaxis effectively prevents infection, it cannot be expected to reduce the recurrence rate of urinary infection after therapy has been discontinued. Stansfeld (1975) conducted a trial of prophylaxis in children using TMP-SMX. All the children were treated for 2 weeks and then were randomized to receive no treatment or 6 months of prophylaxis. Although prophylaxis was highly effective in preventing infection, the rate of recurrent infection after stopping prophylaxis was virtually identical to that observed after 2 weeks of treatment. Similarly, Smellie et al (1976) reported a high recurrence rate (42 per cent) in children with a history of recurrent urinary infections following discontinuation of long-term antimicrobial prophylaxis. In those with cystitis cystica (cystitis follicularis), 80 per cent experienced recurrences within 1 year after 6 to 12 months of continuous prophylaxis (Belman, 1978). Nevertheless, it is helpful to achieve an infection-free period in those children with a history of multiple, symptomatic urinary infections. During this period of time, aggressive efforts should be made to improve the voiding pattern in those children who have clinical evidence of dysfunctional voiding, a common finding in this difficult group of patients. Antimicrobials with proved efficacy in the prevention of recurrent urinary infections include nitrofurantoin (Smellie et al, 1978), TMP-SMX (Smellie et al, 1976), and TMP alone (Lidin-Janson, et al; Smellie et al, 1982; White). Pure SMX is less effective, and synthetic penicillins are particularly poor prophylactic agents because of the frequent emergence of resistant organisms.

Prophylactic doses are generally less than those used to treat acute infection. Smellie et al (1976, 1978) effectively used SMX, 10 mg, plus TMP, 2 mg/kg/day, or nitrofurantoin, 1 to 2 mg/kg/day in one to two doses. My practice is to administer one third to one half of the therapeutic dose once or twice daily. Requesting a twice-daily dose schedule has a pragmatic advantage: If one dose is missed, the child still receives some medication each day; however, in a highly compulsive family, a single nighttime dosage schedule is usually effective. It should be noted that Harding et al reported successful prevention of recurrent infection in preadolescent girls with low-dose TMP-SMX administered only three times per week.

Treatment in Renal Failure

The dynamics of antibiotic detoxification and excretion are usually deranged in the child with renal failure. Antibacterial doses need to be adjusted in such patients to avoid adverse reactions. Certain drugs—those that are dependent on renal function for efficacy—are useless in these patients. The frequency of administration of those drugs that are effective in the face of renal failure—rather than their dosages—should be modified based on the degree of renal insufficiency.

Specific Therapy

In addition to appropriate antimicrobial therapy, other factors must be taken into consideration in patient management. Voiding frequency and control of constipation are the two most common variables that are readily changeable and may be the most important in effecting changes in susceptibility to infection.

Establishing a voiding schedule in small children may be extremely difficult and may provoke conflict in the parent-child relationship. The physician can interject his or her influence by explaining the treatment goal to the child and requesting that a regular voiding pattern be instituted and maintained. These children should be told that they will be reminded by their parents to void regularly and that they should follow this request even if they do not feel the urge to void at that time.

For constipation, an intensive therapeutic approach is often required. Initially, in severe cases, enemas given for several days may be necessary to disrupt a high fecal impaction and relax an overstretched colon. Increased intake of fiber and fluid and regular toilet habits must then be instituted. In refractory cases, regular use of a fiber-based laxative may be necessary. In most cases, these are long-term requirements, and failure to continue this regimen generally results in recurrence of both constipation and urinary tract infection.

The most severe voiding problems in the otherwise normal child are associated with uninhibited bladder activity and *Hinman's syndrome* (non-neuropathic voiding dyssynergia). Recognition and differentiation of this entity from neuropathic disease are mandatory. Treatment with anticholinergics and antibiotic prophylaxis has been demonstrated to be more effective than antibiotics alone, both in reducing the frequency of recurrent urinary infections and in accelerating the resolution of associated reflux (Koff and Murtagh).

The management of infection associated with obstruction is usually determined by the type of obstructive anomaly and is beyond the scope of this chapter. Urinary stasis for any other reason needs to be addressed if infection cannot be otherwise controlled with antibiotic prophylaxis. Causes may include severe reflux with secondary poor bladder emptying (megacystis-megaureter syndrome), dilatation in the absence of obstruction, bladder diverticula, or residual ureteral stumps. Since otherwise unexplained urinary infection is so common, it is incumbent upon the physician to document the influence of any of these entities on infection prior to recommending surgical correction; for example, a specimen for culture may be obtained by needle aspiration of a dilated, nonobstructed upper collecting system to ascertain its involvement prior to surgical revision.

The role of the female urethra in UTI historically was one of the most controversial subjects in pediatric urology. The "mechanical school" advocated that UTI was the result of voiding problems secondary to urethral obstruction, resistance, or turbulence. However, as Graham et al and Immergut and Wahman demonstrated years ago, the urethral caliber of girls with infection is slightly larger than those of age-matched controls. Nevertheless, the practice of urethral dilation, meatotomy, and urethrotomy continues to be practiced by a few.

Hendry et al and Van Gool and Tanagho found that the incidence of recurrence of urinary infection was not affected by urethral dilation. Both reports concluded that a dysfunctioning voiding cycle can be disrupted by overstretching the urethra but that the same results can probably be achieved with control of infection using antibacterials and institution of a regular voiding schedule aided by anticholinergic therapy. Govan et al reported no decreased recurrence rate of urinary infection in a group of girls observed 3 years before and after urethral dilation, and Kaplan et al found

no difference between controls and a group subjected to dilation who both received antibacterial prophylaxis for 3 months. Forbes et al found no change in either voiding patterns or recurrent infection rates in girls subjected to urethral meatotomy alone.

Earlier studies suggested a possible beneficial role for internal urethrotomy in the treatment of girls with recurrent urinary infections. (Halverstadt and Leadbetter; Immergut and Gilbert). However, subsequent blinded, prospective studies have not demonstrated a significant difference in the incidence of urinary infections in girls subjected to urethrotomy compared with those receiving medication alone (Busch et al; Kaplan et al). Therefore, it appears that urethral manipulation in girls is rarely, if ever, necessary. In the absence of significant anatomic abnormalities that necessitate further diagnostic evaluation, the roles of cystoscopy, urethral calibration, dilation, meatotomy, and urethrotomy in the current practice of pediatric urology are minimal.

APPENDIX: ANTIBACTERIAL AGENTS

Sulfonamides

Sulfonamides act by competitively blocking the conversion of para-aminobenzoic acid to folic acid (Feingold). About 75 per cent of the oral dose is absorbed. Free sulfonamide is excreted by filtration and tubular secretion. Although high tissue levels are not achieved, excellent urine levels result. Sulfonamides are most effective against *E. coli* but also may be effective against other gram-negative and gram-positive organisms.

Sulfonamides are well tolerated by children, are inexpensive, and produce few side effects. They affect the gastrointestinal flora when used for long-term prophylaxis but are effective agents for short-term acute therapy of uncomplicated infections. They displace protein-bound bilirubin and hence in the neonate have the potential to interfere with bilirubin excretion and cause jaundice. Once the infant has passed through the period of "physiologic jaundice," these agents can be utilized safely. Some patients are allergic to sulfa, but fortunately most reactions are of a minor cutaneous nature, such as urticaria. There have been some problems with major hypersensitivity reactions, such as the Stevens-Johnson syndrome, but these are rare. The most widely

used agent is sulfisoxazole employed in a dose of 120 to 150 mg/kg of body weight per day, given acutely in four to six divided doses orally (Behrman and Vaughan).

Nitrofurantoin

Nitrofurantoin is quite useful in the treatment of simple cystitis and is also a very effective agent for long-term, low-dose prophylaxis. It is thought to interfere with early stages of the bacterial Krebs cycle (AMA Drug Evaluations). It is well absorbed from the gastrointestinal tract and has minimal effect on bowel flora. Tissue levels are low because it is excreted almost entirely in the urine by glomerular filtration. Urinary levels tend to be quite high. Urinary alkalinization increases urine levels, whereas acidification increases tissue levels. It works well against most *E. coli* and enterococci but is not particularly effective against *Klebsiella, Proteus,* or *Pseudomonas.*

Nausea and vomiting are frequent troublesome side effects in children; however, these can be minimized by administering the agent immediately following a meal or by utilizing nitrofurantoin macrocrystals supplied in capsule form. For the small child, the contents of the capsule can be emptied and administered in potatoes or applesauce.

In neonates nitrofurantoin has the potential to cause a hemolytic anemia because of glutathione instability. Consequently, it should not be used in this age group. Additionally, the drug is ineffective in patients with significant renal impairment. Other side effects are rare but do include peripheral neuropathy and pulmonary infiltrates. The usual dose in children older than 3 months of age is 5 to 7 mg/kg/day given orally in three to four divided doses (Behrman and Vaughan).

Trimethoprim-Sulfamethoxazole

The TMP-SMX combination is useful both in the management of simple cystitis and for long-term antibacterial prophylaxis. This combination has a diminished effect on bowel flora and offers the advantage of trimethoprim entering vaginal secretions in the adult female (Stamey et al, 1977). This latter characteristic appears to be of particular utility in its effectiveness as a prophylactic agent. In addition, trimethoprim has also been shown in vitro to induce phase variation of fimbriated *E. coli* to a non-fimbriated state (Vaisanen et al). This and the high concentration in vaginal secretions work to prevent vaginal and periurethral colonization with organisms that could potentially cause urinary tract infection. Trimethoprim interferes with dihydrofolic acid reductase, and sulfa blocks the conversion of para-aminobenzoic acid to dihydrofolic acid. The combination is effective against many gram-negative as well as gram-positive organisms. It is well absorbed, attains high levels in both serum and urine, and is well tolerated by children. Neutropenia and thrombocytopenia are not uncommon with its use. However, the significance of these changes is unknown (Asmar et al).

The combination is available as a suspension containing 40 mg of trimethoprim and 200 mg of sulfamethoxazole per 5 ml. The dose employed in children over 2 months of age is TMP, 6 to 12 mg, and SMX, 30 to 60 mg/kg/day, in two divided doses (Behrman and Vaughan).

Nalidixic Acid

Nalidixic acid is an antibacterial agent that produces good urinary levels and is effective against gram-negative organisms. It is especially effective against *Proteus*. Previous negative reports regarding the effectiveness of this agent can probably be accounted for by inadequate dosage (Stamey and Bragonzi, 1976). Nalidixic acid is readily absorbed from the gastrointestinal tract and is well tolerated by children. It is rapidly inactivated by the liver. It is thought to interfere with DNA synthesis. The development of pseudotumor cerebri has been reported as a complication of its use in children (Anderson et al). Nalidixic acid is available in both tablet and suspension form. The recommended dose is 55 mg/kg/day in four divided doses (Behrman and Vaughan).

Methenamine Mandelate and Methenamine Hippurate

These agents are readily absorbed from the intestinal tract and remain inactive until they are excreted by the kidney and concentrated in the urine. Methenamine in an acid urine is converted to the bactericidal agent formaldehyde; however, this conversion takes a minimum of 2 hours to achieve adequate bactericidal levels. Mandelic and hippuric acids are urinary acidifiers that have some additional inherent but weak antibacterial effect. Efficacy of methenamine may be enhanced further by supplementary urinary acidification, such as with ascorbic acid. Both can cause dysuria when administered in high doses, and methenamine mandelate has on rare occasions produced hemorrhagic cystitis (Ross and Conway). The recommended dose for these agents initially is 100 mg/kg/day given orally in four divided doses, followed by 50 mg/kg/day in four divided doses (Behrman and Vaughan).

Penicillin

The penicillins as a class are probably the most widely used antibiotics. All act by blocking mucopeptide synthesis in the cell walls so that the bacterium is unprotected from its high internal osmotic pressure (Goodman and Gilman). This effect occurs only in growing cells.

Penicillin G. Extremely high urine levels can be achieved with penicillin G in patients with normal renal function, and under those circumstances this drug may be very effective against both *E. coli* and *Proteus*. Its major toxic effect is allergy manifested by rash or anaphylaxis.

Ampicillin. Ampicillin is the most widely used penicillin in the treatment of urinary tract infections. It is not well absorbed from the gastrointestinal tract; therefore, high fecal levels do occur and diarrhea is common. High serum and urine concentrations are achievable. This agent should not be administered to patients with a known history of penicillin allergy. The usual dose is 50 to 100 mg/kg/day given every 6 hours. It can be administered either orally or intravenously (Behrman and Vaughan).

Amoxicillin. Amoxicillin is a derivative of ampicillin that is absorbed more readily and therefore produces less diarrhea. It is administered orally in a dose of 20 to 40 mg/kg/day every 6 to 8 hours (Behrman and Vaughan).

Carbenicillin. Carbenicillin is an agent that may be useful in the treatment of *Pseudomonas* and indole-positive *Proteus;* however, its usefulness is often diminished by the emergence of resistant strains. It is available as tablets and as a parenteral solution. When it is used parenterally for urinary tract infection in children, the usual dose is 50 to 200 mg/kg/day given every 4 hours; for severe infections, the dose can be increased to 400 to 500 mg/kg/day (Kunin, 1987). The oral form is not predictably effective in children.

Ticarcillin. Ticarcillin is available for parenteral therapy only. Like carbenicillin, it is active against *Pseudomonas* and indole-positive *Proteus,* which may be resistant to other drugs. It is often used with an aminoglycoside for a synergistic effect. This combination may also delay the emergence of resistant strains. Sodium overload is less likely to occur with ticarcillin compared with carbenicillin. The usual dose in children for treatment of urinary tract infection is 50 to 100 mg/kg/day given every 4 to 6 hours. In life-threatening infections, the dose can be increased to 200 to 300 mg/kg/day (Kunin, 1987).

Piperacillin. Piperacillin has essentially the same antimicrobial spectrum as carbenicillin and ticarcillin, but is more effective on a weight basis. Piperacillin may have some advantage in allowing lower doses and therefore less sodium load compared with carbenicillin and ticarcillin. The dosage in children is 50 mg/kg/day given every 4 to 6 hours (Kunin 1987).

Cephalosporins

Cephalosporins are usually effective against most of the gram-negative and many of the gram-positive pathogens. Excretion is by both glomerular filtration and tubular secretion. Although there can be some cross-reactivity in patients who are allergic to penicillin, in general these agents can be cautiously administered to patients with penicillin allergy.

Oral Drugs

Oral cephalexin, a "first-generation" cephalosporin, is well absorbed from the gastrointestinal tract and can be given in a dose of 25 to 50 mg/kg/day every 6 hours (Behrman and Vaughan). Cefaclor, a "second-generation" oral cephalosporin, is somewhat more active against gram-negative bacteria but is more expensive than cephalexin. The dosage is 20 to 40 mg/kg/day given every 8 hours (Behrman and Vaughan). Other oral cephalosporins include cephradine (first generation) and cefadroxil (second generation). A new "third-generation" cephalosporin for oral administration, cefixime, is now available. In addition to broader coverage of gram-negative organisms, an advantage of cefixime is a prolonged half-life, allowing for once or twice daily dosage. The recommended dose for children is 8 mg/kg/day in one or two divided doses (Drug Newsletter).

Parenteral Drugs

Numerous cephalosporins are available for parenteral use. The first-generation cephalosporins (cephalothin, cefazolin, cepharadine, cephapirin) are useful agents for urinary infections caused by most strains of *E. coli, Klebsiella, and Proteus,* but not *Pseudomonas.* As with all cephalosporins, they are inactive against enterococci. The second-generation parenteral cephalosporins (cefamandole, cefoxitin) are more active than the first-generation agents against many enteric gram-negative bacteria, but not *Pseudomonas.* Cefoxitin is the most active cephalosporin against anaerobes, including *Bacteroides fragilis.* There are a number of new third-generation cephalosporins (cefoperazone, cefotaxime, ceftazidime, ceftriaxone). These drugs have been developed because of their relatively greater activity against gram-negative bacteria. Although most retain some activity against gram-positive bacteria, they are much less active than first-generation cephalosporins for staphylococci or other gram-positive bacteria. Ceftriaxone has a longer half-life, allowing for once or twice daily dosage. It is also more active than cefoperazone against most gram-negative bacteria.

There are so many new cephalosporins that it is difficult to choose among them. It is recommended that the physician become familiar with the use of one oral and one parenteral drug in each generation. Dosage in children varies with each cephalosporin.

Aminoglycosides

The aminoglycosides are well tolerated by children and are of special utility in the treatment of complicated gram-negative UTI. They interfere with protein synthesis by binding proteins of the bacterial ribosomes.

Gentamicin. Gentamicin is probably the most widely used of the aminoglycosides in children and is especially effective against *Pseudomonas*. The usual pediatric dose is 5 to 7.5 mg/kg/day parenterally in two divided doses, depending upon age (Behrman and Vaughan). It achieves high tissue concentration and can be ototoxic, particularly to the vestibular cells. Nephrotoxicity also occurs in a small percentage of patients and should be watched for by checking serum creatinine and/or serum gentamicin levels periodically during the course of therapy. Nephrotoxicity occurs particularly frequently when gentamicin is given in combination with cephalosporins. Both ototoxicity and nephrotoxicity are usually transient.

Tobramycin. Tobramycin has the advantage of particular efficacy against *Pseudomonas*. It is said to be less nephrotoxic than gentamicin (Kurnin). The dosage is 4 to 7.5 mg/kg/day given every 8 to 12 hours, depending upon age (Behrman and Vaughan).

Amikacin. A newer aminoglycoside, amikacin, was developed to improve activity against emerging resistant strains of *Pseudomonas*. As with other aminoglycosides, it is potentially both nephrotoxic and ototoxic. The dosage is 15 to 22.5 mg/kg/day given every 8 to 12 hours, depending upon age (Behrman and Vaughan).

Tetracyclines

Tetracyclines should not be used in children under 8 years of age because they stain the permanent teeth. The need for tetracycline is unusual in modern-day pediatrics.

Bibliography

Abbott GD: Neonatal bacteriuria: a prospective study in 1460 infants. Br Med J 1:267, 1972.

Allen TD: The non-neurogenic neurogenic bladder. J Urol 117:232, 1977.

American Medical Association: AMA Drug Evaluations. Chicago, AMA, 1971.

Anderson EE, Anderson B Jr, Nashold BS: Childhood complications of nalidixic acid. JAMA 216:1023, 1971.

Arneil GC, McAllister RA, Kay P: Measurement of bacteriuria by plane dipslide culture. Lancet 1:94, 1973.

Aronson M, Medalia O, Schori L, et al: Prevention of colonization of the urinary tract of mice with *Escherichia coli* by blocking of bacterial adherence with methyl α-D-mannopyranoside. J Infect Dis 139:329, 1979.

Arthur M, Johnson CE, Rubin RH, et al: Molecular epidemiology of adhesin and hemolysin virulence factors among uropathogenic *Escherichia coli*. Infect Immun 57:303, 1989.

Askari A, Belman AB: Vesicoureteral reflux in black girls. J Urol 127:747, 1982.

Asmar BI, Maqbool S, Dajani AS: Hematologic abnormalities after oral trimethoprim-sulfamethoxazole therapy in children. Am J Dis Child 135:1100, 1981.

Austenfeld MS, Snow BW: Complications of pregnancy after reimplantation for vesicoureteral reflux. J Urol 140:1103, 1988.

Avner ED, Inglefinger JR, Herrin JT, et al: Single-dose amoxicillin therapy of uncomplicated urinary tract infections. J Pediatr 102:623, 1983.

Bagley FH, Stewart AM, Jones PF: Diffuse xanthogranulomatous pyelonephritis in children: an unrecognized variant. J Urol 118:434, 1977.

Ball P: Ciprofloxacin: an overview of adverse experiences. J Antimicrob Chemother (Suppl D) 18:187, 1986.

Barry AL, Jones RN, Thornsberry C, et al: Antimicrobial activities of ciprofloxacin, norfloxacin, oxalinic acid, cinoxacin, and nalidixic acid. Antimicrob Agents Chemother 25:633, 1984.

Bar-Sharit Z, Goldman R, Ofek I, et al: Mannose-binding activity of *Escherichia coli:* A determinant of attachment and ingestion of the bacteria by macrophages. Infect Immun 29:417, 1980.

Behrman RF, Vaughan VC III: Nelson Textbook of Pediatrics, 13th ed. Philadelphia, WB Saunders Co, 1987.

Bellinger MF, Duckett JW: Vesicoureteral reflux: a comparison of non-surgical and surgical management. *In* Contributions to Nephrology, Vol 39. Reflux Nephropathy Update 1983. Edited by CJ Hodson, RH Heptinstall, J Winberg. Basel, Karger, 1984.

Belman AB: Clinical significance of cystitis cystica in girls: results of a prospective study. J Urol 127:7474, 1978.

Belman AB: Genitourinary infections: nonspecific infections. *In* Clinical Pediatric Urology, 2nd ed. Edited by PP Kelalis, LR King, AB Belman Philadelphia, WB Saunders Co, 1985.

Ben-Ami T, Rozin M, Hertz M: Imaging of children with urinary tract infection: a tailored approach. Clin Radiol 40:64, 1989.

Bergström T, Larson H, Lincoln K, et al: Studies of urinary tract infections in infancy and childhood. J Pediatr 80:858, 1972.

Bergström T, Lincoln K, Orskov F, et al: Studies of urinary tract infections in infancy and children. VIII. Reinfection vs relapse in recurrent urinary tract infections: Evaluation by means of identification of infection organisms. J Pediatr 72:13, 1967.

Bingham JB, Maisey MN: An evaluation of the use of 99m Tc-dimercapto-succinic acid (DMSA) as a static renal imaging agent. Br J Radiol 51:599, 1978.

Bisset GS, Strife JL, Dunbar JS: Urography and voiding cystourethrography: findings in girls with urinary tract infection. AJR 148:479, 1987.

Blickman JG, Taylor GA, Lebowitz RL: Voiding cystourethrography as the initial radiologic study in the child with urinary tract infection. Radiology 156:659, 1985.

Blumenstock E, Jann K: Adhesion of piliated *Escherichia coli* strains to phagocytes: differences between bacteria with mannose-sensitive pili and those with mannose-resistant pili. Infect Immun 35:264, 1982.

Bolann BJ, Sandberg S, Digranes A: Implications of probability analysis for interpreting results of leukocyte esterase and nitrite test strips. Clin Chem 35:1663, 1989.

Bollgren I, Winberg J: The periurethral aerobic bacterial flora in healthy boys and girls. Acta Paediatr Scand 65:74, 1976a.

Bollgren I, Winberg J: The periurethral aerobic bacterial flora in girls highly susceptible to urinary infections. Acta Paediatr Scand 65:81, 1976b.

Bouissou H, Caujolle D, Caujolle F, et al: Tissus cartilagineux et acide nalidixique. C R Acad Sci (Paris) 286(23):1743, 1978.

Brook I: Urinary tract infections caused by anaerobic bacteria in children. Urology 16:596, 1980.

Busch R, Huland H: Correlation of symptoms and results of direct bacterial localization in patients with urinary tract infections. J Urol 132:282, 1984.

Busch R, Huland H, Kollermann MW, et al: Does internal urethrotomy influence susceptibility to recurrent urinary tract infection? Urology 20:134, 1982.

Caine M, Edwards P: The peripheral control of micturition: a cine-radiographic study. Br J Urol 30:34, 1958.

Carbonetti NH, Boonchai S, Parry SH, et al: Aerobactin-mediated iron uptake by *Escherichia coli* isolates from human extraintestinal infections. Infect Immun 51:966, 1986.

Cardiff-Oxford Bacteriuria Study Group: Sequelae of covert bacteriuria in school children. Lancet 1:889, 1978.

Chan RCY, Bruce AW, Reid G: Adherence of cervical, vaginal and distal urethral normal microbial flora to human uroepithelial cells and inhibition of adherence of gram-egative uropathogens by competitive exclusion. J Urol 131:596, 1984.

Chan RCY, Reid G, Irvin RT, et al: Competitive exclusion of uropathogens from human uroepithelial cells by lactobacillus whole cells and cell wall fragments. Infect Immun 47:84, 1985.

Chick S, Harver MJ, MacKenzie R, et al: Modified method for studying bacterial adhesion to isolated uroepithelial cells and uromucoid. Infect Immun 34:256, 1981.

Clark H, Ronald AR, Turck M: Serum antibody response in renal versus bladder bacteria. J Infect Dis 123:539, 1971.

Conway JJ: Role of scintigraphy in urinary tract infection. Semin Nucl Med 18:308, 1988.

Cordon-Cardo C, Lloyd KO, Sinkstad CL, et al: Immunoanatomic determination of blood group antigens in the human urinary tract: influence of secretor status. Lab Invest 55:444, 1986.

Corman LI, Fosage WS, Kotchmar GS: Simplified urinary microscopy to detect significant bacteriuria. Pediatrics 70:133, 1982.

Corriere JN Jr, McClure JM III, Lipschultz LI: Contamination of bladder urine by urethral particles during voiding: urethrovesical reflux. J Urol 107:399, 1972.

Cox CE, Hinman F Jr: Experiments with induced bacteriuria, vesical emptying, and bacterial growth on the mechanisms of bladder defense to infection. J Urol 86:739, 1961.

Craig WA, Kunin CM, DeGroot J: Evaluation of new urinary screening devices. Appl Microbiol 26:196, 1975.

Dickinson JA: Incidence and outcome of symptomatic urinary tract infection. Br Med J 1:1330, 1979.

Drew JH, Acton CM: Radiological findings in newborn infants with urinary infection. Arch Dis Child 51:628, 1976.

Drug Newsletter. Facts and Comparisons Div., JB Lippincott Co, St. Louis, 8:56, 1989.

Durbin WA Jr, Peter G: Management of urinary tract infections in infants and children. Pediatr Infect Dis 3:564, 1984.

Edwards D, Normand ICS, Prescod N, et al: Disappearance of vesicoureteric reflux during long-term prophylaxis of urinary tract infection in children. Br Med J 2:285, 1977.

Ehrenkranz NJ, Carter MJ: Immunologic studies in urinary tract infections. I. The hemagglutinin response to *Escherichia* O antigen in infections of varying severity. J Immunol 92:798, 1964.

Eichenwald HF: Some aspects of the diagnosis and management of urinary tract infection in children and adolescents. Pediatr Infect Dis 5:760, 1986.

Eisenstein BI: Phase variation of type I fimbriae in *Escherichia coli* is under transcriptional control. Science 214:337, 1981.

Fairley KF, Bond AG, Brown RB: Simple test to determine the site of urinary-tract infection. Lancet 2:427, 1967.

Feingold DS: Antimicrobial chemotherapeutic agents: the nature of their action in selected toxicity. N Engl J Med 269:900, 1963.

Fennell RS, Wilson SG, Garin EH, et al: Bacteriuria in families of girls with recurrent bacteriuria. Clin Pediatr 16:1132, 1977.

Fleidner M, Mehls O, Rauterberg EW, et al: Urinary SIgA in children with urinary tract infection. J Pediatr 109:416, 1986.

Fletcher KS, Bremer EG, Schwarting GA: P blood group regulation of glycosphingolipid levels in human erythrocytes. J Biol Chem 264:11196, 1979.

Forbes PA, Drummond KN, Nogrady MB: Meatotomy in girls with meatal stenosis and urinary tract infection. J Pediatr 75:937, 1969.

Fowler JE Jr, Stamey TA: Studies of introital colonization of women with recurrent urinary tract infections. VI. The role of bacterial adherence. J Urol 117:472, 1977.

Fried FA, Wong RJ: Etiology of pyelonephritis: significance of hemolytic *Escherichia coli*. J Urol 103:718, 1970.

Fussell EN, Kaack MB, Cherry R, et al: Adherence of bacteria to human foreskins. J Urol 140:997, 1988.

Gelbart SM, Chen WT, Reid R: Clinical trial of leukocyte test strips in routine use. Clin Chem 29:997, 1983.

Gerzof SG, Gale ME: Computed tomography and ultrasonography for diagnosis and treatment of renal and retroperitoneal abscesses. Urol Clin North Am 9:1, 1982.

Gillenwater JY: Detection of urinary leukocytes by chemistrip-1. J Urol 125:383, 1981.

Gillenwater JY, Gleason CH, Lohr JA, et al: Home urine cultures by the dipstick method: results in 289 children. Pediatrics 58:508, 1976.

Gillenwater JY, Harrison RB, Kunin CM: Natural history of bacteriuria in school girls. N Engl J Med 301:396, 1979.

Ginsburg CM, McCracken GH: Urinary tract infections in young infants. Pediatrics, 69:409, 1982.

Glauser MP, Lyons JM, Braude AI: Prevention of chronic experimental pyelonephritis by suppression of acute suppuration. J Clin Invest 61:403, 1978.

Goldraich NP, Ramos OL, Goldraich IM: Urography versus DMSA scan in children with vesicoureteral reflux. Pediatr Nephrol 3:1, 1989.

Gordon I: Indications for 99m technetium dimercaptosuccinic acid scan in children. J Urol 137:464, 1987.

Govan DE, Fair WR, Friedlend GW, et al: Management of children with urinary tract infections. Urology 6:273, 1975.

Graham JB, King LR, Kropp KA, et al: The significance of distal urethra narrowing in young girls. J Urol 97:1045, 1967.

Granoff DM, Roskes S: Urinary tract infection due to *Hemophilus influenzae* type B. J Pediatr 84:414, 1974.

Greenfield SP, Montgomery P: Computerized tomography and acute pyelonephritis in children. Urology 29:137, 1987.

Gross GW, Lebowitz RL: Infection does not cause reflux. AJR 137:929, 1981.

Gruneberg RN: Relationship of infecting urinary organisms to fecal flora in patients with symptomatic urinary infection. Lancet 2:766, 1969.

Hahn H, Kaufmann SHE: The role of cell-mediated immunity in bacterial infections. Rev Infect Dis 3:1221, 1981.

Hagberg L, Hull R, Hull S, et al: Contribution of adhesion to bacterial persistence in the mouse urinary tract. Infect Immun 40:265, 1983.

Hagberg L, Jodal U, Korhenen TK, et al: Adhesion, hemagglutination, and virulence of *Escherichia coli* causing urinary tract infections. Infect Immun 31:564, 1981.

Halverstadt DB, Leadbetter GW Jr: Internal urethrotomy in recurrent urinary tract infection in children: results in the management of infection. J Urol 100:297, 1968.

Handmaker H: Nuclear renal imaging in acute pyelonephritis. Semin Nucl Med 12:246, 1982.

Hanson LA, Ahlstedt S, Fasth A, et al: Antigens of *Escherichia coli,* human immune response, and the pathogenesis of urinary tract infections. J Infect Dis 136:S144, 1977.

Hansson S, Jodal U, Noren L, et al: Untreated bacteriuria in asymptomatic girls with renal scarring. Pediatrics 84:964, 1989.

Harding GKM, Buckwold FJ, Marrie TJ, et al: Prophylaxis of recurrent urinary tract infection in female patients. JAMA 242:1975, 1979.

Hart AF, Cherry JD: Cytology of the urine in children after poliovirus vaccine. N Engl J Med 272:174, 1965.

Heale WF, Weldone DP, Hewstone AS: Reflux nephropathy: presentation of urinary infection in children. Med J Aust 1:1138, 1973.

Hellerstein S, Duggan E, Savage B: Urinary lactic acid dehydrogenase activity in the site of urinary tract infections. Pediatr Infect Dis J 7:180, 1988.

Hellerstein S, Duggan E, Welchert E, et al: Serum C-reactive protein in the site of urinary tract infections. J Pediatr 100:21, 1982.

Hellerstein S, Kennedy E, Nussbaum L, et al: Localization of the site of urinary tract infections by means of antibody-coated bacteria in the urinary sediments. J Ped 92:188, 1978.

Hellström M, Jacobsson B, Mårild S, et al: Voiding cystourethrography as a predictor of reflux nephropathy in children with urinary tract infection. AJR 152:801, 1989.

Hellström M, Jodal U, Mårild S, et al: Ureteral dilatation in children with febrile urinary tract infection or bacteriuria. AJR 148:483, 1987.

Hendry WF, Stanton SL, Williams DI: Recurrent urinary tract infections in girls: effects of urethral dilatation. Br J Urol 45:72, 1973.

Hermansson G, Bollgren I, Bergstrom T, et al: Coagulase negative staphylococci as a cause of symptomatic urinary infections in children. J Pediatr 84:807, 1974.

Herzog LW: Urinary tract infections and circumcision. Am J Dis Child 143:348, 1989.

Hinman F: Mechanisms for the entry of bacteria and the establishment of urinary infection in female children. J Urol 96:546, 1966.

Hinman F: Urinary tract damage in children who wet. Pediatrics 54:142, 1974.

Hjelm EM: Local cellular immune response in ascending urinary tract infection: occurrence of T-cells, immunoglobulin-producing cells, and Ia-expressing cells in rat urinary tract tissue. Infect Immun 44:627, 1984.

Hooper DC, Wolfson TS, Ng EY, et al: Mechanism of action and resistance to ciprofloxacin. Am J Med 82(Suppl 4A):12, 1987.

Hopkins GB, Hall RL, Mende CW: Gallium-67 scintigraphy for the diagnosis and localization of perinephric abscesses. J Urol 115:126, 1976.

Horgan JG, Rosenfield NS, Weiss RM, et al: Is renal ultrasound a reliable indicator of a nonobstructed duplication anomaly? Pediatr Radiol 14:388, 1984.

Horwitz MA, Silverstein SC: Influence of *Escherichia coli* capsule on complement fixation and on phagocytosis and killing by human phagocytes. J Clin Invest 65:82, 1980.

Hughes C, Hacker J, Roberts A, et al: Hemolysin production as a virulence marker in symptomatic and asymptomatic urinary tract infections caused by *Escherichia coli.* Infect Immun 39:546, 1983.

Hull S, Clegg S, Svanborg Edén C, et al: Multiple forms of genes in pyelonephritogenic *Escherichia coli* encoding adhesins binding globoseries glycolipid receptors. Infect Immun 47:80, 1985.

Hurwitz SR, Kessler WO, Alazrake NP, et al: Gallium-67 imaging to localize urinary infections. Br J Radiol 49:156, 1976.

Immergut MA, Gilbert EC: Internal urethrotomy in recurring urinary infections in girls. J Urol 109:126, 1973.

Immergut MA, Wahman GE: The urethral caliber of female children with urinary tract infection. J Urol 99:189, 1968.

International Reflux Committee: Medical versus surgical treatment of primary vesicoureteral reflux. Pediatrics 67:392, 1981.

Israele V, Darabi A, McCracken GH Jr: The role of bacterial virulence factors and Tamm-Horsfall protein in the pathogenesis of *Escherichia coli* urinary tract infection in infants. Am J Dis Child 141:1230, 1987.

Iwahi T, Abe Y, Nakao M, et al: Role of type I fimbriae in the pathogenesis of ascending urinary tract infection induced by *Escherichia coli* in mice. Infect Immun 39:1307, 1984.

Jacobson SN, Hammarlind M, Lidefeldt KJ, et al: Incidence of aerobactin-positive *Escherichia coli* strains in patients with symptomatic urinary tract infection. Eur J Clin Microbiol Infect Dis 7:630, 1988.

James GP, Paul KL, Fuller JB: Urinary nitrate in urinary-tract infection. Am J Clin Pathol 70:671, 1978.

Jantausch B, Wiedermann B, Hull S, et al: *Escherichia*

coli virulence factors and 99m Tc-DMSA renal scan in children with febrile urinary tract infection. Submitted for publication.

Jequier S, Forbes PA, Nogrady MB: The value of ultrasound as a screening procedure in first documented urinary tract infection in children. J Ultrasound Med 4:393, 1985.

Jenkins RD, Fenn JP, Matsen JM: Review of microscopy for bacteriuria. JAMA 255:3397, 1986.

Jodal U: The natural history of bacteriuria in childhood. Infect Dis Clin North Am 1:713, 1987.

Jodal U: Host risk factors in pyelonephritis. *In* Dialogues in Pediatric Urology. Vol 13(2). Pyelonephritis: Pathogenesis and Management Update. Edited by HG Rushton, RM Ehrlich. Pearl River, NY, William J Miller Assoc, Inc, 1990.

Jodal U, Lindberg U, Lincoln K: Level diagnosis of symptomatic urinary tract infections in childhood. Acta Paediatr Scand 64:201, 1975.

Kaack MV, Dowling KJ, Patterson GM, et al: Immunology of pyelonephritis. VIII. *E. coli* causes granulocytic aggregation and renal ischemia. J Urol 136:1117, 1986.

Kaijser B: Immunology of *Escherichia coli* K antigen and its relation to urinary tract infections in children. Lancet 1:663, 1977.

Kaijser B, Jodal U, Hanson LA: Studies on antibody response and tolerance to *E. coli* K antigens in immunized rabbits and in children with urinary tract infection. Int Arch Allergy 44:260, 1973b.

Kaijser B, Larsson P, Olling S: Protection against ascending *Escherichia coli* pyelonephritis in rats and significance of local immunity. Infect Immun 20:78, 1978.

Kaijser B, Larrson P, Olling S, et al: Protection against acute, ascending pyelonephritis caused by *Escherichia coli* in rats, using isolated capsular antigen conjugated to bovine serum albumin. Infect Immun 39:142, 1983.

Kallenius G, Mollby R, Svenson SB, et al: The p^k antigen as receptor for the hemagglutination of pyelonephritogenic *Escherichia coli*. FEMS Microbiol Lett 7:297, 1980.

Kallenius G, Svensson SB, Hultberg H, et al: Occurrence of P-fimbriated *Escherichia coli* in urinary tract infections. Lancet 2:1369, 1981.

Kallenius G, Svensson SB, Mollby R, et al: Carbohydrate structures recognized by uropathogenic *E. coli*. Scand J Infect Dis 33 (Suppl 1):52, 1982.

Kallenius G, Winberg J: Bacterial adherence to periurethral cells in girls prone to urinary tract infection. Lancet 2:540, 1978.

Kallings LO: Medicinsk behandling av urinvagsinfekioner (1). Bakteriologisk oversikt. Sven Lakartidn 65 (Suppl III):30, 1968.

Kangarloo H, Gold RH, Fine RN, et al: Urinary tract infection in infants and children evaluated by ultrasound. Radiology 154:367, 1985.

Kaplan GW, Sammons TA, King LR: A blind comparison of dilation, urethrotomy, and medication alone in the treatment of urinary infections in girls. J Urol 109:917, 1973.

Kass EH: Asymptomatic infections of the urinary tract. Trans Assoc Am Phys 69:56, 1956.

Kass EH: Bacteriuria and the diagnosis of infections of the urinary tract. Arch Intern Med 100:709, 1957.

Kass EJ, Majd M, Belman AB: Comparison of the diuretic renogram and the pressure perfusion study in children. J Urol 134:92, 1985.

Kaye D: Antibacterial activity of human urine. J Clin Invest 47:2374, 1968.

Kinane DF, Blackwell CC, Brettle RP, et al: ABO blood group, secretor state and susceptibility to recurrent urinary tract infection in women. Br Med J 285:7, 1982.

Kisielius P, Schwan WR, Amundsen S, et al: In vivo expression and variation of *Escherichia coli* Type 1 and P pili in the urine of adults with acute urinary tract infections. Infect Immun 57:1656, 1989.

Koff SA, Byard MA: The daytime urinary frequency syndrome of childhood. J Urol 140:1280, 1988.

Koff SA, Murtagh DS: The uninhibited bladder in children: Effect of treatment on recurrence of urinary infection and/or vesicoureteral reflux resolution. J Urol 130:1138, 1983.

Koehler PR: The roentgen diagnosis of renal inflammatory masses—special emphasis on angiographic changes. Radiology 112:257, 1974.

Kumar B, Coleman RE, Anderson PO: Gallium citrate Ga-67 imaging in patients with suspected inflammatory processes. Arch Surg 110:1237, 1975.

Kunin CM: Detection, Prevention and Management of Urinary Tract Infections, 4th ed. Philadelphia, Lea and Febiger, 1987.

Kunin CM: The natural history of recurrent bacteriuria in school girls. N Engl J Med 282:1443, 1970.

Kunin CM, Deutscher R, Paquin A Jr: Urinary tract infection in school children: an epidemiologic, clinical and laboratory study. Medicine 4:91, 1964.

Kurnin GD: Clinical nephrotoxicity of tobramycin and gentamicin: a prospective study. JAMA 244:1808, 1980.

Kusumi RK, Grover PJ, Kunin CM: Rapid detection of pyuria by leukocyte esterase activity. JAMA 254:1653, 1981.

Labigne-Roussel AF, Lark D, Schoolnick G, et al: Cloning and expression of a fimbrial adhesin (AFA-I) responsible for P blood group–independent, mannose-resistant hemagglutination from a pyelonephritic *Escherichia coli* strain. Infect Immun 46:251, 1984.

Leadbetter G Jr, Slavins S: Pediatric urinary tract infections: significance of vaginal bacteria. Urol 3:581, 1974.

Lebowitz RL: The detection of vesicoureteral reflux in the child. Invest Radiol 21:519, 1986.

Lebowitz RL, Mandell J: Urinary tract infection in children: putting radiology in its place. Radiology 165:1, 1987.

Leffler H, Svanborg Edén C: Chemical identification of a glycosphingolipid receptor for *Escherichia coli* attaching to human urinary tract epithelial cells and agglutinating human erythrocytes. FEMS Microbiol Lett 8:127, 1980.

Leonidas JC, McCauley RGK, Klauber GC, et al: Sonography as a substitute for excretory urography in children with urinary tract infection. AJR 144:815, 1985.

Lidin-Janson G, Jodal U, Lincoln K: Trimethoprim och nitrofurantoin for profylax mot UVI hos barn. Recip Reflex (Suppl VI):38, 1980.

Lindberg U, Bjure J, Haugstvedt S, et al: Asymptomatic bacteriuria in school girls: III. Relation between residual urine volume and recurrence. Acta Paediatr Scand 64:437, 1975a.

Lindberg U, Claesson I, Hanson LA, et al: Asymptomatic bacteriuria in school girls: I. Clinical and laboratory findings. Acta Paediatr Scand, 64:425, 1975b.

Lindberg U, Claesson I, Hanson LA, et al: Asymptomatic bacteriuria in school girls: VIII. Clinical course during a three-year follow-up. J Pediatr 92:194, 1978.

Lindberg U, Hanson LA, Lidin-Janson G, et al: Asymptomatic bacteriuria in school girls: II. Differences in *E. coli* causing asymptomatic and symptomatic bacteriuria. Acta Paediatr Scand 64:432, 1975c.

Littlewood JM, Kite P, Kite BA: Incidence of neonatal urinary tract infection. Arch Dis Child, 44:617, 1969.

Lomberg H, de Man P, Svanborg Edén C: Bacterial and host determinants of renal scarring. APMIS 97:193, 1989a.

Lomberg H, Hanson LA, Jacobbson B, et al: Correlation of P blood group, vesicoureteral reflux, and bacterial attachment in patients with recurrent pyelonephritis. N Engl J Med 308:1189, 1983.

Lomberg H, Hellström M, Jodal U: Virulence associated traits in Escherichia coli causing first and recurrent episodes of urinary tract infection in children with or without reflux. J Infect Dis 150:561, 1984.

Lomberg H, Hellström M, Jodal U, et al: Secretor state in renal scarring in girls with recurrent pyelonephritis. FEMS Microbiol Immunol 47:371, 1989b.

Longoria CC, Gonzalez GA: FiltraCheck–UTI, a rapid, disposable system for detection of bacteriuria. J Clin Microbiol 25:926, 1987.

Loo SYT, Scottolini AG, Luangphinith MT, et al: Urine screening strategy employing dipstick analysis and selective culture: an evaluation. Am J Clin Pathol 81:634, 1984.

Lorentz WB Jr, Resnick MI: Comparison of urinary lactic dehydrogenase with antibody-coated bacteria in the urine sediment as a means of localizing the site of urinary tract infection. Pediatrics 64:672, 1979.

Low V, David V, Lark D, et al: Gene clusters governing the production of hemolysin and mannose-resistant hemagglutination are closely linked in Escherichia coli serotype O4 and O6 isolates from urinary tract infections. Infect Immun 43:353, 1984.

Madrigal G, Odio CM, Mohs E, et al: Single dose antibiotic therapy is not as effective as conventional regimens for management of acute urinary tract infections in children. Pediatr Infect Dis J 7:316, 1988.

Majd M: Radionuclide imaging in pediatrics: symposium on pediatric radiology. Pediatr Clin North Am 32:1559, 1985.

Majd M, Rushton HG, Jantausch B, et al: Acute febrile urinary infection in children: a prospective clinical, laboratory, and imaging study. J Pediatr 119:578, 1991.

Malek RS, Elder JS: Xanthogranulomatous pyelonephritis: a critical analysis of 26 cases of the literature. J Urol 119:589, 1978.

Mårild S, Jodal U, Mangelus L: Medical histories of children with acute pyelonephritis compared with controls. J Pediatr Infect Dis 8:511, 1989.

Mårild S, Wettergren B, Hellström M, et al: Bacterial virulence and inflammatory response in infants with febrile urinary tract infection or screening bacteriuria. J Pediatr 112:348, 1988.

Marr TJ, Traisman HS: Detection of bacteriuria in pediatric outpatients. Am J Dis Child 129:940, 1975.

Marre R, Hacker J: Role of S and common type I fimbriae of Escherichia coli in experimental upper and lower tract infection. Microbiol Pathog 2:223, 1987.

Mattsby-Baltzer I, Hanson LA, Kaijser B, et al: Experimental Escherichia coli ascending pyelonephritis in rats: changes in bacterial properties and the immune response to surface antigens. Infect Immun 35:639, 1982.

McCabe WR, Kaijser B, Olling S, et al: Escherichia coli in bacteremia: K and O antigens and serum sensitivity of strains from adults and neonates. J Infect Dis 138:33, 1978.

McCracken GH, Ginsburg CM, Namasonthi V, et al: Evaluation of short-term antibiotic therapy in children with uncomplicated urinary tract infection. Pediatrics 67:796, 1981.

McGeachie J: Recurrent infection of the urinary tract: reinfection or recrudescence? Br Med J 1:952, 1966.

McLachlan MSF, Mellar ST, Verrier Jones ER, et al: The urinary tract in school girls with covert bacteriuria. Arch Dis Child 50:253, 1975.

Merrick MV, Uttley WS, Wild SR: The detection of pyelonephritic scarring in children by radioisotope imaging. Br J Med 53:544, 1980.

Miller TE, Scott L, Stewart E, et al: Modification by suppressor cells and serum factors of the cell-mediated immune response in experimental pyelonephritis. J Clin Invest 61:964, 1978.

Moffat M, Embree J, Grimm P, et al: Short-course antibiotic therapy for urinary tract infections in children. Am J Dis Child 142:57, 1988.

Mollby R, Svensson SB, et al: The pk antigen as receptor for hemagglutination of pyelonephritic Escherichia coli. FEMS Microbiol Lett 7:297, 1980.

Morrell RE, Duritz G, Oltorf C: Suprapubic aspiration associated with hematuria. Pediatrics 69:455, 1982.

Nasu Y: The virulence factor of E. coli in genitourinary infections. Nippon Hinyokika Gakkai Zashi 79:1162, 1988.

Nelson JD, Peters PC: Suprapubic aspiration of urine in premature and term infants. Pediatrics 36:132, 1965.

Neumann PZ, deDomenico IJ, Nogrady MB: Constipation and urinary tract infection. Pediatrics 52:241, 1973.

Newcastle Asymptomatic Bacteriuria Research Group: Asymptomatic bacteriuria in school children in Newcastle-upon-Tyne. Arch Dis Child 50:90, 1975.

Norden CW, Kass EH: Bacteriuria of pregnancy—a critical appraisal. Ann Rev Med 19:431, 1968.

Normark S, Lark D, Hull R, et al: Genetics of digalactoside binding adhesin from a uropathogenic Escherichia coli strain. Infect Immun 41:942, 1983.

Nowicki B, Rhen M, Vaisanen-Rhen V: Immunofluorescence study of fimbrial phase variation in Escherichia coli KS71. J Bacteriol 160:691, 1984.

Nowicki B, Svanborg Edén C, Hull R, et al: Molecular analysis and epidemiology of the Dr hemagglutinin of uropathogenic Escherichia coli. Infect Immun 57:446, 1989.

O'Doherty NJ: Urinary tract infection in the neonatal period and later infancy. In Urinary Tract Infection. Edited by F. O'Grady, W. Brumfitt. London, Oxford University Press, 1968.

O'Hanley P, Lark D, Falkow S, Schoolnik G: Molecular basis of Escherichia coli colonization of the upper urinary tract in BALB/c mice. J Clin Invest 75:347, 1985.

Ofek I, Beachey EH: Mannose binding and epithelial cell adherence of Escherichia coli. Infect Immun 22:247, 1978.

Ofek I, Mosek A, Sharon N: Mannose-specific adherence of Escherichia coli freshly excreted in the urine of patients with urinary tract infections and of isolates subcultured from the infected urine. Infect Immun 34:708, 1981.

Olling S, Hanson LA, Holmgren JU, et al: The bactericidal effect of normal human serum on E. coli strains from normals and from patients with urinary tract infections. Infection 1:24, 1973.

O'Regan S, Yazbeck S, Schick E: Constipation, bladder instability, urinary tract infection syndrome. Clin Nephrol 23:152, 1985.

Orskov I, Ferencz A, Orskov F: Tamm-Horsfall protein or uromucoid is the normal urinary slime that traps Type I fimbriated Escherichia coli. Lancet 2:887, 1980.

Orskov F, Orskov I: Summary of a workshop on the clone concept in the epidemiology, taxonomy, and evolution of the Enterobacteriaceae and other bacteria. J Infect Dis 148:346, 1983.

Orskov I, Orskov F, Birch-Andersen A, et al: O, K, H and fimbrial antigens in *Escherichia coli* serotypes associated with pyelonephritis and cystitis. Scand J Infect Dis (Suppl) 33:18, 1982.

Orskov I, Svanborg Edén C, Orskov F: Aerobactin production of serotyped *Escherichia coli* from urinary tract infections. Med Microbiol Immun 177:9, 1988.

Parsons CL, Greenspan C, Moore S, et al: Role of surface mucin in primary antibacterial defense of the bladder. Urology 9:48, 1977.

Parsons CL, Greenspan C, Mulholland SG: The primary antibacterial defense mechanism of the bladder. Invest Urol 13:72, 1975.

Parsons CL, Mulholland SG, Anwar H: Antibacterial activity of bladder surface mucins duplicated by exogenous glycosaminoglycan (heparin). Infect Immun 24:552, 1979.

Parsons CL, Schrom SH, Hanno P, et al: Bladder surface mucin: examination of possible mechanism for its antibacterial effect. Invest Urol 16:196, 1978.

Pecha B, Low D, O'Hanley P: Gal-Gal pili vaccines prevent pyelonephritis by piliated *E. coli* in a murine model. J Clin Invest 83:2102, 1989.

Pedersen JF, Hancke S, Kristensen JV: Renal carbuncle: antibiotic therapy governed by ultrasonically guided aspiration. J Urol 109:777, 1973.

Pere A, Nowicki B, Saxen H, et al: Expression of P, type-1, and type-1c fimbriae of *Escherichia coli* in the urine of patients with acute urinary tract infections. J Infect Dis 156:567, 1987.

Pezzlo M: Detection of urinary tract infections by rapid methods. Clin Microbiol Rev 1:268, 1988.

Polnay L, Fraser AM, Lewis JM: Complications of suprapubic bladder aspiration. Arch Dis Child 50:80, 1975.

Pryles CV, Eliot CR: Pyuria and bacteriuria in infants and children: the value of pyuria as a diagnostic criterion of urinary tract infections. Am J Dis Child 110:628, 1965.

Pryles CV, Luders D: Bacteriology found in infants and children with gastroenteritis. Pediatrics 28:877, 1961.

Pylkkanen J, Vilska J, Koskimes O: The value of level diagnosis of childhood urinary tract infections in predicting renal injury. Acta Paediatr Scand 70:879, 1981.

Rajkumar S, Saxena Y, Rajagopal V, et al: Trimethoprim in pediatric urinary tract infection. Child Nephrol Urol 9:77, 1988–89.

Ransley PG, Risdon RA: Reflux in renal scarring. Br J Radiol (Suppl 14) 51:1, 1978.

Ransley PG, Risdon RA: Reflux nephropathy: effects of antimicrobial therapy on the evolution of the early pyelonephritic scar. Kidney Int 20:733, 1981.

Reid BS, Bender TM: Radiographic evaluation of children with urinary tract infections. Radiol Clin North Am 26:393, 1988.

Rene P, Silverblatt FJ: Serological response to *Escherichia coli* on pyelonephritis. Infect Immun 37:749, 1982.

Ribot S, Gal K, Goldblat M, et al: The role of anaerobic bacteria in the pathogenesis of urinary tract infections. J Urol 126:852, 1981.

Roberts JA: Experimental pyelonephritis in the monkey: III. Pathophysiology of ureteral malfunction induced by bacteria. Invest Urol 13:117, 1975.

Roberts JA: Pathogenesis of pyelonephritis. J Urol 129:1102, 1983.

Roberts JA, Dominique GJ, Martin LN, et al: Immunology of pyelonephritis in the primate model: live versus heat-killed bacteria. Kidney Int 19:297, 1981.

Roberts JA, Hardaway K, Kaack B, et al: Prevention of pyelonephritis by immunization with P-fimbria. J Urol 131:602, 1984.

Roberts JA, Ruth JK Jr, Dominique GJ, et al: Immunology of pyelonephritis in the primate model: V. Effect of superoxide dismutase. J Urol 128:1394, 1982.

Roberts JA, Suarez GM, Kaack B, et al: Experimental pyelonephritis in the monkey: VII. Ascending pyelonephritis in the absence of vesicoureteral reflux. J Urol 133:1068, 1985.

Robins DG, Rogers KB, White RHR: Urine microscopy as an aid to detection of bacteriuria. Lancet 1:476, 1975.

Roomi LGA, Sutton AM, Cockburn F, et al: Amoxycillin and clavulanic acid in the treatment of urinary infection. Arch Dis Child 59:256, 1984.

Ross RR Jr, Conway GF: Hemorrhagic cystitis following an accidental overdosage of methenamine mandelate. Am J Dis Child 119:86, 1970.

Rote AR, Bauer SB, Retik AB: Renal abscess in children. J Urol 119:254, 1978.

Ruberto U, D'Eufemia P, Ferretti L, Giardini O: Effect of 3- vs 10-day treatment of urinary tract infections (letter). J Pediatr 104:483, 1984.

Ruberto U, D'Eufemia P, Martino F, et al: Amoxycillin and clavulanic acid in the treatment of urinary tract infections in children. J Int Med Res 17:168, 1989.

Ruggieri MR, Levin RM, Hanno PM, et al: Defective antiadherence activity of bladder extracts from patients with recurrent urinary tract infection. J Urol 140:157, 1988.

Rushton HG, Majd M, Chandra R, et al: Evaluation of 99m technetium-dimercaptosuccinic acid renal scans in experimental acute pyelonephritis in piglets. J Urol 140:1169, 1988.

Rushton HG, Majd M, Jantausch B, Wiedermann B, Belman AB: Renal scarring following reflux and nonreflux pyelonephritis. J Urol (in press).

Savage DCL, Wilson MI, McHardy M, et al: Covert bacteriuria of childhood: a clinical and epidemiological study. Arch Dis Child 48:8, 1973.

Saxena SR, Collis A, Laurence BM: Bacteriuria in preschool children. Lancet 2:517, 1974.

Schaad UB, Wedgwood-Krucko J: Nalidixic acid in children: retrospective matched controlled study for cartilage toxicity. Infection 15:165, 1974.

Schaeffer AJ, Amundsen SK, Schmidt LN: Adherence of *Escherichia coli* to human urinary tract epithelial cells. Infect Immun 24:753, 1979.

Schaeffer AJ, Chmiel JJ, Duncan JL, et al: Mannose-sensitive adherence of *Escherichia coli* to epithelial cells from women with recurrent urinary tract infections. J Urol 131:906, 1984.

Schaeffer AJ, Jones TM, Dunn JK: Association of in vitro *Escherichia coli* adherence to vaginal and buccal epithelial cells with susceptibility of women to recurrent urinary tract infections. N Engl J Med 304:1062, 1981.

Schardijn G, Statius van Eps LW, Swaak AJG, et al: Urinary beta-2 microglobulin in upper and lower urinary-tract infections. Lancet 1:805, 1979.

Schiff M Jr, Glickman M, Weiss RM, et al: Antibiotic treatment of renal carbuncle. Ann Intern Med 8:305, 1977.

Schluter G: Toxicology of ciprofloxacin. *In* First International Ciprofloxacin Workshop, Proceedings. Vol 61. Edited by HC Neu, H Weuta. Amsterdam, Excerpta Medica, 1986.

Schofer O, Ludwig KH, Mannhardt W, et al: Antibacterial capacity of buccal epithelial cells from healthy donors and children with recurrent urinary tract infections. Eur J Pediatr 147:229, 1988.

Schulman CC, Denis R: Xanthogranulomatous pyelonephritis in childhood (letter). J Urol 117:398, 1977.

Segura JW, Kelalis PP, Martin WJ, et al: Anaerobic bacteria in the urinary tract. Mayo Clin Proc 47:30, 1972.

Shapiro ED: Short course antimicrobial treatment of urinary tract infections in children: a critical analysis. Pediatr Infect Dis 1:294, 1982.

Sheinfeld J, Cordon-Cardo C, Fair WR, et al: Association of type 1 blood group antigens with urinary tract infections in children with genitourinary structural anomalies. J Urol 144:469, 1990.

Sheinfeld J, Schaeffer AJ, Cordon-Cardo C, et al: Association of the Lewis blood group phenotype with recurrent urinary tract infections in women. N Engl J Med 320:773, 1989.

Silver TM, Kass EJ, Thornbury JR, et al: The radiological spectrum of acute pyelonephritis in adults and adolescents. Radiology 118:65, 1976.

Silverblatt FJ, Cohen LS: Antipili antibody affords protection against experimental ascending pyelonephritis. J Clin Invest 64:333, 1979.

Silverblatt FJ, Ofek I: Interaction of bacterial pili and leukocytes. Infection 11:235, 1983.

Silverblatt FJ, Weinstein R, Rene P: Protection against experimental pyelonephritis by antibodies to pili. Scand J Infect Dis (Suppl) 33:79, 1982.

Skoog SJ, Belman AB, Majd M: A nonsurgical approach to the management of primary vesicoureteral reflux. J Urol 138:941, 1987.

Smellie JM, Edwards D, Hunter N, et al: Vesicoureteric reflux and renal scarring. Kidney Int 8:S-65, 1975.

Smellie JM, Gruneberg RN, Leakey A, et al: Long-term low-dosage co-trimoxazole in the management of urinary tract infection in children. J Antimicrob Chemotherap 2:287, 1976.

Smellie JM, Gruneberg RN, Normand ICS, et al: Trimethoprim-sulfamethoxazole and trimethoprim alone in the prophylaxis of childhood urinary tract infection. Rev Infect Dis 4:461, 1982.

Smellie JM, Hodson CJ, Edwards D, et al: Clinical and radiological features of urinary infection in childhood. Br Med J 2:1222, 1964.

Smellie JM, Katz G, Gruneberg RN: Controlled trial of prophylactic treatment in childhood urinary-tract infection. Lancet 2:175, 1978.

Smellie JM, Normand ICS, Katz G: Children with urinary infection: a comparison of those with and those without vesicoureteral reflux. Kidney Int 20:717, 1981.

Smellie JM, Ransley PG, Normand ICS, et al: Development of new renal scars: a collaborative study. Br Med J 290:1957, 1985.

Sohl-Akerlund A, Ahlstedt S, Hanson LA, et al: Antibody responses in urine and serum against Escherichia coli in childhood urinary tract infection. Acta Pathol Microbiol Scand (Sect C) 87:29, 1979.

Stamey TA: The role of introital enterobacteria in recurrent urinary infections. J Urol 109:467, 1973.

Stamey TA: Urinary infections in infancy and childhood. In Pathogenesis and Treatment of Urinary Tract Infections. Baltimore, Williams & Wilkins, 1980.

Stamey TA, Bragonzi J: Resistance to nalidixic acid: a misconception due to underdosage. JAMA 236:1857, 1976.

Stamey TA, Condy M, Mihara G: Prophylactic efficacy of nitrofurantoin macrocrystals and trimethoprim-sulfamethoxazole in urinary infections: biologic effects on the vaginal and rectal flora. N Engl J Med 296:780, 1977.

Stamey TA, Fair WR, Timothy MM, et al: Serum versus urinary antimicrobial concentrations in cure rate of urinary-tract infections. N Engl J Med 291:1159, 1974.

Stamey TA, Govan DE, Palmer JM: The localization and treatment of urinary tract infections: the role of bactericidal urine levels as opposed to serum levels. Medicine 44:1, 1965.

Stamey TA, Timothy MM: Studies of introital colonization in women with recurrent urinary infections: I. The role of vaginal pH. J Urol 114:261, 1975.

Stamm WE: Measurement of pyuria and its relationship to bacteriuria. Am J Med 75(Suppl 1B):53, 1983.

Stamm WE, Counts GW, Running KR, et al: Diagnosis of coliform infection in acutely dysuric women. N Engl J Med 307:463, 1982.

Stansfeld JM: Duration of treatment for urinary tract infections in children. Br Med J 3:65, 1975.

Sty JR, Wells RG, Starshak RJ, et al: Imaging in acute renal infection in children. AJR 148:471, 1987.

Svanborg Edén C, de Man P: Bacterial virulence in urinary tract infections. Infect Dis Clin North Am 1:731, 1987.

Svanborg Edén C, Erikson BA, Hanson LA: Adhesion to normal uroepithelial cells of Escherichia coli from children with various forms of urinary tract infections. J Pediatr 93:398, 1978.

Svanborg Edén C, Hagberg L, Hull R, et al: Bacterial virulence versus host resistance in the urinary tracts of mice. Infect Immun 55:1224, 1987.

Svanborg Edén C, Hanson LA, Jodal U, et al: Variable adherence to normal human urinary tract epithelial cells of Escherichia coli strains associated with various forms of urinary tract infections. Lancet 2:490, 1976.

Svanborg Edén C, Jodal U: Attachment of Escherichia coli to sediment epithelial cells from UTI prone in healthy children. Infect Immun 26:837, 1979.

Svanborg Edén C, Svennerholm AM: Secretory immunoglobulin A and G antibodies prevent adhesion of Escherichia coli to human urinary tract epithelial cells. Infect Immun 22:790, 1978.

Subramanyam BR, Megibow AJ, Raghavendra BN, et al: Diffuse xanthogranulomatous pyelonephritis: analysis by computed tomography and sonography. Urol Radiol 4:5, 1982.

Taylor PW: Bactericidal and bacteriolytic activity of serum against gram-negative bacterias. Microbiol Rev 47:46, 1983.

Thomas D, Simpson K, Ostojic H, et al: Bacteremic epididymo-orchitis due to Hemophilus influenzae type B. J Urol 126:832, 1981.

Thomas SR, Gelfand MJ, Burns GS: Radiation absorbed—dose estimates for the liver, spleen and metaphyseal growth complexes in children undergoing gallium-67 citrate scanning. Radiology 146:817, 1983.

Thomas V, Shelokov A, Forland M: Antibody coated bacteria in the urine and the site of urinary tract infection. N Engl J Med 290:588, 1974.

Timmons JW, Perlmutter AD: Renal abscess: a changing concept. J Urol 115:299, 1976.

Tomisawa S, Kogure T, Kuroume T, et al: P blood group and proneness to urinary tract infections in Japanese children. Scand J Infect Dis 21:403, 1989.

Traisman ES, Conway JJ, Traisman HS, et al: The localization of urinary tract infection with 99mTc glucoheptonate scintigraphy. Pediatr Radiol 16:403, 1986.

Tuttle JP Jr, Sarvas H, Koistinen J: The role of vaginal immunoglobulin A in girls with recurrent urinary tract infections. J Urol 120:742, 1978.

Uehling DT, Jensen J, Balish E: Vaginal immunization against urinary tract infection. J Urol 128:1382, 1982.

Uehling DT, King LR: Secretory immunoglobulin A excretion in cystitis cystica. Urology 1:305, 1973.

Uehling DT, Mizutani K, Balish E: Effect of immunization on bacterial adherence to urothelium. Invest Urol 16:145, 1978.

Uehling DT, Stiehm ER: Elevated urinary secretory IgA in children with urinary tract infection. Pediatrics 47:40, 1971.

Vaisanen V, Lounatama R, Korhonen TK: Effects of sublethal concentrations of antimicrobial agents on the hemagglutination adhesion, and ultrastructure of pyelonephritogenic *Escherichia coli* strains. Antimicrob Agents Chemother 22:120, 1982.

Vaisanen V, Tallgren LG, Makela PH, et al: Mannose-resistant hemagglutination and P antigen recognition are characteristic of *Escherichia coli* causing primary pyelonephritis. Lancet 2:1366, 1981.

Vaisanen-Rhen V, Elo J, Vaisanen E, et al: P-fimbriated clones among uropathogenic *Escherichia coli* strains. Infect Immun 43:149, 1984.

Van Gool J, Tanagho EA: External sphincter activity and recurrent infection in girls. Urology 10:348, 1977.

Waalwijk C, MacLaren DM, deGraaf J: In vivo function of hemolysin in the nephropathogenicity of *Escherichia coli*. Infect Immun 42:245, 1983.

Walten MG, Kunin CM: Significance of borderline counts in screening programs for bacteriuria. J Pediatr 78:246, 1971.

Watson AR, Marsden HB, Cendon M, et al: Renal pseudotumors caused by xanthogranulomatous pyelonephritis. Arch Dis Child 57:635, 1982.

White RHR: Management of urinary tract infection. Arch Dis Child 62:421, 1987.

Wientzen RL, McCracken GH Jr, Petruska ML, et al: Localization and therapy of urinary tract infections of childhood. Pediatrics 63:467, 1979.

Willi U, Treves S: Radionuclide voiding cystography. *In* Interventional Nuclear Medicine. Edited by RP Spencer. Orlando, Grune and Stratton, 1984.

Winberg J, Andersen HJ, Bergstrom T, et al: Epidemiology of symptomatic urinary tract infection in childhood. Acta Paediatr Scand (Suppl) 252:1, 1974.

Winberg J, Andersen HJ, Hanson LA, et al: Studies of urinary tract infections in infancy and childhood: I. Antibody response in different types of urinary tract infections caused by coliform bacteria. Br Med J 2:524, 1963.

Winberg J, Bergström T, Jacobsson B: Morbidity, age and sex distribution, recurrences and renal scarring in symptomatic urinary tract infection in childhood. Kidney Int 8:S-101, 1975.

Winberg J, Bollgren I, Kallenius G, et al: Clinical pyelonephritis and focal renal scarring: a selected review of pathogenesis, prevention, and prognosis. Pediatr Clin North Am 29:801, 1982.

Winter AL, Hardy BE, Alton DJ, et al: Acquired renal scars in children. J Urol 129:1190, 1983.

Winter CC: Rapid miniaturized tests for bacteriuria: Microstix and Bacturcult and urine tests. J Urol 114:755, 1975.

Wiswell TE, Roscelli JD: Corroborative evidence for the decreased incidence of urinary tract infections in circumcised male infants. Pediatrics 78:96, 1986.

Wiswell TE, Smith FR, Bass JW: Decreased incidence of urinary tract infection in circumcised male infants. Pediatrics 75:90, 1985.

Wold AE, Mestecky J, Svanborg Edén C: Agglutination of *E. coli* by secretory IgA—a result of interaction between bacterial mannose-specific adhesins and immunoglobulin carbohydrate? Monogr Allergy 24:307, 1988.

Yazaki T, Ishikawa S, Ogawa Y, et al: Xanthogranulomatous pyelonephritis in childhood: case report and review of English and Japanese literature. J Urol 127:80, 1982.

Young LS, Martin WJ, Meyer RD, et al: Gram-negative rod bacteremia: microbiologic, immunologic, and therapeutic considerations. Ann Intern Med 86:456, 1977.

□ SPECIFIC INFECTIONS OF THE GENITOURINARY TRACT

David E. Hill and Stephen A. Kramer

TUBERCULOSIS

The advent of effective antituberculosis agents has made genitourinary tuberculosis an uncommon occurrence in the Western world. In 1984, 21,197 cases were reported in the United States and nearly 2000 people died of the disease (Weinberg and Boyd). The infection rate in children living in the United States whose parents were born in this country ranges between one and two cases per 10,000 per year. We have seen no new cases of genitourinary tuberculosis in children at the Mayo Clinic since 1956.

Genitourinary tuberculosis accounts for approximately one fifth of the cases of extrapulmonary tuberculosis (Weinberg and Boyd). More cases may be seen in the future with the influx of refugees and the increase in children with acquired immunodeficiency syndrome (AIDS).

Tuberculosis in children occurs most often in lower socioeconomic groups. Case rates are higher in black children and other minorities than in white children. Transmission of tuberculous infection from mother to infant via the placenta or amniotic fluid has been reported in 130 to 200 patients (Smith and Marquis).

Pathogenesis

Mycobacterium tuberculosis, the tubercle bacillus, is a slow-growing, acid-fast organism that is usually acquired through inhalation of respiratory droplets from an infected person. Renal tuberculosis is always preceded by a focus of infection in some other organ system, usually pulmonary (Cotran et al). The tubercle bacilli gain access to the kidneys via hematogenous dissemination, and therefore renal infection must be considered bilateral in nature.

Pathology

Genitourinary tuberculosis occurs in 4 to 15 per cent of patients with tuberculosis (Cinman; Cos and Cockett); it accounts for 73 per cent of the cases of extrapulmonary tuberculosis (García-Rodriguez et al). Renal tuberculosis is a late and uncommon complication of pulmonary disease, which rarely occurs less than 4 to 5 years after primary infection. Predisposing conditions, such as malnutrition, diabetes mellitus, and chronic corticosteroid administration, play a significant role in the development of genitourinary tuberculosis. The tuberculous bacillary emboli are deposited initially in the glomerular and cortical arterioles and cause small tubercles to develop. These tubercles undergo necrosis, with eventual caseation and cavitation of sloughed material into the calyceal walls at the papillary tips. These lesions may extend throughout the renal parenchyma and cause total destruction of the renal pyramids. Rupture of the bacilli into the calyx and collecting system results in dissemination of disease to other calyces, renal pelvis, ureter, and bladder.

Progression of disease results in fibrosis and may lead to stenosis at the calyceal neck, infundibulum, ureteropelvic junction, mid ureter, and ureterovesical junction. Ureteral fibrosis results in straightening and shortening of the ureter and ultimately produces the classic gaping golf-hole ureteral orifice with vesicoureteral reflux. Alternatively, ureteral stricture may produce hydroureteronephrosis and ultimately a nonfunctioning "autonephrectomized" kidney (Murphy et al).

Involvement of the bladder by tubercle bacilli causes ulceration and bleeding with destruction of the vesical mucosa. In the later stages of the disease, progressive fibrosis produces vesical contraction and scarring, which may lead to vesicoureteral reflux or ureterovesical junction obstruction.

Tuberculosis of the genital tract is uncommon in both sexes before puberty. In males, involvement of the genital tract usually occurs either hematogenously or through retrograde passage of infected urine through the posterior urethra in the prostatic ducts. Tuberculous epididymitis or epididymo-orchitis can occur in early childhood and may be the initial method of presentation. In females with genital tuberculosis, the fallopian tubes are involved in approximately 90 per cent of cases, the endometrium in 50 per cent, the ovaries in 20 to 30 per cent, and the cervix in 2 to 4 per cent (Smith and Marquis).

Symptoms

The majority of young children with genitourinary tuberculosis have no symptoms during the initial infection (Ehrlich and Lattimer). The lag time between pulmonary infection and the clinical onset of renal tuberculosis explains why most patients are adolescents at the time of initial presentation. Symptoms of frequency, dysuria, hematuria, and pyuria occur late in the course of disease, when the lesions ulcerate through the calyces and renal pelvis, and tubercle bacilli are disseminated to the bladder. Some children may present with systemic symptoms of generalized malaise, fatigue, low-grade persistent fever, or night sweats. Genitourinary tuberculosis must be suspected in patients with chronic or recurrent urinary tract infections who do not respond to standard antibiotic therapy. Furthermore, in children with sterile pyuria, patients with draining sinuses, and those with a history of tuberculosis elsewhere in the body or in the family, genitourinary involvement should be suspected. One child with a tuberculous vesicovaginal fistula and total urinary incontinence has been reported (Singh et al). With treatment of the tuberculosis, the fistula closed and the incontinence was corrected.

Diagnosis

Microscopic hematuria and pyuria are usually present. Routine urine specimens for culture are often negative; however, 15 to 20 per cent of patients with tuberculous bacilluria may have coexistent bacterial infection. The diagnosis of genitourinary tuberculosis is suggested by the demonstration of acid-fast bacilli in the stained urinary sediment and is confirmed by culture, usually guinea pig inoculation. Collection of fresh morning urine specimens appears to be just as accurate as 24-hour urinary concentrates in providing the diagnosis (Kenney et al). The acid-fast tubercle bacilli are discharged intermittently, and therefore at least three separate specimens should be collected for study. Tetracycline and sulfa medications exert mild bacteriostatic effects on tuberculosis cultures, and these drugs should be discontinued before urine collection (Lattimer et al). Skin tests for tuberculosis (PPD) are usually positive except in cases of overwhelming infection or with human immunodeficiency virus (HIV) infection. The erythrocyte sedimentation rate (ESR) may be increased, and anemia may be seen in advanced disease.

Plain films of the abdomen may reveal punctate calcification overlying the renal parenchyma (Hartman et al). In approximately 10 per cent of patients with renal tuberculosis, calculi are present. The earliest radiographic findings on the excretory urogram may be minimal calyceal dilatation or erosion of the papillary tip. As the infection proceeds, there is increased destruction of the calyces (Fig. 10–23). With advanced disease, there may be cavitation and cicatricial deformity of the collecting system, which may progress to pyonephrosis and nonfunction (Fig. 10–24). Conversely, a normal excretory urogram does not

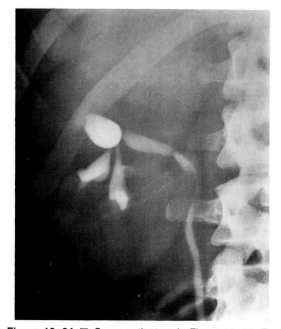

Figure 10–24 □ Same patient as in Figure 10–23. Excretory urogram shows cicatricial deformity of collecting system with amputation of upper pole infundibulum.

rule out active genitourinary tuberculosis. In patients with hydroureteronephrosis or nonfunctioning renal units, ureteral catheterization may be helpful for selective urinary collection and retrograde pyelography may be necessary to provide accurate delineation of pyelocalyceal architecture.

Cystoscopic examination reveals only minimal inflammatory changes in the early stages of disease. With coalescence of the tubercles, there may be areas of white or yellow raised nodules with a halo of hyperemia. With advanced localized disease, bladder capacity may become markedly diminished, with fixed and incompetent ureteral orifices, mucosal ulceration, and diffuse cystitis.

Treatment

The advent of short-course chemotherapy has changed the surgical management of genitourinary tuberculosis (Gow). The current recommendation is for surgery to restore function or to remove irreparable disease. Surgery can be performed 6 weeks after the start of chemotherapy.

Antituberculosis drugs inhibit multiplication of tubercle bacilli and arrest the course of disease progression. Various antituberculosis agents are currently available, as discussed in

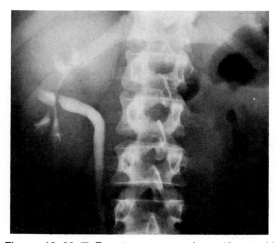

Figure 10–23 □ Excretory urogram in a 19-year-old male demonstrates extensive papillary necrosis involving upper pole of right kidney from renal tuberculosis.

the following paragraphs (American Academy of Pediatrics; Glassroth et al; Smith and Marquis). The efficacy of combination chemotherapy compared with single-drug administration has been well documented. Furthermore, analysis of long-term follow-up demonstrated that therapy with orally administered agents is as effective as parenteral drug administration.

Isoniazid

The dosage of isoniazid (INH) is 10 to 30 mg/kg of body weight per day, up to 300 mg daily, given in one dose. The drug is the most effective of the antituberculosis agents available and remains the keystone of all therapeutic regimens. Isoniazid is metabolized in the liver and is excreted primarily through the kidney. It is available in liquid form (50 mg/5 ml) and in tablets, which may be dissolved in fruit juice or water; this makes drug administration easier in infants and young children. Peripheral neuritis is the most common side effect and is probably caused by inhibition of pyridoxine metabolism. Neurotoxic side effects have not been reported in children younger than 11 years of age, and thus pyridoxine supplementation is not recommended unless nutrition is inadequate. Hepatotoxicity, which is seen often in older patients, rarely occurs in children.

Rifampin

The dosage of rifampin is 10 to 20 mg/kg/day, up to 600 mg daily. Rifampin, one of the newest antituberculosis agents, is extremely effective and virtually nontoxic for administration in children. Rare cases of minor hepatic and renal dysfunction have been reported. This drug is indicated for the initial treatment of genitourinary tuberculosis and for cases requiring re-treatment. Rifampin is excreted in the bile and urine and may cause orange discoloration of urine, tears, and sweat. In older females taking rifampin, contraceptive drugs should be avoided because rifampin changes the kinetics of the estrogen component.

Ethambutol

The dosage of ethambutol is 15 to 20 mg/kg/day, up to 2500 mg daily, divided into two to three doses. This is an extremely effective antituberculosis drug, which has replaced p-aminosalicylic acid for use in most adults. It is rapidly absorbed and excreted in the urine.

Optic neuritis is a major toxic effect of ethambutol, and monthly visual examinations are required. This drug is not recommended for use in small children who are not able to cooperate in examination of visual acuity and color vision.

Streptomycin

The dosage of streptomycin is 20 to 40 mg/kg/day given intramuscularly, up to 1000 mg daily. Although streptomycin is still a useful drug for the treatment of genitourinary tuberculosis, the risk of eighth nerve damage prohibits use of this medication for longer than 12 weeks.

p-Aminosalicylic Acid (PAS)

The dosage of PAS is 200 mg/kg/day, up to 12 g daily. PAS is an effective bactericidal drug for the treatment of renal tuberculosis when used in combination with other antituberculosis medications. However, PAS is not effective when used alone. Major side effects are gastrointestinal problems, including nausea, vomiting, diarrhea, and anorexia. It is best to give PAS after meals and in the form of sodium and potassium PAS to decrease gastrointestinal irritability.

Pyrazinamide

The dosage of pyrazinamide is 15 to 30 mg/kg/day, up to 2 g/day. The drug is bactericidal, seldom hepatotoxic, and well tolerated by children.

Ethionamide

The dosage of ethionamide is 15 to 20 mg/kg/day, up to a maximum of 1 g/day. The drug is well tolerated by children, is bacteriostatic, and occasionally is useful for drug-resistant cases. A physician experienced with this drug should be consulted prior to its use.

Other Drugs

Cycloserine, kanamycin, and capreomycin may be useful in treating drug-resistant cases of genitourinary tuberculosis.

Specific Therapy for Genitourinary Tuberculosis

The accepted treatment for genitourinary tuberculosis is triple-drug chemotherapy administered daily for 2 years (Wechsler and Lattimer). Recently, short-course chemotherapy (6-month treatment regimen) has been advocated in an attempt to (1) increase patient compliance, (2) decrease the cost of medication, (3) lower drug toxicity, and (4) produce an equally successful regimen comparable with the standard therapy (Fox; Gow). Short-course chemotherapy must include rifampin as one of the drugs (Weinberg and Boyd).

The current recommendation of the American Academy of Pediatrics for treatment of genitourinary tuberculosis is 9 months of INH and rifampin. In the first 2 months of therapy, a third drug should be added. This may include pyrazinamide, streptomycin, or ethambutol in children older than 5 years of age. If the infection is associated with HIV infection, treatment should include three drugs and may need to be longer than 9 months (American Academy of Pediatrics).

The majority of relapses occur within the first 2 years. Females in the childbearing years should avoid pregnancy until therapy is completed (Gow and Barbosa). Women who are delivered of a baby while they have genitourinary tuberculosis may infect the infant with tuberculosis (Schaaf et al).

With the rapid bactericidal activity of drugs like rifampin, recent recommendations call for 1-year follow-up unless calcification is seen on abdominal radiographs (Weinberg and Boyd). If calcification is present, the child requires long-term follow-up to be sure that the disease does not progress. During the follow-up period, urinalysis should be performed every 2 months. The upper urinary tracts should be monitored prior to, during, and after treatment to assess for obstruction because strictures are common. Renal ultrasonography is useful for screening, and an intravenous urogram should be performed if any abnormality is noted.

Although aggressive surgical therapy in patients with genitourinary tuberculosis has been recommended (Flechner and Gow; Wong and Lau), the results of chemotherapy are so impressive that surgical intervention should be limited to exceptional cases, such as ureteral stricture (Murphy et al), ureterovesical junction reconstruction, or augmentation cytoplasty in children with small contracted bladders (Zinman and Libertino).

With the introduction of smaller ureteral stents and ureteroscopic instrumentation, children may now benefit from stenting of ureteral strictures, as has been done in adults. This allows stabilization of disease before surgical reconstruction.

AIDS

AIDS was first reported in 1981 by the Centers for Disease Control (McNamara). Since 1982, AIDS has been recognized in children, with the majority of children acquiring the infection by transplacental, intrapartum, or postpartum transmission from an infected mother (Mok). Many more children are HIV-positive, and approximately one third of these are hemophiliacs or recipients of blood components (Davies). AIDS represents one of the most significant public health hazards and has received more attention in the past few years than any other infection.

Pathogenesis

HIV was identified as the virus present in patients with or at risk for AIDS. After transmission of HIV through an infected mother or blood transfusion (the most common forms of transmission in children), HIV selectively infects CD4-positive lymphocytes. A selective depletion of this population of lymphocytes leads to the profound immunodeficiency of AIDS. These CD4-positive helper/inducer T cells are involved in controlling and regulating the immune system through the elaboration of numerous soluble mediators called lymphokines. Induction of growth and differentiation of numerous hematopoietic cell lines is dependent on these mediators, and without them the many immunologic abnormalities associated with the AIDS complex are noted. Other abnormalities include a qualitative defect in proliferative responses to antigens and in lymphokine production, macrophage dysfunctions, and dysfunction of the humoral immune system (McNamara). This leads to an increased susceptibility to opportunistic infections and neoplasms, which is the hallmark of AIDS in adult patients (McNamara). However, children with AIDS more frequently experience recurrent bacterial infections (Albano and Pizzo).

Pathology

Pathologic findings in AIDS relate to the manifestations of the profound lymphoid depletion, infections, and unusual neoplasms. Urologic involvement in AIDS may be related to infectious or neoplastic processes. HIV has been seen in the urinary tract (Miles et al). Cytomegalovirus (CMV) infection has been reported in the adrenal gland, kidneys, bladder, seminal vesicles, and testes. CMV may be seen in the adrenal cortex but is found primarily in the medulla (Reichert et al). Disorders of spermatogenesis have been noted in adult males, and Kaposi's sarcoma has been noted in the epididymis as well as the adrenal glands, prostate, seminal vesicles, bladder, and penis (Miles et al; Reichert et al). Some previously undiagnosed young men with AIDS have presented with testis tumors. These have been mainly B-cell lymphomas (Miles et al).

Symptoms

Children with HIV infection may present with nonspecific signs and symptoms, including failure to thrive, recurrent respiratory infections, chronic diarrhea, unexplained fever, generalized lymphadenopathy, and hepatosplenomegaly (Mok). Recurrent bacterial infections are seen more frequently in pediatric AIDS patients than in adult AIDS patients (Albano and Pizzo). Other signs and symptoms include decrease in size and force of the urinary stream, dysuria, frequency, hesitancy, hematuria, urethral discharge, urinary tract infection (UTI), and dermatologic conditions of the genitalia. Urologic symptoms have been noted in only 16 per cent of patients with AIDS (Miles et al). Of 17 AIDS patients with UTIs, nine had standard bacterial urinary infections, six had CMV, one had *Cryptococcus,* and one had gonorrhea.

AIDS patients may also present with nephrologic manifestations, such as proteinuria, renal insufficiency, and the nephrotic syndrome. Focal and segmental glomerulosclerosis have been documented, and when they are associated with proteinuria and uremia, the prognosis is poor (Miles et al).

Diagnosis

The diagnosis of AIDS is based on the finding of immunosuppression in a previously healthy patient with no known cause for the immunosuppression and a disease that is indicative of a defect in cellular immune function (Reichert et al). The most common opportunistic infections seen in children are *Pneumocystis carinii* pneumonia and *Candida* esophagitis. The presence of HIV is confirmed by a positive antibody test (Bradford et al). HIV antibodies are transferred across the placenta, making the interpretation of a positive antibody test in an infant difficult. Clearance of the antibody can take up to 18 months, so that

children younger than 18 months of age who are positive for HIV antibody are classified as having indeterminate infection, unless there is other evidence for HIV infection (Mok). If urinary tract symptoms are present, urinalysis and sensitivity tests should be done and specimens for urine culture obtained. If hematuria is present and the urine is sterile, an excretory urogram (IVP) and cystoscopy should be performed.

Care must be taken in examining any patient suspected of having AIDS. Universal blood and body fluid precautions should be strictly followed. Cystoscopic equipment used in the evaluation of these patients should be gas sterilized after use.

Treatment

There is no known cure for AIDS, and treatment is directed at the symptoms. With bacterial infections, prompt, aggressive, broad-spectrum antibiotic therapy should be instituted. Administration of parenteral immunoglobulins has been used in an attempt to prevent infection and has been associated with a decreased incidence of serious bacterial infection. Chemoprophylaxis with trimethoprim-sulfamethoxazole may prevent *P. carinii* pneumonia. Experimental methods that attempt to improve the altered immune mechanisms are being studied. Azidothymidine, an antiretroviral agent, has produced some improvement in the defects associated with HIV infection in adult AIDS patients. Trials using azidothymidine in children with AIDS and AIDS-related complex are currently under way (Albano and Pizzo).

FUNGAL DISEASES

Fungal infestation should be considered in the differential diagnosis of children with inflammatory disease of the genitourinary tract. Opportunistic fungal infections in adults and children have increased significantly in recent years. These fungal infections occur most often in patients with obstructive uropathy and in patients with impaired host resistance owing to causes such as extensive burns, blood dyscrasias, collagen vascular disease, and long-term steroid therapy. Glycosuria provides a favorable environment for mycotic growth, and patients with diabetes mellitus, in particular, are at increased risk for fungal involvement of the genitourinary tract.

Candidiasis

Candida albicans and, more rarely, *Candida tropicalis* are yeast forms that may exist as commensals in the mouth, intestinal tract, vagina, and skin of normal persons. *Candida* is the most common of the opportunistic mycoses, and systemic disease occurs almost exclusively in patients with impaired host resistance. *Candida* may also be recoverable in the urine of persons with asymptomatic infection, usually as a result of overgrowth after broad-spectrum antibiotic therapy. Systemic candidiasis may be seen in up to 4 per cent of newborns weighing 1500 g or less and in up to 9 per cent of newborns weighing less than 1000 g (Pappu et al).

Pathogenesis and Pathology

Conditions that predispose to candidemia include prematurity, contamination of intravenous catheters, long-term antibiotic therapy, steroid administration, immunosuppressive agents, impaired T-cell–dependent cellular immunity, cytotoxic drug therapy, blood dyscrasias, burns, and open surgical wounds (MacMillan et al; Pappu et al; Stone et al; van't Wout). In patients with gram-negative bacteremia, antibiotic therapy appears to be one of the most important predisposing factors in the development of subsequent candidemia (Stone et al).

The kidney is usually involved secondary to a generalized systemic candidal infection but may be involved primarily along with the ureters and bladder (Pappu et al). Candiduria may lead to the formation of fungus balls in the collecting system with obstruction, pyelonephritis, or perinephric abscess formation. In up to 88 per cent of patients with disseminated candidiasis, microorganisms are demonstrable within the renal parenchyma.

Symptoms

The most common clinical manifestation is oliguria or anuria (Pappu et al). Patients may present with fever, chills, flank pain or mass, renal colic, hypertension, or urosepsis. Pyelonephritis and ureteral obstruction caused by fungus ball infestation have been reported (Kozinn et al, 1976; Schönebeck et al). Anuria in infants can result from bilateral renal pelvic fungus balls (Eckstein and Kass; Khan; Schmitt and Hsu). In patients with localized candidal cystitis, urinary urgency, frequency, and dysuria are typical findings.

Diagnosis

Schönebeck stated that any number of *Candida* specimens for culture obtained from a mid-stream urine collection in the male or from a catheterized specimen in the female is significant for *Candida* infection. Colony counts greater than 15,000 per ml obtained by mid-stream clean catch or a single urethral catheterization are evidence of renal *Candida* infection (Kozinn et al, 1978; Wise et al, 1976). Conversely, colony counts of more than 100,000 per ml in patients with indwelling urethral catheters appear to have no relationship to upper tract candidal infection.

Criteria for determining significant candidal infection should be based on clinical data, urinary findings, and serum precipitin titers. The presence of agglutinating antibodies and serum precipitins, as detected by agar gel diffusion techniques, provides an accurate index of parenchymal or invasive candidal infection (Dolan and Stried; Everett et al; Wise et al, 1972). In a series of patients with systemic candidiasis, Kozinn et al (1976) reported true-positive precipitin reactions in 65 of 69 patients (94 per cent). Interestingly, fewer than 50 per cent of patients with systemic candidiasis demonstrate positive blood cultures.

The diagnosis can be made at the bedside by portable renal ultrasonography if the infant is too ill to transport. Renal ultrasonograms may show the presence of an echogenic mass within the renal collecting system. Percutaneous nephrostomy tubes can be placed, through which brush biopsy of the mass may confirm the presence of pseudohyphae consistent with *Candida* (Schmitt and Hsu).

The excretory urogram may suggest papillary necrosis, tuberculosis, calculous disease, or neoplasm. A fungus ball may appear as a filling defect in the collecting system and may cause obstructive uropathy or nonvisualization of the kidney. Cystoscopic examination reveals diffuse cystitis with purulent material distributed over the mucosal surface.

Treatment

Candiduria that occurs in healthy patients after long-term, broad-spectrum antibiotic therapy should clear after the antibiotic has been stopped. Localized infections of the kidney or bladder may be controlled and eradicated by irrigation with a solution of 5 per cent amphotericin B (Fungizone) in sterile water via a nephrostomy tube or three-way bladder catheter (Wise et al, 1973, 1982). Infants with renal fungus balls may require emergency pyelotomy and insertion of nephrostomy tubes for irrigation. Continuous irrigation with a slow-drip infusion can be maintained for several days without systemic toxic effects. Alkalinization of the urine to a pH of 7.5 with sodium bicarbonate given orally is recommended.

The treatment of choice for systemic candidiasis is amphotericin B, a nephrotoxic, fungistatic agent that must be given intravenously. Amphotericin B must be administered in 5 per cent dextrose in water. Initially, a test dose of 0.1 mg/kg, up to a total dose of 1 mg, is given over a period of 3 to 4 hours with careful monitoring of temperature, respiration, and blood pressure. The dose should be increased gradually in daily increments of 0.25 mg/kg over a 4-day period until a total dose of 1 mg/kg is achieved. Peak serum levels should be twice the mean inhibitory concentration for the infectious organism, and trough levels should be approximately equal to the mean inhibitory concentration for the fungus. Toxic side effects include fever, nausea and vomiting, generalized malaise, and phlebitis. Decreased renal function is not uncommon, and frequent determinations of serum creatinine values are required. The duration of therapy is dependent on the extent of the infection, but intravenous drug administration is usually required for several weeks to eradicate disseminated disease. Some authors recommend adding flucytosine because of its synergistic effect and low toxic potential (Pappu et al; Polak).

Flucytosine (Ancobon) is a much less toxic agent than amphotericin B and is effective in the treatment of systemic candidiasis (Wheeler et al; Wise et al, 1974). The drug is administered orally and is excreted primarily unchanged in the urine. The dose is 150 mg/kg/day given orally at 6-hour intervals. Adverse side effects are infrequent; however, thrombocytopenia, leukopenia, rash, hepatic dysfunction, and diarrhea may occur, especially in patients with diminished renal function.

Miconazole, an intravenously administered antifungal agent, lacks hepatic and renal toxicity. The use of miconazole in the treatment of genitourinary candidiasis in a newborn has been reported (Noe and Tonkin). The drug is administered intravenously every 8 hours at a dose of 20 to 40 mg/kg. A single infusion should never exceed 15 mg/kg (American

Academy of Pediatrics). There is limited experience with this drug in the clinical setting, however, and amphotericin B and flucytosine remain the initial drugs of choice in children with *Candida* sepsis (Wise).

Ketoconazole is an antimycotic agent that has been shown to be effective for both superficial and deep fungal infections (Graybill et al). It is given as a single oral dose of 3.3 to 6.6 mg/kg and appears to have minimal toxicity (Borgers et al; American Academy of Pediatrics).

Aspergillosis

Aspergillosis is the second most common fungal infection in patients with hematologic malignancies (Hinson et al). *Aspergillus* species are prevalent worldwide and grow on decaying vegetation, in damp hay or straw, and in the soil (Young et al). Most cases of human disease are caused by *Aspergillus fumigatus, Aspergillus flavus,* or *Aspergillus niger* (Levitz).

Pathogenesis and Pathology

The disease is caused by inhalation of fungal spores. The organism is occasionally introduced through an operative wound, via trauma, or from a foreign body such as an intravenous or urinary catheter. Three separate patterns of disease have been described: (1) disseminated hematogenous spread with multiple organ involvement (Levitz; Young et al), (2) involvement limited to the renal pelvis or parenchyma (Comings et al; Eisenberg et al; Godec et al; Warshawsky et al), and (3) panurothelial disease involving the urethra, bladder, ureters, and kidneys (Flechner and McAninch). Renal infection is characterized by vascular invasion, focal microabscess formation, and, occasionally, papillary necrosis.

Symptoms

Microscopic hematuria and pyuria are often present in patients with aspergillosis. Obstructive uropathy from a fungus ball or "aspergilloma" in the renal pelvis may be the initial method of presentation (Comings et al; Eisenberg et al; Melchior et al; Young et al).

Diagnosis

The fungi may be identified as branched septate hyphae on potassium hydroxide preparations of infected material. Results of urine cultures are variable, and positive blood cultures rarely occur. Multiple specimens for culture are often required to identify the organism. Diagnosis of invasive aspergillosis by antibody testing is rarely helpful (Levitz). Testing for *Aspergillus* antigens in sera is under investigation and not yet available, although it does show promise. Skin tests are usually positive but are nondiagnostic. Definitive diagnosis of invasive aspergillosis is established by tissue biopsy or by identification of sloughed tissue and fungus balls per urethra. Excretory urographic findings are nonspecific and may demonstrate filling defects in the renal pelvis secondary to fungus ball infestation.

Treatment

Invasive aspergillosis is usually a rapidly fatal disease, and treatment is generally unsuccessful. Amphotericin B is the most potent and reliable drug available. Flucytosine is inactive against aspergillosis (Bennett). In patients with fungus balls in the kidney, upper tract irrigation through a nephrostomy tube may be indicated (Warshawsky et al). Alternatively, Flechner and McAninch reported successful upper tract irrigation through ureteral catheters by the use of a solution of sterile water with 15 mg of amphotericin B and one ampule of neomycin and polymyxin B administered at 100 ml/hour. Surgery to relieve obstruction may be required in conjunction with medical therapy (Godec et al).

Actinomycosis

Actinomycosis is a prokaryotic, gram-positive organism with variable morphology. *Actinomyces* is either a facultative or a strict anaerobe (Medoff and Kobayashi). Disease in humans is caused by *Actinomyces israelii* and in animals by *Actinomyces bovis*. The organism is normally present in the mouth and throat and may also be found elsewhere in the gastrointestinal tract. Although rare, actinomycotic infection in infants and children has been reported (Drake and Holt; Kretschmer and Hibbs).

Pathogenesis and Pathology

Actinomycosis is a chronic, progressive suppurative disease characterized by multiple abscesses and draining sinuses (Berardi). It is usually not an opportunistic infection and ap-pears to be a cooperative disease between *Actinomyces* and a mixed flora of other bacteria (Medoff and Kobayashi). Progression of disease is associated with pronounced fibrosis and development of spontaneous fistulas. Three major varieties of clinical disease are cervicofacial, abdominal, and thoracic. Genitourinary involvement by actinomycosis has been well documented (Crosse et al; Deshmukh and Kropp; Grierson and Zelas; Isaacson and Jennings). Renal involvement usually occurs as a result of hematogenous dissemination or of direct extension from a pulmonary or gastrointestinal lesion (Robbins and Scott).

Symptoms

Patients with actinomycosis of the kidney may present with a painful flank mass or urosepsis secondary to a perinephric abscess. The bladder may become involved secondarily from direct extension of infection in the appendix, colon, or fallopian tube. Patients with vesical involvement may present with dysuria, urgency, and frequency.

Diagnosis

The demonstration of "sulfur granules" in pus establishes the diagnosis of actinomycosis. A Gram stain reveals a dense reticulum of filaments that stains violet and projects around the periphery of the granule. Specimens for culture must be obtained anaerobically on selective media. Although there have been no serodiagnostic techniques available for the diagnosis of actinomycosis, the recent use of fluorescent antibody reagents has been promising (Holmberg et al).

Excretory urography may demonstrate calyceal erosion and may produce findings that simulate genitourinary tuberculosis. The urogram may also show a mass lesion simulating a parenchymal abscess or neoplasm (Fig. 10–25).

Treatment

Treatment of actinomycosis consists of large doses of penicillin given parenterally over 2 to 4 weeks followed by orally administered antibiotics for 3 to 6 months (Eastridge et al; Medoff and Kobayashi). Tetracycline, erythromycin, lincomycin, chloramphenicol, and clindamycin have been used with successful results (Fass et al; Rose and Rytel). In unresponsive cases and in patients with extensive

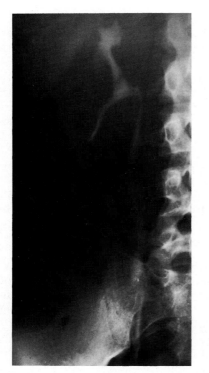

Figure 10–25 □ Right retrograde pyelogram demonstrates calyceal splaying and mass lesion, suggesting renal tumor in a patient with actinomycosis. (From Hunt VC, Mayo C: Actinomycosis of the kidney. Ann Surg 93:501, 1931. By permission of JB Lippincott Company.)

renal parenchymal destruction, surgical drainage and occasionally nephrectomy may be required.

Coccidioidomycosis

Coccidioidomycosis is an infection caused by a dimorphic fungus, *Coccidioides immitis*. Endemic areas are confined to the Western Hemisphere. In the United States, these areas include the Southwest, encompassing western Texas, New Mexico, Arizona, and California. Primary coccidioidal infection is seen most frequently in summer and fall. Person-to-person spread is rare (Libke and Granoff).

Pathogenesis and Pathology

The disease is usually acquired via the respiratory tract. Genitourinary involvement is common with disseminated disease. In an autopsy series of patients with disseminated coccidioidomycosis, renal involvement was recorded in 30 of 50 cases (60 per cent) (Conner et al). Fungal involvement of the kidney appears confined to the cortex as small miliary granulomas or microabscesses. Genital involvement with bilateral epididymitis may be the initial method of presentation (Cheng).

Diagnosis

In disseminated disease, microscopic examination of exudates or biopsy specimens is diagnostic if typical spherules are visualized. Skin tests are helpful and become positive 1 to 3 weeks after exposure to the fungus. Definitive identification requires animal inoculation or special culture techniques. Serologic studies are useful and include serum precipitins and latex agglutination (Drutz and Catanzaro; Weinstein and Farkas). Immunodiffusion and counterimmunoelectrophoresis are alternative methods for the detection of specific coccidioidal antibodies (Aguilar-Torres et al).

The radiographic findings of advanced renal coccidioidomycosis may mimic those of tuberculosis and demonstrate infundibular stenosis, blunted or sloughed calyces, and calcified granulomas.

Treatment

Amphotericin B is the drug of choice for disseminated disease. Ketoconazole is an orally administered active antifungal agent that is undergoing clinical trials. Miconazole has been used successfully in some patients but should probably be reserved for patients who have failed to respond to therapy with amphotericin B and are unable to receive ketoconazole therapy (Libke and Granoff; Stevens et al).

Cryptococcosis

Cryptococcosis is an infectious disease caused by a spherical fungus, *Cryptococcus neoformans*. Cryptococcosis occurs most often in debilitated patients, especially those with Hodgkin's disease.

Pathogenesis

Infection with *C. neoformans* may be acquired by inhalation of infected particles during exposure to pigeon excreta (Wittner). The primary site of disease is pulmonary; however, hematogenous dissemination of the fungus often occurs, and renal involvement is well documented (Lewis and Rabinovich; Randall et al). In a review of autopsy cases of disseminated cryptococcal infection, Salyer and Salyer found that 30 of 39 patients (77 per cent) demonstrated involvement of the kidneys. Cryptococcal involvement of the prostate has been documented at autopsy (Bowman and Ritchey; Cohen and Kaufmann; Salyer and Salyer) and as a cause of lower urinary tract obstruction (Huynh and Reyes; O'Connor et al; Tillotson and Lerner). In rare instances, Addison's disease may be seen secondary to extensive involvement of the adrenal gland (Wittner).

Symptoms

Microscopic hematuria and pyuria occur in the majority of patients with genitourinary cryptococcosis. In patients with diffuse granulomatous involvement of the kidneys, pyelonephritis may be the initial method of presentation.

Diagnosis

The encapsulated yeasts may be demonstrated in urine, pus, or India ink preparations of cerebrospinal fluid. Precise diagnosis, however, depends on identification of the organism by culture techniques. In patients with disseminated cryptococcosis, urine and blood cultures have usually been positive. The latex agglutination test for cryptococcal antigen is highly specific and may have diagnostic and prognostic value (Gordon and Vedder; Wittner).

Treatment

Amphotericin B in combination with 5-fluorocytosine is the treatment of choice for human cryptococcosis. In vitro, these two drugs act synergistically; when these drugs are used in combination, the nephrotoxicity of amphotericin is decreased, possibly because less amphotericin B is required to cure the patient (Wittner).

Blastomycosis

Blastomyces dermatitidis, the etiologic agent of North American blastomycosis, is a dimorphic fungus found in the soil. Endemic sites of disease in the United States include Ohio, the Mississippi and Missouri River valleys, and the area along the western shores of Lake Michigan (Furcolow et al).

Pathogenesis

Infection with blastomycosis usually occurs from inhalation of the fungus, which produces a primary pulmonary focus. Dissemination of the fungus may occur to any organ of the body through hematogenous or lymphogenous routes. Genitourinary involvement occurs in approximately 20 to 30 per cent of cases (Denton et al), and childhood involvement has been documented (Gill and Gerald; Eickenberg et al; Yogev and Davis).

Symptoms

Blastomycosis should be considered in the differential diagnosis of any granulomatous or suppurative disease of the genitourinary tract. The fungus tends to affect males; no female patients with genitourinary involvement were documented in a series of 51 patients recorded by Eickenberg et al. Blastomycosis may involve the kidney, prostate, epididymis, and testes (Bergner et al; Furcolow et al; Macher; Schwarz and Salfelder). Symptoms vary with the organ involved; however, dysuria, urgency, frequency, hematuria, and epididymo-orchitis have been frequent modes of presentation.

Diagnosis

Potassium hydroxide preparations of urine demonstrate the thick-walled, single-budding yeast forms of blastomycosis. Definitive diagnosis is substantiated only by culture or by histologic examination of tissue specimens. Complement fixation, immunodiffusion antibody, and skin sensitivity testing are not sensitive diagnostic aids.

Treatment

Ketoconazole and amphotericin B are both effective in blastomycosis. Ketoconazole may be indicated in mild infections whereas amphotericin B should be used for the more severe cases. Surgical excision of localized lesions may be indicated, particularly in cases of epididymo-orchitis.

Mucormycosis

Mucormycosis is a ubiquitous saprophyte and opportunistic pathogen that may cause rapidly fatal disease in patients with impaired host resistance (Baker; Meyer et al). Of 185 cases of disseminated infection reported, 21 patients are younger than 5 years old (Ingram et al).

Pathogenesis

Mucormycosis develops subsequent to ingestion of fungal elements from decaying food and vegetation. The organism has a tendency for growth in the walls of blood vessels, and its presence may lead to arterial thrombosis and infarction.

Symptoms

Most cases of mucormycosis occur in patients with an underlying malignancy (Ingram et al). Dehydration, acidosis, and shock may predispose infants to mucormycosis (Lloyd and Bolte). Renal abscesses may occur alone (Langston et al; Prout and Goddard) or in conjunction with disseminated disease (Dansky et al). Hematuria has been reported in most patients with genitourinary involvement; obstructive uropathy may be the initial method of presentation.

Diagnosis

For the diagnosis of mucormycosis, morphologic identification of mycotic elements in biopsy tissue or culture of biopsy tissue (Ingram et al) is required. There are no good serologic tests available.

Treatment

Amphotericin B is the drug of choice for disseminated mucormycosis. Acidosis and immunosuppression should both be brought under control. Partial or total nephrectomy may be indicated in selected cases with extensive renal parenchymal involvement.

PARASITIC INFECTIONS

Schistosomiasis

Urinary schistosomiasis, or bilharziasis, is a vascular, parasitic infectious disease caused by the blood fluke *Schistosoma haematobium*. It is estimated that between 200 and 300 million people in Africa, Asia, South America, and the Caribbean area are infected by schistosoma (Hanash and Bissada). The disease is endemic in Egypt. Rare cases are seen in the United States and always originate from an endemic area.

Pathogenesis

The life cycle of *S. haematobium* begins when a person with schistosomiasis urinates and discharges the parasite's egg into the stagnant water of a lake or a river. During warm hours of the day, the egg swells, ruptures, and liberates a miracidium. The miracidium swims toward and penetrates a specific species of fresh-water snail. After penetration, the miracidium matures into a sporocyst. These sporocysts bud and produce thousands of cercariae, which are liberated into the water. The cercariae penetrate the skin or mucous membranes of a human host. After cutaneous penetration, the cercariae become schistosomula, enter the venous and lymphatic systems, and are carried to the right side of the heart. They then migrate to the portal circulation, where copulation between males and females occurs. The male carries the female to the pelvic venules, where the eggs are deposited. These eggs (ova) pass through the vessels and are either buried in the bladder wall or excreted with the urine and thereby complete the life cycle (von Lichtenberg and Lehman).

Pathology

The basic response to schistosome eggs is a pronounced eosinophilic infiltrate, with the formation of granulomas or "pseudotubercles" around the ova. Vigorous antibody and cell-mediated immune responses are provoked in most patients (Kline and Sullivan). In advanced disease, collagen formation occurs, with scarring of the bladder wall, deposition of calcareous material, and calcification sclerosis. In younger patients, there is a greater prevalence of active inflammatory lesions.

Urothelial changes occur in all stages of disease and include mucosal hyperplasia, squamous metaplasia, and epithelial dysplasia. Involvement of the trigone may lead to fibrosis of the bladder neck and cause vesical outlet obstruction. Outlet obstruction with stasis of infected urine predisposes to the formation of bladder calculi in older patients. In children, however, urinary bilharziasis does not appear to play a role in the cause of vesical calculi (Kambal). In patients with long-standing disease, chronic vesical irritation may predispose the bladder to squamous cell carcinoma.

In the ureter, tissue reaction to the ova may result in ureteritis cystica, ureteritis calcinosa, or stricture formation. Vesicoureteral reflux is a result of fibrosis and lateral displacement of the intramural ureter and is seen in up to 50 per cent of patients (Hanna).

The kidneys are involved infrequently with bilharzial infection; however, it has been suggested that glomerulonephritis may result from an immune complex reaction (Hanash and Bissada). Bilharziasis has been reported in five children with xanthogranulomatous pyelonephritis and may be an etiologic factor for xanthogranulomatous pyelonephritis by increasing the incidence of UTI, obstruction, and stone formation (Bazeed et al, 1989).

Symptoms

Humans become infected with *Schistosoma* after coming into contact with contaminated water through drinking, swimming, bathing, or washing clothes. Children of any age are at risk for infection. Acute schistosomiasis occurs between 3 and 9 weeks after infection and coincides with the deposition of eggs in the bladder wall. Terminal hematuria and dysuria are classic findings. Occasionally, bleeding becomes so extensive as to result in anemia. In patients with bladder ulceration, symptoms include urinary urgency, frequency, and severe suprapubic pain.

In the later stages of disease (inactive phase of infection), fibrosis and contracture of the bladder and ureter have the potential to produce obstructive uropathy. The disease process is insidious, and massive hydroureteronephrosis or renal nonfunction may occur before the onset of clinical symptoms. In children with bladder calcification, there is also a higher prevalence of hydronephrosis and hydroureter but the presence of these findings was not related to the intensity of the bilharzial infection (King et al).

Diagnosis

The diagnosis of schistosomiasis is established by the presence of terminal-spined eggs in the urine. There is a diurnal pattern to the excretion of eggs, and to take advantage of that, a urine specimen should be collected between 11 a.m. and 1 p.m.; the sediment is examined under the microscope to look for the classic terminal-spined eggs (Kline and Sullivan). A 24-hour urine collection may be required to make the diagnosis. In the absence of eggs from multiple urine specimens, bladder or rectal biopsy provides a satisfactory method of obtaining the diagnosis (von Lichtenberg and Lehman). Intradermal skin tests and serologic techniques, including fluorescent antibody, latex flocculation, complement fixation, and precipitin tests, have been described (Kagan). Positive test findings indicate prior exposure to schistosome infection, but these studies do not identify the present status of disease and therefore may remain positive in the absence of eggs or living worms.

Peripheral blood examination usually demonstrates eosinophilia. With chronic worm infestation, the patient may be anemic as a result of destruction of erythrocytes by the blood fluke or as a consequence of chronic disease and uremia.

Radiographic and Cystoscopic Evaluation

A plain film of the abdomen may reveal calcification within the urinary tract or in other organs (Hanna). Egg-shell calcification over the bladder in an appropriate clinical setting is likely to indicate chronic urinary schistosomiasis (Fig. 10–26). Excretory urography may demonstrate ureteral strictures, hydronephrosis, or filling defects in the bladder and ureter secondary to polypoid lesions. In chronic disease, vesicoureteral reflux can occur.

Endoscopic evaluation with or without transurethral bladder biopsy may yield characteristic findings. In patients with active lesions, the bilharzial tubercles predominate over the trigone and posterior bladder wall as granular white or yellow lesions with a halo of hyperemia (Hanash and Bissada). Overdistention of the bladder results in bleeding and is reminiscent of interstitial cystitis or hemorrhagic cystitis. Coalescence of these tubercles may form a bilharzioma, which is a multinodular, hypervascular lesion usually attached by a narrow pedicle. In patients with chronic disease, fibrosis and calcification of the tubercles in the submucosa form dull, granular "sandy patches" that resemble grains of sand under water.

Treatment

Historically, antimony-containing compounds—for example, sodium or potassium

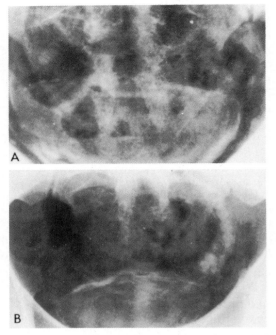

Figure 10–26 □ *A,* Plain film shows curvilinear calcification of the bladder and both distal ureters. *B,* There are numerous calculi in the left ureter. (From Hanash BA, Bissada NK, Lewall DB, et al: Genito-urinary schistosomiasis (bilharziasis): Part 2. Clinical, parasitologic, immunologic, and radiologic diagnosis. King Faisal Specialist Hosp Med J 1:119, 1981. By permission of the King Faisal Specialist Hospital and Research Centre.)

antimonyltartrate (tartar emetic)—formed the basis of medical treatment. These drugs must be given intravenously or intramuscularly and are accompanied by frequent side effects, including nausea, vomiting, peripheral neuritis, joint pains, and diarrhea. Tartar emetic is cardiotoxic and has been associated with ventricular irritability and Adams-Stokes syndrome.

The drug of choice for the treatment of schistosomiasis is praziquantel. For the treatment of *S. haematobium,* a single dose of 40 mg/kg given orally is effective. A dose of 20 mg/kg given three times in a single day is effective treatment for other schistosome species. Toxicity is low and generally resolves within 48 hours of giving the drug (American Academy of Pediatrics; Kline and Sullivan).

Metrifonate is an effective alternative to praziquantel for the treatment of *S. haematobium* infections. The drug is an inexpensive, orally administered agent, which is currently being evaluated in several endemic areas in Africa. The dosage for children is 10 mg/kg administered every other week for three doses (Kline and Sullivan).

Patients should be evaluated monthly to ascertain if living eggs are being passed. Treatment generally causes a marked decrease in the number of eggs excreted, but disappearance of eggs is not mandatory. In fact, persistence of a few living organisms may perpetuate a state of immunity against reinfection (Kline and Sullivan). Dead eggs may be recovered for long periods after therapy and are not necessarily an indication for re-treatment.

Surgical intervention in schistosomiasis should be reserved until the effects of medical management can be assessed. Not infrequently, however, genitourinary schistosomiasis may cause fibrosis and contracture of the bladder, requiring augmentation cystoplasty. Bilharzial strictures of the ureter can produce obstructive uropathy, with damage to the upper tracts, recurrent UTI, and renal calculi. The lower ureter is involved in approximately two thirds of cases, and surgical reconstruction is often required at the ureterovesical junction. Extensive fibrosis of the ureteral wall and vesical mucosa usually precludes ureteroneocystostomy by a submucosal tunnel technique. Partial flap ureteroneocystostomy has produced improved or stabilized upper tracts radiographically in 83 per cent of patients (Bazeed et al, 1982). It is noteworthy that vesicoureteral reflux developed in 30 per cent of the patients postoperatively. In patients requiring surgery, it is important that the urine be sterilized preoperatively and that chemotherapy be continued postoperatively to prevent reinfection.

Echinococcosis

Echinococcosis, or hydatid cyst disease, is an infestation caused by the dog tapeworm *Echinococcus granulosus.* The major endemic sites of echinococcosis occur in sheep-raising areas such as Argentina, Australia, Spain, and Greece.

Pathogenesis

The adult tapeworm inhabits the intestinal tracts of dogs. The dogs become infected by swallowing the parasite scolex, which is encysted in the liver or lungs of sheep. Worm eggs from the dog are then excreted in the feces and may be ingested by sheep, cattle, pigs, and occasionally humans. After human ingestion, larval eggs pass through the intestinal wall and are disseminated throughout the body. Hydatid cysts have been found in virtually all human organs (Hunter et al). In humans, the liver is the primary organ affected. *Echinococcus* gains access to the kidney in approximately 3 per cent of the cases, usually from rupture of hepatic cysts into the peritoneal cavity with subsequent retroperitoneal penetration (Musacchio and Mitchell; Silber and Moyad).

Symptoms

Auldist and Myers reported 114 cases of hydatid cyst disease in children. Children of any age may be affected; however, the disease occurs infrequently in patients younger than 5 years old. Echinococcosis in children has been reported in the kidneys (Gajjar and Sinclair-Smith; Gharbi et al; Sharma et al; Shulman and Morales) and in the bladder (Fuloria et al) and as a cause of bilateral hydronephrosis (Keramidas et al). Echinococcosis has been implicated as a cause of eosinophilic cystitis (Hansman and Brown).

The growth of the hydatid cyst occurs slowly over several years, and the size of the cyst can be extremely large at initial presentation. Hydatid cyst of the kidney usually presents as a painful flank mass, and microscopic hematuria is often present. Rupture of the cyst into the renal pelvis causes acute flank pain and passage of scolices or daughter cysts with hematuria, with or without urinary obstruction (Gilsanz et al).

Diagnosis

A history of contact with sheep dogs in an endemic area is most helpful in diagnosing echinococcosis. The finding of scolices and hooklets in the urine is pathognomonic for echinococcosis. Eosinophilia is present in approximately one third of affected children (Apt and Knierim). A positive Casoni skin sensitivity test is useful, and positive reactions have been reported in approximately 90 per cent of patients at 24 hours (Buckley et al; Hunter et al). Serologic methods are particularly important in the diagnosis of echinococcal infections. The indirect hemagglutination test is the most specific of these techniques and is available through the Centers for Disease Control.

Plain films of the abdomen reveal spherical cysts with peripheral calcification overlying the kidneys. Ultrasonograms showing multiple daughter cysts within a cyst, separation of the membrane, or collapsed cysts are pathognomonic of hydatid disease (Pant and Gupta). Excretory urography demonstrates a calcified renal mass lesion, with or without calyceal distortion, which mimics a renal abscess or neoplasm (Fig. 10–27). Nephrotomography and selective renal arteriography are useful in clarifying the diagnosis (Baltaxe and Fleming).

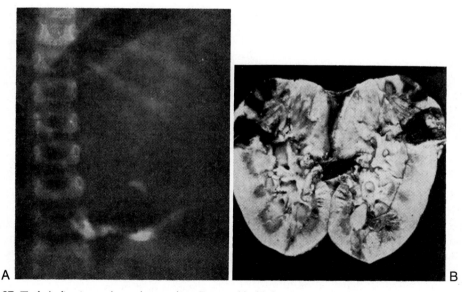

Figure 10–27 □ *A,* Left retrograde pyelogram in a 7-year-old girl demonstrates a large renal mass with distortion of the upper and middle calyces. *B,* Right nephrectomy specimen from a 17-year-old male shows hydatid cyst involving upper calyces. (From Shawket TN, Al-Waidh M: Hydatid cysts of the kidney simulating similar kidney lesions. Br J Urol 43:371, 1974. By permission of the British Association of Urological Surgeons.)

Treatment

Surgical intervention may be required in some patients with hydatid cyst disease. Nephrectomy remains the mainstay of treatment of hydatid disease of the kidney, but partial nephrectomy, simple cyst removal, or ex vivo resection and replantation have been reported (Buckley et al; Tscholl and Ausfeld). Meticulous care is necessary to prevent spillage of the cyst contents, a complication that can produce systemic anaphylactoid symptoms. Excision of the cyst wall is often difficult because of an inadequate plane of cleavage between the renal parenchyma and the fibrous cyst capsule. Marsupialization of the cyst wall or partial nephrectomy may result in spillage of infective scolices and, in turn, increased morbidity. The hydatid fluid should be aspirated and replaced with one of several chemical scolicidal agents before the cyst cavity is opened; hydrogen peroxide, sodium hypochloride, glycerin, and formalin are useful agents. Meymerian and coauthors recommended a solution of hydrogen peroxide (0.1 per cent) and cetrimide (0.005 per cent) as an effective and less toxic agent than formalin. In patients with systemic echinococcosis, mebendazole appears to be an effective antihelminthic agent (Nabizadeh et al).

Chlamydial Infection

Chlamydia trachomatis is an obligate intracellular parasite that may be responsible for 50 per cent of cases of nongonococcal urethritis and up to 66 per cent of cases of pelvic inflammatory disease in women (Rettig and Nelson). *Chlamydia* has only rarely been isolated from the genital tracts of prepubertal children. Rettig and Nelson were able to recover *C. trachomatis* from boys with coexistent or previous anogenital gonorrhea.

Symptoms

Chlamydial infection in males typically presents as urethritis, epididymitis, or Reiter's syndrome and may be a rare cause of prostatitis (Berger et al; Smith et al). The most common symptom is a clear, mucoid urethral discharge with or without urinary urgency and frequency. In females, acute inflammatory changes in the vagina or cervix lead to mucopurulent cervicitis, endometritis, or salpingitis. Conversely, asymptomatic carriage of *Chlamydia* in the endocervix may occur in the absence of urogenital symptoms.

Diagnosis

Chlamydia should be suspected in patients who have persistent urethral or vaginal discharge and a history of anogenital gonorrhea. It has been recommended that a culture for *C. trachomatis* be done for all female children being evaluated for sexual abuse because a positive culture is an excellent marker of sexual contact (Fuster and Neinstein; Ingram et al). Sexually active female adolescents should be screened for *Chlamydia* by the fluorescein-conjugated monoclonal antibody test because 10 to 25 per cent of these patients show positive test findings (Fisher et al). The organism may be visualized in smears with the use of the immunofluorescent antibody-typing test or Giemsa stain. Definitive diagnosis is established through isolation of the organism by inoculation into selected cell culture lines.

Treatment

Sulfonamides, erythromycin, and tetracycline, administered for 10 days to 2 weeks, are effective agents for the treatment of chlamydial infection (Oriel et al). (Tetracycline should not be administered to children younger than 8 years of age.) Cephalosporins have not proved effective in vitro against *Chlamydia* (Ridgway and Oriel). In prepubertal female patients with persistent asymptomatic genitourinary colonization with *Chlamydia*, Rettig and Nelson recommended treatment to prevent possible adverse side effects of prolonged genital carriage. Persistence or recurrence of disease after treatment is not uncommon, and follow-up cultures and prolonged antibiotic therapy may be required.

OTHER DISORDERS

Pinworm Infestation

Pinworm is caused by the nematode *Enterobius vermicularis*. The disease is distributed worldwide and occurs commonly in families.

Pathogenesis

The adult worm lives in the large intestine of the human. The gravid female migrates to the rectum, deposits her eggs on the perianal skin and perineum at night, and then dies. Autoinfection and infection of other persons continue as long as adult gravid females deposit eggs on the perianal skin.

Symptoms

Pinworm infection causes pruritus ani and occasionally pruritus vulvae. *Enterobius* has been implicated as a factor in secondary enuresis and also in acute and chronic UTI (Mayers and Purvis; Sachdev and Howards). In a study of female children, Kropp and co-workers demonstrated that 22 per cent of patients with documented UTI had pinworm infestation in contrast to only 5 per cent of the control population. Although the relationship between female UTI and the presence of introital enteric organisms is well recognized, the association between pinworms and positive introital cultures is also noteworthy. Kropp and co-workers found that the incidence of pinworms recovered from the perineum of females was higher in girls with enteric organisms present on a swab of the introitus than in those with negative introital cultures.

Diagnosis

Enterobius is recovered by application of adhesive tape to the perianal skin to pick up any eggs. The tape is then applied to a glass slide and examined under low-power magnification (Graham). Specimens should be obtained early in the morning before washing of the genitalia.

Treatment

The drugs of choice for enterobiasis are pyrantel pamoate, given orally, 11 mg/kg in a single dose (maximum, 1 g), or mebendazole, as a single 100-mg dose. Both doses should be repeated in 2 weeks. Neither drug is recommended for children younger than 2 years of age. These medications should be administered to all family members (MacPherson).

Trichomoniasis

Trichomonas vaginalis, a flagellate protozoan, often affects the genitourinary tract and may cause significant urologic complications.

Pathogenesis

Vaginal trichomoniasis in the newborn may result from nonsexual transmission via infected mothers to the fetus at the time of delivery (Al-Salihi et al; Krieger; Postlethwaite; Rein). In adolescents, the majority of cases are acquired through sexual intercourse.

Symptoms

Approximately 25 per cent of females with culture-proven *Trichomonas* infection have no symptoms (Rein). Conversely, *Trichomonas* may be responsible for abacterial cystitis or may occur concomitantly with recurrent bacterial UTI. Symptoms of urgency, frequency, pruritus, and vaginal discharge are typically present (Fouts and Kraus).

In males, *T. vaginalis* infection is usually asymptomatic; however, this organism has been implicated as an infrequent cause of nonspecific urethritis, prostatitis, epididymitis, balanoposthitis, and urethral stricture disease, and it may result in infertility (Krieger; Meares).

Diagnosis

The diagnosis of *T. vaginalis* infection is made by direct microscopic examination of a wet-mount specimen or by growth of the trichomonads in a selective culture medium. Recovery of *T. vaginalis* requires meticulous culture techniques under anaerobic conditions with optimal incubation at 37°C (Rothenberg et al). Serologic techniques remain research tools at this time. The association between *Trichomonas* and gonorrhea is well documented, and patients treated for gonorrhea who have persistent urinary symptoms or culture-proven reinfection should be investigated for trichomoniasis. Trichomoniasis in a premenarchal girl should raise the question of sexual abuse.

Treatment

The drug of choice for *T. vaginalis* infection is metronidazole (Flagyl), which is effective in 90 to 95 per cent of patients (Perl and Ragazzoni). Side effects include vertigo, nausea, and headaches. The dosage recommended by the Bureau of Venereal Disease Control is 250 mg given orally three times a day for 7 days, or 2 g given orally as a single dose. In females with neonatal vaginitis, Postlethwaite recommended 50 mg three times a day for 10 days.

Ureaplasma Infection

Ureaplasma urealyticum is a common inhabitant of male and female genital tracts after puberty. Colonization is primarily the result of sexual contact (McCormack et al, 1973a, 1973b). Infants acquire *U. urealyticum* during passage through the birth canal of an infected mother (Klein et al). In prepubertal children, *Ureaplasma* has been recovered infrequently from the urine or external genitalia (Foy et al).

Ureaplasma has been implicated in approximately 20 to 30 per cent of patients with nongonococcal urethritis and may be responsible for cases of postgonococcal urethritis (McCormack et al, 1973a; Taylor-Robinson and McCormack). Microscopic examination of the urethral discharge is essential to rule out gonorrhea. Definitive diagnosis is established by culture techniques.

The treatment of choice is tetracycline, 40 mg/kg over 24 hours in four divided doses for 10 days (Holmes et al; Handsfield). Erythromycin is the preferred antimicrobial agent in children younger than 9 years of age. In adolescent patients, sexual partners should be treated as well.

Cyclophosphamide Cystitis

Cyclophosphamide (Cytoxan) is an effective and widely utilized antineoplastic agent in children. A major side effect of this drug is hematuria, which has been reported in 2 to 40 per cent of patients (Lawrence et al; Texter et al). Although acute hemorrhagic cystitis is usually reversible, extensive chronic bleeding may lead to irreversible changes of vesical fibrosis and contracture. The long-term complications from cyclophosphamide appear to be related to the duration of therapy and the total dose of drug administered (Levine and Richie).

Pathogenesis

The cyclophosphamide molecule itself does not appear to be responsible for damage to the bladder mucosa (Philips et al). Cyclophosphamide is converted by the liver into an active, toxic metabolite, acrolein, which is excreted through the kidneys and produces cell damage by local contact with the urothelium. The bladder is the organ most susceptible to damage because the surface contact with urine is longest here. The entire uroepithelial surface may be affected, however, and lesions of the renal pelvis and ureter have been reported.

Symptoms

Hemorrhagic cystitis can occur after oral or intravenous cyclophosphamide administration. Bleeding may develop soon after intravenous drug injection but more commonly occurs several weeks to months after therapy (Jerkins et al; Liedberg et al). The initial onset of symptoms may be delayed for several years after cyclophosphamide therapy (Kende et al). There appears to be additive toxicity between radiation therapy and cyclophosphamide administration. Children with extensive disease present with urinary urgency, frequency, suprapubic pain, and passage of blood clots. Profuse bleeding has been reported and may be life-threatening.

Diagnosis

Cystoscopic examination demonstrates diffuse erythematous changes with patchy mucosal sloughing and necrosis. Slow oozing of blood is demonstrable from most areas of the bladder. Bladder biopsy demonstrates nonspecific inflammatory changes with edema in the mucosa and submucosa.

Treatment

In an experimental model (Tolley) and in the clinical setting (Primack), *N*-acetylcysteine has been shown to be of value in protecting the bladder from developing hemorrhagic cystitis without impairing the therapeutic efficacy of cyclophosphamide. This agent contains sulfhydryl groups that may bind and inactivate active sites within the toxic metabolites of cyclophosphamide. The recommended dose ratio of *N*-acetylcysteine to cyclophosphamide is 1:1 weight per weight given within 2 hours of drug administration. *N*-acetylcysteine does not appear to speed resolution of the inflammatory changes if given after a course of cyclophosphamide therapy.

Ehrlich and co-workers reported success in preventing cyclophosphamide cystitis by administering sodium 2-mercaptoethane sulfonate. This drug prevents the formation of acrolein, the metabolite of cyclophosphamide responsible for urotoxicity, by attaching to the double bond of acrolein and forming a stable thioether that is harmless.

Hemorrhagic cystitis can be prevented by promoting overhydration and frequent micturition during therapy. An indwelling urethral catheter can be justified in patients in whom frequent voiding is not possible. Adequate hydration and maintenance of vigorous diuresis are recommended in patients with extensive hemorrhagic cystitis (Droller et al). Attempts at bladder fulguration usually prove ineffective because of the diffuse nature of the vesical involvement. In extensive bleeding, various treatment regimens have included instillation of formalin (Shrom et al), phenol (Duckett et al), silver nitrate (Jerkins et al) or prostaglandins (deVries and Freiha; Trigg et al), intravenous vasopressin administration (Pyeritiz et al), bilateral hypogastric artery ligation, and cystectomy with urinary diversion. Rabinovitch reported success with suprapubic cystostomy and continuous bladder irrigation for evacuation of clots.

Eosinophilic Cystitis

Eosinophilic cystitis is an uncommon inflammatory disease of the bladder that is characterized by irritative urinary symptoms, hematuria, and suprapubic pain. This entity has been reported in all age groups (Champion and Ackles; Goldstein; Hellstrom et al; Nkposong and Attah; Tauscher and Shaw). There is often a personal or family history of allergy (Rubin and Pincus).

Pathogenesis and Pathology

No causative agent has been definitively identified, although food allergens, medications, bladder injury, and parasites have been suggested as the cause of the disease. Others have postulated an antigen-immune-complex reaction in the bladder that stimulates eosinophilic infiltration (Hellstrom et al; Littleton et al).

Symptoms

Dysuria, urgency, frequency, and hematuria are usually present, and symptoms last for 1 to 3 weeks. Gross hematuria has been reported (Nkposong and Attah). Physical examination may reveal suprapubic tenderness with or without a palpable pelvic mass. Eosinophilic gastroenteritis may be associated with eosinophilic cystitis (Sutphin and Middleton).

Diagnosis

The differential diagnosis includes bacterial cystitis, interstitial cystitis, parasitic infection of the bladder, and vesical neoplasia. Peripheral eosinophilia is a routine finding in children with eosinophilic cystitis. Results of urinalysis are nonspecific; most patients demonstrate microscopic pyuria and hematuria. Urine culture is negative. Excretory urographic findings range from normal to the demonstration of filling defects in the bladder (Farber and Vawter). Bilateral hydronephrosis may result (Nkposong and Attah). Cystoscopic findings reveal inflammatory mucosal changes with polypoid lesions and thickening of the bladder wall. Bladder biopsy demonstrates intense eosinophilic infiltration of the bladder mucosa and musculature.

Treatment

Steroids, antihistamines, cytotoxic drugs, radiotherapy, and long-term antibiotics have all been advocated in the treatment of eosinophilic cystitis, but most cases of eosinophilic cystitis in children are self-limited and no specific therapy is required (Sutphin and Middleton). Powell and co-workers recommended that these patients be evaluated by an allergist to rule out a specific allergen as the cause of the disease. If the history or laboratory studies suggest a parasitic etiology, specific treatment for this may be indicated. In rare cases of advanced disease, extirpative surgery may be necessary (Sidh et al).

Chronic Granulomatous Disease

Chronic granulomatous disease of infancy is a hereditary disorder of leukocyte metabolism that is associated with chronic and recurrent bacterial infections. The disease is transmitted as a sex-linked disorder in males and as an autosomal recessive disease in females (Young and Middleton).

Pathogenesis

In patients with chronic granulomatous disease, the leukocytes have ineffective bactericidal and fungicidal activity (Lehrer; Rodey et al). One of the normal mechanisms of bacterial destruction involves halogenation of the bacterial cell wall and requires hydrogen peroxide and peroxidase (Klebanoff and White). In children with chronic granulomatous disease, granulocytes are capable of normal ingestion of bacteria; however, hydrogen peroxide production is impaired. Thus, these leukocytes are unable to destroy bacteria that do not produce their own hydrogen peroxide, such as *Staphylococcus aureus* and gram-negative enteric organisms (Elgefors et al; Holmes et al). These defective granulocytes also produce inadequate amounts of superoxide, an agent that shows significant bactericidal activity (Curnutte et al).

Symptoms

Chronic granulomatous disease should be suspected in children who show an increased propensity to infection. The most frequent sites of involvement include the skin, lymphatics, respiratory tract, gastrointestinal system, liver, spleen, and bone. Urologic involvement has been reported and may manifest as xanthogranulomatous pyelonephritis (Johansen et al), cystitis (Young and Middleton), or glomerulonephritis (Frifelt et al).

Diagnosis

The laboratory diagnosis of chronic granulomatous disease is established by the nitroblue tetrazolium dye test (Baehner and Nathan). Ninety per cent of normal leukocytes reduce nitroblue tetrazolium during phagocytosis of latex particles. In children with chronic granulomatous disease, however, only 10 per cent of the leukocytes are capable of reducing nitroblue tetrazolium. Definitive diagnosis of the disease depends on the demonstration of impaired intracellular bactericidal activity.

Treatment

Continuous and long-term prophylactic antibiotic therapy appears indicated in these children (Philippart et al). The frequency and severity of bacterial infections appear to be decreased in children undergoing long-term sulfonamide therapy (Johnston et al).

Gonococcal Urethritis

Gonorrhea is the most common reportable communicable disease in the United States today (Clark). Infection with *Neisseria gonorrhoeae* occurs most commonly in sexually active teenagers and young adults, but prepubertal involvement is not uncommon (Farrell et al; Meek et al). The incidence of gonorrhea has increased in adolescents at a faster rate than in any other age group since 1970 (McGregor).

Pathogenesis

The incubation period of *N. gonorrhoeae* is 2 to 8 days. Urethral infection in males is localized in the glands of Littre. Rectal carriage may occur in the absence of urethral colonization. Transmission of gonorrhea to prepubertal children may occur via nonsexual contact in social settings in which the parents are infected (Shore and Winkelstein). Conversely, Branch and Paxton noted a history of sexual exposure in 43 of 45 children, either from molestation from relatives or from voluntary sexual contact. Potterat and co-workers reported child-to-child transmission of gonorrhea in three children younger than 10 years of age. The majority of cases in infancy are due to exposure or contact during childbirth. Sexually transmitted diseases in children and adolescents should be presumed to be the result of sexual abuse until proven otherwise (Whitner and Anderson).

Symptoms

In adolescent males, gonorrhea is typically associated with dysuria and a profuse, yellow urethral discharge. Occasionally, asymptomatic pyuria may be the initial form of presentation. In younger children, penile swelling and the inability to void may be presenting complaints (Meek et al). Barrett-Connor reported a 23-month-old boy whose presenting symptom was an abscess on the glans penis.

Diagnosis

Specimens should be obtained by stripping the urethra or by gently inserting a swab into the distal urethra. Demonstration of ovoid, gram-negative diplococci on staining is presumptive evidence of gonorrhea. Specimens must be obtained for cultures and should be plated and incubated immediately in a modified Thayer-Martin medium (Kellogg et al). Chocolate agar should also be used because an occasional strain of gonococcus is susceptible to the vancomycin present in modified Thayer-Martin medium. Serologic tests for syphilis should be performed in all patients with urethral discharge. The use of a Papanicolaou-stained urethral smear may aid in the etiologic diagnosis of urethritis, especially if more than one pathogen is involved (Saxena and Feriozi).

Treatment

In males with urethritis, the Centers for Disease Control recommend 75,000 to 100,000 units of aqueous procaine penicillin G per kilogram of body weight given intramuscularly (Meek et al). Amoxicillin, 50 mg/kg given orally to a maximum dose of 3.5 g, is as effective as penicillin G (Nelson et al). Each of these treatment regimens should be preceded by the oral administration of probenecid, 25 mg/kg, to a maximum dose of 1 g. In patients who are allergic to penicillin, alternative therapies for children older than 8 years of age include tetracycline given orally, 25 mg/kg as an initial dose, followed by 40 to 60 mg/kg/day for 7 days (Karney et al). In children younger than 10 years of age, ceftriaxone, 125 mg in a single intramuscular dose, is recommended (American Academy of Pediatrics). Subsequent urethral cultures should be done approximately 1 week after completion of therapy to identify patients infected with penicillinase-producing organisms (Kellogg et al). Infected contacts with gonorrhea should be similarly treated with the dosage regimen described above.

Nongonococcal Urethritis

Nongonococcal urethritis, or nonspecific urethritis, is currently the most common sexually transmitted disease in males (Felman and Nikitas). Nongonococcal urethritis is quite common in the sexually active adolescent male but is rare in children.

Pathogenesis

Chlamydia and *Ureaplasma* have both been implicated as causative organisms in at least 50 to 60 per cent of cases of nonspecific ure-

thritis (Smith et al). In the remaining 30 to 40 per cent of patients who have neither *Chlamydia* nor *Ureaplasma* isolated from the urethra, *Trichomonas vaginalis,* yeasts, or viruses may be the etiologic agents responsible for the urethritis.

Symptoms

The onset of symptoms is usually more gradual in patients with nongonococcal urethritis than in those with gonococcal urethritis. Virtually all patients with gonorrhea have a urethral discharge with or without dysuria. Conversely, Jacobs and Kraus reported that only 38 per cent of patients with nongonococcal urethritis have both dysuria and urethral discharge. Whereas the urethral discharge in patients with gonococcal urethritis is characteristically purulent, the discharge in nongonococcal urethritis is clear, thin, and watery.

Diagnosis

Nonspecific urethritis should be suspected in patients with a clear mucoid urethral discharge, persistent urethral discharge after treatment for gonococcal urethritis, or a history of anogenital gonorrhea. Examination of the first 10 to 15 ml of an early morning voided urine demonstrates increased polymorphonuclear leukocytes and establishes the diagnosis of urethritis. It is imperative to rule out gonococcal urethritis by staining for gram-negative diplococci and obtaining Thayer-Martin specimens for culture. The presence of *C. trachomatis* can be confirmed by using the fluorescent monoclonal antibody tests (Goldenring).

Treatment

Sulfonamides, erythromycin, and tetracycline, administered for 10 days to 2 weeks, are all effective agents for the treatment of chlamydial urethritis (Oriel et al). The drug of choice for *T. vaginalis* is metronidazole (Flagyl). Tetracycline and erythromycin are both effective agents for the treatment of *Ureaplasma* (see *Ureaplasma* Infection earlier in this chapter).

Herpes Simplex Infection

Herpes simplex is an infectious venereal disease caused by *Herpesvirus hominis* that is the most common cause of vesiculoulcerative lesions of the genitalia in males and females.

Pathogenesis

The virus is transmitted via sexual intercourse, oral-genital contacts, or oral-anal contacts. Newborns may acquire infection during passage through a virus-infected birth canal (Nahmias et al, 1967, 1970). The incubation period for herpes is 3 to 14 days for primary infections and 12 to 24 hours for repeat infections.

Symptoms

In adolescent males, herpetic infections present as painful, clear vesicles on the shaft of the penis, scrotum, or thigh. These vesicles eventually coalesce and form pustules with ulceration. Herpesvirus has been implicated as a cause of urethritis.

In female infants and children, contact of the external genitalia with contaminated hands or through sexual abuse may be responsible for vulvovaginitis. In adolescent females, herpetic ulcers may develop at the introitus, within the vagina, or on the cervix. Symptoms of dysuria may be a clue to the diagnosis of herpetic cystitis (Person et al).

The vesiculoulcerative lesions heal spontaneously within 7 to 14 days. The disease is characterized by long latency and repeated recurrent localized lesions, which may remain asymptomatic for long periods.

Diagnosis

The diagnosis of herpes simplex is established by the clinical appearance of the vesicular lesions and the associated history of recurrences or exposure to disease. Herpes simplex virus can be grown in vitro in various tissue cultures, with recovery of the virus in approximately 1 week. Serologic tests are available in some centers. Cytologic techniques involve scraping cells from the base of vesicular lesions and observing multinucleate giant cells and nuclear inclusion bodies.

Concurrent infection with *Treponema pallidum* is not uncommon, and therefore vesicular lesions on the genitalia should be tested by darkfield examination and patients should be observed serologically until recovery is complete (Fiumara et al).

Treatment

There is no effective treatment for herpes simplex virus infection. Acyclovir given orally may shorten the duration of signs and symptoms and decrease viral shedding in primary genital herpes (American Academy of Pediatrics). Topical therapy has proved ineffective, and there is no immunologic vaccine available at this time. Idoxuridine (IDU) has been used to treat superficial keratitis, but it does not decrease the rate of recurrent disease. Photodynamic inactivation by means of tricyclic dyes—for example, neutral red—has been disappointing and may enhance the oncogenic potential of the virus.

Syphilis

Syphilis is caused by infection with the anaerobic spirochete *T. pallidum.* The overall rate of infectious syphilis in the United States has increased significantly since 1958 and parallels the increase in other venereal diseases (Wilfert and Gutman). Reported cases of syphilis increased 41 per cent from 28,607 in 1984 to 40,275 in 1988 (Fiumara). In children, syphilis occurs much less often than gonorrhea.

Pathogenesis

T. pallidum has the ability to invade the intact mucous membrane or open wounds. Sexual contact is the most common method of disease transmission; however, other sites of inoculation include the lips, oral cavity, and abraded areas of skin. After tissue invasion, the organisms multiply and are disseminated by perivascular lymphatics to the systemic circulation (Cotran et al).

Congenital syphilis may result from transplacental infection of the developing fetus or by contact with a primary syphilitic lesion during passage through the birth canal (Taber and Huber). Between 70 and 100 per cent of all pregnant women with untreated syphilis may transmit infection to the fetus. Congenital syphilis may be responsible for up to 25 per cent fetal mortality in utero and an additional 25 to 30 per cent mortality in the perinatal period (Wilfert and Gutman).

Symptoms

The incubation period for syphilis is 9 to 90 days, with an average of 21 days (Fiumara).

The patient initially experiences an inflammatory response to infection at the site of inoculation. The chancre of primary syphilis is characteristically a single, nonpainful, nontender, firm lesion, which occurs most commonly on the penis in males and the vagina or cervix in females. Other sites of involvement include the lips, mouth, face, and abraded areas of skin.

Two to 10 weeks after the primary lesions, the patient may experience secondary disease manifested by maculopapular skin and mucous membrane lesions, fever, pharyngitis, generalized lymphadenopathy, headache, and flat moist lesions around the anus or vagina (condylomata lata). These secondary lesions of the skin and mucous membrane are highly infectious.

Tertiary syphilis develops years after secondary disease and may be characterized by gumma formation and also by neurologic and cardiovascular involvement.

Diagnosis

The primary penile lesions of syphilis must be differentiated from chancroid, lymphogranuloma venereum, granuloma inguinale, herpes, and gangrenous balanitis (see below). The diagnosis is made by direct visualization of the pathogenic spirochetes on darkfield examination of the serous fluid from a syphilitic ulcer. If the chancre has been present for 7 days, the rapid plasma reagin (RPR) test is reactive (Fiumara). This should be confirmed with a fluorescent treponemal antibody absorption (FTA-ABS) test. After treatment, patients should be examined monthly and a quantitative RPR test should be performed. This test should become nonreactive within 12 months of treatment if this was the patient's first infection with syphilis. The FTA-ABS test rarely becomes nonreactive and is used for diagnosis only.

Treatment

Penicillin remains the drug of choice for syphilis. For primary disease, the Centers for Disease Control recommend treatment with either a single intramuscular injection of benzathine penicillin G in a dosage of 2.4 million units or aqueous procaine penicillin G, 600,000 units daily for 8 days. In patients with penicillin allergies, erythromycin and tetracycline are alternative regimens. Infants with congenital syphilis should be treated with aqueous crystalline penicillin G, 50,000 units/kg daily, divided into two doses for at least 10 days.

Early treatment affords a high cure rate with excellent prognosis and minimal relapse. Retreatment is indicated in patients with persistently high serologic titers or in cases of decreasing titers that subsequently increase. Family members should be examined for syphilis, and case reports should be forwarded to local public health officials.

Prostatitis

Bacterial prostatitis is extremely rare in prepubertal children. Mann reported three neonates with prostatic abscesses, each associated with *Staphylococcus aureus*. Children may present with vesical irritative symptoms, urinary retention, or urethral discharge. Physical examination may reveal a cystic prostatic or seminal vesicle swelling that is exquisitely tender to palpation. In the majority of patients with symptoms of prostatitis, specimens for urine culture are negative. In cases in which specific organisms are isolated, gram-negative bacteria and *U. urealyticum* are usually identified. *Trichomonas vaginalis* infection of the prostate has been reported. There also have been rare cases of fungal prostatic infection, which is usually secondary to generalized systemic disease (Meares).

Treatment

The rare case of acute prostatitis in children and adolescents responds well to the initiation of appropriate antimicrobial therapy. Supportive treatment, such as bed rest, hydration, antipyretics, and analgesics, is recommended. Urethral instrumentation and prostatic massage should be avoided in the acute phase of the disease.

Epididymitis

Acute epididymitis is rare in prepubertal boys; most childhood cases occur in adolescents (Amar and Chabra; Doolittle et al). In a retrospective analysis of 136 patients with acute epididymitis, Barker and Raper reported no patients younger than 14 years of age.

Pathogenesis

Infection in the epididymis may result from distal urethral obstruction, ectopic ureter draining into the seminal vesicle or vas deferens, or instrumentation or it may be idiopathic in nature (Coran and Perlmutter; Waldman et al). *Haemophilus influenzae* has been reported to cause simultaneous otitis media and epididymitis. These children present with high fever and a tense, tender scrotum (Greenfield; Weber). Brucellosis has also been associated with episodes of epididymo-orchitis (Ibrahim et al; Khan et al). Although infection with bacteria or viral organisms has been implicated as a cause of epididymitis (Greenfield; Weber), most cases are not associated with UTI (Hodgson and Hasan). Thus, it appears that sterile urine in the epididymis may be sufficient to incite an inflammatory response and clinical symptoms. Epididymal infection usually occurs via abnormal retrograde passage of urine from the prostatic ducts through the vas deferens (Fig. 10–28) (Kiviat et al). Hematogenous spread from an acute staphylococcal infection can occur subsequent to pneumonia, peritonitis, or other systemic infections. Epididymal involvement may also occur as a result of direct extension from a pre-existing orchitis.

Symptoms

Patients with epididymitis have an enlarged and exquisitely tender epididymis and vas deferens. Scrotal edema, pain, and tenderness are

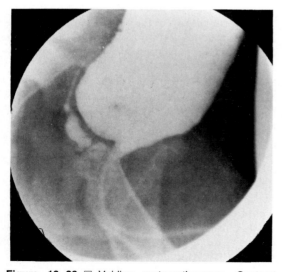

Figure 10–28 ☐ Voiding cystourethrogram. Contrast medium is demonstrated in left seminal vesicle and left vas deferens.

early features of the disease. A reactive hydrocele usually develops with disease progression as a result of inflammatory changes in the tunica vaginalis.

Diagnosis

For prepubertal boys with suspected epididymitis, an excretory urogram should be performed to rule out the presence of an ectopic ureter. The differential diagnosis of epididymitis in children should always include testicular torsion, torsion of a testicular or epididymal appendage, and idiopathic scrotal edema. The onset of pain is usually more insidious in children with epididymitis than in those with testicular torsion. The physical examination in children with epididymitis usually reveals erythema and edema of the scrotum. Epididymal tenderness with or without urethral discharge is usually, but not invariably, present. The presence of a horizontal testicular lie or an absent ipsilateral cremasteric reflex is characteristic of torsion of the testis. Prehn's sign is often unreliable in distinguishing epididymitis from testicular torsion. Urinalysis most often demonstrates pyuria with or without bacteriuria. However, results of urinalysis are abnormal in approximately 10 per cent of patients with testicular torsion (Ransler and Allen). Leukocytosis ($>$ 10,000 leukocytes per μl) occurs in 30 to 50 per cent of children with epididymitis, testicular torsion, and torsion of a testicular appendage and, therefore, is not a helpful discriminator among these entities (Levy et al; Ransler and Allen). The Doppler ultrasonic stethoscope and radionuclide testicular scanning have been utilized to differentiate epididymitis from testicular torsion. Our experience and that of others (Brereton; Ransler and Allen) has been that the Doppler flowmeter is associated with false-negative results. Similarly, although nuclear scrotal scanning has proved to be a highly accurate diagnostic tool in large series of children with acute scrotum (Levy et al; Valvo et al), this method of investigation is not universally available or reliable. It must be remembered that epididymitis is extremely rare in children, and the safe and sure method of resolving the diagnosis of an acute scrotum necessitates scrotal exploration (Kelalis and Stickler).

Treatment

The treatment of acute epididymitis involves administration of broad-spectrum antibiotics (usually on an empiric basis), scrotal support with elevation, bed rest, and application of ice packs to the affected area. Injection of the spermatic cord with lidocaine hydrochloride (1 to 2 ml) may alleviate severe pain (Smith).

Orchitis

Acute infection involving solely the testis is a relatively rare occurrence in boys (Kaplan and King). Malkin and co-authors reported a case of bacterial orchitis in a newborn due to hematogenous spread of *Escherichia coli.* Tuberculosis may spread to the testis from the epididymis and reflects tuberculous infection elsewhere in the body (Cotran et al).

Pathogenesis

In the majority of cases, orchitis develops as a result of extension of inflammation in the epididymis with the production of epididymoorchitis. Less often, orchitis may develop by hematogenous or lymphogenous dissemination. Gram-negative coliforms, streptococci, or staphylococci account for most of the cases of bacterial orchitis. Mumps orchitis, which may occur in up to 20 per cent of adults with the virus, is exceedingly rare before puberty.

Symptoms

Acute pyogenic orchitis presents as a swollen, tender, and sometimes fluctuant testis. The scrotal skin is erythematous and edematous, and there is usually an associated hydrocele caused by inflammation of the tunica vaginalis. Pain may radiate to the inguinal canal and may by associated with nausea and vomiting. The differential diagnosis of acute orchitis includes acute epididymitis, torsion of the testicle or testicular appendages, and strangulated inguinal hernia.

Treatment

Broad-spectrum antibiotics are recommended pending the results of urine cultures. Supportive therapy includes bed rest, scrotal elevation, and hot or cold compresses for symptomatic relief. Aspiration of the associated symptomatic hydrocele may afford considerable relief of pain in selected patients.

Vulvovaginitis

Most female babies have a rather profuse, thick vaginal discharge during the newborn period as a consequence of prenatal stimulation by maternal hormones. This is a limited and physiologic condition for which therapy is not required. Similarly, copious vaginal secretion associated with swelling of the vulvar and vaginal tissues may occur at the time of puberty, as a result of the normal increase in estrogen stimulation. Vaginal discharge may result from an ectopic ureter that inserts into the vagina, and therefore excretory urography is recommended.

Pathogenesis

In premenarchal females, vulvovaginitis occurs most commonly between 2 and 7 years of age. Vulvovaginitis in this age group may be due to specific infections from bacteria, fungi, *Trichomonas, Mycoplasma, Chlamydia, Yersinia enterocolitica,* parasites, or viruses (Heller et al; Rein; Rosenfeld and Clark; Watkins and Quan). Vulvovaginitis may be nonspecific in origin or may be related to chemical or allergic agents or foreign bodies in the vagina. In adolescent females, vulvovaginitis is usually the result of sexual promiscuity.

Specific Vulvovaginitis

The most common causes of specific vulvovaginitis in adolescents are *Gardnerella vaginalis, Candida,* and *Trichomonas. G. vaginalis* is treated with metronidazole or ampicillin (Sanfilippo). Infection with these agents is less common in younger children because the organisms tend to prefer an estrogenic vagina (Arsenault and Gerbie). Gonococcal vulvovaginitis in prepubertal girls may result from sexual abuse or from nonsexual contact with freshly infected material on clothing or towels (Burry; Tunnessen and Jastremski). Rarely, gonococcal vaginitis may be acquired during passage of the newborn through an infected birth canal (Stark and Glode). In prepubertal females, the endocervical glands are not well developed and do not harbor the gonococcus. Thus, prepubertal gonorrhea is limited to the vagina. The majority of adolescent females have no symptoms; however, an occasional patient may present with endometritis and salpingitis.

The child with gonococcal vulvovaginitis may complain of vulvar discomfort, dysuria, frequency, and pain on walking. The vulvar tissues are edematous and hyperemic and are covered by a profuse, thick, yellowish discharge that exudes from the vagina. The diagnosis is established by smears and cultures of urethral, vaginal, and rectal swabs. Endocervical cultures are not recommended in prepubertal females. Penicillin is the treatment of choice (see Gonococcal Urethritis).

Common parasitologic causes of premenarchal vulvovaginitis are *T. vaginalis* and *Enterobius vermicularis* (Gaafar et al), and infants and children may be affected. The disease may be acquired during passage of the newborn through an infected birth canal. Symptoms include vulvar pruritus, and physical examination reveals a grayish-white, frothy vaginal discharge. The diagnosis is established by the presence of numerous leukocytes and trichomonads in saline wet-mount vaginal preparations. The treatment for trichomonal vaginitis is metronidazole, 15 mg/kg/day for 10 days; for *E. vermicularis,* a simple dose of mebendazole, 100 mg, is given orally (Arsenault and Gerbie).

Mycotic infections, particularly those caused by *C. albicans,* may produce vulvovaginitis in infants and children. In most instances, the child will have received antibiotic therapy before the onset of genital symptoms. One should also consider diabetes mellitus or immunodeficiency status in children with severe candidal infection. Children usually have vulvar pruritus. Physical examination reveals diffuse vulvar hyperemia with whitish plaques on the vaginal wall and minimal vaginal discharge. The diagnosis is established by finding leukocytes and mycelia in potassium hydroxide preparations and is confirmed by identifying *C. albicans* in culture. The treatment for mycotic vulvovaginitis is miconazole or clotrimazole, 100 mg intravaginally daily for 7 days. Alternatively, 1 ml of 0.5 per cent aqueous solution of gentian violet may be injected intravaginally with a sterile eye dropper each night for 10 days (Huffman).

Nonspecific Vulvovaginitis

Nonspecific vulvovaginitis may result from pinworm infestation; foreign bodies; irritation by clothing, chemicals, or cosmetics; anaerobic bacteria, such as *Bacteroides* and *Peptococcus* species; *Gardnerella* infection; or upper respiratory infections. Approximately 70 per cent of these cases result from poor perineal hygiene with fecal contamination (Arsenault and Gerbie). There is usually a moderate vaginal discharge, which is whitish gray. Microscopic examination of the discharge demonstrates few leukocytes, and there are epithelial cells coated with small bacteria (clue cells). Vaginal smears and cultures are mandatory to rule out *N. gonorrhoeae* and other specific infections. Therapy is based on good perineal hygiene, including proper cleansing after defecation (Sanfilippo).

Gangrenous Balanoposthitis

Inflammation of the glans penis and foreskin occurs commonly in infants and appears to be related to chronic irritation from wet or soiled diapers and from poor genital hygiene. Mild cases usually respond to local cleansing.

Gangrenous balanoposthitis is a result of an anaerobic fusospirochetal infection of the glans penis. The lesion begins as an ulcer in the region of the corona, beneath a tight and unclean prepuce. Spread of the ulcer produces a foul, profuse discharge with secondary edema of the glans. Gangrenous change may occur in both the glans and the shaft of the penis.

Diagnosis

The diagnosis of gangrenous balanoposthitis is made by clinical appearance and by demonstration of spirochetes and fusiform bacilli in stained smears of the discharge. Darkfield examination is necessary to rule out infection with *T. pallidum*. It is important to remember that hair wrapped around the coronal sulcus may produce gangrenous balanoposthitis.

Treatment

Penicillin is the drug of choice. Hydrogen peroxide soaks are helpful in reversing the anaerobic process. A dorsal slit may be necessary in the acute stage of the disease; circumcision is recommended electively after resolution of edema.

Lymphogranuloma Venereum

Lymphogranuloma venereum is an infectious venereal disease caused by *C. trachomatis,* serotypes L-1, L-2, and L-3 (Fiumara). The disease is characterized by granulomatous ulceration, abscess formation, and fibrosis of the inguinal, perineal, and rectal lymphatics (Abrams). There have been several reports of lymphogranuloma venereum in children (Banov; Levy; Weinstock and Keesal).

Pathogenesis and Pathology

Acquisition of lymphogranuloma venereum in childhood occurs as a result of genital contact and may be transmitted by handling towels or clothes that contain drainage from an ulcerated lesion. In adolescents, the disease is transmitted by sexual intercourse. The incubation period is approximately 7 weeks after exposure (Fiumara).

The initial form of childhood presentation is painful and tender inguinal adenitis with subsequent abscess formation and draining sinuses. Extension of disease into the deep pelvic tissue may result in rectal and colonic strictures and also elephantiasis of the external genitalia.

Diagnosis

Lymphogranuloma venereum should be suspected in persons with acutely painful inguinal lymphadenopathy or with an ulcerative or granulomatous lesion on the vulva or perineum. Definitive diagnosis is established by a positive intradermal skin test (Frei test) with the use of antigens from killed organisms. Serum complement fixation is highly accurate in the detection of initial infections and can be used to observe the course of the disease (Holder and Duncan). Biopsy of involved tissues is indicated to confirm the diagnosis. Patients with lymphogranuloma venereum should be evaluated for concurrent syphilitic infection and for other granulomatous and ulcerative genital diseases.

Treatment

Tetracycline, administered four times daily for 3 weeks, is the treatment of choice. Sulfonamides are also effective. The discharge from ulcerated lesions is infectious, and thus appropriate precautions should be taken to prevent transmission of disease.

Granuloma Inguinale

Granuloma inguinale is a chronic venereal infection of the genital skin and subcutaneous tissues of the perineum (Davis; Lal and Nicholas). The etiologic agent is the encapsulated gram-negative bacillus *Calymmatobacterium granulomatis*. This disease occurs most commonly in the tropics and is relatively unusual in the United States.

Pathogenesis and Pathology

Granuloma inguinale is sexually transmitted; however, children may become infected by coming in contact with contaminated clothing or towels. The initial lesion is a reddish nodule on the penis, groin, vulva, or perineum that develops into a soft mass of granulation tissue (Douglas). A purulent discharge is common, and ulceration occurs with progressive disease. The ulcerative process may extend into the urethra and anus and cause extensive scarring and elephantiasis.

Diagnosis

The initial lesion can appear from 7 to 30 days after exposure (Wysoki et al). The diagnosis of granuloma inguinale is established by identification of Donovan bodies in smears of the affected tissue. Biopsy of the granulation tissue is helpful in confirming the diagnosis. Absence of lymphadenopathy is a diagnostic characteristic (Wysoki et al). The differential diagnosis includes other venereal diseases, and thus darkfield examination and serologic studies for syphilis, smears, biopsy, complement fixation, and skin sensitivity testing are indicated.

Treatment

Tetracycline administered four times daily for 3 weeks or until the lesion has resolved is the treatment of choice. Alternative drugs include chloramphenicol, gentamicin, erythromycin, and trimethoprim-sulfamethoxazole.

Chancroid

Chancroid is an acute ulcerative disease of the external genitalia that occurs infrequently in children (Willcox). The causative agent is the gram-negative bacillus *Haemophilus ducreyi*.

Pathogenesis and Pathology

Chancroid is transmitted by physical contact, most often via sexual intercourse. The incubation period is 1 to 5 days. The initial lesion is a single, painful erythematous ulcer on the corona of the glans in males and on the labia minora or vulva in females. The ulcer multiplies by autoinoculation and forms an erosive lesion with purulent exudate. Inguinal lymphadenitis (buboes) occurs in approximately half the cases. With advanced disease, the inguinal nodes may abscess and produce draining sinuses.

Diagnosis

The diagnosis of chancroid is made by identification of *H. ducreyi* in smears (Gram's or Wright's stain) or cultures and by the histologic appearance of biopsy tissue specimens. Intradermal skin tests with bacillary antigen become positive in 1 to 4 weeks in approximately 75 per cent of patients. Urethral smears and cultures for gonococcus, darkfield examination for spirochetes, and serologic tests for syphilis are indicated to rule out other venereal infections.

Treatment

Chancroidal infection should respond to a 10-day course of sulfonamides (or erythromycin). Fluctuant inguinal abscesses should be aspirated rather than drained openly. Discharge from these buboes is highly infectious, and therefore appropriate precautionary measures should be taken to prevent transmission of disease.

Bibliography

TUBERCULOSIS

American Academy of Pediatrics: Report of the Committee on Infectious Diseases, 21st ed. Elk Grove Village, Ill, American Academy of Pediatrics, 1988.

Cinman AC: Genitourinary tuberculosis. Urology 20:353, 1982.

Cos LR, Cockett ATK: Genitourinary tuberculosis revisited. Urology 20:111, 1982.

Cotran RS, Kumar V, Robbins SL: Robbins Pathologic Basis of Disease, 4th ed. Philadelphia, WB Saunders Co, 1989, pp 374–380.

Ehrlich RM, Lattimer JK: Urogenital tuberculosis in children. J Urol 105:461, 1971.

Flechner SM, Gow JG: Role of nephrectomy in the treatment of non-functioning or very poorly functioning unilateral tuberculous kidney. J Urol 123:822, 1980.

Fox W: The chemotherapy of pulmonary tuberculosis: a review. Chest 76(Suppl):785, 1979.

García-Rodriguez JA, García Sanchez JE, Gómez-García AC, et al: Extrapulmonary tuberculosis in a university hospital in Spain. Eur J Epidemiol 5:154, 1989.

Glassroth J, Robins AG, Snider DE Jr: Letter to the editor. N Engl J Med 303:940, 1980.

Gow JG: Genitourinary tuberculosis. *In* Campbell's Urology, Vol 1, 5th ed. Edited by PC Walsh, RF Gittes, AD Perlmutter, et al. Philadelphia, WB Saunders Co, 1986, pp 1037–1069.

Gow JG, Barbosa S: Genitourinary tuberculosis: a study of 1117 cases over a period of 34 years. Br J Urol 56:449, 1984.

Hartman GW, Segura JW, Hattery RR: Infectious diseases of the genitourinary tract. *In* Emmett's Clinical Urography: An Atlas and Textbook of Roentgenologic Diagnosis, Vol 2, 4th ed. Edited by DM Witten, GH Myers Jr, DC Utz. Philadelphia, WB Saunders Co, 1977, pp 898–918.

Kenney M, Loechel AB, Lovelock FJ: Urine cultures in tuberculosis. Am Rev Respir Dis 82:564, 1960.

Lattimer JK, Vasquez G, Wechsler H: New drugs for treatment of genitourinary tuberculosis: a comparison of efficacy. J Urol 83:493, 1960.

Murphy DM, Fallon B, Lane V, et al: Tuberculous stricture of ureter. Urology 20:382, 1982.

Schaaf HS, Smith J, Donald PR, et al: Tuberculosis presenting in the neonatal period. Clin Pediatr (Phila) 28:474, 1989.

Singh A, Fazal AR, Sinha SK, et al: Tuberculous vesicovaginal fistula in a child. Br J Urol 62:615, 1988.

Smith MHD, Marquis JR: Tuberculosis and other mycobacterial infections. *In* Textbook of Pediatric Infectious Diseases. Vol 1. Edited by RD Feigin, JD Cherry. Philadelphia, WB Saunders Co, 1981, pp 1016–1060.

Wechsler H, Lattimer JK: An evaluation of the current therapeutic regimen for renal tuberculosis. J Urol 113:760, 1975.

Weinberg AC, Boyd SD: Short-course chemotherapy and role of surgery in adult and pediatric genitourinary tuberculosis. Urology 31:95, 1988.

Wong SH, Lau WY: The surgical management of nonfunctioning tuberculous kidneys. J Urol 124:187, 1980.

Zinman L, Libertino JA: Antirefluxing ileocecal conduit. Urol Clin North Am 7(2):503, 1980.

AIDS

Albano EA, Pizzo PA: The evolving population of immunocompromised children. Pediatr Infect Dis J 7(Suppl 5):S79, 1988.

Bradford BF, Abdenour GE Jr, Frank JL, et al: Usual and unusual radiologic manifestations of acquired immunodeficiency syndrome (AIDS) and human immunodeficiency virus (HIV) infection in children. Radiol Clin North Am 26(2):341, 1988.

Davies PA: Paediatric infectious diseases: some recent advances and future priorities. Arch Dis Child 64:1332, 1989.

McNamara JG: Immunologic abnormalities in infants infected with human immunodeficiency virus. Semin Perinatol 13:35, 1989.

Miles BJ, Melser M, Farah R, et al: The urological manifestations of the acquired immunodeficiency syndrome. J Urol 142:771, 1989.

Mok J: HIV infection in children. J R Coll Gen Pract 38:342, 1988.

Reichert CM, O'Leary TJ, Levens DL, et al: Autopsy pathology in the acquired immune deficiency syndrome. Am J Pathol 112:357, 1983.

CANDIDIASIS

American Academy of Pediatrics: Report of the Committee on Infectious Diseases, 21st ed. Elk Grove Village, Ill, American Academy of Pediatrics, 1988.

Borgers M, Van den Bossche H, De Brabander M: The mechanism of action of the new antimycotic ketoconazole. Am J Med 74(Suppl 1B):2, 1983.

Dolan CT, Stried RP: Serologic diagnosis of yeast infections. Am J Clin Pathol 59:49, 1973.

Eckstein CW, Kass EJ: Anuria in a newborn secondary to bilateral ureteropelvic fungus balls. J Urol 127:109, 1982.

Everett ED, LaForce FM, Eickhoff TC: Serologic studies in suspected visceral candidiasis. Arch Intern Med 135:1075, 1975.

Graybill GR, Galgiani JN, Jorgensen JH, et al: Ketoconazole therapy for fungal urinary tract infections. J Urol 129:68, 1983.

Khan MY: Anuria from *Candida* pyelonephritis and obstructing fungal balls. Urology 21:421, 1983.

Kozinn PJ, Galen RS, Taschdjian CL, et al: The precipitin test in systemic candidiasis. JAMA 235:628, 1976.

Kozinn PJ, Taschdjian CL, Goldberg PK, et al: Advances in the diagnosis of renal candidiasis. J Urol 119:184, 1978.

MacMillan BG, Law EJ, Holder IA: Experience with *Candida* infections in burn patients. Arch Surg 104:509, 1972.

Noe HN, Tonkin ILD: Renal candidiasis in the neonate. J Urol 127:517, 1982.

Pappu LD, Purohit DM, Bradford BF, et al: Primary renal candidiasis in two preterm neonates. Am J Dis Child 138:923, 1984.

Polak A: Combination therapy with antifungal drugs. Mycoses 31(Suppl 2):45, 1988.

Schmitt GH, Hsu AS: Renal fungus balls: diagnosis by ultrasound and percutaneous antegrade pyelography and brush biopsy in a premature infant. J Ultrasound Med 4:155, 1985.

Schönebeck J: Studies on *Candida* infection of the urinary tract and on the antimycotic drug 5-fluorocytosine. Scand J Urol Nephrol Suppl 11:1, 1972.

Schönebeck J, Andersson L, Lingårdh G, et al: Ureteric obstruction caused by yeast-like fungi. Scand J Urol Nephrol 4:171, 1970.

Stone HH, Kolb LD, Currie CA, et al: *Candida* sepsis: pathogenesis and principles of treatment. Ann Surg 179:697, 1974.

van't Wout JW: Clinical manifestations of systemic fungal infections. Mycoses 31(Suppl 2):9, 1988.

Wheeler JG, Boyle R, Abramson J: *Candida tropicalis* pyelonephritis successfully treated with 5-fluorocytosine and surgery. J Pediatr 102:627, 1983.

Wise GJ: Renal candidiasis in the neonate (letter). J Urol 128:828, 1982.

Wise GJ, Goldberg P, Kozinn PJ: Genitourinary candidiasis: diagnosis and treatment. J Urol 116:778, 1976.

Wise GJ, Kozinn PJ, Goldberg P: Amphotericin B as a urologic irrigant in the management of noninvasive candiduria. J Urol 128:82, 1982.

Wise GJ, Ray B, Kozinn PJ: The serodiagnosis of significant genitourinary candidiasis. J Urol 107:1043, 1972.

Wise GJ, Wainstein S, Goldberg P, et al: Candidal cystitis: management by continuous bladder irrigation with amphotericin B. JAMA 224:1636, 1973.

Wise GJ, Wainstein S, Goldberg P, et al: Flucytosine in urinary *Candida* infections. Urology 3:708, 1974.

ASPERGILLOSIS

Bennett JE: Chemotherapy of systemic mycoses (second of two parts). N Engl J Med 290:320, 1974.

Comings DE, Turbow BA, Callahan DH, et al: Obstructing *Aspergillus* cast of the renal pelvis: report of a case in a patient having diabetes mellitus and Addison's disease. Arch Intern Med 110:255, 1962.

Eisenberg RL, Hedgcock MW, Shanser JD: Aspergillus mycetoma of the renal pelvis associated with ureteropelvic junction obstruction. J Urol 118:466, 1977.

Flechner SM, McAninch JW: Aspergillosis of the urinary tract: ascending route of infection and evolving patterns of disease. J Urol 125:598, 1981.

Godec CJ, Mielnick A, Hilfer J: Primary renal aspergillosis. Urology 34:152, 1989.

Hinson KFW, Moon AJ, Plummer NS: Broncho-pulmonary aspergillosis: a review and a report of eight new cases. Thorax 7:317, 1952.

Levitz SM: Aspergillosis. Infect Dis Clin North Am 3(1):1, 1989.

Melchoir J, Mebust WK, Valk WL: Ureteral colic from a fungus ball: unusual presentation of systemic aspergillosis. J Urol 108:698, 1972.

Warshawsky AB, Keiller D, Gittes RF: Bilateral renal aspergillosis. J Urol 113:8, 1975.

Young RC, Bennett JE, Vogel CL, et al: Aspergillosis: the spectrum of the disease in 98 patients. Medicine (Baltimore) 49:147, 1970.

ACTINOMYCOSIS

Berardi RS: Abdominal actinomycosis. Surg Gynecol Obstet 149:257, 1979.

Crosse JEW, Soderdahl DW, Schamber DT: Renal actinomycosis. Urology 7:309, 1976.

Deshmukh AS, Kropp KA: Spontaneous vesicocutaneous fistula caused by actinomycosis: case report. J Urol 112:192, 1974.

Drake DP, Holt RJ: Childhood actinomycosis: report of 3 recent cases. Arch Dis Child 51:979, 1976.

Eastridge CE, Prather JR, Hughes FA Jr, et al: Actinomycosis: a 24 year experience. South Med J 65:839, 1972.

Fass RJ, Scholand JF, Hodges GR, et al: Clindamycin in the treatment of serious anaerobic infections. Ann Intern Med 78:853, 1973.

Grierson JM, Zelas P: Actinomycosis involving urachal remnants. Med J Aust 1:849, 1971.

Holmberg K, Nord C-E, Wadström T: Serological studies of *Actinomyces israelii* by crossed immunoelectrophoresis: taxonomic and diagnostic applications. Infect Immun 12:398, 1975.

Isaacson P, Jennings M: Bilateral ureteric obstruction in a patient with ileocaecal Crohn's disease complicated by actinomycosis. Br J Urol 49:410, 1977.

Kretschmer HL, Hibbs WG: Actinomycosis of the kidney in infancy and childhood. J Urol 36:123, 1936.

Medoff G, Kobayashi G: Actinomycosis and nocardiosis. *In* Textbook of Pediatric Infectious Diseases, Vol 1, 2nd ed. Edited by RD Feigin, JD Cherry. Philadelphia, WB Saunders Co, 1987, pp 1080–1082.

Robbins TS, Scott SA: Actinomycosis: the disease and its treatment. Drug Intell Clin Pharm 15:99, 1981.

Rose HD, Rytel MW: Actinomycosis treated with clindamycin (letter). JAMA 221:1052, 1972.

COCCIDIOIDOMYCOSIS

Aguilar-Torres FG, Jackson LJ, Ferstenfeld JE, et al: Counterimmunoelectrophoresis in the detection of antibodies against *Coccidioides immitis*. Ann Intern Med 85:740, 1976.

Cheng SF: Bilateral coccidioidal epididymitis. Urology 3:362, 1974.

Conner WT, Drach GW, Bucher WC Jr: Genitourinary

aspects of disseminated coccidioidomycosis. J Urol 113:82, 1975.

Drutz DJ, Catanzaro A: Coccidioidomycosis. Part I. Am Rev Respir Dis 117:559, 1978.

Libke RD, Granoff DM: Coccidioidomycosis. *In* Textbook of Pediatric Infectious Diseases, Vol 2, 2nd ed. Edited by RD Feigin, JD Cherry. Philadelphia, WB Saunders Co, 1987, pp 1949–1962.

Stevens DA, Levine HB, Deresinski SC: Miconazole in coccidioidomycosis: II. Therapeutic and pharmacologic studies in man. Am J Med 60:191, 1976.

Weinstein AJ, Farkas S: Serologic tests in infectious diseases: clinical utility and interpretation. Med Clin North Am 62(5):1099, 1978.

CRYPTOCOCCOSIS

Bowman HE, Ritchey JO: Cryptococcosis (torulosis) involving the brain, adrenal and prostate. J Urol 71:373, 1954.

Cohen JR, Kaufmann W: Systemic cryptococcosis: a report of a case with review of the literature. Am J Clin Pathol 22:1069, 1952.

Gordon MA, Vedder DK: Serologic tests in diagnosis and prognosis of cryptococcosis. JAMA 197:961, 1966.

Huynh MT, Reyes CV: Prostatic cryptococcosis. Urology 20:622, 1982.

Lewis JL, Rabinovich S: The wide spectrum of cryptococcal infections. Am J Med 53:315, 1972.

O'Connor FJ, Foushee JHS Jr, Cox CE: Prostatic cryptococcosis: a case report. J Urol 94:160, 1965.

Randall RE Jr, Stacy WK, Toone EC, et al: Cryptococcal pyelonephritis. N Engl J Med 279:60, 1968.

Salyer WR, Salyer DC: Involvement of the kidney and prostate in cryptococcosis. J Urol 109:695, 1973.

Tillotson JR, Lerner AM: Prostatism in an eighteen-year-old boy due to infection with *Cryptococcus neoformans.* N Engl J Med 273:1150, 1965.

Wittner M: Cryptococcosis. *In* Textbook of Pediatric Infectious Diseases, Vol 2, 2nd ed. Edited by RD Feigin, JD Cherry. Philadelphia, WB Saunders Co, 1987, pp 1968–1973.

BLASTOMYCOSIS

Bergner DM, Kraus SD, Duck GB, et al: Systemic blastomycosis presenting with acute prostatic abscess. J Urol 126:132, 1981.

Denton JF, McDonough ES, Ajello L, et al: Isolation of *Blastomyces dermatitidis* from soil. Science 133:1126, 1961.

Eickenberg H-U, Amin M, Lich R Jr: Blastomycosis of the genitourinary tract. J Urol 113:650, 1975.

Furcolow ML, Chick EW, Busey JF, et al: Prevalence and incidence studies of human and canine blastomycosis: I. Cases in the United States, 1885–1968. Am Rev Respir Dis 102:60, 1970.

Gill JA, Gerald B: Blastomycosis in childhood. Radiology 91:965, 1968.

Macher A: Histoplasmosis and blastomycosis. Med Clin North Am 64(3):447, 1980.

Schwarz J, Salfelder K: Blastomycosis: a review of 152 cases. Curr Top Pathol 65:165, 1977.

Yogev R, Davis AT: Blastomycosis in children: a review of the literature. Mycopathologia 68(3):139, 1979.

MUCORMYCOSIS

Baker RD: Resectable mycotic lesions and acutely fatal mycoses. JAMA 150:1579, 1952.

Dansky AS, Lynne CM, Politano VA: Disseminated mucormycosis with renal involvement. J Urol 119:275, 1978.

Ingram CW, Sennesh J, Cooper JN, et al: Disseminated zygomycosis: report of four cases and review. Rev Infect Dis 11:741, 1989.

Langston C, Roberts DA, Porter GA, et al: Renal phycomycosis. J Urol 109:941, 1973.

Lloyd TR, Bolte RG: Rhinocerebral mucormycosis in an infant with streptococcal sepsis and purpura fulminans. Pediatr Infect Dis J 5:575, 1986.

Meyer RD, Rosen P, Armstrong D: Phycomycosis complicating leukemia and lymphoma. Ann Intern Med 77:871, 1972.

Prout GR Jr, Goddard AR: Renal mucormycosis: survival after nephrectomy and amphotericin B therapy. N Engl J Med 263:1246, 1960.

SCHISTOSOMIASIS

American Academy of Pediatrics: Report of the Committee on Infectious Diseases, 21st ed. Elk Grove Village, Ill, American Academy of Pediatrics, 1988, pp 376–377.

Bazeed MA, Ashamalla A, Abd-Alrazek A-A, et al: Partial flap ureteroneocystostomy for bilharzial strictures of the lower ureter. Urology 20:237, 1982.

Bazeed MA, Nabeeh A, Atwan N: Xanthogranulomatous pyelonephritis in bilharzial patients: a report of 25 cases. J Urol 141:261, 1989.

Hanash KA, Bissada NK: Genito-urinary schistosomiasis (bilharziasis). Part 1. King Faisal Specialist Hosp Med J 1:59, 1982.

Hanna AAZ: Genitourinary bilharziasis (schistosomiasis). *In* Emmett's Clinical Urography, Vol 2, 4th ed. Edited by DM Witten, GH Myers Jr, DC Utz. Philadelphia, WB Saunders Co, 1977, pp 921–939.

Kagan IG: Current status of serologic testing for parasitic diseases. Hosp Pract 9:157, 1974.

Kambal A: The relation of urinary bilharziasis to vesical stones in children. Br J Urol 53:315, 1981.

King CH, Keating CE, Muruka JF, et al: Urinary tract morbidity in schistosomiasis haematobia: associations with age and intensity of infection in an endemic area of Coast Province, Kenya. Am J Trop Med Hyg 39:361, 1988.

Kline MW, Sullivan TJ: Schistosomiasis. *In* Textbook of Pediatric Infectious Diseases, Vol 2, 2nd ed. Edited by RD Feigin, JD Cherry. Philadelphia, WB Saunders Co, 1987, pp 2125–2134.

von Lichtenberg F, Lehman JS: Parasitic diseases of the genitourinary system. *In* Campbell's Urology, Vol 1, 5th ed. Edited by PC Walsh, RF Gittes, AD Perlmutter, et al. Philadelphia, WB Saunders Co, 1986, pp 983–1024.

ECHINOCOCCOSIS

Apt W, Knierim F: An evaluation of diagnostic tests for hydatid disease. Am J Trop Med Hyg 19:943, 1970.

Auldist AW, Myers NA: Hydatid disease in children. Aust N Z J Surg 44:402, 1974.

Baltaxe HA, Fleming RJ: The angiographic appearance of hydatid disease. Radiology 97:599, 1970.

Buckley RJ, Smith S, Herschorn S, et al: Echinococcal disease of the kidney presenting as a renal filling defect. J Urol 133:660, 1985.

Fuloria HK, Jaiswal MSD, Singh RV: Primary hydatid cyst of bladder. Br J Urol 47:192, 1975.

Gajjar PD, Sinclair-Smith CC: Renal echinococcosis in children: a report of 2 cases. S Afr Med J 54:984, 1978.

Gharbi HA, Ben Cheikh MB, Hamza R, et al: Les localisations rares de l'hydatidose chez l'enfant. (Rare sites of hydatid disease in children.) Ann Radiol (Paris) 20:151, 1977.

Gilsanz V, Lozano F, Jimenez J: Renal hydatid cysts: communicating with collecting system. AJR 135:357, 1980.

Hansman DJ, Brown JM: Eosinophilic cystitis: a case associated with possible hydatid infection. Med J Aust 2:563, 1974.

Hunter GW III, Swartzwelder JC, Clyde DF: Tropical Medicine, 5th ed. Philadelphia, WB Saunders Co, 1976, pp 609–615.

Keramidas DC, Doulas N, Fotis G, et al: Bilateral hydronephrosis and hydroureter due to hydatid cyst in the pouch of Douglas. J Pediatr Surg 15:345, 1980.

Meymerian E, Luttermoser GW, Frayha GJ, et al: Host-parasite relationships in echinococcosis: X. Laboratory evaluation of chemical scolicides as adjuncts to hydatid surgery. Ann Surg 158:211, 1963.

Musacchio F, Mitchell N: Primary renal echinococcosis: a case report. Am J Trop Med Hyg 15:168, 1966.

Nabizadeh I, Morehouse HT, Freed SZ: Hydatid disease of kidney. Urology 22:176, 1983.

Pant CS, Gupta RK: Diagnostic value of ultrasonography in hydatid disease in abdomen and chest. Acta Radiol 28:743, 1987.

Sharma RS, Tiwari DS, Tiwari R: Hydatid cyst of the kidney. Indian J Pediatr 43:211, 1976.

Shulman Y, Morales P: Case profile: renal echinococcosis. Urology 20:452, 1982.

Silber SJ, Moyad RA: Renal echinococcus. J Urol 108:669, 1972.

Tscholl R, Ausfeld R: Renal replantation (orthotopic autotransplantation) for echinococcosis of the kidney. J Urol 133:456, 1985.

CHLAMYDIAL INFECTION

Berger RE, Alexander ER, Monda GD, et al: *Chlamydia trachomatis* as a cause of acute "idiopathic" epididymitis. N Engl J Med 298:301, 1978.

Fisher M, Swenson PD, Risucci D, et al: *Chlamydia trachomatis* in suburban adolescents. J Pediatr 111:617, 1987.

Fuster CD, Neinstein LS: Vaginal *Chlamydia trachomatis* prevalence in sexually abused prepubertal girls. Pediatrics 79:235, 1987.

Ingram DL, White ST, Occhiuti AR, et al: Childhood vaginal infections: association of *Chlamydia trachomatis* with sexual contact. Pediatr Infect Dis J 5:226, 1986.

Oriel JD, Ridgway GL, Tchamouroff S: Comparison of erythromycin stearate and oxytetracycline in the treatment of non-gonococcal urethritis: their efficacy against *Chlamydia trachomatis*. Scott Med J 22:375, 1977.

Rettig PJ, Nelson JD: Genital tract infection with *Chlamydia trachomatis* in prepubertal children. J Pediatr 99:206, 1981.

Ridgway GL, Oriel JD: Activity of antimicrobials against *Chlamydia trachomatis in vitro* (letter). J Antimicrob Chemother 5:483, 1979.

Smith TF, Weed LA, Segura JW, et al: Isolation of *Chlamydia* from patients with urethritis. Mayo Clin Proc 50:105, 1975.

PINWORM INFESTATION

Graham CF: A device for the diagnosis of *Enterobius* infection. Am J Trop Med 21:159, 1941.

Kropp KA, Cichocki GA, Bansal NK: Enterobius vermicularis (pinworms), introital bacteriology and recurrent urinary tract infection in children. J Urol 120:480, 1978.

MacPherson DW: Intestinal parasites. *In* Current Therapy 1990. Edited by RE Rakel. Philadelphia, WB Saunders Co, 1990, pp 486–492.

Mayers CP, Purvis RJ: Manifestations of pinworms. Can Med Assoc J 103:489, 1970.

Sachdev YV, Howards SS: *Enterobius vermicularis* infestation and secondary enuresis. J Urol 113:143, 1975.

TRICHOMONIASIS

Al-Salihi FL, Curran JP, Wang J-S: Neonatal *Trichomonas vaginalis:* report of three cases and review of the literature. Pediatrics 53:196, 1974.

Fouts AC, Kraus SJ: *Trichomonas vaginalis:* reevaluation of its clinical presentation and laboratory diagnosis. J Infect Dis 141:137, 1980.

Krieger JN: Urologic aspects of trichomoniasis. Invest Urol 18:414, 1981.

Meares EM Jr: Prostatitis syndromes: new perspectives about old woes. J Urol 123:141, 1980.

Perl G, Ragazzoni H: Further studies in treatment of female and male trichomoniasis with metronidazole. Obstet Gynecol 22:376, 1963.

Postlethwaite RJ: *Trichomonas* vaginitis and *Escherichia coli* urinary infection in a newborn infant. Clin Pediatr (Phila) 14:866, 1975.

Rein MF: *Trichomonas vaginalis*. *In* Principles and Practice of Infectious Diseases, 3rd ed. Edited by GL Mandell, RG Douglas Jr, JE Bennett. New York, Churchill Livingstone, 1990, pp 2115–2118.

Rothenberg RB, Simon R, Chipperfield E, et al: Efficacy of selected diagnostic tests for sexually transmitted diseases. JAMA 235:49, 1976.

UREAPLASMA INFECTION

Foy H, Kenny G, Bor E, et al: Prevalence of *Mycoplasma hominis* and *Ureaplasma urealyticum* (T strains) in urine of adolescents. J Clin Microbiol 2:226, 1975.

Handsfield HH: Gonorrhea and nongonococcal urethritis: recent advances. Med Clin North Am 62(5):925, 1978.

Holmes KK, Johnson DW, Floyd TM: Studies of venereal disease: III. Double-blind comparison of tetracycline hydrochloride and placebo in treatment of nongonococcal urethritis. JAMA 202:474, 1967.

Klein JO, Buckland D, Finland M: Colonization of newborn infants by mycoplasmas. N Engl J Med 280:1025, 1969.

McCormack WM, Braun P, Lee Y-H, et al: The genital mycoplasmas. N Engl J Med 288:78, 1973a.

McCormack WM, Lee Y-H, Zinner SH: Sexual experience and urethral colonization with genital mycoplasmas: a study in normal men. Ann Intern Med 78:696, 1973b.

Taylor-Robinson D, McCormack WM: The genital mycoplasmas. N Engl J Med 302:1003, 1063, 1980.

CYCLOPHOSPHAMIDE CYSTITIS

deVries CR, Freiha FS: Hemorrhagic cystitis: a review. J Urol 143:1, 1990.

Droller MJ, Saral R, Santos G: Prevention of cyclophosphamide-induced hemorrhagic cystitis. Urology 20:256, 1982.

Duckett JW Jr, Peters PC, Donaldson MH: Severe cyclophosphamide hemorrhagic cystitis controlled with phenol. J Pediatr Surg 8:55, 1973.

Ehrlich RM, Freedman A, Goldsobel AB, et al: The use of sodium 2-mercaptoethane sulfonate to prevent cyclophosphamide cystitis. J Urol 131:960, 1984.

Jerkins GR, Noe HN, Hill D: Treatment of complications of cyclophosphamide cystitis. J Urol 139:923, 1988.

Kende G, Wajsman Z, Thomas PRM, et al: Chronic hematuria and localized bladder damage following combined cyclophosphamide and local radiotherapy. J Surg Oncol 12:169, 1979.

Lawrence HJ, Simone J, Aur RJA: Cyclophosphamide-induced hemorrhagic cystitis in children with leukemia. Cancer 36:1572, 1975.

Levine LA, Richie JP: Urological complications of cyclophosphamide. J Urol 141:1063, 1989.

Liedberg C-F, Ruasing A, Langeland P: Cyclophosphamide hemorrhagic cystitis. Scand J Urol Nephrol 4:183, 1970.

Philips FS, Sternberg SS, Cronin AP, et al: Cyclophosphamide and urinary bladder toxicity. Cancer Res 21:1577, 1961.

Primack A: Amelioration of cyclophosphamide-induced cystitis. J Natl Cancer Inst 47:223, 1971.

Pyeritz RE, Droller MJ, Bender WL, et al: An approach to the control of massive hemorrhage in cyclophosphamide-induced cystitis by intravenous vasopressin: a case report. J Urol 120:253, 1978.

Rabinovitch HH: Simple innocuous treatment of massive cyclophosphamide hemorrhagic cystitis. Urology 13:610, 1979.

Shrom SH, Donaldson MH, Duckett JW Jr, et al: Formalin treatment for intractable hemorrhagic cystitis: a review of the literature with 16 additional cases. Cancer 38:1785, 1976.

Texter JH Jr, Koontz WW Jr, McWilliams NB: Hemorrhagic cystitis as a complication of the management of pediatric neoplasms. Urol Surv 29:47, 1979.

Tolley DA: The effect of N-acetyl cysteine on cyclophosphamide cystitis. Br J Urol 49:659, 1977.

Trigg ME, O'Reilly J, Rumelhart S, et al: Prostaglandin E_1 bladder instillations to control severe hemorrhagic cystitis. J Urol 143:92, 1990.

EOSINOPHILIC CYSTITIS

Champion RH, Ackles RC: Eosinophilic cystitis. J Urol 96:729, 1966.

Farber S, Vawter GF: Clinical pathological conference. J Pediatr 62:941, 1963.

Goldstein M: Eosinophilic cystitis. J Urol 106:854, 1971.

Hellstrom HR, Davis BK, Shonnard JW: Eosinophilic cystitis: a study of 16 cases. Am J Clin Pathol 72:777, 1979.

Littleton RH, Farah RN, Cerny JC: Eosinophilic cystitis: an uncommon form of cystitis. J Urol 127:132, 1982.

Nkposong EO, Attah EB: Eosinophilic cystitis. Eur Urol 4:274, 1978.

Powell NB, Powell EB, Thomas OC, et al: Allergy of the lower urinary tract. J Urol 107:631, 1972.

Rubin L, Pincus MB: Eosinophilic cystitis: the relationship of allergy in the urinary tract to eosinophilic cystitis and the pathophysiology of eosinophilia. J Urol 112:457, 1974.

Sidh SM, Smith SP, Silber SB, et al: Eosinophilic cystitis: advanced disease requiring surgical intervention. Urology 15:23, 1980.

Sutphin M, Middleton AW Jr: Eosinophilic cystitis in children: a self-limited process. J Urol 132:117, 1984.

Tauscher JW, Shaw DC: Eosinophilic cystitis. Clin Pediatr (Phila) 20:741, 1981.

CHRONIC GRANULOMATOUS DISEASE

Baehner RL, Nathan DG: Quantitative nitroblue tetrazolium test in chronic granulomatous disease. N Engl J Med 278:971, 1968.

Curnutte JT, Kipnes RS, Babior BM: Defect in pyridine nucleotide dependent superoxide production by a particulate fraction from the granulocytes of patients with chronic granulomatous disease. N Engl J Med 293:628, 1975.

Elgefors B, Olling S, Peterson H: Chronic granulomatous disease in three siblings. Scand J Infect Dis 10:79, 1978.

Frifelt JJ, Schønheyder H, Valerius NH, et al: Chronic granulomatous disease associated with chronic glomerulonephritis. Acta Paediatr Scand 74:152, 1985.

Holmes B, Page AR, Good RA: Studies of the metabolic activity of leukocytes from patients with a genetic abnormality of phagocytic function. J Clin Invest 46:1422, 1967.

Johansen KS, Borregaard N, Koch C, et al: Chronic granulomatous disease presenting as xanthogranulomatous pyelonephritis in late childhood. J Pediatr 100:98, 1982.

Johnston RB Jr, Wilfert CM, Buckley RH, et al: Enhanced bactericidal activity of phagocytes from patients with chronic granulomatous disease in the presence of sulphisoxazole. Lancet 1:824, 1975.

Klebanoff SJ, White LR: Iodination defect in the leukocytes of a patient with chronic granulomatous disease of childhood. N Engl J Med 280:460, 1969.

Lehrer RI: Measurement of candidacidal activity of specific leukocyte types in mixed cell populations: II. Normal and chronic granulomatous disease eosinophils. Infect Immun 3:800, 1971.

Philippart AI, Colodny AH, Baehner RL: Continuous antibiotic therapy in chronic granulomatous disease: preliminary communication. Pediatrics 50:923, 1972.

Rodey GE, Park BH, Windhorst DB, et al: Defective bactericidal activity of monocytes in fatal granulomatous disease. Blood 33:813, 1969.

Young AK, Middleton RG: Urologic manifestations of chronic granulomatous disease of infancy. J Urol 123:119, 1980.

GONOCOCCAL URETHRITIS

American Academy of Pediatrics. Report of the Committee on Infectious Diseases, 21st ed. Elk Grove Village, Ill, American Academy of Pediatrics, 1988.

Barrett-Connor E: Gonorrhea and the pediatrician. Am J Dis Child 125:233, 1973.

Branch G, Paxton R: A study of gonococcal infections among infants and children. Public Health Rep 80:347, 1965.

Clark DO: Gonorrhea: changing concepts in diagnosis and management. Clin Obstet Gynecol 16(2):3, 1973.

Farrell MK, Billmire ME, Shamroy JA, et al: Prepubertal gonorrhea: a multidisciplinary approach. Pediatrics 67:151, 1981.

Karney WW, Pedersen AHB, Nelson M, et al: Spectinomycin versus tetracycline for the treatment of gonorrhea. N Engl J Med 296:889, 1977.

Kellogg DS Jr, Holmes KK, Hill GA: Laboratory diagnosis of gonorrhea. Cumitech 4:1, 1976.

McGregor JA: Adolescent misadventures with urethritis and cervicitis. J Adolesc Health Care 6:286, 1985.

Meek JM, Askari A, Belman AB: Prepubertal gonorrhea. J Urol 122:532, 1979.

Nelson JD, Mohs E, Dajani AS, et al: Gonorrhea in

preschool- and school-aged children: report of the Pre-pubertal Gonorrhea Cooperative Study Group. JAMA 236:1359, 1976.

Potterat JJ, Markewich GS, King RD, et al: Child-to-child transmission of gonorrhea: report of asymptomatic genital infection in a boy. Pediatrics 78:711, 1986.

Saxena SB, Feriozi D: An evaluation of urethral smear by Papanicolaou stain in men with urethritis. J Adolesc Health Care 9:76, 1988.

Shore WB, Winkelstein JA: Nonvenereal transmission of gonococcal infections to children. J Pediatr 79:661, 1971.

Whitner MS, Anderson MV: Sexually transmitted diseases in children. Health Care for Women International 8:9, 1987.

NONGONOCOCCAL URETHRITIS

Felman YM, Nikitas JA: Nongonococcal urethritis: a clinical review. JAMA 245:381, 1981.

Goldenring JM: Acute urethral syndromes. Semin Adolesc Med 2:125, 1986.

Jacobs NF Jr, Kraus SJ: Gonococcal and nongonococcal urethritis in men: clinical and laboratory differentiation. Ann Intern Med 82:7, 1975.

Oriel JD, Ridgway GL, Tchamouroff S: Comparison of erythromycin stearate and oxytetracycline in the treatment of non-gonococcal urethritis: their efficacy against *Chlamydia trachomatis*. Scott Med J 22:375, 1977.

Smith TF, Weed LA, Segura JA, et al: Isolation of *Chlamydia* from patients with urethritis. Mayo Clin Proc 50:105, 1975.

HERPES SIMPLEX INFECTION

American Academy of Pediatrics: Report of the Committee on Infectious Diseases, 21st ed. Elk Grove Village, Ill, American Academy of Pediatrics, 1988.

Fiumara NJ, Schmidt-Ulrick B, Comite H: Primary herpes simplex and primary syphilis: a description of seven cases. Sex Transm Dis 7(3):130, 1980.

Nahmias AJ, Alford CA, Korones SB: Infection of the newborn with *Herpesvirus hominis*. Adv Pediatr 17:185, 1970.

Nahmias AJ, Josey WE, Naib ZM: Neonatal herpes simplex infection: role of genital infection in mother as the source of virus in the newborn. JAMA 199:164, 1967.

Person DA, Kaufman RH, Gardner HL, et al: Herpesvirus type 2 in genitourinary tract infections. Am J Obstet Gynecol 116:993, 1973.

SYPHILIS

Cotran RS, Kumar V, Robbins SL: Robbins Pathologic Basis of Disease, 4th ed. Philadelphia, WB Saunders Co, 1989, pp 368–371, 1106.

Fiumara NJ: Infections of the genitals. I.: Bacterial and fungal infections. Infect Urol May/June, 1989, p 79.

Taber LH, Huber TW: Congenital syphilis. Prog Clin Biol Res 3:183, 1975.

Wilfert C, Gutman L: Syphilis. *In* Textbook of Pediatric Infectious Diseases, Vol 1, 2nd ed. Edited by RD Feigin, JD Cherry. Philadelphia, WB Saunders Co, 1987, pp 608–621.

PROSTATITIS

Mann S: Prostatic abscess in the newborn. Arch Dis Child 35:396, 1960.

Meares EM Jr: Prostatitis: a review. Urol Clin North Am 2(1):3, 1975.

EPIDIDYMITIS

Amar AD, Chabra K: Epididymitis in prepubertal boys: presenting manifestation of vesicoureteral reflux. JAMA 207:2397, 1969.

Barker K, Raper FP: Torsion of the testis. Br J Urol 36:35, 1964.

Brereton RJ: Limitations of the Doppler flow meter in the diagnosis of the "acute scrotum" in boys. Br J Urol 53:380, 1981.

Coran AG, Perlmutter AD: Mumps epididymitis without orchitis. N Engl J Med 272:735, 1965.

Doolittle KH, Smith JP, Saylor ML: Epididymitis in the prepubertal boy. J Urol 96:364, 1966.

Greenfield SP: Type B *Hemophilus influenzae* epididymo-orchitis in the prepubertal boy. J Urol 136:1311, 1986.

Hodgson NB, Hasan S: Unusual cause of acute scrotal swelling. Society for Pediatric Urology Newsletter, April 9, 1980, p 17.

Ibrahim AIA, Awad R, Shetty SD, et al: Genito-urinary complications of brucellosis. Br J Urol 61:294, 1988.

Kelalis PP, Stickler GB: The painful scrotum: torsion vs epididymo-orchitis. Clin Pediatr (Phila) 15:220, 1976.

Khan MS, Humayoon MS, Al Manee MS: Epididymo-orchitis and brucellosis. Br J Urol 63:87, 1989.

Kiviat MD, Shurtleff D, Ansell JS: Urinary reflux via the vas deferens: unusual cause of epididymitis in infancy. J Pediatr 80:476, 1972.

Levy OM, Gittelman MC, Strashun AM, et al: Diagnosis of acute testicular torsion using radionuclide scanning. J Urol 129:975, 1983.

Ransler CW III, Allen TD: Torsion of the spermatic cord. Urol Clin North Am 9(2):245, 1982.

Smith DR: Treatment of epididymitis by infiltration of spermatic cord with procaine hydrochloride. J Urol 46:74, 1941.

Valvo JR, Caldamone AA, O'Mara R, et al: Nuclear imaging in the pediatric acute scrotum. Am J Dis Child 136:831, 1982.

Waldman LS, Kosloske AM, Parsons DW: Acute epididymo-orchitis as the presenting manifestation of *Hemophilus influenzae* septicemia. J Pediatr 90:87, 1977.

Weber TR: *Hemophilus influenzae* epididymo-orchitis. J Urol 133:487, 1985.

ORCHITIS

Cotran RS, Kumar V, Robbins SL: Robbins Pathologic Basis of Disease, 4th ed. Philadelphia, WB Saunders Co, 1989, p 1106.

Kaplan GW, King LR: Acute scrotal swelling in children. J Urol 104:219, 1970.

Malkin RB, Joshi VV, Koontz WW Jr: Bacterial orchitis, abscess and sepsis in a newborn: a case report. J Urol 112:530, 1974.

VULVOVAGINITIS

Arsenault PS, Gerbie AB: Vulvovaginitis in the preadolescent girl. Pediatr Ann 15(8):577, 1986.

Burry VF: Gonococcal vulvovaginitis and possible peritonitis in prepubertal girls. Am J Dis Child 121:536, 1971.

Gaafar SA, Awadalla Fel-Z, Hassan RR, et al: Study of parasitological causes of vulvovaginitis in Egyptian children. J Egypt Soc Parasitol 18:443, 1988.

Heller RH, Joseph JM, Davis HJ: Vulvovaginitis in the premenarcheal child. J Pediatr 74:370, 1969.

Huffman JW: Gynecologic infections in childhood and adolescence. *In* Textbook of Pediatric Infectious Diseases, Vol 1, 2nd ed. Edited by RD Feigin, JD Cherry. Philadelphia, WB Saunders Co, 1987, pp 555–587.

Rein MF: Current therapy of vulvovaginitis. Sex Transm Dis 8:316, 1981.

Rosenfeld WD, Clark J: Vulvovaginitis and cervicitis. Pediatr Clin North Am 36(3):489, 1989.

Sanfilippo JS: Adolescent girls with vaginal discharge. Pediatr Ann 15(8):509, 1986.

Stark AR, Glode MP: Gonococcal vaginitis in a neonate. J Pediatr 94:298, 1979.

Tunnessen WW Jr, Jastremski M: Prepubescent gonococcal vulvovaginitis. Clin Pediatr (Phila) 13:675, 1974.

Watkins S, Quan L: Vulvovaginitis caused by *Yersinia enterocolitica*. Pediatr Infect Dis J 3:444, 1984.

LYMPHOGRANULOMA VENEREUM

Abrams AJ: Lymphogranuloma venereum. JAMA 205:199, 1968.

Banov L Jr: Rectal lesions of lymphogranuloma venereum in childhood: review of the literature and report of a case in a ten-year-old boy with rectal stricture. Am J Dis Child 83:660, 1952.

Fiumara NJ: Infections of the genitals: I. Bacterial and fungal infections. Infect Urol May/June 1989, p 79.

Holder WR, Duncan WC: Lymphogranuloma venereum. Clin Obstet Gynecol 15(4):1004, 1972.

Levy H: Lymphogranuloma venereum in childhood: review of the literature with report of a case. Arch Pediatr 57:441, 1940.

Weinstock HL, Keesal S: Lymphogranuloma venereum: report of a case in a child. Urol Cutan Rev 50:520, 1946.

GRANULOMA INGUINALE

Davis CM: Granuloma inguinale: a clinical, histological, and ultrastructural study. JAMA 211:632, 1970.

Douglas CP: Lymphogranuloma venereum and granuloma inguinale of the vulva. J Obstet Gynaec Br Common 69:871, 1962.

Lal S, Nicholas C: Epidemiological and clinical features in 165 cases of granuloma inguinale. Br J Vener Dis 46:461, 1970.

Wysoki RS, Majmudar B, Willis D: Granuloma inguinale (donovanosis) in women. J Reprod Med 33:709, 1988.

CHANCROID

Willcox RR: Chancroid (soft sore). *In* Recent Advances in Sexually Transmitted Diseases, Vol 1. Edited by Morton RS, Harris JRW. Edinburgh, Churchill Livingstone, 1975.

11

☐ Enuresis

H. Gil Rushton

The involuntary voiding of urine beyond the age of anticipated control is called enuresis. Nocturnal enuresis refers to nighttime wetting, whereas diurnal enuresis refers to daytime wetting. A more accurate differentiation would be "sleepwetting," a newly coined term by author Alison Mack, versus awake wetting. For instance, many otherwise dry children who wet during the night will also wet during a daytime nap. The term "sleepwetting" may eliminate many of the negative guilt and shame connotations implied by the more commonly used term "bedwetting." Although criteria vary among different authors, a reasonable definition of nocturnal enuresis is persistent sleepwetting more than twice a month past the age of 5 years. Primary enuresis is defined as sleepwetting in patients who have never been dry for extended periods. Secondary enuresis is the onset of wetting after a continuous dry period of more than 6 months.

The literature is replete with reports concerning the epidemiology, etiology, and management of nocturnal enuresis. Despite this, the causes and treatment options for enuresis remain controversial. This is not surprising in view of the multiple factors that influence the manifestation and resolution of this perplexing phenomenon. This chapter provides an overview of the epidemiologic and etiologic factors in enuresis and relates these to the evaluation and treatment of this interesting condition. The author would like to acknowledge the scholarly contribution from the last edition of this text, which served as the foundation for the current chapter (Perlmutter).

EPIDEMIOLOGY

The reported prevalence of enuresis varies substantially among different populations, based to some extent on social mores and its definition by different authors (Fig. 11–1). However, it is generally accepted that nocturnal enuresis occurs in 15 to 20 per cent of 5-year-old children (Miller). An estimated 15 per cent of sleepwetters will achieve nocturnal control each year, such that by age 15, only 1 to 2 per cent of adolescents remain enuretic (DeJonge; Forsythe and Redmond, 1974; Miller). Secondary, or onset, enuresis accounts for approximately 20 to 25 per cent of the enuretic population (DeJonge; Hallgren, 1959; Notschaele). Furthermore, approximately 15 to 20 per cent of young sleepwetters also have diurnal enuresis (wetting while awake), a figure that rapidly decreases in children older than 5 years of age (DeJonge). Sleepwetting occurs more commonly in boys, although daytime frequency and wetting tend to be more common in girls. Enuresis is reported to occur more frequently in lower socioeconomic populations and in larger families (Miller).

ETIOLOGY

Nocturnal enuresis has been attributed to many diverse causes, including maturational lag and/or developmental delay, abnormal sleep patterns, psychopathology, environmental stress, organic urinary tract disease, and abnormalities of the normal circadian rhythm of antidiuretic hormone (ADH) secretion. Enuresis is best viewed as a symptom rather than a disease state. As such, it is a manifestation that can be more or less affected by a number of "etiologic" factors. Efforts to identify specific causes on an individual case basis are often frustrating and have not yet proved to be particularly beneficial in determining management. Nevertheless, awareness of these etiologic factors is fundamental to understanding the basis of the various treatment options available.

Attaining Bladder Control

Although the actual details of the neurophysiologic process by which a child acquires urinary control are not completely understood, various developmental stages have been observed (Duche; MacKeith et al; Muellner; Yeates). In the newborn period, micturition is characterized by reflex voiding occurring at frequent intervals, averaging approximately 20 voidings per day (Goellner et al). Bladder filling results in complete voiding triggered by afferent stimulation of the reflex arc. The efferent response results in detrusor contraction and simultaneous relaxation of the striated muscle (external) urinary sphincter. Prior to micturition, there is progressive constriction of the striated muscle sphincter in response to gradual bladder distention.

After 6 months of age, voiding becomes less frequent as the voided volumes increase. This has been attributed to the development of unconscious inhibition of the voiding reflex (Yeates). Others have suggested, based on the observation that bladder capacity increases and the volume of urine per kilogram per day decreases during this time period, that the decrease in voiding frequency is at least partly due to a growth-related increase in bladder capacity that is proportionately greater than the increase in the urine volume produced (Goellner et al; Koff, 1986). Between 1 and 2 years of age, a conscious sensation of bladder fullness develops, setting the stage for voluntary control of voiding (Yeates). As described by Nash, this process involves three separate developmental events: (1) increase in bladder capacity to allow for adequate storage, (2) voluntary control of the periurethral striated muscle sphincter in order to initiate and terminate voiding, and (3) direct volitional control over the spinal micturition reflex.

Voluntary control of micturition involves a complex and, as yet, incompletely understood interaction of inhibitory and facilitative influences that act on the sacral micturition reflex center (Mahony et al, 1977). The ability to void or inhibit voiding voluntarily at any degree of bladder filling commonly develops in the second and third year of life, such that most children have acquired an adult pattern of urinary control by age 4 (Stein and Susser, 1967). The "typical" sequence for the development of bladder and bowel control has been described as follows: (1) nocturnal bowel control, (2) daytime bowel control, (3) daytime control of voiding, (4) nocturnal control of voiding. However, there is considerable interindividual and intercultural variation from this orderly scheme of events (Brazelton; Craw-

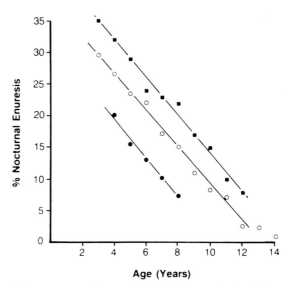

Figure 11–1 □ Rates of nocturnal enuresis in children of three disparate populations. ●, Children in Christchurch, New Zealand, reported by Fergusson et al. ○, Children living in Khartoum, Sudan, surveyed by Rahim and Cederblad. ■, Children of Baltimore, reported by Oppel et al. (From Crawford, JD: Introductory comments. Treatment of nocturnal enuresis. J Pediatr 114(Suppl):687, 1989.)

ford). A more detailed description of the physiology of micturition is provided in Chapter 6.

Maturational Lag/ Developmental Delay

Maturational Lag

The theory that delayed functional maturation of the central nervous system is a cause of enuresis has remained a popular, although not universally accepted, explanation (Bakwin, 1961; Linderholm; MacKeith; Muellner). This hypothesis is largely based on epidemiologic and urodynamic evidence. Certainly, the most convincing argument in favor of a maturational lag is the recognized spontaneous cure rate that allows for the majority of enuretics eventually to gain urinary control. Other indirect evidence comes from children who have both diurnal and nocturnal enuresis. In this group, the sequence of events leading to dryness usually mimics the same pattern typically seen in normal children, that is, daytime control followed by control during sleep. In many children, this maturational lag seems to be related to genetic factors. A positive family history of sleepwetting is one of the most common findings noted by physicians who treat childhood enuresis (Fergusson et al; Hallgren, 1957; Kaffman and Elizur). In one survey, when both parents had a history of enuresis, 77 per cent of children were enuretic; when only one parent had a history of enuresis, 44 per cent of the children were enuretic; and when neither had a history of enuresis, only 15 per cent of the children were affected (Bakwin, 1973).

The neurophysiologic defect involved in this maturational lag may be related to an abnormality in pelvic floor activity (urethral sphincteric guarding reflex) (Mahony et al, 1981; Norgaard 1989a), inadequate central inhibition (Linderholm; Troup and Hodgson), or a defect in sensation resulting in adequate or delayed recognition of bladder filling (Gillison and Skinner; McGuire and Savastano; Yeates). Urodynamic findings of persistent bladder instability of the infantile type and poorly tolerated bladder filling, reported in many enuretics, support this concept of a functional maturational delay. Numerous studies have documented reduced bladder capacities in enuretics when compared with normal controls (Esperanca and Gerrard, 1969a; Hallman; Muellner; Starfield and Mellits; Zaleski et al). The finding that the total bladder capacity in enuretics is actually normal during general anesthesia suggests that the reduced capacity is functional and not structural (Troup and Hodgson).

As many as one fifth of patients with nocturnal enuresis and one third of patients with both nocturnal and diurnal enuresis manifest symptoms of bladder instability, such as daytime frequency and urgency (Hallgren, 1956). Urodynamic findings of persistent bladder instability have been reported in 35 to 90 per cent of enuretic patients (Firlit et al; Giles et al; Hagglund, 1965; Linderholm; Mahony et al, 1981; McGuire and Savastano; Pompeius; Webster et al, 1984a). One study described bladder instability in 15 per cent of those patients with nocturnal enuresis only, compared with 97 per cent with both diurnal and nocturnal enuresis (Whiteside and Arnold). Mahony and associates (1981) have described a mild form of compensated detrusor instability in children who have nocturnal enuresis only. They define this as an intermediate condition of "excitability" of the sacral micturition reflex center. Voluntary inhibition, which is required to control this "excitability," is successful in preventing involuntary detrusor contractions during the daytime. However, voluntary inhibition fails during sleep, resulting in an enuretic episode.

Comparison between studies is hindered by variation in the populations in question as well as methodology (Norgaard, 1989a). Most contain patients with daytime voiding symptoms and/or complicating neurologic or urologic disorders mixed with children who only have nocturnal enuresis. Methodologic variations in urodynamic testing include the type of catheter used (transurethral versus suprapubic), bladder filling rates, and medium used (gas versus liquid). Norgaard (1989a, 1989b) studied a group of children with uncomplicated nocturnal enuresis by performing repetitive awake and sleep cystometry over a 5-day observation period. Strict attention was paid to infusion flow rates. He reported bladder instability in approximately 15 per cent. Although there was considerable individual variation in bladder capacity, functional daytime capacity correlated well with the bladder capacity during sleep. When present, nocturnal unstable bladder contractions did not result in sleepwetting. Instead, enuretic events were triggered by a full bladder and were characterized by a well-coordinated micturition with complete bladder emptying.

Regardless of whether unstable bladder contractions result in enuretic episodes, the underlying defect in sleepwetting and bladder instability of childhood may be related in some cases to a common maturational factor. Children with daytime frequency or enuresis may simply have a more pronounced maturational lag compared with those who wet only during sleep. This is suggested by the frequent association of daytime urgency and frequency in children who are wet. Those children with associated daytime enuresis and frequency or urgency have been shown to have smaller functional bladder capacities than patients who only have nocturnal enuresis. Daytime symptoms are also much more prevalent in younger children with enuresis. As maturation occurs, daytime symptoms in enuretics usually improve prior to attaining nocturnal control, similar to the sequence of events observed in normal toilet training.

Additional evidence for a maturational lag in patients with enuresis comes from electroencephalographic (EEG) studies that have shown an increased incidence in cerebral dysrhythmias (Campbell and Young; Fermaglich; Kaijtor et al). Although the actual clinical significance of these minor abnormalities is not known, they have been attributed by some to a delayed functional maturation of portions of the central nervous system (Edvardsen; Kaijtor et al).

Developmental Delay

Others have argued that enuresis represents a developmental delay that is not the result of a lag in neurophysiologic maturation but, rather, is due to deficient learning of a habit pattern (Lovibond; Lovibond and Coote). Those who challenge the concept of maturational lag argue that the intermittent nature of enuresis seen in many children is proof that neurophysiologic maturity is complete. Behavioralists have also argued that successful response to conditioning therapy is evidence that nocturnal enuresis can be "learned" by operant conditioning and is therefore not dependent upon maturation of the central nervous system (Lovibond and Coote). Additional support for the concept of a developmental delay comes from a retrospective study of 1265 children from New Zealand followed from birth until 8 years of age. In addition to a family history of enuresis and early sleeping patterns, the child's overall developmental level at 1 and 3 years of age was predictive of the age of attainment of bladder control (Fergusson et al).

A developmental basis for enuresis is also suggested by a number of epidemiologic studies implicating a role of environmental factors such as socioeconomic level and stress. Sleepwetting has been reported more frequently in lower socioeconomic populations and larger families (Essen and Peckham; McKendry et al; Miller). The prevalence also appears to be higher in children from broken homes and institutions, environments in which greater stress might be expected (Douglas, 1970; Miller; Stein and Susser, 1966). Conversely, in a study of children from upper middle-class neighborhoods in Boston, 98.5 per cent of children raised in a low-anxiety, supportive environment achieved bladder control by the age of 5 years (Brazelton).

MacKeith states that neurophysiologic maturation is complete by age 5 and has postulated that enuresis may result from a transient episode of stress occurring at a critical period of development (MacKeith et al). He notes that the 2nd to the 4th year of life appears to be a sensitive and perhaps vulnerable period for the acquisition of urinary control. During this time, particularly during the third year, there is a high rate of emergence of nocturnal bladder control compared with the periods preceding and following it. A stressful or anxiety-provoking episode or environment during this critical period could prevent emergence of the behavioral skills necessary for nocturnal urinary control. This concept is supported by the frequent association of secondary-onset enuresis with a stressful event, such as birth of a new sibling or separation from a parent. It is difficult to attribute secondary-onset enuresis to a maturational lag unless one assumes that there is an underlying deficiency in bladder control that is "latent" and susceptible to "exaggerating" or adverse environmental factors (Yeates). Although a higher incidence of stressful events during this "sensitive" period has been reported in some studies (Douglas, 1973), others have not substantiated this association (Fergusson et al; Kaffman and Elizur).

Actually, the two concepts of maturational lag and developmental delay may not be mutually exclusive (Kolvin and Taunch). If there is indeed a "sensitive" period for the emergence of control between ages 2 and 4, either a stressful event or maturational lag during this time period could prevent emergence of nocturnal bladder control. Even MacKeith, who contends that enuresis is developmental, acknowledges that maturational lag may be a contributing factor in children up to age 5 (MacKeith et al). Once a child is past this critical period, subsequent spontaneous control may be less likely to develop even if neurophysiologic "maturation" has occurred.

Antidiuretic Hormone

As early as 1952, Poulton considered relative nocturnal polyuria as a pathogenic factor in enuresis. Later studies with carefully controlled diet and fluid intake demonstrated no difference in the average day/night ratio of urine output in enuretics compared with controls (Vuliamy). Subsequently, little attention was given to this concept until studies reported a circadian variation in normal subjects of the excretion of ADH, demonstrating an increase during nighttime (George et al). Two subsequent studies did *not* show such an increase in nocturnal ADH excretion in enuretic children (Norgaard et al; Puri, 1980a). In a larger study, a group of enuretic children had significantly lower increases in nocturnal mean serum ADH levels when compared with a group of normal controls (Rittig et al, 1989a) (Fig. 11–2). Lower mean nocturnal urine osmolalities and higher mean nocturnal urinary excretion rates were also observed in the enuretic population. No difference was found in the total diurnal urinary volume, osmolality, or tubular capacity for reabsorption of water between enuretics and normal controls. The high volume of urine output during sleep in these enuretic children

exceeded their daytime functional bladder capacity (Norgaard, 1989a). Once bladder capacity was exceeded, an enuretic episode occurred.

The findings reported by this group of investigators suggest a physiologic basis for sleepwetting in some children who have nocturnal enuresis only. The influence of an ADH factor in the enuretic population at large cannot be determined from those studies that have involved only a small, select group of enuretic children. Furthermore, why these and other enuretic children do not awaken to void when the bladder is full is not accounted for by this physiologic explanation. Another unanswered question is whether these children subsequently spontaneously develop a normal circadian rhythm of ADH excretion when they stop wetting. In other words, is the absence of a diurnal pattern of ADH excretion in enuretics due to a maturational delay in this circadian rhythm? It would appear that, although it is probably a contributory factor in some enuretics, this abnormality in ADH excretion is not, by itself, the "physiologic" cause for enuresis.

Sleep Disorders

Historically, bedwetters have been considered "deep sleepers." Certainly, this is one of the most common complaints of parents of enuretics (Wille, 1989). This premise has been questioned by some who suggest that this merely reflects subjective bias resulting from the increased efforts made by parents to awaken enuretic children (Boyd; Graham). Others have not found any significant difference in the waking time of enuretic versus nonenuretic controls (Kaffman and Elizur). It has also been suggested that the difference may only represent an exaggerated state of confusion that may accompany any forceful awakening, even in normal children. In children with various sleep disorders, the intensity of "sleep-drunkenness" does, however, seem to be greater (Lowy).

The development of electroencephalography in the 1950s made more objective studies by sleep monitoring possible. From these studies, two categories of sleep stages were identified: rapid eye movement (REM) and non–rapid eye movement (NREM) sleep. NREM sleep is considered deep sleep and is divided into four progressively deeper sleep stages (stages

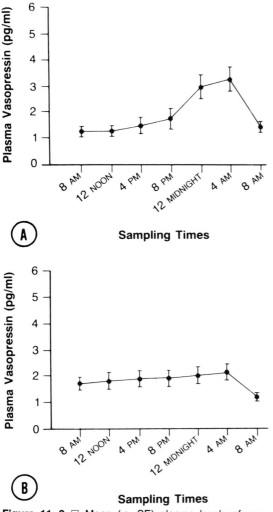

Figure 11–2 □ Mean (± SE) plasma levels of vasopressin in (A) 11 normal and (B) 15 enuretic children. Vasopressin levels are stable in enuretic children throughout the 24-hour period, whereas normal children show an increase at nighttime. (From Norgaard JP, Rittig S, Djurhuus JC: Nocturnal enuresis: an approach to treatment based on pathogenesis. J Pediatr 114(Suppl):705, 1989.)

1 through 4), which are identifiable by specific EEG patterns. REM sleep is associated with increased autonomic activity and dreaming. Normal sleep begins with NREM sleep and consists of cycles of NREM sleep, REM sleep, and occasional awakenings. Children have longer periods of deep sleep (stages 3 and 4), which progressively decrease with aging. In children older than 2 years of age and throughout adulthood, REM sleep occupies approximately 20 to 25 per cent of total sleep time (Rechtschaffen and Kales).

A number of studies in enuretics were reported in the 1960s and early 1970s. Many of these studies reported that enuretic events occur primarily during delta or slow-wave sleep (stages 3 and 4) (Broughton; Evans; Finley). Broughton proposed that bedwetting was a disorder of arousal, suggesting that enuretic episodes originated in delta sleep and were preceded by arousal signals. Typically, the enuretic event occurred within a few minutes as the child shifted into a lighter stage of sleep. Ritvo and colleagues identified a small group of patients with psychopathology who wet during arousal or very light sleep.

Later and more sophisticated sleep research studies have not substantiated the findings of these early reports. In the later studies, enuretic episodes were observed to occur on a random basis throughout the night and occurred in each stage of sleep in proportion to the amount of time spent in that stage (Kales et al; Mikkelsen et al; Norgaard and Rittig). Psychiatrically disturbed enuretics did not differ from nondisturbed enuretics with regard to the distribution of enuretic events of sleep stage. These findings suggested that enuresis is independent of sleep stage and that sleep patterns of enuretics are not appreciably different from those of normal children. However, the question of an arousal disorder remains unanswered. Finley and Wansley consider enuresis a disorder characterized by an elevated arousal threshold that is distinguished from "deep sleep" as defined by EEG monitoring.

Psychologic Factors

Studies in the literature reporting the prevalence and role of emotional disturbances and psychopathology in enuretics vary considerably based on the methodology and study populations. The conclusion of several large reviews is that although a higher proportion of enuretic children are maladjusted and exhibit measurable behavioral symptoms when compared with nonenuretic controls, only a minority of enuretic children have significant underlying psychopathology (Moffatt; Shaffer; Werry). Even in those children with emotional disturbances, there is no specific psychiatric or behavioral disorder associated with enuresis (Kaffman and Elizur; Shaffer). Furthermore, according to psychoanalytic theory, if enuresis were a symptom of underlying emotional problems, resolution of enuresis would likely result in symptom substitution by another maladaptive behavior. Several investigations of this issue have failed to demonstrate that this phenomenon occurs (Behrle et al; Lovibond; Werry and Cohrssen). In one study reporting long-term follow-up of 29 young adults who had been treated 10 years earlier with drug therapy, there was no evidence of maladjustment or significant psychologic disturbances (Bindelglas and Dee). Although studies show that most enuretics do not suffer from psychopathology, several do show that enuretic children tend to be more immature and less self-reliant, ambitious, and secure than nonenuretic controls (Hallgren, 1957; McKendry et al, 1968; Oppel et al, 1968b; Shaffer). In a longitudinal analysis of 161 children living in an Israeli kibbutz and observed for 6 years, enuretics significantly more often displayed lower motivation for achievement, lower adaptability to environmental changes, more aggressive behavior, and greater motor hyperactivity when compared with nonenuretic controls (Kaffman and Elizur).

An important consideration for the clinician is that children who seek help for enuresis are often under greater stress and have more behavioral problems than enuretics who do not (Foxman et al; Hallgren, 1957). In one study of Swedish children, 40 per cent of enuretics referred to a physician were considered "problem children" compared with 26 per cent of their enuretic siblings and 15 per cent of their nonenuretic siblings (Hallgren, 1957). In summary, the bulk of clinical evidence suggests that the majority of enuretics do not have significant underlying psychopathology, although they may manifest more behavioral problems. Certainly, the two can coexist. However, inasmuch as successful treatment of enuresis does not result in symptom substitution, symptomatic treatment is justifiable even in this group of patients.

Infection

An uncommon but clinically important cause of enuresis is urinary tract infection. Overall, increased bacteriuria has been noted in school-aged girls (5.6 per cent) with enuresis compared with those without enuresis (1.5 per cent) (Dodge et al). Urinary infection may be found even more commonly in those children with secondary-onset enuresis. The increased incidence of bacteriuria in the enuretic population may be related to underlying bladder instability in many of these children, particularly those with daytime voiding symptoms. The mechanism for this is thought to be related to the voluntary contraction of the external striated sphincter that a child makes in response to an unstable bladder contraction in an effort to prevent wetting. This leads to increased intravesical pressures and incomplete emptying, both predisposing factors to urinary infection. Therefore, urinary infection must be excluded in all patients who present with enuresis. In those found to be infected, initial therapy should be directed toward eradication of urinary infection. In one study of girls with recurrent infections, 16 of 56 with associated enuresis became dry following successful treatment of the infection. In the remainder, enuresis persisted despite eradication of urinary infection (Jones et al).

EVALUATION

Evaluation and subsequent treatment are contingent upon the pattern of enuresis, the findings on physical examination, and the results of urinalysis and urine culture. A careful history should be obtained, determining the severity and the circumstances under which the child becomes wet. Associated daytime voiding problems, including diurnal enuresis, intermittent or weak stream, urgency, and infrequent voiding, should be noted. Also important are the child's bowel habits and any previous episodes of urinary tract infection. Finally, pertinent psychosocial and family history should be reviewed. Physical examination includes abdominal and genital assessment, observation of the child voiding if the history suggests an abnormal stream, and brief neurologic evaluation. Neurologic evaluation should include checking peripheral reflexes, noting perineal sensation and anal sphincter tone, observing gait, and visually inspecting the lower back for evidence of sacral dimpling or cutaneous anomalies suggestive of a spinal abnormality. Renal or metabolic disorders that might produce obligatory polyuria should be excluded by urinalysis, including determination of urinary glucose and protein levels and specific gravity. In the absence of protein, glucose, or radiopaque contrast, a urine specific gravity (≥ 1.022) indicates adequate concentrating ability (Kassirer and Harrington). A lower urine specific gravity can be further evaluated by testing a concentrated early morning specimen. Microscopic examination of the urinary sediment is also recommended.

On the basis of this initial evaluation, patients can be categorized into *uncomplicated* or *complicated* enuretics (Fig. 11–3) (Rushton). Patients with pure nocturnal enuresis, normal physical findings, normal urinalysis, and negative urine culture have uncomplicated enuresis. Some of these children also have mild daytime frequency or enuresis, a positive family history of enuresis, and perhaps slightly delayed developmental milestones. The incidence of organic uropathology in these children does not appear to be higher than in the normal population (American Academy of Pediatrics; Redmond and Seibert). No further urologic evaluation is indicated in these patients.

In contrast, patients with a positive urine culture or history of urinary tract infection, abnormal neurologic examination, or history of significant voiding dysfunction characterized by either infrequent voiding or severe frequency associated with incontinence, poor urinary stream, and/or encopresis have complicated enuresis. These patients constitute a minority of the enuretic population and should be further evaluated with renal-bladder sonography and voiding cystography (with spine films) to exclude vesicoureteral reflux, a posterior urethral valve, and/or hydroureteronephrosis associated with a thickened, unstable bladder. The latter findings indicate the need for further urologic evaluation, probably to include urodynamic evaluation. If the cause is not clearly identified, neurosurgical evaluation is indicated to exclude sacral pathology or a tethered spinal cord. Those children with an abnormal urinalysis suggesting an underlying metabolic or renal abnormality require further medical or nephrologic evaluation.

TREATMENT

Individual therapy for children with enuresis must be tailored to some extent based on the

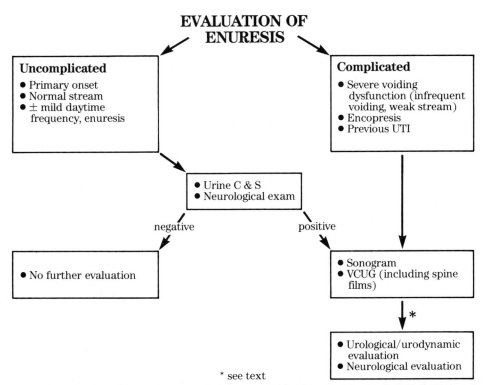

EVALUATION OF ENURESIS

Uncomplicated
- Primary onset
- Normal stream
- ± mild daytime frequency, enuresis

Complicated
- Severe voiding dysfunction (infrequent voiding, weak stream)
- Encopresis
- Previous UTI

- Urine C & S
- Neurological exam

negative

positive

- No further evaluation

- Sonogram
- VCUG (including spine films)

*

- Urological/urodynamic evaluation
- Neurological evaluation

* see text

Figure 11–3 □ Flow chart for evaluation of uncomplicated and complicated enuresis. C & S, Culture and sensitivity testing; UTI, urinary tract infection; VCUG, voiding cystourethrogram. (Modified from Rushton, HG: Nocturnal enuresis: epidemiology, evaluation and treatment. J Pediatr 114(Suppl):691, 1989.)

perceptions of the parent and child toward enuresis and the social structure of the home environment. For example, if the child shares a room with other siblings, conditioning therapy may not be practical. Some families lack the necessary motivation and skills required to implement a program of behavioral modification. Other parents do not consider drug therapy to be a good form of treatment for enuresis (Shelov et al).

The psychologic impact of treatment on a child with enuresis is also a consideration in determining treatment. Psychologic testing of children before and after treatment for enuresis has yielded conflicting results, partly because of variation in methodology, sample size, and experimental design. There appears to be evidence that self-concept in children with enuresis may be improved following successful treatment (Moffatt et al). One concern regarding treatment is that children who fail to improve may suffer adverse emotional effects as a result of failure. Although no studies have specifically addressed this question, Moffatt concluded from a collective review of other studies that there is no evidence that behavior

will deteriorate in those children who fail treatment.

The timing of treatment is important and varies from patient to patient. Treatment should be addressed when wetting becomes a problem to the patient, the family, or both. Rarely will this be necessary prior to age 5 or 6 years. In younger children, treatment may mean simply educating the family as to the causes, commonness, and prognosis of the problem and suggesting a positive reinforcement program. As the child becomes older, more directed therapy may become necessary.

Although there is no objective evidence that withholding fluids in the evening, random awakenings of the child to void, or punitive measures result in significant cessation of enuresis, numerous therapeutic options for uncomplicated nocturnal enuresis are available that may be successful. These include various techniques of behavioral modification treatment (conditioning therapy, motivational counseling, bladder training exercises), pharmacologic therapy, psychotherapy, diet therapy, and hypnotherapy. The reported success of each of these modalities attests in part to the recognized spontaneous cure rate and the response to increased attention directed toward the patient. On the other hand, the evolution of so many different types of therapy clearly suggests that there is no single therapeutic plan that is ideal for all patients.

Behavioral Modification Therapy

A variety of behavioral modification techniques have been employed in the treatment of enuresis. Although these will be described individually, it is important to recognize that these techniques can often be combined to improve the success of the treatment program. Generally, the behavioral modification approach requires greater commitment and involvement of the parents, the physician, and the child when compared with other modalities such as pharmacologic therapy. Therefore, motivation is a key element and must be assessed prior to instituting any program of behavioral modification. This approach will usually be more effective in children older than 7 years of age who have demonstrated significant interest in becoming dry.

Conditioning Therapy

Described by Pfaunder in 1904 and popularized by Mowrer and Mowrer in 1938, conditioning therapy revolves around the use of a signal alarm device that is electrolytically triggered as the child voids. The models of classical conditioning have been used by some to explain the mechanism of action of the moisture alarm (Doleys). This model suggests that if an event (unconditioned stimulus)—the moisture alarm—awakens the child and initiates reflexive inhibition of micturition (unconditioned response) repeatedly following the onset of micturition, then the stimuli that evoked urination (conditioned stimulus)—bladder distention, detrusor contraction, sphincter relaxation—would produce the same inhibitory response and awaken the child (conditioned response). Lovibond (1964, 1970) and others have argued against the model of classical conditioning therapy, contending that it does not adequately account for those children who progress from awakening to the buzzer to remaining dry throughout the night without awakening to urinate. Instead, they attribute the success of moisture alarms to an avoidance response to the noxious stimulation produced by the buzzer.

Regardless of the mechanism of action, initial cure rates ranging from 65 to 100 per cent have been reported following 4 to 6 months of treatment (Dische; Forsythe and Redmond, 1970; Schmitt; Wagner et al). In a compilation of 16 published studies reviewed by Turner, the average initial cure rate was 82 per cent. There is considerable individual variation in the duration of treatment necessary to become dry. One study reported an average of 18 wet nights before achieving dryness in a group of enuretics treated with conditioning therapy (Meadow). Another study of a large number of enuretics reported that the average length of treatment required to achieve dryness was 2½ months (White).

Because success depends on a cooperative and motivated child, behavior modification therapy is generally used in patients older than 7 years of age. Patient dropout may be significant, and results are not as good in children with behavioral disturbances or difficult housing or family relationships (Dische et al). Some children fail to awaken to the alarm, whereas others may be frightened by it. In some children who fail to awaken to the alarm or who awaken in a confused state, a low dose of imipramine in conjunction with the alarm system may be beneficial (Philpott and Flasher). Increasing the intensity of the alarm stimulus may also be helpful in those who fail to awaken or respond slowly (Finley and Wansley; Morgan). Adjunctive measures that increase the effectiveness of the alarm system include positive reinforcement programs with the child receiving a "reward" following a predetermined number of dry nights. The child is encouraged to keep a record of his or her progress such as using a calendar with stars for each dry night. In addition, there should be no delay between the alarm's sounding and the child's getting up to void. Initially, this may require supervision or direct involvement of the parents (Dische).

Relapse occurs in 20 to 30 per cent, but a similarly favorable outcome can be anticipated with retreatment (Dische; Morgan; Turner). Deliberate forcing of fluids toward the end of the course of conditioning therapy invokes the principle of "overlearning" and reduces the relapse rate to under 10 per cent (Brooshank; Morgan). Relapse is less likely after discontinuation of use following a 4-week dry period than when compared with a shorter dry period (Forsythe and Redmond, 1970). Intermittent, as opposed to continuous, use of the alarm has also been reported to decrease the rate of relapse (Morgan).

Numerous systems are available at reasonable costs. Occasional complications have been reported with pad and buzzer systems, such as "buzzer ulcers" of the skin, or alarm failure if the child is not positioned properly on the pad. Transistorized modifications of the alarm system, such as the "Wet-Stop" (Palco Labs, Santa Cruz, California) and Nytone (Medical Products, Inc., Salt Lake City, Utah), use a small sensor that is attached to the child's underwear while the alarm is attached to the child's wrist or pajama collar (Fig. 11–4). These units are compact, safe, and effective and avoid many of the problems associated with a pad and buzzer. A controlled trial comparing a transistorized mini-alarm with a standard pad and buzzer alarm showed similar response rates for each (Fordham and Meadow). However, various models do differ in mechanical reliability (Goel et al).

Despite consistently showing the highest reported cure rates and lowest relapse rates,

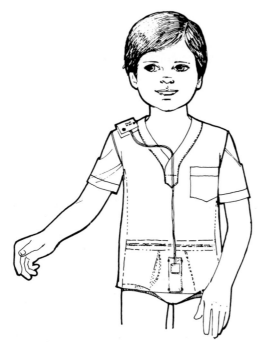

Figure 11–4 ☐ Diagram of miniaturized moisture alarm used in conditioning therapy for nocturnal enuresis. Small moisture sensor in cotton packet of underwear is connected by wires to transistorized alarm attached to the child's pajama top. (Used with permission from Palco Laboratories, Santa Cruz, California.)

conditioning therapy is used by only a small minority (less than 5 per cent) of American primary care physicians for treatment of enuresis (Foxman et al; Shelov et al). This number is in contrast to 32 to 50 per cent of physicians who use medication. Perhaps this difference is due to the delayed success of conditioning therapy, the major commitment required by the physician, parents, and child, and the American need for instant gratification.

Motivational Therapy

Motivational therapy involves a series of counseling interviews during which the child is encouraged to assume responsibility for his or her enuresis and to be an active participant in the treatment program (Marshall et al). This involves a combination of approaches, including reassurance, guilt removal, and emotional support by the physician and parents (Schmitt). It promotes development of a positive relationship between parents and child and provides positive reinforcement ranging from words of praise to actual material rewards. Reassurance is first provided by the physician concerning both the causes and prognosis of enuresis. It is important to clarify that the child is not at fault, and punishment for wetting is discouraged.

One form of this approach is termed responsibility-reinforcement therapy (Marshall et al). Based on principles from "reality therapy" and behavior modification therapy, the child is encouraged to assume responsibility for his or her own learning (Glasser; Skinner). A progress record, such as a gold star on a calendar for each dry night, is kept by the child. "Sensation awareness"—an improved recognition of the sensation of a full bladder—is another responsibility that the child assumes. As the child progresses stepwise toward the ultimate goal of being dry, the parents and physician provide positive reinforcement as a means of "response shaping." This form of behavior modification obviously requires considerable input by supportive physicians and parents.

Although the actual cure rate with motivational counseling is unknown, it is estimated to be about 25 per cent (Schmitt). However, "marked improvement" (defined as a decrease in enuresis of 80 per cent or more) has been reported in more than 70 per cent of patients treated with this modality (Marshall et al). A longer period of treatment is required in comparison with other therapeutic modalities, but the reported relapse rate of approximately 5 per cent is lower. Although motivational counseling has been used as the primary treatment modality for enuresis, many of these same principles can be applied to other treatment programs, including conditioning and pharmacologic therapy.

Bladder Retention Training

Bladder retention training involves conscious attempts at "bladder stretching" by voluntarily prolonging the intervals between voidings. The assumption that improvement in bladder capacity will improve or eliminate enuresis is the basis for this treatment modality. Small bladder capacities and the findings of persistent detrusor instability of the infantile type support this approach. Furthermore, cessation of enuresis, regardless of the method of treatment, is associated with an increased bladder capacity and decreased diurnal frequency (Zaleski et al).

It may be helpful to estimate normal bladder capacity for each age group based on the following formula:

bladder capacity in ounces = age in years + 2

to determine those enuretics with small bladder capacity who might be candidates for this form of therapy (Koff, 1988). Adjunctive measures employed with this technique include conscious stream interruption exercises designed to increase the child's ability to withstand uninhibited bladder contractions. The actual beneficial effect from this particular measure has not been proven. Overtraining by forcing fluids during the daytime may also help to improve bladder capacity, although it is often difficult to convince parents of this. Haaglund (1965) reported an increase in bladder capacity and greater improvement in enuresis in children who were treated by forcing fluids compared with those treated either by fluid restriction and random waking or by supportive psychological therapy. In an uncontrolled study of 83 children treated with bladder retention exercises for 6 months, 66 per cent demonstrated improvement, including 30 per cent who were cured or had only minimal enuresis (Starfield and Mellits). Those who responded were found to have a significantly increased bladder capacity (62.4 ml) when compared with children who were not cured (11.25 ml).

Dry-Bed Training

Azrin and associates have described a technique that combines a variety of behavioral modification techniques referred to collectively as "dry-bed training." This multimodal approach combines conditioning therapy using a moisture alarm with cleanliness training, positive practice, nighttime awakenings, retention control, increased fluid intake, and differential positive reinforcement. In 24 patients treated with this program, dryness was achieved in all in a matter of days. However, 34 per cent relapsed and required retraining. This complicated, multistep approach is quite labor-intensive and has not received widespread acceptance or use.

Pharmacologic Therapy

A number of pharmacologic agents have been used to treat enuresis. There appears to be no benefit from the use of sedatives, stimulants, or sympathomimetic agents. Because treatment with medication may be effective even in children with an organic problem, such as infection or neuropathy, careful evaluation should always precede institution of drug therapy.

Tricyclic Antidepressants

A variety of tricyclic antidepressants, particularly imipramine (Tofranil), have been studied and used most extensively. The exact pharmacologic mechanism of action of tricyclic antidepressants in enuresis is not well understood. Several theories have been proposed to explain their drug actions in enuresis. These are related to the (1) antidepressant action, (2) alterations in arousal and sleep mechanisms, and (3) anticholinergic effects (Blackwell and Currah). Imipramine is also alleged to alter the excretion of ADH (Puri, 1980b).

There is no evidence to suggest that depression plays a significant role as a causative factor in most enuretic children (Werry). Furthermore the antienuretic effects of tricyclic antidepressants are often immediate, whereas the antidepressant effects often take 10 or more days to appear (Rapoport et al). The theory that tricyclic antidepressants work by altering the sleep and arousal mechanisms is based on early sleep research studies linking sleepwetting to REM sleep (Khazan and Sulman;

Pierce et al). They concluded that tricyclic antidepressants work by decreasing the percentage of REM sleep in enuretics. However, results of more recent sleep research studies do not support the existence of a significant relationship between enuretic episodes and sleep stage (Mikkelsen et al). Furthermore, the antienuretic effect of imipramine appears to be independent of its effects on sleep stages (Kales et al; Rapoport et al).

Imipramine has also been demonstrated to exert weak peripheral anticholinergic and antispasmodic effects as well as have a complex effect on sympathetic input to the bladder (Labay and Boyarsky; Sigg; Stephenson). All of these effects may well explain its efficacy in the treatment of enuresis. Support for this theory is provided by one study that documented a 34 per cent increase in bladder capacity in enuretics treated with imipramine compared with a 9 per cent increase in untreated controls (Haaglund and Parkkulainen). However, treatment with other pure anticholinergic or antispasmodic drugs has not been found to be effective in controlling nocturnal enuresis (Lovering et al; Rapoport et al; Wallace and Forsythe).

Imipramine is generally not used to treat enuresis in children younger than age 6 to 7 years, and it should be kept out of the reach of small children because of its extreme toxicity in excessive dosages. Success rates are best in older children, with complete cessation of enuresis reported in 5 to 40 per cent (Bindelglas et al; Blackwell and Currah; General Practitioner Research Group; Haaglund and Parkkulainen; Kardash et al; Kunin et al; Milner and Hills; Pouissant and Ditman; Shaffer et al). Initial success rates in children taking medication range from 10 to 50 per cent (Blackwell and Currah). Combined data from eight controlled double-blind studies revealed a long-term cure rate of 25 per cent (Blackwell and Currah). Some children who are not complete responders will note significant improvement. Many children escape control, requiring an increasingly higher dosage for effectiveness, and the relapse rate following discontinuation is high, particularly when the drug is stopped abruptly or prematurely (Blackwell and Currah; Pouissant and Ditman; Rapoport et al).

The dose of imipramine commonly prescribed is 25 mg taken 1 to 2 hours prior to bedtime for patients 6 to 8 years old and 50 to 75 mg in older children and adolescents. A new sustained-release form (Tofranil PM) may be most effective. The effectiveness of the drug may be influenced by the timing of administration. It has been suggested that children who wet the bed before 1:00 a.m. may benefit from late afternoon administration of the drug (Alderton). Clinical response has been shown to correlate with plasma levels (Jorgenson et al; Rapoport et al). On a weight basis, the usual recommended dosage is 0.9 to 1.5 mg/kg/day (Maxwell and Seldrup). In one study, this dose resulted in a therapeutic plasma level in only 30 per cent of patients (Jorgenson et al). It was estimated that a three-fold to five-fold increase would be necessary to achieve therapeutic levels in all children. However, this would result in nearly toxic levels in a significant number of patients. Other investigators have reported beneficial responses with subtherapeutic plasma levels (Devane).

Although the maximal effects usually occur within the first week of therapy (Blackwell and Currah), it is best to continue therapy for 1 to 2 weeks prior to assessing efficacy and possibly adjusting the dosage. The optimal duration of therapy in those patients who favorably respond is uncertain. A reasonable approach would be to treat for 3 to 6 months, at which time the patient should be "weaned" by gradually reducing the dose and/or frequency, i.e., every other night over 3 to 4 weeks. Should relapse occur, a repeated course of treatment can be started. Often imipramine will work on an as-needed basis, and use may be reserved for a situation when staying dry is particularly important to the child (sleepovers, camp).

Side effects from treatment with imipramine are uncommon but include anxiety, insomnia, dry mouth, nausea, and adverse personality changes (Kardash et al; Shaffer et al). Overdoses have been reported secondary to excess ingestion in both patients and siblings (Goel and Shanks; Herson et al; Parkin and Fraser; Penny); these can cause potentially fatal toxicity with cardiac arrhythmias and conduction blocks (Fouron and Chicoine), hypotension, respiratory complications, and convulsions (Koehl and Wenzel; Rohner and Sanford). Therapeutic doses, however, do not induce electrocardiographic changes (Martin). Treatment of imipramine toxicity includes initial hemodynamic stabilization, continuous cardiac monitoring, serum alkalinization, and specific anti-arrhythmic and anti-convulsant therapy (McGuigan et al). For obtunded patients who present early following ingestion, repeated administration of activated charcoal (through a gastric tube) together with a cathartic enhances total body clearance of tricyclic antidepressants.

Other tricyclic antidepressants also have been used to treat enuresis effectively, including desipramine (Pertofrane), amitriptyline (Elavil), and nortriptyline (Aventyl). Response rates appear similar to those with imipramine when compared with placebo (Pouissant and Ditman; Pouissant et al; Milner and Hills). Evidence is insufficient to determine whether individual drugs within this category differ significantly from each other.

Desmopressin Acetate

Studies have reported promising results from treatment with the antidiuretic hormone desmopressin acetate (DDAVP), an analogue of arginine vasopressin (AVP). This drug was recently approved by the Food and Drug Administration for the treatment of nocturnal enuresis. Created by Zaoral and colleagues in 1967, DDAVP incorporates two modifications of the parent AVP molecule, removal of the amino group of cysteine at position 1 and substitution of D-arginine for L-arginine at position 8. These changes resulted in a marked increase in the antidiuretic activity of DDAVP compared with AVP and almost completely abolished the vasopressor activity of the parent molecule. In addition to its highly specific antidiuretic effect, DDAVP has a prolonged half-life and a long duration of action (Andersson and Arnes). It is the drug of choice in central diabetes insipidus, for which it has been used for more than 15 years with an excellent safety record (Richardson and Robinson).

Desmopressin acetate is rapidly absorbed in the nasal mucosa, achieving maximal plasma concentrations after 40 to 55 minutes. The biologic half-life is usually 4 to 6 hours, and the duration of action varies from 6 to 24 hours (Richardson and Robinson). Desmopressin acetate does not appear to affect the endogenous secretion of vasopressin (Rew and Rundle; Williams et al). Bioavailability of desmopressin via the nasal route is approximately 10 per cent (Harris et al, 1988). Desmopressin acetate is commercially available as a nasal spray pump that delivers an exact dose of 10 μg of desmopressin acetate per spray (Harris et al, 1987). An oral preparation also has been developed but is not commercially available in the United States. In one study, an oral dose of 200 μg/day was almost as effective as an intranasal dose of 20 μg/day (Fjellsted-Paulsen et al). Desmopressin acetate is considerably more expensive than imipramine. However, like imipramine, its effect is usually immediate, and thus, it can be used on a "prn" basis.

The proposed mechanism of action of DDAVP is a reduction in nocturnal urine output to a volume less than the functional bladder capacity of the enuretic child. This mechanism assumes that when children wet at night, they exceed bladder capacity (Norgaard, 1989a). Desmopressin acetate may be particularly effective in a subgroup of enuretics who do not manifest the normal diurnal rhythm of vasopressin excretion, resulting in relatively lower vasopressin excretion levels and therefore higher urine output at night (Puri, 1980a; Rittig et al, 1989a). To date there is no simple and reliable way to differentiate this subgroup from others with enuresis.

A significant improvement in enuresis has been consistently reported in several double-blind, randomized trials with doses of 10 to 40 μg administered intranasally (Aladjem et al; Dimson; Ferrie et al; Fjellsted-Paulsen et al; Pedersen et al; Post et al; Terho and Kekomaki; Tuvemo). Responses have varied from a low of 10 per cent improvement with DDAVP to a high of 65 per cent. Fewer patients achieved complete dryness, which occurred in 12 to 40 per cent of enuretics while taking the medication. The results of three United States multicenter trials demonstrated a less dramatic response of 24 to 35 per cent fewer wet nights in enuretics while taking DDAVP (Klauber). Almost all of these studies involved children who had failed other forms of treatment. As such, they may represent a "hard-core" group of enuretics.

The response to DDAVP appears to be dose-related (Klauber; Post et al). One study reported dryness in 70 per cent of 34 patients treated according to a dose titration protocol (Rittig et al, 1989b). Other studies have reported a response to DDAVP related to urine osmolality (Dimson; Fjellsted-Paulsen et al; Wille, 1986). Significantly better responses were seen in patients whose early morning urine osmolality during treatment was greater than 1000 mOsm/kg.

The initial recommended dosage of the nasal spray for children is 20 μg (one spray in each nostril) at bedtime. Nonresponders and partial responders can be increased to 40 μg/day (two sprays in each nostril). Some patients respond to as little as 10 μg/day. Relapse rates following discontinuation of therapy are high. In one study that compared DDAVP with conditioning therapy, 70 per cent of 24 patients given DDAVP improved compared with 86 per cent of 22 patients treated with the enuresis alarm (Wille, 1986). After 14 weeks of treatment, ten patients treated with DDAVP relapsed compared with only one treated with conditioning therapy.

The optimal duration of treatment using DDAVP is not known because almost all studies have been short-term. One long-term double-blind study used DDAVP for 24 weeks (Rittig et al, 1989b). During a 12-week period following completion of therapy, six patients (21 per cent) remained dry off medication. In another uncontrolled long-term study of 55 children with nocturnal enuresis, 28 (51 per cent) achieved total dryness including 15 (27 per cent) who remained dry after discontinuation of desmopressin therapy (Miller et al). It is noteworthy that of those 15 patients who were dry off medication, eight had required treatment for 12 to 36 months (mean, 24 months). Tapering of the drug was recommended as opposed to abrupt cessation of therapy.

Side effects in patients taking DDAVP, compared with those taking placebo, have been negligible in all of the reported randomized studies. Rhinorrhea and epistaxis have been occasionally reported (Fjellsted-Paulsen et al; Wille). Although transient elevation in plasma renin activity has been observed following intravenous administration of DDAVP (Williams et al), hypertension has not been reported in any children or adults treated for enuresis with intranasal DDAVP. The selective antidiuretic effect of DDAVP could theoretically result in water retention leading to hyponatremia. However, in the treatment of enuresis, the once-nightly use normally allows daytime escape from the effect of the drug by obligatory polyuria (Hilton and Stanton). There have been two case reports of symptomatic hyponatremia in children using DDAVP to treat nocturnal enuresis. One episode occurred in a 13-year-old girl with cystic fibrosis who developed severe water intoxication with convulsions and coma after four doses of DDAVP (Simmonds et al). It is possible that this adverse effect was a result of her underlying disease. The other instance involved a 6-year-old healthy boy who took the drug for 8 days and developed hyponatremia associated with a grand mal seizure (Bamford and Cruickshank).

Anticholinergics

Anticholinergic drugs, specifically oxybutynin (Ditropan), reduce or abolish uninhibited bladder contractions and may be particularly beneficial in patients who have daytime frequency or enuresis associated with uninhibited bladder contractions as manifested by urgency and urge incontinence (Kass et al; Thompson and Laurentz). However, oxybutynin is rarely beneficial for those with exclusively nocturnal enuresis. In a recent prospective double-blind crossover study in 30 such children, there was no difference in response to 10 mg oxybutynin compared with placebo (Lovering et al). The dose in children older than 6 years old is usually 5 mg two to three times a day. Common side effects include dryness of the mouth and facial flushing. Occasionally, hyperpyrexia may occur, particularly when the child is exposed to hot weather. Excessive dosage may result in blurring of vision and hallucinations.

Miscellaneous

Psychotherapy

Varying success has been reported in regard to psychotherapy, but this tool probably does not play a major role in treatment in the majority of those with uncomplicated nocturnal enuresis who do not also have underlying psychopathology (Fraser). Two studies comparing supportive psychotherapy with conditioning therapy failed to demonstrate any significant improvement in those receiving psychotherapy compared with a control "no treatment" group. In both studies, conditioning therapy produced significant improvement compared with the psychotherapy and control groups (De Leon and Mandell; Werry and Cohrssen).

In those patients with complicated enuresis associated with severe voiding dysfunction, including infrequent voiding and encopresis (Hinman's syndrome), a careful family and social history may reveal underlying psychosocial stresses. Treatment of these children is initially directed toward emotional support. Those patients with bladder or upper tract damage secondary to severe voiding dysfunction who do not have an organic neurologic or obstructive lesion may also benefit from timed voidings, anticholinergic therapy, and/or biofeedback therapy (McGuire and Savastano). Occasional renal damage may be so severe as to necessitate a program of intermittent catheterization if bladder emptying cannot be achieved by other means. In some of these cases, psychotherapy may also be warranted.

Diet Therapy

Diet therapy may have a role in a small minority of enuretics. One study reported significant improvement by serially eliminating certain foods such as dairy products, chocolate, cola, citrus fruit and juices, and Kool-Aid from the diets of enuretic children (Esperanca and Gerrard, 1969b). However, the success of such a program has not been substantiated by other investigators and may be based on the attention focused on the patient during therapy.

Hypnotherapy

Although hypnotherapy has not been widely practiced, dramatic improvements have been reported in children with enuresis treated with this modality. In one study 31 of 40 children treated by hypnotherapy were cured and an additional six were improved (Olness). The majority of those cured ceased wetting within the first month of therapy and continued to remain dry during follow-up from 6 to 28 months. Similar success was reported in a group of patients with specific precipitating stresses or a high level of family tension at the onset of enuresis (Collison). Despite this reported success, hypnotherapy is rarely recommended by physicians for treatment of enuresis.

SUMMARY

Enuresis is a symptom and not a disease state, with sleepwetting affecting 15 to 20 per cent of 5-year-olds, 5 to 10 per cent of 10-year-olds, and 1 to 2 per cent of 15-year-olds. Although the etiology of enuresis remains controversial, evidence supports the theory of a maturational lag and/or developmental delay that may be influenced by a number of factors including stress, nocturnal polyuria, genetic predisposition, and infection. Although psychopathology and enuresis may coexist, the majority of enuretics do not suffer from a psychological disorder. However, enuretics often have lower self-esteem and are more likely to underachieve compared with nonenuretics. Recent evidence does not support the theory that enuresis represents a sleep disorder, although the possibility of an arousal disorder independent of sleep stage remains a possibility.

Treatment of childhood enuresis must begin with a careful history, physical examination, urinalysis, and urine culture to determine if one is dealing with uncomplicated or complicated enuresis. The majority of patients have uncomplicated enuresis, and there are a number of treatment options available to the physician that can be tailored to the individual patient. Behavioral modification techniques, specifically conditioning therapy, yield the highest reported long-term cure rates, averaging 80 per cent. This approach, compared with pharmacologic therapy, requires greater commitment and involvement of the physician, parents, and child. Imipramine has been the most commonly used drug. Desmopressin has shown promising results, with similar reported response rates. Both drugs are associated with high relapse rates following discontinuation of treatment. Imipramine is less expensive; however, desmopressin appears to have fewer side effects and toxicity. Anticholinergics may be beneficial in those children who also have daytime frequency or enuresis. Regardless of the choice of treatment, parental support, empathy, and patience are key elements in any successful plan of management of the child with enuresis. Likewise, reassurance, periodic feedback, and encouragement of the parents and child by the physician are necessary for optimal results.

Bibliography

Aladjem M, Wohl R, Boichis H, et al: Desmopressin and nocturnal enuresis. Arch Dis Child 57:137, 1982.

Alderton HR: Imipramine in childhood enuresis: further studies on the relationship of time of administration to effect. Can Med Assoc 102:1179, 1970.

American Academy of Pediatrics, Committee on Radiology: Excretory urography for evaluation of enuretics. Pediatrics 65:644, 1980.

Andersson KE, Arner B: Effects of DDAVP, a synthetic analogue of vasopressin, in patients with cranial diabetes insipidus. Acta Med Scand 192:21, 1972.

Azrin NH, Sneed TJ, Foxx RM: Dry bed: rapid elimination of childhood enuresis. Behav Res Ther 12:147, 1974.

Bakwin H: Enuresis in children. J Pediatr 58:806, 1961.

Bakwin H: The genetics of enuresis. *In* Bladder Control and Enuresis. Edited by I Kolvin, RC MacKeith, SR Meadow. London, W Heinemann Medical Books Ltd, 1973.

Bamford MFM, Cruickshank G: Dangers of intranasal desmopressin for nocturnal enuresis (letter). J R Coll Gen Pract 39:345, 1989.

Behrle FC, Elkin MH, Laybourne PC: Evaluation of a conditioning device in the treatment of nocturnal enuresis. Pediatrics 17:849, 1956.

Bindelglas PM, Dee G: Enuresis treatment with imipramine hydrochloride: a 10-year follow-up study. Am J Psychiatry 135:1549, 1978.

Bindelglas PM, Dee GH, Enos FA: Medical and psychosocial factors in enuretic children treated with imipramine hydrochloride. Am J Psychiatry 1124:1107, 1968.

Blackwell B, Currah J: The psychopharmacology of nocturnal enuresis. *In* Bladder Control and Enuresis. Edited by I Kolvin, RC MacKeith, SR Meadow. London, W Heinemann Medical Books Ltd, 1973.

Boyd MM: The depth of sleep in enuretic children and in non-enuretic controls. J Psychosom Res 4:274, 1960.

Brazelton TB: A child-oriented approach to toilet training. Pediatrics 29:121, 1962.

Brooshank DJ: The conditioning treatment of bed-wetting in secondary school age children. J Adolesc 2:239, 1979.

Broughton RF: Sleep disorders: disorders of arousal? Science 159:1070, 1968.

Campbell EW Jr, Young JD Jr: Enuresis and its relationship to electroencephalographic disturbances. J Urol 96:947, 1966.

Collison PR: Hypnotherapy in the management of nocturnal enuresis. Med J Aust 1:52, 1970.

Crawford JD: Treatment of nocturnal enuresis: introductory comments. J Pediatr 114:687, 1989.

De Jonge DA: Epidemiology of enuresis: a survey of the literature. *In* Bladder Control and Enuresis. Edited by I Kolvin, RC MacKeith, SR Meadow. London, W Heinemann Medical Books Ltd, 1973.

DeLeon G, Mandell W: A comparison of conditioning and psychotherapy in the treatment of functional enuresis. J Clin Psychol 22:326, 1966.

Devane C: Concentrations of imipramine and its metabolites during enuresis therapy. Pediatric Pharmacology 4:245, 1984.

Dimson SB: DDAVP and urine osmolality in refractory enuresis. Arch Dis Child 61:1104, 1986.

Dische S: Management of enuresis. Br Med J 2:33, 1971.

Dische S, Yule W, Corbett HJ, et al: Childhood nocturnal enuresis: factors associated with outcome of treatment with an enuresis alarm. Dev Med Child Neurol 25:67, 1983.

Dodge WF, West EF, Bridgforth EB, Travis LB: Nocturnal enuresis in 6- to 10-year old children. Correlation of bacteriuria, proteinuria and dysuria. Am J Dis Child 120:32, 1970.

Doleys DM: Behavioral treatments for nocturnal enuresis in childhood: a review of the recent literature. Psychol Bull 84:30, 1977.

Douglas JWB: Broken homes and child behavior. J R Coll Physicians Lond 4:203, 1970.

Douglas JWB: Early disturbing events in later enuresis. *In* Bladder Control and Enuresis. Edited by I Kolvin, RC MacKeith, SR Meadow. London, W Heinemann Medical Books Ltd, 1973.

Duche DJ: Patterns of micturition in infancy. *In* Bladder Control and Enuresis. Edited by I Kolvin, RC MacKeith, SR Meadow. London, W Heinemann Medical Books Ltd, 1973.

Edvardsen P: Neurophysiologic aspects of enuresis. Acta Neurol Scand 48:222, 1972.

Esperanca M, Gerrard JW: Nocturnal enuresis: studies in bladder function in normal children and enuretics. Can Med Assoc J 101:269, 1969a.

Esperanca M, Gerrard JW: Nocturnal enuresis: comparison of the effect of imipramine and dietary restriction on bladder capacity. Can Med Assoc J 101:721, 1969b.

Essen J, Peckham C: Nocturnal enuresis in childhood. Dev Med Child Neurol 18:577, 1976.

Evans JI: Sleep of enuretics. Br Med J 3:110, 1971.

Fergusson DM, Hons BA, Horwood LJ, Shannon FT: Factors related to the age of attainment of nocturnal bladder control: an 8-year longitudinal study. Pediatrics 78:884, 1986.

Fermaglich JL: Electroencephalographic study of enuretics. Am J Dis Child 18:473, 1969.

Ferrie BG, MacFarlane J, Glen ES: DDAVP in young enuretic patients: a double blind trial. Br J Urol 56:376, 1984.

Finley W: An EEG study of the sleep of enuretics at three age levels. Clin Electroencephalogr 2:35, 1971.

Finley WW, Wansley RA: Auditory intensity as a variable in the conditioning treatment of enuresis nocturna. Behav Res Ther 15:181, 1977.

Firlit CF, Smey P, King LR: Micturition urodynamic flow studies in children. J Urol 119:250, 1978.

Fjellsted-Paulsen A, Wille S, Harris AS: Comparison of intraanal and oral desmopressin for nocturnal enuresis. Arch Dis Child 62:674, 1987.

Fordham KM, Meadow SR: Controlled trial of standard pad and bell alarm against mini alarm for nocturnal enuresis. Arch Dis Child 64:651, 1989.

Forsythe WI, Redmond A: Enuresis and the electric alarm: a study of 200 cases. Br Med 1:211, 1970.

Forsythe WI, Redmond A: Enuresis and spontaneous cure rate: study of 1129 enuretics. Arch Dis Child 49:259, 1974.

Fouron J, Chicoine R: ECG changes in fatal imipramine (Tofranil) intoxication. Pediatrics 48:777, 1971.

Foxman B, Valdez RB, Brock RH: Childhood enuresis: prevalence, perceived impact, and prescribed treatments. Pediatrics 77:482, 1986.

Fraser MJ: Nocturnal enuresis. Practitioner 208:203, 1972.

General Practitioner Research Group. Imipramine in enuresis. Practitioner 203:94, 1969.

George CPL, Messerli FH, Genest J, et al: Diurnal variation of plasma vasopressin in man. J Clin Endocrinol Metab 41:332, 1975.

Giles GR, Light K, Van Blerk PJP: Cystometrogram studies in enuretic children. S Afr J Surg 16:33, 1978.

Gillison TH, Skinner JL: Treatment of nocturnal enuresis by the electric alarm. Br Med J 2:1268, 1958.

Glasser W: Reality Therapy. New York, Harper & Row, 1965.

Goel KM, Shanks RA: Amitriptyline and imipramine poisoning in children. Br Med J 1:261, 1974.

Goel KM, Thompson RB, Gibb EM, et al: Evaluation of nine different types of enuresis alarms. Arch Dis Child 59:748, 1984.

Goellner MH, Ziegler EE, Foman SJ: Urination during the first three years of life. Nephron 28:174, 1981.

Graham P: Depth of sleep and enuresis: a critical review. *In* Bladder Control and Enuresis. Edited by I Kolvin, RC MacKeith, SR Meadow. London, W Heinemann Medical Books Ltd, 1973.

Haaglund TB: Enuretic children treated with fluid restriction or forced drinking: a clinical and cystometric study. Ann Paediatr Fenn 1:84, 1965.

Haaglund TB, Parkkulainen KV: Enuretic children treated with imipramine (Tofranil): a cystometric study. Ann Paediatr Fenn 11:53, 1965.

Hallgren B: Enuresis: I. A study with reference to the morbidity risk and symptomatology. Acta Psychiatr Neurol Scand 31:379, 1956.

Hallgren B: Enuresis: a clinical and genetic study. Acta Psychiatr Neurol Scand [Suppl] 114:1, 1957.

Hallgren B: Nocturnal enuresis: aetiologic aspects. Acta Paediatr (Uppsala) 118(Suppl):66, 1959.

Hallman N: On the ability of enuretic children to hold urine. Acta Paediatr 39:87, 1950.

Harris AS, Hedner P, Vilhardt H: Nasal administration of desmopressin by spray and drops. J Pharmacol 39:932, 1987.

Harris AS, Ohlin M, Lathagen S, et al: Effects of concentration and volume on nasal bioavailability and biological response to desmopressin. J Pharm Sci 77:337, 1988.

Herson VC, Schmitt BD, Rumack BH: Magical thinking and imipramine poisoning in two school-age children. JAMA 241:1926, 1979.

Hilton P, Stanton SL: The use of desmopressin (DDAVP) in nocturnal urinary frequency in the female. Br J Urol 54:252, 1982.

Jones B, Gerrard JW, Shokeir MK, et al: Recurrent urinary infections in girls: relation to enuresis. Can Med Assoc J 106:127, 1972.

Jorgenson OJ, Lober M, Christansen J, et al: Plasma concentration and clinical effect in imipramine treatment of childhood enuresis. Clin Pharmacokinet 5:386, 1980.

Kaffman M, Elizur E: Infants who become enuretics: a longitudinal study of 161 kibbutz children. Monogr Soc Res Child Dev 42 (2, serial No. 170):1, 1977.

Kaijtor S, Ovary I, Zsandanyi O: Nocturnal enuresis: electroencephalographic and cystometric examinations. Acta Med Acad Sci Hung 23:153, 1967.

Kales A, Kales JM, Jacobson A, et al: Effect of imipramine on enuretic frequency and sleep stages. Pediatrics 60:431, 1977.

Kardash S, Hillman ES, Werry J: Efficacy of imipramine in childhood enuresis: a double blind study with placebo. Can Med Assoc J 99:263, 1968.

Kass EJ, Diokno AC, Montealegue A: Enuresis: principles of management and result of treatment. J Urol 121:794, 1979.

Kassirer JP, Harrington JT: Laboratory evaluation of renal function. In Diseases of the Kidney, 4th ed. Edited by RW Schrier, CW Gottschalk. Boston, Little, Brown & Co, 1988.

Khazan N, Sulman EG: Effects of imipramine on paradoxical sleep in animals with reference to dreaming and enuresis. Psychopharmacologia 10:89, 1966.

Klauber GT: Clinical efficacy and safety of desmopressin in the treatment of nocturnal enuresis. J Pediatr 114(Suppl):719, 1989.

Koehl GW, Wenzel JE: Severe postural hypotension due to imipramine therapy. Pediatrics 47:132, 1971.

Koff SA: Enuresis. In Campbell's Urology, 5th ed. Edited by PC Walsh, RF Gittes, AD Perlmutter, TA Stamey. Philadelphia, WB Saunders Co, 1986.

Koff SA: Estimating bladder capacity in children. Urology 21:248, 1988.

Kolvin I, Taunch J: A dual theory of nocturnal enuresis. In Bladder Control and Enuresis. Edited by I Kolvin, RC MacKeith, SR Meadow. London, W Heinemann Medical Books Ltd, 1973.

Kunin JA, Limbert DJ, Platzker ACG, et al: The efficacy of imipramine in the management of enuresis. J Urol 104:612, 1970.

Labay P, Boyarsky S: The action of imipramine on the bladder musculature. J Urol 109:385, 1973.

Linderholm BE: The cystometric findings in enuresis. J Urol 96:718, 1966.

Lovering JS, Tallett SE, McKendry JBJ: Oxybutynin efficacy in treatment of primary enuresis. Pediatrics 82:104, 1988.

Lovibond SH: Conditioning in Enuresis. New York, Pergamon Press, 1964.

Lovibond SH, Coote MA: Enuresis. In Symptoms of Psychopathology. Edited by CG Costello. New York, John Wiley & Sons, 1970.

Lowy FH: Recent sleep and dream research: clinical implications. Can Med Assoc J 102:1069, 1970.

MacKeith RC: Is maturation delay a frequent factor in the origins of primary nocturnal enuresis? Dev Med Child Neurol 14:217, 1972.

MacKeith RC, Meadow SR, Turner RK: How children become dry. In Bladder Control and Enuresis. Edited by I Kolvin, RC MacKeith, SR Meadow. London, W Heinemann Medical Books Ltd, 1973.

Mack A: Dry All Night. Boston, Little, Brown & Co, 1989.

Mahony DT, Laferte RO, Blais DJ: Integral storage and voiding reflexes. Neurophysiologic concept of continence and micturition. Urology 9:95, 1977.

Mahony DT, Laferte RO, Blais DJ: Studies of enuresis: IX. Evidence of a mild form of compensated detrusor hyperreflexia in enuretic children. J Urol 126:520, 1981.

Marshall S, Marshall HH, Lyons RP: Enuresis: an analysis of various therapeutic approaches. Pediatrics 52:813, 1973.

Martin GI: ECG monitoring of enuretic children given imipramine (letter). JAMA 224:902, 1973.

Maxwell C, Seldrup J: Imipramine in the treatment of childhood enuresis. Practitioner 207:809, 1971.

McGuigan MA, Gaudreault P, Woolf A (eds): Clinical Toxicology Review. Cyclic Antidepressants. Boston, Massachusetts Poison Control System, Vol 13, No. 9, 1991.

McGuire EJ, Savashino JA: Urodynamic studies in enuresis and the non-neurogenic–neurogenic bladder. J Urol 132:299, 1984.

McKendry JBJ, Williams HA, Broughton C: Enuresis—a study of untreated patients. Appl Ther 10:815, 1968.

Meadow SR: How to use buzzer alarms to cure bedwetting. Br Med J 2:1073, 1977.

Mikkelsen EJ, Rapoport JL, Nee L, et al: Childhood enuresis I. Sleep patterns and psychopathology. Arch Gen Psychiatry 37:1139, 1980.

Miller FJW: Children who wet the bed. In Bladder Control and Enuresis. Edited by I Kolvin, RC MacKeith, SR Meadow. London, W Heinemann Medical Books Ltd, 1973.

Miller KM, Goldberg S, Atkins B: Nocturnal enuresis: experience with long term use of intranasally administered desmopressin. J Pediatr 114(Suppl):723, 1989.

Milner G, Hills NF: A double blind assessment of antidepressants in the treatment of 212 enuretic patients. Med J Aust 1:943, 1968.

Moffatt MEK: Nocturnal enuresis: psychologic implications of treatment and nontreatment. J Pediatr 114(Suppl):697, 1989.

Moffatt MEK, Kato C, Pless IB: Improvements in self-concept after treatment of nocturnal enuresis: a randomized clinical trial. J Pediatr 110:647, 1987.

Morgan RTT: Relapse and therapeutic response in the

conditioning treatment of enuresis: a review of recent findings on intermittent reinforcement, overlearning and stimulus intensity. Behav Res Ther 16:278, 1978.

Mowrer OH, Mowrer WM: Enuresis: a method for its study and treatment. Am J Orthopsychiatry 8:436, 1938.

Muellner SR: Development of urinary control in children: some aspects of the cause and treatment of primary enuresis. JAMA 172:1256, 1960.

Nash DFE: The development of micturition control with special reference to enuresis. Ann R Coll Surg Engl 5:318, 1949.

Norgaard JP: Urodynamics in enuresis I: reservoir function. Neurourol Urodynam 8:119, 1989a.

Norgaard JP: Urodynamics in enuretics II: a pressure/flowstudy. Neurourol Urodynam 8:213, 1989b.

Norgaard JP, Pedersen EB, Djurhuus JC: Diurnal antidiuretic-hormone levels in enuretics. J Urol 134:1029, 1985.

Norgaard JP, Rittig S: Recent studies of the pathophysiology of nocturnal enuresis. In Desmopressin in Nocturnal Enuresis. Proceedings of an International Symposium. Edited by SR Meadow. Canwell, Sutton Coldfield, England, Horus Medical Publications, 1989.

Notschaele LA: Vedwateren bij kinderen van de kleuteren lagere school. Tijdschrift voor Social Geneeskunde 42:226, 1964.

Olness K: The use of self-hypnosis in the treatment of childhood nocturnal enuresis. Clin Pediatr 14:273, 1975.

Oppel WC, Harper PA, Rider RV: The age of attaining bladder control. Pediatrics 42:614, 1968a.

Oppel WC, Harper PA, Rider RV: Social, psychological, and neurological factors associated with nocturnal enuresis. Pediatrics 42:627, 1968b.

Parkin JM, Fraser MS: Poisoning as a complication of enuresis. Dev Med Child Neurol 14:7272, 1972.

Pedersen PS, Hejl M, Kjoller SS: Desamino-D-Arginine vasopressin in childhood nocturnal enuresis. J Urol 133:65, 1985.

Penny R: Imipramine hydrochloride poisoning in childhood. Am J Dis Child 116:181, 1968.

Perlmutter AD: Enuresis. In Clinical Pediatric Urology, 2nd ed. Edited by PP Kelalis, LR King, AB Belman. Philadelphia, WB Saunders Co, 1985.

Pfaundler M: Demonstration eines apparatus zuf selsattigen signalisierung Statlgehabter Rettnassung. Verhandlungen der Gesellschaft fur Kinderheilkunde 21:219, 1904.

Philpott MG, Flasher MC: The treatment of enuresis: further clinical experience with imipramine. Br J Clin Pract 24:327, 1970.

Pierce CM, Whitman RM, Mass JW, et al: Enuresis and dreaming: experimental studies. Arch Gen Psychiatry 4:116, 1961.

Pompeius R: Cystometry in pediatric enuresis. Scand J Urol Nephrol 5:222, 1971.

Post EM, Richman RA, Blackett PR, et al: Desmopressin response of enuretic children: effects of age and frequency of enuresis. Am J Dis Child 173:962, 1983.

Poulton EM: Relative nocturnal polyuria as a factor in enuresis. Lancet 2:906, 1952.

Poussaint AF, Ditman KS: A controlled study of imipramine (Tofranil) in the treatment of childhood enuresis. J Pediatr 67:283, 1965.

Poussaint AF, Ditman KS, Greenfield R: Amitriptyline in childhood enuresis. Clin Pharmacol Ther 7:21, 1966.

Puri VN: Urinary levels of antidiuretic hormone in nocturnal enuresis. Indian Pediatr 17:675, 1980a.

Puri VN: Increased urinary antidiuretic hormone excretion by imipramine. Exp Clin Endocrinol 88:112, 1980b.

Rahim SIA, Cederblad M: Epidemiology of nocturnal enuresis in a part of Khartoum, Sudan. I. The extensive study. Acta Pediatr Scand 75:1017, 1986.

Rapoport JL, Mikkelsen EJ, Zavadil A, et al: Childhood enuresis. II. Psychopathology, tricyclic concentration in plasma, and antienuretic effect. Arch Gen Psychiatry 37:1146, 1980.

Rechtschaffen A, Kales A: A manual of standardized terminology, techniques and scoring system for sleep stages of human subjects. Los Angeles, Brain Information Service/Brain Research Institute, University of California, 1968.

Redmond JF, Seibert JJ: The uroradiographic evaluation of the enuretic child. J Urol 122:799, 1979.

Rew DA, Rundle JSV: An assessment of the safety of regular DDAVP therapy in primary nocturnal enuresis. Br J Urol 63:352, 1989.

Richardson DW, Robinson AG: Desmopressin. Ann Intern Med 103:228, 1985.

Rittig S, Knudsen UB, Norgaard JP, et al: Abnormal diurnal rhythm of plasma vasopressin and urinary output in patients with enuresis. Am J Physiol 256(Renal Fluid Electrolytes Physiol 25):F664, 1989a.

Rittig S, Knudsen UB, Sorensen S, et al: Long-term double-blind crossover study of desmopressin intranasal spray in the management of nocturnal enuresis. In Desmopressin in Nocturnal Enuresis: Proceedings of an International Symposium. Edited by SR Meadow. Canwell, Sutton Coldfield, England, Horus Medical Publications, 1989b.

Ritvo ER, Ornitz EM, Gottlieb F, et al: Arousal and nonarousal enuretic events. Am J Psychiatry 126:115, 1969.

Rohner TJ, Sanford EJ: Imipramine toxicity. J Urol 114:402, 1975.

Rushton HG: Nocturnal enuresis: epidemiology, evaluation and currently available treatment options. J Pediatr 114(Suppl):691, 1989.

Schmitt BD: Nocturnal enuresis: an update on treatment. Pediatr Clin North Am 29:21, 1982.

Shaffer D: The association between enuresis and emotional disorder: a review of the literature. In Bladder Control and Enuresis. Edited by I Kolvin, RC MacKeith, SR Meadow. London, W Heinemann Medical Books Ltd, 1973.

Shaffer D, Costello AJ, Hill ID: Control of enuresis with imipramine. Arch Dis Child 43:65, 1968.

Shelov SP, Gundy J, Weiss JC, et al: Enuresis: a contrast of attitudes of parents and physicians. Pediatrics 67:707, 1981.

Sigg EB. Pharmacological studies with Tofranil. Can Psychiatr Assoc J 4:75, 1959.

Simmonds EJ, Mahoney MJ, Little JM : Convulsion and coma after intranasal desmopressin in cystic fibrosis. Br Med J 297:1614, 1988.

Skinner BF: Science and human behavior. New York, Macmilan Co, 1953.

Starfield B, Mellits ED: Increase in functional bladder capacity and improvement in enuresis. J Pediatr 72:483, 1968.

Stein ZA, Susser MW: Nocturnal enuresis as a phenomenon of institutions. Dev Med Child Neurol 8:677, 1966.

Stein ZA, Susser MW: Social factors in the development of sphincter control. Dev Med Child Neurol 9:692, 1967.

Stephenson JD: Physiological and pharmacological basis for the chemotherapy of imipramine. Psychol Med 9:249, 1979.

Terho P, Kekomaki M: Management of nocturnal enuresis with a vasopressin analogue. J Urol 131:925, 1984.

Thompson IM, Lauretz R: Oxybutynin in bladder spasm, neurogenic bladder, and enuresis. Urology 8:452, 1976.

Troup CW, Hodgson NB: Nocturnal functional bladder capacity in enuretic children. J Urol 105:132, 1971.

Turner RK: Conditioning treatment of nocturnal enuresis: present status. *In* Bladder Control and Enuresis. Edited by I Kolvin, RC MacKeith, SR Meadow. London, W Heinemann Medical Books Ltd, 1973.

Tuvemo T: DDAVP in childhood nocturnal enuresis. Acta Paediatr Scand 67:753, 1978.

Vuliamy D: The day and night output of urine in enuresis. Arch Dis Child 31:439, 1956.

Wagner W, Johnson SB, Walker D, et al: A controlled comparison of two treatments of nocturnal enuresis. J Pediatr 101:302, 1982.

Wallace TR, Forsythe W: The treatment of enuresis: a controlled clinical trial of propantheline, propantheline and phenobarbital, and a placebo. Br J Clin Pract 23:207, 1969.

Webster GD, Koefoot RB, Sihelnik SA: Urodynamic abnormalities in neurologically normal children with micturition dysfunction. J Urol 132:74, 1984a.

Werry JS: Enuresis—a psychosomatic entity? Can Med Assoc J 97:319, 1967.

Werry JS, Cohrssen J: Enuresis—an etiologic and therapeutic study. J Pediatr 67:423, 1965.

White M: A thousand consecutive cases of enuresis: results of treatment. Medical Officer 120:151, 1968.

Whiteside CG, Arnold EP: Persistent primary enuresis: urodynamic assessment. Br Med J 1:36, 1975.

Wille S: Comparison of desmopressin and enuresis alarm for nocturnal enuresis. Arch Dis Child 61:30, 1986.

Wille S: Comparison of desmopressin and enuresis alarm for nocturnal enuresis. *In* Desmopressin in Nocturnal Enuresis. Proceedings of an International Symposium. Edited by SR Meadow. Canwell, Sutton Coldfield, England, Horus Medical Publications, 1989.

Williams TDM, Lightman SL, Leadbeater MJ: Hormonal and cardiovascular response to DDAVP in man. Clin Endocrinol (Oxf) 24:19, 1986.

Yeates WK: Bladder function in normal micturition. *In* Bladder Control and Enuresis. Edited by I Kolvin, RC MacKeith, SR Meadow. London, W Heinemann Medical Books Ltd, 1973.

Zaleski A, Gerrard JW, Shokeir MHK: Nocturnal enuresis: the importance of a small bladder capacity. *In* Bladder Control and Enuresis. Edited by I Kolvin, RC MacKeith, SR Meadow. London, W Heinemann Medical Books Ltd, 1973.

Zaoral M, Kole T, Sorm S: Amino acids and peptides, LXXI, synthesis of 1-deamino-8-D-y-amino-uterine vasopressin, 1-deamino-8-D-lysine vasopressin, and 1-deamino-8-D-arginine vasopressin. Collect Czech Chem Commun 32:1250, 1967.

12

□ Urinary Incontinence

Ricardo Gonzalez

Urinary incontinence in children can be a manifestation of serious anatomic or functional problems of the urinary tract, the resolution of which often necessitates complex surgical procedures. This chapter addresses the evaluation and treatment of such problems, leaving aside the more common functional problems of the unstable bladder in childhood, nocturnal enuresis, and infrequent voiding conditions, which are usually treated by behavior modification and pharmacologic agents and, if left untreated, tend to resolve spontaneously. These more common disorders are discussed in other chapters.

As an introduction to evaluation and treatment, it is necessary to review the causes, pathophysiology, and methods of evaluation that guide us in selecting the most appropriate treatment. The normal and abnormal physiology of micturition is described in Chapter 6.

ETIOLOGY

The most common, and not spontaneously reversible, cause of severe incontinence is neurologic deficit. Causes of neurogenic incontinence are myelomingocele, sacral agenesis, and related vertebral malformations as well as neoplastic, inflammatory, and traumatic lesions of the spinal cord. It is important to remember that some seemingly stable lesions of the spinal cord, such as myelomeningocele, may change with time owing to tethering of the spinal cord and the development of syringes and other degenerative changes in the central nervous system.

The diagnosis and treatment of the syndrome of non-neurogenic detrusor-sphincter incoordination (also known as non-neurogenic–neurogenic [neuropathic] bladder or Hinman syndrome) (Hinman) are analogous to that of bladder and sphincteric dysfunctions of neurogenic origin. The non-neurogenic causes of severe incontinence include bladder exstrophy, epispadias, urethral trauma, bilateral ectopic ureters, and female urogenital sinus malformations. The case of an incontinent child with a history of posterior urethral valves presents unique therapeutic challenges, in part because even children with severe forms of incontinence may improve spontaneously after puberty.

Severe urinary incontinence in boys and girls may follow pelvic trauma that results in urethral rupture. Iatrogenic sphincteric incontinence may follow endoscopic manipulations, including internal urethrotomy in girls, endoscopic treatment for posterior urethral valves, and excision of ureteroceles.

In girls, incontinence secondary to an ectopic ureter that is part of a duplicated system may be difficult to diagnose but is easily corrected. The surgical treatment of vesicovaginal fistula, although a rare finding in a child, is fairly straightforward. These disorders are addressed in detail in other chapters.

PATHOPHYSIOLOGY

In general, urinary incontinence results from (1) chronic retention and overflow, (2) insufficient urethral resistance or sphincteric failure, (3) diminished bladder storage capacity, (4) mixed causes, and (5) bypass of normal sphincters. Overflow incontinence may result from an anatomic or functional obstruction or from detrusor atony. Sphincteric failure may result from an anatomic defect or from sphincter denervation. Diminished storage capacity of the bladder may be functional as a result of neurogenic or non-neurogenic detrusor dysfunction, or the child may have an anatomically small bladder (Table 12–1).

384

Table 12–1 □ Mechanism and Causes of Urinary Incontinence in Children

1. Overflow	Detrusor failure	Neurogenic	
		Myogenic	
	Obstruction	Anatomic	Posterior urethral valves Ectopic ureterocele
		Functional (nonrelaxation of sphincters)	Hinman syndrome Neurogenic
2. Insufficient urethral resistance	Neurogenic		
	Anatomic	Bladder exstrophy Urogenital sinus malformations Bilateral single ectopic ureters	
3. Diminished storage capacity of the bladder	Small bladder	Exstrophy—ureteral ectopia Neurogenic, iatrogenic	
	Noncompliant bladder	Posterior urethral valves Neurogenic Exstrophy	
	Uninhibited contractions	Neurogenic Non-neurogenic	
4. Mixed causes			
5. Bypass of normal sphincter mechanisms	Fistulas		
	Ectopic ureter with duplication		
6. Pseudoincontinence	Vaginal voiding		
	Urethral diverticula		

EVALUATION

In an evaluation of the incontinent child, the anatomy of the urinary tract should be precisely defined and the storage and emptying functions of the bladder and the competence of the sphincter mechanisms should then be analyzed in detail.

Medical History and Physical Examination

The careful taking of medical history is essential in establishing the severity of the problem as well as determining the possible physical and psychologic consequences of the incontinence. A detailed voiding history is important in establishing whether or not spontaneous voiding occurs and, if it does, the frequency and volume. The relationship of the incontinence to the voiding episodes and the time of the day or night when incontinence occurs are also important. Polyuria is common in children with compromised renal tubular function even when the serum creatinine level is normal. The history should also include previous medical and surgical treatment for incontinence and their results and any adverse effects. Knowing how well the child and his or her family have accepted prior therapeutic measures, particularly intermittent catheterization, is invaluable. Pseudoincontinence in females results from vaginal voiding. The vagina empties when the child stands and walks. A history of wetting only shortly after voiding is characteristic. Teaching the child to spread the thighs while voiding corrects the problem.

Gastrointestinal tract function and bowel habits in particular should be evaluated. Colonic dysfunction is common in children with neurogenic incontinence as well as in children with functional bladder disorders. In formulating a treatment plan, it is essential to assess the child's degree of emotional and intellectual maturity, manual dexterity, and the ability to ambulate independently.

The physical examination should be exhaustive and should complement the information obtained in the medical history. Of particular importance are the genital, rectal, and neurologic examinations. Nevertheless, it is important to remember that the neurologic findings may not predict the type of bladder and urethral dysfunction, especially in cases of myelomeningocele.

Laboratory Investigations

Laboratory tests are useful in evaluating renal function and in ruling out metabolic acidosis and urinary tract infections.

Imaging Studies

Imaging studies are essential in establishing the integrity of the urinary tract and ruling out obstruction and possible associated malformations. Computed tomography (CT) is invaluable in detecting subtle duplications of the collecting system that may be associated with ectopic ureters. Fluoroscopic micturition cystourethroscopy is performed to determine the presence of vesicoureteral reflux and to outline the bladder contour so that trabeculae or diverticula may be seen. This last test is also important in assessing the competence of the bladder neck and, occasionally, the external sphincter.

Endoscopy

Endoscopy is used to evaluate the anatomy of the bladder and urethra and to rule out fistulas and obstruction.

Urodynamic Studies

Urodynamic studies are an indispensable complement to the medical history, physical examination, and imaging and endoscopic studies. Although these other components of the evaluation often yield important clues as to the mechanism of incontinence, in general it is not appropriate to proceed with pharmacologic or surgical treatment without having performed urodynamic studies.

In patients who can void spontaneously, a urinary flow study must precede catheterization to measure residual urine volume and to obtain a sample of urine for culture.

Cystometrography with simultaneous recording and subtraction of the intrarectal pressure provides information on the relationship between bladder filling and intravesical pressure and allows for the determination of bladder capacity and compliance, the presence of uninhibited contractions, and the ability of the detrusor to generate a sustained and effective contraction. The cystometric evaluation of bladder capacity and compliance in patients with incompetent sphincters often requires the use of a balloon catheter to occlude the bladder outlet (Woodside and McGuire).

The competence of the sphincters, in general, is more difficult to establish. A history of incontinence despite good bladder capacity and compliance, absence of uninhibited detrusor contractions, and good bladder emptying suggests sphincteric incompetence. Also, urinary leakage when the bladder is not full in a patient with neurogenic incontinence and a capacious, atonic bladder in a patient who performs intermittent catheterization (IC) indicate sphincteric incontinence.

As mentioned earlier, fluoroscopic cystography with the patient in the upright position during stress and relaxation is the best way to evaluate the competence of the bladder neck. Needle electromyography is useful for patients with neurogenic incontinence to evaluate the innervation of the external sphincter and to determine whether there is an upper or lower motor neuron lesion (Gonzalez and Sidi).

Video-urodynamic studies are elegant and sometimes essential in determining the precise mechanism of incontinence. Urethral profilometry is favored by some to evaluate urethral resistance. Measurement of the leak point pressure also gives a rough estimate of the resistance offered by the sphincters (Wang et al).

TREATMENT

Principles

The ideal goal of all treatments for urinary incontinence is to re-establish normal, periodic, complete, spontaneous, and voluntary micturition with dry intervals between voidings. This goal can be reached for most cases of incontinence resulting from an ectopic ureter or a fistula, urogenital sinus malformations, or traumatic injury to the sphincters and in many cases of bladder exstrophy. In most other instances, however, the patient must live with reasonably long dry intervals between catheterizations to empty the bladder. To this end, the urologist must achieve sufficient bladder storage capacity at low pressure and a urethral resistance that exceeds bladder pressure during the filling phase.

Whenever possible, restoring the normal anatomy should be the first step in the treatment. If this is not feasible, the evaluation described in the preceding section will permit the patient to be placed in one of the categories depicted in Figure 12–1. This categorization assists in the formulation of a rational treatment plan. In the most general terms, treatment (Fig. 12–1) attempts to improve bladder emptying, increase outlet resistance, and restore bladder storage capacity. In the following sections, specific therapeutic measures are described.

Measures to Improve Bladder Emptying

Surgical removal of an obstruction, such as posterior urethral valves or an ectopic ureterocele, should be the initial form of treatment, when appropriate. However, in most children with urinary retention of neurogenic origin and in children without neurologic deficits in whom previous therapeutic maneuvers to increase bladder outlet resistance have resulted in chronic urinary retention, IC is the principal therapeutic measure to facilitate bladder emptying (Lapides et al).

The wide acceptance of clean intermittent catheterization (CIC) has drastically changed the philosophy on the treatment of urinary incontinence. Intermittent catheterization has made supravesical diversion the exception and has allowed bladder augmentation to be performed and the artificial urinary sphincter to be placed in patients who are unable to void spontaneously and who formerly were considered unsuitable for such treatments (Diokno and Sonda; Sidi et al, 1987a). For many cases of neurogenic incontinence when there is a capacious, complaint bladder and a modicum of urethral resistance, the only treatment required to restore dryness is IC (Wang et al).

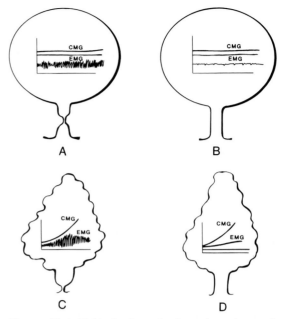

Figure 12–1 □ Mechanism of urinary incontinence in children with neurologic deficits.

A, Atonic bladder with adequate urethral resistance. Treatment by intermittent catheterization.

B, Compliant bladder with good capacity and insufficient urethral resistance. Treatment should increase outlet resistance without diminishing bladder capacity, i.e., implantation of an artificial urinary sphincter with or without intermittent catheterization or fascial sling and intermittent catheterization.

C, Incontinence caused by impaired storage capacity of the bladder with adequate urethral resistance. Treatment with anticholinergic and smooth muscle–relaxing medications or augmentation cystoplasty.

D, Incontinence of mixed origin. If bladder capacity and compliance can be improved pharmacologically, implantation of an artificial sphincter or a fascial sling and intermittent catheterization are sufficient. If an augmentation cystoplasty is required, the options to increase bladder outlet resistance also include bladder neck tubularization procedures (Kropp or Young-Dees-Leadbetter).

(Adapted from Gonzalez R, Guzman JM: Evaluación y tratamiento del niño mielodisplástico. Pediatria 5:29, 1981.)

In children with neurogenic urinary retention resulting from a nonrelaxing sphincter, IC is preferred to external sphincterotomy. Fitting of external collection devices in children is unsatisfactory; IC is preferable, even when it must be performed by the child's caregiver. I perform transurethral external sphincterotomy in exceptional cases of children with urinary retention and a functioning artificial sphincter who are unable to perform catheterization because of uncorrectable urethral abnormalities (Koleilat et al).

Measures to Increase Outlet Resistance

In general, pharmacologic treatments to increase urethral resistance in children are not very effective but alpha-adrenergic agents are sometimes effective in boys with posterior urethral valves if the primary cause of incontinence is low urethral resistance. In this case, pharmacologic treatment is justified, since urethral resistance is expected to improve at puberty.

When ineffective urethral closure results from a correctable congenital anomaly, the first therapeutic measure should be surgery to restore normal anatomy. Such is the case for girls whose incontinence results from urogenital sinus malformations. In these patients, distal urethral reconstruction using the anterior vaginal wall and vaginoplasty with available labial tissue or with a gluteal flap will restore continence, provided there is no associated neurologic deficit (Fig. 12–2) (Hendren). In children with bladder exstrophy and epispadias, bladder neck reconstruction using the modified Young-Dees-Leadbetter operation should be the initial treatment, provided that bladder capacity is adequate (Lepor and Jeffs).

For most patients, including all those with neurogenic sphincteric incompetence, the restoration of normal anatomy is not possible; however, several procedures are available to increase outlet resistance. These procedures fall into two general categories:

1. Placement of the artificial urinary sphincter, which provides urethral occlusion that can be controlled by the patient (Gonzalez et al, 1989a).

2. Procedures that produce a fixed and constant increase in outlet resistance by providing external compression (i.e., slings [McGuire et al] or the periurethral injection of polytef paste or collagen [Politano]) or by creating a continence mechanism with the bladder neck (i.e., the Young-Dees-Leadbetter operation [Leadbetter] and its variations, the creation of an anterior bladder tube as described by Tanagho and Smith, or the creation of a valvular mechanism with a bladder tube, as described by Kropp and Angwafo). These procedures usually require the use of IC, particularly in patients with neurogenic incontinence.

The following sections describe indications and technical aspects of some of these procedures as well as their advantages and disadvantages.

The Artificial Urinary Sphincter

The artificial urinary sphincter is the only method available to increase outlet resistance that may obviate the need for IC in patients with a neurogenic bladder and sphincteric dysfunction who are capable of spontaneous voiding.

This device is the result of more than 15 years of development and clinical experience (Gonzalez and DeWolf; Gonzalez et al, 1989a;

A **Pre-op**

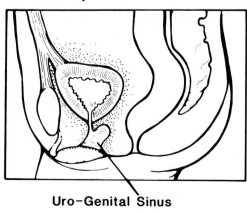

Uro–Genital Sinus

B **Post-op**

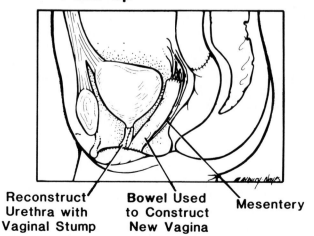

Reconstruct Urethra with Vaginal Stump

Bowel Used to Construct New Vagina

Mesentery

Figure 12–2 □ Example of surgical correction of urinary incontinence by anatomic reconstruction in a 4-year-old girl presenting with diurnal and nocturnal incontinence. *A,* Anatomic abnormalities included unilateral renal agenesis, urogenital sinus malformation with proximal vaginal atresia, short and wide urethra. *B,* Reconstruction of the urethra using the existing urogenital sinus and vaginal reconstruction with sigmoid colon were sufficient to achieve normal urinary control.

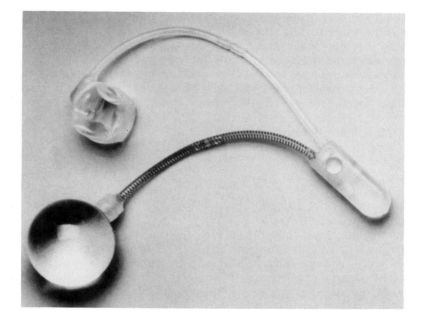

Figure 12–3 ☐ Implantable artificial urinary sphincter AS800. The device consists of an inflatable sphincter cuff, a pressure-regulating balloon and a control unit that contains a pump to open the sphincter cuff, and the necessary resistors and valve mechanisms that allow automatic closing of the sphincter as well as the deactivation mechanism.

Scott et al). The model AS800 (American Medical Systems, Minneapolis), currently in use, consists of a cuff that is placed around the urethra or bladder neck, a pressure-regulating balloon, and a pumping and valve mechanism that is implanted in the scrotum or labium (Fig. 12–3). The inflatable cuff has a strong backing to direct the compression to the urethra and is internally lubricated to increase durability. The cuffs are 2 cm wide and are available in lengths or circumferences from 4.5 to 11 cm. The elasticity of the pressure-regulating balloon allows it to maintain a preselected pressure, although the volume of fluid it contains varies within a certain range. The balloons are available in pressure ranges of from 51 to 60 cm of water up to 71 to 80 cm of water when inflated with 22 ml of fluid. The AS800 pump assembly contains the mechanism and valves that allow transfer of fluid from the cuff to the balloon. This transfer of fluid opens the urethra to allow voiding or catheterization. At rest, the passive return of fluid to the cuff equilibrates the pressure in the cuff and the balloon and closes the urethra automatically within a few minutes. A locking mechanism can interrupt the fluid flow to the cuff. This allows the device to be deactivated in the open position and is used to keep the sphincter open in the postoperative period and at other desired times. The device is reactivated by a single, firm compression of the pump assembly. In small children, I have implanted a modified AS800 pump that is separate from

the valve and locking mechanism. This smaller pump is appropriate for young girls and for boys with a small scrotum. The separate valve unit is implanted in the subcutaneous tissue (Fig. 12–4).

At the University of Minnesota, implantation of the artificial urinary sphincter is the initial form of treatment for patients with neurogenic sphincteric incompetence. These patients represent 80 per cent of the total. In patients with exstrophy or epispadias, the

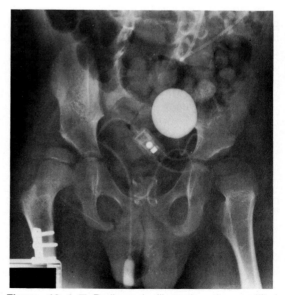

Figure 12–4 ☐ Radiograph illustrating the modified AS800 sphincter with the valve mechanisms separate from the pump.

sphincter is implanted if bladder neck reconstruction has been unsuccessful. It is used for rare cases of posterior urethral valves when persistent incontinence is clearly the result of sphincteric incompetence. The sphincter has also been implanted in patients with sphincteric incompetence resulting from urethral trauma, bilateral ectopic ureters, and iatrogenic sphincteric trauma.

The following are prerequisites for artificial sphincter implantation: (1) sterile urine samples, (2) competent ureterovesical junction, (3) ability to perform IC, and (4) adequate bladder capacity with good compliance and no uninhibited contractions. A history of recurrent urinary tract infections is not a contraindication to implantation of an artificial sphincter, but the urine must be sterile at the time of implantation surgery. Vesicoureteral reflux must be corrected prior to sphincter implantation. If ureteral dilatation is not pronounced, the extravesical (Lich-Gregoir) technique (Gregoir and Schulman) avoids opening of the bladder.

If the preoperative evaluation indicates diminished compliance by end filling pressures greater than 40 cm of water at volumes well below the expected bladder capacity for the child's age or if there are uninhibited bladder contractions, the patient is given oxybutinin (0.2 to 0.5 mg/kg/day) for 4 weeks and cystometrography is repeated. If the response to the medication is adequate and the incontinence persists, an artificial sphincter can be implanted. If the response is not adequate, the patient should undergo enterocystoplasty prior to or at the time of artificial sphincter implantation.

Most patients with sphincteric incompetence have reduced bladder capacity. In our experience, if the end filling pressure is low and the capacity is 60 per cent or greater of the capacity expected for the child's age, patients do well with the artificial sphincter alone in an average follow-up for more than 5 years after sphincter implantation. In contrast, one half of the children with a bladder capacity of less than 60 per cent of the predicted volume but low end filling pressures required bladder augmentation an average of 14 months after sphincter implantation. However, since one half of these children did well without enterocystoplasty, it is reasonable to implant a sphincter initially and observe the patient carefully (Gonzalez et al, 1990).

In children, the artificial sphincter cuff is always implanted around the bladder neck. In my experience, the cuff was placed around the bulbous urethra in only one postpubertal male, in whom there was a previous bladder neck erosion.

For artificial sphincter implantation, the patient is placed supine on the operating table with access to the urethral meatus in the surgical field. In females, the interior of the vagina is prepared as well. A small balloon catheter is inserted into the bladder, and the bladder is emptied. The skin incision is transverse, with a slight cephalad concavity 2 to 3 cm above the pubic symphysis. Skin and subcutaneous tissue flaps are elevated cephalad and caudally. The aponeurosis is incised vertically in the midline, and the retropubic space is exposed by blunt dissection. The spaces lateral to the bladder neck are exposed and dissected. Large veins running in approximately longitudinal direction indicate the anterior aspect of the seminal vesicles in males and the anterior vaginal wall in females. In the course of the dissection, some of these veins may need to be fulgurated. A plane of dissection is created between these veins and the bladder neck. The dissection is carried out bilaterally, and the correctness of the plane is verified repeatedly by digital palpation. The last few millimeters of retrovesical dissection must be performed with particular care so as not to injure the posterior bladder wall. When the space surrounding the bladder neck is developed, a vessel loop is passed around it.

The bladder is now filled with a methylene blue solution to rule out the possibility that the bladder neck was inadvertently injured. If the bladder neck has been injured during dissection, the bladder should be opened in the midline, away from the bladder neck, and the laceration is repaired in two layers. The inexperienced surgeon may choose to perform an elective cystotomy, away from the site at which the cuff will be implanted, to guide in the dissection around the bladder neck. The circumference of the bladder neck is measured with the cuff sizer provided with the sphincter. The cuff, which is prefilled with fluid but collapsed, is passed around the bladder neck, and its connecting tube is brought to the subcutaneous space through a stab wound in the fascia.

The manufacturer's instructions on filling of the sphincter components with fluid must be followed meticulously. A pocket is created between the anterior abdominal wall and the peritoneum, usually on the left side, to contain the pressure-regulating balloon. The connecting tube for the balloon is also brought subcutaneously through the fascia. The wound is irrigated with an antibiotic solution, and the aponeurosis of the recti is closed. A space is created in the right hemiscrotum or the labium to contain the sphincter pump. The appropriate connections are made, the sphincter is tested and left deactivated, and the subcutaneous tissue and the skin are closed. A compressive dressing is applied over the incision to prevent a seroma (Fig. 12–5).

One hour before the operation, the patient receives ampicillin (25 mg/kg per dose) and gentamicin (1 mg/kg per dose). These antibiotics are administered every 8 hours for the next 5 days. The urethral catheter is left indwelling for 2 days. If the patient was able to void spontaneously before sphincter implantation, residual urine volume is measured occasionally to rule out the possibility of retention. If the patient has performed IC before the operation, this procedure is resumed.

Six weeks after implantation, the sphincter is activated and renal ultrasonography is performed to rule out the possibility of hydronephrosis. The patient or the parents are thoroughly instructed on the use of the device. Renal and bladder ultrasonography are repeated in 6 months and at yearly intervals thereafter. Cystometrography is performed 3 and 6 months after surgery and then yearly.

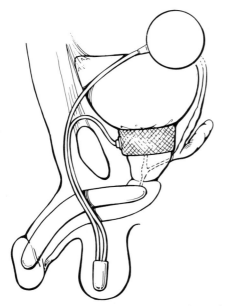

Figure 12–5 □ Diagrammatic representation of the AS800 implanted in a male around the bladder neck not encircling the seminal vesicles or ejaculatory ducts.

Voiding cystourethrography is performed if the intravesical pressure is elevated.

Overall, 85 per cent of patients achieve a satisfactory degree of continence (Barrett and Parulkar; Gonzalez et al, 1989a). The best results are obtained for patients with neurogenic sphincteric incompetence when the artificial sphincter is the first surgical treatment used. In these patients, good results for the artificial sphincter alone or in combination with IC, anticholinergic medications, and, occasionally, enterocystoplasty are the rule. Sixty per cent of our patients use IC, 40 per cent take oxybutinin, and approximately one third have required enterocystoplasty. This procedure can be performed prior to, at the time of, or following sphincter implantation with equally good results (Gonzalez et al, 1989b). Other authors have reported a success rate of 69 per cent for the sphincter in patients who have previously undergone reconstructive surgery for bladder exstrophy (Light and Scott).

When prepubertal males who void spontaneously reach puberty, growth of the prostate, which is partially encircled by the cuff, may cause obstruction and urinary retention, which can then be treated by IC or replacement of the cuff.

The most frequent complication associated with the artificial sphincter is loss of fluid from the system and subsequent recurrence of incontinence. (Although the mean longevity of the AS800 sphincter has not been established, we and others have reported a significant improvement in contrast to previous models of the device.) If this occurs, all components should be replaced. Intraoperative testing to locate the leak point is unreliable, and, in general, operations to replace all components offer few technical difficulties. All components can be located by following the connecting tubes rather than by trying to identify anatomic structures because of the fibrous sheath that surrounds the components.

Sphincter malfunctions that result from kinks in the tubes generally reflect a technical error during implantation but may develop later as a result of the child's growth.

Infection of the prosthesis necessitates removal of the entire device. With proper technique and patient preparation, the infection rate should be less than 2 per cent.

Over the last several years, erosion of the tissues in contact with the sphincter (i.e., bladder neck, scrotum, or vulva) has occurred exclusively in patients who have previously undergone surgery on the eroded area. Therefore, implantation of the artificial sphincter should be considered the first choice for surgical treatment rather than a salvage operation (Gonzalez et al, 1989a). Despite the potential for erosion, a success rate of 73 per cent for sphincter implantation was reported for a series of patients who had previously undergone surgery for incontinence (Aliabadi and Gonzalez).

The finding that previous operations on the area in contact with the sphincter predispose to erosion suggests that poor vascularization of the tissues, rather than infection, is an important factor in the pathogenesis of erosion.

Bladder neck erosion occurs almost always in the first year after implantation and is manifested by hematuria, infection, or recurrent incontinence. The treatment consists of removal of the device and establishment of an alternative treatment.

Changes in bladder function leading to decreased compliance and high storage pressure, recurrence of incontinence, vesicoureteral reflux, and deterioration of the upper urinary tract occur in some patients who use an artificial urinary sphincter (Bauer et al; Light and Pietro). These changes occur most commonly in patients with neurogenic bladder dysfunction and mandate lifelong follow-up. The possible causes of these changes include (1) preexisting hyperreflexia or decreased bladder compliance not detected preoperatively, (2) changes in the detrusor in response to the obstruction created by the sphincter, (3) neurologic changes caused by tethering of the spinal cord, and (4) progressive, chronic urinary retention in patients who void spontaneously but not completely.

In our experience at the University of Minnesota, upper tract deterioration occurred in three of approximately 75 children followed after artificial sphincter implantation. In these three patients, the presenting symptom was recurrent urinary incontinence; however, the possibility that reflux and hydronephrosis develop without symptoms cannot be ruled out. Treatment for upper tract deterioration includes deactivation of the sphincter and a period of catheter drainage that is followed by the use of IC, administration of smooth muscle relaxants, and, when needed, augmentation cystoplasty.

When a patient with an artificial sphincter presents with persistent or recurrent incontinence, the differential diagnosis includes (1) loss of fluid from the system; (2) inadvertent deactivation of the device; (3) incomplete bladder emptying; (4) urinary retention in a patient who previously voided spontaneously; (5) noncompliance with the recommended use of the device or with the program of IC; (6) tube kinks; (7) changes in detrusor function; (8) tissue atrophy, which results in the loosening of the cuff and ineffective compression of the urethra; and (9) urethral or bladder neck erosion. A thorough physical examination along with imaging, urodynamic studies, and endoscopy leads to an accurate diagnosis and treatment in all cases.

Procedures That Produce a Fixed Increase in Outlet Resistance

Alternatives to the artificial sphincter for the treatment of sphincteric incontinence have received well-deserved attention.

Slings

The most viable alternative treatment is the periurethral fascial sling for bladder neck suspension and urethral compression (McGuire et al). An advantage of the sling procedure for postpubertal females is that the dissection between the urethra and the vagina can be performed transvaginally, an approach considered by many to be simpler than pelvic dissection. The fascial sling can be used as a free graft or can remain attached at one end (Fig. 12–6). It is important to verify during the operation that the sling is not tight and that IC will still be possible after the sutures are tied. Of course, when this procedure is performed in a male or prepubertal female, pelvic dissection of the retrourethral space is necessary and the dissection is identical to that for implantation of an artificial sphincter. For children with neurogenic incontinence, patient selection criteria are similar, if not identical, to those used for implantation of an artificial sphincter. All the considerations regarding bladder compliance and capacity discussed previously for implantation of the artificial sphincter apply to the urethral sling. Of course, in a patient with neurogenic incontinence, bladder emptying after construction of a sling is always by intermittent catheterization.

The success of urethral slings in females with neurogenic incontinence has been reported to be in the neighborhood of 85 per cent, but most reports concern a small series of patients and the follow-up is short. Bloom (personal

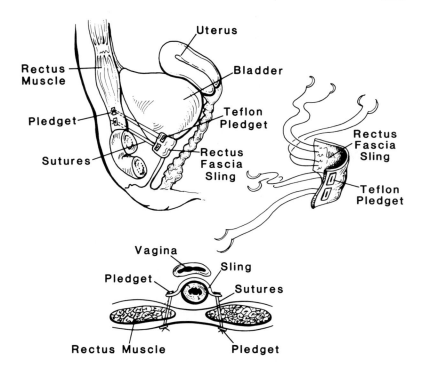

Figure 12–6 □ Urethral fascial sling used to increase outlet resistance. In patients with neurogenic incontinence, emptying is accomplished by intermittent catheterization. The sling should not angulate the urethra, making catheterization difficult or impossible.

communication, 1990) reported success for 11 of 13 females; Peters and Bauer reported success with the initial operation for seven of nine girls whose mean age was 13 years. Four of these patients required augmentation cystoplasty, and one required reoperation to tighten the sling. Elder reported on eight females, all of whom also underwent enterocystoplasty, for whom the results, in general, were good. McGuire et al reported their experience with eight females, of unspecified age, with myelomeningocele who achieved continence after construction of a pubovaginal sling, but the length of follow-up was not stated. Fascial slings appear to be less reliable for males, and the numbers reported are even smaller than for females. Elder reported success for three of four males and Raz et al (1986b) reported success for four males aged 10 to 22 years who underwent bladder augmentation and construction of a fascial sling. However, Bloom noted considerably less success for males than for females. Others have reported similar success rates using other types of bladder neck suspensions in combination with enterocystoplasty (Gearhart and Jeffs). This combination of treatments and the lack of controls make it difficult to evaluate the effectiveness of the bladder neck suspension when used alone. I reserve the sling procedure for cases in which the artificial sphincter has failed. Fascial slings

may be an ideal treatment in parts of the world where the artificial sphincter is not available.

Bladder Neck Tubularization

The Young-Dees-Leadbetter bladder neck tubularization is the initial treatment of choice for an incontinent child with the exstrophy-epispadias complex (Lepor and Jeffs). Sidi et al (1987b) reported that seven of 11 patients with neurogenic incontinence achieved a satisfactory level of continence with this procedure (Fig. 12–7). In this case, the tube is made quite long and narrow and emptying is accomplished by catheterization. The disadvantage of this procedure for a patient with myelomeningocele is that the significant reduction in bladder capacity results in the frequent need for reoperations to correct problems with catheterization. Sidi et al (1987b) reported that seven of 11 patients achieved an initial satisfactory level of continence.

Periurethral Substances

The injection of periurethral substances to increase urethral resistance continues to undergo clinical trials. The use of polytef paste in children is discouraged because of its uncertain success and the possibility of long-term complications resulting from migration of

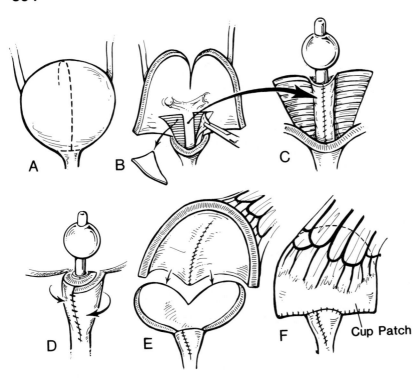

Figure 12–7 □ *A–F*, Technique for bladder neck tubularization modified from the technique described by Young, Dees and Leadbetter. In patients with neurogenic incontinence, the tube should be sufficiently long to cause urinary retention. This requires ureteral reimplantation and augmentation cystoplasty in most patients. Emptying is accomplished by intermittent catheterization. (See Leadbetter, J Urol 91:261, 1964.)

polytef particles to distant organs (Malizia et al). The use of collagen may avoid this risk, but the long-term effectiveness remains open to question.

Procedures That Create a Valve Mechanism

In 1986, Kropp and Angwafo described a procedure to create a valve mechanism at the bladder neck that permits IC but prevents urine flow from the bladder to the urethra. A tube is constructed from the anterior bladder wall and is then tunneled under the mucosa of the posterior bladder wall between the ureteral orifices (Fig. 12–8). The mechanism is similar to that which is achieved after tunneled reimplantation of the ureters to prevent vesicoureteral reflux. Nill and associates reported results

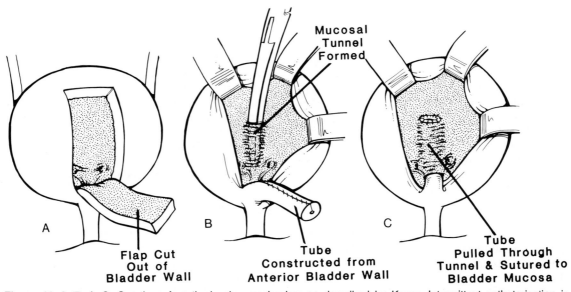

Figure 12–8 □ *A–C*, Creation of urethral valve mechanism as described by Kropp. Intermittent catheterization is required in all patients, and bladder augmentation is generally necessary.

for the first 25 patients who have undergone this procedure. Approximately one half of the patients had been observed for 5 or more years. Of the patients, 22 had neurogenic incontinence and 20 patients had previously undergone bladder augmentation or underwent bladder augmentation at the time the valve mechanism was constructed.

In 80 per cent of the patients, a good result was achieved. Seventeen of the 24 patients have achieved an excellent level of continence, and three have experienced rare episodes of wetness. Complications have included vesicoureteral reflux in ten patients; in eight of these patients, corrective surgery was required. Eleven patients experienced transient difficulty with IC and two have had persistent difficulties. In eight patients bladder calculi developed, and in nine there was a clinical suspicion of an episode of bladder rupture. Of the 24 patients, 19 have required a total of 34 reoperations.

Belman and Kaplan reported on a modification of the Kropp procedure, which may reduce the incidence of catheterization problems.

Summary of Procedures That Increase Outlet Resistance

In patients with anatomic defects that result in incontinence, restoration of normal anatomy should always be the first step in treatment. For patients with exstrophy or epispadias, bladder neck reconstruction using the Young-Dees-Leadbetter technique yields the best results.

When selecting a procedure to increase bladder outlet resistance in a patient with neurogenic sphincteric incontinence, the surgeon must take the following into account: (1) the present need for IC to empty the bladder, (2) the predicted need for bladder augmentation, and (3) previous anti-incontinence operations. For patients with good bladder capacity and compliance who void spontaneously, the artificial sphincter is the ideal treatment. For patients who depend on IC, the artificial sphincter also provides excellent results and does not create new difficulties with catheterization. Females who use IC may also benefit from urethral suspension using a pubovaginal fascial sling. The patient who requires bladder augmentation can easily undergo the simultaneous implantation of an artificial sphincter without risk of increased complications. The creation of a fascial sling may be a reasonable alternative treatment to the sphincter for females who require bladder augmentation. For these patients, the Kropp procedure also can be contemplated. The disadvantage of this and other tubularization procedures lies in the potential difficulty of catheterizing the tubularized urethra. Furthermore, because the Kropp procedure produces a servomechanism in which increased bladder pressure enhances closure of the valve, the risk of bladder perforation may be increased in a patient with an augmented bladder who does not comply with the prescribed schedule of catheterization.

With the procedures described above, a success rate of approximately 80 to 85 per cent can reasonably be expected. The artificial sphincter yields the best results when implanted around a virgin bladder neck. Patients for whom one or more of these operations fails and patients whose urethras do not permit catheterization are candidates for a continent urinary diversion, with the Mitroffanoff principle being used whenever possible (Duckett and Snyder). A second alternative for these patients is the creation of a continent ileal stoma (Guzman et al).

Measures to Enhance the Storage Capacity of the Bladder

Anticholinergic drugs and, preferably, smooth muscle relaxants, such as oxybutinin and dicyclomine, can enhance continence in patients with reduced bladder compliance and in patients with uninhibited detrusor contractions. The results of pharmacologic treatment can usually be assessed clinically if the patient has an adequate bladder resistance; however, if the incontinence has a mixed urethral and bladder origin, evaluation of the response requires cystometrography. Children are initially given oxybutinin, 0.2 to 0.5 mg/kg/day in two divided doses. The dose can be increased, if needed, as long as side effects do not develop.

Patients who fail to respond to pharmacologic treatment are candidates for bladder augmentation. Although increasing bladder capacity and compliance without the use of an intestinal segment—especially the gastrointestinal mucosa—is the ideal, enterocystoplasty is the only proven method of achieving these goals. Excision of the detrusor, as described by Cartwright and Snow, is a promising technique and has produced clinical improvement of incontinence; unfortunately, however, urodynamic documentation of its effectiveness is lacking (Fig. 12–9). Perivesical denervation is an intriguing method for improving bladder storage capacity, but it is difficult to evaluate. For example, in the report by Raz et al (1988a), all patients also underwent enterocystoplasty.

Bladder augmentation is described in detail in another chapter. This portion of the chapter briefly discusses some general principles of enterocystoplasty that pertain to the treatment of incontinence.

It is now well established that an intestinal segment used to enlarge the bladder should be reconfigured to maximize the volume for a given surface area and to minimize the occurrence of volume-dependent mass contractions (Sidi et al, 1986). The reconfiguration of the ileum described by Goodwin (Gonzalez, 1991) can be used very successfully for the sigmoid and descending colon (Fig. 12–10). Because of the larger diameter, a given length of colon yields a greater capacity than the same length of small bowel. I continue to favor the use of the sigmoid colon in neurogenic patients because of its large diameter, close anatomic

proximity to the bladder, and the lack of alterations of intestinal function of the remaining colon in the intestinal tract. Nevertheless, the intestinal segment chosen probably is of less importance than the configuration used and volume achieved. However, in patients with neurogenic incontinence, the use of the ileocecal segment should be avoided. The exclusion of the ileocecal valve from the intestinal tract can accelerate transit and produce diarrhea and fecal incontinence because these patients rely on well-formed stools for rectal continence (Cabral and Gonzalez). Because all patients who undergo cystoplasty must use IC for emptying, it is imperative to establish that catheterization can be performed by the patient or caregiver and that a sufficiently large catheter can be introduced so that urine and mucus can be evacuated quickly. Enterocystoplasty invariably causes some degree of metabolic acidosis, but it is seldom clinically significant except in patients with compromised renal function. In these patients, as well as in those with a short bowel or previous colonic operations, gastocystoplasty (Fig. 12–11) is indicated (Adams et al).

Chronic bacteriuria invariably is present following enterocystoplasty, but in the absence of reflux it seldom produces symptoms (Gonzalez and Reinberg). In patients with symptomatic bacteriuria, daily irrigations with an antibiotic solution are often effective. Daily irrigations of the augmented bladder also help to minimize the problems caused by mucus and help to prevent stone formation.

Spontaneous rupture of the augmented bladder is a life-threatening complication of cystoplasty (Elder et al; Rushton et al). It occurs most frequently in patients with neurogenic incontinence who have effective continence mechanisms and who do not comply with the prescribed schedule of catheterization. Of 75 children who have undergone sigmoid cystoplasty in the pediatric urology service at the University of Minnesota, in only one was there a bladder perforation.

The long-term risk of cancer in patients with enteric or gastric augmentation is unknown, but all patients should be observed for life (Filmer and Spencer).

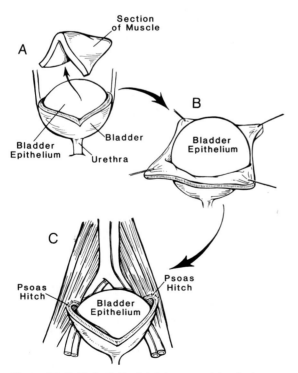

Figure 12–9 ☐ *A–C*, Partial detrusor excision (autoaugmentation) in an attempt to increase bladder capacity and compliance without using a portion of the gastrointestinal tract.

CONCLUSIONS

The management of the child with severe urinary incontinence presents a unique challenge to the pediatric urologist. A careful evaluation

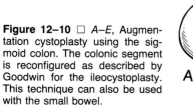
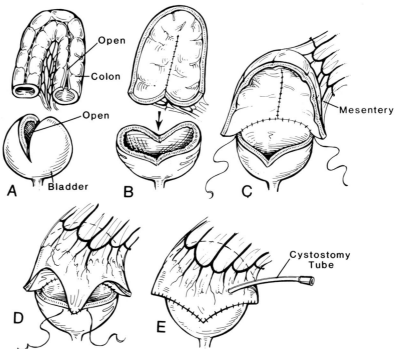

Figure 12–10 □ *A–E*, Augmentation cystoplasty using the sigmoid colon. The colonic segment is reconfigured as described by Goodwin for the ileocystoplasty. This technique can also be used with the small bowel.

of the patient allows a precise definition of the pathophysiology of the incontinence and the implementation of therapeutic measures directed at solving the existing problems. Surgical measures to enhance urethral resistance and improve bladder storage capacity are effective but should be used in concert with other forms of treatment, including medications and IC. Life-long follow-up of these patients is essential.

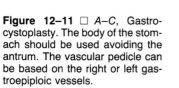
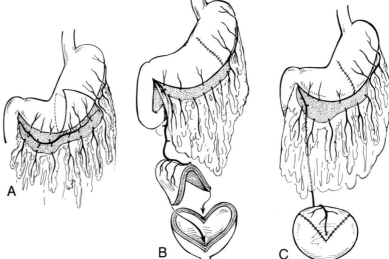

Figure 12–11 □ *A–C*, Gastrocystoplasty. The body of the stomach should be used avoiding the antrum. The vascular pedicle can be based on the right or left gastroepiploic vessels.

References

Adams MC, Mitchell ME, Rink RC: Gastrocystoplasty: an alternative solution to the problem of urological reconstruction in the severely compromised patient. J Urol 140:1152, 1988.

Aliabadi H, Gonzalez R: Success of the artificial urinary sphincter after failed surgery for incontinence. J Urol 143:987, 1990.

Barrett DM, Parulkar BG: The artificial sphincter (AS800): experience in children and young adults. Urol Clin North Am, 16:119, 1989.

Bauer SB, Reda EF, Colodny AH, et al: Detrusor instability: a delayed complication in association with the artificial urinary sphincter. J Urol 135:1212, 1986.

Belman AB, Kaplan GW: Experience with the Kropp antiincontinence procedure. J Urol 141:1160, 1989.

Cabral B, Gonzalez R: Rectal continence after enterocystoplasty in patients with neurogenic bladder. Dialogues in Pediatric Urology 10:4, 1987.

Cartwright PG, Snow BW: Bladder auto augmentation: partial detrusor excision to augment the bladder without the use of bowel. J Urol 139:524, 1988a.

Diokno AC, Sonda LP: Compatibility of genitourinary prostheses and intermittent self-catheterization. J Urol 125:659, 1981.

Duckett JW, Snyder HM III: Continent urinary diversion: variation on the Mitrofanoff principle. J Urol 146:58, 1986.

Elder JS: Pubovaginal and puboprostatic sling repair. Dialogues in Pediatric Urology 12:5, 1989.

Elder JS, Snyder HM, Hulbert WC, et al: Perforation of the augmented bladder in patients undergoing clean intermittent catheterization. J Urol 140:1159, 1988.

Filmer BR, Spencer JR: Malignancies in bladder augmentations and intestinal conduits. J Urol 143:671, 1990.

Gearhart JP, Jeffs RD: Suprapubic bladder neck suspensions. Dialog Pediat Urol 12:2, 1989.

Gonzalez R: Undiversion. In Urologic Surgery, 4th ed. Edited by JF Glenn. Philadelphia, JB Lippincott, 1991, p 1069.

Gonzalez R, de Badiola F, Austin C, et al: Prediction for the need for enterocystoplasty before artificial sphincter implantation in patients with neurogenic sphincter incontinence (abstr). J Urol 143:277A, 1990.

Gonzalez R, DeWolf WC: The artificial bladder sphincter AS721 for the treatment of incontinence in patients with neurogenic bladder. J Urol 121:71, 1979.

Gonzalez R, Koleilat N, Austin C, et al: The artificial sphincter AS800 in congenital urinary incontinence. J Urol 142:512, 19891.

Gonzalez R, Nguyen DH, Koleilat N, et al: Compatibility of enterocystoplasty and the artificial urinary sphincter. J Urol, 142:502, 1989b.

Gonzalez R, Reinberg Y: Localization of the bacteriuria in patients with enterocystoplasty and nonrefluxing conduits. J Urol 138:1104, 1987.

Gonzalez R, Sidi AA: Preoperative prediction of continence after enterocystoplasty or undiversion in children with neurogenic bladder. J Urol 134:705, 1985.

Gregoir W, Schulman CC: Die extravesikale antireflux plastik. Urologe A 16:124, 1977.

Guzman JM, Ercole CJ, Montes de Oca L, et al: Modification of the Benchoukrun continent ileal stoma. J Urol 142:1431, 1989.

Hendren WH: Construction of a female urethra from the vaginal wall and a perineal flap. J Urol 123:657, 1980.

Hinman F: Nonneurogenic-neurogenic bladder (the Hinman syndrome)—15 years later. J Urol 136:729, 1986.

Koleilat N, Sidi AA, Gonzalez R: Urethral false passage as a complication of intermittent catheterization. J Urol 142:1216, 1989.

Kropp KA, Angwafo FF: Urethral lengthening and reimplantation for neurogenic incontinence in children. J Urol 135:533, 1986.

Lapides J, Diokno AC, Silber SJ, et al: Clean intermittent catheterization in the treatment of urinary tract disease. J Urol 107:458, 1971.

Leadbetter GW Jr: Surgical correction of total urinary incontinence. J Urol 91:261, 1964.

Lepor H, Jeffs RD: Primary bladder closure and bladder neck reconstruction in classical bladder exstrophy. J Urol 130:1142, 1983.

Light JK, Pietro T: Alteration of detrusor behavior and the effect on renal function following insertion of the artificial sphincter. J Urol 136:632, 1986.

Light JK, Scott FB: Treatment of epispadias—exstrophy complex with AS792 artificial urinary sphincter. J Urol 129:738, 1983.

Malizia AA Jr, Reiman HM, Myers RP, et al: Migration and granulomatous reaction after periurethral injection of polytef (Teflon). JAMA 251:3277, 1984.

McGuire EJ, Wang SC, Usitalo H, et al: Modified pubovaginal sling in girls with myelodysplasia. J Urol, 135:94, 1986.

Nill TG, Peller PA, Kropp KA: Management of urinary incontinence by bladder tube urethral lengthening and submucosal reimplantation. J Urol 144:559, 1990.

Peters CA, Bauer SB: Urethral suspension procedures. Dialog Pediatr Urol 12:3, 1989.

Politano VA: Periurethral polytetra fluoroethylene injection for urinary incontinence. J Urol 127:439, 1982.

Raz S, Erlich RM, Zeidman EJ, et al: Surgical treatment of the incontinent female patient with myelomeningocele. J Urol 139:524, 1988a.

Raz S, McGuire EJ, Erlich RM, et al: Fascial sling to correct male neurogenic sphincter incompetence: the McGuire/Raz approach. J Urol 139:528, 1988b.

Rushton HG, Woodward JR, Parrott TS, et al: Delayed bladder rupture after augmentation enterocystoplasty. J Urol 140:344, 1988.

Scott FB, Bradley WE, Timm GW, et al: Treatment of incontinence secondary to myelodysplasia by an implantable prosthetic urinary sphincter. South Med J 66:987, 1973.

Sidi AA, Aliabadi H, Gonzalez R: Enterocystoplasty in the reconstruction and management of the pediatric neurogenic bladder. J Pediatr Surg 22:153, 1987a.

Sidi AA, Reinberg Y, Gonzalez R: Comparison of artificial sphincter implantation and bladder neck incontinence. J Urol 138:1120, 1987b.

Sidi AA, Reinberg Y, Gonzalez R: Influence of intestinal segment and configuration on the outcome of augmentation enterocystoplasty. J Urol 136:1201, 1986.

Tanagho EA, Smith DR: Clinical evaluation of a surgical technique for the correction of complete urinary incontinence. J Urol 107:402, 1972.

Wang SC, McGuire EJ, Bloom DA: A bladder pressure management system for myelodysplasia: clinical outcome. J Urol 140:1499, 1988.

Woodside JR, McGuire EJ: Technique for detection of detrusor hypertonia in the presence of urethral sphincter incompetence. J Urol 127:740, 1982.

13

☐ Neuropathology of the Lower Urinary Tract

Stuart B. Bauer

At least 25 per cent of the clinical problems in pediatric urology are caused by neurologic lesions that affect lower urinary tract function. The advent of clean intermittent catheterization (CIC), introduced in the early 1970s by Dr. Jack Lapides (Lapides et al), and the refinements in the techniques of urodynamic studies in children (Blaivas, 1979; Blaivas et al; Gierup and Ericson) dramatically changed the way these children were managed (Smith). As a result, a greater understanding of the pathophysiology of the many diseases that primarily affect children is now known. Functional assessment of the lower urinary tract is currently an essential element in the evaluation process and is as important as x-ray visualization in characterizing and managing these abnormal conditions (McGuire et al). Because urodynamic testing is such an integral part of any discussion on the subject, this chapter first defines the testing process as it applies to children, its pitfalls and advantages, and then elaborates on the various neurourologic abnormalities that are prevalent in children.

ASSESSMENT

Initially, all children with overt or suspected neuropathic bladder dysfunction should undergo evaluation as outlined in Table 13–1. Of paramount importance in the work-up of children with neuropathic bladder dysfunction are the history and physical examination. The child's voiding habits prior to any injury and the current pattern of bladder emptying should be delineated. It is imperative to note whether the child voids voluntarily, spontaneously, or only with a Credé maneuver. Does the child have periods of dryness between voiding, or is there constant urinary leakage? Is the incontinence characterized by urgency and an inability to get to the bathroom on time? Does

the urine flow with a good stream or only dribble out during emptying? Does leakage occur with crying or laughing? Has the child had a urinary infection? How much urine is produced each day? What is the pattern of bowel function?

A careful assessment is made of perianal and perineal sensation, anal sphincter tone, and the presence of bulbocavernosus and anocutaneous reflexes. The bulbocavernosus reflex is elicited by placing one's finger just at or slightly inside the external anal sphincter and briskly squeezing the glans penis or compressing the clitoris. If the reflex is present, the external anal sphincter should contract. The anocutaneous reflex is elicited by scratching

Table 13–1 ☐ Evaluation of Children with Neuropathic Bladder Dysfunction

History
Bowel and bladder habits
Pattern of incontinence
Birth and development

Physical Examination
Spine
Lower extremities
  Reflexes
  Muscle mass
  Gait
  Perineal sensation/tone/reflexes

Laboratory
Urine analysis/culture
Urine specific gravity
Serum creatinine level

Radiography
Excretory urography (or renal sonography)
Voiding cystourethrography
Spine radiograph

Urodynamics
Flow rate
Residual urine
Cystometrogram
External urethral sphincter electromyography
Static/filling/voiding urethral pressure profile

the pigmented skin directly adjacent to the anal opening, which results in a contraction of the perianal muscle. In children with suspected neuropathic bladder dysfunction, complete evaluation of the back, including looking for agenesis of the sacrum or a cutaneous manifestation of an underlying occult spinal dysraphism, is an important diagnostic aid (Bauer, 1983; Mandell et al). Examination of the lower extremities, comparing muscle mass and strength of each leg, eliciting deep tendon reflexes, and observing the gait, may provide clues to the presence of an occult spinal dysraphism affecting not only the sacral but the lumbar cord as well.

Technique of Urodynamic Studies

Before a urodynamic study is performed, it is important that the child and family have full knowledge of the procedure. One must try to reproduce the natural act of voiding in the laboratory in order to avoid any misunderstandings regarding what is observed and recorded. Unfortunately, urodynamics is an invasive procedure. Currently, no reliable indirect methods exist to assess bladder and sphincter function accurately. Therefore, an explanation of the test and a questionnaire are sent to each family prior to their appointment. A booklet is provided so that parents know what to expect, and can explain the test to their child. If old enough, the individual can read about it. Attempts are made to minimize the anxiety level in those children who are old enough to understand what will happen. The questionnaire tries to elicit information about the child's birth and development, current bladder and bowel habits, and any other information that might be pertinent.

Sometimes, in very anxious children older than 1 year of age, meperidine, 1 mg/kg of body weight, is administered intramuscularly to reduce their discomfort and anxiety level; this does not alter the child's cooperativeness nor responsiveness (Ericsson et al). If feasible, however, no medication is given, but the child is conscientiously attended to, in order to minimize his or her fears. When possible, the child is instructed to come to the urodynamic suite with a full bladder in order to obtain an initial, representative uroflowmetry. This enables the nurse to record a reliable residual urine volume when catheterizing the child after voiding. The flowmeter is located in a private bathroom that contains a one-way mirror so that voiding can be viewed unobtrusively. This allows the investigator to see if a Credé or a Valsalva maneuver is employed by the individual to help empty the bladder and to determine the presence of stress incontinence when the child coughs.

When voiding takes place, peak and mean flow rates and volume voided are recorded; in addition, the characteristics of the urinary flow are assessed on a DANTEC (DANTEC Medical, Inc., Santa Clara, California) uroflowmeter. For those children who have no control, either a reflex bladder contraction is attempted or Credé voiding is used to empty the bladder and determine an estimate of residual urine volume.

Next, the nurse reviews the test and shows the child all the equipment in an attempt to make him or her as comfortable as possible. Then the child is catheterized with either a 7 Fr. or an 11 Fr. triple-lumen urodynamic catheter (Bard Urologic, Murray Hill, N.J.) after a small amount of liquid xylocaine is injected into the urethra and held in place for a moment or two. The contents in the bladder drain into a graduated container so the residual urine can be carefully measured. Sometimes it is necessary to aspirate the catheter to get an accurate volume of residual urine, especially if the bladder is hypotonic (particularly if the child is taking anticholinergic medication) or has been previously augmented and secretes mucus, in which case complete drainage may then not occur following catheter insertion (Bauer, 1983).

A small balloon catheter is passed into the rectum at this time to measure intra-abdominal pressure during the cystometrogram in order to identify artifacts of motion and monitor increases in abdominal pressure during the filling and emptying phases of the study (Bates et al; Bauer, 1979). Uninhibited contractions can be clearly differentiated by this maneuver.

Prior to filling the bladder, one may obtain a urethral pressure profile by infusing saline through the side-hole channel at a rate of 2 ml/minute as the catheter is withdrawn at a rate of 2 mm/second (Yalla et al, 1980). Some urodynamicists advocate using a balloon or microtipped transducer catheter to measure urethral resistance instead of saline infusion (Tanagho). When the maximum resistance is known, the catheter is positioned so that the urethral pressure port is located at that or any other point of interest. This area can then be monitored throughout the urodynamic study.

Urethral pressure profilometry (UPP) measures the passive resistance of a particular point within the urethra to stretch (Gleason et al, 1974). Many factors contribute to this resistance, including the elastic properties of the tissues surrounding the lumen and the tension generated by the smooth and skeletal muscles of the urethra that are constantly changing during the micturition cycle (Fig. 13–1) (Abrams; Evans et al). Thus, the static urethral pressure profile is a measure of the resistance under a specific set of circumstances (Yalla et al, 1979). It is difficult to extrapolate data when the bladder is empty and apply them to a time when (1) the bladder is full, (2) it responds to increases in abdominal pressure, or (3) emptying takes place (Fig. 13–2). Failure to recognize this problem will lead to false assumptions and improper treatment.

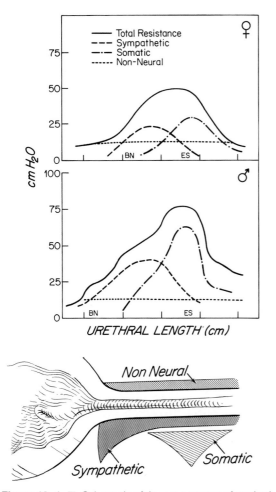

Figure 13–1 □ Schematic of the components of urethral wall tension according to their geographic distribution and effect along the urethra in males and females. BN, bladder neck; ES, external sphincter.

External urethral sphincter electromyography (EMG) is recorded using a 24-gauge concentric needle electrode (Blaivas et al, 1977b; Diokno et al) inserted perineally in males or paraurethrally in females (Fig. 13–3), and advanced into the skeletal muscle component of the sphincter until individual motor unit action potentials are seen and/or heard on a standard electromyographic recorder (TECA Corporation, Pleasantville, N.Y.).

When the electrode is in the muscle, characteristic motor unit action potentials are seen on the oscilloscope and heard from the audio output channel. Permanent recordings can be made on light-sensitive photographic paper using an electron beam display. Artifacts that are not readily discernible on a graphic recorder with a heat stylus pen can be easily detected and eliminated by observing the oscilloscopic screen, listening to the audio channel, and studying the recordings made on the photographic paper (Bauer, 1983; Blaivas, 1979a). This method allows for accurate assessment of the degree of denervation involving the striated muscle component of the external urethral sphincter. Evidence of both acute and chronic denervation involving the sacral cord is easily discernible. Repositioning the needle allows the investigator to determine variations in the degree of denervation on one side of the external sphincter versus the other.

Alternatively, perineal (Maizels and Firlit) or abdominal patch electrodes (Koff and Kass), perineal wire electrodes (Scott et al), or anal plugs (Bradley et al) have been used to record the bioelectric activity in the sphincter muscle. Disagreements exist as to the accuracy of these surface electrode measurements versus those obtained via needle electrodes, particularly during voiding. The intactness of sacral cord function is easily measured with needle electrodes by (1) looking at the characteristic wave form of individual motor unit action potentials when the patient is relaxed and the bladder empty, (2) performing and recording responses to bulbocavernosus and anal stimulation, and Credé and Valsalva maneuvers, (3) asking the patient to contract and relax the external sphincter voluntarily, and (4) seeing the reaction of the sphincter to filling and emptying of the bladder (Fig. 13–4) (Blaivas, 1979b; Blaivas et al, 1977a).

The rate of bladder filling is usually set by determining the child's predicted capacity (average capacity (ml) = (age [years] + 2) × 30) (Koff) and dividing by 10. This estimation

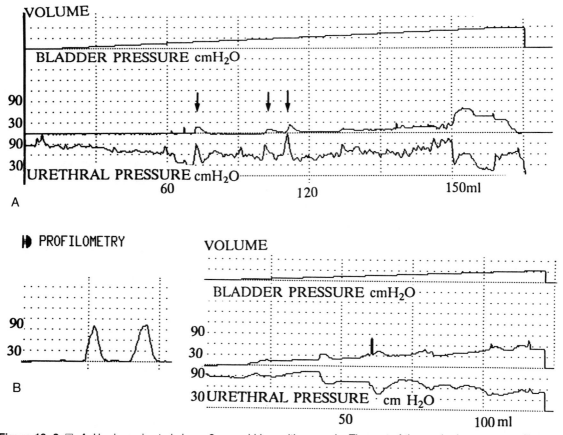

Figure 13–2 □ *A*, Urodynamic study in an 8-year-old boy with enuresis. The port of the urethral pressure profilometry multichannel urodynamic catheter is positioned in the mid-urethra. Note urethral resistance is adequate at the start of filling, but it decreases just prior to each uninhibited contraction and then increases during the contraction *(arrows)*. At capacity, the resistance is very high, but then it equals bladder pressure during voiding. *B*, This 7-year-old girl with myelomeningocele demonstrates a very good level of resistance when a urethral pressure profile is performed initially. During bladder filling with the catheter positioned in the mid-urethra, urethral resistance drops from 90 to 58 cm H_2O at capacity.

of bladder capacity is only accurate for children older than 2 years of age. Bladder capacity has been measured in newborns and infants up to 2 years and a formula for determining capacity devised—capacity (ml) = 7.0 × weight (kg) (Fairhurst et al). Again, the rate of infusion is set at 10 per cent of the calculated capacity.

It has been shown that more rapid filling rates may yield falsely low levels of detrusor compliance and minimize uninhibited contractions (Joseph and Duggan; Turner-Warwick). In an attempt to avoid this problem, one fills the bladder slowly with saline warmed to 37°C. When it is important to determine very mild degrees of hypertonicity, even slower rates of filling are employed. During filling, it is helpful to try to divert the child's attention by asking unrelated questions, reading him or her a story, or showing a video tape cartoon. If the

examiner wishes to elicit uninhibited contractions, the child is asked to cough (Mayo); alternatively, a cold solution may be instilled at a rapid rate.

The study is not considered complete unless the child urinates and the voiding pressures are measured. The small size of the urodynamic catheter does not seem to adversely affect the micturition pressures, even in very young children. The normal voiding pressure in boys varies between 55 and 80 cm H_2O, and between 30 and 65 cm H_2O in girls (Blaivas, 1979a; Blaivas et al, 1977b; Gierup et al). Sometimes it is difficult to get the child to void; patience and a great deal of time are needed to accomplish this. Placing a bedpan under the buttocks, if the child is supine, or dripping tepid water on the genital area will often stimulate the child sufficiently to begin

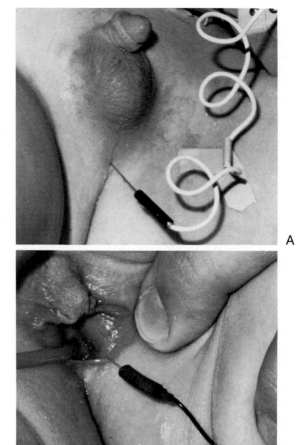

Figure 13–3 □ *A*, Placement of the electromyography (EMG) electrode in the male perineum. *B*, The EMG electrode in the female is inserted paraurethrally. In both sexes, the needle is advanced until the external sphincter muscle is reached as judged by the sound output and oscilloscopic picture on the EMG amplifier.

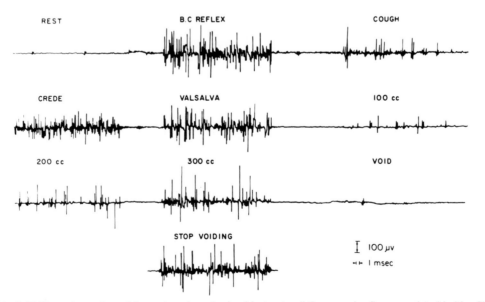

Figure 13–4 □ Normal reaction of the external urethral sphincter to all the sacral reflexes and to bladder filling and emptying.

urinating. Having the child listen to the audio channel of the EMG amplifier machine while he or she tightens and relaxes the sphincter provides a means of biofeedback training to encourage voiding. Once the child has voided, analyzing the pressure curve to see if it is sustained until voiding is complete, determining if abdominal pressure has been used to facilitate the emptying process, monitoring both intravesical and intraurethral pressures to see if there is any increased resistance to flow, listening to the change in EMG activity of the sphincter, noting the flow rate characteristics and voided volume, and observing for aftercontractions are all important factors. When voiding actually begins, the child is asked to stop urinating to determine how strongly he or she can block the micturition reflex.

It has been demonstrated convincingly that CO_2 cystometry does not give results comparable to water cystometry, especially during voiding (Gleason et al, 1977). Carbon dioxide, being a gas, exhibits a property common to all gases; when pressure is applied, its volume contracts. Therefore, it is difficult to measure a detrusor contraction accurately with CO_2 because a damping effect is produced from the diminishing volume of the gas. In addition, it is painful to void out the gas, and the sensation is foreign to children. Oftentimes they stop voiding as a result. Therefore the use of CO_2 is relegated to those babies whose urethra will only accept a 5 Fr. feeding tube, with filling

and pressure monitoring occurring through the solitary channel.

It is often appropriate to see the effects of drug administration, and so studies are repeated under similar circumstances several weeks to months later. This is especially true when one is trying to treat detrusor hypertonicity medically. To determine the maximal effect of most drugs, their usual dose is taken 2 to 3 hours before the test is performed a second time. The most commonly used drugs that affect lower urinary tract function are listed in Table 13–2 along with their appropriate dosage ranges.

CLASSIFICATION OF NEUROPATHIC BLADDER

The classification of neuropathic bladder dysfunction used in this chapter is that which has been adopted by the Urology Section of the American Academy of Pediatrics in conjunction with the Urodynamic Society's classification.

Under normal conditions, all portions of the lower urinary tract (detrusor, bladder neck, and external sphincter mechanism) function as a coordinated unit for adequate storage and efficient evacuation of urine. When a neurourologic lesion exists, these components usually fail to act in unison. A classification has been adopted based on dysfunction of a specific area

Table 13–2 □ Drug Therapy in Neuropathic Bladder Dysfunction

Type	Minimum Dosage	Maximum Dosage
Cholinergic		
Bethanechol (Urecholine)	0.7 mg/kg t.i.d.	0.8 mg/kg q.i.d.
Anticholinergic		
Propantheline (Pro-Banthine)	0.5 mg/kg b.i.d.	0.5 mg/kg q.i.d.
Oxybutynin (Ditropan)	0.2 mg/kg b.i.d.	0.2 mg/kg q.i.d.
Glycopyrrolate (Robinul)	0.01 mg/kg b.i.d.	0.03 mg/kg t.i.d.
Hyoscyamine (Levsin)	0.03 mg/kg b.i.d.	0.1 mg/kg q.i.d.
Sympathomimetic		
Phenylpropanolamine (alpha)	2.5 mg/kg b.i.d.	2.5 mg/kg t.i.d.
Ephedrine (alpha)	0.5 mg/kg b.i.d.	1.0 mg/kg t.i.d.
Pseudoephedrine (alpha)	0.4 mg/kg b.i.d.	0.9 mg/kg t.i.d.
Sympatholytic		
Prazosin (alpha) (Minipress)	0.05 mg/kg b.i.d.	0.1 mg/kg t.i.d.
Phenoxybenzamine (alpha)	0.3 mg/kg b.i.d.	0.5 mg/kg t.i.d.
Propranolol (beta)	0.25 mg/kg b.i.d.	0.5 mg/kg b.i.d.
Smooth Muscle Relaxant		
Flavoxate (Urispas)	3.0 mg/kg b.i.d.	3.0 mg/kg t.i.d.
Dicyclomine (Bentyl)	0.1 mg/kg t.i.d.	0.3 mg/kg t.i.d.
Other		
Imipramine (Tofranil)	0.7 mg/kg b.i.d.	1.2 mg/kg t.i.d.

of the vesicourethral unit rather than on a specific etiology (Table 13–3).

Improper storage may be related to an alteration in detrusor function or an inadequate urethral closure mechanism. The bladder may have increased tone secondary to loss of elasticity of the muscle, overactivity from excessive or unopposed sympathetic discharges, or hyperreflexia due to a central nervous system lesion above the sacral cord (see Figs. 13–12 and 13–22) that prevents the normal inhibitory centers from influencing the sacral reflex arc. Incontinence may occur with any one of these conditions despite a normal level of resistance in the bladder neck and urethra. Alternatively, incontinence may occur when the bladder neck and external sphincter areas do not provide adequate resistance during filling of the bladder or do not generate a reciprocal increase in outflow resistance as abdominal pressure is raised (see Fig. 13–23). An injury to the spinal cord or nerve roots affecting the sympathetic, parasympathetic, or sacral somatic nervous systems may alter both bladder neck and urethral tone. Periodic relaxation of the external urethral sphincter during filling of the bladder, the result of loss of central nervous system inhibition, may also lead to urinary incontinence (see Fig. 13–27).

Incomplete evacuation of the bladder may be due to a hypoactive or an areflexic detrusor muscle. Central nervous system lesions affecting the parasympathetic efferents may be responsible. However, nonsynchronous relaxation of the bladder neck or external sphincter area mechanisms (dyssynergia) (Fig. 13–5) resulting from a lesion in the central nervous system above the sacral cord—e.g., the pontine center or the cerebral cortex—can produce a similar effect. Myogenic failure occurs as the detrusor muscle hypertrophies and then decompensates owing to persistent outflow resistance (see Fig. 13–29A). Eventually, this mechanism may produce an overflow type of incontinence.

In general, medical treatment of neuropathic bladder dysfunction is based on the functional impairment produced by the specific neurourologic defect (see Table 13–2). Inadequate storage capacity may be enhanced by lowering detrusor tone or abolishing uninhibited contractions with anticholinergic medication, such as oxybutynin, glycopyrrolate, hyoscyamine, or propantheline. These drugs block cholinergic receptor sites in the detrusor muscle, diminishing its tone and suppressing involuntary contractions of the bladder. Other drugs, for example, flavoxate, act directly on the smooth muscle cells and lower detrusor tone without affecting contractility. Failure of drug therapy to increase bladder capacity and lower detrusor tone results in the need for subtotal cystectomy and augmentation cystoplasty to enhance bladder storage capability. This procedure is satisfactory as long as outflow resistance is normal or increased.

If inadequate urethral resistance is the primary reason for impaired storage of urine, the bladder neck mechanism or the external sphincter area, or both, may be responsible. Alpha-sympathomimetic agents, such as ephedrine sulfate, pseudoephedrine, and phenylpropanolamine, stimulate receptors in the bladder neck area to enhance the tone of the muscles in this region. No drugs are commercially available that will increase the tone of denervated skeletal muscle in the external sphincter region.

Incomplete emptying of the bladder may also be due to an areflexic bladder, unsustained detrusor contractions, or uncoordinated activity at the bladder neck or external sphincter area. Emptying may be facilitated by cholinergic drugs, such as bethanechol chloride or alpha-sympatholytic agents, or skeletal muscle relaxants. Although conflicting reports have been published regarding the efficacy of bethanechol, it does seem to improve emptying of the bladder in most instances. It should be

---

Table 13–3 □ Functional Classification of Vesicourethral Dysfunction

Storage
Detrusor Tone
Normal
Increased
    Nonelastic
    Overactive
    Hyperreflexic
    Decreased
Urethral Closing Mechanism
Incompetent
    Bladder neck
    External sphincter
    Nonreciprocal
    Periodic hypoactivity

Evacuation
Detrusor Contraction
Normoactive
Underactive
    Areflexic (nonreactive)
    Hypoactive (unsustained)
Urethral Closing Mechanism
Nonsynchronous
    Bladder neck
    External sphincter

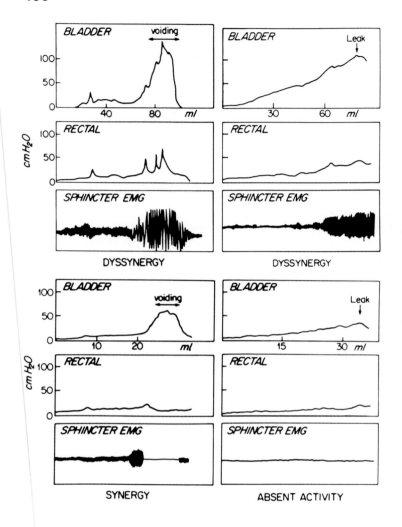

Figure 13–5 □ Various patterns of urodynamic findings in newborns with myelodysplasia. Note that a hypertonic detrusor with a nonrelaxing sphincter is also labeled dyssynergy. (From Bauer SB: Early evaluation and management of children with spina bifida. *In* Urologic Surgery in Neonates and Young Infants. Edited by LR King. Philadelphia, WB Saunders Co, 1988, pp 252–264.)

administered with alpha-sympatholytic agents because bethanechol also increases urethral resistance at the bladder neck. Alpha-sympathomimetic agents such as phenoxybenzamine or prazosin act primarily in the bladder neck area, whereas diazepam and baclofen diminish skeletal muscle tone at the external sphincter region to lower outlet resistance to voiding.

Most neurologic conditions affecting vesicourethral function in children, including myelomeningocele, lipomeningocele, sacral agenesis, and occult lesions, are congenital neurospinal dysraphisms (Table 13–4). Occasionally, bladder dysfunction is seen in conjunction with other neurologic lesions. Cerebral palsy is an acquired nonprogressive form of dysfunction occurring in the perinatal period as a consequence of cerebral anoxia from a variety of conditions. Other traumatic causes of spinal cord or cerebral dysfunction resulting

Table 13–4 □ Etiologic Classification of Vesicourethral Dysfunction

Neuropathic	Neuropathic (cont.)
Spinal Cord	***Peripheral***
Congenital	Trauma
Neurospinal dysraphism	Tumor
Other anatomic	Degenerative
Acquired	Guillain-Barré syndrome
Trauma	
Tumor	**Non-neuropathic**
Infection	Anatomic
Vascular	Myopathic
Miscellaneous	Psychological
Supraspinal Cord	Endocrinologic
Anatomic/congenital	Toxic
Trauma	
Tumor	
Infection	
Vascular	
Degenerative	
Miscellaneous	
Temporary	

in neuropathic bladder are rare and are not dealt with in any detail in this chapter. Indications for evaluation, however, are proposed for each specific type of dysfunction.

Children without obvious neurologic disease may have a voiding abnormality on a functional or maturational basis. Most children gain urinary control before age 5. Persistent day and night incontinence without a prolonged period of dryness or the recurrence of wetting lasting into puberty are indications for urodynamic evaluation in neurologically normal children. Although an overwhelming number have normal findings, a significant percentage may have a dysfunctional voiding state. The types of abnormalities are discussed separately along with individual approaches to therapy.

NEUROSPINAL DYSRAPHISMS

Myelodysplasia

The most common etiology of neuropathic bladder dysfunction in children is secondary to abnormal spinal column development. Formation of the spinal cord and vertebrae begins about the 18th day of gestation. The canal closes in a caudal direction from the cephalad end, and is complete by 35 days. Although the exact mechanism causing a dysraphism is unknown at present, numerous factors have been implicated. The incidence has been reported to be 1 per 1000 births in the United States (Stein et al) but there has been a definite decrease in this occurrence in the last 10 years (Laurence). If spina bifida is already present in one member of a family, there is a 2 to 5 per cent chance of a second sibling being born with the same condition (Scarff and Fronczak). The incidence doubles when more than one family member has a neurospinal dysraphism (Table 13–5).

Pathogenesis

Myelodysplasia is an all-inclusive term used to describe the various abnormal conditions of the vertebral column that affect spinal cord function. More specific labels regarding each abnormality include the following:

- A *meningocele* occurs when just the meninges extend beyond the confines of the vertebral canal without any neural elements contained inside of it.

Table 13–5 □ Familial Risk of Myelodysplasia in the United States per 1000 Live Births

Relationship	Incidence (%)
General population	0.7–1.0
Mother with one affected child	30–50
Mother with two affected children	100
Patient with myelodysplasia	40
Mother older than 35 years	30
Sister of mother with affected child	10
Sister of father with affected child	3
Nephew who is affected	2

Adapted from Kroovand RL: Myelomeningocele. *In* Campbell's Urology, 5th ed. Edited by Walsh PC, et al. Philadelphia, WB Saunders Co, 1986.

- A *myelomeningocele* implies that neural tissue, either nerve roots and/or portions of the spinal cord, have evaginated with the meningocele.
- A *lipomyelomeningocele* denotes that fatty tissue has developed with the cord structures and both are protruding into the sac.

Myelomeningocele accounts for over 90 per cent of all the open spinal dysraphic states (Stark). Most spinal defects occur at the level of the lumbar vertebrae, with the sacral, thoracic and cervical areas affected in decreasing order of frequency (Table 13–6) (Bauer et al, 1977). An overwhelming number of meningoceles are directed posteriorly, but on rare occasions, the meningocele may protrude anteriorly, particularly in the sacral area. Usually the meningocele is made up of a flimsy covering of transparent tissue, but it may be open and leaking cerebrospinal fluid. For this reason, urgent repair is necessary, with sterile precautions being followed in the interval between birth and closure. In 85 per cent of affected children there is an associated Arnold-Chiari malformation, in which the cerebellar tonsils have herniated down through the foramen magnum, obstructing the fourth ventricle and preventing the cerebrospinal fluid from

Table 13–6 □ Spinal Level of Myelomeningocele

Location	Incidence (%)
Cervical–high thoracic	2
Low thoracic	5
Lumbar	26
Lumbosacral	47
Sacral	20

Adapted from Kroovand RL: Myelomeningocele. *In* Campbell's Urology, 5th ed. Edited by Walsh PC, et al. Philadelphia, WB Saunders Co, 1986.

entering the subarachnoid space surrounding the brain and spinal cord.

The neurologic lesion produced by this condition can be quite variable. It depends on what neural elements, if any, have everted with the meningocele sac. The bony vertebral level often gives little or no clue as to the exact neurologic level or lesion that is produced. The height of the bony level and the highest extent of the neurologic lesion may vary from one to three vertebrae in one direction or another (Bauer et al, 1977). There may be differences in function from one side of the body to the other at the same neurologic level, and from one neurologic level to the next, as a result of asymmetry of affected neural elements. In addition, 20 per cent of affected children have a vertebral bony or intraspinal abnormality occurring more cephalad from the vertebral defect and meningocele, which can affect function in those additional portions of the cord as well. Children with thoracic and upper lumbar meningoceles often have complete reconstitution of their spine in the sacral area and these individuals will frequently have intact sacral reflex arc function involving the sacral spinal roots. In fact, it is more likely for children with upper thoracic or cervical lesions to have just a meningocele and no myelocele. Finally, the differential growth rates between the vertebral bodies and the elongating spinal cord add a factor of dynamicism in the developing fetus that further complicates the picture. Superimposed on all this is the Arnold-Chiari malformation that may have profound effects on the brain stem and pontine center, which are involved in the control over lower urinary tract function.

Thus, the neurologic lesion produced by this condition influences lower urinary tract function in a variety of ways and cannot be predicted just by looking at the spinal abnormality or the neurologic function of the lower extremities. Even careful assessment of the sacral area may not provide sufficient information to make a concrete inference. As a result, urodynamic evaluation in the neonatal period is now recommended at most pediatric centers in the United States because it not only provides a clear picture of the function of the sacral spinal cord and lower urinary tract but also has predictive value regarding babies at risk for future urinary tract deterioration and progressive neurologic change (Bauer et al, 1984; McGuire et al, 1981; Sidi et al, 1986; VanGool et al).

Newborn Assessment

Ideally, it would be best to perform urodynamic testing immediately after the baby is born, but the risk of spinal infection and the exigency for closure has not made this a viable option at this time. In a 1990 study, however, preoperative testing was accomplished, and it showed that less than 5 per cent of children experience a change in their neurologic status as a result of the spinal canal closure (Kroovand et al). Therefore, renal ultrasonography and a measurement of residual urine are performed as early as possible after birth, either prior to or immediately after the spinal defect is closed, with urodynamic studies delayed until it is safe to transport children to the urodynamic suite and place them on their back or side for the test. For infants who cannot empty their bladder following a spontaneous void or with a Credé maneuver, intermittent catheterization is begun, even before urodynamic studies are conducted. If a Credé maneuver is effective in emptying the bladder, it is performed instead of CIC on a regular basis. The normal bladder capacity in the newborn period is between 10 and 15 ml; thus, an acceptable residue of urine is less than 5 ml. Other tests that should be performed in the neonatal period include a urine analysis and culture, and determination of serum creatinine level.

Once the spinal closure has healed sufficiently, either excretory urography or renal ultrasonography and renal scintigraphy are performed to reassess upper urinary tract architecture and function. Following this, voiding cystourethrography and a urodynamic study are conducted. These studies fulfill several objectives (Bauer, 1984b; Bauer et al, 1984; McGuire et al, 1981; Sidi et al, 1986):

- They provide baseline information about the radiologic appearance of the upper and lower urinary tract, as well as the condition of the sacral spinal cord and the central nervous system.
- The studies can then be compared with later assessments, so that early signs of deteriorating urinary tract drainage and function, or of progressive neurologic denervation, can be detected.
- They help to identify babies at risk for urinary tract deterioration as a result of detrusor hypertonicity or outflow obstruction from detrusor sphincter dyssynergy,

which then allows prophylactic measures to be initiated before the changes actually take place.

- They help the physician to counsel parents with regard to their child's future bladder and sexual function.

Findings

Ten to 15 per cent of newborns have an abnormal radiologic appearance to their urinary tract when first evaluated (Bauer, 1985); 3 per cent have hydroureteronephrosis secondary to spinal shock, probably from the closure procedure (Chiaramonte et al), whereas 10 per cent have abnormalities that developed in utero as a result of abnormal lower urinary tract function in the form of outlet obstruction.

Urodynamic studies in the newborn period have shown that 57 per cent of infants with myelomeningocele have bladder contractions. This is especially true in children with upper lumbar or thoracic lesions who have sparing of the sacral spinal cord, 83 per cent of whom have detrusor contractions (Keating et al). Forty-three per cent have an areflexic bladder; compliance during bladder filling is either good (25 per cent) or poor (18 per cent) in this subgroup (Bauer et al, 1984). Electromyographic assessment of the external urethral sphincter demonstrates an intact sacral reflex arc with no evidence of lower motor neuron denervation in 47 per cent of newborns, whereas partial denervation is seen in 24 per cent, and complete loss of sacral cord function is noted in 29 per cent (Spindel et al).

Combining bladder contractility and external sphincter activity results in three categories of lower urinary tract dynamics: synergic; dyssynergic, with and without detrusor hypertonicity; and complete denervation (see Fig. 13–5) (Bauer et al, 1984; Sidi et al, 1986). Dyssynergy occurs when the external sphincter fails to decrease, or actually increases its activity during a detrusor contraction or a sustained increase in intravesical pressure, as the bladder is filled to capacity (Blaivas et al, 1986). Frequently, a poorly compliant bladder with high intravesical pressure is seen in conjunction with a dyssynergic sphincter, resulting in a bladder that empties only at high intravesical pressures (Sidi et al, 1986; VanGool et al). Synergy is characterized by complete silencing of the sphincter during a detrusor contraction or when capacity is reached at the end of filling. Voiding pressures are usually within the

normal range. Complete denervation is noted when no bioelectric potentials are detectable in the region of the external sphincter at any time during the micturition cycle or in response to a Credé maneuver or sacral stimulation.

Categorizing lower urinary tract function in this way has been extremely useful because it has defined which children are at risk for urinary tract changes, who should be treated prophylactically, who needs close surveillance, and who can be followed at greater intervals. Seventy-one per cent of newborns with dyssynergy had, on initial assessment or subsequent studies, urinary tract deterioration within the first 3 years of life, whereas only 17 per cent of synergic children and 23 per cent of completely denervated individuals developed similar changes (Fig. 13–6). The infants in the synergic group who deteriorated did so only after they converted to a dyssynergic pattern of sphincter function. Among the infants with complete denervation, the only babies who deteriorated were those who had elevated levels of urethral resistance, presumably due to fibrosis of the skeletal muscle component of the external sphincter. Thus, it appears that outlet obstruction is a major contributor to the development of urinary tract deterioration in

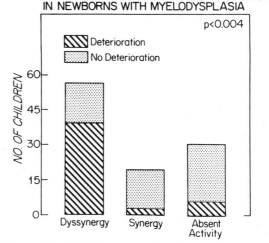

URINARY TRACT CHANGES IN RELATION TO EXTERNAL URETHRAL SPHINCTER FUNCTION IN NEWBORNS WITH MYELODYSPLASIA

Figure 13–6 □ Urinary tract deterioration is related to outflow obstruction and most often associated with dyssynergy. Children with synergy converted to dyssynergy and patients with complete denervation developed fibrosis with a fixed high-outlet resistance in the external sphincter, before any changes occurred in the urinary tract. (From Bauer SB: Early evaluation and management of children with spina bifida. *In* Urologic Surgery in Neonates and Young Infants. Edited by LR King. Philadelphia, WB Saunders Co, 1988, pp 252–264.)

these children (Fig. 13–7). Bladder tonicity plays an important but somewhat less critical role in this regard (McGuire et al, 1981), although detrusor compliance seems to be worse in children with high levels of outlet resistance (Ghoniem et al). Recently, Bloom and associates noted an improvement in compliance when outlet resistance was lowered following gentle urethral dilation in these children; however, the reasons for this are unclear and the long-term effect of this maneuver remains uncertain.

Recommendations

Because expectant treatment has revealed that infants with outlet obstruction in the form of detrusor-sphincter dyssynergy are at considerable risk for urinary tract deterioration, the idea of prophylactically treating the children has emerged as an important alternative. When CIC is begun in the newborn period, it becomes easy for parents to master, even in uncircumcised boys, and for children to accept as they grow older (Joseph et al). Complications of meatitis, epididymitis, or urethral injury are rarely encountered, and urinary infection occurs in less than 30 per cent (Kasabian et al).

Clean intermittent catheterization alone or in combination with anticholinergic agents, when detrusor filling pressures are greater than 40 cm H_2O and voiding pressures reach levels higher than 80 to 100 cm H_2O, has resulted in only an 8 to 10 per cent incidence of urinary tract deterioration (Geraniotis et al; Kasabian et al). This represents a significant drop in the occurrence of detrimental changes when compared with the group of children followed expectantly (Bauer et al, 1984; McGuire et al, 1981; Sidi et al, 1986). Oxybutynin hydrochloride is administered in a dose of 1.0 mg per year of age, every 12 hours in order to help lower detrusor filling pressure. In neonates or children younger than 1 year of age, the dose is lowered to below 1.0 mg in relation to the child's age at the time and increased proportionately as he or she approaches 1 year. Side effects have not manifested themselves when oxybutynin has been administered according to this schedule (Joseph et al; Kasabian et al). When a hyperreflexic or hypertonic bladder fails to respond to these measures, a cutaneous vesicostomy may need to be performed (Fig. 13–8) (Duckett; Mandell et al).

Neurologic Findings and Recommendations

Although it has been suspected for a long time, it has not been well documented until recently that the neurourologic lesion in myelodysplasia is a dynamic disease process with changes taking place throughout childhood (Epstein; Reigel; Venes and Stevens), especially in early infancy (Spindel et al), and then

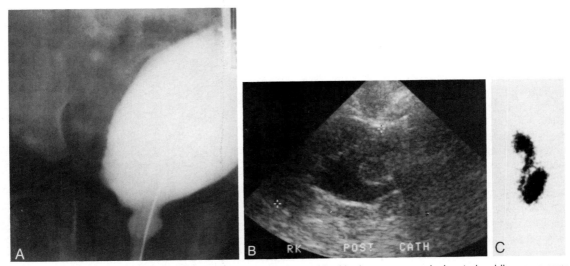

Figure 13–7 □ *A,* A voiding cystourethrogram in a newborn girl with dyssynergy and elevated voiding pressures demonstrates no reflux and a smooth-walled bladder. Her initial renal echogram was normal. She was started on clean intermittent catheterization and oxybutynin (Ditropan) but did not respond. Within 1 year, she had right hydronephrosis *(B)* and severe reflux on a radionuclide cystogram *(C).*

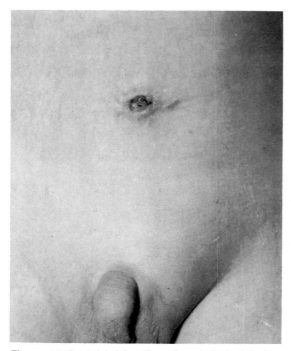

Figure 13–8 □ Administration of oxybutynin failed to lower bladder filling and detrusor contractile pressures in a 6-month-old boy with a myelomeningocele and detrusor sphincter dyssynergy. Because his lower ureters showed increasing dilation on ultrasonography and a poor response to medication in lowering intravesical pressure, a vesicostomy was performed. The dome of the bladder is brought through the anterior abdominal wall midway between the umbilicus and pubis.

at puberty (Begger et al), when the linear growth rate accelerates again. When a change is noted on neurologic, orthopedic, or urodynamic assessment, radiologic investigation of the central nervous system often reveals (1) tethering of the spinal cord, (2) a syrinx or hydromyelia of the cord, (3) increased intracranial pressure due to a shunt malfunction, or (4) partial herniation of the brain stem and cerebellum. Children with completely intact or only partially denervated sacral cord function are particularly vulnerable to progressive changes. Today, magnetic resonance imaging (MRI) is the test of choice because it reveals beautiful anatomic details of the spinal column and central nervous system. However, it is not a functional study, and when used alone, it cannot provide exact information with regard to a changing neurologic lesion.

Sequential urodynamic testing on a yearly basis beginning in the newborn period and continuing until 5 years of age provides the means for carefully following these children to detect signs of change, thus offering the hope that early detection and neurosurgical intervention may help to arrest or even reverse a progressive pathologic process. Changes occurring in a group of newborns followed in this manner involved both the sacral reflex arc as well as the pontine-sacral reflex interaction (Fig. 13–9) (Spindel et al). Most children who change tend to do so in the first 3 years of life (Fig. 13–10). Seven of 15 children who exhibited a worsening in their neurologic picture underwent a second neurosurgical procedure. Most had a beneficial effect from the surgery, with 4 of these 7 showing improvement in urethral sphincter function (Spindel et al).

As a result of these developments, all babies with myelodysplasia should be observed according to the guidelines set forth in Table 13–7. It is not enough to look at just the radiologic appearance of the urinary tract; critical scrutiny of the functional status of the lower urinary tract is important as well. In addition to the reasons cited above, it may be necessary to repeat a urodynamic study when the upper urinary tract dilates secondary to impaired drainage from a hypertonic detrusor.

Management of Reflux

Vesicoureteral reflux occurs in 3 to 5 per cent of newborns with myelodysplasia, usually in association with detrusor hypertonicity and/or dyssynergia. It is rare to find reflux in any neonate with a spinal cord lesion without dyssynergy or poor compliance (Bauer 1984a; Geraniotis et al). If left untreated, the incidence of reflux in these at-risk infants increases with time until 30 to 40 per cent are afflicted by 5 years of age (Bauer, 1984a).

In children with reflux, grades I to III (international classification), who void spontaneously or who have complete lesions with little or no outlet resistance and empty their bladder completely, management consists of antibiotic prophylaxis to prevent recurrent infection. When these children have high-grade reflux, grade IV or V, intermittent catheterization is begun to ensure complete emptying. Children who cannot empty their bladder spontaneously, regardless of the grade of reflux, are catheterized intermittently to ensure complete emptying. Children with detrusor hypertonicity, with or without hydroureteronephrosis, are also treated with oxybutynin to lower intravesical pressure and ensure adequate upper urinary tract decompression. When reflux has been managed in this manner, a dramatic response has resulted, with reflux

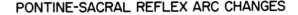

PONTINE-SACRAL REFLEX ARC CHANGES

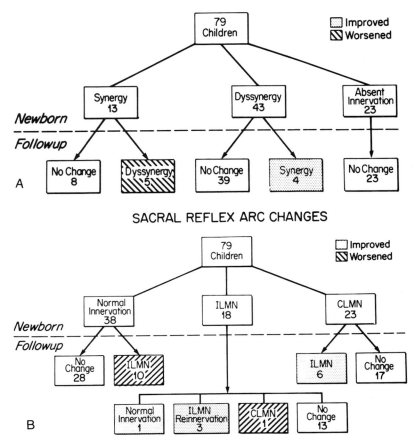

Figure 13–9 ☐ The changes in innervation of the pontine-sacral *(A)* and purely sacral *(B)* reflex arc pathways that occurred in a group of children with myelodysplasia followed with sequential urodynamic studies between the newborn period and a subsequent time. ILMN, incomplete lower motor neuron lesion; CLMN, complete lower motor neuron lesion. (From Bauer SB: Early evaluation and management of children with spina bifida. *In* Urologic Surgery in Neonates and Young Infants. Edited by LR King. Philadelphia, WB Saunders Co, 1988, pp 252–264.)

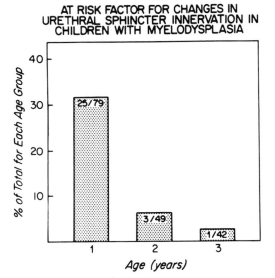

Figure 13–10 ☐ The propensity for a change in urethral sphincter innervation is greatest in the first year of life. (From Bauer SB: Early evaluation and management of children with spina bifida. *In* Urologic Surgery in Neonates and Young Infants. Edited by LR King. Philadelphia, WB Saunders Co, 1988, pp 252–264.)

resolving in 30 to 55 per cent of individuals (Bauer, 1984a; Joseph et al; Kass et al). Although bacteriuria can be seen in as many as 56 per cent of children on intermittent catheterization, generally it is not harmful except in the presence of high-grade reflux because symptomatic urinary infection and renal scarring rarely occur with the lesser grades of reflux (Kass et al).

Credé voiding is to be avoided in children with reflux, especially those with a reactive external sphincter. Under these conditions, the Credé maneuver results in a reflex response in the external sphincter that increases urethral resistance and raises the pressure needed to expel urine from the bladder (Fig. 13–11) (Barbalias et al). This has the effect of aggravating the degree of reflux and accentuating the water hammer effect of regurgitation on the kidneys. Vesicostomy drainage (Duckett; Mandell et al) is reserved for (1) those infants who have such severe reflux that intermittent catheterization and anticholinergic medication fail to improve upper urinary tract drainage,

Table 13–7 ☐ Surveillance in Infants with Myelodysplasia*

Sphincter Activity	Recommended Tests	Frequency
Intact—synergic	Post-voiding residual	Every 4 months
	IVP or renal echo	Every 12 months
	UDS	Every 12 months
Intact—dyssynergic†	IVP or renal echo	Every 12 months
	UDS	Every 12 months
	VCUG or RNC‡	Every 12 months
Partial denervation	Post-voiding residual	Every 4 months
	IVP or renal echo	Every 12 months
	UDS§	Every 12 months
	VCUG or RNC‡	Every 12 months
Complete denervation	Post-voiding residual	Every 6 months
	Renal echo	Every 12 months

*Until age 5.
†Patients on intermittent catheterization and anticholinergic agents.
‡If detrusor hypertonicity or reflux already present.
§Depending on degree of denervation.
Abbreviations: IVP, intravenous pyelography; echo, sonography; UDS, urodynamic study; VCUG, voiding cystourethrography; RNC, radionuclide cystography.

or (2) those whose parents cannot adapt to the catheterization program.

The indications for antireflux surgery today are not very different from those for children with normal bladder function and include re-current symptomatic urinary infection while on adequate antibiotic therapy and appropriate catheterization techniques, persistent hydro-ureteronephrosis despite effective emptying of the bladder and lowering of intravesical pres-

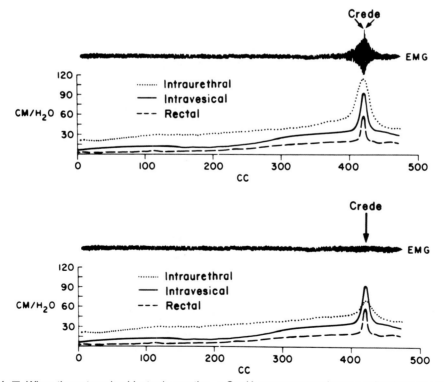

Figure 13–11 ☐ When the external sphincter is reactive, a Credé maneuver produces a reflex increase in electromyo-graphic (EMG) activity of the sphincter and a concomitant rise in urethral resistance, resulting in high "voiding" pressure. A child whose sphincter is denervated and nonreactive will not have a corresponding rise in EMG activity, urethral resistance, or "voiding" pressure. A Credé maneuver here will not be detrimental. (From Bauer SB: Early evaluation and management of children with spina bifida. *In* Urologic Surgery in Neonates and Young Infants. Edited by LR King. Philadelphia, WB Saunders Co, 1988, pp 252–264.)

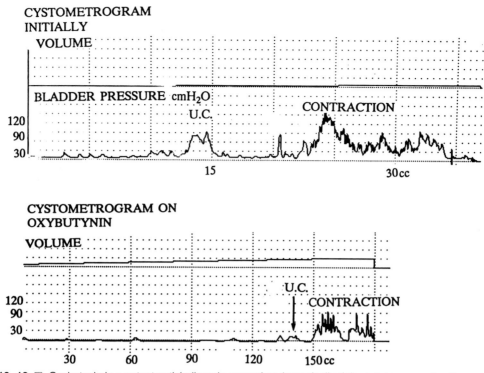

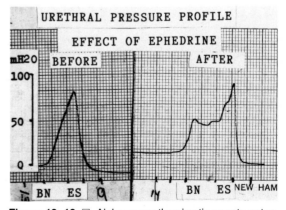

Figure 13–12 □ Oxybutynin is a potent anticholinergic agent that dramatically delays detrusor contractions and lowers contraction pressure, as demonstrated on these two graphs from a 6-month-old girl with myelodysplasia. U.C., uninhibited contraction.

sure, severe reflux with an anatomic abnormality at the ureterovesical junction, and reflux persisting into puberty. In addition, children with any grade of reflux who are being considered for implantation of an artificial urinary sphincter or any other procedure designed to increase bladder outlet resistance should have the reflux corrected at the time or prior to the anti-incontinence surgery.

Jeffs and colleagues noted that antireflux surgery could be very successful in children with neuropathic bladder dysfunction as long as it is combined with measures to ensure complete bladder emptying. Before this observation was made, the results of ureteral reimplantation were so dismal that most physicians treating these children advocated urinary diversion as a means of managing their reflux (Cass; Smith). Since the advent of intermittent catheterization, success rates for antireflux surgery have approached 95 per cent (Bauer et al, 1982; Kaplan and Firlit; Kass et al; Woodard et al).

Continence

Urinary continence is becoming an increasingly important issue to deal with at an early age as parents try to mainstream their handicapped children. Initial attempts at achieving continence include CIC and drug therapy designed to maintain a low intravesical pressure and a reasonable level of urethral resistance (Figs. 13–12 and 13–13). Although this approach can be conducted on a trial-and-error basis, it is more efficient to have exact treat-

Figure 13–13 □ Alpha-sympathomimetic agents potentially have their greatest effect in the bladder neck region, where the highest concentration of alpha receptor sites exist. They can raise outlet resistance and improve continence in many individuals.

ment protocols based on specific urodynamic findings. As a result, urodynamic testing is performed if initial attempts with CIC and oxybutynin fail to achieve continence. Without urodynamic studies, it is hard to know whether (1) a single drug is effective, (2) the drug dosage should be increased, or (3) a second drug should be added to the regimen.

At this point, if detrusor hypertonicity or uninhibited contractions have not been dealt with effectively (see Table 13–2), another anticholinergic agent may be combined with or given instead of the oxybutynin. Although glycopyrrolate is the most potent oral anticholinergic drug available today, it may have the typical belladonna-like side effects common to all these drugs. Hyoscyamine, although less effective, seems to produce fewer side effects.

If urodynamic testing reveals that urethral resistance is inadequate to maintain continence because there is either a failure of the sphincter to react to increases in abdominal pressure or a drop in resistance with bladder filling (see Fig. 13–2B), then alpha-sympathomimetic agents are added to the regimen (see Table 13–2); phenylpropanolamine is the most effective drug in this regard.

Surgery becomes a viable option when this program fails to achieve continence. In general, this alternative is not undertaken until the child is about 5 years of age and ready to start school. Persistent hypertonicity and/or hyperreflexia may be treated with either enterocystoplasty (Mitchell and Piser; Sidi et al, 1987) or autoaugmentation (Cartwright and Snow, 1989a, 1989b). First, sigmoid, then cecum, and lastly, small intestine have been used to enlarge the bladder. Although the ileocecal segment is a favored source for bladder replacement in adults, it is avoided here because removing it might aggravate the bowel dysfunction so often a factor in these children already. Detubularization of the bowel is needed to minimize intrinsic contractions of the intact segment, which may cause intractable incontinence once it has been added to the bladder (Goldwasser et al, Hinman, 1988). More recently, gastrocystoplasty has been advocated when considering a bowel augment because it has fewer intrinsic contractions, provides an acid milieu, and is free of mucus secretions, which can lead to repeated urinary infection (Adams et al).

If bladder neck or urethral resistance is insufficient to allow for an adequate storage capability, several operations are available to improve this continence mechanism. Bladder neck reconstruction can be undertaken in a variety of ways, including the Young-Dees (Dees; Young) or Leadbetter (Leadbetter) procedures, or the operation described by Kropp (Kropp and Angwafo). Fascial sling operations to suspend the bladder neck and buttress it up against the undersurface of the pubis have been advocated with enthusiasm by several individuals (McGuire et al, 1986; Peters et al; Raz et al). Each of these operations necessitates the use of CIC to empty the bladder postoperatively. The artificial sphincter (Barrett and Furlow; Light et al) also increases bladder outlet resistance while its mechanism of opening allows for emptying at low urethral pressures. Any person who could empty his or her bladder before the device was implanted should be able to do so afterwards without the need for CIC. Because long-term results with the artificial sphincter are lacking (Bosco et al), many people do not yet consider this to be a viable alternative for children.

Diversion and Undiversion

Urinary diversion, once considered a panacea for children with myelodysplasia, has turned out to be a Pandora's box of new clinical problems (Schwarz and Jeffs; Shapiro et al). Pyelonephritis and renal scarring, calculi, ureterointestinal obstruction, strictures of the conduit, and stomal stenosis are problems often encountered in children who are followed on a long-term basis. Although antirefluxing colon conduits seem to have fewer complications, they are still not ideal. There have been very successful attempts to undivert the urinary tract in children who probably would not have had a diversion performed today (Hendren, 1973, 1976). Few children, if any, are undergoing urinary diversion now; if they are, it is in the form of a continent stoma.

Several operations have been devised, but the ones that have achieved the most publicity are the Kock pouch in adults (Kock; Skinner et al) and the Indiana reservoir in children (Rowland et al). Mitrofanoff created a continence mechanism by tunneling one end of the vermiform appendix into the bladder just as one would reimplant the ureter to prevent reflux, with the other end being brought to the skin as a catheterizable stoma (Mitrofanoff). This principle has been extended to the ureter, which is transected at approximately the pelvic brim. Following this, a proximal transureteroureterostomy is performed, while the cut end of the distal segment is brought to the skin as a stoma (Duckett and Snyder); again, the continence mechanism is provided for by the intramural tunnel of the ureter. Other narrow structures, i.e., Fallopian tube, a rolled strip of stomach, or a tapered ileal segment, have been implanted either into the native bladder or along the tinea of a detubularized portion of sigmoid or cecum acting as a urinary reservoir (Bihrle et al; Riedmiller et al; Woodhouse et al). The success rate for achieving continence has been excellent primarily as a result of the flap valve effect of the intramural tunnel (Hinman, 1990) and the active peristalsis of the conduit itself (Tutrone et al).

Sexuality

Sexuality in this population is becoming an increasingly important issue to deal with as more and more individuals are reaching adulthood and wanting either to marry or to have meaningful long-term relationships with the opposite sex (Cromer et al). Investigators are looking into the concerns, fears, and desires of emerging teenagers and the ability of males to procreate and females to bear children. Few studies are available, however, that critically look at sexual function in these patients.

In one study, researchers interviewed a group of teenagers and reported that at least 28 per cent of them had one or more sexual encounters, and almost all had a desire to marry and ultimately bear children (Cromer et al). Another study revealed that 70 per cent of myelodysplastic women were able to become pregnant and have an uneventful pregnancy and delivery, although urinary incontinence in the latter stages of gestation and cesarean section were common (Cass et al). In the same study, 17 per cent of males claimed they were able to father children. It is more likely for males to have problems with erectile and ejaculatory function because of the frequent neurologic involvement of the sacral spinal cord, whereas reproductive function in the female, which is under hormonal control, is not affected.

As important as knowing what the precise sexual function is in an individual, sexuality or the ability to interact with the opposite sex in a meaningful and lasting way is just as important. Until recently, however, this subject was not addressed. Sexual identity, education, and social mores are issues that have been taken out of the realm of secrecy and are now openly discussed and taught to handicapped people. Boys reach puberty at an age similar to that for normal males, whereas breast development and menarche tend to start as much as 2 years earlier than usual in myelodysplastic females. The etiology of this early hormonal surge is uncertain, but it may be related to pituitary function changes in girls secondary to their hydrocephalus (Hayden).

Lipomeningocele and Other Spinal Dysraphisms

Diagnosis

A group of congenital defects affect the formation of the spinal column but do not result in an open vertebral canal (Table 13–8) (James and Lassman). These lesions may be very subtle with no obvious outward signs, but in more than 90 per cent of cases, the children manifest a cutaneous abnormality overlying the lower spine (Anderson). This may vary from a small dimple or skin tag to a tuft of hair, a dermal vascular malformation, or a very noticeable subcutaneous lipoma (Fig. 13–14). In addition, on careful inspection of the legs, one may note a high arched foot or feet; alterations in the configuration of the toes, with hammer or claw digits being seen; a discrepancy in muscle size and strength between the legs with weakness at the ankle; and/or a gait abnormality, especially in older children, as a result of shortness of one leg (Dubrowitz et al; Weissert et al). Absent perineal sensation and back pain are not uncommon symptoms in older children or young adults (Linder et al; Weissert et al; Yip et al). Lower urinary tract function is abnormal in 40 per cent of affected individuals (Mandell et al). The child may experience difficulty with toilet training, urinary incontinence after an initial period of dryness once toilet training

Table 13–8 □ Types of Occult Spinal Dysraphisms

Lipomeningocele
Intradural lipoma
Diastematomyelia
Tight filum terminale
Dermoid cyst/sinus
Aberrant nerve roots
Anterior sacral meningocele
Cauda equina tumor

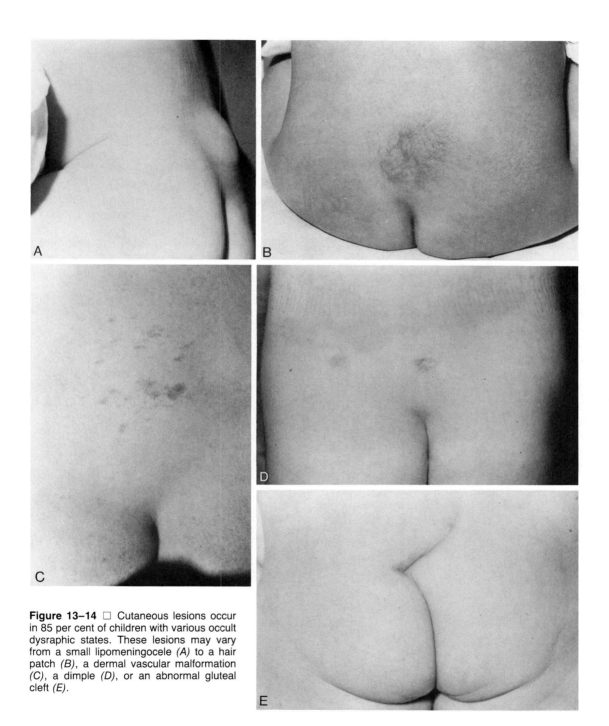

Figure 13–14 □ Cutaneous lesions occur in 85 per cent of children with various occult dysraphic states. These lesions may vary from a small lipomeningocele (A) to a hair patch (B), a dermal vascular malformation (C), a dimple (D), or an abnormal gluteal cleft (E).

has been mastered (especially during the pubertal growth spurt), recurrent urinary infection, and/or fecal soiling.

Findings

When these children are evaluated in the newborn or early infancy period, the majority have a perfectly normal neurologic examination. Urodynamic testing, however, will reveal abnormal lower urinary tract function in about one third of the babies younger than the age of 1½ years (Fig. 13–15) (Keating et al). In fact, these studies may provide the only evidence for a neurologic injury involving the lower spinal cord (Foster et al; Keating et al). When present, the most likely abnormality is an upper motor neuron lesion characterized by detrusor hyperreflexia and/or hyperactive sacral reflexes, with mild forms of detrusor-sphincter dyssynergy being noted rarely. Lower motor neuron signs with denervation potentials in the sphincter, or detrusor areflexia, occur in only 10 per cent of young children.

In contrast, practically all individuals in the group older than 3 years of age who have not been operated on or have been belatedly diagnosed as having an occult dysraphism will have either an upper motor neuron and/or lower motor neuron lesion on urodynamic testing (92 per cent) (Figure 13–15), or neurologic signs of lower extremity dysfunction (Keating et al; Kondo et al; Yip et al). There does not seem to be a preponderance for one type of lesion over the other (upper versus lower motor neuron); each occurs with equal frequency, and often the child manifests signs of both (Hellstrom et al; Kondo et al).

Pathogenesis

The reason for this difference in neurologic findings may be related to (1) compression on the cauda equina or sacral nerve roots by an expanding lipoma or lipomeningocele (Yamada et al, 1983), or (2) tension on the cord from tethering secondary to differential growth rates between the bony and neural elements (Dubrowitz et al). Under normal circumstances, the conus medullaris ends just below the L-2 vertebra at birth and should recede upward to T-12 by adulthood (Barson). When the cord does not "rise" secondary to one of these lesions, ischemic injury may ensue (Yamada et al, 1981). Correction of the lesion in infancy has resulted in not only stabilization but improvement in the neurologic picture in some instances (Fig. 13–16). Sixty per cent of the babies with abnormal urodynamic findings preoperatively reverted to normal postoperatively, with improvement noted in 30 per cent, whereas 10 per cent worsened with time. In the older child, there is a less dramatic change following surgery, with only 27 per cent becoming normal, 27 per cent improving, 27 per cent stabilizing, but 19 per cent actually worsening with time (Fig. 13–16) (Keating et al). Older individuals with hyperreflexia tend to improve, while those with areflexic bladders do not (Flanigan et al; Hellstrom et al; Kondo et al). Finally, less than 5 per cent of the children operated on in early childhood developed secondary tethering when observed for several years, suggesting that early surgery has both a beneficial and sustaining effect with these conditions.

As a result of these findings, it is apparent that urodynamic testing may be the only way to document that an occult spinal dysraphism

OCCULT SPINAL DYSRAPHISM

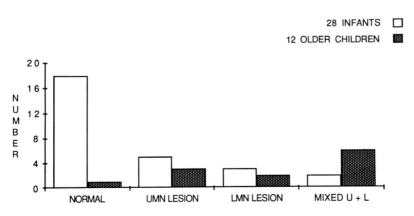

28 INFANTS □
12 OLDER CHILDREN ■

Figure 13–15 □ Most newborns with a covered spinal dysraphism have normal lower urinary tract function, whereas older children tend to have both upper and lower motor neuron lesions. UMN, upper motor neuron; LMN, lower motor neuron; U+L, upper and lower motor neuron.

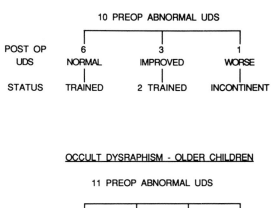

OCCULT DYSRAPHISM - INFANTS

10 PREOP ABNORMAL UDS

POST OP UDS	6 NORMAL	3 IMPROVED	1 WORSE
STATUS	TRAINED	2 TRAINED	INCONTINENT

OCCULT DYSRAPHISM - OLDER CHILDREN

11 PREOP ABNORMAL UDS

POST OP UDS	3 NORMAL	3 IMPROVED	3 STABLE	2 WORSE

1 NORMAL REMAINED SO

Figure 13–16 □ The potential for recoverable function is greatest in infants (6 of 10 [60 per cent]) and less in older children (3 of 11 [27 per cent]). The risk of damage to neural tissue at the time of exploration to those with normal function is small (2 of 19 [11 per cent], not shown).

is actually affecting lower spinal cord function (Keating et al; Khoury et al). Some investigators have shown that posterior tibial somatosensory evoked potentials are even a more sensitive indicator of tethering and should be an integral part of the urodynamic evaluation (Roy et al). The implication of this recommendation is that early detection and intervention are associated with both a reversibility to the lesion that is lost in the older aged child (Kaplan et al; Tami et al; Yamada et al, 1981, 1983) and a degree of protection from subsequent tethering, which seems to be a frequent occurrence when the lesion is not dealt with expeditiously in infancy (Seeds and Jones).

Recommendations

Consequently, in addition to MRI (Tracey and Hanigan), urodynamic testing should be conducted in everyone who has a questionable skin or bony abnormality of the lower spine (Campobasso et al; Hall et al; Packer et al). If the child is younger than 4 to 6 months of age, ultrasonography may be useful to image the spinal canal before the vertebral bones have had a chance to ossify (Raghavendra et al; Scheible et al). In the past, these conditions were usually treated by removing only the superficial skin lesions without delving further

into the spinal canal to remove or repair the entire abnormality. Today, most neurosurgeons advocate laminectomy and removal of the intraspinal process as completely as possible without injuring the nerve roots or cord, in order to release the tethering and to prevent further injury that occurs with subsequent growth (Foster et al; Kaplan et al; Kondo et al; Linder et al).

Sacral Agenesis

Sacral agenesis has been defined as absence of part or all of two or more lower vertebral bodies. Although the etiology of this condition is still uncertain, teratogenic factors may play a role inasmuch as insulin-dependent mothers have a 1 per cent chance of giving birth to a child with this disorder. In addition, 16 per cent of children with sacral agenesis have a diabetic mother (Guzman et al; Passarge and Lenz). The mothers often may have only gestational, insulin-dependent diabetes. Sacral agenesis has been reproduced in chicks when exposed as embryos to insulin (Landauer; White and Klauber). Maternal insulin-antibody complexes have been noted to cross the placenta; their concentration in the fetal circulation directly correlated with macrosomia (Menon et al). It is possible that a similar cause-and-effect phenomenon is occurring in sacral agenesis.

Diagnosis

The diagnosis is often delayed until failed attempts at toilet training bring the child to the attention of a physician. Sensation, including perianal dermatomes, is usually intact, and lower extremity function is normal (Jakobson et al; Koff and DeRidder). Because these children have normal sensation and little or no orthopedic deformity involving the lower extremities (although high arched feet and/or claw or hammer toes may be present), the underlying lesion is often overlooked. In fact, 20 per cent of children escape detection until age 3 or 4, when parents begin to question their ability to train their child (Guzman et al). The only clue, requiring a high index of suspicion, is flattened buttocks and a low short gluteal cleft (Fig. 13–17) (Bauer). Palpation of the coccyx will detect the absent vertebrae (White and Klauber). The diagnosis is most easily confirmed with a lateral film of the lower

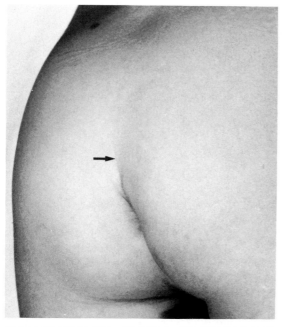

Figure 13–17 □ Characteristically, the gluteal crease is short and seen only inferiorly (below *arrow*) as a result of the flattened buttocks in sacral agenesis.

spine, because this area is often obscured by the overlying gas pattern on an anteroposterior projection (Fig. 13–18) (Guzman et al; White and Klauber). MRI has been used to visualize the spinal cord in these cases; a sharp cutoff of the conus opposite the T-12 vertebra seems to be a consistent finding (Fig. 13–19).

Urodynamic Findings

When urodynamic studies are undertaken, almost an equal number of individuals will manifest an upper or lower motor neuron lesion (35 per cent versus 40 per cent, respectively), whereas 25 per cent have no signs of denervation at all (Guzman et al). The upper motor neuron lesion is characterized by detrusor hyperreflexia, exaggerated sacral reflexes, absence of voluntary control over sphincter function, detrusor-sphincter dyssynergy, and no electromyographic evidence of denervation potentials in the urethral sphincter (Guzman et al; Koff and DeRidder; White and Klauber).

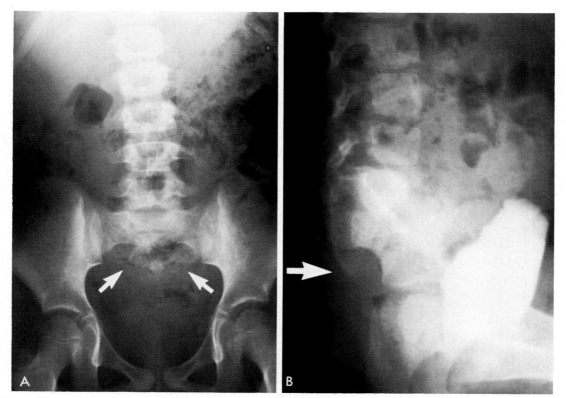

Figure 13–18 □ The diagnosis is easily confirmed on an anteroposterior *(A)* or lateral *(B)* film of the spine (the latter is performed if bowel gas obscures the sacral area).

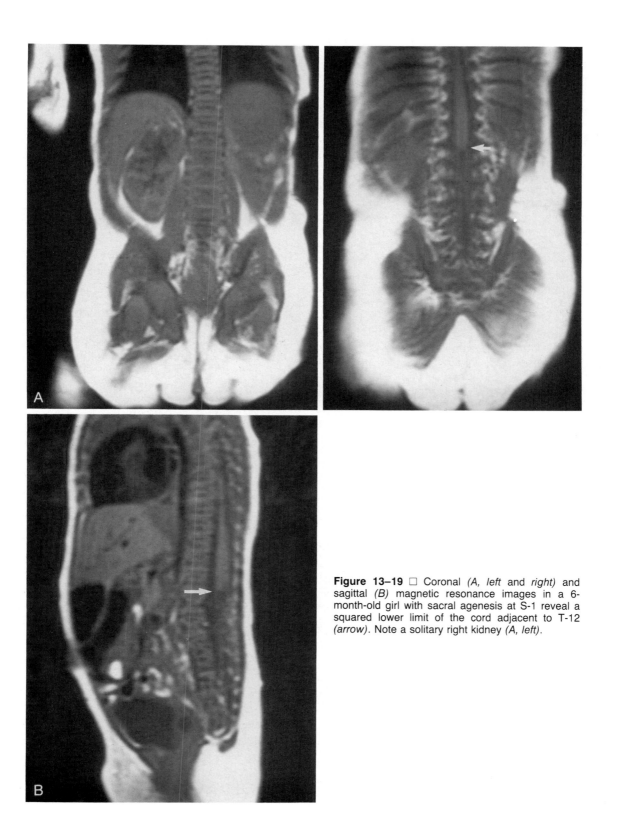

Figure 13–19 □ Coronal *(A, left* and *right)* and sagittal *(B)* magnetic resonance images in a 6-month-old girl with sacral agenesis at S-1 reveal a squared lower limit of the cord adjacent to T-12 *(arrow)*. Note a solitary right kidney *(A, left)*.

A lower motor neuron lesion is noted when detrusor areflexia and partial or complete denervation of the external urethral sphincter with diminished or absent sacral reflexes are seen. The number of affected vertebrae does not seem to correlate with the type of motor neuron lesion present (Fig. 13–20). The lesion usually appears to be stable without signs of progressive denervation.

Recommendations

Management depends on the specific type of neurourologic dysfunction seen on urodynamic testing. Anticholinergic agents should be given to those children with upper motor neuron findings of uninhibited contractions, whereas intermittent catheterization and alpha-sympathomimetic medication may need to be initiated in individuals with lower motor neuron deficits who can neither empty their bladder nor stay dry between catheterizations. The bowel manifests a similar picture of dysfunction and needs as much characterization and treatment as the lower urinary tract. It is important to identify these individuals as early as possible so they can be rendered continent and out of diapers at an appropriate age, thus avoiding the social stigmata of fecal and/or urinary incontinence.

Associated Conditions

Imperforate Anus

Imperforate anus is a condition that can occur alone or as part of a constellation of anomalies that has been called the VATER or VACTERL syndrome (Barry and Auldist).

This mnemonic stands for all the organs that possibly can be affected (V = Vertebral, A = Anal, C = Cardiac, TE = Tracheo-Esophageal fistula, R = Renal, L = Limb). Urinary incontinence is not common unless the spinal cord is involved or the pelvic floor muscles and/or nerves are injured during the imperforate anus repair. A plane film of the abdomen and an ultrasonographic scan of the spine and kidneys are obtained in the neonatal period in all children regardless of the level of the rectal atresia, once the child has either stabilized or has had a colostomy performed (Karrer et al; Tunnell et al). Vertebral bony anomalies often signify an underlying spinal cord abnormality. Because the vertebral segments have not fully calcified at this time, ultrasonography can readily image the spinal cord. Any hint of an abnormality on these studies or the presence of a lower midline skin lesion overlying the spine warrants MRI to delineate any pathologic intraspinal process (Fig. 13–21) (Barnes et al). If the radiologic images demonstrate an abnormality, urodynamic studies are conducted in the first few months of life. Urodynamic studies are also indicated prior to repair in the child with a high imperforate anus who has undergone an initial colostomy. Abnormal findings may provide a reason to explore and treat any intraspinal abnormality in order to improve the child's chances at becoming continent of both feces and urine; in addition, they furnish a baseline for comparison, especially if incontinence should become a problem in the future, particularly in those children needing extensive repair of their imperforate anus.

Electromyographic studies of the perianal musculature at this time help to define the optimal location of the future anus. Before the

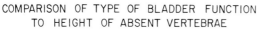

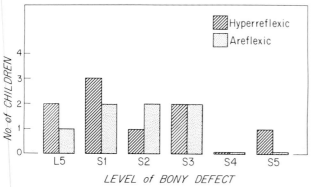

COMPARISON OF TYPE OF BLADDER FUNCTION TO HEIGHT OF ABSENT VERTEBRAE

Figure 13–20 □ Bladder contractility is unrelated to the number of absent vertebrae.

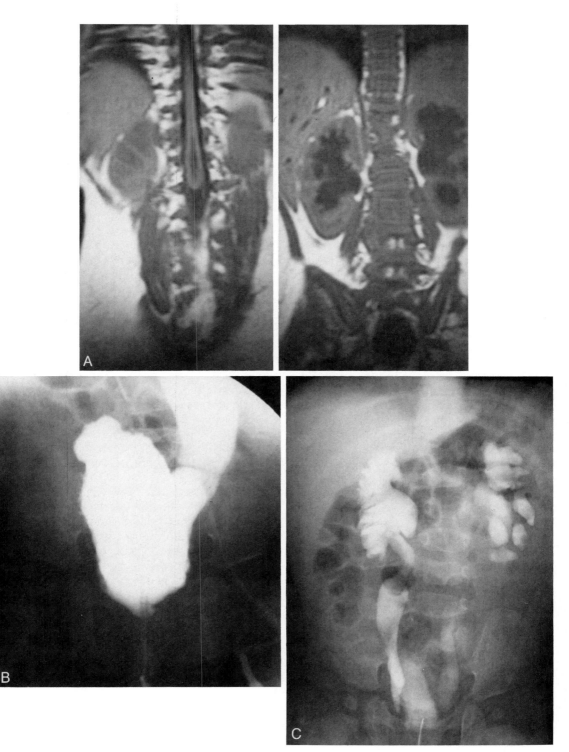

Figure 13–21 □ *A, Right* and *Left,* This 1-year-old girl with an imperforate anus and bony vertebral abnormalities has bilateral hydronephrosis and a tethered cord on this MRI scan. *B,* Her voiding cystourogram reveals significant trabeculation and reflux on the left, whereas her excretory urogram *C* demonstrates bilateral hydronephrosis secondary to the reflux on the left and a ureterovesical junction obstruction on the right. Her urodynamic study manifested detrusor hypertonicity and dyssynergy.

Peña operation, which utilizes a posterior midline approach, was developed to correct high imperforate anus, rectal incontinence was thought to be due to an injury involving the pelvic nerves that innervate the levator ani muscles (Parrott and Woodard; Peña; Williams and Grant). Because the dissection is confined to the midline area, this procedure has reduced the chance of traumatizing the nerve fibers that course laterally and around the bony pelvis from the spine to the sphincter muscles. Urodynamic and perianal EMG studies are repeated after the imperforate anus repair, if fecal and/or urinary continence has not been achieved by a reasonable age or if incontinence develops secondarily.

Thirty to 45 per cent of these children have a spinal abnormality even though they may not have any other associated anomalies (Carson et al; Uehling et al). This abnormality may range from tethering of the spinal cord secondary to an intraspinal dysraphism, which produces an upper motor neuron type of dysfunction involving the bladder and external urethral sphincter (see Fig. 13–21), to an atrophic abnormality of the conus medullaris, which leads to a partial or complete lower motor neuron lesion involving the lower urinary tract (Greenfield and Fera). In these circumstances, urinary and fecal incontinence might be the child's only complaints. Because lower extremity function may be totally normal, an examination of the legs alone can be misleading (Carson et al). In one review, 20 per cent of children with neuropathic bladder dysfunction and imperforate anus had a normal bony spine, suggesting that postnatal spinal ultrasonography should be performed in all newborns with imperforate anus (Sheldon et al).

CENTRAL NERVOUS SYSTEM INSULTS

Cerebral Palsy

Etiology

Cerebral palsy is a nonprogressive injury to the brain in the perinatal period that produces a neuromuscular disability or a specific symptom complex of cerebral dysfunction. Its incidence is approximately 1.5 per 1000 births but may be increasing as more smaller and younger premature infants are surviving in intensive care units. It is usually due to a perinatal infection or period of anoxia (or hypoxia) that affects the central nervous system (Naeye et al; Nelson and Ellenberg). It most commonly appears in babies who were premature, but it may be seen following a seizure, infection, or intracranial hemorrhage in the neonatal period.

Diagnosis

Affected children have delayed gross motor development, abnormal fine motor performance, altered muscle tone, abnormal stress gait, and exaggerated deep tendon reflexes. These findings can vary substantially from being very obvious to exquisitely subtle with no discernible lesion present unless a careful neurologic examination is performed. Among the more overtly affected individuals, spastic diplegia is the most common of the five types of dysfunction that characterize this disease, accounting for nearly two thirds of the cases.

Findings

Most children with cerebral palsy develop total urinary control. Incontinence is a feature in some, but the exact incidence has never been truly determined (Decter et al; McNeal et al). The presence of incontinence is not related to the extent of the physical impairment, although the physical handicap may prevent the individual from getting to the bathroom before he or she has an episode of wetting. A number of children have such a severe degree of mental retardation that they are not trainable, but the majority have sufficient intelligence to learn basic societal protocol with patient and persistent handling. Oftentimes, continence is achieved at a later than expected age. Therefore, urodynamic evaluation is reserved for children who appear trainable and do not seem to be hampered too much by their physical impairment, but who have not achieved continence by late childhood or early puberty.

One review reports on urodynamic studies that were performed in 57 children with cerebral palsy (Table 13–9) (Decter et al). Forty-nine (86 per cent) presented the expected picture of a partial upper motor neuron lesion type of dysfunction, with exaggerated sacral reflexes, detrusor hyperreflexia and/or detrusor-sphincter dyssynergia (Fig. 13–22), even though they manifested voluntary control over

Table 13–9 □ Lower Urinary Tract Function in Cerebral Palsy*

Type of Dysfunction	No. (%)
Upper motor neuron lesion	49 (86)
Mixed upper and lower motor neuron lesion	5 (9.5)
Incomplete lower motor neuron lesion	1 (1.5)
No urodynamic lesion	2 (3)

*Study included 57 children.

Table 13–10 □ Urodynamic Findings in Cerebral Palsy*

Finding	Number
Upper Motor Neuron	
Uninhibited contractions	35
Detrusor-sphincter dyssynergy	7
Hyperactive sacral reflexes	6
No voluntary control	3
Small-capacity bladder	2
Hypertonia	2
Lower Motor Neuron	
Excessive polyphasia	5
Increased amplitude and increased duration potentials	4

*Study included 57 children; some exhibited more than one finding.

voiding. Six of the 57 (11 percent), however, had evidence of both upper and lower motor neuron denervation with detrusor areflexia and/or abnormal motor unit potentials on sphincter electromyographic assessment (Table 13–10). When their records were analyzed on a retrospective basis, most of the children who exhibited these latter findings had experienced an episode of cyanosis in the perinatal period (Table 13–11). Thus, a lower motor neuron lesion may be seen in addition to the expected upper motor neuron dysfunction.

Recommendations

Treatment usually centers around abolishing the uninhibited contractions with anticholinergic medication, but residual urine volume must be monitored closely to ensure complete evacuation with each void. Intermittent catheterization may be required for those who cannot empty their bladder.

Traumatic Injuries to the Spine

Despite the exposure and potential for a traumatic spinal cord injury, this condition is rarely encountered in children. When an injury does occur, it is most likely to happen as a result of a motor vehicle accident, a gunshot wound, or a diving incident (Cass et al). It has also occurred iatrogenically following surgery to correct scoliosis, kyphosis, or other intraspinal processes as well as congenital aortic anomalies or patent ductus arteriosus (Cass et al). Newborns are particularly prone to hyperextension injuries during a high forceps delivery (Adams et al; Lanska et al). The lower urinary tract dysfunction that ensues is not likely to be an isolated event, but rather, it is usually associated with loss of sensation and paralysis of the lower limbs. Radiologic investigation of the spine may not reveal any bony abnormality even though momentary subluxation of osseous structures due to elasticity of vertebral ligaments can result in a neurologic injury (Pollack et al). Myelography and computed

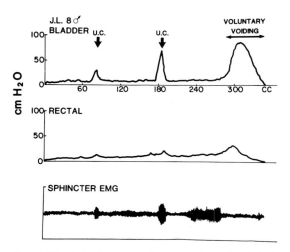

Figure 13–22 □ An 8-year-old boy with spastic diplegia has a typical partial upper motor neuron lesion–type bladder with uninhibited contractions (U.C.'s) associated with increased sphincter activity but normal voiding dynamics at capacity. Wetting is due to these contractions when unaccompanied by the heightened sphincter activity.

Table 13–11 □ Perinatal Risk Factors in Cerebral Palsy

Factor	UMN	LMN
Prematurity	10	1
Respiratory distress/arrest/apnea	9	2
Neonatal seizures	5	
Infection	5	
Traumatic birth	5	
Congenital hydrocephalus	3	
Placenta previa/abruption	2	2
Hypoglycemia with or without seizures	2	
Intracranial hemorrhage	2	
Cyanosis at birth	1	3
No specific factor noted	15	

Abbreviations: UMN, upper motor neuron lesion; LMN, lower motor neuron lesion.

tomography (CT) will show swelling of the cord below the level of the lesion (Adams et al; Lanska et al). Many times, what appears initially as a permanent lesion turns out instead to be a transient phenomenon. Although sensation and motor function in the lower extremities may be restored relatively soon, the dysfunction involving the bladder and rectum may persist for a considerable period of time.

If urinary retention occurs immediately following the injury, an indwelling Foley catheter is passed into the bladder and left in place for as short a period of time as possible, until intermittent catheterization can be started safely on a regular basis (Barkin et al; Guttmann and Frankel). When the child starts voiding again, the timing of catheterization can be such that it is used as a means of measuring the residual urine volume after a spontaneous void. Residual urine volumes of 25 ml or less are considered safe enough to allow for reduction of the frequency and even stopping the catheterization program (Barkin et al). After 2 to 3 weeks, however, if there is no improvement in lower urinary tract function, urodynamic studies are conducted to determine if this condition is the result of spinal shock or actual nerve root or spinal cord injury. Detrusor areflexia is not uncommon under these circumstances (Iwatsubo et al). On the other hand, electromyographic recording of the sphincter often reveals normal motor units without fibrillation potentials, but absent sacral reflexes and a nonrelaxing sphincter with bladder filling, a sign that transient spinal shock has occurred (Iwatsubo et al). The outcome from this condition is guarded but good, inasmuch as most cases resolve completely as edema of the cord in response to the injury subsides, leaving no permanent damage (Fanciullacci et al; Iwatsubo et al).

Most permanent traumatic injuries involving the spinal cord produce an upper motor neuron type lesion with detrusor hyperreflexia and detrusor-sphincter dyssynergia. The potential danger from this outflow obstruction is obvious (Donnelly et al). Substantial residual urine volumes, high pressure reflux, urinary infections, and their sequelae are the leading cause of long-term morbidity and mortality in spinal cord–injured patients. Urodynamic studies willl identify those patients at risk (Barkin et al). Early identification and proper management may prevent the signs and effects of outlet obstruction before they become apparent on x-ray examination of the urinary tract (Ogawa et al; Pearman).

FUNCTIONAL VOIDING DISORDERS

Enuresis is defined as inappropriate voiding at an age when urinary control is expected. It is difficult, however, to say when this should occur. Studies of large groups of children have provided some guidelines for expectations, but there are no absolute milestones for the individual child (Bellman; Fergusson et al). Girls tend to become trained before boys, and daytime continence is achieved before nighttime control. Although the possibility exists, it is rare to achieve control before 1 1/2 years of age (Yeats). From that time onward, urinary control is gained by approximately 20 per cent of children for each year of life up to 4 1/2, with a smaller percentage of the population attaining complete continence every year after that. By age 10, about 5 per cent of children still have some nocturnal wetting; this diminishes, however, to 2 per cent after puberty (MacKeith et al).

The evaluation of the incontinent child begins with a comprehensive history, including details of the mother's pregnancy and delivery, family history of enuresis, developmental milestones, school performance, fine and gross motor coordination, previous continence, social setting and sibling interaction, parental expectations, and characterization of the wetting episodes. If there is a suspicion of an ectopic ureter in a girl (someone who voids normally but is constantly damp both day and night), then excretory urography (preferably) or renal ultrasonography is performed. Boys who have a question of outflow obstruction (urgency or urge incontinence and enuresis beyond age 5) are evaluated by voiding cystography. The indications for performing urodynamic studies are as follows: any suspicion of a neurologic condition, diurnal incontinence with no associated pathology, nocturnal enuresis in a pubertal child who is resistant to conventional therapy, fecal and urinary incontinence at any age, persistent voiding difficulties long after a urinary infection has been treated, recurrent urinary infection despite continuous antibiotics, and bladder trabeculation and/or "sphincter spasm" on voiding cystography (Fig. 13–23).

When urodynamic studies are performed on a group of children who have these findings without an obvious neurologic or systemic disorder, a spectrum of voiding pattern abnormalities emerges (Table 13–12) (Bauer et al).

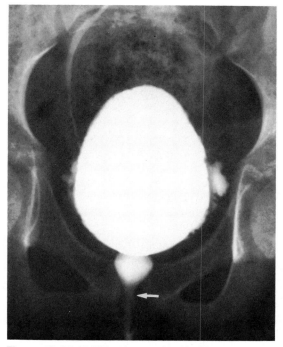

Figure 13–23 □ This 10-year-old girl with recurrent urinary tract infections has spasm of the sphincter during voiding with "narrowing" in the distal urethra demonstrated on the voiding cystourethrogram *(arrow)*. Note grade 2/5 right-sided reflux.

Classification and a detailed description of these disorders help one to understand and treat each condition specifically.

Small-Capacity Hypertonic Bladder

Children with recurrent urinary infection without an anatomic abnormality may have symptoms of voiding dysfunction, including frequency, urgency, urge incontinence, staccato voiding, nocturia and/or enuresis, and dysuria, long after the infection has cleared. Sometimes, persistence of these symptoms with their associated abnormal voiding dynamics can lead to repeated infections (Hansson et al).

An inflammatory reaction in the bladder

Table 13–12 □ Patterns of Voiding Dysfunction in Neurologically Normal Children

Small-capacity bladder
Detrusor hyperreflexia
Infrequent voider–lazy bladder syndrome
Psychologic non-neuropathic bladder (Hinman syndrome)

wall may produce an irritability that affects the sensory threshold and increases the need to void sooner than anticipated. If the detrusor muscle is affected as well, the increased irritability may lead to instability of the muscle and eventually to poor compliance (Mayo and Burns). When the child attempts to hold back urination because it is either painful or inappropriate to void, he or she may actually tighten or only partially or intermittently relax the external sphincter muscle during voiding, producing a form of outflow obstruction and disrupting the laminar flow pattern that normally exists (Fig. 13–24) (Hansson et al; Tanagho et al; VanGool and Tanagho). The stop-and-start voiding (Fig. 13–25) leads to recurrent infection because bacteria can be carried back up into the bladder from the meatus as a result of the "milk back" phenomenon occurring within the urethra when urination is interrupted in this manner (Webster et al). Theoretically, if unrecognized or left untreated in young girls, this may become the forerunner of interstitial cystitis seen in many adult females and may even be the precursor of prostatitis in males.

Radiologic investigation often reveals a normal upper urinary tract, but the bladder may be small and have varying degrees of trabeculation on routine excretory urography or a thickened wall on ultrasonography (Bauer et al; Lebowitz and Mandell). During the voiding phase of cystourethrography, the posterior urethra may show signs of intermittent dilatation at its upper end, with a uniform narrowing occurring toward the external sphincter region. In girls, this "spinning top" deformity has raised the question of an obstructed meatus (see Fig. 13–23) (Tanagho et al; VanGool and Tanagho), whereas in boys, it has often been mistaken for posterior urethral valves. This appearance is due to failure of complete relaxation of the external sphincter and persistence of a relative obstruction at the distal end of the posterior urethra in an attempt by the child to suppress voiding (Saxton et al).

Urodynamic studies demonstrate a bladder of small capacity (when adjusted for age) and elevated detrusor pressure during filling (Fig. 13–26) (Bauer et al; VanGool and Tanagho). At capacity, the child has an uncontrolled urge to void and sometimes cannot suppress urination, despite contracting the external sphincter. The bladder contraction is usually sustained, with pressures reaching higher than normal values. Emptying may not always be complete despite these high pressures. The

INTERMITTENCY

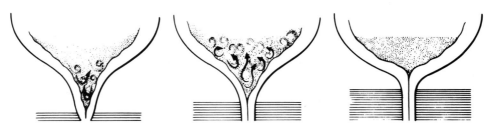

Figure 13–24 □ Nonlaminar flow secondary to periodic tightening and relaxation of the external sphincter leads to eddy currents and the "milk back" phenomenon, which can carry bacteria colonized at the urethral meatus up into the bladder and cause infection of the residual urine.

baseline sphincter EMG activity is normal at rest, but there may be complex repetitive discharges (pseudomyotonia) (Dyro et al) or periodic relaxation of the muscle during filling, contributing to the sense of urgency or actual incontinent episodes. During voiding, the sphincter may relax intermittently or even completely at first, but then contract in response to discomfort, preventing complete emptying (Fig. 13–26) (Hansson et al; Rudy and Woodside).

Treatment is based on trying to eliminate the recurrent infections, to minimize any possible environmental influences that predispose the individual to infection, and to improve both the child's voiding pattern and bathroom habits. Girls should learn to take showers instead of baths, or at least bathe alone without other siblings, to wipe from front to back, to

try to completely relax when they void so that a steady stream is produced, and to take the time to completely empty each time they urinate (Hansson et al). In some instances, biofeedback training to teach individuals to relax the sphincter when they void has been used with success (Masek).

In addition to antibiotics, antispas-

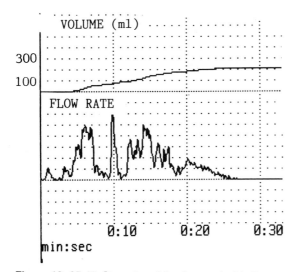

Figure 13–25 □ Staccato voiding is seen in this 8-year-old girl with recurrent infection.

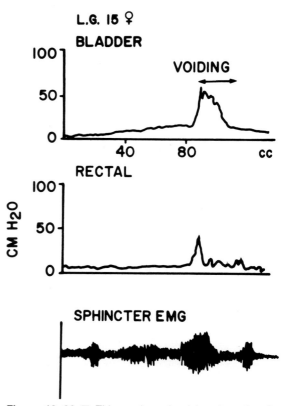

Figure 13–26 □ This urodynamic picture in a female teen-ager with recurrent infections reveals a small-capacity bladder and a hypertonic sphincter that relaxes only partially during voiding.

modic/anticholinergic agents (flavoxate, hyoscyamine, dicyclomine) are administered. On rare occasions when cystoscopy is performed, an intense inflammatory reaction may be noted in the trigone region, contributing to the symptomatology. If this reaction is present, fulguration of this area will prove beneficial in some children (personal observation).

Detrusor Hyperreflexia

Children with long-standing symptoms of daytime frequency, urgency, or sudden incontinence and squatting, in addition to nocturia and/or enuresis, may have detrusor hyperreflexia. Vincent's curtsy, a characteristic posturing by these children in an attempt to prevent voiding, is a commonly described behavior pattern (Kondo et al; Vincent). The child's parents or siblings often relate a personal history of delayed control over micturition. These affected family members may compensate for their own abnormality by displaying continued daytime frequency or nocturia, or both. Although the child's physical examination may be normal, hyperactive deep tendon reflexes in the lower and/or upper extremities, ankle clonus, posturing with a stress gait, or difficulty with tandem walking and mirror movements (similar motion in the contralateral hand when the individual is asked to rapidly pronate and supinate one hand) may be evident. Left-handedness, left-footedness, or left-eyedness in a family in which all other members are right-handed may signify crossed dominance from a previously unrecognized perinatal insult. Carefully questioning the parents about perinatal events or reviewing birth history records may uncover such an insult that has affected the central nervous system and caused these findings.

X-ray evaluation usually reveals no abnormality other than a mildly trabeculated or thick-walled bladder. Urodynamic studies demonstrate uninhibited contractions of the bladder during filling, which the child may or may not sense and/or abolish by increasing the activity of the external urethral sphincter (see Fig. 13–22) (Bauer et al; Rudy and Woodside). Alternatively, periodic relaxation of the sphincter, the initial phase of an uninhibited contraction, which leads to a sense of urgency or to an episode of leaking, may be the only clue to a hyperreflexic bladder (Fig. 13–27). During filling, capacity may be reached sooner than expected, at which time a normal detrusor

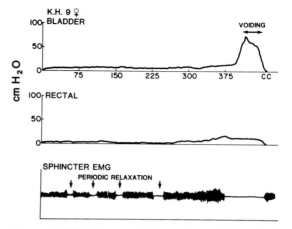

Figure 13–27 □ Some children only manifest periodic relaxation of the sphincter without a rise in detrusor pressure as an early phase of a hyperreflexic bladder producing urgency and incontinence.

contraction occurs with a sustained relaxation of the sphincter, resulting in complete emptying. Some children will not be able to suppress this contraction even though the bladder has not been filled to capacity. Sometimes, uninhibited contractions may only be elicited following a cough or strain, or when the child assumes a change in posture (Kondo et al). The uninhibited contractions are thought to be responsible for the symptoms (McGuire and Savastano).

These findings may be the result of a cerebral insult, however mild, in the neonatal period, but they are linked more commonly to delayed maturation of the reticulospinal pathways and the inhibitory centers in the midbrain and cerebral cortex. Thus, total control over vesicourethral function may be lacking (MacKeith et al; Mueller; Yeats). Several investigators have found a similar urodynamic picture in a significant number of adults with nocturnal enuresis and/or daytime symptoms (Torrens and Collins). Parents who exhibit the same behavior pattern as their children may have a genetically determined delayed rate of central nervous system maturation.

On occasion, children with profound constipation develop uninhibited contractions of the bladder and urinary incontinence secondary to them (O'Regan et al, 1985). The etiology of this condition is unclear, but treatment of the bowel distention has resulted in a dramatic improvement in the bladder dysfunction (O'Regan et al, 1986).

Sometimes, repeated urinary infection may produce an identical urodynamic picture. Detrusor hyperreflexia occurs as a result of the inflammatory response in the bladder wall that irritates the receptors located in the submucosa and/or detrusor muscle layers (Koff and Murtagh). Therefore, all these children should be screened for infection. It has been postulated that a hyperactive detrusor may lead to inappropriate voiding. When the child realizes what is happening, he or she tightens the sphincter to reverse this process, which shuts the distal urethra first and the bladder neck second, causing the "milk back" phenomenon and the potential for urinary infection, as presented in the previous discussion, to occur (Koff and Murtagh; Webster et al).

Anticholinergic medication (oxybutynin, propantheline, glycopyrrolate) and imipramine alone or in combination have been used successfully to manage this condition (Kondo et al). If infection is present, it should be eradicated and antibacterial prophylaxis should be employed (Bauer et al; Buttarazzi; Firlit et al; Kass et al; Mayo and Burns).

The Infrequent Voider–Lazy Bladder Syndrome

Most children urinate four to five times per day, and defecate daily or at least every other day. Some children, primarily girls, may void only twice a day, once in the morning (either at home or after they are in school), and again at night (DeLuca et al). It is not uncommon to find children who do not void at all while in school. These children exhibited normal voiding patterns as infants, but after toilet training, they learned to withhold micturition for extended periods of time. Their parents may have instilled in them, however unintentionally, the idea that it is bad to wet or soil themselves. As a result, a few develop a fear of strange bathrooms or mimic their mother's pattern of infrequent urination and defecation (Bauer et al). Others have experienced an aversive event or had an infection associated with dysuria around the time of training, which led to the infrequent pattern of micturition. Some children are excessively neat or have a fetish for cleanliness that causes them to avoid bathrooms. Often, they only void enough to relieve the pressure to urinate and do not empty their bladder completely.

The infrequent voiding and incomplete emptying produce an ever-increasing bladder capacity and a diminished stimulus to urinate (Webster et al). The chronically distended bladder is prone to urinary infection and/or overflow or stress incontinence. Sometimes, these signs are the first manifestations of the abnormal voiding pattern. When the child is carefully questioned, the aberrant micturition is easily detected. More often, the problem is diagnosed following voiding cystourethrography when a larger than normal capacity (for age) is noted and the residual urine volume on initial catheterization is measured, with the child being questioned afterwards about his or her voiding habits (Fig. 13–28 A, B) (Webster et al). The cystogram usually reveals a smooth-walled bladder without reflux.

Urodynamic studies demonstrate a very large capacity, highly compliant bladder with either normal, unsustained, or absent detrusor contractions (Fig. 13–29A) (Bauer et al). Straining to void is a common form of emptying. Sphincter EMG reveals normal motor unit potentials at rest and normal responses to various sacral reflexes, bladder filling, and attempts at emptying. The urinary flow rate may be intermittent, with sudden peaks coinciding with straining, or it may be normal but short lived, secondary to an unsustained detrusor contraction (Webster et al). Unless strongly encouraged, the child will not completely empty his or her bladder during voiding (Fig. 13–29B) (Bauer et al). This picture is consistent with myogenic failure from chronic distention (Koefoot et al).

Changing the child's voiding habits is the first approach to therapy. Keeping to a rigid schedule of toileting and encouraging the child to empty each time he or she voids are mandatory (Masek). Behavioral therapy techniques to encourage compliance are helpful. Occasionally, bethanechol chloride is administered to increase the sensitivity to regular voiding. Rarely, intermittent catheterization may be necessary to allow the detrusor muscle to regain its contractility and ability to empty. Antibiotics are needed when urinary infection is present; they are continued until the voiding pattern improves.

Psychological Nonneuropathic Bladder (Hinman Syndrome)

A group of children demonstrate an apparent "syndrome" of voiding dysfunction that mimics neuropathic bladder disease but that may be a learned disorder. At first, this syndrome was believed to be caused by an isolated neu-

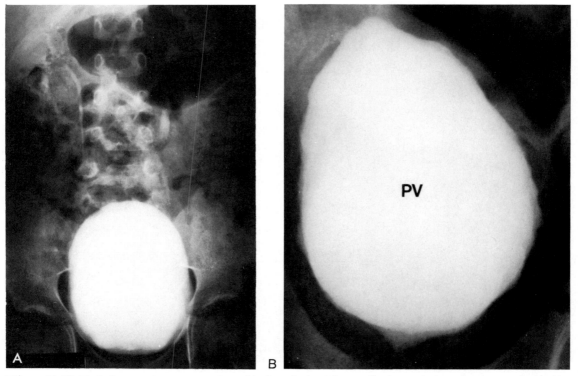

Figure 13–28 □ *A,* An excretory urogram in a girl who urinates infrequently demonstrates a large-capacity bladder with a normal upper urinary tract. *B,* Her post-voiding (PV) residual is quite large.

rologic lesion (Johnston and Farkas; Mix; Williams et al), but now it is felt to be an acquired abnormality (Allen; Allen and Bright; Bauer et al; Hinman, 1974). It is produced by an active contraction of the sphincter during voiding, creating a degree of outflow obstruction. Some investigators think that this phenomenon may be the result of persistence of the transitional phase of gaining control in which the child learns to prevent voiding by voluntarily contracting the external urethral sphincter (Allen; Rudy and Woodside), whereas others think that this pattern results from the child's normal response to uninhibited contractions (McGuire and Savastano). This behavior becomes habitual because the child has difficulty distinguishing between involuntary and voluntary voiding; as a consequence, the inappropriate sphincter activity occurs all the time (Bauer et al).

These children have urgency, urge and/or stress incontinence, infrequent voluntary voiding, intermittent urination associated with straining, recurrent urinary infection, and irregular bowel movements, with fecal soiling in between times (Bauer et al). Most striking is the similarity in the pattern of family dynamics that is disclosed on carefully observing and questioning the family (Table 13–13) (Allen and Bright). The parents, especially the father, tend to be domineering, exacting, unyielding, and intolerant of weakness or failure. Divorce and alcoholism are common threads that only exacerbate the situation. Wetting is perceived as immature, defiant, and purposeful behavior that the parents feel must be counteracted with stern reprimands. The children are often punished, both mentally and physically, for their ineptness. Confusion, depression, and withdrawal for fear of wetting with its added punitive response become the children's prevalent attitudes because they do not know how to nor can they prevent this provocative behavior. They try to withhold urination and defecation further by keeping the sphincter muscle tight, aggravating the situation. Thus, wetting becomes more commonplace, and abdominal pain from chronic constipation is likely.

X-ray evaluation reveals profound changes within the urinary tract. Hydroureteronephrosis with or without pyelonephritic scarring from recurrent infection occurs in two thirds of the children (Fig. 13–30 *A*) (Bauer et al). Fifty per

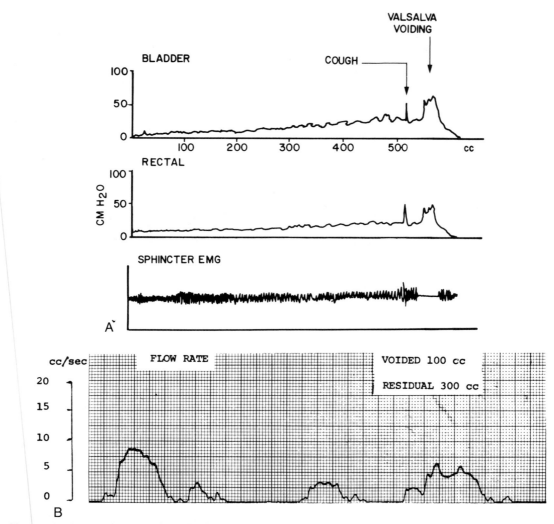

Figure 13–29 □ *A*, Urodynamic evaluation reveals a very-large-capacity, low-pressure bladder. She empties entirely by straining after relaxing the sphincter with no apparent detrusor contraction. EMG, electromyography. *B*, Her intermittent urinary flow rate is characteristic of this effort to empty and leads to a considerable volume of residual urine.

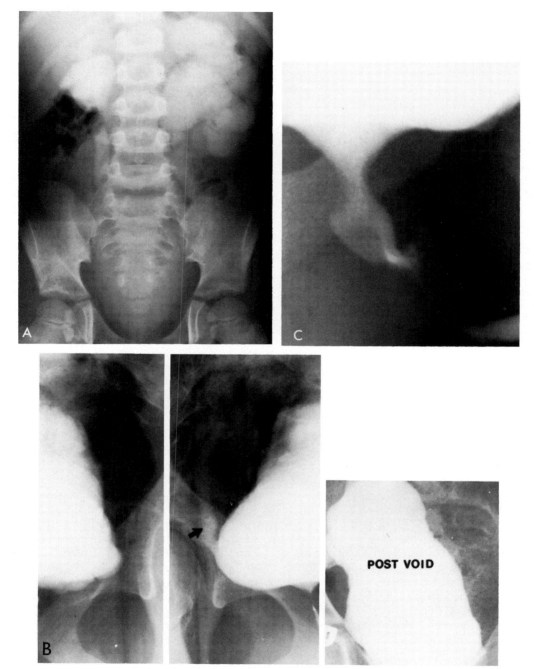

Figure 13–30 □ *A,* Excretory urogram in a 14-year-old male with day and nighttime incontinence and encopresis. Note the impression of faintly opacified distended bladder. *B,* His voiding cystourethrogram reveals trabeculation, mild right vesicoureteral reflux *(arrow),* and a large post-voiding residual urine volume. *C,* A film during voiding demonstrates intermittent relaxation of the external sphincter area.

Table 13–13 □ Psychological Non-neuropathic Bladder (Hinman Syndrome)

Clinical Features
Day and night wetting
Encopresis/constipation/impaction
Recurrent urinary tract infections
Parental characteristics
    Domineering/exacting
    Divorce
    Alcoholism
    Punishments (mental and physical) inflicted for wetting
Previous surgery
    Ureteral reimplantation
    Bladder neck plasty
    Diversion

Radiologic Features
Hydronephrosis, with or without pyelonephritis
Reflux: III/V in degree
Large-capacity, trabeculated bladder
Large residual volume
Posterior urethra sometimes dilated with narrowing at
    external sphincter
Heavily loaded colon

Urodynamic Features
Elevated detrusor and voiding pressures
Ineffective detrusor contractions
High resting sphincter electromyography
Unsustained sphincter relaxation during voiding
Large residual volume

Treatment—Individualized!
Bladder retraining
    Behavioral modification
    Double voiding
    Biofeedback techniques for sphincter relaxation
Drugs
    Oxybutynin
    Flavoxate
    Bethanechol
    Prazosin
    Diazepam
Bowel reregulation program
    Stool softeners
    Bulking agents
    Laxatives, enemas

cent have severe vesicoureteral reflux. Nearly every child has a grossly trabeculated, large-capacity bladder with a considerable post-voiding residual urine volume (Fig. 13–30B). Voiding films show either persistent or intermittent narrowing in the region of the external sphincter in almost half the children (Fig. 13–30C). Finally, the scout film from the excretory urogram displays considerable fecal material in the colon, consistent with chronic constipation.

Urodynamic studies demonstrate a large-capacity bladder with poor compliance, uninhibited contractions, and either high pressure or ineffective detrusor contractions during voiding (Fig. 13–31A) (Bauer et al; Kass et al). Sometimes, Valsalva voiding is needed to empty the bladder. The urinary flow rate is often intermittent as a result of the failure of the external sphincter to relax (Fig. 13–31B). The bethanechol supersensitivity test may be positive; in the past, it was this response that led to the belief that these children had neuropathic bladder dysfunction (Williams et al). EMG recordings, however, reveal normal external urethral sphincter innervation and exclude the possibility of a sacral spinal cord lesion. The sphincter fails to relax completely and may actually tighten episodically once voiding commences (Rudy and Woodside); this finding, along with the uninhibited contractions, suggests an upper motor neuron lesion, but usually, no other signs are present to confirm this urodynamic hypothesis. Recently, spinal canal imaging with magnetic resonance has failed to reveal any intraspinal process as a cause for the voiding dysfunction in these children (Hinman, 1986).

The dyssynergy created by the incoordination between the bladder and sphincter muscles leads to high voiding pressures initially and later, to ineffective detrusor contractions (Rudy and Woodside). Depending on which point of the spectrum one is at, a low or intermittent flow rate and either a minimal or significant post-voiding residual urine volume are noted.

Before this "syndrome" was recognized and the pathophysiology elucidated, many children underwent multiple operations to improve bladder emptying and correct vesicoureteral reflux. Failure of these procedures to succeed led to urinary diversion in a number of instances. Some of these individuals were eventually able to be undiverted at an older age after they outgrew the conditions that caused their dysfunction in the first place. Today, an entirely different approach is taken. Treatment is focused on improving the child's ability to empty the bladder and bowel and alleviating the psychosocial pressures that contribute to the aggravation of the voiding dysfunction (see Table 13–13) (Hinman, 1986; Masek). A frequent emptying schedule accompanied by biofeedback techniques to relax the sphincter during voiding, anticholinergic drugs to abolish uninhibited contractions, and improved bowel emptying regimes are instituted (Bauer et al). Bethanechol chloride and prazosin (an alpha-blocking agent) may be added if the detrusor exhibits poor contractility. Despite these measures, intermittent catheterization may be needed in children who fail to respond and in

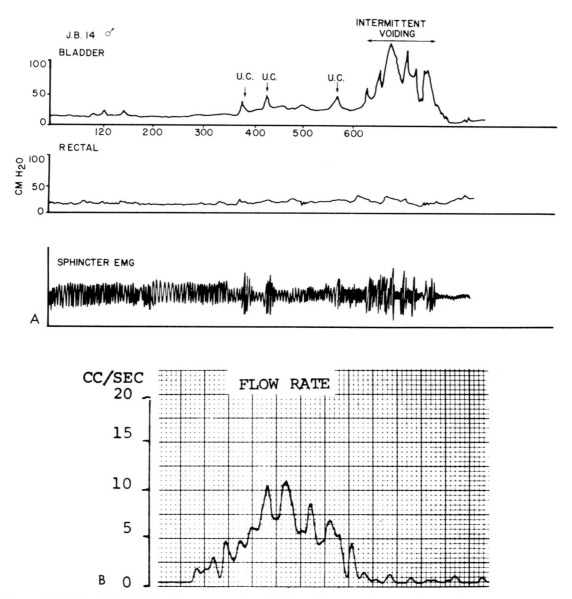

Figure 13–31 □ A, Uninhibited detrusor contractions (U.C.) and increases in external urethral sphincter electromyography (EMG) activity are noted as the bladder is filled. During voluntary voiding, very high bladder pressures (above 100 cm H$_2$O) are generated owing to increased activity and then intermittent relaxation of the external sphincter. B, The urinary flow rate reflects the voiding pattern seen on urodynamic evaluation.

those individuals who require immediate decompression of their upper urinary tract (Snyder et al). In some cases, the outflow obstruction may have produced severe renal damage and even chronic kidney failure, which must be managed accordingly.

Psychotherapy is an integral part of the rehabilitative process to re-educate both the child and the parents in appropriate voiding habits. Punishments are stopped and a reward system initiated in order to improve the child's self-image and confidence (Masek).

Bibliography

INTRODUCTION

Blaivas JG: A critical appraisal of specific diagnostic techniques. *In* Clinical Neurourology. Edited by RJ Krane, MB Siroky. Boston, Little, Brown & Co, 1979, pp 69–110.

Blaivas JG, Labib KB, Bauer SB, Retik AB: Changing concepts in the urodynamic evaluation of children. J Urol 117:777, 1977.

Gierup J, Ericsson NO: Micturition studies in infants and children: intravesical pressure, urinary flow and urethral resistance in boys with intravesical obstruction. Scand J Urol Nephrol 4:217, 1970.

Lapides J, Diokno AC, Silber SJ, Lowe BS: Clean intermittent self-catheterization in the treatment of urinary tract disease. J Urol 107:458, 1972.

McGuire EJ, Woodside JR, Borden TA, Weiss RM: The prognostic value of urodynamic testing in myelodysplastic patients. J Urol 126:205, 1981.

Smith ED: Urinary prognosis in spina bifida. J Urol 108:115, 1972.

ASSESSMENT

Abrams PH: Perfusion urethral profilometry. Urol Clin North Am 6:103, 1979.

Bates CP, Whiteside CG, Turner-Warwick RT: Synchronous cine/pressure/flow/cystourethrography with special reference to stress and urge incontinence. Br J Urol 42:714, 1970.

Bauer SB: Pediatric neurourology. *In* Clinical Neurourology. Edited by RJ Krane, MB Siroky. Boston, Little, Brown & Co, 1979, pp. 275–294.

Bauer SB: Urodynamics in children: indications and methods. *In* Controversies in Neuro-urology. Edited by DM Barrett, AJ Wein. New York, Churchill Livingstone, 1983, pp 193–202.

Blaivas JG: A critical appraisal of specific diagnostic techniques. *In* Clinical Neurourology. Edited by RJ Krane, MB Siroky. Boston, Little, Brown & Co, 1979a, pp 69–110.

Blaivas JG: EMG: other uses. *In* Controversies in Neuro-urology. Edited by DM Barrett, AJ Wein. Churchill Livingstone, 1979b, pp 103–116.

Blaivas JG, Labib KB, Bauer SB, Retik AB: A new approach to electromyography of the external urethral sphincter. J Urol 117:773, 1977a.

Blaivas JG, Labib KB, Bauer SB, Retik AB: Changing concepts in the urodynamic evaluation of children. J Urol 117:777, 1977b.

Bradley WE, Timm GW, Scott FB: Sphincter electromyography. Urol Clin North Am 1:69, 1974.

Diokno AC, Koff SA, Bender LF: Periurethral striated muscle activity in neurogenic bladder dysfunction. J Urol 112:743, 1974.

Ericsson NO, Hellstrom B, Negardth A, Rudhe U: Micturition urethrocystography in children with myelomeningocele. Acta Radiol [Diagn] (Stockh) 11:321, 1971.

Evans AT, Felker JR, Shank RA, Sugarman SR: Pitfalls of urodynamics. J Urol 122:220, 1979.

Fairhurst JJ, Rubin CME, Hyde I, et al: Bladder capacity in infants. J Pediatr Surg 26:55, 1991.

Gierup J, Ericsson NO, Okmain L: Micturition studies in infants and children. Scand J Urol Nephrol 3:1, 1969.

Gleason DM, Bottacini MR, Reilly RJ: Comparison of cystometrograms and urethral pressure profiles with gas and water media. Urology 9:155, 1977.

Gleason DM, Reilly RJ, Bottacini MR, Pierce MJ: The urethral continence zone and its relation to stress incontinence. J Urol 112:81, 1974.

Joseph DB, Duggan ML: The effects of fast and slow saline infusion on hypertonicity and peak/leak pressure during cystometrogram evaluation of infants and children with myelodysplasia. Presented at Section on Urology, Annual Meeting, American Academy of Pediatrics, October 21, 1989, Chicago.

Koff SA: Estimating bladder capacity in children. Urology 21:248, 1982.

Koff SA, Kass EJ: Abdominal wall electromyography: a noninvasive technique to improve pediatric urodynamic accuracy. J Urol 127:736, 1982.

Maizels M, Firlit CF: Pediatric urodynamics. Clinical comparison of surface vs. needle pelvic floor/external sphincter electromyography. J Urol 122:518, 1979.

Mandell J, Bauer SB, Hallett M, et al: Occult spinal dysraphism: a rare but detectable cause of voiding dysfunction. Urol Clin North Am 7:349, 1980.

Mayo ME: Detrusor hyperreflexia: the effect of posture and pelvic floor activity. J Urol 119:635, 1978.

Scott FB, Quesada EM, Cardus D: Studies on the dynamics of micturition. J Urol 92:455, 1964.

Tanagho EA: Membrane and microtransducer catheters. Their effectiveness for profilometry of the lower urinary tract. Urol Clin North Am 6:110, 1979.

Turner-Warwick RT: Some clinical aspects of detrusor dysfunction. J Urol 113:539, 1975.

Yalla SV, Rossier AB, Fam B: Vesico-urethral pressure recordings in the assessment of neurogenic bladder functions in spinal cord injury patients. Urol Int 32:161, 1979.

Yalla SV, Sharma GVRK, Barsamian EM: Micturitional static urethral pressure profile method of recording urethral pressure profiles during voiding and implications. J Urol 124:649, 1980.

MYELODYSPLASIA

Adams MC, Mitchell ME, Rink RC: Gastrocystoplasty: an alternative solution to the problem of urological reconstruction in the severely compromised patient. J Urol 140:1152, 1988.

Barbalias GA, Klauber GT, Blaivas JG: Critical evaluation of the Credé maneuver: A urodynamic study of 207 patients. J Urol 130:720, 1983.

Barrett DM, Furlow WL: The management of severe urinary incontinence in patients with myelodysplasia by implantation of the AS791/792 urinary sphincter device. J Urol 128:44, 1982.

Bauer SB: Bladder neck reconstruction. *In* Urologic Surgery. Edited by JF Glenn, SD Graham. Philadelphia, JB Lippincott Co, 1990, pp 509–522.

Bauer SB: Early evaluation and management of children with spina bifida. *In* Urologic Surgery in Neonates and Young Infants. Edited by LR King. Philadelphia, WB Saunders Co, 1988, pp 252–264.

Bauer SB: Evaluation and management of the newborn with myelomeningocele. *In* Common Problems in Urology. Edited by ET Gonzales, DR Roth. St Louis, Mosby Year Book Inc, 1991, pp 169–180.

Bauer SB: The management of spina bifida from birth onwards. *In* Paediatric Urology. Edited by RH Whitaker, JR Woodard. London, Butterworths, 1985, pp 87–112.

Bauer SB: Myelodysplasia: newborn evaluation and management. *In* Spina Bifida: A Multidisciplinary Approach. Edited by RL McLaurin. New York, Praeger, 1984b, pp 262–267.

Bauer SB: Vesico-ureteral reflux in children with neurogenic bladder dysfunction. *In* International Perspectives in Urology, Vol 10. Edited by JH Johnston. Baltimore, Williams & Wilkins, 1984a, pp 159–177.

Bauer SB, Colodny AH, Retik AB: The management of vesico-ureteral reflux in children with myelodysplasia. J Urol 128:102, 1982.

Bauer SB, Hallet M, Khoshbin S, et al: The predictive value of urodynamic evaluation in the newborn with myelodysplasia. JAMA 152:650, 1984.

Bauer SB, Labib KB, Dieppa RA, et al: Urodynamic evaluation in a boy with myelodysplasia and incontinence. Urology 10:354, 1977.

Bauer SB, Reda EF, Colodny AH, Retik AB: Detrusor instability: a delayed complication in association with the artificial sphincter. J Urol 135:1212, 1986.

Begger JH, Meihuizen de Regt MJ, Hogen Esch I, et al: Progressive neurologic deficit in children with spina bifida aperta. Z Kinderchir 41(Suppl 1):13, 1986.

Bihrle R, Klee LW, Adams MC, et al: Transverse colon–gastric tube composite reservoir. Urology 37:36, 1991.

Blaivas JG, Sinka HP, Zayed AH, et al: Detrusor-sphincter dyssynergia: a detailed electromyographic study. J Urol 125:545, 1986.

Bloom DA, Knechtel JM, McGuire EJ: Urethral dilation improves bladder compliance in children with myelomeningocele and high leak point pressures. J Urol 144:430, 1990.

Bosco PJ, Bauer SB, Colodny AH, et al: Long-term results of artificial urinary sphincters in children. J Urol 146:396, 1991.

Cartwright PC, Snow BW: Bladder autoaugmentation: early clinical experience. J Urol 142:505, 1989a.

Cartwright PC, Snow BW: Bladder autoaugmentation: partial detrusor excision to augment bladder without use of bowel. J Urol 142:1050, 1989b.

Cass AS: Urinary tract complications of myelomeningocele patients. J Urol 115:102, 1976.

Cass AS, Bloom BA, Luxenberg M: Sexual function in adults with myelomeningocele. J Urol 136:425, 1986.

Chiaramonte RM, Horowitz EM, Kaplan GA, et al: Implications of hydronephrosis in newborns with myelodysplasia. J Urol 136:427, 1986.

Cromer BA, Enrile B, McCoy K, et al: Knowledge, attitudes and behavior related to sexuality in adolescents with chronic disability. Dev Med Child Neurol 32:602, 1990.

Dees JE: Congenital epispadias with incontinence. J Urol 62:513, 1949.

Duckett JW: Cutaneous vesicostomy in childhood. Urol Clin North Am 1:485, 1974.

Duckett JW, Snyder HM III: Continent urinary diversion: variations of the Mitrofanoff principle. J Urol 136:58, 1986.

Epstein F: Meningocele: pitfalls in early and late management. Clin Neurosurg 30:366, 1982.

Geraniotis E, Koff SA, Enrile B: Prophylactic use of clean intermittent catheterization in treatment of infants and young children with myelomeningocele and neurogenic bladder dysfunction. J Urol 139:85, 1988.

Ghoniem GM, Bloom DA, McGuire EJ, Stewart KL: Bladder compliance in meningocele children. J Urol 141:1404, 1989.

Goldwasser B, Barrett DM, Webster GD, Kramer SA: Cystometric properties of ileum and right colon after bladder augmentation, substitution and replacement. J Urol 138:1007, 1987.

Hayden P: Adolescents with meningomyelocele. Pediatr Rev 6:245, 1985.

Hendren WH: Reconstruction of the previously diverted urinary tracts in children. J Pediatr Surg 8:135, 1973.

Hendren WH: Urinary diversion and undiversion in children. Surg Clin North Am 56:425, 1976.

Hinman F Jr: Functional classification of conduits for continent diversion. J Urol 144:27, 1990.

Hinman F Jr: Selection of intestinal segments for bladder substitution: physical and physiological characteristics. J Urol 139:519, 1988.

Jeffs RD, Jones P, Schillinger JF: Surgical correction of vesico-ureteral reflux in children with neurogenic bladder. J Urol 115:449, 1976.

Joseph DB, Bauer SB, Colodny AH, Mandell J, Retik AB: Clean intermittent catheterization in infants with neurogenic bladder. Pediatrics 84:78, 1989.

Kaplan WE, Firlit CF: Management of reflux in myelodysplasic children. J Urol 129:1195, 1983.

Kasabian NG, Bauer SB, Dyro FM, et al: The value of prophylactic therapy in neonates and infants with myelodysplasia at risk for urinary tract deterioration. Presented at Annual Meeting of the Urology Section of the American Academy of Pediatrics, Boston, October 6, 1990, abstract No. 11.

Kass EJ, Koff SA, Lapides J: Fate of vesico-ureteral reflux in children with neuropathic bladders managed by intermittent catheterization. J Urol 125:63, 1981.

Keating MA, Bauer SB, Krarup C, et al: Sacral sparing in children with myelodysplasia. Presented at the Annual Meeting of the American Urological Association. Anaheim, May 18, 1987.

Khoury AE, Hendrick EB, McLorie GA, et al: Occult spinal dysraphism: clinical and urodyanmic outcome after division of the filum terminale. J Urol 144:426, 1990.

Kock NG: Ileostomy without external appliances: a survey of 25 patients provided with intra-abdominal intestinal reservoir. Ann Surg 173:545, 1971.

Kroovand RL, Bell W, Hart LJ, Benfeld KY: The effect of back closure on detrusor function in neonates with myelodysplasia. J Urol 144:423, 1990.

Kropp KA, Angwafo FF: Urethral lengthening and reimplantation for neurogenic incontinence in children. J Urol 135:533, 1986.

Lapides J, Diokno AC, Silber SJ, Lowe BS: Clean intermittent self-catheterization in the treatment of urinary tract disease. J Urol 107:458, 1972.

Laurence KM: A declining incidence of neural tube defects in U.K. Z Kinderchir 44(Suppl 1):51, 1989.

Leadbetter GW Jr: Surgical correction for total urinary incontinence. J Urol 91:261, 1964.

Light JK, Hawila M, Scott FB: Treatment of urinary incontinence in children: the artificial sphincter vs. other methods. J Urol 130:518, 1983.

Light JK, Scott FB: Use of the artificial urinary sphincter in spinal cord injury patients. J Urol 130:1127, 1983.

Mandell J, Bauer SB, Colodny AH, Retik AB: Cutaneous vesicostomy in infancy. J Urol 126:92, 1981.

McGuire EJ, Wang CC, Usitalo H, Savastano J: Modified pubovaginal sling in girls with myelodysplasia. J Urol 135:94, 1986.

McGuire EJ, Woodside JR, Borden TA, Weiss RM: The prognostic value of urodynamic testing in myelodysplastic patients. J Urol 126:205, 1981.

McLorie GA, Perez-Morero R, Csima AL, Churchill BM: Determinants of hydronephrosis and renal injury in patients with myelomeningocele. J Urol 140:1289, 1986.

Mitchell ME, Piser JA: Intestinocystoplasty and total bladder replacement in children and young adults: follow-up of 129 cases. J Urol 138:1140, 1987.

Mitrofanoff P: Cystometrie continente trans-appendiculaire dans le traitement de vessies neurologiques. Chir Pediatr 21:297, 1980.

Peters CA, Bauer SB, Colodny AH, et al: The use of rectus fascia to manage urinary incontinence. J Urol 142:516, 1989.

Raz S, Ehrlich RM, Ziedman EJ, et al: Surgical treatment of the incontinent female patient with myelomeningocele. J Urol 139:524, 1988.

Reigel DH: Tethered spinal cord. Concepts Pediatr Neurosurg 4:142, 1983.

Riedmiller H, Burger R, Muller S, et al: Continent appendix stoma: a modification of the Mainz pouch technique. J Urol 143:1115, 1990.

Rinck C, Berg J, Hafeman C: The adolescent with myelomeningocele: a review of parent experiences and expectations. Adolescence 24:699, 1989.

Roth DR, Vyas PR, Kroovand RL, Perlmutter AD: Urinary tract deterioration associated with the artificial urinary sphincter. J Urol 135:528, 1986.

Rowland RG, Mitchell ME, Birhle R, et al: Indiana continent urinary reservoir. J Urol 137:1136, 1987.

Scarff TB, Fronczak S: Myelomeningocele: a review and update. Rehab Literature 42:143, 1981.

Schwarz GR, Jeffs RD: Ileal conduit urinary diversion in children: computer analysis of follow-up from 2 to 16 years. J Urol 114:285, 1975.

Shapiro SR, Lebowitz RL, Colodny AH: Fate of 90 children with ileal conduit urinary diversion a decade later: analysis of complications, pyeloplasty, renal function and bacteriology. J Urol 114:289, 1975.

Sidi AA, Aliabadi H, Gonzalez R: Enterocystoplasty in the management and reconstruction of the pediatric neurogenic bladder. J Pediatr Surg 22:153, 1987.

Sidi AA, Dykstra DD, Gonzalez R: The value of urodynamic testing in the management of neonates with myelodysplasia: a prospective study. J Urol 135:90, 1986.

Skinner DG, Lieskovsky G, Boyd SD: Construction of a continent ileal reservoir (Kock pouch) as an alternative to cutaneous urinary diversion: an update after 250 cases. J Urol 137:1140, 1987.

Smith ED: Urinary prognosis in spina bifida. J Urol 108:115, 1972.

Spindel MR, Bauer SB, Dyro FM, et al: The changing neuro-urologic lesion in myelodysplasia. JAMA 258:1630, 1987.

Stark GD: Spina bifida: problems and management. Oxford, Blackwell Scientific Publications, 1977.

Stein SC, Feldman JG, Freidlander M, et al: Is myelomeningocele a disappearing disease? Pediatrics 69:511, 1982.

Steinhardt GF, Goodgold HM, Samuels LD: The effect of intravesical pressure on glomerular filtration rates in patients with myelomeningocele. J Urol 140:1293, 1986.

Torrens M, Abrams P: Cystometry. Urol Clin North Am 6:79, 1979.

Tutrone RF, Bauer SB, Peters CA, et al: Physiologic basis for continence in the Mitrofanoff principle. Presented at the Annual Meeting of the American Urological Association, Toronto, June 3, 1991.

VanGool JD, Kuijten RH, Donckerwolcke RA, Kramer PP: Detrusor-sphincter dyssynergia in children with myelomeningocele: a prospective study. Z Kinderchir 37:148, 1982.

Venes JL, Stevens SA: Surgical pathology in tethered cord secondary to meningomyelocele repair. Concepts Pediatr Neurosurg 4:165, 1983.

Woodard JR, Anderson AM, Parrott TS: Ureteral reimplantation in myelodysplastic children. J Urol 126:387, 1981.

Woodhouse CRJ, Malone PR, Cumming J, Reilly TM: The Mitrofanoff principle for continent urinary diversion. Br J Urol 63:53, 1989.

Woodside JR, McGuire EJ: Techniques for detection of detrusor hypertonia in the presence of urethral sphincter incompetence. J Urol 127:740, 1982.

Young HH: An operation for the cure of incontinence of urine. Surg Gynecol Obstet 28:84, 1919.

LIPOMENINGOCELE AND OTHER SPINAL DYSRAPHISMS

Anderson FM: Occult spinal dysraphism: a series of 73 cases. Pediatrics 55:826, 1975.

Barson AJ: The vertebral level of termination of the spinal cord during normal and abnormal development. J Anat 106:489, 1970.

Campobasso P, Galiani E, Verzerio A, et al: A rare cause of occult neuropathic bladder in children: the tethered cord syndrome. Pediatr Med Chir 10:641, 1988.

Dubrowitz V, Lorber J, Zachary RB: Lipoma of the cauda equina. Arch Dis Child 40:207, 1965.

Flanigan RF, Russell DP, Walsh JW: Urologic aspects of tethered cord. Urology 33:80, 1989.

Foster LS, Kogan BA, Cogan PH, Edwards MSB: Bladder function in patients with lipomyelomeningocele. J Urol 143:984, 1990.

Hall WA, Albright AL, Brunberg JA: Diagnosis of tethered cord by magnetic resonance imaging. Surg Neurol 30(Suppl 1):60, 1988.

Hellstrom WJ, Edwards MS, Kogan BA: Urologic aspects of the tethered cord syndrome. J Urol 135:317, 1986.

James CM, Lassman LP: Spinal dysraphism: spina bifida occulta. New York, Appleton-Century-Crofts, 1972.

Kaplan WE, McLone DG, Richards I: The urologic manifestations of the tethered spinal cord. J Urol 140:1285, 1988.

Keating MA, Rink RC, Bauer SB, et al: Neuro-urologic implications of changing approach in management of occult spinal lesions. J Urol 140:1299, 1988.

Khoury AE, Hendrick EB, McLorie GA, et al: Occult spinal dysraphism: clinical and urodynamic outcome after division of the filum terminale. J Urol 144:426, 1990.

Kondo A, Kato K, Kanai S, Sakakibara T: Bladder dysfunction secondary to tethered cord syndrome in adults: is it curable? J Urol 135:313, 1986.

Linder M, Rosenstein J, Sklar FH: Functional improvement after spinal surgery for the dysraphic malformations. Neurosurgery 11:622, 1982.

Mandell J, Bauer SB, Hallett M, et al: Occult spinal dysraphism: a rare but detectable cause of voiding dysfunction. Urol Clin North Am 7:349, 1980.

Packer RJ, Zimmerman RA, Sutton LN, et al: Magnetic resonance imaging of spinal cord diseases of childhood. Pediatrics 78:251, 1986.

Raghavendra BN, Epstein FJ, Pinto RS, et al: The tethered spinal cord: diagnosis by high-resolution real-time ultrasound. Radiology 149:123, 1983.

Roy MW, Gilmore R, Walsh JW: Evaluation of children and young adults with tethered spinal cord syndrome: utility of spinal and scalp recorded somatosensory evoked potentials. Surg Neurol 26:241, 1986.

Scheible W, James HE, Leopold GR, Hilton SW: Occult spinal dysraphism in infants: screening with high-resolution real-time ultrasound. Radiology 146:743, 1983.

Seeds JW, Jones FD: Lipomyelomeningocele: prenatal diagnosis and management. Obstet Gynecol 67(Suppl):34, 1986.

Tami S, Yamada S, Knighton RS: Extensibility of the lumbar and sacral cord. Pathophysiology of the tethered cord in cats. J Neurosurg 66:116, 1987.

Tracey PT, Hanigan WC: Spinal dysraphism: use of magnetic resonance imaging in evaluation. Clin Pediatr 29:228, 1990.

Weissert M, Gysler R, Sorensen N: The clinical problem of the tethered cord syndrome—a report of 3 personal cases. Z Kinderchir 44:275, 1989.

Yamada S, Knierim D, Yonekura M, et al: Tethered cord syndrome. J Am Paraplegia Soc 6(Suppl 3):58, 1983.

Yamada S, Zincke DE, Sanders D: Pathophysiology of "tethered cord syndrome." J Neurosurg 54:494, 1981.

Yip CM, Leach GE, Rosenfeld DS, et al: Delayed diagnosis of voiding dysfunction: occult spinal dysraphism. J Urol 124:694, 1985.

SACRAL AGENESIS

Bauer SB: Urodynamics in children. *In* Pediatric Urology. Edited by KW Ashcraft. Orlando, Grune & Stratton, 1990, pp 49–76.

Guzman L, Bauer SB, Hallett M, et al: The evaluation and management of children with sacral agenesis. Urology 23:506, 1983.

Jakobson H, Holm-Bentzen M, Hald T: Neurogenic bladder dysfunction in sacral agenesis and dysgenesis. Neurourol Urodynam 4:99, 1985.

Koff SA, DeRidder PA: Patterns of neurogenic bladder dysfunction in sacral agenesis. J Urol 118:87, 1977.

Landauer W: Rumplessness of chicken embryos produced by the injection of insulin and other chemicals. J Exp Zool 98:65, 1945.

Menon RK, Cohen RM, Sperling MA, et al: Transplacental passage of insulin in pregnant women with insulin-dependent diabetes mellitus. N Engl J Med 323:309, 1990.

Passarge E, Lenz K: Syndrome of caudal regression in infants of diabetic mothers: observations of further cases. Pediatrics 37:672, 1966.

White RI, Klauber GT: Sacral agenesis: analysis of twenty-two cases. Urology 8:521, 1976.

IMPERFORATE ANUS

Barnes PD, Lester PD, Yamanashi WS, Prince JR: MRI in infants and children with spinal dysraphism. Am J Radiol 147:339, 1986.

Barry JE, Auldist AW: The Vater syndrome. Am J Dis Child 128:769, 1974.

Carson JA, Barnes PD, Tunell WP, et al: Imperforate anus: the neurologic implication of sacral abnormalities. J Pediatr Surg 19:838, 1984.

Greenfield SP, Fera M: Urodynamic evaluation of the imperforate anus patient: a prospective study. J Urol 146:539, 1991.

Karrer FM, Flannery AM, Nelson MD Jr, et al: Anal rectal malformations: evaluation of associated spinal dysraphic syndromes. J Pediatr Surg 23:45, 1988.

Parrott T, Woodard J: Importance of cystourethrography in neonates with imperforate anus. Urology 13:607, 1979.

Peña A: Posterior sagittal approach for the correction of anal rectal malformations. Adv Surg 19:69, 1986.

Sheldon C, Cormier M, Crone K, Wacksman J: Occult neurovesical dysfunction in children with imperforate anus and its variants. J Pediatr Surg 26:49, 1991.

Tunnell WP, Austin JC, Barnes TP, Reynolds A: Neuroradiologic evaluation of sacral abnormalities in imperforate anus complex. J Pediatr Surg 22:58, 1987.

Uehling DT, Gilbert E, Chesney R: Urologic implications of the VATER syndrome. J Urol 129:352, 1983.

Williams DI, Grant J: Urologic complications of imperforate anus. Br J Urol 41:660, 1969.

CEREBRAL PALSY

Decter RM, Bauer SB, Khoshbin S, et al: Urodynamic assessment of children with cerebral palsy. J Urol 138:1110, 1987.

McNeal DM, Hawtrey CE, Wolraich ML, Mapel JR: Symptomatic neurogenic bladder in a cerebral-palsied population. Dev Med Child Neurol 25:612, 1983.

Naeye RL, Peters EC, Bartholomew M, Landis R: Origins of cerebral palsy. Am J Dis Child 143:1154, 1989.

Nelson KB, Ellenberg JH: Antecedents of cerebral palsy. N Engl J Med 315:81, 1986.

TRAUMATIC INJURIES TO THE SPINE

Adams C, Babyn PS, Logan WJ: Spinal cord birth injury: value of computed tomographic myelography. Pediatr Neurol 4:109, 1988.

Barkin M, Dolfin D, Herschorn S, et al: The urologic care of the spinal cord injury patient. J Urol 129:335, 1983.

Cass AS, Luxenberg M, Johnson CF, Gleich P: Management of the neurogenic bladder in 413 children. J Urol 132:521, 1984.

Donnelly J, Hackler RH, Bunts RC: Present urologic status of the World War II paraplegic: 25-year follow-up comparison with status of the 20-year Korean War paraplegic and 5-year Vietnam paraplegic. J Urol 108:558, 1972.

Fanciullacci F, Zanollo A, Sandri S, Catanzaro F: The neuropathic bladder in children with spinal cord injury. Paraplegia 26:83, 1988.

Guttmann L, Frankel H: The value of intermittent catheterization in the early management of traumatic paraplegia and tetraplegia. Paraplegia 4:63, 1966.

Iwatsubo E, Iwakawa A, Koga H, et al: Functional recovery of the bladder in patients with spinal cord injury—prognosticating programs of an aseptic intermittent catheterization. Acta Urologica Japonica 31:775, 1985.

Lanska MJ, Roessmann U, Wiznitzer M: Magnetic resonance imaging in cervical cord birth injury. Pediatrics 85:760, 1990.

Ogawa T, Yoshida T, Fujinaga T: Bladder deformity in traumatic spinal cord injury patients. Acta Urologica Japonica 34:1173, 1988.

Pearman JW: Urologic follow-up of 99 spinal cord injury patients initially managed by intermittent catheterization. Br J Urol 48:297, 1976.

Pollack IF, Pang D, Sclabassi R: Recurrent spinal cord injury without radiographic abnormalities in children. J Neurosurg 69:177, 1988.

FUNCTIONAL VOIDING DISORDERS

Bauer SB, Retik AB, Colodny AH, et al: The unstable bladder of childhood. Urol Clin North Am 7:321, 1980.

Bellman N: Encopresis. Acta Paediatr Scand 70(Suppl 1):1, 1966.

Fergusson DM, Hons BA, Horwood LJ, Shannon FT: Factors related to the age of attainment of nocturnal bladder control: an eight year longitudinal study. Pediatrics 78:884, 1986.

MacKeith RL, Meadow SR, Turner RK: How children become dry. *In* Bladder Control and Enuresis. Edited by I Kolvin, RL MacKeith, SR Meadow. Philadelphia, JB Lippincott, 1973, pp 3–15.

Yeats WK: Bladder function in normal micturition. *In* Bladder Control and Enuresis. Edited by I Kolvin, RL MacKeith, SR Meadow. Philadelphia, JB Lippincott, 1973, pp 28–41.

SMALL-CAPACITY HYPERTONIC BLADDER

Bauer SB, Retik AB, Colodny AH, et al: The unstable bladder of childhood. Urol Clin North Am 7:321, 1980.

Dyro FM, Bauer SB, Hallett M, Khoshbin S: Complex repetitive discharges in the external urethral sphincter in a pediatric population. Neurourol Urodynam 2:39, 1983.

Hansson S, Hjalmas K, Jodal U, Sixt R: Lower urinary tract dysfunction in girls with untreated asymptomatic or covert bacteriuria. J Urol 143:333, 1990.

Lebowitz RL, Mandell J: Urinary tract infection in children: putting radiology in its place. Radiology 165:1, 1987.

Masek BJ: Behavioral management of voiding dysfunction in neurologically normal children. Dialog Pediatr Urol 8:7, 1985.

Mayo ME, Burns MW: Urodynamic studies in children who wet. Br J Urol 65:641, 1990.

Rudy DC, Woodside JR: Non-neurogenic neurogenic bladder: the relationship between intravesical pressure and the external sphincter EMG. Neurourol Urodynam 10:169, 1991.

Saxton HM, Borzyskowski M, Mundy AR, Vivian GC: Spinning top deformity: not a normal variant. Radiology 168:147, 1988.

Tanagho EA, Miller EA, Lyon RP: Spastic striated external sphincter and urinary tract infection in girls. Br J Urol 43:69, 1971.

VanGool JD, Tanagho EA: External sphincter activity and recurrent urinary tract infection in girls. Urology 10:348, 1977.

Webster GD, Koefoot RB, Sihelnik S: Urodynamic abnormalities in neurologically normal children with micturition dysfunction. J Urol 132:74, 1984.

HYPERREFLEXIC BLADDER

Bauer SB, Retik AB, Colodny AH, et al: The unstable bladder of childhood. Urol Clin North Am 7:321, 1980.

Buttarazzi PJ: Oxybutynin chloride (Ditropan) in enuresis. J Urol 118:46, 1977.

Firlit CF, Smey P, King LR: Micturition: urodynamic flow studies in children. J Urol 119:250, 1978.

Kass EJ, Diokno AC, Montealegre A: Enuresis: principles of management and results of treatment. J Urol 121:794, 1979.

Koff SA, Murtagh DS: The uninhibited bladder in children. Effect of treatment on recurrence of urinary infection and vesico-ureteral reflux. J Urol 130:1158, 1983.

Kondo A, Kobayashi M, Otani T, et al: Children with unstable bladder: clinical and urodynamic observation. J Urol 129:88, 1983.

MacKeith RL, Meadow SR, Turner RK: How children become dry. In Bladder Control and Enuresis. Edited by I Kolvin, RL MacKeith, SR Meadow. Philadelphia, JB Lippincott, 1973, pp 3–15.

Mayo ME, Burns MW: Urodynamic studies in children who wet. Br J Urol 65:641, 1990.

McGuire EJ, Savastano JA: Urodynamic studies in enuresis and non-neurogenic bladder. J Urol 132:299, 1984.

Mueller SR: Development of urinary control in children. JAMA 172:1256, 1960.

O'Regan S, Yazbeck S, Hamburger B, Schick E: Constipation: a commonly unrecognized cause of enuresis. Am J Dis Child 140:260, 1986.

O'Regan S, Yazbeck S, Schick E: Constipation, unstable bladder, urinary tract infection syndrome. Clin Nephrol 5:154, 1985.

Rudy DC, Woodside JR: Non-neurogenic neurogenic bladder: the relationship between intravesical pressure

and the external sphincter EMG. Neurourol Urodynam 10:169, 1991.

Torrens MJ, Collins CD: The urodynamic assessment of adult enuresis. Br J Urol 47:433, 1975.

Vincent SA: Postural control of urinary incontinence. The curtsy sign. Lancet 2:631, 1966.

Webster GD, Koefoot RB, Sihelnik S: Urodynamic abnormalities in neurologically normal children with micturition dysfunction. J Urol 132:74, 1984.

Yeats WK: Bladder function in normal micturition. In Bladder Control and Enuresis. Edited by I Kolvin, RC MacKeith, SR Meadow. Philadelphia, JB Lippincott, 1973, pp 28–41.

THE INFREQUENT VOIDER—LAZY BLADDER SYNDROME

Bauer SB, Retik AB, Colodny AH, et al: The unstable bladder of childhood. Urol Clin North Am 7:321, 1980.

DeLuca FG, Swenson O, Fisher JH, Loutfi AH: The dysfunctional "lazy" bladder syndrome in children. Arch Dis Child 37:117, 1962.

Koefoot RB, Webster GD, Anderson EE, Glenn JF: The primary megacystis syndrome. J Urol 125:232, 1981.

Masek BJ: Behavioral management of voiding dysfunction in neurologically normal children. Dial Pediatr Urol 8:7, 1985.

Webster GD, Koefoot RB, Sihelnik S: Urodynamic abnormalities in neurologically normal children with micturition dysfunction. J Urol 132:74, 1984.

PSYCHOLOGIC NON-NEUROPATHIC BLADDER (HINMAN SYNDROME)

Allen TD: The non-neurogenic bladder. J Urol 117:232, 1977.

Allen TD, Bright TC: Urodynamic patterns in children with dysfunctional voiding problems. J Urol 119:247, 1978.

Bauer SB, Retik AB, Colodny AH, et al: The unstable bladder of childhood. Urol Clin North Am 7:321, 1980.

Hinman F: Non-neurogenic bladder (the Hinman syndrome) fifteen years later. J Urol 136:769, 1986.

Hinman F: Urinary tract damage in children who wet. Pediatrics 54:142, 1974.

Johnston JH, Farkas A: Congenital neuropathic bladder: practicalities and possibilities of conservational management. Urology 5:719, 1975.

Kass EJ, Diokno AC, Montealegre A: Enuresis: principles of management and results of treatment. J Urol 121:794, 1979.

Masek BJ: Behavioral management of voiding dysfunction in neurologically normal children. Dial Pediatr Urol 8:7, 1985.

McGuire EJ, Savastano JA: Urodynamic studies in enuresis and non-neurogenic bladder. J Urol 132:299, 1984.

Mix LW: Occult neuropathic bladder. Urology 10:1, 1977.

Rudy DC, Woodside JR: Non-neurogenic neurogenic bladder: its relationship between intravesical pressure and the external sphincter EMG. Neurourol Urodynam 10:169, 1991.

Snyder H McC, Caldamone AA, Wein AJ, Duckett JW Jr: The Hinman syndrome—alternatives for treatment. Presented at the Annual Meeting of the American Urological Association, Kansas City, May 16, 1982.

Williams DI, Hirst G, Doyle D: The occult neuropathic bladder. J Pediatr Surg 9:35, 1975.

14

☐ Vesicoureteral Reflux

Stephen A. Kramer

HISTORICAL REVIEW

Vesicoureteral reflux (VUR) is the abnormal flow of urine from the bladder into the upper urinary tract. Reflux was recognized as early as medieval times by Galen and Leonardo da Vinci (Lines; Polk). Semblino first demonstrated reflux experimentally in 1883 (Levitt and Weiss). In 1893, Pozzi was the first to observe reflux in humans when he noted urine flow from the cut end of the distal ureter after nephrectomy (Walker). In 1898, Young and Wesson concluded that patients with a normal ureterovesical junction did not have VUR. Sampson observed, in 1903, that the normal obliquity of the ureter through the bladder prevented reflux (Walker). Hutch's classic studies on the pathophysiology of reflux in paraplegic patients demonstrated the relationship between reflux and chronic pyelonephritis and led the way for the widespread use of the voiding cystourethrogram (VCU) in the evaluation of patients with unexplained hydronephrosis or recurrent urinary tract infections (UTIs), or both (Hutch, 1952).

Tanagho and associates (1965) performed experiments on the ureteral trigonal complex in dogs and demonstrated that incision of the trigonal musculature distal to the ureteral orifice produced VUR. Ransley and Risdon (1975b) showed that resection of the roof of the submucosal tunnel in piglets consistently resulted in VUR. Kiruluta et al showed that maturation of the adrenergic fibers in the bladder has a role in the presence or absence of reflux.

INCIDENCE AND EPIDEMIOLOGY

The prevalence of VUR in healthy children is probably less than 1 per cent and varies depending on race and country of origin. Politano (1960) and Lich et al (1964) found no evidence of reflux in large series of patients undergoing cystograms. Ransley found only seven instances of reflux in a series of 535 VCUs performed in presumably normal neonates, infants, and children. Iannaccone and Panzironi reported only one instance of reflux in a series of 50 assessable infants without urologic disease who underwent voiding cystourethrography. Jones and Headstream found reflux in only 1 of 100 children evaluated.

Manley suggested that reflux occurs more commonly in children with fair skin, blond hair, and blue eyes (Walker). Conversely, others have found a higher incidence of reflux only in red-headed children. Askari and Belman noted that reflux occurred 10 times more frequently in white girls with UTI than in black girls with infections. Peters et al found no instances of reflux in 56 black children who underwent cystography.

DIAGNOSIS OF VESICOURETERAL REFLUX

Clinical Presentation

Infants and young children frequently present with nonspecific symptoms related to both UTI and reflux. These symptoms may include fever, lethargy, anorexia, nausea, vomiting, and failure to thrive. Older children usually present with lower tract symptoms such as dysuria or with flank pain and tenderness secondary to acute pyelonephritis. The symptomatic presentation of VUR is almost always in conjunction with an associated UTI. Sterile reflux is a rare and unusual cause of flank pain.

Fever is the single most important symptom to differentiate children with upper tract (pyelonephritis) from those with lower tract (cystitis) infections (Govan and Palmer). Woodard and Holden evaluated 350 children with UTI and found that 90 per cent of children with reflux had a temperature greater than 38.5° C. Conversely, only 40 per cent of children without reflux had similar temperature increases.

The widespread use of obstetric ultrasonography and early screening of infants at risk for urinary tract abnormalities has led to detection of a significant number of fetuses with hydronephrosis. VUR can be suspected in utero secondary to bilateral hydronephrosis on ultrasonography and confirmed postnatally by voiding cystourethrography (Paltiel and Lebowitz; Philipson et al; Scott, 1987; Stelle et al).

RADIOLOGIC EVALUATION OF LOWER TRACT

Voiding Cystourethrography

Any infant or child with a first UTI, with or without fever, should undergo radiographic assessment of the urinary tract. The diagnosis of VUR is established accurately by use of a VCU with fluoroscopy. In a study of 350 children with UTI, 10 per cent of those with documented reflux were afebrile at presentation, and the diagnosis of reflux would have been missed if patients without fever had been excluded from voiding cystourethrography (Woodard and Holden).

Vesicoureteral reflux may occur with bladder filling or during voiding, or both. Conway et al observed reflux during bladder filling three times more frequently than during voiding. The rate of urinary flow has been shown to have an effect on the presence or absence of VUR. High flow rates are associated with an increase in the frequency and magnitude of ureteral peristalsis, which prevents VUR (Briggs et al). Conversely, low flow rates, secondary to either dehydration or poor renal function, may increase the possibility of detecting VUR.

Reflux may be diagnosed with the patient in either the awake or the anesthetized state (Lyon, 1977; Poznanski and Poznanski; Timmons et al; Woodard and Filardi). Anesthesia results in a reduction in glomerular filtration rate and, consequently, in urinary flow rates (Mazze et al). Cystograms in awake patients may result in artificially increased bladder pressures secondary to straining to resist bladder filling (King, 1976). Intravesical pressure is also an important factor in producing reflux, and minimal degrees of reflux may occur only at high intravesical pressures, such as occur with detrusor contractions.

This author prefers that voiding cystourethrography be performed with the patient awake. The dynamic VCU clearly delineates the bladder outline, bladder neck, and urethral anatomy and gives an accurate estimation of bladder capacity. Sleep cystograms can be useful in selected individuals (Timmons et al; Woodard and Filardi), but this technique should be reserved for those individuals who require cystoscopy under the same anesthetic. Contrast material should be warmed if necessary and instilled by slow to moderate infusion through a small urethral catheter. Friedland postulated that trigonal irritation secondary to instillation of contrast material at room temperature may account for transient VUR. The optimal hydrostatic pressure for a VCU is still controversial. Gravity flow should be used at no greater than 70 to 100 cm H_2O, controlled by the height of the infusion bottle above the bladder (Levitt and Weiss). The key to a successful VCU is an experienced pediatric uroradiologist and gentle and confident personnel. It often helps to have the parents with the child when the study is performed.

The timing of the VCU in relation to the presence or absence of UTI is an important consideration. Acute cystitis may result in edema at the ureterovesical junction or produce an increase in intravesical pressure and cause transient VUR (Van Gool and Tanagho). Bacteriuria may produce ureteral atony and decreased peristalsis and may also be responsible for VUR (Jeffs and Allen; Kaveggia et al). Therefore, many physicians defer voiding cystourethrography for at least 3 to 4 weeks after the urine is sterile. However, some children will have reflux only during an acute infection (Kaplan; Walker). In these selected patients, it is important to document reflux that occurs only during a UTI because this would justify placing the patient on suppressive antibiotic therapy. There is little risk of performing a VCU in the presence of reflux and bacteriuria, if the patient is covered adequately with parenteral antibiotics for a few days prior to the study.

Radionuclide Cystography

Radionuclide cystography is ideal for the patient who may require repeated or longitudinal studies on an annual basis and for screening siblings (Conway et al; Nasrallah et al; Weiss and Conway). This test offers two advantages: it subjects the patient to less radiation exposure and is more sensitive than the standard VCU. A dose of 0.5 mCi of technetium 99m pertechnetate in isotonic saline is instilled into the bladder. This provides a gonadal radiation dose of only 4 to 5 $\times$ 10^{-5} Gy, which is significantly less than the exposure with conventional voiding cystourethrography with fluoroscopy (Blaufox et al). In addition to minimizing the risk from radiation, this technique allows for prolonged observation under the gamma camera, thereby enhancing the sensitivity of the test by providing a delayed cystogram (Stewart).

Indirect Cystography

The use of indirect cystography by scanning the bladder at the time of a radionuclide renal scan is grossly inaccurate and cannot be recommended to detect VUR accurately. Compared with conventional direct radionuclide cystography, this technique is associated with at least a 50 per cent false-negative rate (Levitt and Weiss) and is particularly unreliable with milder grades of reflux. Furthermore, gonadal radiation exposure may be higher with indirect radionuclide cystography than with direct radioisotope cystograms, because radiation exposure increases further when a prolonged period is required to induce voiding.

Ultrasonography

Ultrasonography has been proposed as an in-office technique for follow-up of patients with reflux or to detect reflux in siblings. Pfister and co-workers instilled a carbonated solution into the bladder and were able to detect CO_2 bubbles in the upper urinary tract by sonography (Levitt and Weiss). Ultrasonographers claim that they can detect reflux by observing distention of the ureters and pelvicalyceal system in patients with moderately severe reflux. Although this is an easy technique and eliminates ionizing radiation, the study is associated with a significant incidence of false-negative results in patients with low-grade reflux and cannot be recommended as a routine test for the detection of VUR.

RADIOLOGIC EVALUATION OF UPPER TRACT

Excretory Urography

Assessment of upper tract anatomy is performed after voiding cystourethrography. Excretory urography has been the standard for the evaluation of upper tract anatomy in children with febrile UTI. This study should be performed in all patients with documented VUR to assess the renal parenchyma, calyceal architecture, presence or absence of duplication, and renal atrophy. Excretory urographic signs suggestive of VUR include pyelonephritic scarring, ureteral dilatation (particularly the lower ureter), longitudinal striations or folds of the renal pelvis or upper ureters, and renal growth retardation. Ginalski et al studied a group of 141 children undergoing surgery for VUR and found that preoperative excretory urography demonstrated signs suggestive of reflux in 68 per cent of refluxing renal units. Interestingly, in 21 per cent of renal units, renal growth retardation was the only radiographic sign; therefore, patients with renal growth retardation indicated by excretory urography should undergo voiding cystourethrography to rule out reflux. In patients undergoing excretory urography who have evidence of pyelonephritic scarring without obstruction, reflux may be found on voiding cystourethrography in up to 85 per cent of patients (Claësson and Lindberg; Filly et al; Govan et al; Scott and Stansfeld; Shah et al; Smellie et al, 1975). Delayed emptying of the ureter after voiding suggests an abnormal distal ureteral segment and concomitant ureterovesical obstruction, which may occur in up to 10 per cent of ureters with reflux (Weiss and Lytton).

Excretory urography should be done approximately 3 to 4 weeks after an acute UTI has cleared, because infection with coliform organisms may result in ureteral stasis, and an excretory urogram performed during infection may show dilated ureters (Teague and Boyarsky) (Fig. 14-1). However, children with a UTI who have persistent fever and symptoms despite antibiotic therapy should undergo excretory urography emergently to rule out obstruction.

Ultrasonography

Ultrasonography is a safe, accurate, and noninvasive test to study upper tract anatomy. This test can detect hydronephrosis, renal duplication in the presence of an obstructed upper pole segment, and gross renal scars. Renal ultrasonography should be done in children with UTI and negative results on a VCU.

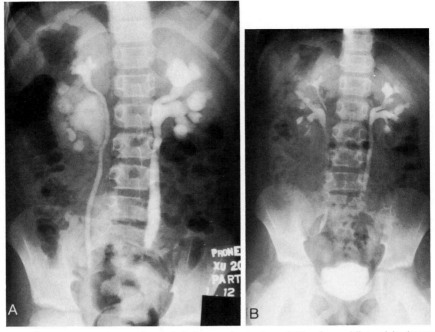

Figure 14–1 □ *A*, Excretory urogram performed during acute pyelonephritis shows bilateral hydroureteronephrosis and duplication of right collecting system. *B*, Excretory urogram performed 6 weeks after pyelonephritis shows resolution of hydroureteronephrosis bilaterally.

Isotope Renography

Radioisotopic renal scanning is a useful adjunct to the excretory urogram for evaluating patients with VUR. Technetium 99m diethylenetriaminepenta-acetic acid (DTPA) can be used to assess glomerular and tubular function, whereas technetium 99m dimercaptosuccinic acid (DMSA) is the best agent for visualizing cortical tissue and evaluating the presence or absence of renal scarring (see Chapter 4).

CLASSIFICATION AND GRADING OF REFLUX

The major etiologic categories of VUR include (1) primary VUR secondary to congenital malimplantation of the ureter with lateral ectopia; (2) chronic infection with edema and distortion of the ureterovesical angle; (3) bladder outlet obstruction with decompensation of the bladder and ureterovesical junction, such as posterior urethral valves and urethral stricture; (4) neuropathic bladder dysfunction with concomitant malfunction of ureterovesical junction, such as myelomeningocele or paraplegia;

and (5) traumatic reflux, which may occur after basket extraction of a ureteral calculus or surgical disruption of the ureterovesical junction.

Several proposed grading systems have been based on the severity of reflux as seen on VCU with contrast material (Dwoskin and Perlmutter; Heikel and Parkkulainen; Rolleston et al, 1970), the ureteral caliber and pelvicalyceal dilation (Bridge and Roe; Edelbrock and Mickelson; Howerton and Lich), or the grade of reflux according to bladder pressure (Lattimer et al; Melick et al; Smellie et al, 1975) (Table 14–1). The grading system used by the International Reflux Study Group (Fig. 14–2) proposes a standard classification for more objective comparison of therapeutic modalities and places particular emphasis on the anatomy of the fornices and calyces. Reflux is graded I through V, and there are subtle variations within each grade (Fig. 14–3).

URODYNAMIC EVALUATION

Urodynamic evaluation, including cystometrography, electromyelography, urethral pressure profiles, urinary flow studies, and occa-

Table 14–1 □ Comparison of the Heikel-Parkkulainen (1966) and Dwoskin-Perlmutter (1973) Reflux Classification Systems

Heikel-Parkkulainen System	Dwoskin-Perlmutter System
Grade I—Reflux confined to lower ureter	Grade 1—Reflux into ureter only
Grade II—Reflux into a renal pelvis of normal size	Grade 2A—Reflux to kidney; no dilation of calyces
Grade III—Reflux with slightly dilated ureter and pelvis	Grade 2B—Mild dilation of ureter with mild calyceal blunting
Grade IV—Reflux into moderately dilated ureter and pelvis	Grade 3—Severe dilation of collecting system and ureteral tortuosity
Grade V—Massive reflux into grossly dilated ureter and pelvis	Grade 4—Massive reflux with megaureter

From Walker RD: Vesicoureteral reflux. *In* Adult and Pediatric Urology, Vol 2. Edited by JY Gillenwater, JT Grayhack, SS Howards, et al. Chicago, Year Book Medical Publishers, 1987, pp 1676–1708.

sionally video-urodynamics, may be helpful in selected patients with VUR. Preoperative urodynamic studies should be done in patients with urgency, frequency, urge incontinence (uninhibited detrusor contractions), squatting maneuvers, or encopresis, all of which may suggest an occult neuropathic bladder with secondary reflux. These studies are also important in children with a sacral dimple, hairy patch, decreased perineal sensation, or decreased rectal tone, or in children in whom the radiographic studies show sacral agenesis, dysgenesis, or a thick-walled or vertical bladder with diverticula. Urodynamic evaluation should also be performed in the patient with persistent VUR after a technically successful ureteroneocystostomy (Mesrobian et al).

Cystometric studies are more difficult to interpret in children with high grades of reflux. In these patients, it is often necessary to place Fogarty catheters into the ureteral orifice to prevent reflux at the time of cystometrography (Woodside and Borden). Patients with detrusor instability or detrusor-sphincter dyssynergia may require frequent or timed voiding,

double voiding, anticholinergic therapy, or intermittent catheterization prior to surgical correction of reflux (Koff and Murtagh). Patients with high-pressure voiding and decreased detrusor compliance may require pharmacologic therapy, intermittent catheterization, or augmentation cystoplasty in conjunction with ureteral reimplantation. (See discussion of Antireflux Surgery in the Neuropathic Bladder.)

ETIOLOGY AND PATHOGENESIS OF PRIMARY REFLUX

The anatomic features that characterize the normal valve mechanism of the ureterovesical junction include an oblique entry of the ureter into the bladder (Harrison), an adequate length of the intramural ureter, especially of its submucosal segment (Johnston, 1962; King et al, 1974), and support of the detrusor muscle (King, 1976) (Fig. 14–4). The extravesical ureter consists of three muscle layers: an inner longitudinal, a middle circular, and an outer

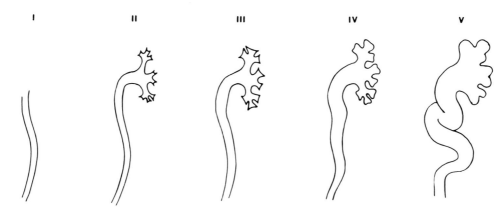

Figure 14–2 □ International Reflux Classification. (From Walker RD: Vesicoureteral reflux. *In* Adult and Pediatric Urology, Vol 2. Edited by JY Gillenwater, JT Grayhack, SS Howards, et al. Chicago, Year Book Medical Publishers, 1987, pp 1676–1708.)

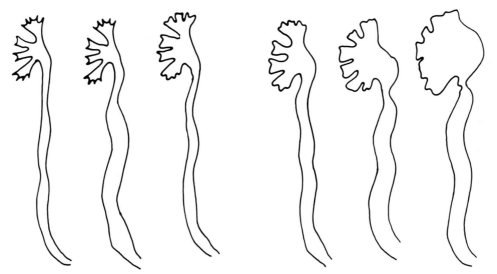

Figure 14–3 □ Variations with grades III and IV of the International Reflux Classification. (From Walker RD: Vesicoureteral reflux. *In* Adult and Pediatric Urology, Vol 2. Edited by JY Gillenwater, JT Grayhack, SS Howards, et al. Chicago, Year Book Medical Publishers, 1987, pp 1676–1708.)

longitudinal layer. The ureteral adventitia and circular muscle layer continue into the bladder wall in the upper part of the ureteral hiatus to form Waldeyer's sheath, which attaches the ureter to the hiatus. This attachment is lax, and during bladder filling, the hiatus can slide along the extravesical ureter. Within the bladder, the circular layer disappears and the longitudinal muscle fibers continue distally be-

yond the ureteral orifice into the trigone and intertwine with fibers from the contralateral ureter, forming Bell's muscle of the trigone and the posterior urethra (Fig. 14–5) (Mathisen). This complex acts as a single functional unit, and experimental interruption of this unit results in incompetence of the ureterovesical angle and VUR (Tanagho et al, 1965). The well-established continuity between the ureter

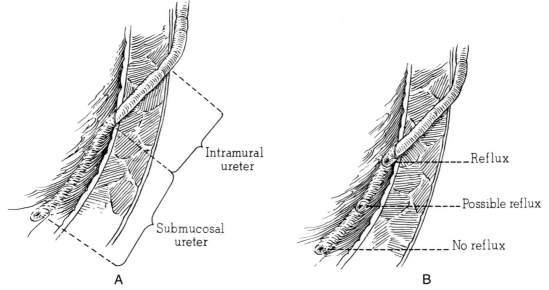

Figure 14–4 □ *A*, Normal ureterovesical junction. Demonstration of length of intravesical submucosal ureteral segment. *B*, Refluxing ureterovesical junction. Same anatomic features as nonrefluxing orifice, except for inadequate length of intravesical submucosal ureter, are shown. Some orifices reflux intermittently with borderline submucosal tunnels. (From Politano VA: Vesicoureteral reflux. *In* Urologic Surgery, 2nd ed. Edited by JF Glenn. New York, Harper & Row Publishers, 1975, pp 272–293.)

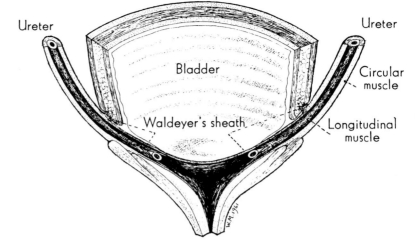

Figure 14–5 □ The passage of the ureter through the ureteral hiatus in the bladder wall. The drawing illustrates how Bell's muscle is a direct continuation of the longitudinal muscle of the ureter. (From Mathisen W: Vesicoureteral reflux and its surgical correction. Surg Gynecol Obstet 118:965, 1964. By permission of Surgery, Gynecology and Obstetrics.)

and the trigone (ureterotrigonal complex) prevents excessive mobility of the orifice by fixing it in position.

With bladder filling, the ureteral lumen is flattened between the bladder mucosa and the detrusor muscle, thereby creating a flap-valve mechanism that prevents VUR. This "valve mechanism" is probably more passive than active (Tanagho et al, 1965; Young and Wesson). The passive nature of the mechanism of the ureterovesical angle is well demonstrated by the fact that reflux cannot be produced in the postmortem specimen (Kelalis, 1985). During micturition, contraction of the detrusor muscle results in an increase in intravesical pressure, which may herniate the ureteral orifice through the wall of the bladder. This herniation does not occur with normal and adequate fixation of the ureterovesical junction, but it is likely to occur with maldevelopment of the trigonal region and lateral displacement of the ureteral orifice. The ureterotrigonal longitudinal muscles close the ureteral meatus and submucosal tunnel during a detrusor contraction and provide the "active" component of the ureterovesical junction (Stephens and Lenaghan; Tanagho et al, 1969).

The single most important factor in maintaining the one-way characteristic of the ureterovesical junction is the occlusion of the ureteral lumen as the increase in intravesical pressure compresses it against the detrusor muscle. The ureteral orifice must be immobile and therefore must have adequate detrusor support. Paraureteral diverticula tend to enlarge and obliterate the submucosal tunnel by displacing the intramural ureter extravesically,

resulting in incompetence of the ureterovesical junction.

Primary VUR is a congenital condition resulting from an inadequate valvular mechanism and deficiency of the longitudinal muscle of the submucosal ureter. The degree of deficiency usually correlates with the degree of incompetence of the ureterovesical junction. There is no obstruction or neuropathic bladder component. The ratio of the submucosal tunnel length to the ureteral diameter is the primary factor that determines the effectiveness of this valve mechanism (Paquin; Stephens and Lenaghan). Paquin found that in normal children without reflux, the ratio of tunnel length to ureteral diameter was 5:1, whereas in children with reflux, the same ratio was 1.4:1. Cussen documented the relationship among intravesical ureteral length, submucosal ureteral length, and ureteral diameters in normal children (Table 14–2). The length of the intravesical ureter (intramural plus submucosal segments) has been estimated to average 1.3 cm in adults and 0.5 cm in neonates (Hutch, 1961).

In 1969, Lyon et al described four basic orifice shapes: cone, stadium, horseshoe, and golf-hole. The position (Fig. 14–6) and shape (Fig. 14–7) of the ureteral orifice correlate well with the length of the intramural tunnel. Orifices that were placed laterally showed a higher incidence of reflux and most likely had shorter submucosal tunnels. Lyon found a 4 per cent prevalence of reflux in patients with a normal orifice configuration, 28 per cent incidence of reflux in those with a stadium orifice, 83 per cent in those with a horseshoe shape, and 100 per cent when the orifice was golf-hole in

Table 14–2 □ Mean Ureteral Tunnel Lengths and Diameters in Normal Children

Age (Years)	Intravesical Ureteral Length (mm)	Submucosal Ureteral Length (mm)	Ureteral Diameter at Ureterovesical Junction (mm)
1–3	7	3	1.4
3–6	7	3	1.7
6–9	9	4	2.0
9–12	12	6	1.9

Adapted from Cussen LJ: Dimensions of the normal ureter in infancy and childhood. Invest Urol 5:164–178, 1967. By permission of Williams & Wilkins Company.

appearance. Heale confirmed Lyon's earlier observations and reported a higher prevalence and grade of reflux, as well as renal scarring, with more laterally placed and abnormally shaped orifices. Stephens subsequently described another orifice configuration that he termed the "lateral pillar defect" (Fig. 14–7). This orifice lies midway between a horseshoe and golf-hole configuration.

Although orifice shape and position can be assessed accurately during cystoscopy, the degree of bladder filling must be taken into account in describing the shape of the orifice and its position. Because reflux often occurs with a full bladder at voiding, it is important to assess the configuration and shape of the orifice during moderate bladder distention. Progressive bladder filling displaces the orifice laterally and changes its appearance toward a more abnormal type. Many orifices that appear normal at initial observation clearly become incompetent with progressive bladder filling.

King et al (1974) emphasized submucosal tunnel length as an important prognostic measurement for predicting the likelihood of spontaneous resolution of VUR. The length of the submucosal tunnel can be measured accurately with a graduated ureteral catheter (Fig. 14–8). Even though King's results indicate an almost linear relationship between tunnel length at time of diagnosis and likelihood of eventual cessation of reflux (Fig. 14–9), Duckett and Bellinger reported inconsistencies with the measurement of submucosal tunnel length and resolution of reflux.

Abnormal location and configuration of the

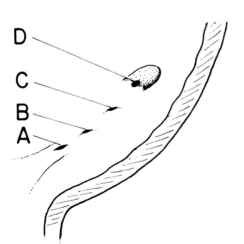

Figure 14–6 □ Diagram showing four different orifice positions. *A*, Normal position. *B*, Moderately lateral. *C*, Very lateral. *D*, Orifice at the mouth of a diverticulum. (From Glassberg KI, Hackett RE, Waterhouse K: Congenital anomalies of the kidney, ureter, and bladder. *In* Urology, Vol 1. Edited by AR Kendall, L Karafin, HS Goldsmith. Philadelphia, Harper & Row, 1987. By permission of the authors.)

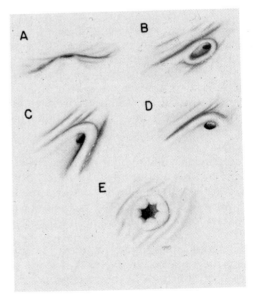

Figure 14–7 □ Orifice morphology. *A*, Normal cone or volcanic orifice. *B*, Stadium orifice. *C*, Horseshoe orifice. *D*, Lateral pillar defect orifice. *E*, Golf-hole orifice. (From Glassberg KI, Hackett RE, Waterhouse K: Congenital anomalies of the kidney, ureter, and bladder. *In* Urology, Vol 1. Edited by AR Kendall, L Karafin, HS Goldsmith. Philadelphia, Harper & Row, 1987. By permission of the authors.)

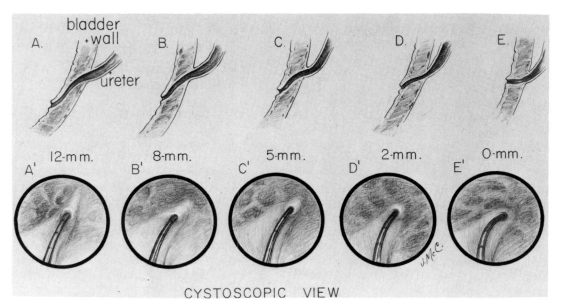

Figure 14–8 □ The cystoscopic appearance of the ureterovesical junction. A ureteral catheter is used to estimate the length of the submucosal tunnel. The ureter is drawn as normal in diameter to emphasize the appearance of the flap elevated by the catheter.

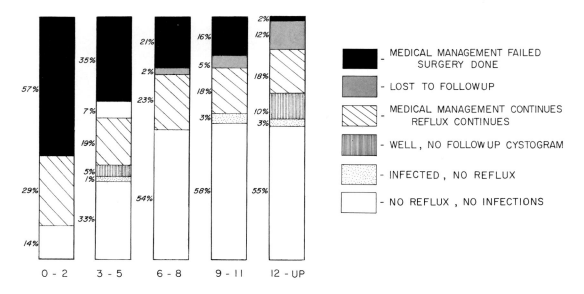

LENGTH OF INTRAMURAL URETER IN MILLIMETERS

Figure 14–9 □ This graph depicts the relationship between the estimated length of the intravesical ureter at the time of diagnosis and the outcome of a trial of nonoperative management in 247 refluxing units in which the tunnel length was estimated in patients followed for 4 to 10 years. There is a nearly linear relationship between original tunnel length and eventual cessation of reflux, indicating the importance of this parameter.

ureteral orifice may be associated with developmental renal anomalies. The "ureteral bud theory" proposed by Mackie and Stephens attempted to correlate renal morphology, based on a quantitative scale of hypoplasia and dysplasia, with the position of the ureteral orifice. These authors postulated that when the ureteral bud did not arise from the appropriate segment of the wolffian duct, the ureteral orifice was located in an abnormally lateral position on the trigone (Mackie and Stephens). The eventual point of contact between the mesonephric duct and the nephrogenic blastema would be similarly ectopic, making it less likely to differentiate normally. More severe degrees of displacement of the orifice correlated well with high scores on the hypoplasia/dysplasia scale (Fig. 14–10). Sommer and Stephens showed correlation between an abnormal position of the ureteral orifice with reflux and associated renal dysplasia and scarring in children. Conversely, other investigators have not found a high prevalence of renal dysplasia in kidneys with VUR and renal scarring (Ambrose et al).

RELATIONSHIP OF VESICOURETERAL REFLUX AND RENAL SCARRING

Experimental Studies

Although some studies suggest that renal scarring may occur on a congenital basis (Mackie and Stephens; Sommer and Stephens), the majority of evidence supports the concept that renal scarring is an acquired phenomenon. The importance of intrarenal reflux in the pathogenesis of pyelonephritic scarring has been demonstrated experimentally. Intrarenal reflux is defined as the extension of refluxed urine into the collecting tubules of the nephrons. This theory provides a readily apparent mechanism by which urinary microorganisms may

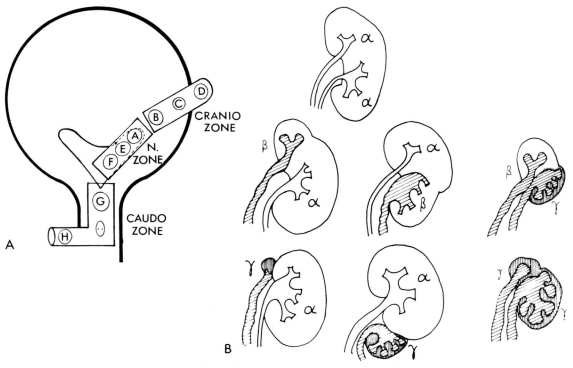

Figure 14–10 ☐ *A*, Possible sites of ureteral orifices. Dissection of stillborn material reveals that orifices on the trigone in the normal position A or in the E and F positions are associated with normal (α) kidneys. Refluxing orifices in the B, C, or D positions are associated with hypoplastic (β) or dysplastic (γ) kidneys shown in *B*. The more lateral the orifice, the worse the renal segment, as development in utero is apparently impaired if the ureteral bud arises from an abnormal position. *B*, The renal segment in duplicated systems. A shaded ureter indicates reflux. (From Mackie GG, Awang H, Stephens FD: The ureteric orifice: the embryologic key to radiologic status of duplex kidneys. J Pediatr Surg 10:473, 1975.)

gain access to the renal parenchyma and produce renal scarring.

Ransley and Risdon (1975b) studied effects of experimentally induced VUR on the papillary anatomy in piglets. Because the pig possesses renal papillary morphology similar to that in humans, this animal model is ideal to study the mechanisms of intrarenal reflux and renal scarring (Ransley and Risdon, 1975a). They studied the effect of low-pressure and high-pressure reflux under both sterile and infected conditions (Ransley and Risdon, 1978). The ureter of young Welsh pigs was cannulated and contrast medium was instilled through the catheter into the renal pelvis at a predetermined peak pressure (Ransley). The areas of renal parenchyma susceptible to intrarenal reflux and subsequent scarring were drained by papillae with flat or concave area cribrosa and large papillary ducts (Fig. 14–11). These concave papillae occurred predominantly in the polar regions of the kidney. Voiding cystourethrography confirmed that intrarenal reflux occurred exclusively at the upper and lower poles. Conversely, papillae in the middle areas of the renal medulla were cone-shaped with slit-like papillary ducts that closed with increased intrarenal pressure. These orifices opened obliquely onto the surface, so that an increase in pressure would tend to occlude the orifice and prevent intrarenal reflux. Scarring occurred only in areas of renal parenchyma exposed to both intrarenal reflux and infected urine. Scarring did not occur in any animal subjected to either high-pressure or low-pressure sterile reflux. These elegant studies support the hypothesis that the development of new renal scars essentially occurs only in the presence of UTI, VUR, and intrarenal reflux (Edwards et al; Ransley and Risdon, 1978; Torres et al, 1984).

The only exception to this statement is the study by Hodson et al (1975b) of sterile reflux in Sinclair miniature piglets. They placed a silver wire ring around the urethra to produce high intravesical pressures and promote intrarenal reflux. These experiments documented that sterile VUR could result in renal scarring experimentally, but only in the presence of severe outlet obstruction. Intrarenal reflux was essential for scar formation, and the severity and duration of intrarenal reflux correlated well with the degree of renal scarring (Hodson and Edwards).

Torres et al (1984) studied the effect of bacterial immunization on experimental reflux nephropathy in piglets. These authors used the experimental model of reflux nephropathy described by Hodson et al (1975b) and modified by Ransley and Risdon (1978). Male piglets underwent surgical creation of VUR at 2 weeks of age. Between the ages of 2 and 6 weeks, half of the piglets received subcutaneous injections of formalin-killed alum-precipitated *Escherichia coli* in incomplete Freund's adjuvant and half received incomplete Freund's adjuvant and vehicle alone. At 6 weeks of age all piglets were infected with an identical strain of *E. coli* introduced by suprapubic puncture. All animals were killed 6 weeks after introduction of the infecting organisms. Immunized animals tended to have less renal scarring, better renal tubular uptake of DMSA, significantly lower serum creatinine values, and less mesangial cell proliferation in glomeruli than their nonimmunized counterparts. The authors concluded that previous exposure to a specific bacterial strain and bacterial immunization had at least a mild protective effect on the development of reflux nephropathy. In a subsequent study, Torres et al (1985) reviewed various pathogenic factors that were thought to be important in the development of reflux nephropathy. The three independent risk factors studied were (1) radiographic evidence of intrarenal reflux, (2) P-fimbriation of the bacterial strain, and (3) absence of previous immunization. Animals with no or only one risk

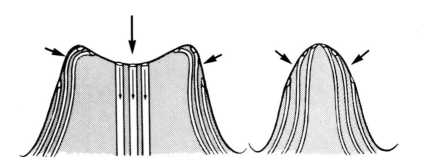

Figure 14–11 □ Anatomy of confluent and simple papillae. (From Ransley PG: Intrarenal reflux: anatomical, dynamic and radiological studies—Part I. Urol Res 5:61, 1977. By permission of Springer-Verlag.)

factor had significantly less scarring, fewer glomerular lesions, and lower serum creatinine values than those animals with two or three factors present. The authors concluded that in the experimental animal, several independent pathogenetic factors appear to have a synergistic effect on the development of reflux nephropathy.

The initial immunologic response in acute renal infection and the early formation of renal scars have been studied in rat models by direct inoculation of *E. coli* into the kidneys or into the systemic circulation or bladder in combination with transient ureteral obstruction. Active production of antibodies against the invading organism occurs systemically and in the kidney. During these inoculations, there is a depression of the cell-mediated immunity to nonspecific stimulants that is secondary to the generation of a suppressor-lymphocyte population in response to renal infection. Many of the basic observations in the rat and pig models of pyelonephritis have been reproduced, expanded, and brought closer to the human disease in a primate model developed by Roberts et al (1985). They postulated that the final determinant of renal scarring is that intrarenal reflux, in the presence of infection, causes an exudative reaction with the release of oxygen free radicals and proteolytic enzymes that develop in fibrosis and scarring. These investigators injected a bacterial inoculum into the renal pelvis of primates and produced intrarenal reflux, demonstrating that infected urine could produce renal scarring in the absence of VUR or obstruction.

Superoxide, an enzyme toxic to the renal tubular cells, is produced by neutrophils during the process of phagocytosis of bacteria. Roberts et al (1982) postulated that the pathogenesis of renal scarring was the result of the inflammatory response itself and that superoxide was responsible for renal parenchymal damage. Administration of superoxide dismutase, an antagonist of superoxide, prevented tubular cell damage without interfering with phagocytosis of bacteria.

Urinary extravasation in the renal interstitium may provoke renal damage either by directly eliciting fibrosis or by initiating an autoimmune reaction against Tamm-Horsfall protein (THP), even in the absence of urinary infection (Cotran and Pennington). This mucoprotein, a normal constituent of urine, is produced in high concentration by the tubular epithelial cells of the loop of Henle and distal nephron and is a primary constituent of renal tubular casts. Immunofluorescent techniques have demonstrated extratubular THP in the interstitium of kidneys with VUR and intrarenal reflux. Such deposits of the protein are associated with inflammatory infiltrates and fibrosis. Although extratubular THP may serve as a marker for urinary extravasation, further investigations regarding the role of THP and extratubular urinary extravasation are warranted.

Clinical Studies

Hodson (1959) was the first to recognize the frequent occurrence of renal scars in children with recurrent UTI. Ninety-seven per cent of children with renal scars showed radiographic evidence of VUR. Hodson et al (1975b) proposed that segmental scarring in chronic atrophic pyelonephritis was due to the reflux of urine into the tubules of the kidney, which either carried infection into the parenchyma or damaged the kidney by urodynamic forces. Hodson and Edwards observed that the scars were most often polar in location and associated with calyceal clubbing.

In 1973, Bailey coined the term "reflux nephropathy" to describe the radiologic abnormality of renal scarring in the presence of VUR. Hinman and Baumann introduced the terms "high-pressure reflux" and "low-pressure reflux" to indicate reflux that occurred during bladder filling (low-pressure) and reflux that occurred during voiding (high-pressure).

Studies of papillary morphology in human kidneys indicate that at least two thirds of papillae are "concave" and allow intrarenal reflux (Ransley and Risdon, 1978). Intrarenal reflux has been observed in 5 to 15 per cent of neonates and infants with VUR (Rose et al). Rolleston et al (1974) detected intrarenal reflux only in children younger than age 5 years and only in those with moderate to severe degrees of reflux. Rolleston et al (1970) observed that infants with severe reflux were more likely to have renal damage than children with lesser degrees of reflux. Furthermore, there was a significant correlation between the presence of intrarenal reflux and the subsequent development of renal scarring in the affected area.

The characteristic scarring associated with reflux nephropathy is frequently present at the time of the initial diagnosis. Renal scars usually develop during the first few years of life and rarely after the age of 5 years (Rolleston et al, 1974; Smellie and Normand). The studies by Ransley and Risdon (1978, 1981), among others (Cremin; Funston and Cremin; Tamminen and Kaprio), provided a possible explanation for this development of scars early in life. Those areas of the kidney that are drained by compound papillae are susceptible to intrarenal reflux and vulnerable to the damaging effects of VUR of infected urine (Ransley and Risdon, 1978, 1981). During the first weeks of life, small amounts of pressure in the renal pelvis can produce intrarenal reflux into these vulnerable areas of the kidney. Thereafter, increasing amounts of pressure are necessary to produce a similar effect (Funston and Cremin). Scars develop in these areas at the time of the first urinary infection during infancy, whereas the remaining areas drain by nonrefluxing papillae and remain unscarred despite persistence of the VUR and recurrent UTI. Marginally refluxing papillae may be transformed into refluxing papillae by (1) high-pressure voiding, (2) hydronephrosis, or (3) scarring and associated contraction from other susceptible areas of the kidney. This sequence of events accounts for the diffusely scarred kidney sometimes seen on excretory urography.

Becu et al proposed a different mechanism for the pathogenesis of renal scarring. These authors studied 27 kidneys from children with a diagnosis of primary nonobstructive reflux who underwent nephrectomy. They concluded that the decreased size of deformities present in patients with reflux nephropathy was the result of either a dysplastic developmental arrest or a primary dwarfism with focal segmental tubular atrophy and glomerular obsolescence rather than an inflammatory response.

Synopsis of Experimental and Clinical Studies

Experimental evidence and clinical observation suggest that the pathogenesis of reflux nephropathy is multifactorial. An integrative view of the different mechanisms that have been proposed to explain the pathogenesis of reflux nephropathy and the more rare development of progressive renal insufficiency is illustrated in Figure 14–12. Some of these mechanisms are hypothetical and obviously not all are of equal importance. Although the clinical relevance of some of the proposed mechanisms remain controversial, the multifactorial concept of the pathogenesis of reflux nephropathy helps us to understand the spectrum of clinical observations.

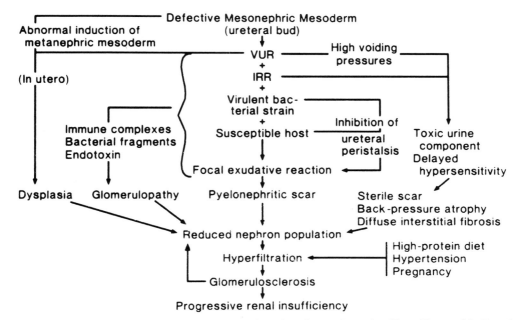

Figure 14–12 □ Integrative view of pathogenetic mechanisms in reflux nephropathy. (From Kramer SA: Experimental vesicoureteral reflux. Dialogues Pediatr Urol 7:1, 1984. By permission of William J. Miller Associates.)

VESICOURETERAL REFLUX AND GROWTH

Renal Growth

The effect of reflux on growth of the kidney is related to the presence of a normal or an abnormal contralateral kidney, infection of the urinary tract, and the grade of VUR in the affected kidney. Children with VUR and recurrent UTI are clearly at increased risk for renal scars and renal growth retardation (Hannerz et al).

Various methods have been used to evaluate renal growth, including determinations of renal length, renal area, and parenchymal thickness (Currarino; Gatewood et al; Klare et al). Even though excretory urography can show evidence of renal scarring, sequential measurements of renal length by excretory urography are inaccurate and unreliable (Hodson, 1979; Hodson et al, 1975a; Redman et al). Scar formation occurs predominantly at the renal poles, and this contracture combined with intervening hypertrophy of normal parenchyma makes interpretation of renal size by using renal length alone inaccurate and unreliable. Hodson (1979) and colleagues (1975a) recommended calculating the ratio of bipolar parenchymal thickness to total renal length. Lyon (1973) and Redman et al used bipolar renal measurements and observed a subnormal rate of renal growth in the presence of VUR without documented UTI. In a study of patients with renal duplication, Hannerz et al found parenchymal thickness to be a more accurate predictor of renal growth than either renal length or renal area.

Claësson et al (1981b) used linear measurements on a urogram to compare observed and expected renal mass. This technique is called "computerized planimetry" and involves tracing the renal parenchymal outline as well as the calyceal system to measure total renal parenchymal area in units of square centimeters. Using these measurements, Claësson et al (1981a) found compensatory hypertrophy in the contralateral normal kidney in patients with unilateral reflux and scarring. The authors devised a nomogram that allows one to determine whether or not a particular kidney or segment of kidney has appropriate mass for somatic size (Fig. 14–13).

Smellie et al (1981a) studied the effects of VUR on renal growth in a series of 76 children with various degrees of reflux. Renal growth was impaired in only those patients with documented UTI and higher grades of reflux (Tables 14–3 and 14–4). Kelalis (1971) showed that successful medical treatment of UTI in patients with VUR may be associated with resumption of renal growth.

Several authors reported accelerated renal growth after successful antireflux surgery (Atwell and Vijay; Ginalski et al; McRae et al; Willscher et al, 1976b). Scott and Stansfeld reported that successful ureteral reimplantation produced a significant increase in renal growth compared with medical management. In a series of 22 patients with a unilateral atrophic kidney and VUR, significant growth of the atrophic kidney was observed in 15 of 22 patients (68 per cent) after ureteral reimplantation (Carson et al). In 7 of 22 children (32 per cent), the small kidney grew proportionally to its mate, suggesting that preservation of small atrophic kidneys is more appropriate than nephrectomy.

Hagberg et al studied renal growth after ureteral reimplantation for gross reflux in infancy. In infants in whom the kidneys had already had significant parenchymal loss at presentation, an early antireflux operation did not influence renal growth significantly. However, kidneys that had minimal parenchymal reduction at presentation showed normal growth postoperatively, but did not "catch up" to normal kidney size.

Willscher et al (1976b) reported on 94 children who underwent antireflux surgery and found that refluxing kidneys that had not demonstrated radiographic evidence of pyelonephritic scarring demonstrated accelerated growth postoperatively. In children with bilateral parenchymal scars, there was also increased growth postoperatively. Interestingly, however, in patients with unilateral renal scarring, renal growth did not increase postoperatively.

There may be no ultimate difference in rates of renal growth whether VUR is treated medically or surgically (Atwell; Birmingham Reflux Study Group, 1983, 1987; Claësson et al, 1981a; Scott et al). Although renal growth may be greater in patients undergoing surgical correction than in those treated medically, accelerated renal growth is known to occur during puberty in medically treated patients and, therefore, these differences may not be significant in long-term follow-up (Claësson et al, 1981a). Both spontaneous resolution of reflux and surgical correction will increase renal

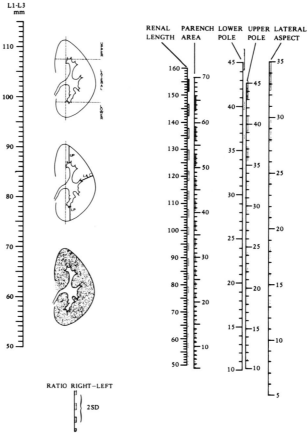

L1-L3
mm

RATIO RIGHT—LEFT

2SD

1 SD denoted by one
coloured segment + one

Figure 14–13 □ Nomogram for measuring renal parenchymal thickness and area. (From Winberg J, Claesson I, Jacobsson B, et al: Renal growth after acute pyelonephritis in childhood: an epidemiological approach. *In* Reflux Nephropathy. Edited by CJ Hodson, P Kincaid-Smith. New York, Masson Publishing USA, 1979, pp 309–322.)

blood flow, decrease voiding pressure effects on the kidney, and allow the small kidney to resume growth. Evidence from the Birmingham Reflux Study Group showed that when patients were allocated on a random basis to either medical treatment or surgery, there was no significant difference in renal growth or renal parenchymal scarring between the treatment groups (Birmingham Reflux Study Group, 1983, 1987).

Table 14–3 □ Renal Growth in 111 Kidneys With Vesicoureteral Reflux Related to Recurrence of Infection During 791 Kidney-Years of Observation*

Renal Growth	Infection	No Infection	Total
Normal	20	80	100
Slow	10	1	11

From Smellie JM, Edwards D, Normand ICS, et al: Effect of vesicoureteric reflux on renal growth in children with urinary tract infection. Arch Dis Child 56:593–600, 1981.

*$\chi^2 = 25.3$, df = 1, $P = 0.001$.

Somatic Growth

Elimination of VUR may also result in an increase in somatic growth (Merrell and Mowad; Sutton and Atwell). Smellie et al (1983) documented normal somatic growth in 51 girls

Table 14–4 □ Renal Growth in 111 Kidneys With Vesicoureteral Reflux Related to Grade of Reflux on First Diagnosis*

Renal Growth	Vesicoureteral Reflux†		Total
	Grades 1–3	Grade 4	
Accelerated or normal	88	12‡	100
Slow	5	6§	11

From Smellie JM, Edwards D, Normand ICS, et al: Effect of vesicoureteric reflux on renal growth in children with urinary tract infection. Arch Dis Child 56:593–600, 1981.

*$\chi^2 = 13.20$, df = 1, $P = 0.001$.

†Grade 1 reflux was minimal, grades 2 and 3 extended up to the kidney without dilatation, grade 2 on voiding only. Grade 4 included all reflux with dilatation of the ureter or renal pelvis.

‡Three kidneys were scarred.

§Five kidneys were scarred; all six were exposed to infection.

with VUR who were maintained on low-dose prophylactic antibiotic therapy. None of these patients underwent surgical treatment. Merrell and Mowad showed that physical growth of prepubertal children with VUR is accelerated after successful antireflux surgery. Sutton and Atwell studied a series of children with primary VUR. Patients undergoing medical treatment were observed during 1 year of treatment and patients undergoing surgical correction were observed for 2 years postoperatively. Patients undergoing successful surgical correction of reflux showed a moderate but significant increase in height and weight compared with patients undergoing medical treatment alone (Hodson, 1959).

VESICOURETERAL REFLUX AND URINARY TRACT INFECTIONS

Hodson and Edwards showed that reflux occurred more commonly in children with UTI than in those with sterile urine. VUR has been documented in 29 to 50 per cent of children with UTI undergoing voiding cystourethrography (Kunin et al; Levitt and Weiss; Savage et al; Shopfner; Walker et al; Wein and Schoenberg). In children with UTI, the prevalence of VUR is inversely proportional to age (Baker et al; Smellie et al, 1975). Infants are more commonly found to have VUR in association with UTI than are older children. In a group of patients with UTI, reflux occurred in 70 per cent of those younger than 1 year of age, 25 per cent of children at 4 years of age, 15 per cent of children at 12 years of age, and 5.2 per cent of adults (Baker et al). Walker et al studied a group of young girls with asymptomatic bacteriuria and found that reflux occurred in 29 per cent of pre–school-age children but only 23 per cent of school-age children.

Govan and Palmer showed that children with reflux tended to present with UTI approximately 2 years earlier than children with UTI and no reflux. Conversely, others (Smellie et al, 1981b) found no age difference at presentation among children with UTI with or without VUR.

Of patients investigated for renal insufficiency and found to have radiographic features of reflux nephropathy, 30 to 40 per cent have no definite history of UTI (Bakshandeh et al). These observations may be explained in that UTIs in infants and children are underdiagnosed and scarring often occurs early in life when the history is obscure and the presenting symptoms of infection may be mistaken for another febrile illness. Transient febrile illnesses with nonspecific symptomatology are generally not considered indications for urinary culture in the usual pediatric practice.

Calculi

The occurrence of primary VUR and urinary calculi in infants and children has been reported infrequently (Malek and Kelalis). The incidence of VUR in patients with calculi is approximately 8 per cent, whereas 0.5 per cent of patients with VUR have calculi (Roberts and Atwell). Voiding cystourethrography should be performed routinely in children with staghorn calculi (Lue et al; Malek).

SECONDARY VESICOURETERAL REFLUX

Infectious

UTI can produce VUR (Jeffs and Allen; Kaveggia et al; Schoenberg et al), and infection may delay spontaneous resolution of reflux (Roberts and Riopelle). Transient reflux may occur in a marginally competent ureterovesical orifice secondary to bladder inflammation or infection. Reflux secondary to UTI will generally resolve spontaneously with treatment of the infection and disappearance of the inflammatory changes at the ureterovesical junction. VUR may predispose children to UTI by contributing to increased residual urine, which acts as a fertile incubation medium for urinary pathogens in susceptible children.

Neuropathic

Neuropathic dysfunction is an important cause of secondary VUR (Allen, 1985; Hinman and Baumann). Reflux can occur in conjunction with neuropathic bladder in 15 to 60 per cent of patients (Sidi et al; Woods and Atwell). Neuropathic vesical dysfunction can be an acquired phenomenon secondary to abnormal voiding and can produce VUR in patients with a previously normal VCU.

The association of infection, reflux, and uninhibited bladder contractions in neurologically normal children has been well documented (Koff and Murtagh; Nasrallah and Simon; Seruca). Interestingly, the peak incidence of VUR occurs in children 3 to 5 years of age, which is also the peak age for dysfunctional voiding (Allen, 1985). The most common urodynamic abnormality in patients with VUR is uninhibited bladder contractions, and this correlates well with urge incontinence, urgency, frequency, and nocturnal enuresis (Homsy et al; Taylor). Taylor et al showed that 75 per cent of girls with reflux had evidence of uninhibited bladder contractions. Allen (1979) and Koff and Murtagh observed reflux in approximately 50 per cent of children undergoing urodynamic evaluation for an abnormal voiding pattern. Dysfunctional voiding secondary to detrusor-sphincter dyssynergia and uninhibited detrusor contractions may result in high intravesical pressure, UTI, and VUR (Kondo et al). Patients with detrusor-sphincter dyssynergia and VUR are at increased risk for pyelonephritis and renal scarring (King, 1983).

Koff and Murtagh treated 62 neurologically normal children with VUR with and without uninhibited bladder contractions. They found that patients with uninhibited contractions treated with anticholinergic therapy showed a statistically significant improvement in resolution of recurrent UTI and reflux compared with a control group of children with normal cystometric findings. Homsy et al and Seruca reported equally good success in treating children with voiding dysfunction with anticholinergic therapy. They observed significant resolution or reduction in stage of reflux, or both, in the majority of children treated. Clearly, bladder instability can be an important factor in causing and perpetuating reflux, and therapy directed at decreasing intravesical pressures can decrease the incidence of UTI and VUR.

Historically, patients with neuropathic bladder secondary to myelomeningocele and associated high-grade reflux were treated by urinary diversion. The acceptance and effectiveness of clean intermittent catheterization as a means to drain the bladder and the use of anticholinergic medication to lower bladder pressures has obviated the need for urinary diversion in the majority of these children (Bauer et al). Most low-grade reflux in patients with neuropathic bladder resolves with intermittent catheterization and pharmacologic therapy (Nasrallah and Simon; Taylor). In a large series of children with reflux and neuropathic bladder, 124 of 200 (62 per cent) either ceased to have reflux or the reflux was downgraded while the patient was maintained on intermittent catheterization and antibiotic suppression (Kaplan and Firlit).

Even though intermittent catheterization, anticholinergics, and antibiotic suppression should be the first line of treatment in patients with neuropathic bladder and VUR, some children may require ureteroneocystostomy. Indications for antireflux surgery in these patients are similar to those of patients with primary reflux and include breakthrough UTI despite intermittent catheterization, anticholinergics, antibiotic suppression, and the development of progressive renal scarring. Ureteral reimplantation has been shown to be an effective method for correcting reflux in children with neuropathic bladder dysfunction (Bauer et al; Evans et al). However, efforts to correct reflux surgically without regard for abnormal bladder dynamics will ultimately lead to failure and persistent reflux. These patients must be maintained on anticholinergic medication and intermittent catheterization postoperatively to keep bladder pressures low.

A select group of patients with neuropathic bladder and high voiding pressure may require augmentation cystoplasty in addition to ureteroneocystostomy. Enterocystoplasty effectively lowers bladder pressures, and the success of ureteral reimplantation into either the bladder or bowel segment has been well documented. The use of enterocystoplasty alone may normalize detrusor pressure and correct reflux without the necessity of performing ureteral reimplantation (Nasrallah and Aliabadi).

VESICOURETERAL REFLUX AND PREGNANCY

Physiologic changes of the urinary tract during pregnancy include hydroureteronephrosis, ureteral tortuosity, and decreased peristalsis. These changes are attributed most often to ureteral obstruction from the gravid uterus and from secretion of prostaglandins and progesterone-like hormones. The prevalence of asymptomatic bacteriuria during pregnancy is between 4 and 6 per cent. Pyelonephritis occurs in 20 to 40 per cent of pregnant women with asymptomatic bacteriuria (Heidrick et al; Whalley and Cunningham).

Williams et al evaluated 100 women with asymptomatic bacteriuria during pregnancy, all of whom were treated with an acute course of antibiotic therapy. Cystograms performed 4 to 6 months post partum showed VUR in 21 patients. The incidence of bacteriuria after delivery was higher in patients with reflux (62 per cent) than in those without reflux (16 per cent). Furthermore, the incidence of renal scarring was also higher in women with reflux (48 per cent) than in those without reflux (9 per cent). Bacteriuria was more difficult to clear during pregnancy despite antibiotic therapy in patients with reflux (33 per cent) compared with those without reflux (67 per cent) ($P < .0005$) (Williams et al).

These studies and others (Heidrick et al; Hutch, 1961) have shown a disproportionately high incidence of acute pyelonephritis during pregnancy in women with recurrent bacteriuria and reflux compared with women without reflux. Furthermore, bacteriuria in the presence of VUR may be more difficult to eradicate with a single course of antibiotics and tends to persist more frequently post partum than in patients without reflux. Because it is not possible to predict in which pregnant women bacteriuria will develop, most authors continue to recommend surgical correction of reflux when it persists beyond puberty in girls.

Austenfeld and Snow reviewed the records of 67 women who had undergone surgical correction of reflux by ureteroneocystostomy and had a minimum of 15 years of follow-up. Thirty women became pregnant, for a total of 64 pregnancies. During pregnancy, 17 of 30 women (57 per cent) had one or more UTIs and 5 of 30 (17 per cent) had one or more episodes of pyelonephritis. The incidence of pyelonephritis during pregnancy (17 per cent) was statistically higher than the 4 per cent incidence of pyelonephritis in these women prior to pregnancy. There were eight spontaneous abortions. These results suggest that women with surgically corrected reflux are at greater risk for pyelonephritis compared to controls. However, a weakness of this study was that the authors did not compare patients who had undergone ureteroneocystostomy with a control group of women with reflux who had not undergone ureteral reimplantation.

Pregnancy has been shown to affect renal function adversely in long-term studies of women with moderate renal failure (Becker et al). The outcome of pregnancy in women with reflux nephropathy is dependent on the degree of renal impairment and the presence of hypertension and proteinuria (Jungers et al; Weaver and Craswell). Women with hypertension and moderate renal insufficiency in the initial stages of pregnancy are at risk for hypertension and accelerated decline in renal function during pregnancy. Kincaid-Smith and Fairley noted that 36 per cent of women with moderate renal insufficiency developed hypertension, and 8 per cent had accelerated decline in renal function throughout pregnancy.

VESICOURETERAL REFLUX AND URETEROPELVIC JUNCTION OBSTRUCTION

The coexistence of VUR and ureteropelvic junction obstruction is well documented (DeKlerk et al; Lebowitz and Blickman; Maizels et al; Whitaker). The incidence of reflux in large series of patients with ureteropelvic junction obstruction ranges from 5 to 24 per cent (Hollowell et al; Kelalis and Kramer, 1987; Lebowitz and Blickman). Maizels et al found VUR in 11 of 124 patients (9 per cent) undergoing pyeloplasty. In a retrospective series of 200 children with ureteropelvic junction obstruction, Lebowitz and Blickman found 10 per cent had associated VUR. In a study of 120 patients with ureteropelvic junction obstruction undergoing voiding cystourethrography, Hollowell et al found that 17 (14 per cent) demonstrated VUR. In each of these studies, the majority of patients had incidental reflux that resolved spontaneously over time.

The incidence of ureteropelvic junction obstruction in patients with VUR ranges from 0.8 to 14 per cent (Hollowell et al; Lebowitz and Blickman; Leighton and Mayne). In a retrospective review of 2800 patients with VUR, Lebowitz and Blickman found ureteropelvic junction obstruction in 0.8 per cent. "Apparent" ureteropelvic junction obstruction is suggested at voiding cystourethrography when there is significant ureteral dilatation and pelvic dilatation. However, the ureter drains well on antegrade studies. Voiding cystourethrography with fluoroscopy and appropriate post-voiding drainage films and antegrade studies (i.e., excretory urography with a catheter draining the bladder to prevent reflux) are necessary to rule out ureteropelvic junction obstruction secondary to VUR. Patients with significant VUR and concomitant ureteropelvic junction obstruction secondary to fixed kinks should undergo primary pyeloplasty (Maizels et al). Primary ureteral reimplantation may provoke an acute ureteropelvic junction decompensation and obstruction that requires subsequent pyeloplasty (Hollowell et al; Leighton and Mayne). Ureteral reimplantation should be reserved for those patients with persistent high-grade reflux after successful pyeloplasty (Kelalis and Kramer, 1987).

VESICOURETERAL REFLUX IN SIBLINGS

The familial incidence of VUR among siblings of patients with reflux ranges from 8 to 45 per cent (Tobenkin; Van den Abbeele et al). This compares with a prevalence of less than 1 per cent spontaneous VUR cases in the general population. Although the pattern of genetic transmission is undetermined, investigators favor a polygenic or multifactorial mode of inheritance (Burger and Burger; Levitt and Weiss). Dwoskin found 26.5 per cent of siblings to have VUR from 125 families of probands with reflux. Jerkins and Noe screened 104 siblings of 78 patients who had VUR with a VCU while they were awake and found 34 (33 per cent) had reflux. Interestingly, 25 (74 per cent) of these siblings did not have evidence of either UTI or voiding dysfunction. The highest incidence of reflux was found in the siblings of patients with radiographic evidence of renal scarring. These authors recommended that all siblings younger than 5 years of age should undergo voiding cystourethrography.

In a follow-up report, Noe studied a group of children with reflux and dysfunctional voiding. Twenty per cent of siblings of these patients demonstrated reflux. In another group of patients without symptoms of bladder dysfunction, 38 per cent of siblings had reflux. In both groups, reflux in siblings occurred irrespective of grade, scarring, frequency of infections, or age of the index case. Noe recommended that all siblings younger than 10 years of age undergo screening cystography.

Most authors concur with these recommendations and obtain a radionuclide VCU in siblings of index patients with reflux. In siblings with documented reflux, upper tract evaluation with either excretory urography, ultrasonography, or isotope renography is recommended.

VESICOURETERAL REFLUX IN BOYS

Decter et al reviewed the records of 86 boys with primary VUR. This group represented approximately 13.5 per cent of the authors' total population with primary reflux. More than a third of the cases were diagnosed during the first year of life, and younger children tended to have the most severe reflux at presentation. Two thirds of patients were evaluated because of UTI, whereas 15 per cent had symptoms of voiding dysfunction without infection. Approximately 20 per cent of patients had renal scars at diagnosis.

Boys with low-grade reflux who presented with UTI were treated initially with antibiotics, but the therapy was discontinued as they grew older. Older boys with low-grade reflux who had not presented with a UTI were simply observed. These patients were assumed to be at minimal risk for scarring subsequent to urinary infection, and long-term antibiotic therapy and aggressive follow-up were not necessary. Unfortunately, the study suffers from the fact that more than half of the patients treated medically did not have adequate follow-up.

Decisions for surgery were based on persistent reflux and the cystoscopic assessment of the orifice position, configuration, and tunnel length. Seventy-three per cent of boys underwent surgery because of high-grade reflux or abnormal location of the orifice on cystoscopy. Thirteen per cent had reimplantation because of breakthrough UTI, 10 per cent because of age, and 3.3 per cent because of progressive scarring.

MEDICAL MANAGEMENT OF REFLUX

Natural History

There is a natural tendency for VUR to improve or resolve spontaneously over time, and this observation should warrant initial medical management of most patients with low-grade reflux. There is a strong inverse correlation between the severity of reflux at the time of initial diagnosis and the likelihood of spontaneous resolution. Resolution or persistence of reflux is directly related to the location and configuration of the ureterovesical junction.

Elongation of the submucosal tunnel with growth increases the ratio between the length of the submucosal tunnel and the diameter of the ureter and tends to correct the abnormality of the valve mechanism (King et al, 1974; Stephens and Lenaghan).

Several objective criteria can be used to predict the chance of resolution of VUR. The presence of ureteral dilatation, abnormal position and configuration of the ureteral orifice, and a periureteral diverticulum, particularly when the ureter enters the diverticulum, all suggest the need for surgical intervention. Smellie and Normand observed spontaneous resolution of VUR in 80 per cent of kidneys with undilated ureters on voiding cystourethrography (grades I and II). Edwards et al found that reflux ceased spontaneously in 85 per cent of children with ureters of normal caliber. Conversely, only 41 per cent of kidneys with ureteral dilatation and grade III, IV, or V reflux underwent spontaneous resolution of reflux (Smellie and Normand).

In a large retrospective series, Skoog et al showed that reflux resolved in approximately 90 per cent of those with grade I reflux, 80 per cent with grade II, 50 per cent with grade III, 10 per cent with grade IV, and essentially none with grade V. In a surveillance study of children with VUR observed for 4 to 10 years, King et al (1974) reported no cases of spontaneous cure of reflux when the orifice was golf-hole in shape and when there was absence of an intravesical ureter. In Duckett's series, reflux resolved spontaneously in 63 per cent of patients with grade II, 53 per cent of those with grade III, and 33 per cent of those with grade IV reflux. Although reflux into the lower pole moiety of a completely duplicated collecting system may resolve with medical management alone, spontaneous resolution of reflux occurred in only 22 per cent of patients followed nonoperatively during a 13-year period of observation (Kaplan et al, 1978).

It had been suggested that spontaneous resolution of reflux most often occurs within the first few years after diagnosis and the rate of reflux resolution remains constant throughout childhood—approximately 10 to 15 per cent per year (Smellie and Normand). Puberty has not been associated with an increased rate of spontaneous cessation of reflux (Edwards et al). A study of a large series of children with VUR suggested that moderate grades of VUR almost always resolve within a 4-year period of observation; reflux was not likely to resolve

after that interval (McLorie et al). A group of 112 patients (86 female and 26 male) with grades III, IV, and V reflux (International Classification) was observed nonoperatively. Sixty-one patients had grade III, 38 had grade IV, and 13 had grade V reflux. Of the patients with grade III reflux, 21 per cent had resolution of reflux in an average of 2.6 years. Ninety-two per cent of patients who had resolution of reflux did so within 4 years. Grade IV reflux resolved in only one patient in 2.9 years of follow-up, and 86 per cent of patients with grade IV reflux ultimately required surgery. Patients with grade V reflux clearly benefited from early surgical repair.

Renal Scarring

Approximately 30 to 50 per cent of patients with VUR have renal scarring on initial evaluation. Huland and Busch observed new renal scars in only 7 of 213 patients (3 per cent) with UTI and reflux. Smellie et al (1975) studied 233 children with VUR, UTI, and previously normal kidneys and found that renal scars developed in only 10 (4 per cent). In a later and expanded series of patients with normal kidneys, Smellie and Normand reported that new renal scars developed in 83 of 1720 (5 per cent). Eighty of these 83 children had a history of reflux and 79 of 83 had UTI.

Although the majority of patients with reflux in whom renal scars develop show them at an early age, renal scarring is not confined exclusively to the young child as has been suggested previously. Smellie et al (1985) documented newly diagnosed renal scars in 34 of 87 patients (39 per cent) who were older than 5 years of age when scarring developed. In many of these patients, treatment of UTI was delayed, which may explain the progression of renal scarring documented subsequently.

The presence or absence of renal scarring is directly related to continuous low-dose antibiotic therapy to maintain sterile urine. Children with uncomplicated primary reflux in whom continuous low-dose chemoprophylaxis is successful in maintaining sterile urine rarely have scars. Smellie and Normand followed a large group of children with VUR and reported that new scarring developed in only two patients while on continuous low-dose chemoprophylaxis in a 7- to 15-year follow-up. Both of these patients had breakthrough UTI and moderate to severe reflux. Lenaghan et al used *intermittent* short courses of antibacterial drugs for the treatment of recurrent infections in children with reflux. Of 76 kidneys that were initially normal, renal scarring developed in 16 (21 per cent). Of 44 kidneys with established scars, additional scarring developed in 66 per cent (Weaver and Craswell). All patients with new or progressive scarring had intercurrent infections.

Rolleston et al (1974) showed that in infants with *intrarenal* reflux who underwent surgical treatment, there was no progression of renal scarring, whereas progression or development of scars was observed in patients treated medically. Surgical correction of reflux failed to prevent progression of renal scarring in the study by Filly et al. Randomized prospective studies have shown no significant difference between medical and surgical treatment with respect to development of new scars or progression of pre-existing scars (Birmingham Reflux Study Group, 1987). The Birmingham Reflux Study Group (1987) found 10 new developing scars in a long-term follow-up of more than 5 years. These new scars affected 3.8 per cent of operated renal units and 4.5 per cent of spontaneously resolved VUR. All scars developed within the first 2 years after randomization in the study. Because the complete formation of radiologically visible scars can take up to 2 years, the 3.8 per cent incidence of scarring found postoperatively may be causally related to ascending UTI preoperatively (Beetz et al).

In 1980, an international prospective randomized clinical trial was initiated among a group of major teaching hospitals in the United States and Europe (Levitt and Weiss). Patients with primary grade IV (International Classification) reflux were accepted into the trial as well as patients with grade III reflux beyond infancy in the European group. The aims of this ongoing study are to compare the effects of successful antireflux surgery performed at the time of diagnosis with effective continuous low-dose antibiotic prophylaxis. This therapeutic trial was designed to examine whether sterile high-grade reflux itself was deleterious and to compare the differences, if any, between surgery and medical treatment of reflux and their effects on renal growth, new scars, and progression of established scars. The study also attempts to examine the incidence of recurrent UTI and hypertension in surgically versus medically treated patients.

Long-term follow-up in adults with corrected or uncorrected VUR has been reported (De Sy et al; Hawtrey et al; Malek et al, 1983a, 1983b; Nativ et al; Neves et al; Torres et al, 1983; Zucchelli and Gaggi). Malek et al (1983b) studied 67 adults with primary VUR and found a significant correlation between the severity of reflux and the extent of renal scarring. The age of the patients at the time of the first recognized UTI and the frequency and pattern of subsequent infections did not correlate with the severity of renal scarring.

Hypertension

Reflux nephropathy is the most common disorder leading to severe hypertension in children. The variability of hypertension in reflux nephropathy is affected by the degree of parenchymal damage, the involvement of one or both kidneys, the degree of renal insufficiency, and the age of the patient. Inasmuch as hypertension may develop several years after renal damage, blood pressure measurements should be performed frequently in these children for the rest of their lives.

Hypertension develops in between 10 and 20 per cent of children with VUR and renal scars with long-term follow-up (Smellie et al, 1975). In a series of 189 patients with VUR observed for a mean of 10.8 years, Beetz et al found that 61 patients (32 per cent) had renal scars. In 7 of those 61 patients (11.5 per cent), moderate arterial hypertension developed. Wallace et al reported hypertension in 11.3 per cent of patients with unilateral renal scarring and in 18.5 per cent of children with bilateral renal scars who were observed more than 10 years after ureteroneocystostomy for correction of VUR.

Hypertension is a well-known long-term complication in children and young adults with reflux nephropathy in whom end-stage renal failure develops (Torres et al, 1983). In an analysis of 100 children with severe hypertension, Gill et al found 14 children with reflux nephropathy. Holland reviewed the literature and found 177 patients with hypertension associated with reflux and renal scarring. The overwhelming majority of patients were female and most patients had a history of prior UTI (Table 14–5).

Malek et al (1983a) reported a 34 per cent incidence of hypertension in long-term follow-up of adults with reflux nephropathy. This incidence of hypertension is approximately twice that expected in a normal white population. Hypertension developed in 3 of 67 pa-

Table 14–5 ☐ Hypertension Associated With Reflux and Renal Scarring

Diagnosis	No. of Cases	Female:Male Ratio	Prior History of UTI (%)	Prevalence of VUR No. with VUR / No. of VCUs Done (%)	
Chronic pyelonephritis	99	4:1	66	36/43	(84)
Segmental hypoplasia	49	5:1	8	9/21	(43)
Primary interstitial nephritis	15	4:1	—	10/11	(91)
Reflux nephropathy	8	8:0	75	8/8	(100)
Ask-Upmark kidney	6	6:0	50	2/2	(100)

Modified from Holland NH: Reflux nephropathy and hypertension. *In* Reflux Nephropathy. Edited by CJ Hodson, P Kincaid-Smith. New York, Masson Publishing USA, 1979, pp 257–262.
Abbreviations: UTI, urinary tract infection; VUR, vesicoureteral reflux; VCU, voiding cystourethrogram.

tients (4 per cent) with unilateral scarring and 19 of 67 (28 per cent) of those with bilateral renal scarring (Torres et al, 1983). Moreau et al found hypertension in 4.9 per cent of the 15- to 25-year-old patients with renal scarring and normal renal function. Up to the age group of 46 to 66 years, the prevalence increased to 41 per cent. Kincaid-Smith et al reported a prevalence of 45.3 per cent in adult women with renal scarring. Interestingly, spontaneous resolution of reflux or surgical correction by ureteral reimplantation did not protect against the development of hypertension (Malek et al, 1983a; Stecker et al; Stickler et al).

In patients with hypertension in association with a poorly functioning renal unit, unilateral nephrectomy or partial nephrectomy has been used to cure hypertension. In these selected patients, renal vein renin studies should be obtained preoperatively. It is often necessary to obtain "segmental" renal vein renin measurements to determine accurately the source of the affected renal segment. Patients with unilateral renal scarring and localized increased renal vein renin ratios of greater than 1.5 most often achieve cure or significant improvement of their hypertension after unilateral nephrectomy (Levitt and Weiss). Conversely, patients with asymmetric bilateral renal scarring and localized increased renal vein renin ratios are less successfully treated by unilateral nephrectomy.

Renal Insufficiency

Vesicoureteral reflux is or has been present in 30 to 40 per cent of children who have renal failure before the age of 16 years and in 20 per cent of adults who have renal failure before the age of 50 years. Reflux nephropathy and renal insufficiency are often detected during the course of diagnostic evaluation for hyper-

tension or proteinuria in older children. Significant proteinuria has been a constant finding in patients with reflux and progressive deterioration of renal function (Malek et al, 1983a; Torres et al, 1983). The glomerular lesion of reflux nephropathy will vary depending on the degree of proteinuria and alteration in renal function (Torres et al, 1980a). In patients with significant proteinuria, segmental sclerotic lesions similar to idiopathic focal sclerosing glomerulonephrosis have been documented.

Genetic markers such as HLA-B12 in female patients, HLA-B8 in combination with HLA-A9 or HLA-Bw15 in male patients, and HLA-Bw15 in patients of both sexes have been found with end-stage renal disease secondary to reflux nephropathy (Torres et al, 1980a). It has been postulated that these markers may be a link to a gene that confers susceptibility to renal damage by VUR.

The role of antireflux surgery in patients with advanced reflux nephropathy and compromised renal function remains controversial (Torres et al, 1980b). Salvatierra and Tanagho recommended surgical correction of bilateral reflux even in older children and adolescents with reflux nephropathy and compromised renal function. They believed that successful surgical correction may (1) retard the rate of progression toward end-stage renal failure, (2) prevent the accelerated deterioration that sometimes occurs in patients with reflux nephropathy after an episode of acute pyelonephritis, and (3) maximize somatic growth in this subset of patients. Benefits in correcting reflux in patients with end-stage renal disease include (1) less severe anemia in those who retain their native kidneys and are on renal dialysis, (2) decreased threat to life from pyelonephritis secondary to reflux in an immunosuppressed patient, and (3) decreased need for bilateral nephrectomies in preparation for renal transplantation (Salvatierra and Tanagho).

In long-term follow-up of 67 adults (mean age, 29 years) with primary bilateral VUR who underwent bilateral ureteroneocystostomy, Torres et al (1983) found that renal insufficiency occurred only in those patients with bilateral renal scarring. The presence or absence of proteinuria was an excellent prognostic indicator, and significant proteinuria was found almost exclusively in patients with renal insufficiency. In a subsequent series of papers, the authors showed that surgical correction of reflux in adults with severely damaged kidneys and significant proteinuria did not prevent the progression of renal insufficiency (Malek et al, 1983a; Neves et al; Torres et al, 1980b). Patients with mean serum creatinine values greater than 2.75 mg/dl often progressed to renal failure despite successful surgical correction of reflux (Torres et al, 1980b).

Antibiotic Prophylaxis

The main goal in the management of VUR is the prevention of ascending UTI and renal scarring. Prospective studies have shown clearly that parenchymal damage can be prevented by long-term continuous chemoprophylaxis or a successful reflux operation. Medical management of VUR consists of preventing UTI through proper wiping techniques, frequent voiding, avoidance of constipation, ensuring low-pressure voiding, and continuous low-dose chemoprophylaxis until reflux has resolved on radiographic studies. Long-term antibacterial therapy is usually safe and well tolerated by the majority of children. Despite rare side effects in isolated patients, most children tolerate long-term antibacterial therapy for years without sequelae. Chemoprophylactic agents should achieve high urinary concentrations and have activity against a broad spectrum of urinary pathogens. Antibacterial therapy is usually prescribed in a liquid form and calculated to be one half of the standard therapeutic dose. The prophylactic medication should be given once daily at bedtime, because that is the time when the child will retain urine longest and infection will likely develop.

Either trimethoprim-sulfamethoxazole (Septra) or nitrofurantoin macrocrystals (Macrodantin) is an excellent initial choice for antibiotic therapy. Septra is contraindicated in children younger than 1 month of age. Sulfa and trimethoprim-sulfa combinations have been associated with blood dyscrasias, Stevens-Johnson syndrome, gastrointestinal symptoms, and central nervous system abnormalities. A complete blood cell count should be done at 6-month intervals to rule out leukopenia and thrombocytopenia.

Rare side effects of nitrofurantoin include interstitial pneumonitis or pulmonary fibrosis, exfoliative dermatitis, hemolytic anemia, and peripheral neuropathies. It may cause gastrointestinal disturbance and is best given in combination with food or drink. This drug is contraindicated in patients with renal insufficiency, because it may result in peripheral neuropathy. Nitrofurantoin should not be used in children younger than 2 months of age. Children allergic to sulfa or nitrofurantoin are candidates for cephalosporins, trimethoprim, nalidixic acid (NegGram), or methenamine mandelate (Mandelamine)–ascorbic acid.

After reflux has been diagnosed, specimens for urine culture should be obtained by catheter every 3 to 4 months in girls and midstream specimens should be obtained in boys to rule out occult UTI. Home culture programs allow the parents to culture the urine at frequent intervals (1 to 3 months) at a fraction of the cost of coming to the clinic. Negative cultures are usually reliable; however, positive cultures should be confirmed in the clinic with a specimen obtained by catheter, and treatment should be altered accordingly.

Inasmuch as resolution of reflux is approximately 10 to 15 per cent per year, a radionuclide cystogram should be obtained at 12-month intervals. Evaluation of the upper tract is done annually with either a DMSA renal scan or renal ultrasonography. Antibiotics should be continued until reflux resolves. Some investigators recommend two sequential normal VCUs before assuming that reflux has resolved. I believe that antibiotic therapy can be discontinued whenever the VCU shows resolution of reflux. If the child develops febrile infections and becomes symptomatic, additional studies are performed at that time.

SURGICAL MANAGEMENT

Ureteral reimplantation for correction of VUR is a highly successful procedure in more than 95 per cent of children thus treated. The choice of technique should be individualized for the patient and will be biased by the surgeon's preference and experience. Although various surgical procedures have been advocated for the correction of VUR, all successful reimplantations involve the development of an adequate length of submucosal ureter as it courses into the bladder. This maneuver permits physiologic valve-like flattening or closing of the distal ureteral segment during periods of increased intravesical pressure such as are encountered with a full bladder and during voiding. Prevention of reflux may also be dependent on shortening of the muscular fibers of the trigone, which in turn elongates and constricts the intramural and intravesical portion of the distal ureter (Tanagho et al, 1965).

Absolute indications for surgical correction of reflux include: (1) persistent pyelonephritis despite antibiotic chemoprophylaxis, (2) noncompliance with medical management or breakthrough infections during medical treatment, (3) a refluxing ureter that opens into a bladder diverticulum, (4) ureteral obstruction in association with reflux, and (5) the cystoscopic observation of a golf-hole orifice with no submucosal tunnel. Successful surgical correction of reflux decreases the risk of pyelonephritis, eliminates progressive renal scarring, and has been associated with resumption of renal growth. Even though successful antireflux surgery prevents recurrent infections in up to 80 per cent of children, 20 to 40 per cent of patients have persistent cystitis despite correction of reflux (Beetz et al; Willscher et al, 1976a, 1976b). Interestingly, postoperative UTI has been noted to occur equally with all grades of reflux (Wacksman et al). These lower tract infections should not affect renal growth or renal function.

GENERAL SURGICAL PRINCIPLES

Endoscopy

Cystoscopic examination should be accomplished with anesthesia, most often at the time of planned ureteral reimplantation. This study serves to exclude the presence of urethral pathology, infravesical obstruction, cystitis cystica, bladder trabeculation, and vesical diverticula. The position and configuration of the ureteral orifices are assessed. Primary VUR is most likely to be associated with some degree of ureterovesical angle incompetence or measurable deficiencies of the submucosal tunnel, or both. Cystoscopic examination may accurately predict which child is likely to have

permanent reflux and, therefore, require surgical intervention.

Preliminary treatment of associated pathology such as persistent UTI or bladder-outlet obstruction should precede ureteral reimplantation. Ureteral reimplantation should be done in the absence of infection and not sooner than several weeks after an acute UTI has been eliminated. Mucosal edema from residual infection will compromise an already delicate operation and increase the chance of surgical failure.

Surgical Technique

The initial step in successful ureteral reimplantation surgery in children is the administration of excellent anesthesia, preferably by a pediatric anesthesiologist. Preoperative enemas are not necessary in most patients; however, those with neuropathic bladders or a history of constipation may benefit from preoperative bowel cathartics. A rolled towel placed under the buttocks and lower sacrum displaces the pelvis anteriorly and provides better exposure. The hips are abducted and the knees are flexed slightly.

A transverse crease incision is made two finger-breadths above the pubic symphysis just to the lateral borders of the rectus muscle. This classical Pfannenstiel incision will permit further lateral extension if necessary. The anterior rectus sheath is divided transversely to achieve adequate exposure. The rectus muscles are retracted laterally and the peritoneum is swept superiorly to provide access to the bladder. Extravesical dissection should be limited because extensive bladder mobilization can result in injury to adjacent vessels or produce vesical dysfunction and a secondary neuropathic bladder. The bladder is opened vertically in the midline down to 2 cm above the bladder neck. Manipulation of the interior of the bladder with sponges or suction is avoided to prevent edema and mucosal bleeding. The Dennis-Brown retractor provides excellent exposure. Saline-soaked sponges are placed beneath each blade of the retractor to prevent mucosal hemorrhage and edema.

A successful reimplantation involves straightening any kinks or angulation of the terminal ureter, decreasing the caliber of a dilated ureter to allow an appropriate length-to-width ratio for reimplantation, mobilization of the ureter to release any fibrous attachments, and prevention of injury to the surrounding peritoneal envelope or intraperitoneal viscera. The bladder mucosa should be handled carefully and with atraumatic instruments. Tagging sutures of fine silk and fine chromic catgut on atraumatic pop-off needles are used to secure the superior and inferior aspects of the ureteral meatus for traction and orientation. The ureter is intubated with a 3 Fr. or 5 Fr. feeding tube.

Mucosal incisions are made around the ureteral meatus with either a knife blade or pinpoint electrocautery. Dissection should continue close to the ureter to preserve the bladder mucosa. A deep 6 o'clock incision through the bladder wall divides the ureterotrigonal continuity and affords access to the retroperitoneal space. Dissection can then be continued in this plane easily and safely. All muscle bundles should be cut and coagulated well away from the ureter. The ureter should be completely freed from its muscle attachments. Use of a vein retractor placed through the ureteral hiatus allows visualization of the peritoneum so that it can be swept well away from the posterior bladder wall.

Periureteral bleeding should be isolated carefully with fine vascular forceps and gently electrofulgurated or suture ligated. Any portion of the ureter that appears to have a compromised blood supply should be excised back to normal tissue.

Division and spatulation of the ureter should be done with tenotomy scissors. Mucosal flaps should be developed widely to allow the ureter to reside clearly in its submucosal tunnel. Any muscular bleeding encountered during development of the submucosal flaps should be controlled carefully with electrocautery or sutures, or both. The ureteral hiatus should be closed snugly to establish a competent ureterovesical angle. Stents are optional, but if used, they should be soft and nonreactive. Stents are probably indicated when the ureter has been excised and tapered, in cases of extensive dissection, particularly with a great deal of edema, and in reoperative cases.

Urinary diversion in girls is accomplished through a urethral Foley catheter. In boys, a suprapubic cystostomy tube is used to avoid a catheter within the urethra. Suprapubic tubes should be placed high on the dome of the bladder to avoid irritation of the trigone. In patients with a history of neuropathic vesical dysfunction, the suprapubic catheter should be clamped in order to assess bladder function

and residual urine volume prior to catheter removal. Drains are not used except in patients who undergo excision and ureteral tapering for megaureter. Postoperative caudal or epidural analgesia is used routinely.

Most children leave the hospital on the 4th or 5th postoperative day. Appropriate antibiotic coverage should be maintained during hospitalization and followed by prolonged chemotherapy for several months postoperatively with either sulfonamides, nitrofurantoin, or another form of antibacterial treatment. The initial radiographic studies are made at 3 to 4 months and include a radionuclide cystogram and radiographic imaging of the upper tracts. If initial studies show no obstruction or reflux, subsequent studies include upper tract evaluation with an ultrasonogram or DMSA scanning at intervals of 12 months, 36 months, and 5 years postoperatively. Although rare, late obstruction or reappearance of reflux may occur several years after an apparently successful operation; therefore, periodic upper tract evaluations are necessary through puberty (Mesrobian et al).

SURGICAL OPTIONS: OPEN SURGICAL PROCEDURES

Suprahiatal Repairs

Hutch-1

Hutch popularized antireflux surgery in the early 1950s by introducing the concept of constructing an antireflux valve by elongating the intravesical portion of the ureter (Hutch, 1952). The transvesical approach of the Hutch-1 technique involves incising the mucosa cephalad and lateral to the original hiatus and developing submucosal flaps bilaterally (Hutch, 1963) (Fig. 14–14). The detrusor musculature is closed under the ureter, and the overlying mucosa is closed over the ureter. This technique leaves the orifice in an abnormal lateral position. It is also not possible to correct any ureteral kinks or adhesions or to perform ureteral tapering. The technique should be applied only to the normal or slightly dilated ureter. The distal ureteral continuity and blood supply are not interrupted, and therefore, this procedure may be applicable to patients in whom the blood supply of the ureter has been compromised superiorly from a previous pyelostomy or ureterostomy.

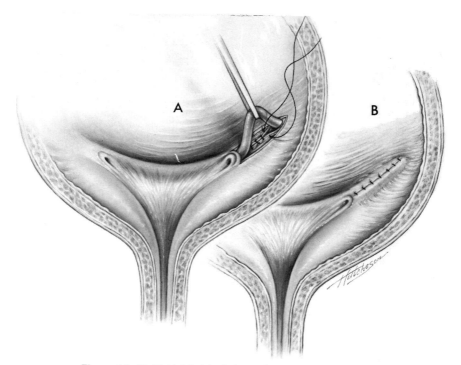

Figure 14–14 □ Hutch-1 technique of ureteroneocystostomy.

Lich-Grégoir

Advantages of this extravesical antireflux procedure include the fact that the bladder is not opened, eliminating the risk of urinary contamination of the wound. Because the ureters are not reimplanted, they do not need stenting (Grégoir and Van Regemorter; Lich et al, 1961). The operation can be performed in a relatively short time and requires minimal hospitalization.

The ureters are identified and isolated, and the lateral umbilical ligaments are ligated and transected. The posterior aspect of the bladder, where the antireflux plasty is to be performed, is freed from the peritoneal pouch. The incision of the bladder muscle is performed cephalad and lateral to the ureteral hiatus and along the natural course of the ureter (Fig. 14–15). The incision is made through the serosal and muscular layer down to the mucosal layer. The muscular coat is

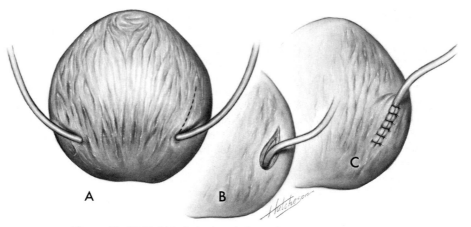

Figure 14–15 □ Lich-Grégoir technique of ureteroneocystostomy.

undermined sufficiently to create an adequate bed for the ureter. The extension of the incision depends on the diameter of the ureter. The ureter is placed into the mucosal bed, and the overlying muscle is closed with running absorbable sutures. It is important that the tunnel be fashioned vertically on the posterior wall and that the incision not interfere with the ureterotrigonal continuity (Marberger et al).

Various authors have used this technique with success rates of greater than 90 per cent (Arap et al; Beetz et al; Brühl et al; Grégoir and Schulman; Palken). The Lich-Grégoir procedure has particular advantages and applicability in the renal transplant population. Although this operation has been applied successfully in patients with ureteral duplication and periureteral diverticula, others (Linn et al) believe that a Hutch diverticulum is a contraindication for this procedure.

Detrusorrhaphy

Zaontz et al repopularized the technique of detrusorrhaphy described by Daines and Hodgson (Fig. 14–16). The bladder is rotated to expose the involved ureter and its detrusor hiatus. The ureter is dissected circumferentially at the ureteral hiatus so that the ureter is attached only with the bladder mucosa. An incision is made in the bladder muscle both proximally and distally from the ureteral hiatus to create a muscular defect. Submucosal flaps are developed. The ureteral orifice is advanced onto the trigone toward the vesical neck with

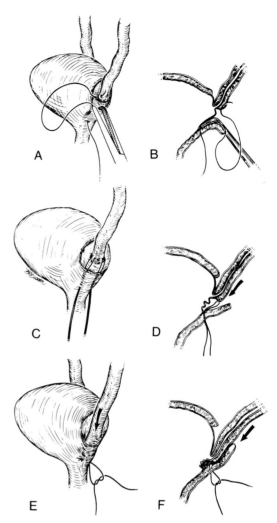

Figure 14–17 □ *A*, Bladder mucosa is elevated off bladder wall muscle, and Vest-type sutures are placed. *B*, Sagittal section shows suture passing between undermined mucosa and detrusor. *C*, Alignment of Vest sutures after placement. *D*, Sagittal section demonstrates appropriate positioning of sutures. *E*, Tying Vest sutures advances and anchors ureter onto trigone. *F*, Sagittal section of ureteromeatal advancement. (From Zaontz MR, Maizels M, Sugar EC, et al: Detrusorrhaphy: extravesical ureteral advancement to correct vesicoureteral reflux in children. J Urol 138:947, 1987. By permission of Williams & Wilkins Company.)

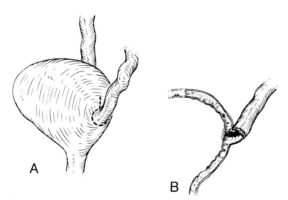

Figure 14–16 □ Detrusorrhaphy. *A*, After ureteral mobilization, detrusor is incised *(dotted lines)* at level of ureteral hiatus. *B*, Sagittal section demonstrates ureteral hiatus. (From Zaontz MR, Maizels M, Sugar EC, et al: Detrusorrhaphy: extravesical ureteral advancement to correct vesicoureteral reflux in children. J Urol 138:947, 1987. By permission of Williams & Wilkins Company.)

a pair of "Vest-type" sutures. Sutures are placed through the distal detrusor and ureteral muscle such that tying the pair of Vest sutures advances and anchors the ureteral orifice distally and creates a new long submucosal tunnel (Figs. 14–17 and 14–18). The procedure has been successful in more than 90 per cent of patients, and morbidity has been negligible (Wacksman and Sheldon; Zaontz et al).

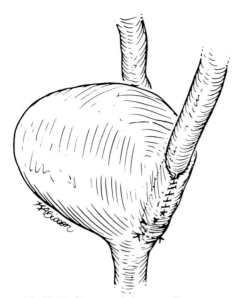

Figure 14–18 □ Closure of detrusor flaps over ureter allows for long submucosal tunnel and completes detrusorrhaphy. (From Zaontz MR, Maizels M, Sugar EC, et al: Detrusorrhaphy: extravesical ureteral advancement to correct vesicoureteral reflux in children. J Urol 138:947, 1987. By permission of Williams & Wilkins Company.)

Politano-Leadbetter

One of the most widely used surgical techniques for ureteroneocystostomy was described by Politano and Leadbetter. This technique achieves most of the basic objectives of ureteroneocystostomy and can be applied to ureteral kinks and dilated ureters in which reduction of the caliber of the ureter is required. A circumferential incision is made around the ureteral orifice, and the ureter is freed from the ureterotrigonal continuity. The ureter is mobilized intravesically. It is then passed extravesically and brought inside the bladder through a new hiatus that lies superior and lateral to the original ureteral hiatus. It is imperative that the peritoneum be swept superiorly away from the ureter prior to bringing the ureter through its new hiatus (Fig. 14–19). It is important not to kink the ureter at the level of the new hiatus and to prevent inadvertent transposition of the ureter around the lateral umbilical ligament through the peritoneal cavity or perhaps through bowel itself (Fig. 14–20).

Currently, most surgeons prefer to combine an extravesical approach with the intravesical approach to be sure that the ureter has a straight course without kinks and that the peritoneal cavity has not been entered. The

lateral umbilical ligaments should be ligated initially to prevent kinking of the ureter. Once the ureter is brought through its new superior and lateral hiatus, a submucosal tunnel is developed from the site of the new hiatus inferiorly down to the site of the original ureteral hiatus. The distal terminal ureter is discarded to remove any obstructive component or mucosa traumatized from placement of tagging sutures. A long intravesical ureteral segment is created in which the ureter lies submucosally and is supported by intact and unincised detrusor muscle.

Paquin

The Paquin ureteroneocystostomy procedure combines transvesical and extravesical approaches and allows correction of normal size ureters or megaureters (Paquin; Woodard and Keats) (Fig. 14–21). This technique differs from the Politano-Leadbetter procedure in that the bladder wall is split open posterior and lateral to the chosen site of the new hiatus.

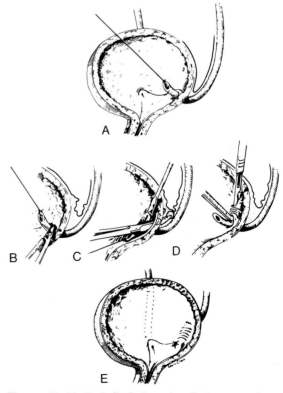

Figure 14–19 □ A–E, Politano-Leadbetter procedure. (From Walker RD: Vesicoureteral reflux. *In* Adult and Pediatric Urology, Vol 2. Edited by JY Gillenwater, JT Grayhack, SS Howards, et al. Chicago, Year Book Medical Publishers, 1987, pp 1676–1708.)

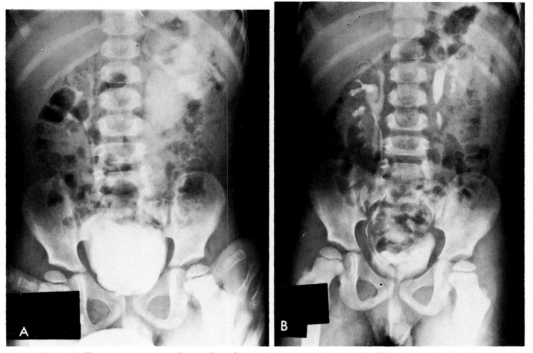

Figure 14–20 □ *A*, Excretory urogram 3 months after ureteroneocystostomy. Left hydronephrosis. At operation, left ureter was found to traverse lumen of sigmoid. Secondary ureteroneocystostomy. *B*, Postoperative urogram.

Figure 14–21 □ *A, B*, Paquin procedure. (From Walker RD: Vesicoureteral reflux. *In* Adult and Pediatric Urology, Vol 2. Edited by JY Gillenwater, JT Grayhack, SS Howards, et al. Chicago, Year Book Medical Publishers, 1987, pp 1676–1708.)

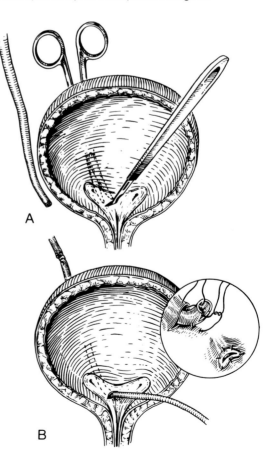

In his original description, Paquin divided the distal terminal ureter and left it in place. I prefer to mobilize the ureter completely and develop a submucosal tunnel from the ureter's new superior point of entry to just below and medial to the original ureteral orifice. The cut end of the ureter may be everted to form a cuff or nipple before it is sutured in place. This maneuver is optional.

We have used a modified Paquin procedure frequently for secondary repairs in which extravesical mobilization is necessary and the ureter is short and wide (Mesrobian et al). A psoas hitch is an important adjunct to this technique. The bladder should be opened obliquely on its anterolateral surface. The corresponding side of the bladder is brought up to the psoas muscle and sutured with Vicryl or polydioxanone sutures lateral to the iliac vessels (Prout and Koontz). Care should be taken to avoid the genitofemoral nerve. This maneuver allows a long intravesical ureter and maintains the new ureteral hiatus at a fixed point so that neither kinking nor obstruction may occur.

Infrahiatal Repairs

Mathisen

Mathisen described a combined extravesical and intravesical procedure that advanced the ureter down onto the trigone (Fig. 14–22). This procedure has wide applicability and is associated with minimal complications and excellent success.

Glenn-Anderson

The advantage of the Glenn-Anderson advancement technique is that the ureter enters the bladder through the normal ureteral hiatus and therefore, the chance of kinking or obstruction—"J-hooking"—of the ureter because of a high ureteral hiatus is virtually eliminated (Glenn and Anderson, 1967). The infrahiatal principle is most applicable to patients in whom the ureteral orifice is placed laterally and there is enough space between the original ureteral hiatus and the bladder neck to reimplant the new intravesical ureter. Ureteral length is gained by dissecting and freeing the intravesical ureter. Once the ureter is freed transvesically, a submucosal tunnel is developed from the ureteral hiatus distally toward the bladder neck (Fig. 14–23). Crea-

tion of the tunnel distally may be difficult at times, and it is acceptable to incise the bladder mucosa in the direction of the tunnel in order to elevate the submucosal flaps bilaterally. The underlying detrusor muscle is closed with a running suture of Vicryl with the knots tied in an inverted fashion. The ureter is placed onto the bladder musculature, and the mucosa is sutured over it. The technique is simple, can be accomplished rapidly, and avoids extravesical dissection. It places the ureter in its proper physioanatomic position on the trigonal musculature.

In 1978, Glenn and Anderson offered a modification of their original technique (Glenn and Anderson, 1978). Whereas the original procedure described mobilization of only the terminal 2 to 3 cm of ureter, the modified technique allows extension of the ureteral hiatus superiorly to achieve a longer tunnel (Fig. 14–24). The modified technique involves the development of a larger hiatus, which provides visibility of the extravesical and extraperitoneal space, peritoneum, and contiguous structures. The development of this large hiatus permits mobilization of at least 8 to 10 cm of distal ureter. Subsequent closure of the enlarged hiatus distal to the point of bladder entry of the ureter creates a longer submucosal tunnel and diminishes the necessity of extensive submucosal dissection onto the trigone. Success of the original and modified repairs has been greater than 90 per cent (Glenn and Anderson, 1978; Gonzales et al).

Cohen

The Cohen technique is simple, safe, and effective for the prevention of VUR (Cohen). It is the most widely used procedure in Europe and perhaps the United States today. Advantages of this technique include the fact that there is minimal angulation at the ureteral hiatus (Fig. 14–25). The ureters are mobilized transvesically, and separate submucosal tunnels are created for each ureter across the bladder base so that each ureter opens on the opposite side from its hiatus. It was previously thought that the ureteral meatus must be brought down onto the immobile portion of the bladder base (trigone) to achieve a satisfactory antireflux mechanism. It is now clear that the ureters can be crisscrossed anywhere on the bladder floor with good results.

Wacksman used this procedure routinely to correct all grades of reflux and reported suc-

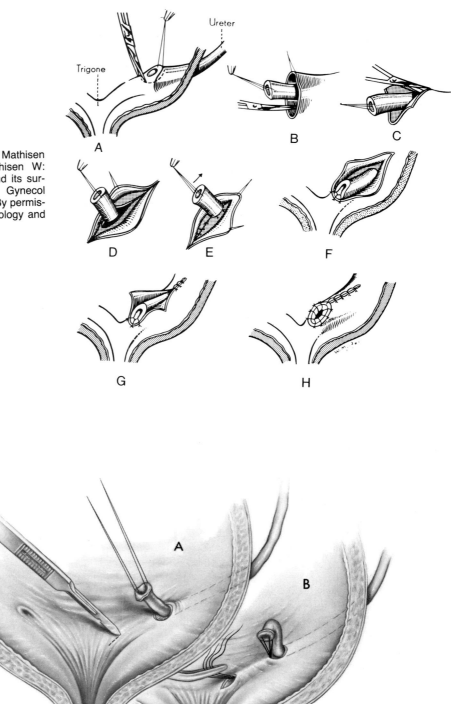

Figure 14–22 □ *A–H,* Mathisen procedure. (From Mathisen W: Vesicoureteral reflux and its surgical correction. Surg Gynecol Obstet 118:965, 1964. By permission of Surgery, Gynecology and Obstetrics.)

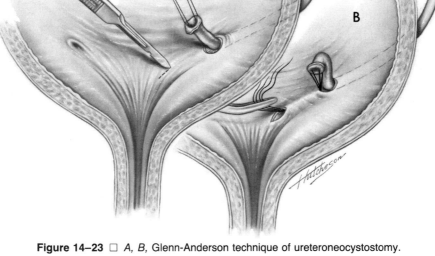

Figure 14–23 □ *A, B,* Glenn-Anderson technique of ureteroneocystostomy.

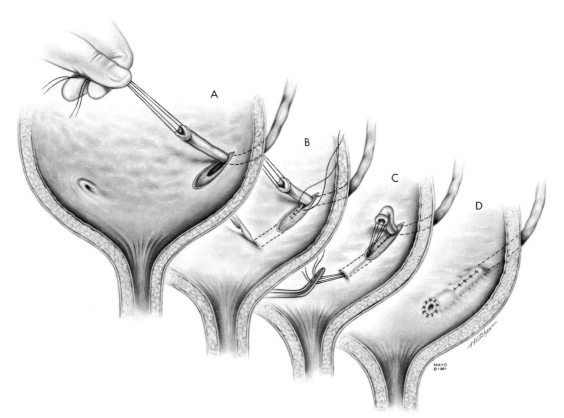

Figure 14–24 □ *A–D,* Modification of Glenn-Anderson technique.

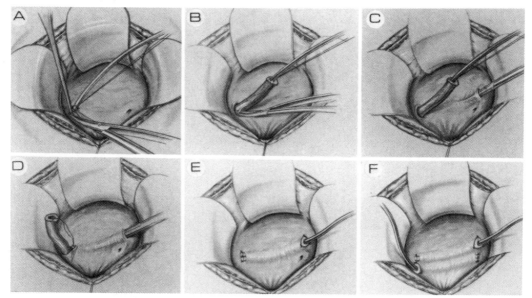

Figure 14–25 □ Cohen technique.

A, Circumferential incision is made around ureteral orifice.

B, Ureter is freed with sharp dissection, always staying close to it and not straying into extraneous planes.

C, Site for new orifice is chosen at point superior and lateral to contralateral orifice. Mucosa at this site is incised and submucosal tunnel is fashioned cephalad to trigone with semi-pointed scissors.

D, Ureter is advanced through tunnel.

E, Ureter is sewn in place, making sure that at least one or two sutures have incorporated a good bite of bladder muscle. Detrusor in previously dissected hiatus is closed inferiorly with care taken not to compromise ureter. Mucosa is closed as a separate layer.

F, In cases of bilateral reimplantation, a separate submucosal tunnel is fashioned within the trigone. The new orifice for the second ureter is placed either at the inferior aspect of the closed contralateral ureteral hiatus or inferior and lateral to it.

(From Glassberg KI, Laungani G, Wasnick RJ, et al: Transverse ureteral advancement technique of ureteroneocystostomy (Cohen reimplant) and a modification for difficult cases (experience with 121 ureters). J Urol 134:304, 1985. By permission of Williams & Wilkins Company.)

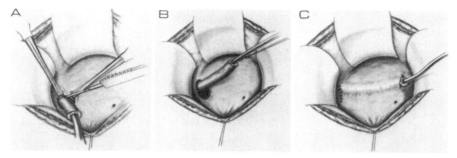

Figure 14–26 □ Modified technique for difficult cases (for example, infant bladders and dilated ureters).

A, Posterior wall of bladder is lifted off ureter and, with cautery, incised superolaterally, taking care not to injure ureter or peritoneum.

B, Note that the ureter now enters the bladder at a more superior and lateral position. Retroperitoneum is visualized better through newly enlarged hiatus, which also facilitates tailoring.

C, A longer submucosal tunnel can be fashioned, inasmuch as the tunnel is made in a wider area of the bladder, well above the trigone.

(From Glassberg KI, Laungani G, Wasnick RJ, et al: Transverse ureteral advancement technique of ureteroneocystostomy (Cohen reimplant) and a modification for difficult cases (experience with 121 ureters). J Urol 134:304, 1985. By permission of Williams & Wilkins Company.)

cessful results in more than 95 per cent of patients. Kondo and Otani reported a 100 per cent success rate for correction of primary reflux and 89 per cent for secondary reflux. Ehrlich (1982) described a 98 per cent success rate in 229 ureters reimplanted for primary reflux and a 95 per cent success rate in 109 ureters corrected for secondary reflux or obstructive megaureter. Glassberg et al recommended a modification of the original technique for patients with dilated ureters and small bladders. This modified technique involves incising the bladder at the superolateral margin of the hiatus and mobilizing the peritoneum superiorly. This incision allows the ureter to enter the bladder in a more superior and lateral position, thus creating a longer tunnel (Figs. 14–26 and 14–27).

Because of the crisscross positioning of the ureteral meatus, problems may arise if retrograde ureteral catheterization becomes necessary (Lamesch). Historically, a Cystocath was placed within the bladder and cystoscopy was performed. The ureters were catheterized through the Cystocath trocar while a second observer directed the catheters cystoscopically. Because difficulty with catheterizing these ureters postoperatively has been lessened with the introduction of a flexible-tip, manually controllable retrograde catheter (Cook Urological, Spencer, Indiana), the suprapubic approach is no longer necessary.

Gil-Vernet

In 1984, Gil-Vernet described a technique based on the principle that the intrinsic mus-

cular fibers of the transmural ureter may provide sphincteric action in preventing reflux. This technique involved advancing the ureters across the trigone by placing a nonabsorbable mattress suture at the base of each ureter, including the periurethral sheath of Waldeyer and the intrinsic ureteral musculature, and tying the suture in the midline. This technique advances the ureters and approximates them in the midline, thereby increasing the intramural length of each distal ureter (Fig. 14–28). The nonabsorbable suture is buried by

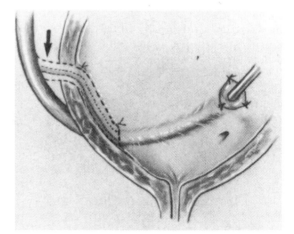

Figure 14–27 □ Gentle curve of ureter in Cohen technique compared with hitch that can occur when ureter *(dotted lines)* is passed through new hiatus *(arrow)* as in Politano-Leadbetter procedure. (From Glassberg KI, Laungani G, Wasnick RJ, et al: Transverse ureteral advancement technique of ureteroneocystostomy (Cohen reimplant) and a modification for difficult cases (experience with 121 ureters). J Urol 134:304, 1985. By permission of Williams & Wilkins Company.)

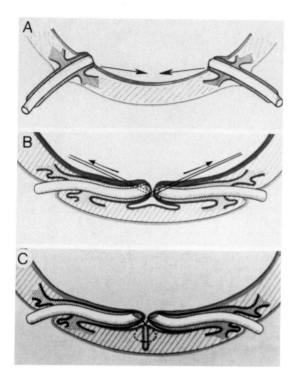

Figure 14–28 □ Schematic representation of Gil-Vernet technique. *A*, Principle involves advancing ureters across trigone. *B*, Traction sutures are used to demonstrate desired result. *C*, On completion, ureteral orifices are in close proximity near midline and submucosal length of ureter has been increased, preserving intrinsic and extrinsic periureteral musculature. (From Gil-Vernet JM: A new technique for surgical correction of vesicoureteral reflux. J Urol 131:456, 1984. By permission of Williams & Wilkins Company.)

placing absorbable sutures through the bladder mucosa and musculature.

Solok and co-workers reported success in 94 per cent of renal units with grades II, III, and IV VUR by using this procedure. Carini and associates also stressed the ease and simplicity of the Gil-Vernet technique and reported successful results in 13 of 14 patients undergoing surgical treatment for reflux. These authors modified the technique and used two or three absorbable sutures in the midline rather than a nonabsorbable suture.

Criticisms of the technique include the fact that it may not be possible to establish sufficient transmural length to prevent reflux in patients with higher grades of reflux. In addition, the nonabsorbable suture may migrate to the mucosal surface and provide a focus for infection or a nidus for stone formation.

Combined Suprahiatal and Infrahiatal Repair

Kelalis (1985) described a technique in which the ureteral hiatus is created posteromedially on a relatively immobile part of the bladder. The submucosal tunnel is lengthened by advancing the ureteral orifice distally. The principle is diagrammatically depicted in Figure 14–29. The operation is performed transvesically; however, if there is any doubt about the proper position of the ureteral hiatus, extravesical dissection should be accomplished. The ureter must be mobilized sufficiently to prevent acute angulation as it enters its new course into the bladder. This technique has the advantage of creating a tunnel that has good support and places the ureter into a position in the bladder that will change little with bladder filling. This prevents intermittent or permanent ureteral obstruction, known as "J-hooking" of the ureter.

The ureter is intubated with a 5 Fr. Stamey catheter, and traction sutures of fine silk and chromic catgut are placed inferomedially and superolaterally to the orifice (Fig. 14–30). These tagging sutures allow the operator to apply tension to the ureter without grasping the ureter itself. They also identify the proper anatomic orientation of the orifice and thus avoid twisting the ureter after its transposition into the bladder. The mucosal cuff around the orifice is outlined circumferentially by using electrocautery or scissor dissection. The plane of cleavage is established between the adventitia of the ureter and the fibers of the bladder. Sufficient mobilization of the ureter is easily achieved by using both blunt and sharp dissection. The base of the bladder is elevated with

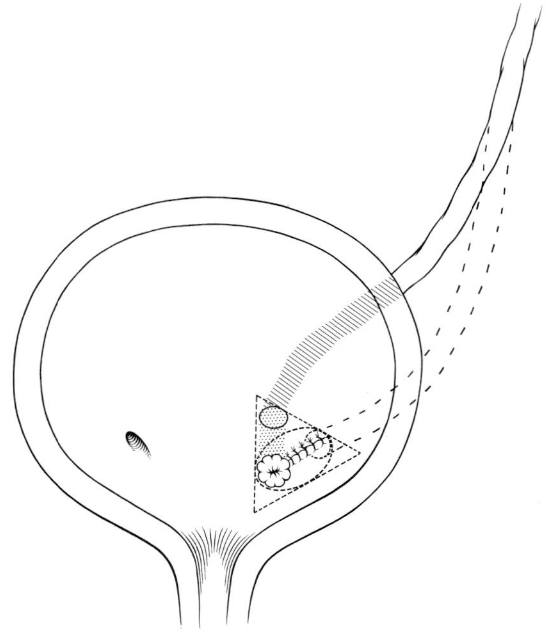

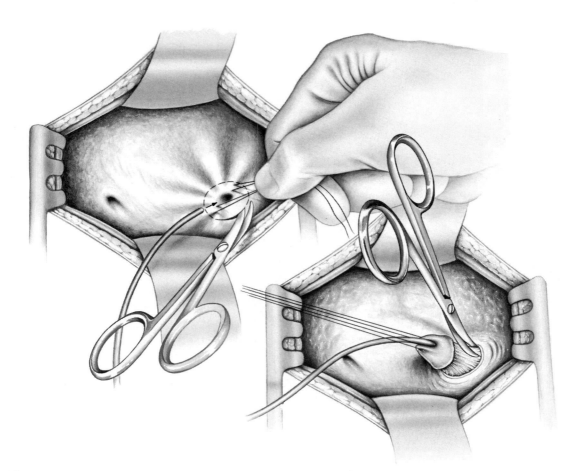

Figure 14–29 □ Principle of combined suprahiatal and infrahiatal repair. (From Kelalis PP: The present status of surgery for vesicoureteral reflux. Urol Clin North Am 1:457, 1974.)

Figure 14–30 □ Tagging sutures are used to secure the superior and inferior aspects of the ureteral meatus for traction and orientation. A mucosal cuff around the orifice is outlined circumferentially with scissor dissection.

a vein retractor, and the peritoneal reflection is pushed superiorly from the bladder base (Fig. 14–31). This ensures that there is no obstruction in the new course of the ureter as it re-enters the bladder. A right-angle clamp is passed from the old ureteral hiatus outside the bladder to the point where the new hiatus is to be created (Fig. 14–32). Once the tip of the clamp appears in the bladder and the new hiatus is stretched to avoid subsequent narrowing, a second clamp is attached to its tip and guided into the bladder to such a position that it can grasp the traction sutures and pull the ureter into the bladder via the new hiatus (Fig. 14–33). The defect in the original hiatus musculature is closed with running polyglactin 910 (Vicryl) sutures (Fig. 14–34). Submucosal flaps are developed, and a submucosal tunnel is constructed. The ureter is brought through this tunnel into the anteromedial portion of the mucosal defect (Fig. 14–35). It is occasionally necessary to inject saline submucosally to facilitate creation of the tunnel. It is important to reinsert a ureteral catheter into the reimplanted ureter and advance it all the way to the kidney to exclude any obstruction or angulation of the ureter. The distal end of the ureter is removed routinely inasmuch as this end is often stenotic and aperistaltic, or it may be traumatized during dissection.

The mucosal cuff of the ureter is sutured to the mucosa of the bladder with several interrupted sutures of fine Vicryl or chromic catgut. The most distal suture should encompass bladder muscle as well as mucosa because this stitch serves to anchor the ureter into position and reestablish the ureterotrigonal continuity. The remaining ureteral mucosal sutures can be stitched to the bladder mucosa only. The bladder mucosa overlying the original ureteral hiatus is closed in a linear fashion with running absorbable sutures.

Submucosal Injection Techniques

The principle of endoscopic injection is identical to that of a formal open ureteroneocystostomy: to create solid support behind the refluxing intravesical ureter. The success of the procedure depends on the ability of the surgeon to place the implant within the lamina propria at a position just proximal to the

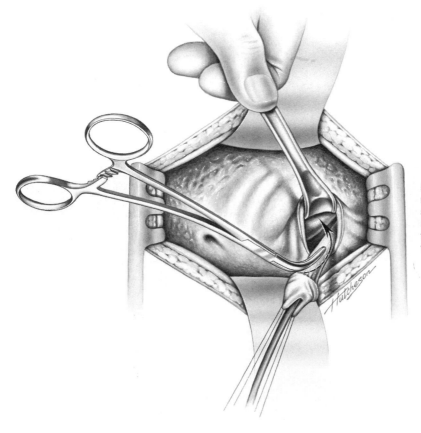

Figure 14–31 □ The ureter is mobilized by using both blunt and sharp dissection. Use of a vein retractor placed through the ureteral hiatus allows visualization of the peritoneum.

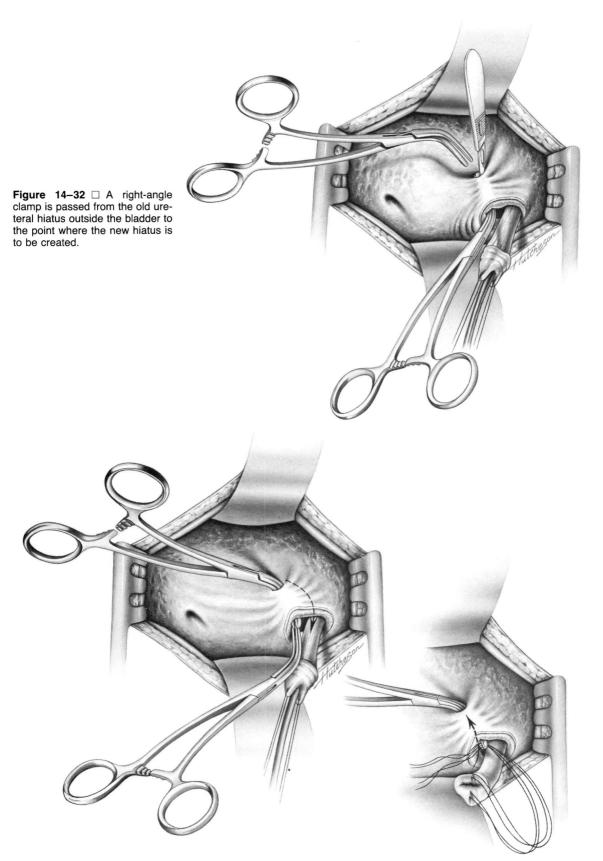

Figure 14–32 ☐ A right-angle clamp is passed from the old ureteral hiatus outside the bladder to the point where the new hiatus is to be created.

Figure 14–33 ☐ The ureter is pulled into the bladder via the new hiatus.

477

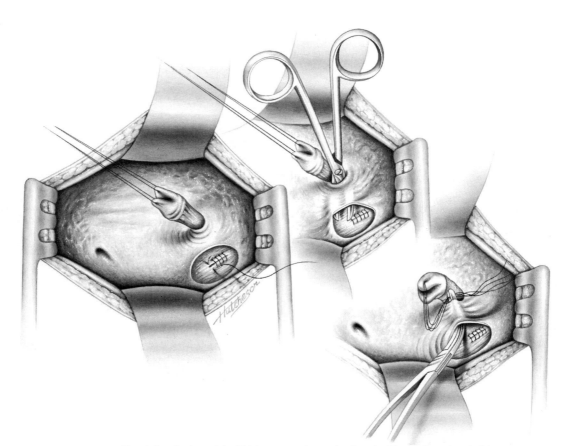

Figure 14–34 □ The defect in the original hiatus musculature is closed with running absorbable sutures.

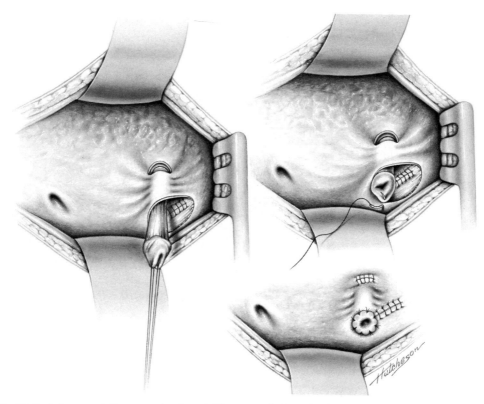

Figure 14–35 □ Submucosal flaps are developed. The ureter is brought through this tunnel into the anteromedial portion of the mucosal defect. (From Kelalis PP: The present status of surgery for vesicoureteral reflux. Urol Clin North Am 1:457, 1974.)

ureteral orifice. This injection elevates the ureteral orifice on a "hillock" and causes the orifice to assume an inverted crescentic appearance. If the needle is not placed correctly, the injection may occur into the ureteral lumen or detrusor musculature and result in implantation that extrudes superficially into the bladder lumen, deeply into the bladder wall, or perhaps extravesically.

Polytetrafluoroethylene

Polytef paste is a sterile mixture of polytetrafluoroethylene (Teflon), glycerin, and polysorbate (Malizia et al, 1984). Injection of this substance has been used for many years to enlarge displaced or deformed vocal cords in patients with dysphonia (Arnold). The subureteric injection of polytetrafluoroethylene for correction of VUR was first utilized in 1981 by Matouschek and applied to both the bladder neck and ureter by Politano et al. In 1984, an experimental study (Puri and O'Donnell) and its clinical application in children (O'Donnell and Puri, 1984) demonstrated that it was possible to correct VUR by the endoscopic injection of polytetrafluoroethylene under the submucosal ureter. The polytef particles stimulate an ingrowth of fibroblasts at the site of injection, which tends to hold the particles within the tissues (O'Donnell and Puri, 1984).

The injection technique is straightforward, can be performed as an outpatient procedure, and requires approximately 5 to 15 minutes under anesthetic. The bladder must be nearly empty to keep the ureteral orifice flat rather than displaced laterally, as occurs during bladder filling. The needle is composed of a 5 Fr. nylon catheter onto which is wedged a 21-gauge needle or a rigid needle of the same dimensions. The Wolf 9.5 Fr. or 11 Fr. cysto-

scope (Richard Wolf Medical Instruments, Rosemont, Ill.) with offset lens is used (Fig. 14–36). The needle is introduced 3 to 4 mm distal to the orifice and as the injection proceeds, the distal ureter flattens and the orifice closes, assuming a slit-like configuration at the conclusion of the procedure (Fig. 14–37). Some authors have advocated the use of a 4 Fr. ureteral catheter or Fogarty catheter to elevate the ureteral orifice during injection to help prevent perforation of the ureteral wall while avoiding the detrusor muscle. When the needle is positioned properly, approximately 0.4 to 0.6 ml of Teflon paste is injected to provide a subureteric buttress (Fig. 14–38).

O'Donnell and Puri (1986) used Teflon in 103 children followed for 3 to 23 months and reported a 75 per cent success rate after one injection of polytef paste. Fourteen additional patients required 2 to 4 injections to correct reflux. There were no instances of obstruction. Sweeny and Thomas reported that 99 of 153 ureters (65 per cent) had absence of reflux on postmicturition voiding cystourethrography after Teflon injection. Schulman et al reported 100 per cent initial success and 91 per cent success at 12 months in 35 children after Teflon injection.

Farkas et al reported their experience with Teflon in 115 ureters with reflux. Of patients with primary reflux, 96 per cent had their reflux corrected after an initial Teflon injection. Reflux into duplex ureters was corrected in 82 per cent of patients after the first injection and in 93 per cent of patients after repeated injections. Patients with dilated ureters and golfhole orifices did not respond to endoscopic Teflon injection therapy.

Subureteric injection of Teflon has been particularly appealing in children with high-grade reflux and neuropathic vesical dysfunc-

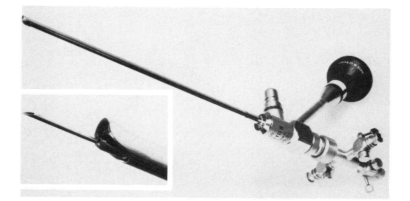

Figure 14–36 □ The Wolf 11 Fr. cystoscope with offset lens. Note the bevel on the tip of the needle that has been inserted through the scope *(inset)*.

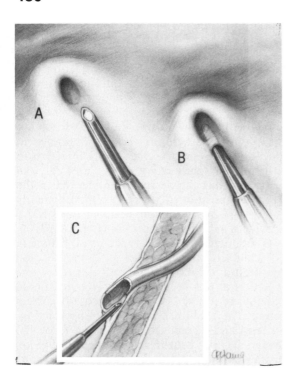

Figure 14–37 □ Subureteric needle placement. *A*, Needle positioned at 6 o'clock position, bevel up. *B*, Needle inserted in subureteric space. Lever up on needle to ensure superficial placement. *C*, Cut-away view to indicate superficial subureteric placement of needle prior to injection.

tion (Wacksman and Sheldon). Kaplan et al (1987) reported improvement or resolution of reflux in 84 per cent of patients with neuropathic bladder who underwent a single subureteric injection of Teflon; success improved to 87 per cent after a second Teflon injection.

Patients with ureteral duplication have been more difficult to treat, and only 50 per cent of these patients have achieved successful results (Quinlan and O'Donnell). Periureteral diverticula are extremely difficult to correct because of lack of adequate detrusor muscle support.

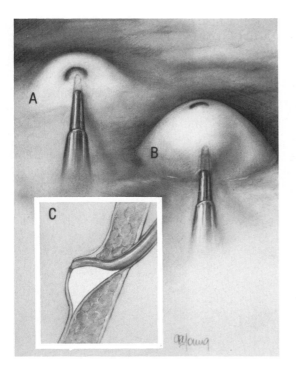

Figure 14–38 □ Injection of paste. *A*, Injection of 0.1 to 0.2 ml of paste, with creation of initial hillock. *B*, Then 0.3 to 0.4 ml of paste is injected at completion of the procedure. Note crescentic appearance of orifice. Final result should look like a volcano. *C*, Side view of completed procedure to indicate support and lengthening of ureter on bead, with only minor compression of distal segment.

Ultrasonography, computed tomographic (CT) scanning, and magnetic resonance imaging (MRI) have been used to determine the size and location of the Teflon mass after subureteric injection (Gore et al; Kaplan; Mann et al). Sonographically, the Teflon paste at the injection site appears as a hyperechoic focus within the bladder wall with distal shadowing (Mann et al). On CT scanning, Teflon was seen in various locations relative to the bladder wall, and the location did not correlate with success or failure of the submucosal injection procedure (Gore et al). Kaplan reported that the injected volume of the Teflon bead remained constant at 2 years with follow-up MRI.

Despite encouraging success rates with this procedure, there remains concern regarding the safety of injectable polytef substance in children. Although the urologic use of Teflon paste has been widespread, recent data from animal experiments demonstrated migration of small Teflon particles beyond the injection site. Malizia et al (1984) studied periurethral polytef injection in animals and found distant migration of Teflon particles to the pelvic lymph nodes, lungs, brain, kidneys, and spleen of monkeys 10.5 months after injection. The Teflon particle size ranged from 4 to 100 μm, with more than 90 per cent of the particles smaller than 40 μm. Particle diameter in currently marketed polytef paste ranges from 4 to 100 μm. The previous belief was that particles would not migrate if they were larger than 50 μm. However, the experiment showed migration of particles as large as 80 μm. At the site of injection, each aggregate was surrounded by a pronounced chronic inflammatory reaction in which histiocytes had phagocytized the outer particles and coalesced to form giant cells.

A similar study performed with smaller injection volumes, placed subureterically in monkeys, showed local migration around the bladder and distal migration to the periaortic and pelvic nodes and the testicles in male monkeys (Malizia et al, 1988). Furthermore, the subureteric injection sites have been monitored with both CT scanning and MRI, and the granulomas enlarge over time. Longer-term follow-up in monkeys demonstrated persistent masses (granulomas) radiographically and at autopsy. A Teflon granuloma has been reported after particle migration to the lung in a patient treated with periurethral injection of polytef paste (Mittleman and Marraccini).

Most recently, Elder reported two unusual complications after the injection of polytef paste. The paste was found inside the corpora cavernosa of a patient with exstrophy who had undergone periurethral injection in an attempt to attain continence. There was moderate scarring within the spongy tissue, and histologic examination confirmed a marked giant cell reaction. In the second patient, a scrotal abscess and a urethrocutaneous fistula developed after periurethral injection of polytef paste. Elder thought that these two complications were a direct result of injecting into periurethral scar tissue.

Brown compared open ureteroneocystostomy to the subureteric injection of polytef paste for primary treatment of VUR. Surgical reimplantation cured reflux in 98 per cent of 76 ureters, whereas endoscopic procedures were successful in only 70 per cent of 40 ureters. Patients undergoing endoscopic surgery required more hospital admissions, more anesthetics, and more VCUs than did those in the surgically reimplanted group. Brown concluded that open reimplantation remains the procedure of choice if surgery is indicated for patients with VUR.

The development of local granulomas and distant migration raise concern about the use of Teflon paste in children and young adults. Until more information is gained about migration and the long-term tissue reaction to this material, many pediatric urologists have significant concerns about the continued use of Teflon. At the time of this writing, the Food and Drug Administration has not approved Teflon paste for urologic use. Further research studies are necessary to develop a safer material that is biocompatible, permanent, causes little inflammatory response, and does not migrate from the injection site.

Collagen

Cross-linked bovine collagen has been used widely for years for hemostatic agents, in cardiac valves, and in the injectable form as a soft-tissue substitute. Glutaraldehyde cross-linked bovine collagen preparation (Zyplast, Collagen Corporation, Palo Alto, Calif.) is a bovine corium collagen that is solubilized by exposure to pepsin in acetic acid and purified by ultrafiltration and ion-exchange chromatography (Gearhart). After purification, the collagen is reconstituted in a neutral solution, harvested, and resuspended in saline to provide non–cross-linked collagen. It is important to distinguish the cross-linked agent from the non–cross-linked substance (Zyderm, Collagen Corporation, Palo Alto, Calif.). Zyplast demonstrates 90 to 100 per cent wet weight persistence as a stable implant in subdermal and suburothelial injection in animals (Gearhart). Zyderm, which has been used to correct reflux with poor success, has a wet weight persistence of less than 50 per cent at 4 months.

Zyplast (glutaraldehyde cross-linked bovine collagen) is a safe and effective alternative to Teflon paste for the endoscopic treatment of VUR. In a series of 50 patients (92 ureters) from Johns Hopkins, there was an overall success rate of 74 per cent 1 month after injection and 60 per cent 1 year postoperatively (Canning et al). Thirty per cent of patients required two injections, and 3 per cent required three injections. In seven patients for whom Zyplast injection failed, open surgical correction for VUR was done. In all seven cases, the reimplantation procedure was not hindered by the presence of the collagen implantation (Leonard et al). Histologically, there was no significant foreign body giant cell reaction in response to the implanted collagen, and the amount of inflammation, neovascularization, and fibroblastic ingrowth was relatively minimal.

In this same series, the initial grades of reflux influenced the cure rates (Canning et al; Leonard et al). Patients with low-grade reflux (grades I, II, and III) had a cure rate of 80 per cent at 1 month. Ureters with higher-grade reflux (grades IV and V) had cure rates of only 40 per cent at 1 month. Patients with nonduplicated primary refluxing systems had a 1-month cure rate of 79 per cent, whereas those with duplicated systems had a cure rate of only 54 per cent. Zyplast is less viscous than polytef paste, which allows for easier injection through a 23- or 25-gauge needle. Importantly, Zyplast elicits little local tissue reaction and no granuloma formation when injected beneath the urothelium in rabbits and humans (Gearhart).

Other Products

Investigators at the Hospital for Sick Children in Toronto compared the use of Ivalon particles to autologous cartilage injected submucosally into rabbit bladders for the prevention of reflux (Merguerian et al). Because autologous cartilage underwent early reabsorp-

tion without evidence of a fibrotic reaction at the injection site, it would not be suitable for the long-term prevention of VUR. Conversely, polyvinyl alcohol foam (Ivalon) was found to be biocompatible, permanent, and caused minimal inflammatory responses at the injection site.

In dogs, the endoscopic injection of blood has been used to correct reflux with variable success. The animal's blood was heparinized, injected subureterically, and then thrombin and protamine were added to form a clot (Kohri et al).

The submucosal injection of any substance for the treatment of VUR should be limited to specific clinical situations, and the risks and unanswered long-term concerns should be discussed thoroughly with the patient's parents. Endoscopic injection therapy for reflux appears to be attractive for correction of reflux after failed ureteral reimplantation in selected patients with neuropathic bladder dysfunction in whom open surgical techniques are less likely to produce a successful result, or in those with persistent reflux after complicated augmentation or reconstruction procedures.

ANTIREFLUX SURGERY IN THE NEUROPATHIC BLADDER

Patients with urinary urgency, frequency, urge incontinence, or abnormal physical findings should be evaluated preoperatively with urodynamic studies. Voiding cystourethrography may show a thick-walled and trabeculated bladder with increased capacity and large postvoiding residual. Reimplantation is more difficult and the results are less satisfactory than in patients with primary VUR.

It is important to recognize voiding dysfunction prior to embarking on surgical treatment of reflux because voiding dysfunction may result in postoperative failure. Methods to improve bladder emptying such as timed and double voiding, intermittent catheterization, anticholinergic therapy to lower bladder pressures, or other maneuvers to reduce bladder outlet resistance may improve the success rate of antireflux surgery (Kaplan; Kass et al). Techniques that involve bringing the ureter through a new hiatus (suprahiatal ureteroneocystostomy) have not been associated with as successful results as those involving infrahiatal advancement procedures. In patients with a neuropathic bladder, contralateral reflux after ureteral reimplantation may occur in up to 50 per cent (Johnston et al).

One of the most important reasons for failure in patients undergoing ureteral reimplantation is undiagnosed occult neuropathic bladder secondary to detrusor-sphincter dyssynergia. Failures may occur late and are often the result of ureterovesical junction obstruction secondary to abnormalities in bladder dynamics with increased intravesical pressures.

VESICOURETERAL REFLUX AND URETERAL DUPLICATION

Vesicoureteral reflux is the most common abnormality associated with complete ureteral duplication. Lower pole reflux in patients with a duplicated collecting system most often persists and is unlikely to abate with growth (Kelalis, 1971). Kelalis (1971) recommended early surgical correction of reflux in patients with duplicated systems. Kaplan et al (1978) followed a group of children with renal duplication and reflux managed conservatively and found that 48 per cent either had spontaneous resolution of reflux or were medically stable. However, only 22 per cent of patients actually had resolution of reflux. Kaplan's group recommended evaluating each patient individually and cystoscopically to assess the position and location of the ureteral orifice prior to committing all patients with duplication and reflux to surgery.

Ben-Ami et al recently compared a series of children with grades I, II, and III reflux into the lower pole of a duplicated collecting system with a control group of children with reflux into a single collecting system. There were no significant differences between the two groups with respect to resolution of reflux or incidence of new parenchymal scars. These authors concluded that reflux into the lower pole of a duplex kidney did not constitute an absolute indication for early surgical intervention.

Approximately 10 per cent of children undergoing antireflux surgery have complete or incomplete duplication of the collecting system (Kelalis, 1985). In patients with a "Y" incomplete ureteral duplication, a single ureteral orifice enters the bladder but reflux affects both components of the duplication. These patients should undergo conventional ureteroneocystostomy.

In rare cases, the duplicated ureters adjoin in the juxtavesical region and form a "V-type" duplication. If operative intervention is indicated, it is preferable that the two ureters be converted into complete duplication by resecting the common stem and reimplanting both ureters as a unit through a single submucosal tunnel. Simple reimplantation without excision of the distal ureter may accentuate the functional obstruction at the union of the two ureters. This may result in ureteroureteral reflux and produce hydroureteronephrosis (Scott, 1963).

When complete ureteral duplication is present, reflux essentially always involves the lower segment orifice. Several surgical alternatives are available for correcting this type of reflux. Reimplanting the ureters via a common submucosal tunnel after the two ureters have been mobilized in their common sheath generally produces satisfactory results, provided that the lower pole ureter is not greatly dilated relative to the normal upper pole ureter (Fig. 14–39) (Fehrenbaker et al). This technique eliminates reflux in the lower ureter without disturbing the function of the upper segment. Disadvantages of this procedure are that the larger ureter may obstruct the smaller one.

In the presence of significant ureteral dilatation of the lower pole ureter, distal ureteroneoureterostomy has been proposed as a method to treat reflux (Bracci et al; Duthoy et

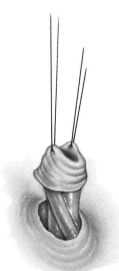

Figure 14–39 □ Ureteroneocystostomy in complete ureteral duplication. (From Fehrenbaker LG, Kelalis PP, Stickler GB: Vesicoureteral reflux and ureteral duplication in children. J Urol 107:862, 1972. By permission of Williams & Wilkins Company.)

al). This procedure converts a duplex system into a bifid system and allows removal of the refluxing ureteral stump (Fig. 14–40*A, B*) (Ahmed and Boucaut; Bockrath et al). The procedure can be accomplished without opening the bladder; it is simple and associated with a high degree of success even in the presence of a dilated ureter.

Another technique to bypass the ureterovesical junction is pyeloureterostomy, in which the renal pelvis is anastomosed end to side into the upper pole ureter (Fig. 14–40*C*). The anastomosis must be angled correctly and be approximately 2 cm in length so that the end result is similar to the naturally occurring bifid renal pelvis. This flank approach allows examination and biopsy of the involved renal segment (Belman et al).

Patients undergoing either a ureteroureterostomy or pyeloureterostomy must have one normal draining nonrefluxing unit. This anastomosis may be difficult if the caliber of the recipient ureter is small. In either case, the anastomotic area is drained and no stents are used.

In some patients with lower pole reflux, the lower pole–involved renal segment may be dysplastic and require lower pole heminephrectomy. Total nephrectomy is almost never justified. In patients undergoing lower pole heminephrectomy, the lower pole ureter is dissected as far down as safely possible, taking care to preserve the blood supply to the intact upper pole ureter. The ureteral stump may be left open with appropriate paravesical drainage for a few days, or the ureter may be split open down to the bladder. It is most unusual for the ureteral stump to be associated with postoperative infection or to act as a vesical diverticulum.

USE OF CATHETERS AND STENTS

This author routinely uses catheters in patients undergoing ureteroneocystostomy. In boys, I prefer a suprapubic cystostomy to avoid placing a catheter into the urethra and risking iatrogenic stricture. In girls, I use a urethral catheter to avoid a second abdominal scar. Patients are continued on pediatric belladonna and opium (B & O) suppositories as necessary. The use of continuous postoperative epidural analgesia or postoperative caudal analgesia has been quite effective in relieving pain from

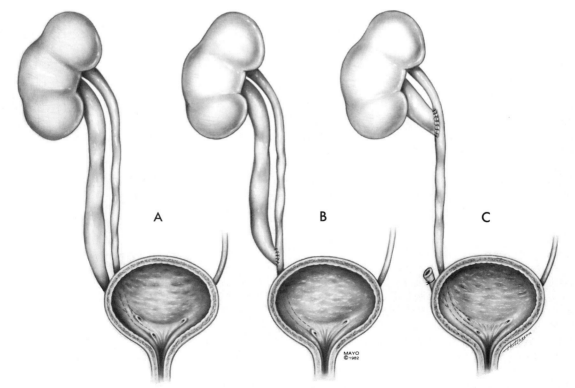

Figure 14–40 □ *A,* Complete duplication with reflux in lower segment. *B,* Ureteroureterostomy. *C,* Pyeloureterostomy.

bladder spasms. Urethral catheters are usually left in place for 2 to 3 days until the urine becomes clear. Early removal of the catheter shortens hospital stay considerably, and most patients are sent home by the fourth or fifth day postoperatively. So et al recommended using neither vesical nor urethral catheters but simply paravesical drainage postoperatively. None of the postoperative complications in their study were directly attributed to the absence of catheters.

The use of stents in patients undergoing ureteroneocystostomy, as in other types of ureteral surgery, is a matter of debate. Most series show that morbidity and operative failure are comparable between stented and non-stented groups (Fort et al). I do not feel that patients undergoing routine ureteroneocystostomy require ureteral stents. Indwelling ureteral stents may be used to avoid possible obstruction by circumventing the edema at the ureteral orifice and to maintain ureteral fixation. Small stents can be troublesome because the lumen of the stent may become occluded with blood, which may then occlude the ureter. Stenting is probably advisable in patients who are undergoing reoperative procedures, those with difficult and perhaps traumatic dissections, and in patients undergoing ureteral caliber reduction with formal excision and tapering of the ureter. When stenting a ureter, I use Silastic tubing of appropriate size and length, small feeding tubes, or single J catheters. Stents are brought out through separate stab wounds in the bladder and through the skin, and are removed a few days after operation. Stents seldom do harm but may lengthen the hospitalization and will not in themselves prevent subsequent complications when a suitable anatomic reconstruction cannot be achieved.

PRELIMINARY DRAINAGE

Rarely do children with vesicoureteral reflux present with diminished renal function or azotemia with acute urinary sepsis. In these patients, it is probably wise to place a urethral catheter temporarily and treat the infection appropriately. In small infants with significant ureteral dilatation, megacystis, and UTI, either intermittent catheterization or a cutaneous vesicostomy may be preferable to initial ureteroneocystostomy. Intermittent catheterization or cutaneous vesicostomy may be continued for 1 to 2 years, at which time ureteral

reimplantation can be accomplished more successfully. I prefer closing the cutaneous vesicostomy initially, allowing the bladder mucosa and muscle to return to normal. A second VCU is obtained a few months later and if reflux persists, I proceed with a ureteroneocystostomy.

POSTOPERATIVE RESULTS

The two criteria for judging the success of ureteroneocystostomy are the elimination of VUR and the absence of obstructive hydroureteronephrosis. The literature is replete with series documenting greater than 90 per cent success after various reimplantation techniques (Gonzales et al; Palken; Politano, 1963; Woodard and Keats). The incidence of clinical pyelonephritis is markedly decreased after successful antireflux surgery. Govan and Palmer reported a decrease in pyelonephritis from 50 per cent to less than 10 per cent after successful ureteroneocystostomy. Willscher et al (1976a) reported that even though UTI recurred postoperatively in approximately 20 per cent of patients, less than 2 per cent had clinical pyelonephritis. Bacteriuria may occur in up to 30 per cent of patients postoperatively and does not correlate with either the preoperative urographic appearance or the severity of the reflux (Wacksman et al). Interestingly, this is approximately the same incidence of bacteriuria as found in children with no reflux and in those with reflux who are being treated conservatively and nonoperatively.

COMPLICATIONS

Complications after ureteral reimplantation result from either preoperative planning errors or errors in intraoperative technique. UTI should be eliminated before operation. Cystitis and mucosal edema compromise the ability to achieve a sufficient submucosal tunnel and increase the risk of postoperative ureteral obstruction. An occult neuropathic bladder may contribute to failure of ureteral reimplantation. It is important that children with reflux and diurnal enuresis, squatting maneuvers, constipation, or encopresis be evaluated thoroughly with complete urodynamic studies before surgery to rule out detrusor-sphincter dyssynergia. In patients with a neuropathic bladder, it is important to normalize detrusor dynamics as much as possible preoperatively; this may include frequent or timed voiding, intermittent catheterization, and anticholinergic therapy.

Excessive tissue handling during ureteral mobilization may contribute to postoperative edema or devascularization of the ureter. Technical errors intraoperatively include ureteral perforation, ureteral transection or avulsion during mobilization, ureteral obstruction secondary to creation of a too tight detrusor hiatus, passing the ureter through a peritoneal fold or intraperitoneal structure, and placement of the neohiatus too cephalad and lateral on the posterior surface of the bladder.

Early perioperative complications include bleeding, catheter obstruction or dislodgment, sepsis, ureteral obstruction, anuria, and prolonged ileus. Postoperative gross hematuria usually resolves within 36 to 48 hours, but it may require catheter irrigation. Hematuria beyond 3 to 4 days may be the result of irritation from the catheter and can be corrected by removal of the urethral catheter.

Occasionally, ileus develops postoperatively in children secondary to anticholinergic and narcotic therapy. These situations respond quite adequately to either glycerin or bisacodyl (Dulcolax) suppositories. Prolonged ileus usually reflects ureteral obstruction, subtle sepsis, retroperitoneal leakage of urine, retroperitoneal hematoma, or passage of a ureter through the peritoneum or a segment of intestine. Ileus that lasts more than 48 hours postoperatively is of concern and should prompt a careful review of kidneys, ureters, and bladder and upright studies.

Interval Management

Early postoperative ureteral obstruction is most often secondary to detrusor edema. Ureteral obstruction may present with oliguria, anuria if bilateral, flank pain, nausea and vomiting, sepsis, or prolonged ileus. Hydronephrosis secondary to ureteral obstruction is confirmed by renal ultrasonography. The options for interval management for patients with early postoperative ureterovesical junction obstruction include observation, placement of percutaneous nephrostomy tubes, or internal ureteral stents. In patients with mild obstruction but with good urine output, observation alone may be indicated. If significant obstruction exists, as evidenced by severe hydrone-

phrosis or delayed visualization on isotope renography, percutaneous nephrostomy tubes can be placed temporarily until the edema resolves. It is best to postpone reoperation for at least 3 months to allow the edema and postsurgical reaction to subside. Periodic nephrostograms can be performed during this interval to reassess ureteral patency, and occasionally, an obstructed system will open up during this interval. Endoscopic visualization and catheterization of the recently reimplanted ureters in the immediate postoperative period is often quite difficult.

Obstruction

The incidence of ureterovesical junction obstruction requiring reoperation ranges between 1.2 and 4 per cent. Obstruction after ureteral reimplantation may occur as a result of one of three major causes.

Mechanical Factors. Mechanical obstruction may result from the presence of paravesical scar tissue, ureteral kinking and angulation, and an intraperitoneal course of the ureter with resultant angulation at the point of entry or exit from the peritoneum. Frequently, this obstruction is intermittent and it results from angulation of the ureter at its new hiatus—"J-hooking"—when the entrance has been placed too high and laterally on the bladder wall. In these instances, a film taken with the bladder full will show hydroureteronephrosis; with the bladder empty, it will show regression of hydroureteronephrosis (Fig. 14–41).

Ischemia. Devascularization of the lower ureter can occur with subsequent stricture formation.

Neuropathic Bladder. Unrecognized "neuropathic bladder" may produce obstruction secondary to a thick-walled trabeculated and scarred detrusor. The level of the obstruction may be either extravesical, intravesical, or at the bladder wall. Extravesical obstruction can be prevented by avoiding injury to blood vessels contiguous to the ureter (i.e., uterine artery), which might result in bleeding and hematoma with subsequent ureteral scarring and compression of the distal ureter. Penetration of the peritoneum may occur during development of a new hiatus and should be avoided by adequate visualization during dissection. Kinking and "J-hooking" of the ureter should be prevented by choosing a more medial hiatus in the posterior, less expansile por-

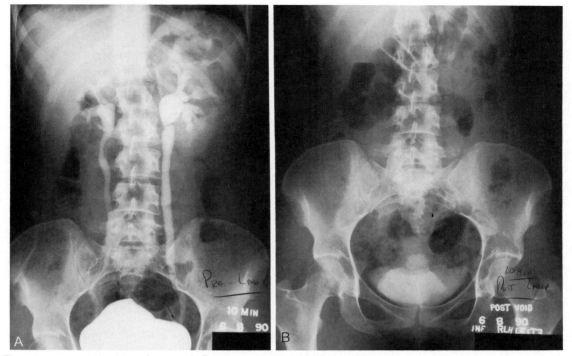

Figure 14–41 □ J-hooking of ureter. *A,* Excretory urogram with bladder full. *B,* With bladder empty. Note regression of dilatation of ureter and straightening of its course. (No reflux demonstrated.)

tion of the bladder. When the bladder wall is thick and trabeculated, it is preferable to reimplant the ureter by one of the techniques that does not require creation of a new hiatus. Finally, distal ureteral ischemia can be prevented by avoiding aggressive dissection of the ureter during intravesical mobilization. Ischemia may also develop by creation of a too tight ureteral hiatus or from twisting of the distal ureteral segment.

Reflux

The incidence of persistent VUR requiring reoperation ranges between 1 and 3 per cent. The mechanisms of failure in patients in whom VUR develops include either a short submucosal tunnel or an unrecognized neuropathic bladder. A short submucosal tunnel is usually secondary to malposition of the ureteral orifice or to its retraction after inadequate trigonal fixation. An unrecognized neuropathic bladder is described above.

VUR that appears on the initial VCU within a few months after surgery does not always signify failure. It may take several months for inflammatory changes to resolve and the antireflux flap-valve mechanism to become com-

petent (Willscher et al, 1976a). Rarely, high-grade reflux that persists after a technically satisfactory ureteral reimplantation may resolve spontaneously several months after reimplantation (Siegelbaum and Rabinovitch).

Contralateral Reflux

The incidence of contralateral reflux after ipsilateral ureteral reimplantation varies between 3 and 30 per cent (Hanani et al; Quinlan and O'Donnell). Contralateral reflux may occur as a result of disturbance of the ureterotrigonal continuity on the contralateral side during surgical dissection but is more likely the result of an incompetent contralateral ureteral orifice that was not reimplanted. Parrott and Woodard found contralateral reflux in eight of 40 children (20 per cent) undergoing unilateral reimplantation. Fifty per cent of these patients had an abnormal-appearing orifice at the time of cystoscopy prior to ipsilateral reimplantation. Warren et al found an abnormal orifice in 4 of 11 patients (36 per cent) in whom contralateral reflux developed. Furthermore, contralateral reflux occurred in an additional 9 of 20 patients (45 per cent) with a previous history of reflux on that side but no reflux at the time of ipsilateral reimplantation. Contralateral reflux most often resolves with prolonged follow-up, and the incidence of *persistent* contralateral reflux in patients undergoing unilateral ureteroneocystostomy is 3 to 5 per cent (Hanani et al; Parrott and Woodard).

In patients with unilateral reflux, bilateral reimplantation should be considered in those who have a history of prior reflux in the now nonrefluxing side and an abnormal location and configuration of the "nonrefluxing" orifice. The additional morbidity of bilateral reimplantation for unilateral reflux in this select group of patients is low.

Definitive Management

The options for definitive management include nonsurgical, endoscopic, and open repairs.

1. *Nonsurgical repair.* The treatment of failed ureteral reimplantation secondary to an occult or primary neuropathic bladder should be directed at the bladder alone. This may consist of anticholinergic therapy, clean intermittent catheterization, or both. Behavioral modification with the institution of proper voiding habits must be incorporated into the overall treatment plan.

2. *Endoscopic repair.* Endoscopic dilation of ureteral strictures has been reported sporadically with variable success (King et al, 1984; Witherington and Shelor). Early dilation has been associated with better long-term results (Hulbert et al; Mesrobian and Kelalis). Balloon dilation may be a reasonable alternative to open surgical repairs if the obstruction is discovered early and if the stricture to be dilated is short (Shore et al).

3. *Open surgical procedures.* The majority of failed ureteral reimplantations can be salvaged by using well-described techniques. In our experience, failure secondary to ureteral vesical junction obstruction has been most reliably treated with a Paquin ureteral reimplantation combined with a psoas hitch (Table 14–6) (Mesrobian et al). This technique allows construction of a long submucosal tunnel and immobilizes the new hiatus. Failed ureteral reimplantation secondary to VUR can be managed effectively by using various ureteral advancement techniques. Although transureteroureterostomy has not been extensively used in our series, this is an excellent surgical option, especially when bilateral reimplantation becomes necessary into a small and scarred bladder.

Table 14–6 □ Results of Reoperation for Ureterovesical Junction Obstruction and Vesicoureteral Reflux

	Renal units		Success	
Procedure	*Number*	*%*	*Number*	*%*
Ureterovesical Junction Obstruction				
Modified Paquin	32	65	25	78
Modified Politano-Leadbetter	15	31	8	53
Advancement	2	4	1	50
Totals	49	100	34	69
Vesicoureteral Reflux				
Modified Paquin	15	31	13	87
Modified Politano-Leadbetter	17	36	17	100
Advancement	14	29	11	79
Transureteroureterostomy	2	4	2	100
Totals	48	100	43	90

From Mesrobian H-GJ, Kramer SA, Kelalis PP: Reoperative ureteroneocystostomy: review of 69 patients. J Urol 133:388–390, 1985. By permission of the Williams & Wilkins Company.

Occasionally, the ureter can become atonic, scarred, and shortened after multiple attempts at reimplantation. Selected patients may require an augmentation cystoplasty to alter bladder dynamics or for reimplantation of the refluxing ureter into the bowel segment.

The overall success after reoperation for ureterovesical junction obstruction or VUR is approximately 80 per cent. Surgery is more likely to be successful in patients with persistent VUR than for persistent ureterovesical junction obstruction (Mesrobian et al). This finding may be the result of a higher proportion of patients in the obstructed group who have a "neuropathic bladder" as the primary cause of failure of the original reimplantation.

It is imperative that patients be followed carefully after ureteral reimplantation. Twenty per cent of patients in Mesrobian's series (Mesrobian et al) demonstrated failure between 4 and 10 years after initial ureteroneocystostomy. This suggests the need for careful monitoring of the reimplanted ureter through and beyond puberty. Conceivably, the growth spurts and hormonal changes at puberty may change the configuration of the ureterovesical junction. Because obstruction rather than reflux is likely to be the late serious complication, periodic ultrasonographic examinations of the urinary tract are advised during this interval.

MEGAURETER

Congenital megaureter may occur as a result of primary VUR, primary ureterovesical junction obstruction, posterior urethral valves, prune-belly syndrome, neuropathic bladder, ectopic ureterocele, or an iatrogenic cause, often the result of failed ureteroneocystostomy (Kelalis and Kramer, 1983). Patients with obstructive or refluxing megaureter require reduction in the ureteral caliber at the time of ureteral reimplantation. This is done to achieve an adequate length-to-width ratio in the new intravesical ureter, to relieve ureteral dilatation, to allow effective ureteral peristalsis, and to eliminate residual urine within the ureter. Interestingly, some megaureters show both reflux and obstruction (Whitaker and Flower).

Refluxing ureters, larger than 1 cm in diameter, almost always require reduction in ureteral caliber because there is often a relatively aperistaltic distal segment (Tanagho). Conversely, in patients with obstructive megaureter, transection and excision of the distal ureteral segment may be all that is necessary, and ureteral reimplantation alone may suffice. Surgical correction for obstructive megaureter responds well to various techniques (Rabinowitz et al), whereas surgical results in refluxing megaureters have been less satisfactory (Johnston and Farkas).

Excision and Tapering

Approximately 10 to 12 cm of distal ureter should be mobilized transvesically. The entire tapering procedure and reimplantation can be performed intravesically without the need to transpose the ureter into the paravesical space. One must pay meticulous attention to the blood supply of the ureter during dissection. The ureter has a medial mesentery from the kidney to the pelvic brim, but the blood supply is lateral in the true pelvis. The tortuous ureter is straightened, and the lower redundant portion is excised. The lower third of the ureter should be reduced in caliber to encompass not only the submucosal tunnel but also a few centimeters proximal to the ureteral hiatus (Johnston, 1967). Hanna has advocated a one-stage total remodeling of the dilated and tortuous ureter, but this is rarely necessary in the majority of patients.

The segment of the ureter to be removed can be marked with Babcock clamps, which are used to trap the ureteral catheter in the segment of the ureter to be preserved (Fig. 14–42). Caliber reduction is achieved by excis-

ing the antimesenteric ureter. The intact ureter that is left behind is subsequently closed in two layers with fine continuous absorbable and interrupted sutures. There should be a gradual transition between the reduced ureteral caliber and the dilated proximal ureter. A 10 Fr. ureteral catheter should fit loosely within the ureter. A ureteroneocystostomy is accomplished, and any excessive ureteral length after tapering is removed.

Hodgson and Thompson described an innovative technique of reductive ureteroplasty in which no instruments were used on the ureter to decrease risk of damage to its wall and blood supply (Fig. 14–43). After the ureter has been circumscribed and mobilized from the bladder, an indwelling Silastic tube is inserted all the way to the renal pelvis. A running horizontal mattress absorbable suture is placed on the antimesenteric border of the ureter to mold the lumen to the catheter. The redundant ureter is excised and a second layer of running suture is used to create a watertight seal and to achieve hemostasis. The ureteroneocystostomy is performed in the usual fashion. This technique avoids the possibility of excessive removal of the ureteral wall.

Ureteral Folding

The ureteral folding technique, first reported by Kaliciński et al and modified by Starr, involves reduction of ureteral caliber without excision of the ureteral wall (Figs. 14–44 and 14–45). The lateral excluded ureteral lumen is folded either anteriorly or posteriorly with multiple interrupted sutures along the medial wall. The reduction of the ureteral caliber should extend for a few centimeters proximal to the bladder wall. A ureteroneocystostomy by one of the accepted techniques is performed. The bulk of the folded ureter usually does not interfere with placement into the submucosal tunnel. However, in some patients, the ureter is too wide and bulky, and formal excision and tapering should be accomplished. This technique has the advantage of preserving blood supply, and it reduces the chance of suture line leakage; therefore, it does not require prolonged ureteral stenting. Stents are optional with this procedure, but if used, they are usually removed within 48 to 72 hours. This technique has produced excellent results with a low incidence of complications (Ehrlich, 1985).

Text continued on page 494

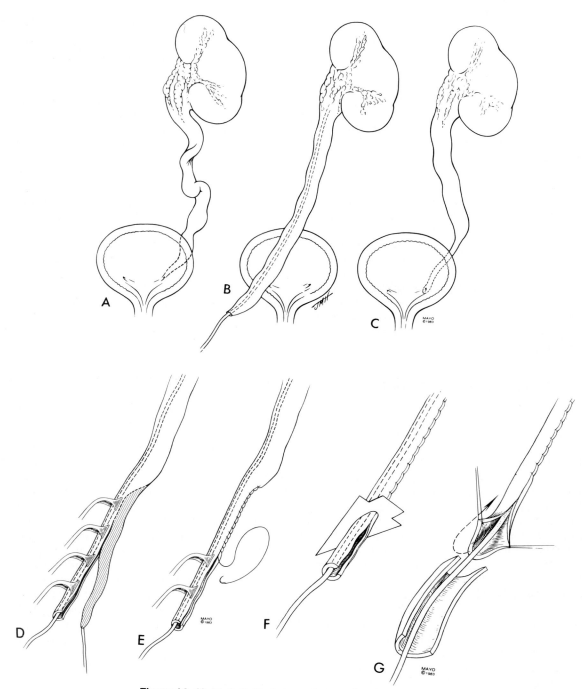

Figure 14–42 □ *A–G*, Technique of ureteral caliber reduction.

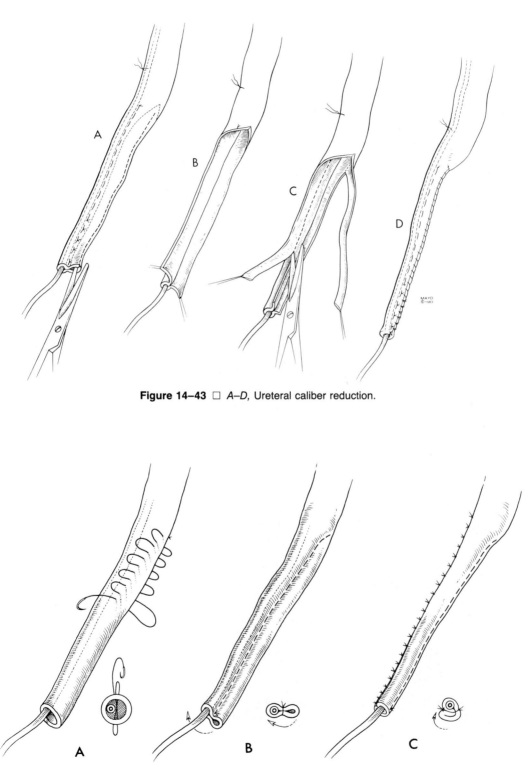

Figure 14–43 □ *A–D*, Ureteral caliber reduction.

Figure 14–44 □ *A–C*, Ureteral folding.

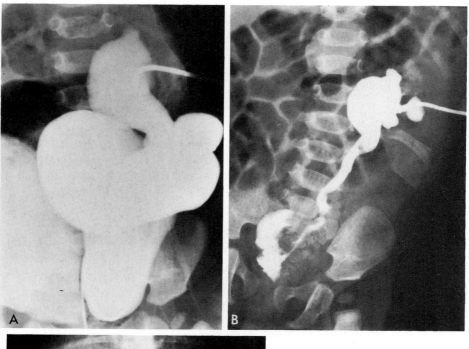

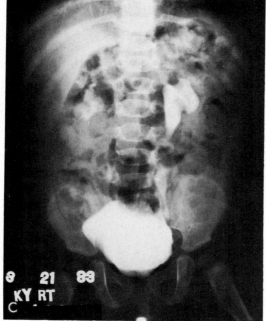

Figure 14–45 ☐ Ureteral folding technique. *A*, Percutaneous nephrostogram. Massive dilatation and tortuosity of ureter. *B*, Same, after excision of redundant ureter, folding of distal portion, and ureteroneocystostomy immediately postoperatively. *C*, Excretory urograms 3 months after operation. Resolution of left hydroureteronephrosis with good function.

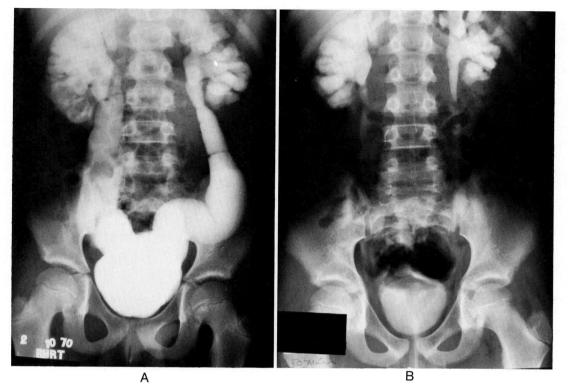

A
B

Figure 14–46 □ Reflux megaureter. Excretory urograms before *(A)* and 1 year after *(B)* ureteral caliber reduction.

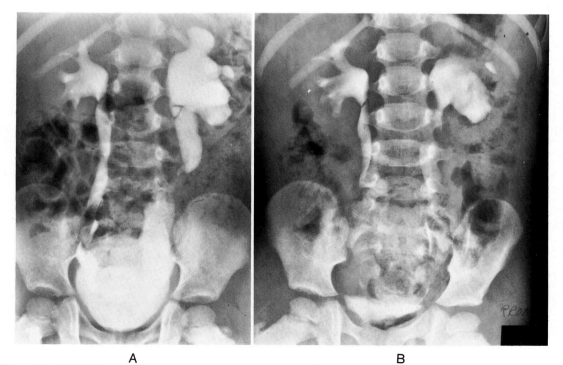

A
B

Figure 14–47 □ Primary obstructive megaureter. Excretory urograms before *(A)* and 5 months after *(B)* left ureteral reduction.

The results of ureteral caliber reduction, either excising or folding, should not be based exclusively on the appearance of the excretory urogram (Figs. 14–46 and 14–47); they should also include renal growth and function and elimination of pyelonephritis. In neonates with bilateral refluxing megaureters and megacystis, preliminary diversion by cutaneous vesicostomy may be indicated. In neonates and infants with bilateral obstructive megaureters and a small bladder capacity, a unilateral ureteral caliber reduction, which uses up most of the bladder base, and transureteroureterostomy of the contralateral ureter may be technically easier than bilateral ureteral reimplantation with ureteral tapering.

Bibliography

Ahmed S, Boucaut HA: Vesicoureteral reflux in complete ureteral duplication: surgical options. J Urol 140:1092, 1988.

Allen TD: Vesicoureteral reflux as a manifestation of dysfunctional voiding. *In* Reflux Nephropathy. Edited by CJ Hodson, P Kincaid-Smith. New York, Masson Publishing USA, 1979, pp 171–180.

Allen TD: Vesicoureteral reflux and the unstable bladder (letter). J Urol 134:1180, 1985.

Ambrose SS, Parrott TS, Woodard JR, et al: Observations on the small kidney associated with vesicoureteral reflux. J Urol 123:349, 1980.

Arap S, Abrão EG, Menezes de Góes G: Treatment and prevention of complications after extravesical antireflux technique. Eur Urol 7:263, 1981.

Arnold GE: Alleviation of aphonia or dysphonia through intrachordal injection of Teflon paste. Ann Otol Rhinol Laryngol 72:384, 1963.

Askari A, Belman AB: Vesicoureteral reflux in black girls. J Urol 127:747, 1982.

Atwell JD: Primary reflux and renal growth. Int Perspectives Urol 10:40, 1984.

Atwell JD, Vijay MR: Renal growth following reimplantation of the ureters for reflux. Br J Urol 50:367, 1978.

Austenfeld MS, Snow BW: Complications of pregnancy in women after reimplantation for vesicoureteral reflux. J Urol 140:1103, 1988.

Bailey RR: The relationship of vesico-ureteric reflux to urinary tract infection and chronic pyelonephritis—reflux nephropathy. Clin Nephrol 1:132, 1973.

Baker R, Maxted W, Maglath J, et al: Relation of age, sex and infection to reflux: data indicating high spontaneous cure rate in pediatric patients. J Urol 95:27, 1966.

Bakshandeh K, Lynne C, Carrion H: Vesicoureteral reflux and end stage renal disease. J Urol 116:557, 1976.

Bauer SB, Colodny AH, Retik AB: The management of vesicoureteral reflux in children with myelodysplasia. J Urol 128:102, 1982.

Becker GJ, Ihle BU, Fairley KF, et al: Effect of pregnancy on moderate renal failure in reflux nephropathy. Br Med J 292:796, 1986.

Becu L, Quesada EM, Medel R, et al: Small kidney associated with primary vesicoureteral reflux in children: a pathological overhaul. Eur Urol 14:127, 1988.

Beetz R, Schulte-Wissermann H, Tröger J, et al: Long-term follow-up of children with surgically treated vesicorenal reflux: postoperative incidence of urinary tract infections, renal scars and arterial hypertension. Eur Urol 16:366, 1989.

Belman AB, Filmer RB, King LR: Surgical management of duplication of the collecting system. J Urol 112:316, 1974.

Ben-Ami T, Gayer G, Hertz M, et al: The natural history of reflux in the lower pole of duplicated collecting systems: a controlled study. Pediatr Radiol 19:308, 1989.

Birmingham Reflux Study Group: Prospective trial of operative versus non-operative treatment of severe vesicoureteric reflux: two years' observation in 96 children. Br Med J 287:171, 1983.

Birmingham Reflux Study Group: Prospective trial of operative versus non-operative treatment of severe vesicoureteric reflux in children: five years' observation. Br Med J 295:237, 1987.

Blaufox MD, Gruskin A, Sandler P, et al: Radionuclide scintigraphy for detection of vesicoureteral reflux in children. J Pediatr 79:239, 1971.

Bockrath JM, Maizels M, Firlit CF: The use of lower ipsilateral ureteroureterostomy to treat vesicoureteral reflux or obstruction in children with duplex ureters. J Urol 129:543, 1983.

Bracci U, Miano L, Laurenti C: Ureteroureterostomy in complete ureteral duplication. Eur Urol 5:347, 1979.

Bridge RAC, Roe CW: The grading of vesicoureteral reflux: a guide to therapy. J Urol 101:821, 1969.

Briggs EM, Constantinou CE, Govan DE: Dynamics of the upper urinary tract: the relationship of urine flow rate and rate of ureteral peristalsis. Invest Urol 10:56, 1972.

Brown S: Open versus endoscopic surgery in the treatment of vesicoureteral reflux. J Urol 142:499, 1989.

Brühl P, van Ahlen H, Mallmann R: Antireflux procedure by Lich-Gregoir: indications and results. Eur Urol 14:37, 1988.

Burger RH, Burger SE: Genetic determinants of urologic disease. Urol Clin North Am 1:419, 1974.

Canning DA, Leonard MP, Peters CA, et al: Endoscopic injection of glutaraldehyde cross-linked bovine dermal collagen for correction of vesicoureteral reflux. Presented at annual meeting, Kimbrough Urologic Seminar, December 3–8, 1989, San Antonio, Texas.

Carini M, Selli C, Lenzi R, et al: Surgical treatment of vesicoureteral reflux with bilateral medialization of the ureteral orifices. Eur Urol 11:181, 1985.

Carson CC III, Kelalis PP, Hoffman AD: Renal growth in small kidneys after ureteroneocystostomy. J Urol 127:1146, 1982.

Claësson I, Jacobsson B, Jodal U, et al: Compensatory kidney growth in children with urinary tract infection and unilateral renal scarring: an epidemiologic study. Kidney Int 20:759, 1981a.

Claësson I, Jacobsson B, Olsson T, et al: Assessment of renal parenchymal thickness in normal children. Acta Radiol Diagn 22:305, 1981b.

Claësson I, Lindberg U: Asymptomatic bacteriuria in schoolgirls: VII. A follow-up study of the urinary tract in treated and untreated schoolgirls with asymptomatic bacteriuria. Radiology 124:179, 1977.

Cohen SJ: Ureterozystoneostomie: Eine neue antireflux technik. Aktuel Urol 6:1, 1975.

Conway JJ, King LR, Belman AB, et al: Detection of vesicoureteral reflux with radionuclide cystography: a comparison with roentgenographic cystography. Am J Roentgen Radium Ther Nuc Med 115:720, 1972.

Cotran RS, Pennington JE: Urinary tract infection, pyelonephritis, and reflux nephropathy. *In* The Kidney, Vol 2, 2nd ed. Edited by BM Brenner, FC Rector Jr. Philadelphia, WB Saunders Co, 1981, pp 1571–1632.

Cremin BJ: Observations on vesico-ureteric reflux and intrarenal reflux: a review and survey of material. Clin Radiol 30:607, 1979.

Currarino G: Roentgenographic estimation of kidney size in normal individuals with emphasis on children. Am J Roentgenol 93:464, 1965.

Cussen LJ: Dimensions of the normal ureter in infancy and childhood. Invest Urol 5:164, 1967.

Daines SL, Hodgson NB: Management of reflux in total duplication anomalies. J Urol 105:720, 1971.

De Sy WA, de Meyer JM, Oosterlinck W, et al: Antireflux in adults: a long-term follow-up. Eur Urol 12:395, 1986.

Decter RM, Roth DR, Gonzales ET Jr: Vesicoureteral reflux in boys. J Urol 140:1089, 1988.

DeKlerk DP, Reiner WG, Jeffs RD: Vesicoureteral reflux and ureteropelvic junction obstruction: late occurrence of ureteropelvic obstruction after successful ureteroneocystostomy. J Urol 121:816, 1979.

Duckett JW: Vesicoureteral reflux: a "conservative" analysis. Am J Kidney Dis 3:139, 1983.

Duckett JW, Bellinger MF: A plea for standardized grading of vesicoureteral reflux. Eur Urol 8:74, 1982.

Duthoy EJ, Soucheray JA, McGroarty BJ: Ipsilateral ureteroureterostomy for vesicoureteral reflux in duplicated ureters. J Urol 118:826, 1977.

Dwoskin JY: Sibling uropathy. J Urol 115:726, 1976.

Dwoskin JY, Perlmutter AD: Vesicoureteral reflux in children: a computerized review. J Urol 109:888, 1973.

Edelbrock HH, Mickelson JC: Selection of children for vesicoureteroplasty. J Urol 104:342, 1970.

Edwards D, Normand ICS, Prescod N, et al: Disappearance of vesicoureteric reflux during long-term prophylaxis of urinary tract infection in children. Br Med J 2:285, 1977.

Ehrlich RM: Success of the transvesical advancement technique for vesicoureteral reflux. J Urol 128:554, 1982.

Ehrlich RM: The ureteral folding technique for megaureter surgery. J Urol 134:668, 1985.

Elder JS: Complications of periurethral Teflon injection. Society for Pediatric Urology Newsletter 41–42, August 25, 1988.

Evans RJ, Raezer DM, Shrom SH: Surgical treatment of reflux in neurologically impaired child. Urology 28:31, 1986.

Farkas A, Moriel EZ, Lupa S: Endoscopic correction of vesicoureteral reflux: our experience with 115 ureters. J Urol 144:534, 1990.

Fehrenbaker LG, Kelalis PP, Stickler GB: Vesicoureteral reflux and ureteral duplication in children. J Urol 107:862, 1972.

Filly R, Friedland GW, Govan DE, et al: Development and progression of clubbing and scarring in children with recurrent urinary tract infections. Radiology 113:145, 1974.

Fort KF, Selman SH, Kropp KA: A retrospective analysis of the use of ureteral stents in children undergoing ureteroneocystotomy. J Urol 129:545, 1983.

Friedland GW: The voiding cystourethrogram: an unreliable examination. *In* Reflux Nephropathy. Edited by CJ Hodson, P Kincaid-Smith. New York, Masson Publishing USA, 1979, pp 93–99.

Funston MR, Cremin BJ: Intrarenal reflux—papillary morphology and pressure relationships in children's necropsy kidneys. Br J Radiol 51:665, 1978.

Gatewood OMB, Glasser RJ, Vanhoutte JJ: Roentgen evaluation of renal size in pediatric age groups. Am J Dis Child 110:162, 1965.

Gearhart JP: Endoscopic management of vesicoureteral reflux. *In* Problems in Urology, Vol 4, No. 4. Edited by DF Paulson, SA Kramer, Guest Editor. Philadelphia, JB Lippincott, 1990, pp 639–647.

Gil-Vernet JM: A new technique for surgical correction of vesicoureteral reflux. J Urol 131:456, 1984.

Gill DB, da Costa BM, Cameron JS, et al: Analysis of 100 children with severe and persistent hypertension. Arch Dis Child 51:951, 1976.

Ginalski J-M, Michaud A, Genton N: Renal growth retardation in children: sign suggestive of vesicoureteral reflux? AJR 145:617, 1985.

Glassberg KI, Laungani G, Wasnick RJ, et al: Transverse ureteral advancement technique of ureteroneocystostomy (Cohen reimplant) and a modification for difficult cases (experience with 121 ureters). J Urol 134:304, 1985.

Glenn JF, Anderson EE: Distal tunnel ureteral reimplantation. J Urol 97:623, 1967.

Glenn JF, Anderson EE: Technical considerations in distant tunnel ureteral reimplantation. J Urol 119:194, 1978.

Gonzales ET, Glenn JF, Anderson EE: Results of distal tunnel ureteral reimplantation. J Urol 107:572, 1972.

Gore MD, Fernbach SK, Donaldson JS, et al: Radiographic evaluation of subureteric injection of Teflon to correct vesicoureteral reflux. AJR 152:115, 1989.

Govan DE, Fair WR, Friedland GW, et al: Management of children with urinary tract infections: the Stanford experience. Urology 6:273, 1975.

Govan DE, Palmer JM: Urinary tract infection in children: the influence of successful antireflux operations in morbidity from infection. Pediatrics 44:677, 1969.

Grégoir W, Schulman CC: Die extravesikale antirefluxplastik. Urologe [A] 16:124, 1977.

Grégoir W, Van Regemorter G: Le reflux vésico-urétéral congénital. Urol Int 18:122, 1964.

Hagberg S, Hjälmå SK, Jacobsson B, et al: Renal growth after antireflux surgery in infants. Z Kinderchir 39:52, 1984.

Hanani Y, Goldwasser B, Jonas P, et al: Management of unilateral reflux by ipsilateral ureteroneocystostomy—is it sufficient? J Urol 129:1022, 1983.

Hanna MK: New surgical method for one-stage total remodeling of massively dilated and tortuous ureter: tapering in situ technique. Urology 14:453, 1979.

Hannerz L, Wikstad I, Celsi G, et al: Influence of vesicoureteral reflux and urinary tract infection on renal growth in children with upper urinary tract duplication. Acta Radiol 30:391, 1989.

Harrison R: On the possibility and utility of washing out the pelvis of the kidney and the ureters through the bladder. Lancet 1:463, 1888.

Hawtrey CE, Culp DA, Loening S, et al: Ureterovesical reflux in an adolescent and adult population. J Urol 130:1067, 1983.

Heale WF: Age of presentation and pathogenesis of reflux nephropathy. *In* Reflux Nephropathy. Edited by CJ Hodson, P Kincaid-Smith. New York, Masson Publishing USA, 1979, pp 140–146.

Heidrick WP, Mattingly RF, Amberg JR: Vesicoureteral reflux in pregnancy. Obstet Gynecol 29:571, 1967.

Heikel PE, Parkkulainen KV: Vesico-ureteric reflux in children. A classification and results of conservative treatment. Ann Radiol 9:37, 1966.

Hinman F, Baumann FW: Vesical and ureteral damage

from voiding dysfunction in boys without neurologic or obstructive disease. J Urol 109:727, 1973.

Hodgson NB, Thompson LW: Technique of reductive ureteroplasty in the management of megaureter. J Urol 113:118, 1975.

Hodson CJ: The radiological diagnosis of pyelonephritis. Proc R Soc Med 52:669, 1959.

Hodson CJ: Reflux nephropathy: scoring the damage. In Reflux Nephropathy. Edited by CJ Hodson, P Kincaid-Smith. New York, Masson Publishing USA, 1979, pp 29–38.

Hodson CJ, Davies Z, Prescod A: Renal parenchymal radiographic measurement in infants and children. Pediatr Radiol 3:16, 1975a.

Hodson CJ, Edwards D: Chronic pyelonephritis and vesicoureteric reflux. Clin Radiol 11:219, 1960.

Hodson CJ, Maling TMJ, McManamon PJ, et al: The pathogenesis of reflux nephropathy (chronic atrophic pyelonephritis). Br J Radiol Suppl 13:1, 1975b.

Holland NH: Reflux nephropathy and hypertension. In Reflux Nephropathy. Edited by CJ Hodson, P Kincaid-Smith. New York, Masson Publishing USA, 1979, pp 257–262.

Hollowell JG, Altman HG, Snyder H McC III, et al: Coexisting ureteropelvic junction obstruction and vesicoureteral reflux: diagnostic and therapeutic implications. J Urol 142:490, 1989.

Homsy YL, Nsouli I, Hamburger B, et al: Effects of oxybutynin on vesicoureteral reflux in children. J Urol 134:1168, 1985.

Howerton LW, Lich R Jr: The cause and correction of ureteral reflux. J Urol 89:672, 1963.

Huland H, Busch R: Pyelonephritic scarring in 213 patients with upper and lower urinary tract infections: long-term followup. J Urol 132:936, 1984.

Hulbert JC, Hunter D, Castaneda-Zuniga W: Classification and techniques for the reconstitution of acquired strictures in the region of the ureteropelvic junction. J Urol 140:468, 1988.

Hutch JA: Vesico-ureteral reflux in the paraplegic: cause and correction. J Urol 68:457, 1952.

Hutch JA: Theory of maturation of the intravesical ureter. J Urol 86:534, 1961.

Hutch JA: Ureteric advancement operation: anatomy, technique and early results. J Urol 89:180, 1963.

Iannaccone G, Panzironi PE: Ureteral reflux in normal infants. Acta Radiol 44:451, 1955.

Jeffs RD, Allen MS: The relationship between ureterovesical reflux and infection. J Urol 88:691, 1962.

Jerkins GR, Noe HN: Familial vesicoureteral reflux: a prospective study. J Urol 128:774, 1982.

Johnston JH: Vesico-ureteric reflux: its anatomical mechanism, causation, effects and treatment in the child. Ann R Coll Surg Engl 30:324, 1962.

Johnston JH: Reconstructive surgery of mega-ureter in childhood. Br J Urol 39:17, 1967.

Johnston JH, Farkas A: The congenital refluxing megaureter: experiences with surgical reconstruction. Br J Urol 47:153, 1975.

Johnston JH, Shapiro SR, Thomas GG: Anti-reflux surgery in the congenital neuropathic bladder. Br J Urol 48:639, 1976.

Jones BW, Headstream JW: Vesicoureteral reflux in children. J Urol 80:114, 1958.

Jungers P, Forget D, Henry-Amar M, et al: Chronic kidney disease and pregnancy. Adv Nephrol 15:103, 1986.

Kaliciński ZH, Kansy J, Kotarbińska B, et al: Surgery of megaureters—modification of Hendren's operation. J Pediatr Surg 12:183, 1977.

Kaplan WE: Early evaluation and treatment of children with meningomyelocele. In Problems in Urology, Vol 4, No 4. Edited by DF Paulson, SA Kramer, Guest Editor. Philadelphia, JB Lippincott, 1990, pp 676–689.

Kaplan WE, Dalton DP, Firlit CF: The endoscopic correction of reflux by polytetrafluorethylene injection. J Urol 138:953, 1987.

Kaplan WE, Firlit CF: Management of reflux in the myelodysplastic child. J Urol 129:1195, 1983.

Kaplan WE, Nasrallah P, King LR: Reflux in complete duplication in children. J Urol 120:220, 1978.

Kass EJ, Koff SA, Diokno AC: Fate of vesicoureteral reflux in children with neuropathic bladders managed by intermittent catheterization. J Urol 125:63, 1981.

Kaveggia L, King LR, Grana L, et al: Pyelonephritis: a cause of vesicoureteral reflux? J Urol 95:158, 1966.

Kelalis PP: Proper perspective on vesicoureteral reflux. Mayo Clin Proc 46:807, 1971.

Kelalis PP: Surgical correction of vesicoureteral reflux. In Clinical Pediatric Urology, 2nd ed. Edited by PP Kelalis, LR King, AB Belman. Philadelphia, WB Saunders Co, 1985, pp 381–419.

Kelalis PP, Kramer SA: Complications of megaureter surgery. Urol Clin North Am 10:417, 1983.

Kelalis PP, Kramer SA: Anomalies of renal ectopy and fusion. In Pediatric and Adult Reconstructive Urologic Surgery, 2nd ed. Edited by JA Libertino. Baltimore, Williams & Wilkins, 1987, pp 102–108.

Kincaid-Smith P, Fairley KF: Renal disease in pregnancy. Three controversial areas: mesangial IgA nephropathy, focal glomerular sclerosis (focal and segmental hyalinosis and sclerosis), and reflux nephropathy. Am J Kidney Dis 9:328, 1987.

Kincaid-Smith PS, Bastos MG, Becker GJ: Reflux nephropathy in the adult. Contrib Nephrol 39:94, 1984.

King LR: Vesicoureteral reflux: history, etiology and conservative management. In Clinical Pediatric Urology, Vol 1. Edited by PP Kelalis, LR King, AB Belman. Philadelphia, WB Saunders Co, 1976, pp 342–365.

King LR: Sphincter dyssynergia in children with reflux. J Urol 129:217, 1983.

King LR, Coughlin PWF, Ford KK, et al: Initial experiences with percutaneous and transurethral ablation of postoperative ureteral strictures in children. J Urol 131:1167, 1984.

King LR, Kazmi SO, Belman AB: Natural history of vesicoureteral reflux: outcome of a trial of nonoperative therapy. Urol Clin North Am 1:441, 1974.

Kiruluta HG, Fraser K, Owen L: The significance of the adrenergic nerves in the etiology of vesicoureteral reflux. J Urol 136:232, 1986.

Klare B, Geiselhardt B, Wesch H, et al: Radiological kidney size in childhood. Pediatr Radiol 9:153, 1980.

Koff SA, Murtagh DS: The uninhibited bladder in children: effect of treatment on recurrence of urinary infection and on vesicoureteral reflux resolution. J Urol 130:1138, 1983.

Kohri K, Kataoka K, Akiyama T, et al: Treatment of vesicoureteral reflux by endoscopic injection of blood. Urol Int 43:324, 1988.

Kondo A, Kobayashi M, Otani T, et al: Children with unstable bladder: clinical and urodynamic observation. J Urol 129:88, 1983.

Kondo A, Otani T: Correction of reflux with the ureteric crossover method: clinical experience in 50 patients. Br J Urol 60:36, 1987.

Kunin CM, Deutscher R, Paquin A Jr: Urinary tract infections in school children: an epidemiologic, clinical and laboratory study. Medicine (Baltimore) 43:91, 1964.

Lamesch AJ: Retrograde catheterization of the ureter

after antireflux plasty by the Cohen technique of transverse advancement. J Urol 125:73, 1981.

Lattimer JK, Apperson JW, Gleason DM, et al: The pressure at which reflux occurs, an important indicator of prognosis and treatment. J Urol 89:395, 1963.

Lebowitz RL, Blickman JG: The coexistence of ureteropelvic junction obstruction and reflux. AJR 140:231, 1983.

Leighton DM, Mayne V: Obstruction in the refluxing urinary tract—a common phenomenon. Clin Radiol 40:271, 1989.

Lenaghan D, Whitaker JG, Jensen F, et al: The natural history of reflux and long-term effects of reflux on the kidney. J Urol 115:728, 1976.

Leonard MP, Canning DA, Gearhart JP, et al: Local tissue reaction to suburothelial injections of glutaraldehyde cross-linked bovine collagen (Zyplast) in humans. Presented at annual meeting of American Academy of Pediatrics, Section of Urology, October 21–23, 1989, Chicago, Illinois.

Levitt SB, Weiss RA: Vesicoureteral reflux. Natural history, classification, and reflux nephropathy. *In* Clinical Pediatric Urology, 2nd ed. Edited by PP Kelalis, LR King, AB Belman. Philadelphia, WB Saunders Co, 1985, pp 355–380.

Lich R Jr, Howerton LW, Davis LA: Recurrent urosepsis in children. J Urol 86:554, 1961.

Lich R Jr, Howerton LW Jr, Goode LS, et al: The ureterovesical junction of the newborn. J Urol 92:436, 1964.

Lines D: 15th century ureteric reflux. Lancet 2:1473, 1982.

Linn R, Ginesin Y, Bolkier M, et al: Lich-Gregoir antireflux operation: a surgical experience and 5–20 years of follow-up in 149 ureters. Eur Urol 16:200, 1989.

Lue TF, Macchia RJ, Pastore L, et al: Vesicoureteral reflux and staghorn calculi. J Urol 127:247, 1982.

Lyon RP: Renal arrest. J Urol 109:707, 1973.

Lyon RP: What does urethral dilation really do? Birth Defects 13:439, 1977.

Lyon RP, Marshall S, Tanagho EA: The ureteral orifice: its configuration and competency. J Urol 102:504, 1969.

Mackie GG, Stephens FD: Duplex kidneys: a correlation of renal dysplasia with position of the ureteral orifice. J Urol 114:274, 1975.

Maizels M, Smith CK, Firlit CF: The management of children with vesicoureteral reflux and ureteropelvic junction obstruction. J Urol 131:722, 1984.

Malek RS: Urolithiasis. *In* Clinical Pediatric Urology, Vol 2. Edited by PP Kelalis, LR King, AB Belman. Philadelphia, WB Saunders Co, 1976, p 870.

Malek RS, Kelalis PP: Pediatric nephrolithiasis. J Urol 113:545, 1975.

Malek RS, Svensson J, Neves RJ, et al: Vesicoureteral reflux in the adult: III. Surgical correction: risks and benefits. J Urol 130:882, 1983a.

Malek RS, Svensson JP, Torres VE: Vesicoureteral reflux in the adult: I. Factors in pathogenesis. J Urol 130:37, 1983b.

Malizia AA Jr, Reiman HM, Myers RP, et al: Migration and granulomatous reaction after periurethral injection of polytef (Teflon). JAMA 251:3277, 1984.

Malizia AA Jr, Woodard JR, Rushton HG, et al: Intravesical/suburetic injection of polytef: serial radiologic imaging (abstr). J Urol 139:185A, 1988.

Mann CI, Jequier S, Patriguin H, et al: Intramural Teflon injection of the ureter for treatment of vesicoureteral reflux: sonographic appearance. AJR 151:543, 1988.

Marberger M, Altwein JE, Straub E, et al: The Lich-Gregoir antireflux plasty: experiences with 371 children. J Urol 120:216, 1978.

Mathisen W: Vesicoureteral reflux and its surgical correction. Surg Gynecol Obstet 118:965, 1964.

Matouschek E: Die behandlung des vesikorenalen refluxes durch transurethrale einspritzung von teflonpaste. Urologe [A] 20:263, 1981.

Mazze RI, Schwartz FD, Slocum HC, et al: Renal function during anesthesia and surgery: 1. Effects of halothane anesthesia. Anesthesiology 24:279, 1963.

McLorie GA, McKenna PH, Jumper BM, et al: High grade vesicoureteral reflux: analysis of observational therapy. J Urol 144:537, 1990.

McRae CU, Shannon FT, Utley WLF: Effect on renal growth of reimplantation of refluxing ureters. Lancet 1:1310, 1974.

Melick WF, Brodeur AE, Karellos DN: A suggested classification of ureteral reflux and suggested treatment based on cineradiographic findings and simultaneous pressure recordings by means of the strain gauge. J Urol 88:35, 1962.

Merguerian PA, McLorie GA, Khoury AE, et al: Submucosal injection of polyvinyl alcohol foam in rabbit bladder. J Urol 144:531, 1990.

Merrell RW, Mowad JJ: Increased physical growth after successful antireflux operation. J Urol 122:523, 1979.

Mesrobian H-GJ, Kelalis PP: Ureterocalicostomy: indications and results in 21 patients. J Urol 142:1285, 1989.

Mesrobian H-GJ, Kramer SA, Kelalis PP: Reoperative ureteroneocystostomy: review of 69 patients. J Urol 133:388, 1985.

Mittleman R, Marraccini JV: Pulmonary Teflon granulomas following periurethral Teflon injection for urinary incontinence (letter to the editor). Arch Pathol Lab Med 107:611, 1983.

Moreau JF, Grenier P, Grünfeld JP, et al: Renal clubbing and scarring in adults: a retrospective study of 110 cases. Urol Radiol 1:129, 1979–1980.

Nasrallah PF, Aliabadi HA: Bladder augmentation in patients with neurogenic bladder and vesicoureteral reflux. J Urol 146:563, 1991.

Nasrallah PF, Simon JW: Reflux and voiding abnormalities in children. Urology 24:243, 1984.

Nasrallah PF, Conway JJ, King LR, et al: Quantitative nuclear cystogram: aid in determining spontaneous resolution of vesicoureteral reflux. Urology 12:654, 1978.

Nativ O, Hertz M, Hanani Y, et al: Vesicoureteral reflux in adults: a review of 95 patients. Eur Urol 13:229, 1987.

Neves RJ, Torres VE, Malek RS, et al: Vesicoureteral reflux in the adult. IV. Medical versus surgical management. J Urol 132:882, 1984.

Noe HN: The relationship of sibling reflux to index patient dysfunctional voiding. J Urol 140:119, 1988.

O'Donnell B, Puri P: Treatment of vesicoureteric reflux by endoscopic injection of Teflon. Br Med J 289:7, 1984.

O'Donnell B, Puri P: Endoscopic correction of primary vesicoureteric reflux. Br J Urol 58:601, 1986.

Palken M: Surgical correction of vesicoureteral reflux in children: results with the use of a single standard technique. J Urol 104:765, 1970.

Paltiel HJ, Lebowitz RL: Neonatal hydronephrosis due to primary vesicoureteral reflux: trends in diagnosis and treatment. Radiology 170:787, 1989.

Paquin AJ Jr: Ureterovesical anastomosis: the description and evaluation of a technique. J Urol 82:573, 1959.

Parrott TS, Woodard JR: Reflux in opposite ureter after successful correction of unilateral vesicoureteral reflux. Urology 7:276, 1976.

Peters PC, Johnson DE, Jackson JH Jr: The incidence of

vesicoureteral reflux in the premature child. J Urol 97:259, 1967.

Pfister RR, Biber RJ, Rose JS, et al: Monitoring ureteral reflux with ultrasound. Presented at the Urologic Section of the 51st American Academy of Pediatrics meeting, October 6, 1982.

Philipson EH, Wolfson RN, Kedia KR: Fetal hydronephrosis and polyhydramnios associated with vesico-ureteral reflux. J Clin Ultrasound 12:585, 1984.

Politano VA: Vesicoureteral reflux in children. JAMA 172:1252, 1960.

Politano VA: One hundred reimplantations and five years. J Urol 90:696, 1963.

Politano VA, Leadbetter WF: An operative technique for the correction of vesicoureteral reflux. J Urol 79:932, 1958.

Politano VA, Small MP, Harper JM, et al: Periurethral Teflon injection for urinary incontinence. J Urol 111:180, 1974.

Polk HC Jr: Notes on Galenic urology. Urol Survey 15:2, 1965.

Poznanski E, Poznanski AK: Psychogenic influences on voiding: observations from voiding cystourethrography. Psychosomatics 10:339, 1969.

Prout GR Jr, Koontz WW Jr: Partial vesical immobilization: an important adjunct to ureteroneocystostomy. J Urol 103:147, 1970.

Puri P, O'Donnell B: Correction of experimentally produced vesicoureteric reflux in the piglet by intravesical injection of Teflon. Br Med J 289:5, 1984.

Quinlan D, O'Donnell B: Unilateral ureteric reimplantation for primary vesicoureteric reflux in children. Br J Urol 57:406, 1985.

Rabinowitz R, Barkin M, Schillinger JF, et al: Surgical treatment of the massively dilated primary megaureter in children. Br J Urol 51:19, 1979.

Ransley PG: Vesicoureteric reflux: continuing surgical dilemma. Urology 12:246, 1978.

Ransley PG, Risdon RA: Renal papillary morphology in infants and young children. Urol Res 3:111, 1975a.

Ransley PG, Risdon RA: Renal papillary morphology and intrarenal reflux in the young pig. Urol Res 3:105, 1975b.

Ransley PG, Risdon RA: Reflux and renal scarring. Br J Radiol Suppl 14:1, 1978.

Ransley PG, Risdon RA: Reflux nephropathy: effects of antimicrobial therapy on the evolution of the early pyelonephritic scar. Kidney Int 20:733, 1981.

Redman JF, Scriber LJ, Bissada NK: Apparent failure of renal growth secondary to vesicoureteral reflux. Urology 3:704, 1974.

Roberts JA, Riopelle AJ: Vesicoureteral reflux in the primate: III. Effect of urinary tract infection on maturation of the ureterovesical junction. Pediatrics 61:853, 1978.

Roberts JA, Roth JK Jr, Domingue G, et al: Immunology of pyelonephritis in the primate model. J Urol 128:1394, 1982.

Roberts JA, Suarez GM, Kaack B, et al: Experimental pyelonephritis in the monkey. VII. Ascending pyelonephritis in the absence of vesicoureteral reflux. J Urol 133:1068, 1985.

Roberts JP, Atwell JD: Vesicoureteric reflux and urinary calculi in children. Br J Urol 64:10, 1989.

Rolleston GL, Maling TMJ, Hodson CJ: Intrarenal reflux and the scarred kidney. Arch Dis Child 49:531, 1974.

Rolleston GL, Shannon FT, Utley WLF: Relationship of infantile vesicoureteric reflux to renal damage. Br Med J 1:460, 1970.

Rose JS, Glassberg KI, Waterhouse K: Intrarenal reflux and its relationship to renal scarring. J Urol 113:400, 1975.

Salvatierra O Jr, Tanagho EA: Reflux as a cause of end stage kidney disease: report of 32 cases. J Urol 117:441, 1977.

Savage DCL, Wilson MI, Ross EM, et al: Asymptomatic bacteriuria in girl entrants to Dundee Primary Schools. Br Med J 3:75, 1969.

Schoenberg HW, Beisswanger P, Howard WJ, et al: Effect of lower urinary tract infection upon ureteral function. J Urol 92:107, 1964.

Schulman CC, Simon J, Pamart D, et al: Endoscopic treatment of vesicoureteral reflux in children. J Urol 138:950, 1987.

Scott JD, Blackford HN, Joyce MRL, et al: Renal function following surgical correction of vesico-ureteric reflux in childhood. Br J Urol 58:119, 1986.

Scott JE: Ureteric reflux in the duplex kidney. Acta Urol Belg 31:73, 1963.

Scott JES: Fetal ureteric reflux. Br J Urol 59:291, 1987.

Scott JES, Stansfeld JM: Ureteric reflux and kidney scarring in children. Arch Dis Child 43:468, 1968.

Seruca H: Vesicoureteral reflux and voiding dysfunction: a prospective study. J Urol 142:494, 1989.

Shah KJ, Robins DG, White RHR: Renal scarring and vesicoureteral reflux. Arch Dis Child 53:210, 1978.

Shopfner CE: Vesicoureteral reflux: five-year re-evaluation. Radiology 95:637, 1970.

Shore N, Bartone FF, Miller A, et al: Balloon dilation of upper ureteral strictures in primates. J Urol 136:342, 1986.

Sidi AA, Peng W, Gonzalez R: Vesicoureteral reflux in children with myelodysplasia: natural history and results of treatment. J Urol 136:329, 1986.

Siegelbaum MH, Rabinovitch HH: Delayed spontaneous resolution of high grade vesicoureteral reflux after reimplantation. J Urol 138:1205, 1987.

Skoog SJ, Belman AB, Majd M: A nonsurgical approach to the management of primary vesicoureteral reflux. J Urol 138:941, 1987.

Smellie J, Edwards D, Hunter N, et al: Vesico-ureteric reflux and renal scarring. Kidney Int 8(Suppl 4):65, 1975.

Smellie JM, Edwards D, Normand ICS, et al: Effect of vesicoureteric reflux on renal growth in children with urinary tract infection. Arch Dis Child 56:593, 1981a.

Smellie JM, Normand C: Reflux nephropathy in childhood. In Reflux Nephropathy. Edited by CJ Hodson, P Kincaid-Smith. New York, Masson Publishing USA, 1979, pp 14–20.

Smellie JM, Normand ICS, Katz G: Children with urinary infection: a comparison of those with and those without vesicoureteric reflux. Kidney Int 20:717, 1981b.

Smellie JM, Preece MA, Paton AM: Normal somatic growth in children receiving low-dose prophylactic co-trimoxazole. Eur J Pediatr 140:301, 1983.

Smellie JM, Ransley PG, Normand ICS, et al: Development of new renal scars: a collaborative study. Br Med J 290:1957, 1985.

So EP, Brock WA, Kaplan GW: Ureteral reimplantation without catheters. J Urol 125:551, 1981.

Solok V, Erözenci A, Kural A, et al: Correction of vesicoureteral reflux by the Gil-Vernet procedure. Eur Urol 14:214, 1988.

Sommer JT, Stephens FD: Morphogenesis of nephropathy with partial ureteral obstruction and vesicoureteral reflux. J Urol 125:67, 1981.

Starr A: Ureteral plication: a new concept in ureteral tailoring for megaureter. Invest Urol 17:153, 1979.

Stecker JF Jr, Read BP, Poutasse EF: Pediatric hypertension as a delayed sequela of reflux-induced chronic pyelonephritis. J Urol 118:644, 1977.

Stelle BT, Robitaille P, DeMaria J, et al: Follow-up evaluation of prenatally recognized vesicoureteric reflux. J Pediatr 115:95, 1989.

Stephens FD: Ureteric configurations and cystoscopy schema. Soc Ped Urol Newsletter, Jan 23, 1980, p 2.

Stephens FD, Lenaghan D: The anatomical basis and dynamics of vesicoureteral reflux. J Urol 87:669, 1962.

Stewart CM: Delayed cystograms. J Urol 70:588, 1953.

Stickler GB, Kelalis PP, Burke EC, et al: Primary interstitial nephritis with reflux. Am J Dis Child 122:144, 1971.

Sutton R, Atwell JD: Physical growth velocity during conservative treatment and following subsequent surgical treatment for primary vesicoureteric reflux. Br J Urol 63:245, 1989.

Sweeny LE, Thomas PS: Evaluation of sub-ureteric Teflon injection as an antireflux procedure. Ann Radiol (Paris) 30:478, 1987.

Tamminen TE, Kaprio EA: The relation of the shape of renal papillae and of collecting duct openings to intrarenal reflux. Br J Urol 49:345, 1977.

Tanagho EA: Ureteral tailoring. J Urol 106:194, 1971.

Tanagho EA, Guthrie TH, Lyon RP: The intravesical ureter in primary reflux. J Urol 101:824, 1969.

Tanagho EA, Hutch JA, Meyers FH, et al: Primary vesicoureteral reflux: experimental studies of its etiology. J Urol 93:165, 1965.

Taylor CM: Unstable bladder activity and the rate of resolution of vesico-ureteric reflux. Contrib Nephrol 39:238, 1984.

Taylor CM, Corkery JJ, White RHR: Micturition symptoms and unstable bladder activity in girls with primary vesicoureteric reflux. Br J Urol 54:494, 1982.

Teague N, Boyarsky S: The effect of coliform bacilli upon ureteral peristalsis. Invest Urol 5:423, 1968.

Timmons JW, Watts FB, Perlmutter AD: A comparison of awake and anesthesia cystography. Birth Defects 13:364, 1977.

Tobenkin MI: Hereditary vesicoureteral reflux. South Med J 57:139, 1964.

Torres VE, Kramer SA, Holley KE, et al: Effect of bacterial immunization on experimental reflux nephropathy. J Urol 131:772, 1984.

Torres VE, Kramer SA, Holley KE, et al: Interaction of multiple risk factors in the pathogenesis of experimental reflux nephropathy in the pig. J Urol 133:131, 1985.

Torres VE, Malek RS, Svensson JP: Vesicoureteral reflux in the adult. II. Nephropathy, hypertension and stones. J Urol 130:41, 1983.

Torres VE, Moore SB, Kurtz SB, et al: In search of a marker for genetic susceptibility to reflux nephropathy. Clin Nephrol 14:217, 1980a.

Torres VE, Velosa JA, Holley KE, et al: The progression of vesicoureteral reflux nephropathy. Ann Intern Med 92:776, 1980b.

Van den Abbeele AD, Treves ST, Lebowitz RL, et al: Vesicoureteral reflux in asymptomatic siblings of patients with known reflux: radionuclide cystography. Pediatrics 79:147, 1987.

Van Gool J, Tanagho EA: External sphincter activity and recurrent urinary tract infection in girls. Urology 10:348, 1977.

Wacksman J: Initial results with the Cohen cross-trigonal ureterocystotomy. J Urol 129:1198, 1983.

Wacksman J, Anderson EE, Glenn JF: Management of vesicoureteral reflux. J Urol 119:814, 1978.

Wacksman J, Sheldon C: Results of the "re-newed"

extravesical reimplant—a quantum leap forward in the surgical management of vesicoureteral reflux. Abstract #350 presented at AUA meeting, May 13–17, 1990, New Orleans.

Walker RD: Vesicoureteral reflux. In Adult and Pediatric Urology, Vol 2. Edited by JY Gillenwater, JT Grayhack, SS Howards, et al. Chicago, Year Book Medical Publishers, 1987, pp 1676–1708.

Walker RD, Duckett J, Bartone F, et al: Screening school children for urologic disease. Pediatrics 60:239, 1977.

Wallace DMA, Rothwell DL, Williams DI: The long-term follow-up of surgically treated vesicoureteric reflux. Br J Urol 50:479, 1978.

Warren MM, Kelalis PP, Stickler GB: Unilateral ureteroneocystostomy: the fate of the contralateral ureter. J Urol 107:466, 1972.

Weaver E, Craswell P: Pregnancy outcome in women with reflux nephropathy—a review of experience at the Royal Women's Hospital Brisbane, 1977–1986. Aust N Z J Obstet Gynaecol 27:106, 1987.

Wein AJ, Schoenberg HW: A review of 402 girls with recurrent urinary tract infection. J Urol 107:329, 1972.

Weiss RM, Lytton B: Vesicoureteral reflux and distal ureteral obstruction. J Urol 111:245, 1974.

Weiss S, Conway JJ: The technique of direct radionuclide cystography. Appl Radiol Nucl Med 4:133, 1975.

Whalley PJ, Cunningham FG: Short-term versus continuous antimicrobial therapy for asymptomatic bacteriuria in pregnancy. Obstet Gynecol 49:262, 1977.

Whitaker RH: Reflux induced pelvic-ureteric obstruction. Br J Urol 48:555, 1976.

Whitaker RH, Flower CDR: Ureters that show both reflux and obstruction. Br J Urol 51:471, 1979.

Williams GL, Davies DKL, Evans KT, et al: Vesicoureteric reflux in patients with bacteriuria in pregnancy. Lancet 2:1202, 1968.

Willscher MK, Bauer SB, Zammuto PJ, et al: Infection of the urinary tract after anti-reflux surgery. J Pediatr 89:743, 1976a.

Willscher MK, Bauer SB, Zammuto PJ, et al: Renal growth and urinary infection following antireflux surgery in infants and children. J Urol 115:722, 1976b.

Witherington R, Shelor WC: Treatment of postoperative ureteral stricture by catheter dilation: a forgotten procedure. Urology 16:592, 1980.

Woodard JR, Filardi G: The demonstration of vesicoureteral reflux under general anesthesia. J Urol 116:501, 1976.

Woodard JR, Holden S: The prognostic significance of fever in childhood urinary infections: observations in 350 consecutive patients. Clin Pediatr (Phila) 15:1051, 1976.

Woodard JR, Keats G: Ureteral reimplantation: Paquin's procedure after 12 years. J Urol 109:891, 1973.

Woods C, Atwell JD: Vesico-ureteric reflux in the neuropathic bladder with particular reference to the development of renal scarring. Eur Urol 8:23, 1982.

Woodside JR, Borden TS: Determination of true intravesical filling pressure in patients with vesicoureteral reflux by Fogarty catheter occlusion of ureters. J Urol 127:1149, 1982.

Young HH, Wesson MB: The anatomy and surgery of the trigone. Arch Surg 3:1, 1921.

Zaontz MR, Maizels M, Sugar EC, et al: Detrusorrhaphy: extravesical ureteral advancement to correct vesicoureteral reflux in children. J Urol 138:947, 1987.

Zucchelli P, Gaggi R: Vesicoureteral reflux and reflux nephropathy in adults. Contrib Nephrol 61:210, 1988.

15

□ Anomalies

□ ANOMALIES OF THE KIDNEY

Michael Ritchey

EMBRYOLOGY

Anomalies of the urogenital tract are among the most common of all organ systems. It has been estimated that almost 10 per cent of the population has some type of urogenital anomaly (Dees, 1941), but this prevalence was derived from symptomatic patients evaluated with excretory urograms. Using real-time ultrasonography as a screening test in healthy infants, Steinhardt et al found that 3.2 per cent of infants had an abnormality of the genitourinary tract and half of these required surgical intervention.

A complete understanding of the embryologic development of the urinary tract is a prerequisite for the evaluation and management of a child with a congenital genitourinary malformation. The development of the urinary tract can be divided into two segments, the *nephric system* and the *vesicourethral system* (Gray and Skandalakis).

There are three stages in the formation of the nephric system. The two intermediate stages are the *pronephros,* which completely disappears, and the *mesonephros.* Although the mesonephros undergoes degeneration, its duct persists and extends caudally to communicate with the anterior cloaca. Vestigial remnants of the mesonephric tubules occur in both sexes and are associated with the reproductive tract. Early in the 4th to 5th weeks, the ureteral bud begins to develop from the distal end of the mesonephric duct near its junction with the cloaca. The cranial end of the ureter then ascends to meet the nephrogenic cord of the intermediate mesoderm. This begins to develop into the *metanephros* and continues its cephalad migration. The cranial end of the ureteral bud begins a series of branchings to form the renal pelvis, the calyces, and a por-

tion of the collecting ducts (Osathanondh and Potter). This branching is associated with the simultaneous differentiation of the metanephrogenic cap, which becomes arranged around the branching collecting ducts.

The kidneys undergo cephalad migration from their site of origin. The ascent of the kidneys occurs in part due to true migration and also secondary to differential somatic growth of the lumbar portion of the body. They reach their final level by the end of the 8th week of fetal life (Fig. 15–1). The kidney also undergoes axial rotation medially of 90 degrees during the 7th and 8th weeks before it assumes its final position. During ascent, each kidney receives its blood supply from the neighboring vessels. Initially, this is from the middle sacral artery, then the common iliac and inferior mesenteric arteries, and finally the aorta. The different renal anomalies encountered may be the result of an arrest in development or a malformation of normal renal development.

ANOMALIES IN NUMBER

Supernumerary Kidney

The supernumerary kidney is an uncommon anomaly with little more than 60 cases reported in the literature (Antony; N'Guessan and Stephens; Wulfekuhler and Dube). The embryologic basis shares some similarities with that found in ureteral duplication. There are either two ureteral buds arising from the mesonephric duct, leading to double ureters, or a branching of the ureteral bud, which results in a bifid collecting system. It is believed that the two ureteral buds then join two separate metanephros or that a splitting of the nephrogenic

500

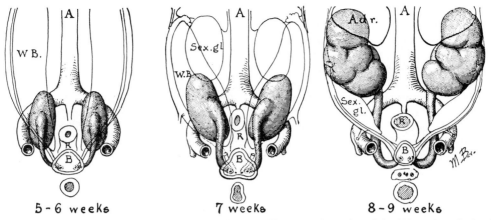

Figure 15–1 □ Ascent and rotation of kidneys during fetal life. The normal rotation of the kidney from facing forward to facing medially is shown. A, aorta; R, rectum; B, bladder; Adr, adrenal gland; Sex gl, sex gland. (From Campbell MF: Clinical Pediatric Urology. Philadelphia, WB Saunders Co, 1951.)

blastema occurs. This later develops into twin metanephros after induction by the two ureteral buds. It is not believed to be necessary for the two ureteral buds to be widely divergent (N'Guessan and Stephens).

The supernumerary kidney is caudal to the ipsilateral kidney in 60 per cent of cases (Fig. 15–2). When the supernumerary kidney is as-

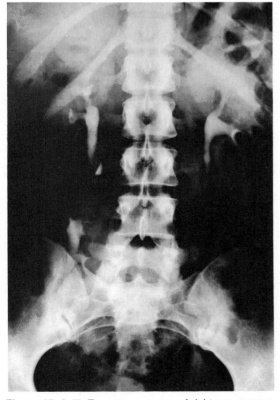

Figure 15–2 □ Excretory urogram of right supernumerary kidney, which lies opposite the fourth and fifth lumbar vertebrae.

sociated with complete ureteral duplication, the supernumerary kidney is more likely to be cranial. There is generally one extra kidney, but as many as five separate renal masses have been reported. This anomaly occurs more frequently on the left side. The extra kidney has its own renal capsule and blood supply. The supernumerary kidney is smaller than the ipsilateral kidney one third of the time and exhibits other pathologic changes (e.g., hydronephrosis, pyelonephritis) in another one third of patients. Renal function is frequently decreased in the smaller hypoplastic unit. The ureter of the anomalous kidney joins the ipsilateral ureter about as commonly as it enters the bladder separately, but only rarely is the ureter ectopic.

Most cases are diagnosed after the third decade of life. Presenting complaints are usually related to urinary obstruction or infection. Patients may experience pain or fever or may be found to have an abdominal mass on examination. However, many patients remain asymptomatic throughout life and 20 per cent of reported cases have been discovered at autopsy (Carlson).

Unilateral Renal Agenesis

Renal agenesis results from a failure of induction of the metanephric blastema by the ureteral bud. This could result from failure of the ureteral bud or wolffian duct to develop, failure of the ureteral bud to reach the blastema, or absence or abnormality of the metanephric blastema. The reported incidence of this condition varies between series of patients collected from either clinical or autopsy data.

Doroshow and Abeshouse estimated that unilateral renal agenesis (URA) is found in one of every 1100 autopsies. The clinical incidence found on excretory urogram is one in 1500, suggesting that most cases are diagnosed during life (Longo and Thompson). There is a slight male predominance, and the condition occurs more frequently on the left side. This male predominance may reflect the earlier differentiation of the wolffian duct that takes place close to the time of ureteral bud formation. The ureteral bud is more likely to be influenced by abnormalities of the wolffian duct than that of the müllerian duct, which occurs later.

Associated Anomalies

The ipsilateral ureter is absent in 50 to 87 per cent of cases (Ashley and Mostofi; Collins) and only partially developed in the other patients (Fig. 15–3). On cystoscopy, a hemitrigone will be present in those patients with ureteral agenesis. Fifteen per cent of cases show anomalies of the contralateral kidney, with malrotation and ectopia most commonly

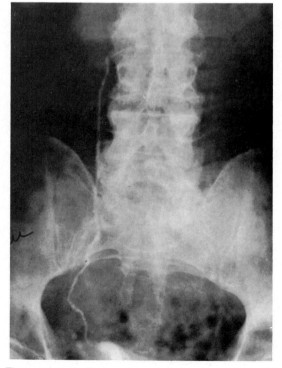

Figure 15–3 □ Retrograde ureterogram in a patient with known unilateral renal agenesis demonstrates hypoplastic ureter to level of the renal fossa.

discovered (Longo and Thompson). Limakeng and Retik found an increased incidence of contralateral abnormality if there was a hypoplastic ureter associated with the absent kidney. The ipsilateral adrenal was found to be absent on autopsy in 8 per cent of patients with URA (Ashley and Mostofi). One report noted ipsilateral agenesis of the adrenal in two of seven patients with URA examined with abdominal ultrasonography (Nakada et al).

The most common associated abnormalities are those of the genitalia. Fortune noted genital anomalies in 69 per cent of females and in 21 per cent of males. Other authors report a 20 to 40 per cent incidence of genital anomalies for both sexes (Doroshow and Abeshouse; Thompson and Lynn). This lower incidence is seen in clinical series. These patients were studied with cystoscopy, excretory urography, and physical examination, with many abnormalities of the internal genitalia going undetected. In the female, these anomalies often assume greater clinical importance, leading to earlier evaluation and diagnosis of the absent kidney. The most common problems involve the uterus and vagina. There is often a unicornuate or bicornuate uterus (Fig. 15–4), and the ipsilateral horn and fallopian tube may be rudimentary or absent (Schumacker). A duplex uterus can result from incomplete midline fusion of the müllerian ducts and may be associated with a duplicated or septate vagina (Fortune). Complete absence or hypoplasia of the vagina, the Mayer-Rokitansky-Kuster-Hauser syndrome, is frequently associated with agenesis of the kidney (Downs et al; Griffin et al). Unilateral renal agenesis is associated with several other syndromes, including Turner's, Poland's (Mace et al), and Klippel-Feil syndromes (Moore et al).

Most of these genital anomalies that occur in female patients with URA are asymptomatic. However, these patients may have increased problems during pregnancy. Obstruction of the genital tract can also occur, leading to hydrocolpos or hematocolpos, which will present as a pelvic mass or pain (Yoder and Pfister). Patients with complete müllerian arrest can undergo reconstruction to achieve adequate sexual function but will be infertile.

In the male, absence of the vas deferens, seminal vesicle, and ejaculatory duct approaches an incidence of 50 per cent (Charney and Gillenwater). Conversely, in those patients presenting with an absent vas, renal agenesis is infrequently discovered. Goldstein

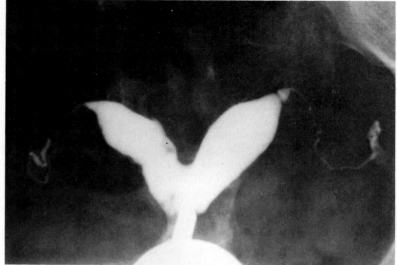

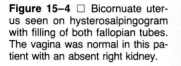

Figure 15–4 □ Bicornuate uterus seen on hysterosalpingogram with filling of both fallopian tubes. The vagina was normal in this patient with an absent right kidney.

and Schlossberg used computed tomography (CT) to evaluate 26 men with absence of the vas deferens. Unilateral renal agenesis was noted in only four men, and in all of these men the seminal vesicle was absent. An earlier report had suggested a higher incidence of associated renal agenesis in men with absence of the vas deferens (Ochsner et al). Cysts of the seminal vesicle associated with URA or dysgenesis and an ectopic ureter have also been reported (Roehrborn et al). The ipsilateral testis is usually present. Collins found the testis absent in fewer than 1 per cent of patients in his series, although Radasch reported a 7 per cent incidence of absence of the ipsilateral testis associated with URA.

Approximately 25 to 40 per cent of patients with URA have other associated congenital anomalies. In such patients, the organ systems frequently involved include cardiovascular (30 per cent), gastrointestinal (25 per cent), and musculoskeletal (14 per cent) anomalies (Emanuel et al). Malformations of the lower rectum and anus and abnormalities of the lower spine are frequently found in both sexes. This may represent a regional disturbance causing maldevelopment of structures arising from the posterior portion of the cloaca and the adjacent mesonephric duct. Duhamel describes this as the "caudal regression syndrome." The fact that the genital defects in the male are most severe near the bladder and diminish toward the testis supports the theory of a disturbance in the caudal portion of the embryo involving the wolffian duct. There is a

greater frequency of such genital malformations in the female, and the caudal portion of the müllerian ducts (uterus and vagina) are also more likely to be malformed. The müllerian duct represents a later development than the wolffian duct, and hence its chance of being involved in malformations is greater (Fortune).

Diagnosis

Absence of the kidney may be suspected on a plain film of the abdomen if the gas pattern of the splenic or hepatic flexure of the colon is displaced into the renal fossa (Curtis et al; Mascatello and Lebowitz). This finding is nonspecific and is also noted in patients in whom the kidney is surgically removed. The diagnosis can be confirmed on excretory urography, which reveals an absent kidney and compensatory hypertrophy of the contralateral kidney. Ultrasonography can also establish the diagnosis, but the hypertrophied adrenal gland can be mistaken for the kidney (McGahan and Myracle). In these cases, the adrenal gland loses its "Y" and "V" configuration and becomes more elliptical in shape. Renal ultrasound scanning has been recommended for screening of parents and siblings of children born with renal agenesis. In this group, Roodhooft et al reported a 9 per cent incidence of asymptomatic renal malformations, with URA being the most common abnormality found. Ultrasonography is also useful for examining the internal genital structures in females with a diagnosis of renal agenesis. Generally, the uterus and cervix can be visualized in both infants and older girls.

Radionuclide scanning is helpful in confirming the diagnosis of renal agenesis. It can detect other conditions in which the kidney has markedly decreased function and clearly shows absence of flow in renal agenesis. Renal arteriography is rarely necessary in the evaluation of the patient with URA.

The majority of cases of congenital solitary kidney are diagnosed in those younger than 5 years of age. This is primarily due to the complete evaluation in the neonatal period of children with multiple organ system anomalies. Of interest, recent follow-up of children with multicystic dysplastic kidneys with serial renal ultrasonography shows that complete disappearance of the dysplastic kidney can occur (Avni et al; Pedicelli et al). It may be that some cases of URA diagnosed in past years were in fact spontaneous regression of a multicystic dysplastic kidney.

Prognosis

For years, physicians have assumed that patients with a normal solitary kidney were not at increased risk for future urologic problems (Dees 1960). However, experimental evidence suggests that hyperfiltration of remnant nephrons in animals may have an adverse effect on renal function (Hostetter et al; Shimamura and Morrison). There are also several reports of focal glomerulosclerosis occurring in humans with URA (Gutierrez-Millet et al; Kiprov et al). Further information is needed regarding the prognosis of patients with a solitary kidney. Whether restriction of dietary protein or other measures to lower glomerular pressures should be recommended in the child with a solitary kidney in an attempt to prevent future glomerular injury is unclear.

Bilateral Renal Agenesis

The incidence of bilateral renal agenesis (Potter's syndrome) is approximately 1 per 4000 births (Potter). There is a slight male predominance (the male-to-female ratio is 2.5:1). A familial tendency has been reported (Rizza and Downing), and the risk of recurrence in subsequent pregnancies is 2 to 5 per cent. These infants have a characteristic facies (Fig. 15–5) that is found in conditions in which there is an absence of intrauterine renal function. The

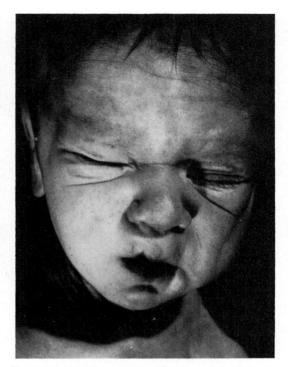

Figure 15–5 □ Potter facies. (Courtesy of Dr. Catherine Poole, University of Miami, Florida.)

most constant finding is a prominent epicanthal fold that extends onto the cheek. The skin of these infants is very loose, particularly over the hands. Oligohydramnios during pregnancy is profound, except in rare instances. This causes intrauterine compression of the fetus, which results in other characteristic external features of these infants (bowed legs, clubbed feet). The most significant sequelae of the oligohydramnios is pulmonary hypoplasia. This is the result of compression of the thoracic cage, preventing lung expansion; lack of pulmonary fluid stenting the airways; or absence of renal factors, such as proline production (Adzick et al).

Approximately 40 per cent of these infants are stillborn, and the remainder rapidly succumb to respiratory failure associated with the pulmonary hypoplasia. This poor prognosis has led to the recommendation of therapeutic abortion if the diagnosis can be made early in gestation.

The antenatal ultrasonogram of a fetus with bilateral renal agenesis reveals oligohydramnios, absence of the kidneys, and nonvisualization of the bladder. Because fetal imaging is very difficult in severe oligohydramnios, nonvisualization of the urinary bladder is a more reliable indication of fetal renal nonfunction than the inability to identify the fetal kidneys. The bladder area is examined intermittently over a 2-hour period, and if the urinary bladder is not seen during this time, 10 mg of furosemide is administered to the mother (Wladimiroff). Persistent failure to image the bladder reportedly confirms fetal anuria. Caution must be used in accepting the antenatal diagnosis of bilateral renal agenesis because false-positive diagnoses have been made (Romero et al).

The ureter is absent in 90 per cent of cases and only partially developed in the remaining individuals (Ashley and Mostofi). The bladder is either absent or severely hypoplastic as a result of the absence of urine flow. The adrenal glands are rarely absent or malpositioned (Davidson and Ross). External genital development is usually normal except when bilateral renal agenesis occurs in a sirenomelic monster. Testicular absence has been reported in up to 10 per cent of cases (Ashley and Mostofi), but the vas is present in most cases. The presence of the vas suggests that this anomaly is not due to failure of the wolffian duct to develop. The organs most often abnormal in the female are derived from the müllerian structures. In both sexes, there is an increased incidence of gastrointestinal malformations, with imperforate anus the most common problem, and an increased incidence of spina bifida. This suggests that a regional disturbance affecting the posterior portion of the cloaca and the adjacent mesonephros and müllerian ducts is responsible for this problem (Potter).

ANOMALIES OF ROTATION

Abnormal rotation, or *malrotation,* is most commonly associated with an ectopic or fused kidney but may also occur in kidneys that undergo complete ascent. The normal orientation of the adult kidney is a medial position of the renal pelvis, with the calyces pointing laterally. The fetal kidneys undergo a 90-degree rotation during the 6th to 8th weeks of embryonic development, which results in this final position (see Fig. 15–1). The rotation of the fetal kidney has been proposed to be the result of differential growth, with more tubules being formed on the ventrolateral side than on the dorsomedial side (Priman). This theory does not explain all of the abnormalities of rotation. Weyrauch suggested that the ureteral bud makes more lateral contact with the renal

blastema. This latter theory may explain an anomalous initial position of the kidney but does not explain normal renal rotation. Campbell (1970) reported only 17 cases of renal malrotation among 32,834 autopsies on adults. Smith and Orkin found an incidence of 1 in 390 and stated that malrotation accounts for 10 per cent of upper urinary tract anomalies. The true incidence of this type of anomaly is probably understated because in many patients there are no clinical manifestations.

The different types of malrotation are depicted in Figure 15–6. The most common is an *incomplete rotation,* or nonrotation (Fig. 15–7). The renal pelvis is in the anterior position or some variation between the fetal anterior and normal medial position in the adult. Other major types of anomalous rotation are *reverse rotation* and *hyperrotation* (excessive rotation) in which the kidney faces laterally (Weyrauch). These are exceedingly rare and cannot be distinguished by excretory urography alone (Fig. 15–8). In reverse rotation, the renal pelvis rotates laterally and the renal vessels cross the kidney anteriorly to reach the hilum (Fig. 15–9). In excessive rotation, the kidney

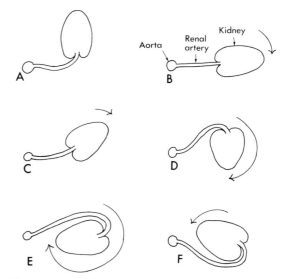

Figure 15–6 □ Rotation of the kidney during its ascent from the pelvis. The left kidney (with its renal artery) and the aorta are viewed in transverse section to show normal and abnormal rotation during its ascent to the adult site. *A,* Primitive embryonic position, hilus faces ventrad (anterior). *B,* Normal adult position, hilus faces mediad. *C,* Incomplete rotation. *D,* Hyperrotation, hilus faces dorsad (posterior). *E,* Hyperrotation, hilus faces laterad. *F,* Reverse rotation, hilus faces laterad. (From Gray SW, Skandalakis JE: Embryology for Surgeons. Philadelphia, WB Saunders Co, 1972.)

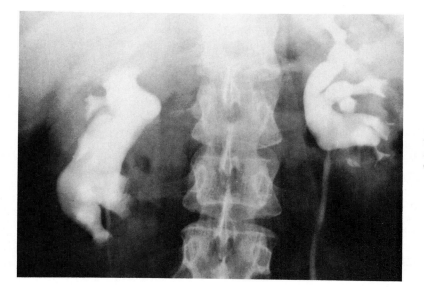

Figure 15–7 □ Incomplete rotation of the right kidney with an anterior pelvis and the lower pole calyces point medial.

rotates more than 180 degrees but less than 360 degrees. The pelvis faces laterally, but the renal vessels are carried posteriorly to the kidney. Less severe hyperrotation may leave the renal pelvis in a dorsal position (Gray and Skandalakis).

Malrotation is usually discovered incidentally during imaging of the kidney, and the degree of rotation is minimal in normally situated kidneys. The condition may be unilateral or bilateral. When symptoms occur, they are most often related to hydronephrosis and con-

sist of vague abdominal pain and vomiting. The obstruction may be secondary to compression of the ureter from an anomalous accessory vessel or other obstructive lesions that also occur in normally rotated kidneys. It is important to establish the correct diagnosis to exclude other pathologic conditions that can produce similar distortion of the kidney. The upper third of the ureter may be displaced laterally and the renal pelvis may appear elongated, suggesting obstruction or effacement by an extrinsic mass. The calyces are often dis-

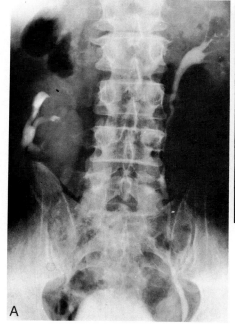

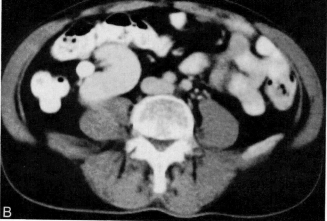

Figure 15–8 □ An example of excessive rotation of the right kidney. *A,* Excretory urogram. *B,* CT scan.

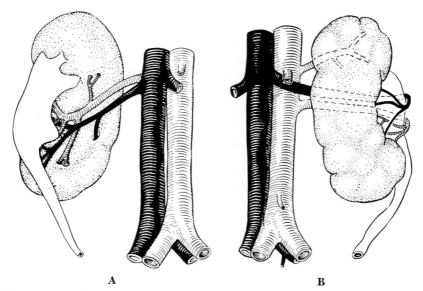

Figure 15–9 □ Abnormal renal rotation. *A*, Reverse rotation. *B*, Hyperrotation. (After Weyrauch HM: Anomalies of renal rotation. Surg Gynecol Obstet 69:183, 1939. By permission of Surgery, Gynecology & Obstetrics.)

torted even without any associated obstruction. Gross inspection of the kidney may also reveal an unusual appearance with a discoid or oval shape and a flattened elongated parenchyma. There are often persistent fetal lobulations present. Additional diagnostic imaging, such as retrograde pyelography, ultrasonography, or CT, may be necessary to confirm the diagnosis. Treatment of malrotation is reserved for alleviation of associated obstruction, calculi, or infection secondary to poor drainage.

ANOMALIES OF ASCENT

Renal Ectopy

Renal ectopy is the term used to describe a kidney that lies outside the renal fossa. As stated previously, the kidney migrates cephalad early in gestation to arrive at its normal position. Failure of the kidney to complete its ascent can be due to a number of factors: abnormality of the ureteral bud or metanephric blastema, genetic abnormalities, teratogenic causes, or anomalous vasculature acting as a barrier to ascent (Malek et al). During ascent, the kidney receives its blood supply from the middle sacral artery, iliac artery, and finally the aorta. The anomalous blood supply that is invariably present is dependent on the final position of the kidney and

is probably not the cause of the malposition. However, the blood vessels are frequently short, rendering surgical mobilization or a change of renal position very difficult.

The incidence of renal ectopy in postmortem studies varies from 1 in 500 (Campbell, 1930) to 1 in 1290 (Thompson and Pace). The incidence of ectopic kidney is higher in autopsy series than in clinical studies, suggesting that many cases remain unrecognized throughout life (Malek et al; Thompson and Pace). There is a slight predilection for the left side, and 10 per cent of cases are bilateral. *Simple renal ectopy* refers to a kidney that remains in the ipsilateral retroperitoneal space. The most common position is in the pelvis (sacral or pelvic kidney) opposite the sacrum and below the aortic bifurcation (Thompson and Pace) (Fig. 15–10). The lumbar or iliac ectopic kidney is one that is fixed above the crest of the ileum but below the level of L2 and L3 (Fig. 15–11). *Crossed renal ectopy* refers to a kidney that crosses the midline (see discussion on anomalies of fusion later in the text).

The differentiation between a *ptotic kidney* and renal ectopia can be difficult, but there are several discerning features. The length of the ureter may be helpful. In renal ectopy, the ureter is short, corresponding to the location of the kidney; in a ptotic kidney, it appears redundant. The ptotic kidney is mobile and usually can be manipulated into its normal position. Lastly, malrotation frequently accompanies renal ectopy (Fig. 15–11).

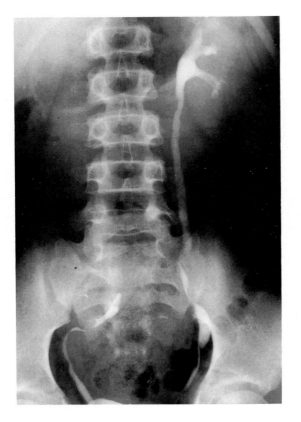

Figure 15–10 □ Ectopic right pelvic kidney with relatively short ureter.

Figure 15–11 □ Malrotated ectopic kidney opposite lower lumbar vertebrae.

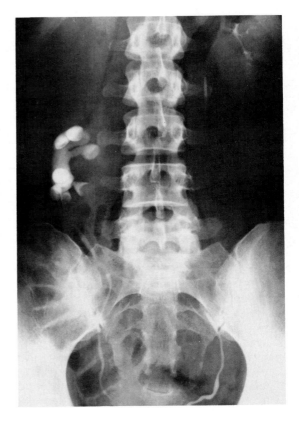

Diagnosis

Most cases of renal ectopy diagnosed in childhood are associated with symptoms attributed to either the genitourinary or gastrointestinal system. Patients have vague abdominal pain or renal colic secondary to ureteropelvic junction obstruction or stone formation. Urinary tract infection is a common presentation found in 30 per cent of children. The ectopic kidney may also be noted incidentally in the evaluation of the other frequently associated anomalies. Modern imaging techniques have increased the frequency of diagnosis of these lesions. For example, in a child undergoing cardiac catheterization, the renal abnormality may be detected on fluoroscopy of the abdomen. Less commonly, the ectopic kidney can be detected as an abdominal mass on physical examination.

Pelvic kidneys may be difficult to recognize on excretory urography because they overlie the bony structures. Oblique films may be quite helpful in visualizing the pelvic kidney (Fig. 15–12). It has been suggested that the short ureter drains the kidney rapidly, preventing complete filling of the collecting system. Whenever a kidney is absent on excretory urography, the pelvic area should be carefully examined for evidence of a ureter from an ectopic kidney. Voiding cystourethrography is recommended in all children with a diagnosis of pelvic kidney to exclude vesicoureteral reflux, which is frequently associated with an ectopic kidney (Fig. 15–13) (Kramer and Kelalis). Poor visualization of the pelvic kidney on excretory urogram may also be due to diminished function secondary to obstruction or other pathologic conditions. Obstruction in the ectopic kidney is often related to a high insertion of the ureter on the renal pelvis with associated hydronephrosis (Fig. 15–14). Retrograde pyelography can be used to opacify the collecting system in those cases with inadequate excretion of contrast (Fig. 15–15).

Confirmation of the diagnosis of an ectopic kidney can be made with ultrasonography in most cases. The abnormal calyces and pelvis are readily visible on the ultrasound scan. Diuretic renography may be needed to distin-

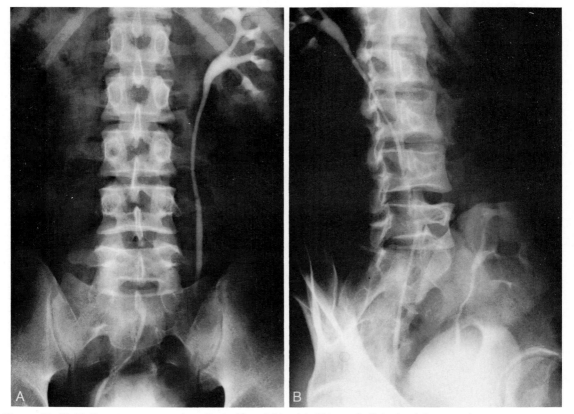

Figure 15–12 □ Excretory urogram in patient with a right pelvic kidney. A, Only the right ureter is seen overlying the bony structures. B, Oblique film allows much better visualization of collecting system and renal outline.

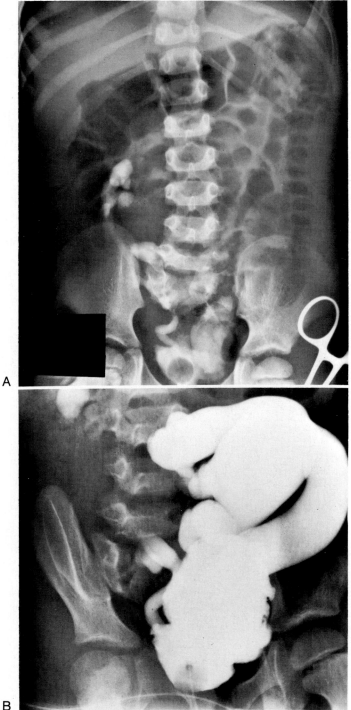

A

B

Figure 15–13 □ Vesicoureteral reflux in ectopic kidney. *A,* Excretory urogram shows dilated left ureter, probably from reflux of contrast medium from the bladder. *B,* Retrograde cystogram shows bilateral vesicoureteral reflux, massive into the left system. (From Kelalis PP, Malek RS, Segura JW: Observations on renal ectopia and fusion in children. J Urol 110:588–592, 1973. © 1973, The Williams & Wilkins Company, Baltimore.)

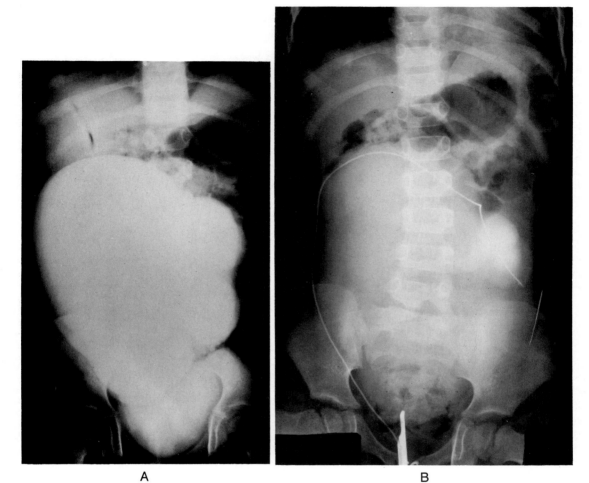

A   B

Figure 15–14 □ Ectopic solitary pelvic kidney in a 6-year-old boy with gross hematuria. *A,* Excretory urogram shows giant hydronephrosis. *B,* Retrograde pyelogram shows catheter in ureter with high insertion into pelvis.

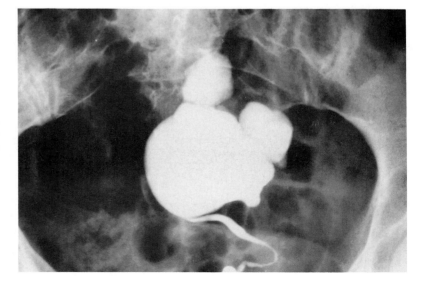

Figure 15–15 □ Retrograde pyelogram in a patient with a symptomatic ureteropelvic junction obstruction in a left pelvic kidney.

guish these abnormal pyelocalyceal patterns from ureteropelvic junction obstruction. The ectopic kidney can be clearly shown on the renal scan, but the gamma camera should be placed anteriorly to obtain better images (Fig. 15–16). Renal arteriography is seldom performed in the patient with an ectopic kidney for diagnostic purposes, but when surgery is planned, it may be helpful in delineating the vascular supply (Fig. 15–17). Most often the kidney is supplied by multiple vessels that arise from the distal aorta, aortic bifurcation, or the iliac artery. More recently, the use of CT and magnetic resonance imaging (MRI) has greatly enhanced the evaluation of these patients. The latter technique can also provide information about the vascular supply (Fig. 15–18).

Associated Anomalies

The contralateral kidney may be abnormal in up to 50 per cent of patients (Malek et al). There is a 10 per cent incidence of contralateral renal agenesis. Kramer and Kelalis found associated vesicoureteral reflux in 70 per cent of children with a pelvic kidney. The adrenal gland is in its normal position in most cases of renal ectopy. Genital anomalies are also seen quite frequently, with an incidence ranging

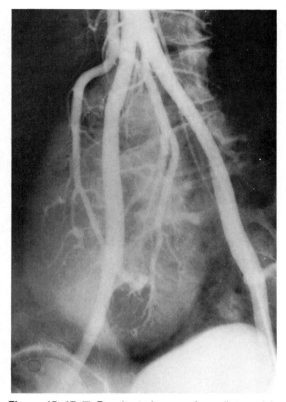

Figure 15–17 □ Renal arteriogram of a solitary pelvic kidney demonstrates multiple anomalous renal vessels arising from distal aorta and common iliac artery.

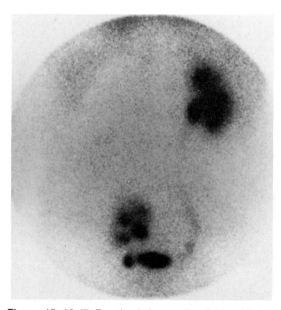

Figure 15–16 □ Renal scintigram of a right pelvic kidney. The camera was placed anteriorly in this patient with bilateral pyelocaliectasis.

from 15 per cent of males to 75 per cent of females (Downs et al; Thompson and Pace). In males, the most common abnormalities are hypospadias and undescended testes (Malek et al). Anomalies of the reproductive organs are seen most frequently in the female: duplication of the vagina, bicornuate uterus, and hypoplasia or agenesis of the uterus or vagina (Griffin et al). These abnormalities have significance, in that there are often problems with pregnancy, which may necessitate cesarean section (Downs et al).

Anomalies of other organ systems also occur with increased frequency. Skeletal anomalies occur in up to 50 per cent of children. The most common abnormalities include asymmetry of the skull, rib abnormalities, dysplastic vertebrae, and absent bones. Cardiovascular lesions were noted in nine of the 21 children studied by Malek et al, and gastrointestinal abnormalities are found in one third of patients. However, Downs et al reported a lower incidence of associated extragenitourinary anomalies.

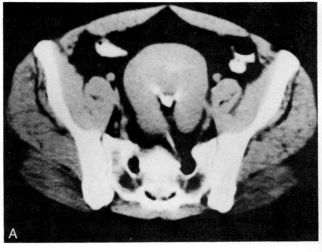

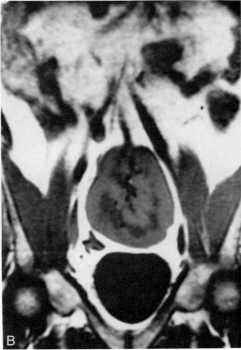

Figure 15–18 □ Solitary left pelvic kidney in a patient diagnosed with a "pelvic mass." *A,* CT scan. *B,* Coronal view with MRI, which is able to demonstrate the renal vessels entering the pelvic kidney.

Management

Although many patients with renal ectopy remain undiagnosed throughout life, surgical intervention is frequently needed in those patients whose condition becomes clinically apparent. Overall, renal disease develops in 40 per cent of patients with a solitary pelvic kidney (Downs et al). The most common problem is that of ureteropelvic junction obstruction. This may be due to the malrotation and high ureteral insertion, or it may be secondary to an anomalous vessel that partially obstructs the collecting system. Treatment should be individualized, but in most cases a transabdominal approach for pyeloplasty is required. The goal of surgery is to achieve dependent drainage, and in some cases ureterocalycostomy may be necessary. Renal stones may also develop in these kidneys (Fig. 15–19). In the past, these were managed with open removal but now may be amenable to extracorporeal shock wave lithotripsy or endourologic techniques.

An important consideration in the management of these patients is that the contralateral kidney is frequently abnormal and every effort should be made to salvage the kidney. Removal of the kidney may lead to significant renal compromise. Even more disastrous

would be the inadvertent removal of a solitary ectopic kidney. Unfortunately, this event has occurred on several occasions when the kidney was mistaken for a pelvic mass (Downs et al).

Thoracic Kidney

Excessive cranial migration of the kidney results in a thoracic kidney. N'Guessan et al prefer to call this a "superior ectopic kidney" because some high kidneys actually lie below the diaphragm. An intrathoracic kidney occurs when there is either a portion or all of the kidney that extends above the diaphragm. This accounts for fewer than 5 per cent of the cases of renal ectopy with an incidence of 1 in 13,000 autopsies (Campbell, 1930). The left side is more commonly involved and there is a male predominance. In rare instances, the condition can be bilateral (N'Guessan et al).

Renal ascent is normally complete by the 8th week of gestation. An intrathoracic kidney may be the result of accelerated ascent prior to diaphragmatic closure or delayed closure of the diaphragmatic anlage, allowing continued ascent (Burke et al; N'Guessan et al). The renal vascular supply often arises from the normal site of origin on the aorta (Lundius) but may arise more superiorly. The kidney

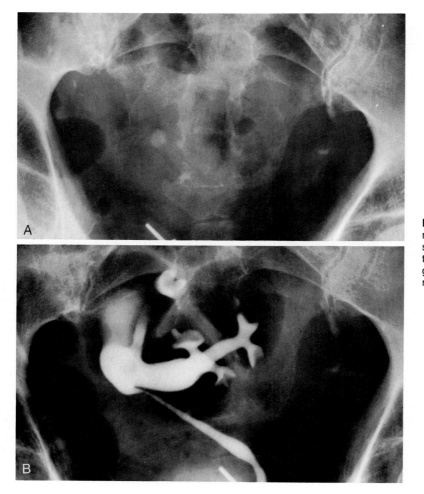

Figure 15–19 □ Left pelvic kidney. *A,* Kidney-ureter-bladder (KUB) study revealed opaque calculus in true pelvis. *B,* Retrograde pyelogram confirms stone to be within renal pelvis of the pelvic kidney.

appears normal otherwise and generally has completed rotation.

In most cases, the kidney is actually subdiaphragmatic in location. A thin membranous portion of the diaphragm overlying the kidney has been described in those patients examined at thoracotomy or necropsy. A completely supradiaphragmatic kidney in which there is a well-formed and muscularized diaphragm is much less common. In the supradiaphragmatic kidney, the ureter and hilar vessels enter through the foramen of Bodchalek. The adrenal gland frequently remains caudal to the kidney in its normal location (N'Guessan et al). A superior ectopic kidney in association with a Bodchalek hernia is uncommon. In this circumstance, there is herniation of other viscera through the diaphragm and the kidney is mobile and can be easily withdrawn from the thorax.

In general, the thoracic kidney functions normally and most patients are asymptomatic.

The condition is often detected on routine chest radiographs as a suspected mediastinal mass (Fig. 15–20). Excretory urography confirms the diagnosis (Fig. 15–21).

ANOMALIES OF FUSION

The congenital renal anomaly that produces some of the most bizarre excretory urograms (IVPs) is the result of fusion of two or more kidney masses. Several mechanisms that could lead to development of this anomaly are proposed. During ascent of the kidneys out of the pelvis, they cross the umbilical arteries. Malposition of the umbilical arteries may cause the developing nephrogenic blastemas to come together. Fusion of the nephrogenic masses in the midline would result in a horseshoe kidney. If, during ascent, one kidney advances slightly ahead of the other, the inferior pole may come in contact with the superior pole of the trailing

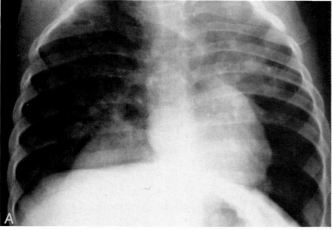

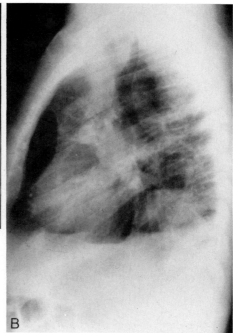

Figure 15–20 □ *A, B,* Routine roentgenograms of chest in a patient with intrathoracic kidney.

kidney. This results in crossed ectopia with fusion. A single nephrogenic mass induced by ureteral buds from both sides may also result in crossed fused renal ectopia (Cook and Stephens). This latter theory, with the ureters crossing the midline, explains a solitary or bilaterally crossed ectopic kidney. Fusion of the two masses occurs early in embryogenesis, and malrotation is present in all cases.

Horseshoe Kidney

The horseshoe kidney represents the most common type of renal fusion. In this anomaly,

two renal masses lie on either side of the midline and are joined at the lower pole in more than 90 per cent of cases (Fig. 15–22). The isthmus crossing the midline joining the two kidneys may consist of renal parenchyma or fibrous tissue. The horseshoe kidney is usually positioned low in the abdomen, with the isthmus lying just below the junction of the inferior mesenteric artery and aorta. It is postulated that the inferior mesenteric artery obstructs the isthmus and prevents further ascent. Although the isthmus usually passes anterior to the great vessels, it may pass posterior to the aorta and/or inferior vena cava (Dajani).

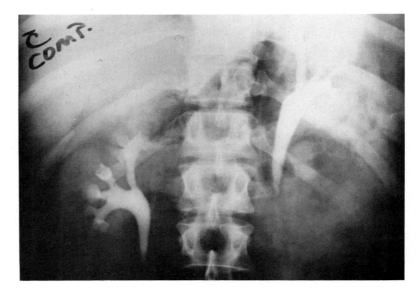

Figure 15–21 □ Excretory urogram of a patient with left intrathoracic kidney.

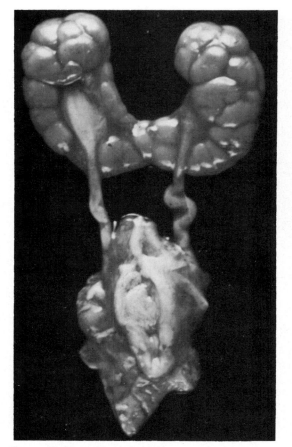

Figure 15–22 □ Horseshoe kidney, postmortem specimen.

The reported incidence of horseshoe kidney varies from 1 in 400 (Glenn) to 1 in 1800 (Campbell, 1970). The abnormality is more common in males. In autopsy series, this anomaly is found more commonly in children (Campbell, 1970) and is attributed to the higher incidence of associated congenital anomalies contributing to the demise of such children. One report found that 78 per cent of stillborn infants with horseshoe kidney had associated congenital malformations (Zondek and Zondek). This is in contrast to the 3.5 per cent incidence of associated congenital malformation in adults discovered to have horseshoe kidneys. Horseshoe kidneys have been reported in identical twins (Bridge) and in several siblings within the same family (David).

Diagnosis

The diagnosis of the horseshoe kidney may be suspected from a plain radiograph of the abdomen if one can visualize the renal outlines in their abnormal position. However, it is excretory urography that allows an accurate diagnosis (Fig. 15–23).

Malrotation of the kidney is invariably present. This is attributed to very early fusion of the kidneys before rotation is complete. The renal pelves remain anterior, with the ureter crossing the isthmus. The orientation of the calyces is generally anteroposterior, but the lowermost calyces invariably point toward the midline, medial to the ureter. These lower calyces often overlie the vertebral column as if in an attempt to reach each other. The renal axis appears to be vertical or even shifted outward, with the lower poles lying closer together than the upper poles. The course of the ureters is variable, but they often lie anterior to the pelvis. The upper ureter appears to be laterally displaced by a midline mass. Other pertinent urographic findings are low-lying kidneys, and the lower outer border of the kidney appears to continue across the midline. The radiographic appearance of a horseshoe kidney is frequently altered by associated abnormalities such as hydronephrosis and/or diminished renal function (Fig. 15–24).

The diagnosis of a horseshoe kidney can be confirmed by a variety of imaging techniques, including renal ultrasonography, CT, or MRI. The fusion of the kidneys generally can be clearly visualized with any of these studies (Fig. 15–25). In the past, renal arteriography was frequently performed, not only to establish the diagnosis of the horseshoe kidney but also to delineate the vascular blood supply. In the majority of cases, there are multiple renal vessels. The blood supply to the isthmus is particularly variable, often supplied by a separate vessel. This may arise from the aorta, common iliac, or inferior mesenteric arteries. Prior to surgery, it may be necessary to assess the function of the isthmus, particularly if symphysiotomy is being considered. This can be accomplished with radionuclide imaging of the kidneys (Fig. 15–26). It is also of value in the neonate to confirm the diagnosis when other imaging modalities may be inconclusive (Grandone et al).

Associated Anomalies

There is a frequent association of other anomalies in children with horseshoe kidney. The incidence of these anomalies is much higher if the horseshoe kidney is discovered in

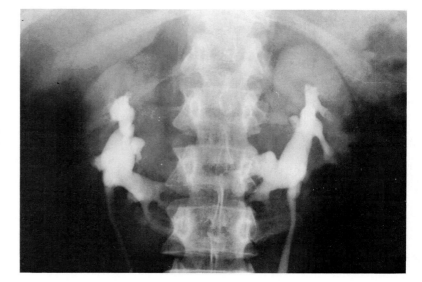

Figure 15–23 □ Typical appearance of horseshoe kidney on excretory urogram.

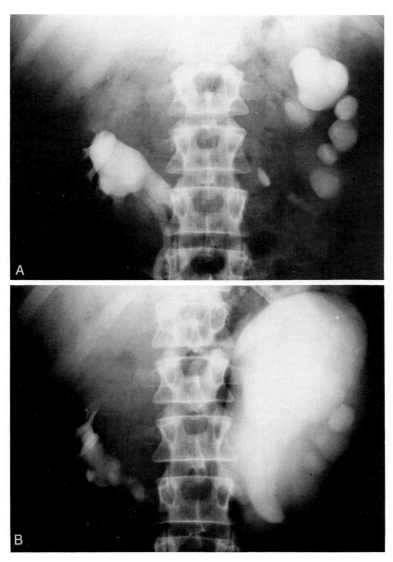

Figure 15–24 □ Horseshoe kidney. *A, B,* Excretory urogram shows severe hydronephrosis with delayed excretion of left renal segment secondary to ureteropelvic obstruction.

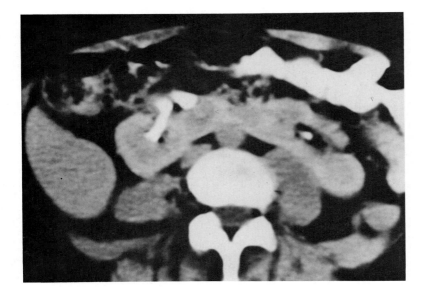

Figure 15–25 □ Fusion of the lower poles over the great vessels seen on CT scan.

the newborn period. Zondek and Zondek examined the postmortem records of 99 individuals with horseshoe kidneys. Of those infants who were stillborn or who died within the first year of life, 78 per cent had malformations of other organ systems. These most commonly involved the central nervous system, gastrointestinal tract, and the skeletal and cardiovascular systems. Boatman et al reported that one third of patients with horseshoe kidney had at least one other abnormality.

Horseshoe kidneys have been found with increased frequency with several well-known

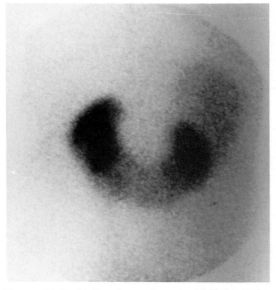

Figure 15–26 □ Renal scan in patient with horseshoe kidney showing minimal function of the isthmus.

syndromes, including trisomy 18, which is associated with a 21 per cent incidence of fused kidneys (Boatman et al; Warkany et al). More than 60 per cent of patients with Turner's syndrome have renal abnormalities, including horseshoe kidneys, ureteral duplication, or other minor abnormalities (Smith). One study noted a 7 per cent incidence of horseshoe kidneys in patients with Turner's syndrome who were evaluated with renal ultrasound scanning (Lippe et al). There is also an increased incidence of horseshoe kidneys in patients with neural tube defects (Whitaker and Hunt).

Other genitourinary abnormalities are also encountered with increased frequency in these patients. Ten per cent of patients have ureteral duplication, and vesicoureteral reflux has been found in 10 (Pitts and Muecke) to 80 per cent of children who undergo evaluation (Fig. 15–27) (Segura et al). Multicystic dysplasia (Novak et al) and adult polycystic kidney disease have also been reported (Pitts and Muecke). Hypospadias and undescended testes occur in 4 per cent of the males, bicornuate uterus or septate vagina in 7 per cent of females (Boatman et al). Retrocaval ureter has been found in association with a horseshoe kidney in six patients (Fernandes et al).

Prognosis

The presence of a horseshoe kidney does not adversely affect survival. Nearly one third of patients with a horseshoe kidney remain

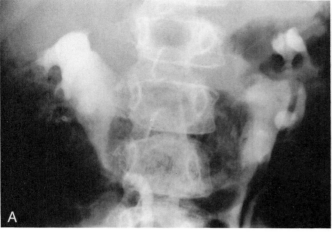

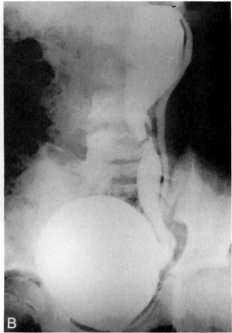

Figure 15–27 □ Horseshoe kidney. *A,* Excretory urogram reveals mild hydronephrosis on left. *B,* Voiding cystourethrogram demonstrates high-grade vesicoureteral reflux into both segments of a complete ureteral duplication.

undiagnosed throughout life (Glenn; Pitts and Muecke). Many women are able to go through pregnancy and delivery without adverse effects (Bell). Of children who survive infancy, 60 per cent require some form of surgical intervention. In those patients with problems, symptoms are most often secondary to hydronephrosis, urinary tract infection, or urolithiasis. These patients generally present with vague abdominal pain. The classic finding of abdominal pain and nausea with hyperextension of the spine—Rovsing syndrome—presumably resulting from stretching of the isthmus is uncommon. Operations to divide the isthmus were once performed to relieve pain, but this procedure has no merit (Glenn; Pitts and Muecke).

Ureteropelvic junction obstruction is the most common cause of hydronephrosis (Fig. 15–28) occurring in 30 per cent of patients diagnosed during life. The obstruction may be caused by a high ureteral insertion or an anomalous renal vessel. It must be recognized that the calyces may have an abnormal appearance as a result of the malrotation alone and that not all of these kidneys are obstructed. Additionally, the upper urinary tract dilatation may be secondary to vesicoureteral reflux (see Fig. 15–27) and should be excluded in all children with a horseshoe kidney.

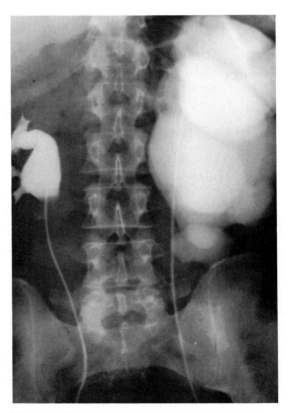

Figure 15–28 □ Bilateral retrograde pyelogram shows massive hydronephrosis on left secondary to ureteropelvic junction obstruction.

More than 100 cases of renal malignancy have been reported in patients with horseshoe kidney (Buntley), with a number of hypernephromas arising from the isthmus (Blackard and Mellinger). There appears to be an increased incidence of renal pelvic tumors and nephroblastoma compared with that in the general population (Blackard and Mellinger; Dische and Johnston). Wilms' tumor is the second most common tumor found in horseshoe kidneys. In a review of National Wilms' Tumor Study patients, Mesrobian et al found that there was a seven-fold increased risk of a Wilms' tumor developing in patients with a horseshoe kidney. In many cases, the diagnosis of horseshoe kidney was missed preoperatively when the distorted pyelogram was presumed to be secondary to the renal mass. No recommendation was made regarding periodic screening with renal ultrasonography to detect occult malignancies.

Management

Correction of ureteropelvic junction obstruction is the most frequent indication for surgical intervention in a patient with a horseshoe kidney. The goal of dependent drainage following pyeloplasty may be difficult to achieve in these patients. Routine division of the isthmus was once recommended to avoid having the ureter cross the isthmus. Before division of the isthmus is undertaken, the increased risk of bleeding, urine leak, and renal infarction should be considered. The isthmus can be divided between two rows of mattress sutures of absorbable material placed for hemostasis (Fig. 15–29). The anomalous blood supply must be identified carefully to avoid injury. Many authors believe that the isthmus does not contribute to the obstruction and should not be routinely divided (Donahoe and Hendren). They report that following symphysiotomy the kidneys often fall back into their preoperative position because of fixation by the abnormal vasculature. However, nephropexy can be a useful adjunct in selected cases to correct the malrotation and to help achieve a successful surgical outcome (Fig. 15–30). An extraperitoneal flank approach is utilized for unilateral operations. In those patients requiring bilateral procedures, a transperitoneal approach may be preferable in order to allow operation on both sides at once.

Ureterocalycostomy is an excellent alternative to achieve dependent drainage of the urinary tract (Mollard and Braun). The ureter can be anastomosed to a lower pole calyx, particularly in a patient with severe hydronephrosis that demonstrates thinning of the renal parenchyma.

Urolithiasis develops in 20 per cent of patients with a horseshoe kidney (Fig. 15–31). Stasis secondary to hydronephrosis may increase the chance of stone formation, but metabolic factors should not be overlooked (Evans and Resnick). Most patients with renal stone disease can be managed with extracorporeal shock wave lithotripsy. Horseshoe kidneys have been successfully treated with this modality, thus avoiding open surgical procedures (Smith et al).

Crossed Renal Ectopia

Crossed renal ectopia is the second most common fusion anomaly after horseshoe kidney. The crossed ectopic kidney crosses the midline to lie on the opposite side from the ureteral insertion into the bladder (Fig. 15–32). The four varieties of crossed renal ectopia are illustrated in Figure 15–33.

The incidence of crossed ectopia has been placed at 1 in 7000 autopsies (Abeshouse and Bhisitkul). Crossed renal ectopia with fusion is the most common type and accounts for 85 per cent of the cases. Crossed ectopia without fusion represents less than 10 per cent of all cases, and solitary crossed ectopia and bilateral crossed ectopia are exceedingly rare (Kakei et al; McDonald and McClellan). With all of these abnormalities, there is a slight male predominance and crossing from left to right occurs more frequently than right to left.

There are many variations in the extent of the fusion that can produce bizarre radiographic pictures. Determining the exact type of crossed ectopia may be a difficult task. McDonald and McClellan described six different varieties of crossed ectopia with fusion (Fig. 15–34). The most common form is *unilateral fused type* with inferior ectopia, in which the upper pole of the crossed kidney is fused to the lower pole of the normally positioned kidney. The renal pelves remain in their anterior position, representing a failure to complete rotation. The second most common type is the *sigmoid*, or S-shaped, *kidney*. The crossed kidney is inferior, but both kidneys have completed their rotation so that the two renal pelves face in opposite directions. The

Text continued on page 525

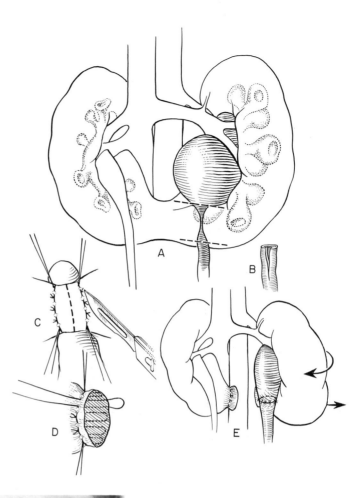

Figure 15–29 ☐ Surgical treatment of horseshoe kidney. Symphysiotomy and revision of ureteropelvic junction. The ureteropelvic junction is excised *(A)*, and after the ureter is spatulated *(B)*, the anastomosis is performed. After division of the isthmus *(C)*, closure is accomplished with mattress sutures *(D)*. The kidney is rotated and fixed to the posterior abdominal wall *(E)*.

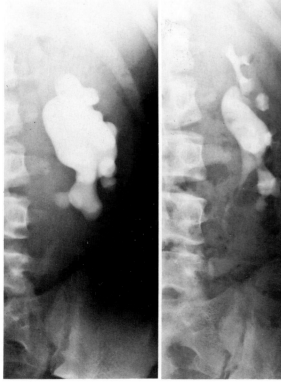

Figure 15–30 ☐ *A,* Preoperative excretory urogram showing left segment hydronephrosis. *B,* Postoperative excretory urogram after left ureteropyelostomy and symphysiotomy.

A   B

521

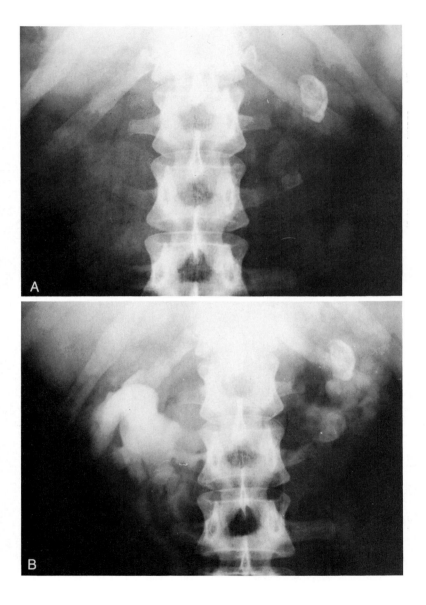

Figure 15–31 □ Horseshoe kidney. *A,* Two large renal stones seen on plain film of abdomen. *B,* Excretory urogram confirms horseshoe kidney with marked decrease in function of left kidney.

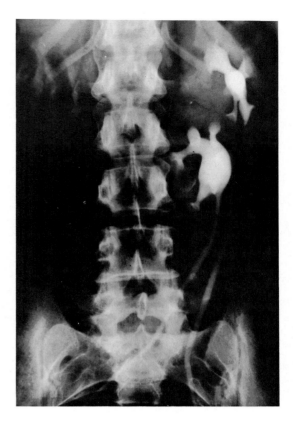

Figure 15–32 □ Crossed ectopia, with right kidney crossing midline and fused to lower pole of left kidney.

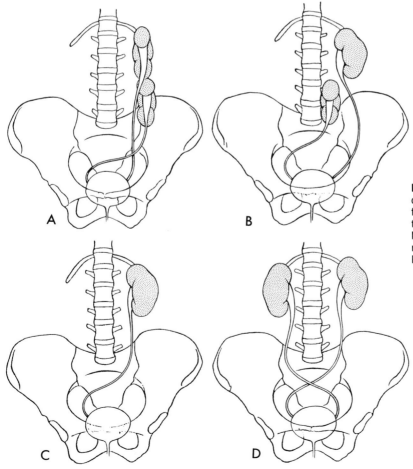

A

B

C

D

Figure 15–33 □ Four varieties of crossed renal ectopia. *A,* With fusion. *B,* Without fusion. *C,* Solitary. *D,* Bilateral. (Redrawn from McDonald JH, McClellan DS, as reproduced by Abeshouse BS, Bhisitkul I. Urol Int 9:63, 1959.)

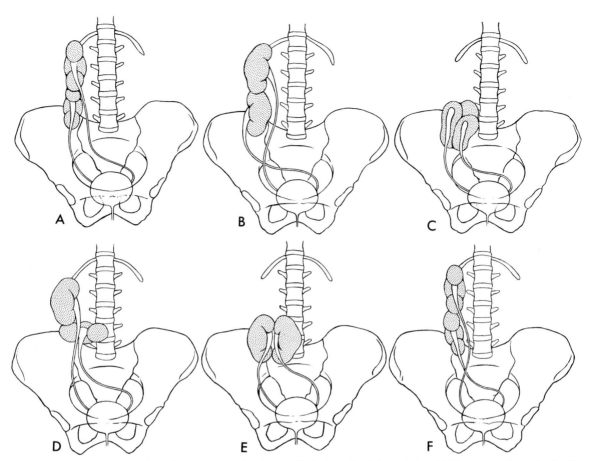

Figure 15–34 □ Six varieties of crossed renal ectopia with fusion. *A,* Unilateral fused kidney, superior ectopia. *B,* Sigmoid or S-shaped kidney. *C,* "Lump" kidney. *D,* L-shaped kidney. *E,* "Disk" kidney. *F,* Unilateral fused kidney, inferior ectopia. (Redrawn from McDonald JH, McClellan DS, as reproduced by Abeshouse BS, Bhisitkul I. Urol Int 9:63, 1959.)

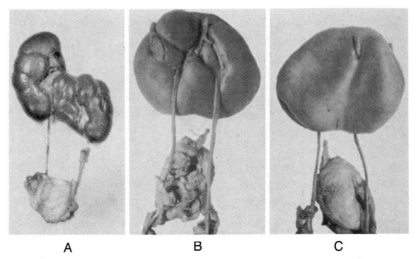

Figure 15–35 □ Renal fusion. *A,* L-shaped kidney from 1-year-old child. A considerable portion of the left renal segment lies across the lower lumbar spinal column. On each side, the pelvic outlet faces anteriorly. *B,* Lump kidney showing the usual anatomy, with the anterior blood supply coming from above the ureters leaving from below. *C,* Posterior view of *B,* with the blood supply entering from above and a deep grooving of the parenchyma indicating where the kidney pressed against the spine. (Courtesy of Dr. H.S. Altman.) (From Campbell MF: Clinical Pediatric Urology. Philadelphia, WB Saunders Co, 1951.)

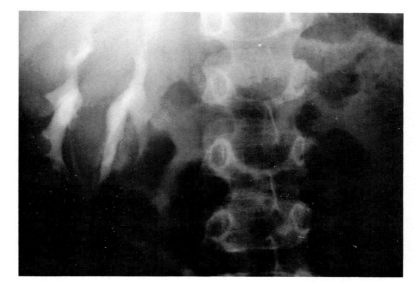

Figure 15–36 □ Crossed renal ectopy with fusion in which both kidneys have ascended to the right renal fossa.

fusion of the two kidneys probably occurs later after axial rotation is completed.

The other four types of fusion are much less common. The *lump,* or "cake," *kidney* and the *disk kidney* both involve extensive fusion of the two renal masses (Fig. 15–35). In an *L-shaped kidney,* the crossed kidney assumes a transverse position. The least common type is the *superior ectopic kidney,* in which the crossed ectopic kidney lies superior to the normal kidney. The two kidneys may also fuse side to side and ascend together to the renal fossa (Fig. 15–36).

Diagnosis

The classification described above was devised in order to stratify the patients in some logical fashion. There is obviously a spectrum of abnormalities, and it is often difficult to categorize patients based on urographic findings. It can be difficult to distinguish between crossed ectopia with fusion from crossed renal ectopy without fusion. This distinction may be possible on excretory urography if the two renal masses are widely separated (Fig. 15–37). In the past, many cases were confirmed by findings at surgical exploration or necropsy. At the present time, the use of CT and MRI should enable one to establish the correct diagnosis.

The vascular supply to these kidneys is quite variable. If surgical intervention is contemplated, renal arteriography often demonstrates multiple anomalous branches to both kidneys arising from the aorta, or common iliac artery. Rarely will the renal artery cross the midline

to supply the crossed kidney (Rubinstein et al).

Associated Anomalies

There is an increased incidence of malformations of other organ systems, including or-

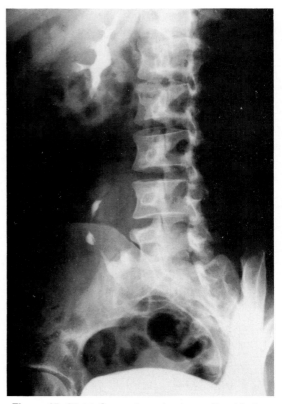

Figure 15–37 □ Crossed renal ectopy without fusion.

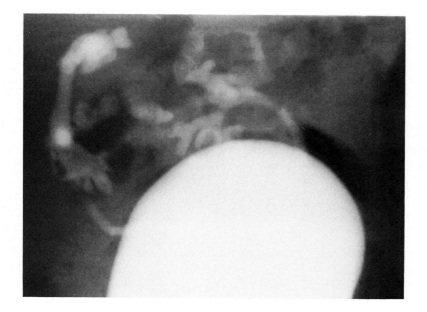

Figure 15–38 ☐ Voiding cysto-urethrogram reveals bilateral vesicoureteral reflux in a patient with crossed renal ectopy with fusion.

Figure 15–39 ☐ Crossed ectopic left kidney is fused to right kidney, with associated ureteropelvic obstruction.

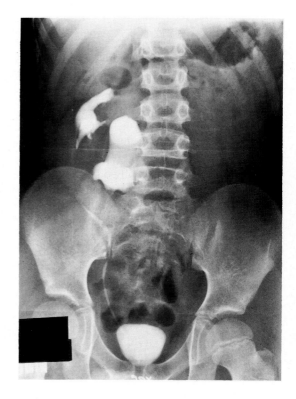

thopedic or skeletal anomalies, imperforate anus, and cardiovascular anomalies (Abeshouse and Bhisitkul). In patients with solitary crossed ectopia, there is a higher incidence of genital abnormalities but this is probably related to the renal agenesis (Kakei et al).

The ureter in the crossed ectopic kidney usually enters the bladder and is only rarely ectopic (Abeshouse and Bhisitkul). The most commonly associated abnormality is that of vesicoureteral reflux (Fig. 15–38) (Kramer and Kelalis). Voiding cystourethrography should be performed in all of these patients. Other uncommon problems encountered in these patients include multicystic dysplasia (Nussbaum et al) and renal tumors (Gerber et al).

Prognosis

Most patients with crossed renal ectopia are discovered incidentally and are asymptomatic. When symptoms do occur, they are often related to infection and obstruction. Abeshouse and Bhisitkul reported that one third of patients had pyelonephritis and one fourth had hydronephrosis (Fig. 15–39). The calyceal dilatation and distortion may be secondary to the malrotation or the presence of vesicoureteral reflux and not due to obstruction. Urolithiasis has been found in up to one third of patients (Boatman et al). Mininberg et al re-

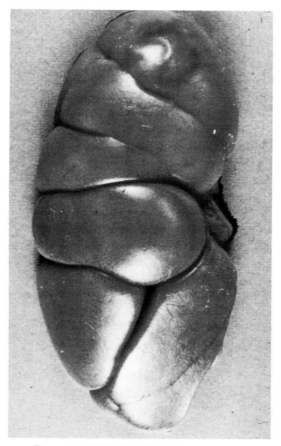

Figure 15–41 □ Fetal lobulation of kidney.

ported one infant who presented with hypertension secondary to a vascular lesion. Other patients may be found to have an abdominal mass on physical examination or during surgical exploration. It is particularly pertinent in the patient with a fused pelvic kidney (Fig. 15–40) to recognize that this is the total functioning renal parenchyma. Inadvertent removal of this "mass" would leave the patient anephric.

Fetal Lobulation

Fetal lobulation is a condition commonly found in children and represents a persistence of normal fetal development (Fig. 15–41). Another term used to describe this is "renal" lobation because it designates the larger renal lobe (pyramid plus surrounding cortex) rather than the lobule (medullary ray and surrounding glomeruli). Campbell (1970) found fetal lobulation at autopsy in 17.6 per cent of children and in 3.9 per cent of adults. This condition is of no clinical importance, except that

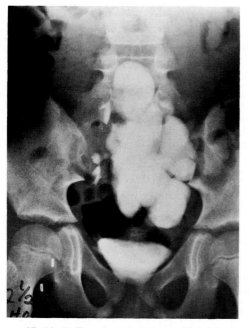

Figure 15–40 □ Fused pelvic kidney with left hydronephrosis secondary to ureteropelvic obstruction.

it should be recognized as a variant of normal renal form. Radiographically, this may appear as small notches in the renal margin that are placed midway between the calyces.

Bibliography

Abeshouse BS, Bhisitkul I: Crossed renal ectopia with and without fusion. Urol Int 9:63, 1959.

Adzick N, Harrison MR, Flake AW, et al: Experimental pulmonary hypoplasia and oligohydramnios: relative contributions of lung fluid and fetal breathing movements. J Pediatr Surg 19:658, 1984.

Antony J: Complete duplication of female urethra with vaginal atresia and supernumerary kidney. J Urol 118:877, 1977.

Ashley DJB, Mostofi FK: Renal agenesis and dysgenesis. J Urol 83:211, 1960.

Avni EF, Thova Y, Lalmand B, et al: Multicystic dysplastic kidney: natural history from in utero diagnosis and postnatal follow-up. J Urol 138:1420, 1987.

Bell R: Horseshoe kidney in pregnancy. J Urol 56:159, 1946.

Blackard CE, Mellinger GT: Cancer in a horseshoe kidney: a report of two cases. Arch Surg 97:616, 1968.

Boatman DL, Kolln CP, Flocks RH: Congenital anomalies associated with horseshoe kidney. J Urol 107:205, 1972.

Bridge RAC: Horseshoe kidneys in identical twins. Br J Urol 32:32, 1960.

Buntley D: Malignancy associated with horseshoe kidney. Urology 8:146, 1976.

Burke EC, Wenzl JE, Utz DC: The intrathoracic kidney: report of a case. Am J Dis Child 113:487, 1967.

Campbell MF: Renal ectopy. J Urol 24:187, 1930.

Campbell MF: Anomalies of the kidney. In Urology, Vol 2, 3rd ed. Edited by MF Campbell, JH Harrison. Philadelphia, WB Saunders Co, 1970, p 1416.

Carlson HE: Supernumerary kidney: a summary of fifty-one reported cases. J Urol 64:224, 1950.

Charney CW, Gillenwater JY: Congenital absence of the vas deferens. J Urol 93:399, 1965.

Collins DC: Congenital unilateral renal agenesia. Ann Surg 95:715, 1932.

Cook WA, Stephens FD: Fused kidneys: morphologic study and theory of embryogenesis. Birth Defects 13:327, 1977.

Curtis JA, Sadhu V, Steiner RM: Malposition of the colon in right renal agenesis, ectopia, and anterior nephrectomy. Am J Roentgenol 129:845, 1977.

Dajani AM: Horseshoe kidney: a review of twenty-nine cases. Br J Urol 38:388, 1966.

David RA: Horseshoe kidney: a report of one family. Br Med J 4:571, 1974.

Davidson WM, Ross GM: Bilateral absence of the kidneys and related congenital anomalies. J Pathol Bacteriol 68:459, 1954.

Dees JE: Clinical importance of congenital anomalies of the upper urinary tract. J Urol 46:659, 1941.

Dees JE: Prognosis of the solitary kidney. J Urol 83:550, 1960.

Dische MR, Johnston R: Teratoma in horseshoe kidneys. Urology 13:435, 1979.

Donahoe PK, Hendren WH: Pelvic kidney in infants and children: experience with 16 cases. J Pediatr Surg 15:486, 1980.

Doroshow LW, Abeshouse BS: Congenital unilateral solitary kidney: report of 37 cases and a review of the literature. Urol Survey 11:219, 1961.

Downs RA, Lane JW, Burns E: Solitary pelvic kidney: its clinical implications. Urol 1:51, 1973.

Duhamel B: From the mermaid to anal imperforation: the syndrome of caudal regression. Arch Dis Child 36:152, 1961.

Emanuel B, Nachman R, Aronson N, et al: Congenital solitary kidney: a review of 74 cases. Am J Dis Child 127:17, 1974.

Evans WP, Resnick MI: Horseshoe kidney and urolithiasis. J Urol 125:620, 1981.

Fernandes M, Scheuch J, Seebode JJ: Horseshoe kidney with retrocaval ureter: a case report. J Urol 140:362, 1988.

Fortune CH: The pathological and clinical significance of congenital one-sided kidney defect with the presentation of three new cases of agenesia and one of aplasia. Ann Intern Med 1:377, 1927.

Gerber WL, Culp DA, Brown RC, et al: Renal mass in crossed-fused ectopia. J Urol 123:239, 1980.

Glenn JF: Analysis of 51 patients with horseshoe kidney. N Engl J Med 261:684, 1959.

Goldstein M, Schlossberg S: Men with congenital absence of the vas deferens often have seminal vesicles. J Urol 140:85, 1988.

Grandone CH, Haller JD, Berdon WE, et al: Asymmetric horseshoe kidney in the infant: value of renal nuclear scanning. Radiology 154:366, 1985.

Gray SW, Skandalakis JE: The kidney and ureter. In Embryology for Surgeons. Philadelphia, WB Saunders Co, 1972, pp 443–518.

Griffin JE, Edwards C, Madden JD, et al: Congenital absence of the vagina: the Mayer-Rokitansky-Kuster-Hauser syndrome. Ann Intern Med 85:224, 1976.

Gutierrez-Millet R, Nieto J, Praga M, et al: Focal glomerulosclerosis and proteinuria in patients with solitary kidneys. Arch Intern Med, 146:705, 1986.

Hostetter TH, Olson JL, Rennke HG: Hyperfiltration in remnant nephrons: a potentially adverse response to renal ablation. Am J Physiol 241:F85, 1981.

Kakei H, Kondo H, Ogisu BI, et al: Crossed ectopia of solitary kidney: a report of two cases and a review of the literature. Urol Int 31:470, 1976.

Kiprov DD, Colvin RB, McClusky RT: Focal and segmental glomerulosclerosis and proteinuria associated with unilateral renal agenesis. Lab Invest 46:275, 1981.

Kramer SA, Kelalis PP: Ureteropelvic junction obstruction in children with renal ectopy. Journal d'urologie 5:331, 1984.

Limakeng ND, Retik AB: Unilateral renal agenesis with hypoplastic ureter: observations on the contralateral urinary tract and report of 4 cases. J Urol 108:149, 1972.

Lippe BL, Geffner ME, Dietrich RB, et al: Renal malformation in patients with Turner's syndrome: imaging in 141 patients. Pediatrics 83:852, 1988.

Longo VJ, Thompson GJ: Congenital solitary kidney. J Urol 68:63, 1952.

Lundius B: Intrathoracic kidney. Am J Roentgenol 125:678, 1975.

Mace JM, Kaplan JM, Schanberger JE, et al: Poland's syndrome: report of seven cases and review of the literature. Clin Pediatr 11:98, 1972.

Malek RS, Kelalis PP, Burke EC: Ectopic kidney in children and frequency of association with other malformations. Mayo Clin Proc 46:461, 1971.

Mascatello V, Lebowitz RL: Malposition of the colon in left renal agenesis and ectopia. Radiology 120:371, 1976.

McDonald JH, McClellan DS: Crossed renal ectopia. Am J Surg 93:995, 1957.

McGahan JP, Myracle MR: Adrenal hypertrophy: possible pitfall in the sonographic diagnosis of renal agenesis. J Ultrasound Med 5:265, 1986.

Mesrobian HJ, Kelalis PP, Hrabovsky E, et al: Wilms' tumor in horseshoe kidneys: a report from the National Wilms' Tumor Study. J Urol 133:1002, 1985.

Mininberg DT, Roze S, Yoon HJ, et al: Hypertension associated with crossed renal ectopia in an infant. Pediatrics 48:454, 1971.

Mollard P, Braun P: Primary ureterocalycostomy for severe hydronephrosis in children. J Pediatr Surg 15:87, 1980.

Moore WB, Matthews TJ, Rabinowitz R: Genitourinary anomalies associated with Klippel-Feil syndrome. J Bone Joint Surg (Am) 57:355, 1975.

Nakada T, Furuta H, Kazama T, et al: Unilateral renal agenesis with or without ipsilateral adrenal agenesis. J Urol 140:933, 1988.

N'Guessan G, Stephens FD: Supernumerary kidney. J Urol 130:649, 1983.

N'Guessan G, Stephens FD, Pick J: Congenital superior ectopic (thoracic) kidney. Urol 24:219, 1984.

Novak ME, Baum NH, Gonzales ET Jr: Horseshoe kidney with multicystic dysplasia associated with ureterocele. Urology 10:456, 1977.

Nussbaum AR, Hartman DS, Whitley N, et al: Multicystic dysplasia and crossed renal ectopia. AJR 149:407, 1987.

Ochsner MG, Brannan W, Goodier EH: Absent vas deferens associated with renal agenesis. JAMA 222:1055, 1972.

Osathanondh V, Potter EL: Development of human kidney as shown in microdissection—3 parts. Arch Pathol 76:271, 1963.

Pedicelli G, Jequier S, Bowen A, et al: Multicystic dysplastic kidneys: spontaneous regression demonstrated with ultrasound. Radiology 161:23, 1986.

Pitts WR Jr, Muecke EC: Horseshoe kidneys: a 40 year experience. J Urol 113:743, 1975.

Potter EL: Bilateral absence of ureters and kidneys: a report of 50 cases. Obstet Gynecol 25:3, 1965.

Priman J: A consideration of normal and abnormal positions of the hilum of the kidney. Anat Rec 42:355, 1929.

Radasch HE: Congenital unilateral absence of the urogenital system and its relation to the development of the wolffian and müllerian ducts. Am J Med Sci 136:111, 1908.

Rizza JM, Downing SE: Bilateral renal agenesis in two female siblings. Am J Dis Child 121:60, 1971.

Roehrborn CG, Schneider HJ, Rugendorff EW, et al: Embryological and diagnostic aspects of seminal vesicle cysts associated with upper urinary tract malformation. J Urol 135:1029, 1986.

Romero R, Cullen M, Grannum P, et al: Antenatal diagnosis of renal anomalies with ultrasound: III. Bilateral renal agenesis. Am J Obstet Gynecol 151:38, 1985.

Roodhooft AM, Birnhalz JC, Holmes LB: Familial nature of congenital absence and severe dysgenesis of both kidneys. N Engl J Med 310:1341, 1984.

Rubinstein ZJ, Heitz M, Shahin N, et al: Crossed renal ectopia: angiographic findings in six cases. Am J Roentgenol 126:1035, 1976.

Schumacker HB Jr: Congenital anomalies of the genitalia associated with unilateral renal agenesis with particular reference to true unicornuate uterus: report of cases and review of the literature. Arch Surg 37:586, 1938.

Segura JW, Kelalis PP, Burke EC: Horseshoe kidney in children. J Urol 108:333, 1972.

Shimamura T, Morrison AB: A progressive glomerulosclerosis occurring in partial five-sixths nephrectomized rats. Am J Pathol 79:95, 1975.

Smith DW: Recognizable patterns of human malformation: genetic, embryologic, and clinical aspects. *In* Major Problems in Clinical Procedures. Philadelphia, WB Saunders Co, 1970, p 57.

Smith EC, Orkin LA: A clinical and statistical study of 471 congenital anomalies of the kidney and ureter. J Urol 53:11, 1945.

Smith JE, Arsdalen KN, Hanno PM, et al: Extracorporeal shock wave lithotripsy treatment of calculi in horseshoe kidneys. J Urol 142:683, 1989.

Steinhardt JM, Kuhn JP, Eisenberg B, et al: Ultrasound screening of healthy infants for urinary tract abnormalities. Pediatrics 82:609, 1988.

Thompson DP, Lynn HB: Genital anomalies associated with solitary kidney. Mayo Clin Proc 41:538, 1966.

Thompson GJ, Pace JM: Ectopic kidney: a review of 97 cases. Surg Gynecol Obstet 64:935, 1937.

Warkany J, Passarge E, Smith LB: Congenital malformations in autosomal trisomy syndromes. Am J Dis Child 112:502, 1966.

Weyrauch HM Jr: Anomalies of renal rotation. Surg Gynecol Obstet 69:183, 1939.

Whitaker RH, Hunt GM: Incidence and distribution of renal anomalies in patients with neural tube defects. Eur Urol 13:322, 1987.

Wladimiroff JW: Effect of furosemide on fetal urine production. Br J Obstet Gynecol 82:221, 1975.

Wulfekuhler WV, Dube VE: Free supernumerary kidney: report of a case. J Urol 106:802, 1971.

Yoder IC, Pfister RC: Unilateral hematocolpos and ipsilateral renal agenesis: report of two cases and review of the literature. Am J Roentgenol 127:303, 1976.

Zondek LH, Zondek T: Horseshoe kidney in associated congenital malformations. Urol Int 18:347, 1964.

ANOMALIES OF THE RENAL PELVIS AND URETER

Edmond T. Gonzales, Jr.

Abnormal development of the ureter is a common cause for urologic symptoms and a need for urologic intervention. A clear insight into normal ureteral embryology as well as the abnormal embryology associated with various anomalies of the ureter is important in understanding the pathophysiology resulting from these anomalies and, in some cases, may be essential in planning appropriate surgical management.

GENERAL EMBRYOLOGIC CONSIDERATIONS

The ureter first appears in the 3- to 5-mm stage as an outpouching on the mesonephric duct at the point where the mesonephric duct bends sharply in a ventral direction just before it enters the cloaca. This site of acute angulation is called the knee of the mesonephric duct. The segment of mesonephric duct from the site of origin of the ureter to the primitive cloaca is known as the common excretory duct. During differentiation of the bladder and urethra, this segment of the mesonephric duct widens as it is incorporated into the developing bladder base and proximal urethra, so that by the 9- to 15-mm stage, the ureter and the remaining mesonephric duct (the future vas deferens in the male) have separate openings into the urogenital sinus (Fig. 15–42). This absorption of the common excretory duct into the urogenital sinus occurs in such a way that the original meatus of the mesonephric duct migrates in a cephalad and lateral direction.

Progressive development of the bladder, bladder neck, and urethra results in a continued lateral and cephalad migration for the urethral orifice and a more medial and caudal migration for the opening of the mesonephric duct. In the male, this terminal end of the mesonephric duct that was proximal to the ureteral bud develops the ejaculatory duct, which normally enters into the distal and posterior aspect of the prostatic urethra at the verumontanum. Muscular bands persist between the ureteral orifice and the openings of the ejaculatory ducts and form the superfi-

cial muscular layer of the trigone. When infravesical obstruction is present, these bands undergo hypertrophy and can be clearly seen as they radiate laterally and cephalad from the verumontanum toward the ureteral orifices. It is believed that hypertrophy of these muscular bands may have been misinterpreted originally as type II posterior urethral valves in the first classification of valves described by Young. In the female, further differentiation of the mesonephric duct ceases and the structure, for the most part, involutes, although segments may persist as Gartner's duct lying along the anterolateral vaginal wall and uterus and within the broad ligament. This development results in the anatomically defined trigone of the normal bladder. Embryologically, then, the region of the trigone is mesodermal in origin (derived primarily from the mesonephric duct) whereas the remainder of the bladder is endodermal in origin.

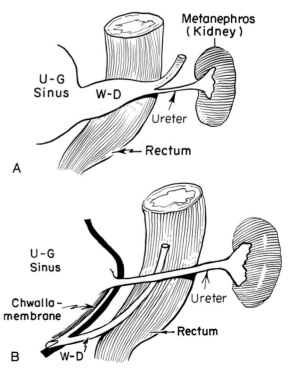

Figure 15–42 □ *A, B,* Incorporation of wolffian (mesonephric) duct (W-D) into urogenital sinus (U-G).

Ureteral development progresses simultaneously during formation of the trigone and proximal urethra. As the ureter grows toward the metanephric blastema, it undergoes a series of dichotomous divisions, ultimately resulting in the complex pattern of infundibula, calyces, and collecting ducts in the mature metanephric kidney. The ureteral bud is responsible for the entire collecting system, including the collecting ducts, which contribute to the parenchyma of the mature kidney. For the purposes of this discussion, though, only the portion of the collecting system from the calyces to the ureterovesical junction are considered.

THE BIFID COLLECTING SYSTEM

More than one ureteral limb may be present anywhere from the bladder to just before the ureter normally separates into the individual infundibula and calyces. Incomplete duplication of the ureter (a single ureteral orifice) is much more common than complete ureteral duplication (two or more ureteral orifices) by a ratio of about 5 to 1. (Incomplete duplication occurs in about one in every 125 individuals; complete duplication is present in about 1 in every 500 to 600 individuals [Campbell, 1951].) However, the incidence of ureteral duplication is as high as 8 per cent in children who are being evaluated for urinary infection (Bisset

and Strife; Hartman and Hodson; Nation; Nordmark).

The incidence of bilaterality with ureteral duplication is high (39 per cent in a series presented by Timothy et al), and there is a familial tendency—perhaps as high as 1 in 8 (Whitaker and Danks). The degree of duplication and/or ectopia, however, may vary significantly among various family members (Babcock et al; Musselman and Barry).

Incomplete Ureteral Duplication

Incomplete duplication is thought to result from early dichotomous branching of a single ureteral bud, resulting in a common distal stem but two (rarely three) ureteral segments impinging on the metanephric blastema. This anomaly can be as mild as having a bifid renal pelvis only, or the anomaly can be almost complete, in which case the common distal stem is very short as it enters the bladder.

The duplex kidney tends to be larger than a kidney with a single ureter, and the separate renal segments can be anatomically (Fig. 15–43) and histologically (Fig. 15–44) diverse. A bifid renal pelvis is very common and is not known to cause any clinical abnormalities. In fact, a bifid renal pelvis might be considered normal, representing one of the many variations in development of the pelvicalyceal system in the human kidney. In fact, distinguish-

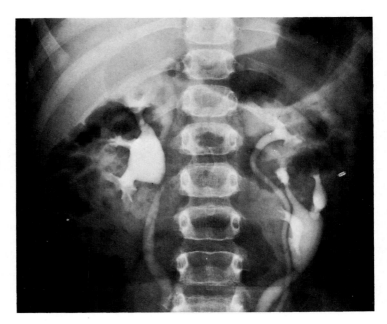

Figure 15–43 □ Excretory urogram. Duplication on left, with malrotation of lower segment.

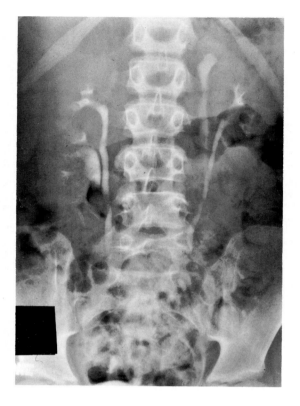

Figure 15–44 □ Bilateral duplex kidney. Right upper segment is normal. Left upper segment is dysplastic and is associated with ectopic ureter.

ing between a bifid (or a trifid) renal pelvis and multiple, long extrarenal infundibula is not always possible.

Incomplete duplication of the ureter is only occasionally associated with distinct clinical symptoms, but two recognized problems are seen with sufficient frequency with incomplete ureteral duplication to warrant discussion: ureteropelvic junction (UPJ) obstruction and retrograde (yo-yo) ureteral peristalsis.

Ureteropelvic junction obstruction occurs occasionally in duplex systems and, for all practical purposes, always affects the collecting system of the lower moiety (Fig. 15–45) (Amis). In the past, this abnormality was commonly mistaken for an intrarenal neoplasm of the lower portion of the kidney because the upper moiety generally functioned well on intravenous urography and mimicked the effaced intrarenal collecting system associated with Wilms' tumor. Today ultrasound scanning suggests the diagnosis accurately in the majority of cases. If the lower pole is salvageable, a pyeloureterostomy is the preferred surgical procedure in nearly all cases (Fig. 15–46). If the duplication is very short, the entire lower segment system can be incorporated into the upper pole ureter. If the duplicated segment is very long, a primary anastomosis of the lower pole pelvis to upper pole ureter, with excision of the remaining portion of the lower pole ureter, is preferred. Although a primary pyeloplasty can be done in many cases, this leaves the duplicated segment intact and incurs the possibility of the development of "yo-yo reflux," which is described below.

In some cases of incomplete ureteral duplication, partial obstruction may exist where the two ureters join (Fig. 15–47) (Kaplan and Elkin). In most instances, this obstruction appears to be a functional disorder resulting from disordered peristalsis and is commonly called yo-yo reflux (O'Reilly et al). Campbell (1967) reported that retrograde peristalsis occurred in 84 per cent of his series of incomplete duplications when the normally propagated peristaltic wave reached the bifurcation. This to-and-fro movement of urine within the ureteral system seems to increase as the branching is positioned closer to the bladder, but it is rare when the bifurcation is within the intramural tunnel (Lenaghan). Patients with yo-yo reflux may present because of urinary infection or flank pain, or they may be found to have incidental hydronephrosis when studied for unrelated symptomatology.

Perhaps the most difficult situation, from a treatment point of view, is determining

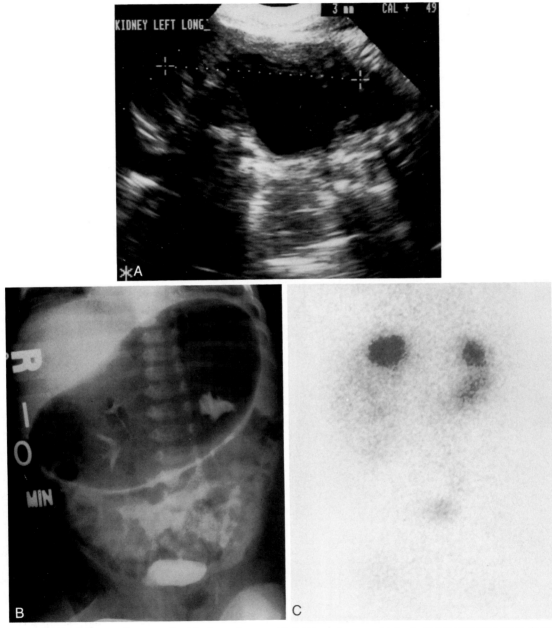

Figure 15–45 □ Prenatally recognized hydronephrosis of left kidney in a newborn. *A,* Renal ultrasonogram demonstrates dilatation of left kidney, but more normal renal parenchyma is present in upper pole. *B,* Excretory urogram shows excellent opacification of apparent upper pole structures on left, displaced superiorly and laterally. A normal duplex ureter on the right suggests a duplex anomaly on the left. *C,* Radioisotope renal scan demonstrates reduced function in hydronephrotic lower pole on the left.

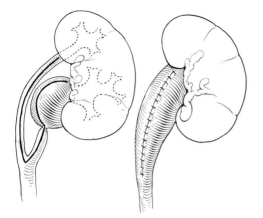

Figure 15–46 □ Surgical treatment of duplication with ureteropelvic obstruction of lower segment. (From Culp OS: Management of ureteropelvic obstruction. Bull NY Acad Med 43:355–377, 1967.)

whether a patient who presents with mild, vague flank pain and incomplete ureteral duplication with ureterectasis is symptomatic because of this finding. Even when definite dilatation of one ureteral limb is present, it can often be difficult to duplicate the patient's

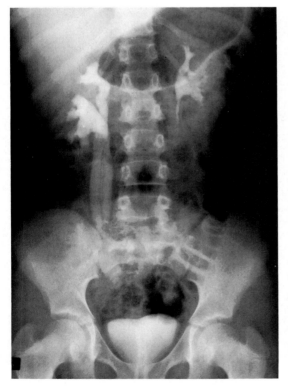

Figure 15–47 □ "Yo-yo reflux" in a 6-year-old female with mild dilatation of the two branches of upper ureter, presumed secondary to to-and-fro peristalsis in an incomplete duplication.

complaint, even during periods of diuretic-induced high urinary flow. Surgical treatment of this anomaly, therefore, should be cautious and selective. Once it is determined that the patient's symptomatology is a result of the partial ureteral duplication, the majority of these patients are best managed with a pyeloureterostomy (preserving the more normal ureter) and complete excision of the discarded ureter (Fig. 15–48) (Sole et al). Care must be taken at the site of the bifurcation not to excise too much ureteral wall, since that could result in the development of a ureteral stricture. An alternative surgical approach in a situation in which the bifurcation is very low would be to do a reimplantation of both ureters in the traditional common sheath technique.

Occasionally, one segment of a bifid ureter may be atretic (Coughlan). The ureter either may end blindly without any apparent attachment to the renal parenchyma or may be in continuity with dysplastic parenchyma by means of a thin fibrous cord (Fig. 15–49). These anomalies may be confused with ureteral diverticula but can be differentiated from them by employing the criteria proposed by Culp. He considered a blind-ending structure to be an aborted bifid ureter when the anomaly joined the functioning ureter at a distinct angle, in which its length was twice its width, and when the histologic features were similar to those of ureters. Other structures arising from the lumen of the ureter would more typically be considered ureteral diverticula. Blind-ending bifid ureters may occur with incomplete ureteral duplication as well as in cases of complete ureteral duplication (Keane and Fitzgerald; Marshall and McLoughlin; Muller et al). In the latter anomaly, the bifid ureter is often discovered at the time of cystoscopy, when an additional ureteral orifice is encountered unexpectedly. Retrograde pyelography confirms the abnormality. During cystography, reflux may occur into a blind-ending ureteral stump, suggesting a paraureteral diverticulum.

The management of these blind-ending ureters is governed by the symptoms they seem responsible for as well as associated anatomic abnormalities (reflux, significant dilatation). Not all small, nondilated blind-ending ureters cause symptoms or sufficient stasis to result in urinary infection. As in all cases of ureteral duplication, the responsible surgeon must carefully assess the pathophysiology before recommending surgical excision.

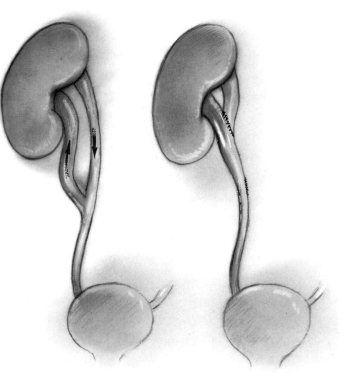

Figure 15–48 □ Surgical treatment of ureteroureteral reflux.

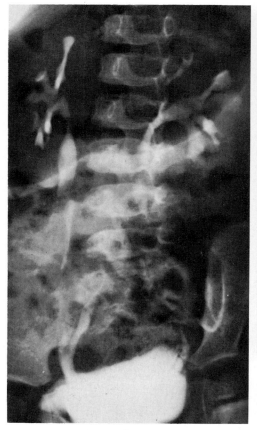

A

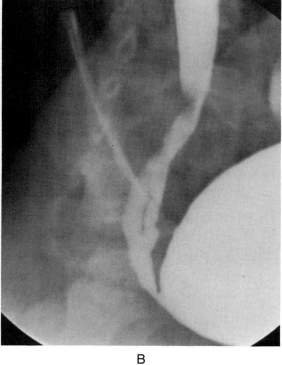

B

Figure 15–49 □ Blind-ending bifid ureter. *A*, Excretory urogram outlines blind-ending bifid ureter on right side. *B*, Voiding cystourethrogram shows reflux and bifurcation.

Complete Ureteral Duplication

Complete ureteral duplication occurs in about one in every 500 individuals. Most often the ureters function normally and the anomaly is not a clinical problem and does not result in an increased risk of urinary infection. A thorough understanding of the embryology of complete ureteral duplication, though, is essential to a clear understanding of many of the disorders of the urinary system that may cause urologic symptoms and require surgical intervention (Weiss, 1988). Extensive studies by Macki and Stephens have suggested a relationship between ureteral orifice position, vesicoureteral reflux, and renal parenchymal dysplasia based on the location of the primitive ureteral bud (or buds) on the mesonephric duct.

Complete ureteral duplication is thought to result from the development of two separate ureteral buds presenting on the mesonephric duct. During absorption and migration of the distal portion of the mesonephric duct into the developing bladder, the orifice of the ureter draining the lower segment of the kidney migrates more cephalad and lateral than the orifice of the ureter draining the upper segment of the kidney. This constant embryologic relationship, whereby the orifice of the upper segment ureter always enters the bladder more medial and caudal than the lower segment orifice, is known as the Weigert-Meyer law (Fig. 15–50) (Meyer; Weigert). When both ureteral buds develop close to one another at the normal location at the bend in the mesonephric duct, both ureteral orifices end up in a satisfactorily normal location on the trigone and function normally. If the ureteral buds are widely separated on the mesonephric duct and displaced from the usual position, migration of the abnormal bud during bladder development results in the orifice to that segment being abnormally positioned in the bladder or the urethra and vesicoureteral reflux or ureteral obstruction may result. If the ureter to the lower segment buds closer to the urogenital sinus than normal, the orifice migrates more lateral and cephalad; therefore, this segment is more likely to be associated with vesicoureteral reflux. When the ureter to the upper segment is displaced more proximally on the mesonephric duct than normal, the ureteral orifice will be distally ectopic in location and may open at the level of the bladder neck or even more distally into the urethra, vestibule,

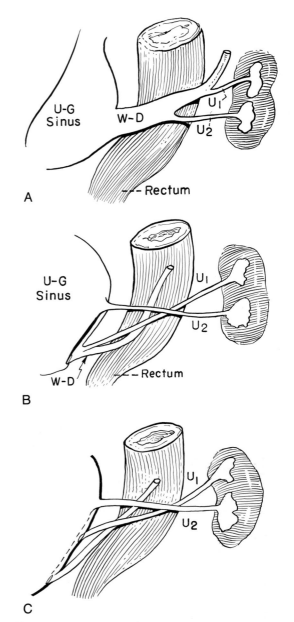

Figure 15–50 □ A–C, Development of ectopic ureter. U-G, urogenital; W-D, wolffian duct; U, ureter.

or vagina. Ectopic ureters may experience reflux but more often are obstructed. Exceptions to the Weigert-Meyer law are exceedingly uncommon (Pope; Lund).

The location of the ureteral bud is also thought to be instrumental in the development of the renal parenchyma. Mackie and Stephens proposed that the metanephric blastema is an elongated structure but noted that only the midregion of this primitive tissue is able to be induced to form normal renal parenchyma. If

Figure 15–51 □ This diagram depicts how the position of the ureteral bud on the wolffian duct (mesonephric duct) will correspond to the final position of the ureteral orifice in the bladder. Ureteral buds that originate at the E position and more proximally on the wolffian duct will tend to hit less normal metanephric blastema and therefore induce dysplastic tissue. (Reprinted with permission from Mackie GG, Stephens FD: Duplex kidneys. A correlation of renal dysplasia with position of the ureteral orifice. J Urol 114:274, 1975. © by Williams & Wilkins, 1975.)

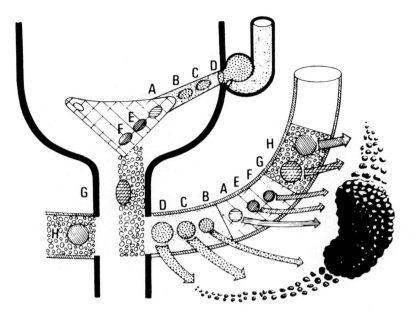

a ureteral bud impinges on the more cephalad or more caudal ends of the metanephric blastema, dysplastic tissue rather than normal renal parenchyma is likely to develop (Fig. 15–51). Although exceptions to this theory occur (Kesavan et al), the observation that final location of the ureteral orifice correlates with the degree of renal dysplasia is consistent enough that this concept of abnormal embryology is embraced today as the most likely explanation for the high incidence of renal dysplasia seen in association with ureteral abnormalities.

Ureteral Duplication and Vesicoureteral Reflux

Vesicoureteral reflux is the most common abnormality seen in association with complete ureteral duplication. For the reasons noted above, the ureter to the lower segment has a more laterally placed orifice and a shortened submucosal tunnel. Thus, reflux occurs much more frequently to the lower segment than it does to the upper segment (Fig. 15–52). In one series of children who presented with urinary tract infection and were found to have complete ureteral duplication with upper tract imaging, vesicoureteral reflux was present in more than two thirds of the patients (Fehrenbaker et al). A similar incidence was reported

more recently by Bisset and Strife (1987). Clearly, cystourethrography should be a routine part of the evaluation of all children who have infection and ureteral duplication.

Reflux is not commonly found in the ureter draining the upper segment because the submucosal segment of distally ectopic ureters is long and much less likely to undergo reflux. When reflux occurs into an upper segment ureter, the ureteral orifice will often be found to be positioned right at the bladder neck (Fig. 15–53) (Stephens, 1958). Occasionally, reflux is seen into both ureters simultaneously. In this situation, there is usually a single ureteral orifice with a very short common stem within the shortened segment of submucosal ureter (Fig. 15–54).

The principles of management of vesicoureteral reflux associated with complete ureteral duplication do not differ substantially from those for management of reflux into single ureteral systems (see Chapter 14). The responsible physician makes decisions regarding indications for surgery using the same criteria as for single ureters (Peppos). The only noted difference is that the anatomy of the ureterovesical junction is more likely to be substantially abnormal when reflux is associated with complete ureteral duplication; for that reason, children with duplex systems more often undergo operative correction of vesicoureteral reflux.

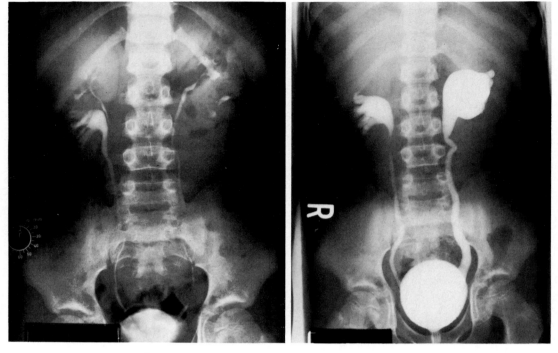

Figure 15–52 □ Ureteral duplication. *A,* Excretory urogram shows mild dilatation of lower right segment and severe atrophy of lower left segment. *B,* Cystogram shows bilateral reflux into both lower segments of duplication.

URETERAL ECTOPIA

The ureter that enters in a distal ectopic position is thought to result from a ureteral bud that develops more cranially on the mesonephros than normal. At this location, absorption of the ureteral orifice into the developing bladder and urethra is delayed and thus the orifice comes to lie in a position caudal to the normal insertion of the ureter on the trigone. As noted above, ectopically positioned ureters are more often obstructed, although they may on occasion also be associated with vesicoureteral reflux. Ureteral ectopia can be associated with both a single ureter as well as a duplex system, but is much more common in association with complete ureteral duplication (Fig. 15–55). The location of the ectopic ureteral orifice is always along the pathway of normal development of the mesonephric system (Fig. 15–56). In the male, ectopic ureteral orifices are found at the level of the bladder neck, within the prostatic urethra to the level of the orifice of the ejaculatory duct and, in more severe degrees of ectopia, along the course of the male genital ductal system, even to the

epididymis (Jona et al). Unusual anomalies of the ureter and vasal system, where a common orifice within the bladder drains both the ureter and the vas deferens, have been described.

In the female, ectopic ureters draining at the bladder neck or within the urethra are easy to explain embryologically. However, when a ureter drains into the vagina, uterus, or, on occasion, fallopian tube, the abnormality in development responsible for the ureteral ectopia is not as clearly defined. Except for the distal portion of the vagina, the entire female internal ductal structures are developed from the müllerian system. The ureter is not a normal bud from the müllerian structures. However, vestigial segments of the mesonephric system lie in an anterolateral position along the vagina and uterus and within the broad ligaments supporting the fallopian tubes (Arey). These structures are commonly known as Gartner's ducts in the obstetric literature. Although this ductal structure is usually not readily apparent, segments of these ducts may encyst and present as clinically significant masses (Gartner's duct cyst). It is believed that ureters ultimately are able to drain into the

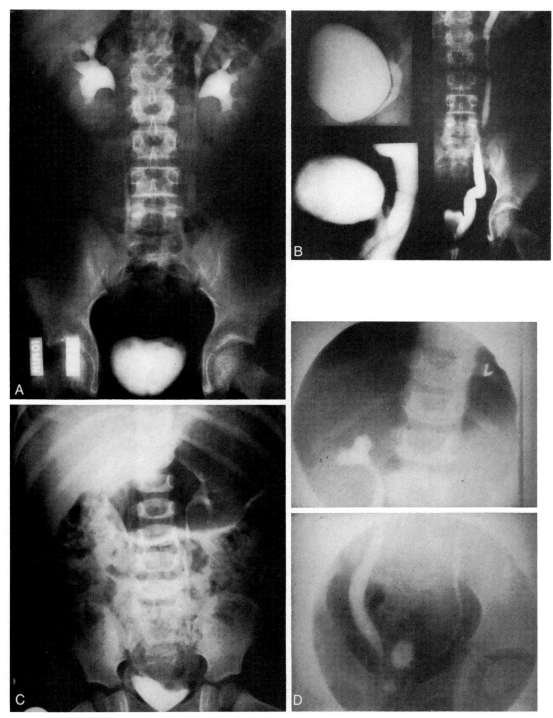

Figure 15–53 □ Reflux into an upper-segment ureter in two patients.
First patient: A, Excretory urogram demonstrates duplex left collecting system. Upper pole system functions well but is dysmorphic. B, Voiding cystourethrogram shows reflux into upper system with insertion of upper segment ureter at the bladder neck.
Second patient: C, Excretory urogram demonstrates duplex right ureter. D, Voiding cystourethrogram shows reflux into the upper pole system, with the ureter inserting right at the bladder neck. Left reflux is also present into a single system.

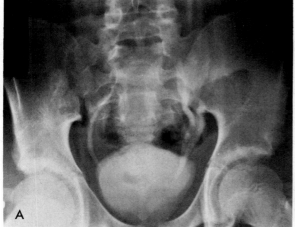

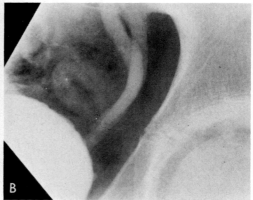

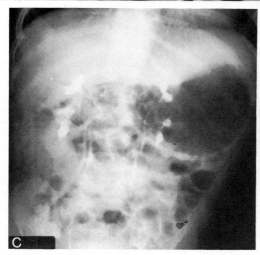

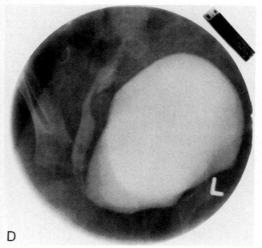

Figure 15–54 □ *First patient:* Incomplete duplication on left, with vesicoureteral reflux into common stem. *A,* Excretory urogram. *B,* Voiding cystourethrogram. *Second patient:* complete duplication, but with both orifices sitting side by side. *C,* Excretory urogram shows bilateral ureteral duplication. *D, E,* Reflux into both ureters on the right.

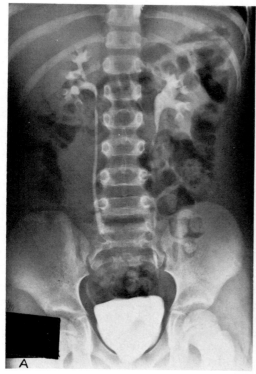

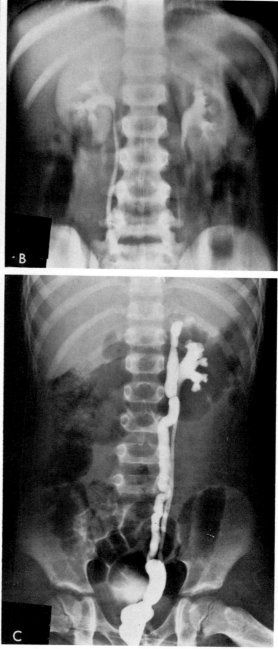

Figure 15–55 □ Ectopic ureter, with duplication on left. *A,* Excretory urogram. Decrease in number of calyces on left. *B,* Same, with tomographic cuts. Upper, renal parenchyma evidently is not supplied by calyces. *C,* Ureterogram, showing ectopic left ureter.

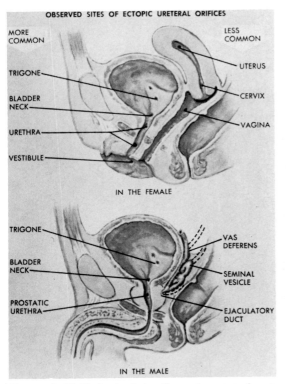

OBSERVED SITES OF ECTOPIC URETERAL ORIFICES

MORE COMMON / LESS COMMON

TRIGONE — / — UTERUS
BLADDER NECK — / — CERVIX
URETHRA — / — VAGINA
VESTIBULE —

IN THE FEMALE

TRIGONE — / — VAS DEFERENS
BLADDER NECK — / — SEMINAL VESICLE
PROSTATIC URETHRA — / — EJACULATORY DUCT

IN THE MALE

Figure 15–56 □ Anatomic locations where ectopic ureters can be expected.

müllerian structures when a segment of Gartner's duct into which the ectopic ureter drains is either absorbed or perhaps ruptures into the developing müllerian systems.

Ureteral ectopy into the rectum usually is discovered incidentally at autopsy. This anomaly is thought to result from either a mesonephric duct misplaced into an abnormally posterior location on the cloaca or a faulty division of the cloaca by the urorectal septum (Uson and Schulman).

Ureteral ectopy occurs in both males and females but is much more common in the female at a ratio of about 6 to 1. About 70 per cent of ectopic ureters are associated with complete ureteral duplication. However, in the male, the incidence of single system ectopia is much more common than in the female. In addition to showing findings consistent with obstruction, ectopic systems are also commonly associated with a very high incidence of renal parenchymal dysplasia in the renal segment drained by the ectopic ureter. There is also a high incidence of contralateral duplication of varying degree, reported to be as high as 80 per cent (Malek et al).

In the male, ectopic ureters usually are discovered during an evaluation for urinary tract infection. When the ureter enters the genital ducts, epididymo-orchitis is a common finding at presentation. Occasionally, the physician might suspect an ectopic ureter when a mass representing either a dilated ureter or a dilated seminal vesicle is palpated on rectal examination. Rarely, grossly purulent material may present through the urethra.

In the female, ectopic ureters present in more varied ways. Many infant girls with ureteral ectopia also present because of urinary tract infection. However, if the ureter does not drain into the urinary tract, urinary infection may not occur and ectopia may be missed until urinary incontinence is noted in later childhood (Fig. 15–57). If the ectopic system drains in an extraurethral location and is so poorly functional that little or no urine is produced, the patient may present with intermittent vaginal discharge or unexplained fevers from pyonephrosis (Fig. 15–58).

The urinary incontinence associated with ureteral ectopia in the female is classically described as total constant urinary dampness in a child otherwise normally toilet trained and voiding with a normal number of micturition episodes. In the classic case, one often sees urine gradually welling up from the vaginal vault during office examination. Occasionally, however, the large dilated ureter associated with the ectopic orifice will pool urine when the child is in a recumbent position, and urinary incontinence may mimic the more typical leakage seen with uninhibited bladder contractions or stress incontinence.

Diagnosis of the Ectopic Ureter

Diagnosis of suspected ureteral ectopia may be relatively easy or can be one of the more subtle and difficult diagnoses in pediatric urology. If the involved segment of renal tissue functions sufficiently to excrete contrast material, the ectopic ureter may be visualized on standard excretory urography (IVP). When an ectopic upper system is very dilated, the functioning lower segment system is often displaced inferiorly and laterally (Figs. 15–59 and 15–60). At other times, though, the involved renal segment, particularly in duplex ureters, is very small and the visualized portion of kidney may look deceptively normal (Fig. 15–61). One can

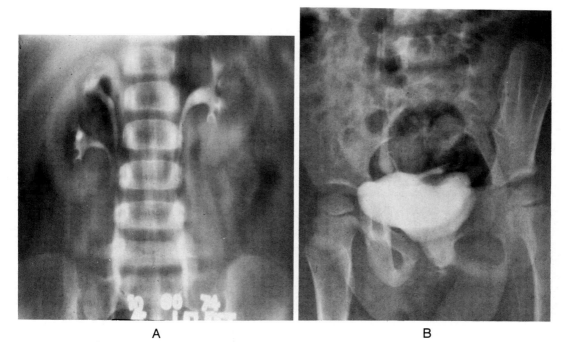

A   B

Figure 15–57 □ Ectopic ureter in a 4-year-old girl with incontinence, demonstrated by excretory urograms. *A,* Duplication on right. *B,* Pooling of medium into vagina from ectopic ureter.

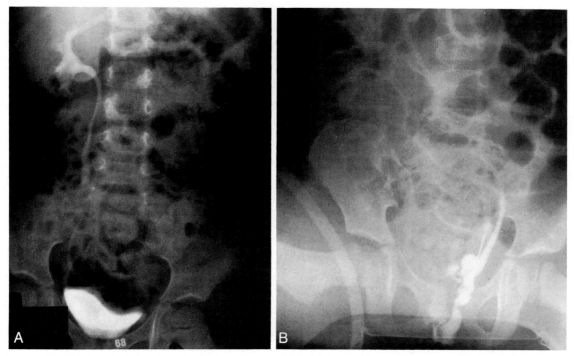

Figure 15–58 □ Vaginal insertion of ectopic ureter (single system) in a 3-year-old girl being evaluated for recurring vaginal discharge. No history of urinary incontinence was evident. *A,* Excretory urogram reveals a solitary right kidney. At cystoscopy, there was a right hemitrigone. The bladder base on the left was elevated; a cystic structure was present of the left vaginal wall. *B,* Transvesical needle puncture of suspected lesion reveals ectopic ureter draining into the vagina.

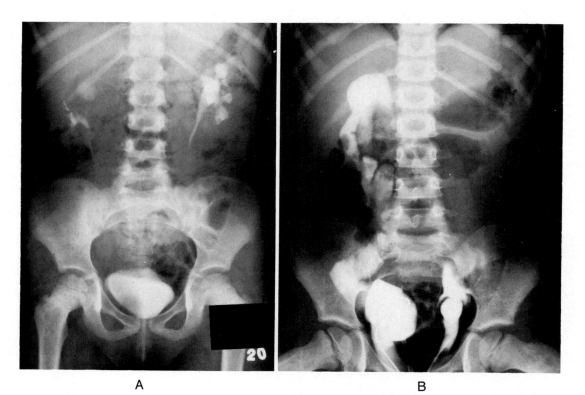

A   B

Figure 15–59 □ Bilateral duplication with ectopic ureters. *A,* Excretory urogram shows poorly functioning hydronephrotic upper right segment and functionless upper left segment. *B,* Bilateral ureterograms with catheters in ectopic ureteral orifices.

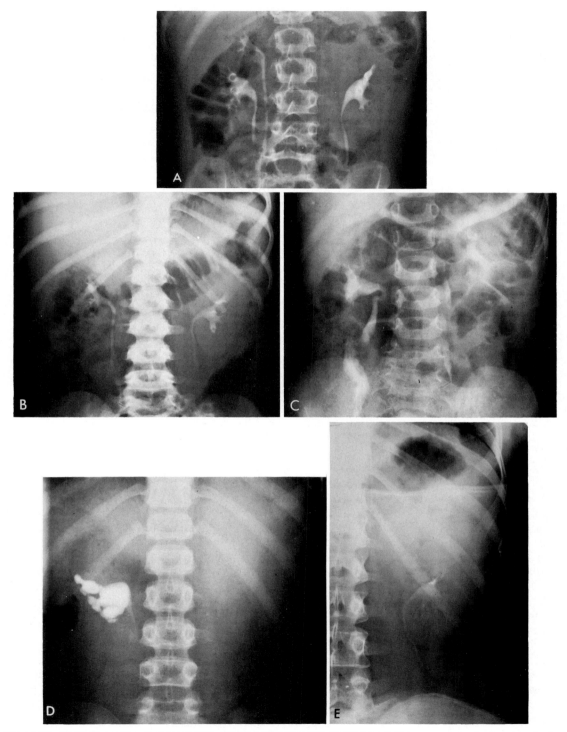

Figure 15–60 □ Examples of characteristic lateral and downward displacement of lower segment when functionless upper pole pelvis is dilated. *A,* Functionless upper left segment. *B,* Poorly functioning upper right segment and functionless upper left segment, with characteristic displacement of both lower segment pelves. *C, D,* Functionless upper right segment and displacement of lower segment. *E,* Functionless upper left segment simulating tumor in upper pole.

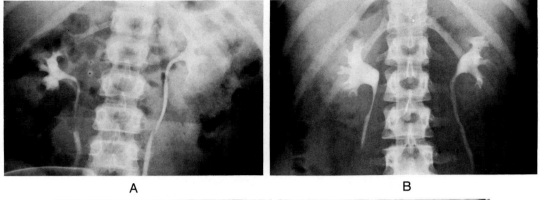

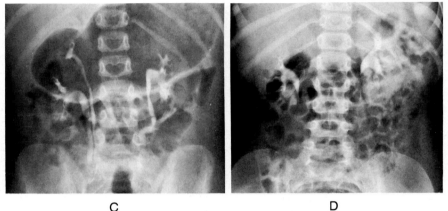

Figure 15–61 ☐ Appearance of lower pole pelvis when the upper pole is functionless and nondilated. *A,* Functionless upper right segment. Calyceal system of lower segment is smaller but relatively normal. *B,* Functionless upper pole on left, with decrease in number of calyces of lower segment. *C,* Functionless upper left segment, with apparent increase in renal substance of upper pole on left. *D,* Functionless upper right segment, with apparent increase in renal substance thickness on medial side of upper pole.

be suspicious of the presence of a large, non-visualized but dilated ureter draining an upper segment when the ureter from the lower segment is noted to be displaced and tortuous along its course toward the bladder (Fig. 15–62). Occasionally, one might suspect a subtle duplication anomaly when the normal medially positioned upper segment calyx is not visualized and when there seems to be an abnormally thickened upper medial pole, especially if there is duplication on the other side (Fig. 15–63). Today, ultrasonography clearly defines the abnormal fluid-filled ureter in most cases and may actually be able to trace the ureter into the pelvis and into an abnormally low position beyond the bladder (Fig. 15–64). Similarly, computed tomography (CT) of the abdomen can help to differentiate a very abnormal system—particularly if the lower pole of a duplex anomaly is significantly dilated also and the large, tortuous ureters tend to overlap and intermingle.

At times reflux occurs into the abnormally positioned upper segment, especially if it is positioned at the bladder neck or in the proximal urethra, and cystography may define the abnormality. A contrast voiding cystourethrogram should be obtained routinely in any patient suspected of having an ectopic ureter. A patulous orifice at the bladder neck is occasionally catheterized directly during attempted cystography (Fig. 15–65).

When standard imaging studies do not clearly define the anatomy and one still suspects that an ectopic ureter is present, the physician can improve the likelihood of establishing a diagnosis by utilizing various dye tests. One example might be to place a dental roll or cotton ball in the vagina and then fill the bladder with contrast dye. The catheter can then be removed and the child allowed to ambulate for a period. If there is no leakage of the colored urine or continued dampness from the vagina, the diagnosis of an ectopic

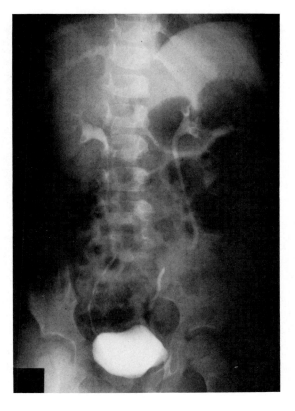

Figure 15–62 □ Ectopic, obstructed nonvisualizing left upper pole in a 2-year-old girl. Note the tortuosity and deviation of the opacified left lower segment ureter.

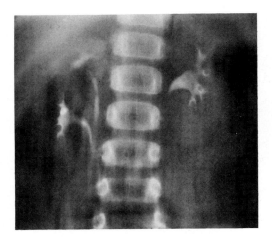

Figure 15–63 □ Excretory urogram. Functionless upper segment on left. Considerable upper-pole parenchyma is not served by calyx. Clue to diagnosis is duplication on right side.

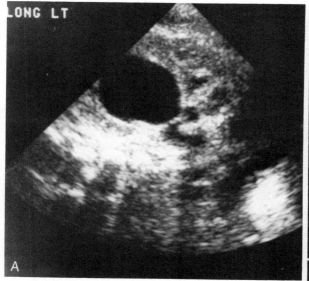

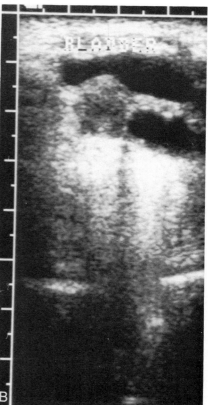

Figure 15–64 ☐ The patient is a newborn female with an abnormal prenatal ultrasonogram. *A,* Renal ultrasonogram reveals dilated left upper pole segment. *B,* Transvesical scan demonstrates a dilated ureter passing behind the bladder.

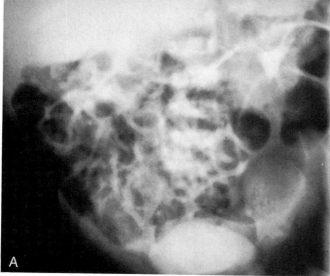

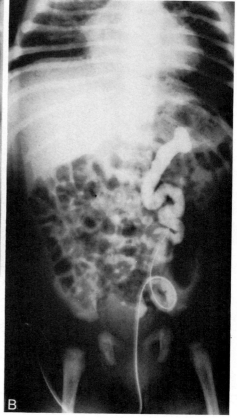

Figure 15–65 ☐ *A,* Excretory urogram reveals an inferiorly displaced group of calyces on the left in a 4-month-old being evaluated for purulent perineal drainage. *B,* During catheterization to obtain a cystogram, the catheter inadvertently slipped up the upper segment ureter.

ureter is almost ensured. Another approach is to place a dental roll in the vagina and give the patient an injection of indigo carmine or methylene blue. After a period of time, the dental roll can be removed. It is preferable during this interval that the child does not void, since this would stain the outer margin of the dental roll. If staining is limited to the upper edge of the dental roll, once again a vaginal ureteral orifice is virtually ensured. This procedure is dependent on function of the ectopic segment. At times this segment functions so poorly that it cannot adequately concentrate the dye to make visualization possible.

It is unusual for the diagnosis to be made only at cystoscopy. The ectopic ureteral orifice within the urethra is not particularly difficult to localize. However, an orifice in the vagina is exceedingly hard to identify with any certainty. These orifices are nearly always present along the anterior and lateral portion of the vagina where one would expect Gartner's duct to be, and it is important for the cystoscopist to be aware of precisely where one is likely to expect to find such an orifice. The author has had experience with two cases in which the only abnormal finding was a small cystic structure in the vagina (Fig. 15–66). When this was unroofed, the ureteral lumen was identified and could be catheterized and the diagnosis of an ectopic ureter was confirmed by retrograde ureterography.

The availability today of quality ultrasound evaluations has significantly altered the sequence of diagnostic maneuvers in the assessment of children with suspected ureteral ectopia. Because the ectopic system is often dilated and ultrasonography is not function-dependent, initial screening with renal ultrasonography seems most appropriate in every case. Even in cases of single-system ureteral ectopia, in which the kidney is often small, abnormally positioned, and difficult to localize with ultrasonography, the ureter is likely to be dilated— particularly in its lower segment, where it passes behind the bladder.

In the male, voiding cystourethrography is more likely to demonstrate reflux if the ureter drains into the prostatic urethra but it may also demonstrate retrograde flow of contrast material down the ejaculatory mechanism. At cystoscopy the ejaculatory duct may be anomalous and wide and relatively easy to catheterize, allowing for performance of a direct vasogram, which would likely reflux into the ectopic ureter (Schulman).

Ectopic Ureter in a Duplex System

The management of the upper segment ectopic renoureteral unit most often involves surgical excision. In the majority of situations, the renal parenchyma is developmentally abnormal and often severely affected from the ravages of pyelonephritis. Excision of this abnormal renal parenchyma and most of the involved ureter is generally curative (Fig. 15–67). In most cases, the distal segment of ureter behind the bladder and as it passes immediately beneath the bladder neck is left in situ. It is unusual to have to excise the entire ureter; in fact, aggressive dissection to remove the entire ureter in the female, or the dilated seminal vesical in the male, risks injury to associated structures (vagina, rectum), may damage the continence mechanisms, and is rarely necessary. However, the distal stump should be left as short as safely possible. In infants, this can usually be done through a single, generous flank incision; older children may require a separate suprapubic incision. In select cases with well-preserved parenchyma of the upper pole, a pyeloureterostomy (upper segment ureter to lower segment pelvis) might be preferable to partial nephrectomy.

Ectopic Ureter in a Single System

Ectopia of a single system is more common in the male than in the female (Fig. 15–68). In the female, though, it occupies an area of special interest, because the ectopic kidney is often small, poorly functional, and very difficult to localize and at cystoscopy a hemitrigone is all that is seen (Fig. 15–69). In the past, the incidence of unilateral single ectopic ureters was often not recognized and the disorder was thought to be rare. Weiss and associates (1984) suggested that the ectopic system may be much more common than previously thought and encouraged a more aggressive diagnostic effort in any female who presents with urologic symptoms and is found to have only a single functioning renal unit associated with an ipsilateral hemitrigone.

When both ureters are ectopic in the female (bilateral single-system ectopia), unique developmental abnormalities and management concerns are present. Because the ureters have not migrated into their normal position within

Text continued on page 554

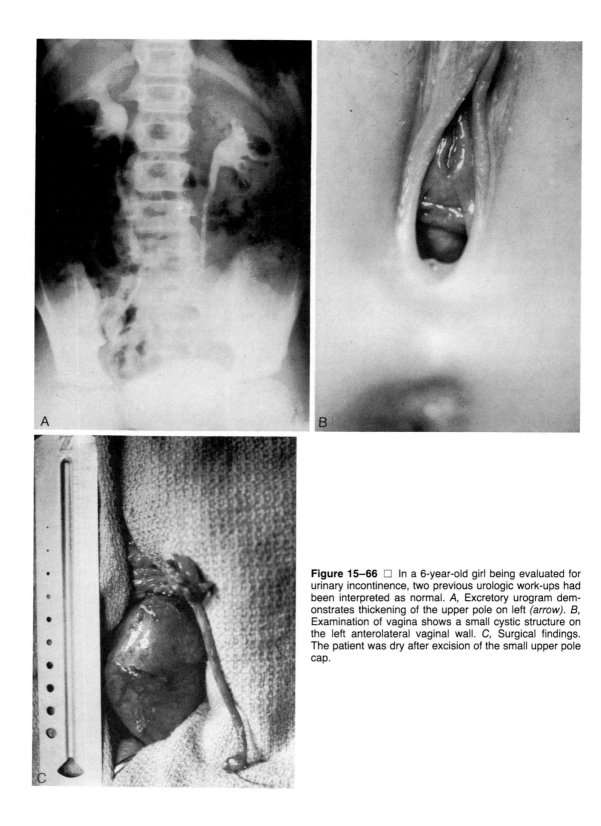

Figure 15–66 □ In a 6-year-old girl being evaluated for urinary incontinence, two previous urologic work-ups had been interpreted as normal. *A,* Excretory urogram demonstrates thickening of the upper pole on left *(arrow). B,* Examination of vagina shows a small cystic structure on the left anterolateral vaginal wall. *C,* Surgical findings. The patient was dry after excision of the small upper pole cap.

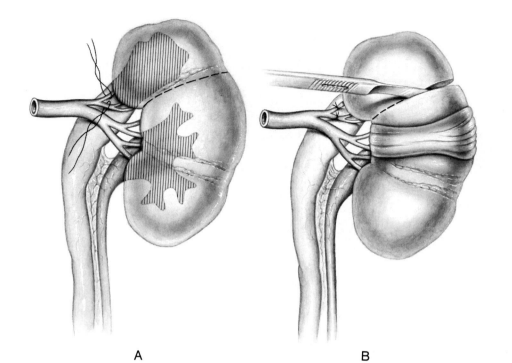

A

B

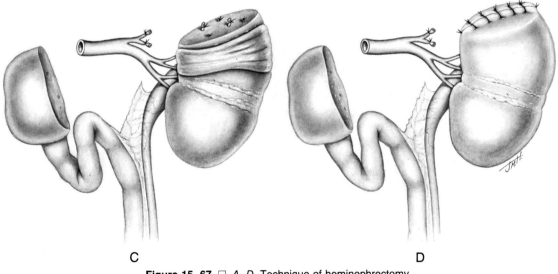

C

D

Figure 15–67 □ *A–D*, Technique of heminephrectomy.

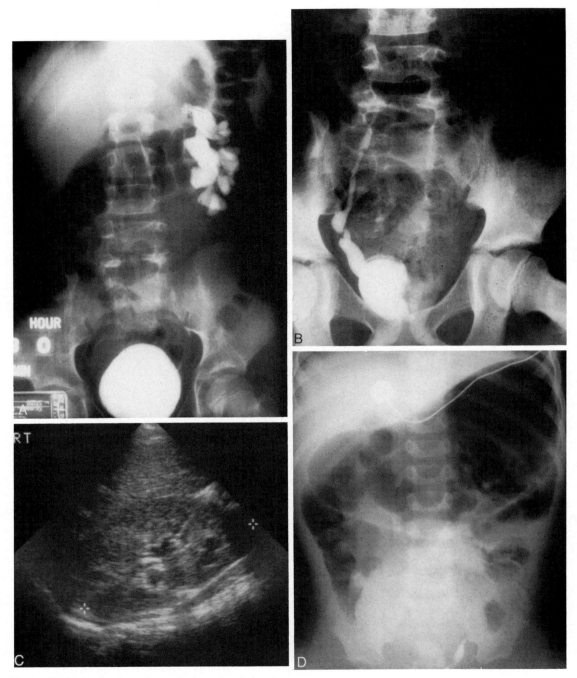

Figure 15–68 □ Single-system ectopic ureters in two boys.
First patient: A, Excretory urogram demonstrates solitary functioning left kidney with mild ureteropelvic junction changes. B, Injection of ectopic system after endoscopic needle puncture of fullness at bladder base.
Second patient: Recurrent urinary tract infection in a 2-year-old boy. C, Renal ultrasonogram demonstrates only a right kidney. D, Retrograde injection of ectopic orifice is found in the prostatic urethra.

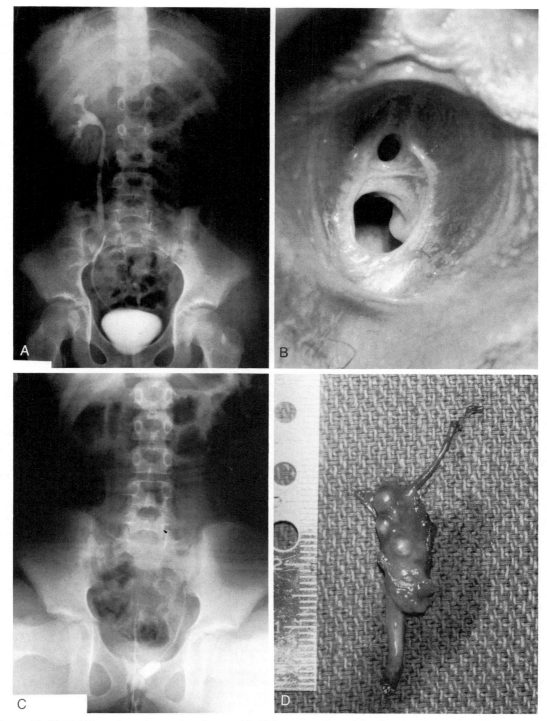

Figure 15–69 □ Urinary incontinence in a 5-year-old girl first seen at age 3 for the same symptoms. No work-up was done at that time. *A,* Excretory urogram shows solitary, normal right kidney. *B,* Inspection of vagina reveals a cystic structure on left anterolateral wall. *C,* Retrograde injection after cyst was "uncapped" and ectopic ureter was catheterized. *D,* Surgical specimen—dysplastic left kidney.

the bladder, the bladder neck and trigone never fully develop (Cox and Hutch). During cystography, the bladder neck is often seen to be widened and V-shaped and obviously incompetent. In addition, the bladder in this unusual situation has never had to store urine because urine leaks directly from the urethra to the outside (Fig. 15–70). Developmentally, then, the bladder is small in capacity and is very thin-walled. Severe bilateral renal dysplasia may be present and renal failure can result. Simple ureteral reimplantation is usually not sufficient to manage this problem. Reconstructive procedures may be necessary at the bladder neck in order to achieve urinary continence. Bladder capacity may never be adequate, and augmentation of the bladder may be necessary. Reconstruction in the child with bilateral single ectopic systems must take all these considerations into account.

Bilateral single-system ectopia is much more common in girls and appears to be a more serious defect than in boys. Presumably, the better-developed external sphincter in boys allows some flow of urine into the bladder, stimulating bladder capacity (Williams and Lightwood, 1972).

URETEROCELES

Ureteroceles represent cystic dilatation of the intravesical segment of the ureter. Children with ureteroceles present with a broad spectrum of abnormalities with a wide diversity of effects on the upper and the lower urinary tracts (Fig. 15–71). Ureteroceles may be associated with either a single ureter or with a duplex ureter (usually involving the upper segment ureter) and may vary considerably in size. Ureteroceles may obstruct the drainage of the other ureters, may prolapse into the bladder neck and impede voiding, or may distort the trigone, resulting in reflux. Ureteroceles are commonly associated with varying degrees of renal dysplasia of the affected segment, but there is, in addition, likely to be obstructive parenchymal atrophy and pyelonephritic damage to all segments in the urinary tract.

Embryology of Ureteroceles

The embryology of ureteroceles remains poorly understood, and it is unlikely that a single abnormality explains the etiology of all ureteroceles. The most accepted theories for the development of ureteroceles are (1) primary ureteral meatal obstruction, (2) incomplete muscularization of the distal ureter, and (3) excessive dilatation or widening of the distal aspect of the ureter as it is absorbed into the developing urogenital sinus and bladder neck.

Some ureteroceles are tense, and the ureteral orifice, if identified, is often pinpoint in size. This observation has prompted the suggestion that some ureteroceles result from ureteral meatal stenosis—probably a result of incomplete dissolution of Chwalla's membrane (Chwalla). This anatomic description is more often seen with the single-system ureterocele and is especially common for those lesions wholly contained within the bladder. In other cases, the orifice is patulous in appearance and it is possible for a catheter or even the cystoscope to be passed into the ureterocele and distal ureter. These findings are present more often when the orifice is at the level of the bladder neck or proximal urethra. Whether or not meatal obstruction plays a role in the development of these ureteroceles is unclear, although Stephens has proposed that some degree of obstruction may result where the abnormal ureter passes through the vesical sphincters (Stephens, 1971). In either situation, endoscopic incision of the ureterocele usually results in a significant reduction in ureteral caliber, suggesting that obstruction was at least a factor in the development of the associated hydronephrosis and, perhaps, of the ureterocele itself. Ureteroceles can be present in the absence of a functioning kidney (so called "blind ureteroceles")—demonstrating that urinary flow is not necessary for persistence of the cystic intravesical mass (Fig. 15–72) (Passerini et al).

In some cases, incomplete muscularization or abnormal muscular differentiation of the lower ureter may be responsible for intrinsic weakness of the lower ureter, allowing it to expand out of proportion to the rest of the ureteral caliber (Fig. 15–73). Tokunaka and associates have described absent or histologically dysplastic muscle in more than 90 per cent of specimens taken from ureteroceles of both single and duplicated systems. Stephens (1983) demonstrated similar findings in his careful gross anatomic and histologic studies. Caldamone et al compared the degree of muscularization of the distal ureter of patients with

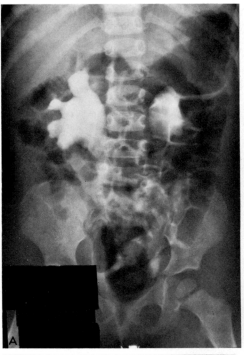

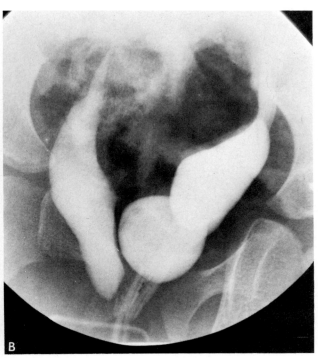

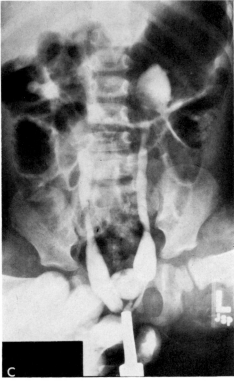

Figure 15–70 □ Bilateral single ectopic ureters. *A,* Excretory urogram. *B,* Cystogram. Reflux into ectopic ureters. Dysplastic bladder. *C,* Anatomy well demonstrated by injection into urethral meatus.

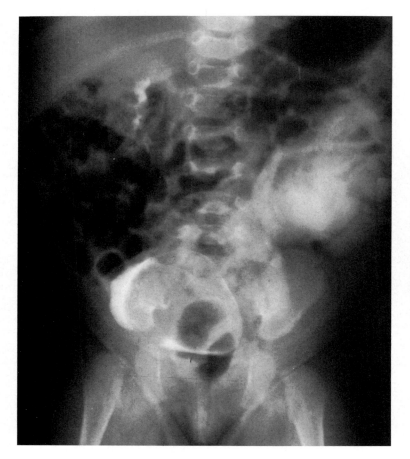

Figure 15–71 □ A 3-month-old girl presented with a palpable left upper quadrant mass. The ureterocele subtending the left upper pole moiety is clearly seen as a filling defect in the bladder. The left lower pole is hydronephrotic because its ureter is being obstructed by the ureterocele. No reflux was seen on the voiding cystourethrogram. (From King LR: Urologic Surgery in Neonates and Young Infants. Philadelphia, WB Saunders Co, 1989.)

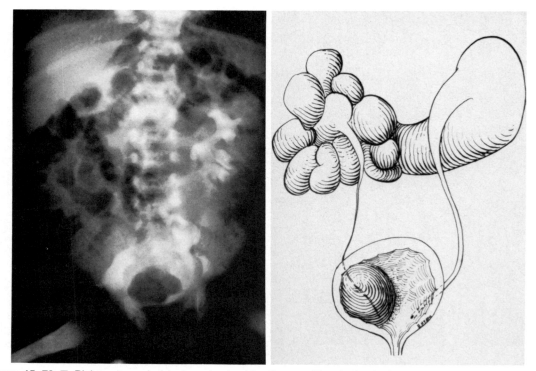

Figure 15–72 □ Right ureterocele (single system) subtending a multicystic dysplastic kidney—so-called blind ureterocele.

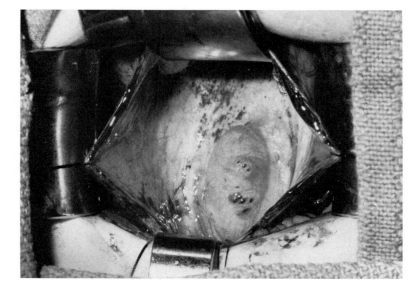

Figure 15–73 □ This ureterocele, which one sees in the open bladder, shows punctate spots that correspond to areas of abnormal muscularization in which ureteral mucosa coapts the vesical mucosa. (From King LR: Urologic Surgery in Neonates and Young Infants. Philadelphia, WB Saunders Co, 1989.)

ureteroceles with those with ectopic ureters without ureteroceles. They found that the ureters associated with ureteroceles consistently have less well-developed musculature.

The most widely accepted theory, though, explains ureterocele formation on abnormal development of the segment of the mesonephric duct between the site of the ureteral bud and the insertion of the duct into the primitive urogenital sinus (the common excretory duct or the trigone precursor). During normal embryogenesis, this segment widens as it is absorbed into the differentiating vesicourethral canal. If this expansion extends too proximally onto the distal ureter, persisting bulbous dilation of the lower ureter (a ureterocele) may result.

Tanagho (1976) and Stephens (1983) propose subtle differences in their concepts of the origin of ureteroceles. Both authors theorize that the position of the ureteral bud on the mesonephric duct is farther from the urogenital sinus than normal. In Tanagho's view, the excessive widening involves primarily the trigone precursor as well as the distal aspect of the ureter itself. Because the ureteral bud is positioned proximally, the ureter reaches the bladder later than normal and some of the expansion is incompletely absorbed, thereby accounting for the ureterocele. Stephens (1971) suggests that ureteroceles develop because the ureter arrives at the urogenital sinus later than normal and is thereby involved in the process of expansion of the vesicourethral canal, an event that generally begins after the migration of the ureter itself. Stephens supports his theory with the observation that ureters which drain into the distal urethra, introitus, or müllerian system are rarely found to have excessive dilatation of the terminal end of the ureter. He suggests that these ureters, with an even more proximal origin on the mesonephric duct, never reach the urogenital sinus and therefore are not affected by the normal expansion of this segment of the primitive bladder. Both of these theories explain best the ureterocele with an ectopically positioned orifice rather than the ureterocele positioned completely intravesically.

Perhaps the most difficult aspect of ureteroceles to explain is the discrepancy in the male-to-female ratio between single and duplex systems. In my own experience of 58 children with ureteroceles, 12 of 13 single-system ureteroceles were found in males. It is not known why this occurs, but it is interesting to speculate that the more complex development of the male bladder neck and genital ductal structures might, on occasion, "hold up" migration of even a normal ureter, subsequently allowing the ureter to become caught up in the expansion of the primitive vesicourethral canal.

Abnormal embryologic development is also felt to be responsible for much of the renal parenchymal abnormalities associated with ureteroceles. In the past, it was felt that the parenchymal changes were secondary to the obstruction from the ureterocele. Currently, the ureteral bud theory proposed by Macki and Stephens (1975) provides a better explanation of the many facets of renal parenchymal maldevelopment associated with these lesions. These ectopically positioned ureteral buds are more likely to impinge on the periphery of the metanephric blastema and thereby induce development of only abnormal (dysplastic) tissue.

Classification of Ureteroceles

A universal classification scheme for ureteroceles has never been accepted (Glassberg et al). In most series, ureteroceles have been grouped according to their association with single systems (so-called orthotopic or simple ureteroceles) or with duplex systems (almost always subtending the upper segment and generally described as ectopic ureteroceles) Ericsson). This classification, though, is clearly inaccurate because not all single-system ureteroceles are really in an orthotopic position, nor are all duplex ureterocele orifices positioned beyond the confines of the trigone. This classification fails to emphasize the great diversity in anatomic variability and presentation seen with ureteroceles and implies, incorrectly, a primary difference between single-

Table 15–1 □ Classification System of
F. Douglas Stephens

1. Stenotic	Orifice located inside the bladder and is the presumed site of obstruction.
2. Sphincteric	Orifice of the ureterocele may be normal or even patulous but lies in the floor of the urethra, so that the ureter leading to it is obstructed by the internal sphincteric mechanism.
3. Sphinctero-stenotic	A combination of 1 and 2.
4. Cecoureterocele	A ureterocele that extends beneath the mucosa of the trigone and urethra; its orifice is large and incompetent, and the lumen of the ureterocele extends beyond the orifice.
5. Blind ureterocele	A ureterocele with no orifice or kidney above the proximal extension of its ureter.
6. Nonobstructed ureterocele	A ureterocele with a large orifice that is not in the grip of the sphincter mechanism.

system and duplex-system lesions. Other classification schemes by Gross and Clatworthy (1950) and by Uson (1961) are complex and not used by the majority of clinicians. Stephens (1971) has grouped ureteroceles by presumed etiology, taking into account the many facets of abnormal embryology involved in ureterocele formation (Table 15–1).

I believe that the location of the orifice of the ureterocele is more important than whether it is associated with a single or duplex system, and orifice position can be described simply as intravesical or extravesical. Ureteral status (single, duplex) and presumed etiology (per Stephens) are secondary factors in the description of the ureterocele. This approach emphasizes the postulate that ureteral orifice location dictates the extent of abnormal embryology, which ultimately determines the severity in most cases of parenchymal maldevelopment in the affected segment as well as the degree of distortion of the bladder neck and proximal urethra.

Presentation

Ureteroceles present in numerous ways. In the past, urinary tract infection or a palpable abdominal mass was usually the first indication for urologic evaluation (Assadi et al). Today, these lesions are being recognized with increasing frequency on prenatal ultrasonography, allowing for appropriate evaluation, management decisions, and necessary surgery before infection or persisting obstruction aggravate the renal damage (Fig. 15–74) (Caione et al).

Cystic masses presenting at the urethral meatus are another manifestation of ureteroceles seen occasionally in the young female infant. These may represent either a prolapse of the ureterocele through the lumen of the urethra (Fig. 15–75) or a suburethral extension of the ureterocele with a blind distal sac (cecoureterocele). In most cases, the former condition is suggested by a tense, congested, ecchymotic lesion (Fig. 15–76) whereas the latter is often a simple cystic structure that is easily mistaken for a vaginal or periurethral cyst (Fig. 15–77).

Evaluation of the Infant with a Ureterocele

Ultrasonography is generally the initial screening study for children with urologic symptoms.

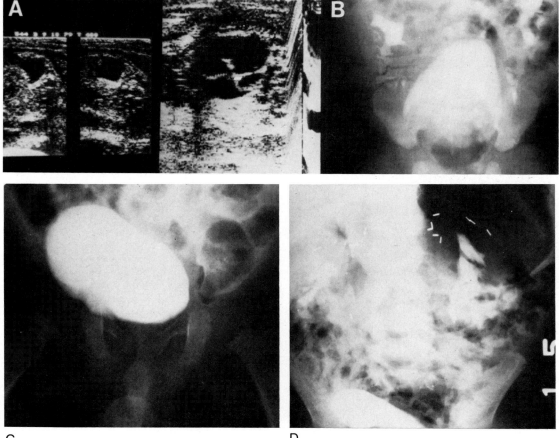

Figure 15–74 □ *A,* Prenatal ultrasonogram. On the left, one can see dilated kidneys bilaterally. On the right of the ultrasound scan, septations in the bladder, representing the walls of the ureteroceles, are evident. *B,* Postnatal excretory urogram shows absence of function in both upper poles and filling defects in the bladder. These proved to be ureteroceles associated with bilateral duplications. *C,* Postnatal cystogram in same patient as in *A.* The cystogram shows no evidence of vesicoureteral reflux. *D,* Postoperative excretory urogram, after bilateral upper pole heminephrectomy and partial ureterectomy, demonstrates good function of both lower segments. Both ureteroceles have collapsed. The patient had been observed for 7 years without further surgery. (From King LR: Urologic Surgery in Neonates and Young Infants. Philadelphia, WB Saunders Co, 1989.)

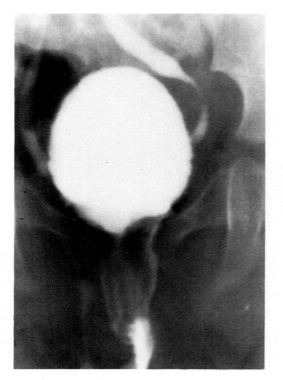

Figure 15–75 ☐ Prolapsing ureterocele. (From Hartman GW, Hodson CJ: The duplex kidney and related abnormalities. Clin Radiol 20:387–400, 1969. By permission of Dr. C. T. Hodson and E & S Livingstone.)

Figure 15–76 ☐ This figure demonstrates the congested, tense, and somewhat ecchymotic prolapsed ureterocele presenting as an interlabial mass. (From King LR: Urologic Surgery in Neonates and Young Infants. Philadelphia, WB Saunders Co, 1989.)

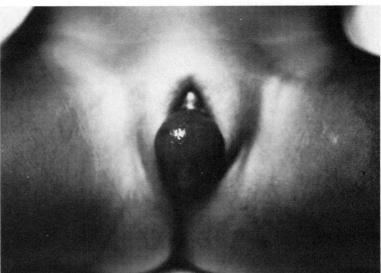

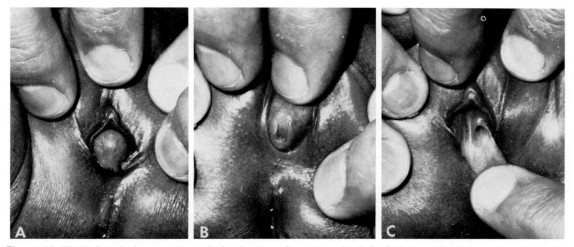

Figure 15–77 □ A typical cecoureterocele is shown as it presents in *A*. In *B*, it is pushed upward, revealing the hymenal ring below it. In *C*, one can see the urethra above the ureterocele. This ureterocele has a more natural coloration and demonstrates contrast between a prolapsed ureterocele and a cecoureterocele. (From King LR: Urologic Surgery in Neonates and Young Infants. Philadelphia, WB Saunders Co, 1989.)

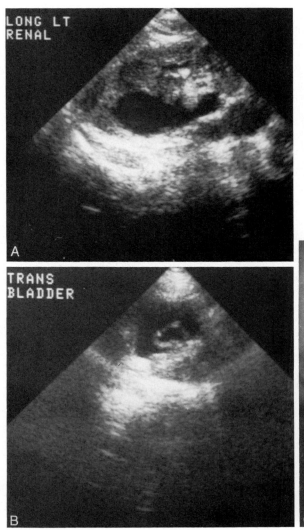

Figure 15–78 □ *A*, Renal ultrasonogram shows hydronephrosis of left upper segment in a 3-month-old girl admitted with urinary infection. *B*, Ultrasonogram of bladder clearly demonstrates dilated lower ureter and ureterocele. *C*, Excretory urogram suggests a left duplex ureter with a dilated upper segment but does not demonstrate the ureterocele nearly as well as the ultrasound scan.

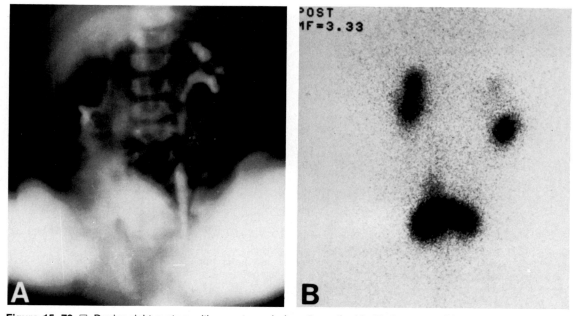

Figure 15–79 ☐ Duplex right system with a ureterocele in a 5-month-old girl. A tomographic cut of the intravenous pyelogram (A) shows typical nonvisualization of the right upper pole. Posterior view of a glucoheptanate renal scan (B) of the same patient shows poor function of the right upper pole. Also noted is an indentation in the base of the bladder that represents the ureterocele, which is not filled with radiopharmaceutical material. (From King LR: Urologic Surgery in Neonates and Young Infants. Philadelphia, WB Saunders Co, 1989.)

With this modality, a ureterocele can be clearly identified as a well-defined cystic mass within the bladder and often can be followed into a dilated ureter deep within the bony pelvis (Fig. 15–78) (Nussbaum et al; Seeds et al). The extent of hydronephrosis and the presence of a double collecting system are also generally visualized well on ultrasonography, and the thickness and echogenicity of the renal paren-chyma can be ascertained. (Cystic dysplasia is suggested by increased echogenicity when compared to normals for that age group.) Further diagnostic studies should include void-ing cystourethrography for the identification of vesicoureteral reflux into other ureteral seg-ments to assess whether the ureterocele has good detrusor backing and for evaluation of bladder neck obstruction. This study should be conducted with a straight catheter because the filled balloon on a Foley catheter can obscure or can be confused with the ureterocele. Renal scans should be obtained to assess function of all renal segments, but especially the renal unit associated with the ureterocele (Geringer et al). Isotopes that "fix" to the renal tubules (DMSA* or glucoheptonate) are preferred over agents handled entirely by filtration alone (DTPA†) because the former compounds

more clearly define focal areas of reduced or absent function in the kidney (Fig. 15–79).

Management

Management of ureteroceles in children is sur-gical in nearly all cases. Although some sur-geons pursue a specific operative approach because of personal bias, numerous options have been described because of the variety in pathology seen in association with ureteroceles (Scholtmeijer). Management might involve surgery at the renal level as well as surgery at the bladder level. The procedures may be done simultaneously or may be staged. A staged procedure may be planned, but it might also involve a "wait-and-see" approach in regard to whether the second procedure is necessary. Most large ureteroceles present in very young infants. Enthusiasm for aggressive, total recon-struction in this age group is often tempered by the technical considerations of an extensive dissection of a large ureterocele in a small, thin-walled bladder as well as by the fact that it is a lengthy procedure. In other cases, the ureterocele may obstruct the bladder neck and the patient may have a thickened, hypertro-phied detrusor muscle along with significant hydronephrosis. If ureteral reimplantation is

---

*DMSA, dimercaptosuccinic acid.

†DTPA, diethylenetriamine pentaacetic acid.

necessary in these situations, ureteral remodeling is likely to be required, substantially lengthening the operative time and increasing the possibility of postoperative complications (King). These concerns have generated different, and occasionally conflicting, opinions regarding management of ureteroceles in young children. A summary of all options is described below.

Management of the renal parenchymal abnormality (i.e., excision or salvage) is dependent primarily on the presence of a functioning renal parenchyma. This is influenced by the degree of dysplasia, hydronephrotic damage, and post-infectious atrophy and is determined preoperatively by the presence or absence of significant function on radionuclide scanning.

Single-System Ureteroceles

Most single-system ureteroceles are completely intravesical (Figs. 15–80 to 15–82). They generally subtend hydronephrotic, but salvageable, renal units. Traditionally, these anomalies in children have been managed by open transvesical excision of the ureterocele with ureteral reimplantation. For years, endoscopic incision has been the preferred approach in the adult, but since this procedure in children often resulted in the development of vesicoureteral reflux, its use was not popular in the pediatric age group (Sen and Ahmed; Snyder and Johnson). More recent experience,

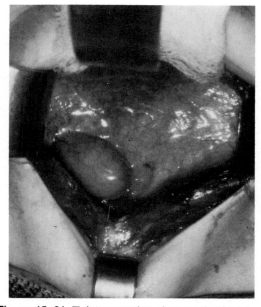

Figure 15–81 □ Intraoperative photograph of bilateral simple ureterocele.

though, with endoscopic incision has necessitated rethinking this traditional approach for the large single-system ureterocele. Even if reflux results after endoscopic incision, obstruction is relieved and there is usually a

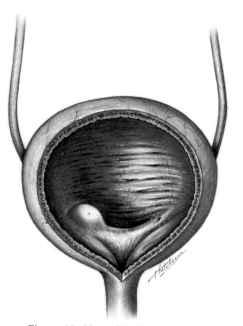

Figure 15–80 □ Simple ureterocele.

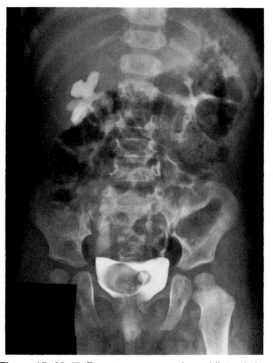

Figure 15–82 □ Excretory urogram shows bilateral simple ureteroceles associated with single systems.

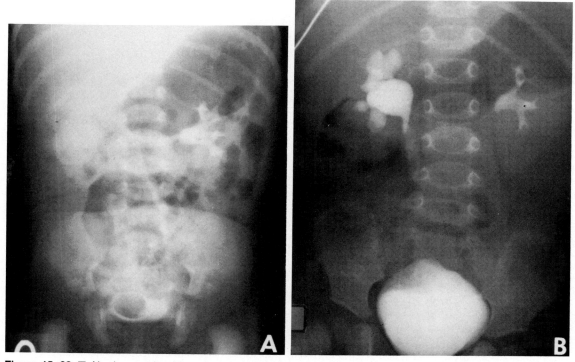

Figure 15–83 ☐ Newborn male with an intravesical, single system right ureterocele. *A,* Excretory urogram shows a hydronephrotic poorly visualized right collecting system with an obvious ureterocele in the bladder. *B,* After transurethral incision of the ureterocele, the hydronephrosis and visualization of the system have improved considerably. (From King LR: Urologic Surgery in Neonates and Young Infants. Philadelphia, WB Saunders Co, 1989.)

dramatic decrease in the dilatation of the obstructed ureter (Fig. 15–83). The risk of infection can be reduced, if not entirely eliminated, with maintenance chemoprophylaxis while reflux persists. If ureteral reimplantation is ultimately necessary, ureteral caliber is likely to be near normal and ureteral remodeling then may not be necessary.

However, vesicoureteral reflux is not inevitable after endoscopic incision (Monfort et al). Improved instrumentation now permits the surgeon to carefully incise the ureterocele on its side rather than in the midline in such a way that a flap is created which helps to prevent vesicoureteral reflux (Fig. 15–84) (Rich et al). In children, I now believe that intravesical single-system ureteroceles are best managed initially by endoscopic incision in nearly all cases in which there is an obstructed but salvageable kidney.

In most instances, the kidney functions promptly on renal scan and there is no question regarding whether this unit should be salvaged or not. In those unusual situations in which it is difficult to be sure how much function is present or how much recoverability is possible

after relieving obstruction, I believe endoscopic incision allows good drainage and time for recovery of the renal unit, is safe, and is preferable to other forms of temporary diver-

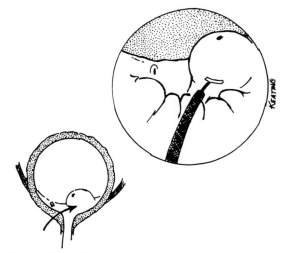

Figure 15–84 ☐ Endoscopic management of single-system ureteroceles. (From Rich MA, Keating MA, Snyder HM, Duckett JW: Low transurethral incision of single system intravesical ureteroceles in children. J Urol *144:*120, 1990. © by Williams & Wilkins, 1990.)

sion (loop cutaneous ureterostomy or percutaneous nephrostomy) or primary ureteral reimplantation. If sufficient recoverability does not occur, it may be that no further therapy will be required if reflux is not present or, alternatively, a simple nephroureterectomy can be done later.

When a single-system ureterocele is extravesical in location, the associated kidney is often dysplastic (poorly functioning or non-

functioning on renal scan) and nonsalvageable. In most cases, a simple nephroureterectomy without opening the bladder is sufficient to collapse the ureterocele and relieve any bladder outlet obstruction that may be present (Fig. 15–85). More complex ureteroceles may present as cystic lesions within the prostatic urethra necessitating innovative management if the lesion is significantly obstructive (Fig. 15–86). In most instances, these lesions should

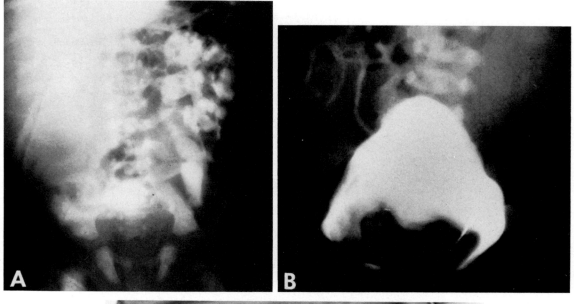

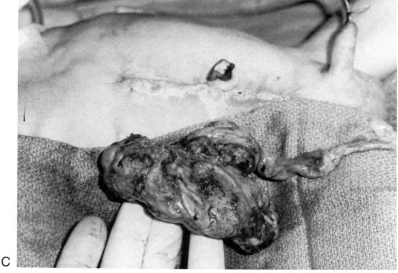

Figure 15–85 □ Newborn male with large, single system ureterocele on the right side. *A,* Excretory urogram shows poor visualization of the right collecting system and a hydronephrotic left side. *B,* Cystogram of same patient shows a large ureterocele filling the bladder and extending through the bladder neck. *C,* At operation, the kidney was shown to be grossly dysplastic and hydronephrotic. A nephroureterectomy was performed with extravesical dissection of the single system ureterocele.

Illustration continued on following page

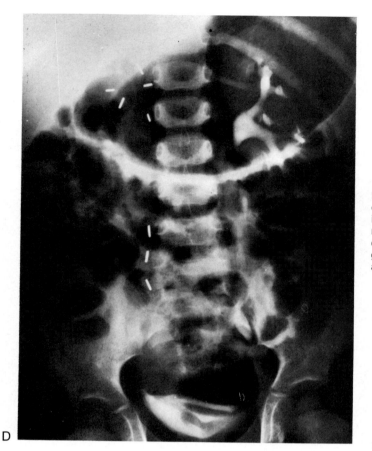

D

Figure 15–85 ☐ *Continued D*, The postoperative excretory urogram shows significant improvement of the left-sided hydronephrosis after the ureterocele has collapsed. (From King LR: Urologic Surgery in Neonates and Young Infants. Philadelphia, WB Saunders Co, 1989.)

collapse with a nephroureterectomy and extravesical decompression alone. If the urethral component remains distended and causes persisting urethral obstruction, endoscopic incision may be necessary. In this case, the surgeon must be very careful not to leave a lip of tissue on the distal margin of the ureterocele that can act like a urethral valve.

Ureteroceles Associated with Duplicated Systems

Several options are available for treating the ureterocele associated with complete ureteral duplication. These procedures can be conveniently divided into two broad areas: management of the renal anomaly and upper ureter,

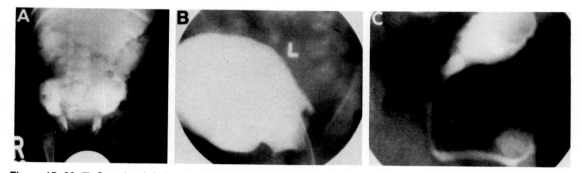

Figure 15–86 ☐ Complex, left single system, extravesical ureterocele in a newborn male. Excretory urogram *(A)* shows nonvisualization of the left kidney and hydronephrosis on the right. A filling cystogram *(B)* and voiding urethrogram *(C)* reveal a ureterocele with both intravesical and extravesical components. The left kidney was dysplastic. (From King LR: Urologic Surgery in Neonates and Young Infants. Philadelphia, WB Saunders Co, 1989.)

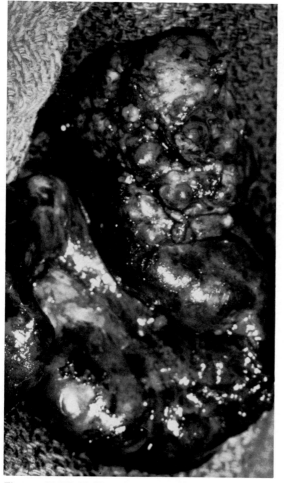

Figure 15–87 □ The obvious cystic dysplasia of the upper pole of this kidney is easily perceived upon inspection. (From King LR: Urologic Surgery in Neonates and Young Infants. Philadelphia, WB Saunders Co, 1989.)

and management of the lower ureter and ureterocele.

Management of the renal parenchymal anomaly is dependent primarily on the extent of renal dysplasia, which is present to some degree in a majority of children with ureteroceles (Fig. 15–87) (Mandell et al). Preoperatively, significant dysplasia can be suggested on IVP (nonfunction) or ultrasonography (hyperechoic renal tissue) but is best evaluated by DMSA or glucoheptonate radionuclide scanning. Visual inspection, with biopsy in some cases at the time of surgery, is ultimately the final determining factor. Although there is universal agreement that a nonfunctioning dysplastic segment should be excised (by upper segment nephrectomy), there is continuing

controversy regarding the appropriate management of a functioning but hydronephrotic upper polar unit. Salvaging renal tissue is attractive, and ureteropyelostomy (or ureteroureterostomy) is an accepted and generally successful procedure (Fig. 15–88). However, these abnormal upper segments represent a very small portion of the patient's total renal mass. In addition, the upper segment ureter is often very dilated and anastomosis of this large, thick-walled ureter to a delicate lower segment pelvis or ureter can be quite difficult. Surgery to save a small upper segment can risk the larger and usually healthy lower pole if a ureteral stricture develops at the anastomosis. For this reason, I prefer to perform an upper segment nephrectomy in the majority of children with duplication anomalies. Caldamone and associates have reported a similar experience and management philosophy with uniform success.

During upper segment nephrectomy, it may be necessary to mobilize the kidney substantially to adequately isolate the segmental renal blood supply and to control bleeding from the cut surface of the renal parenchyma. During this dissection it is important not to stretch the renal pedicle excessively. In the young infant, especially, intimal tears can sometimes occur, resulting in subintimal dissection and arterial thrombosis with eventual atrophy of the entire kidney (Fig. 15–89).

The main controversy in managing ureteroceles subtending an upper pole segment involves the question of whether anything need be done to the distal segment of upper pole ureter and collapsed ureterocele after heminephroureterectomy. Ordinarily, after only an upper segment nephrectomy, bladder outlet obstruction abates and secondary ureteral dilatation improves (Fig. 15–90). Even vesicoureteral reflux may resolve, although that is inconsistent and not to be expected. The patient may do well with no further surgery. However, not all of these ureteroceles have strong detrusor backing and some of them appear on cystography, when collapsed, like a bladder diverticulum. Urinary infection can be a continuing problem, and further reconstruction may be necessary. Because of these uncertainties, several options in management have been proposed:

1. An initial endoscopic unroofing of the ureterocele with secondary total reconstruction (management of the upper renal segment,

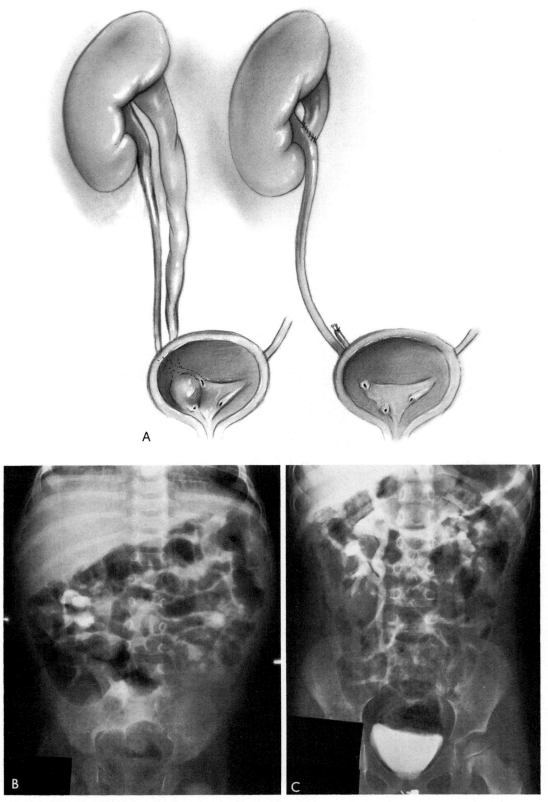

Figure 15–88 □ *A,* Ureteropyelostomy for treatment of ectopic ureterocele. *B,* Excretory urogram. Bilateral duplication and ectopic ureteroceles. Poorly functioning hydronephrosis, upper segment on right, salvageable according to DMSA scan. *C,* Excretory urogram after right ureteropyelostomy, left upper heminephrectomy, and bilateral subtotal ureterectomy. Note return of function in upper segment on right and collapse of both ureteroceles.

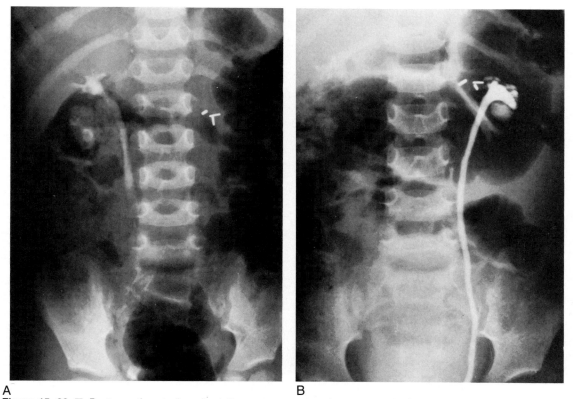

A   B

Figure 15–89 □ Postoperative studies after left upper segment nephrectomy and partial ureterectomy. The excretory urogram *(A)* does not show any contrast excretion by the remaining lower pole of the kidney, which had been well visualized prior to surgery. A retrograde pyelogram *(B)* demonstrates a shrunken unobstructed lower pole moiety. This is an example of a vascular injury to a lower pole moiety at the time of upper pole heminephrectomy. (From King LR: Urologic Surgery in Neonates and Young Infants. Philadelphia, WB Saunders Co, 1989.)

excision of ureterocele remains, reconstruction of the bladder defect, ureteral reimplantation), or

2. An initial upper (renal) procedure, usually a partial nephrectomy, and one of the following:
   a. Subtotal ureterectomy only,
   b. Total ureterectomy and partial excision of the ureterocele extravesically, or
   c. Primary total reconstruction.

Each of these concepts is discussed individually, as each approach has separate advantages and disadvantages.

Endoscopic incision of a ureterocele (or, occasionally, direct incision when the ureterocele is prolapsed through the urethra) is an easy and effective way to decompress the upper urinary tract in infants (Cobb et al; Gerridzen and Schillinger). Its main drawback is that a previously "obstructed" system is almost always converted into a massively refluxing one—into a very dilated, atonic, and dysplastic ureter (Fig. 15–91). Because of this, uretero-

cele incision has not been looked upon favorably in the recent past by most surgeons interested in this problem. Tank, however, has reported a series of children in whom internal decompression (endoscopic incision or open unroofing) of ureteroceles was performed routinely as initial management and was ultimately associated with very favorable results. Although reflux occurred in most, as expected, infection was readily controlled with chemoprophylaxis after decompression and reconstruction of the ureterocele defect was accomplished, when indicated, electively and in an older child. Of particular interest was the observation that one half of the renal segments that showed no function initially on IVP demonstrated some excretion of contrast material after internal decompression. Although uncontrolled, the data suggest that endoscopic incision in the very young infant allows for recovery of renal function in some instances and might therefore encourage salvage of some obstructed upper poles that otherwise might have been removed. Unfortunately, radio-

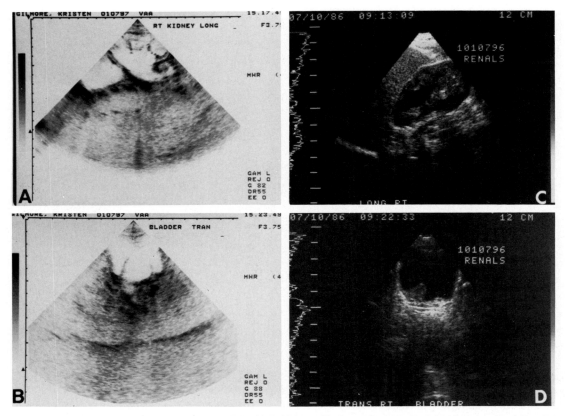

Figure 15–90 □ Preoperative ultrasonogram of the right kidney *(A)* shows hydronephrosis of both segments of the kidney. The bladder view of this ultrasound examination *(B)* shows the wall of the ureterocele clearly. Postoperatively, after right upper pole heminephrectomy, the hydronephrosis of the lower pole moiety has considerably improved *(C)* and the ureterocele has collapsed down to be only a small remnant that one can visualize in the bladder view *(D)*. (From King LR: Urologic Surgery in Neonates and Young Infants. Philadelphia, WB Saunders Co, 1989.)

nuclide scans were not obtained routinely in these children and evidence of excretion of intravenous radiographic contrast material does not always correlate well with the level of renal function.

Despite this encouraging report, one must be cautioned, I believe, about using this procedure routinely, because once vesicoureteral reflux is established, essentially all of these infants will some day require a lower, complete reconstruction of the bladder with excision of the ureterocele and ureteral reimplantations—procedures I believe are not necessary in every case. Perhaps some day, endoscopic correction of reflux will lessen this need for open surgery, although this particular anti-reflux procedure is not yet universally accepted (Diamond and Boston). I believe that this approach should be reserved for the very young infant with sepsis that is unresponsive to intensive antibiotic therapy, for the infant with a prolapsing ureterocele, or for associated massive vesico-

ureteral reflux into an ipsilateral lower pole ureter or into contralateral ureters. In these situations, it has been my experience that complete reconstruction of the ureterocele anomaly is ultimately necessary in nearly all cases. Primary endoscopic decompression does allow the surgeon to delay this major repair in a very young infant.

Total ureterocele excision and reconstruction of the bladder neck may become a formidable, lengthy operation in a baby. In addition to the fact that bilateral ureteral reimplantations are commonly necessary and may necessitate tailoring, the ureterocele often extends well down into the urethra. If the ureterocele is not totally incised and if the bladder mucosa is not carefully repaired, a free flap along the posterior urethra may be created that functions like a urethral valve and obstructs voiding (Ashcraft and Hendren). On the other hand, aggressive ureterocele excision may damage the bladder neck and urethral

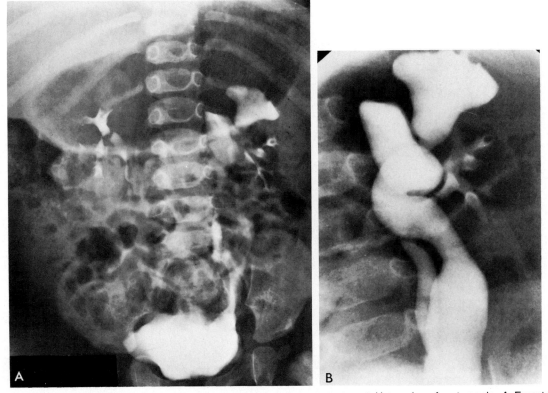

Figure 15-91 □ Duplication on left, with ectopic ureterocele in upper segment. Uncapping of ureterocele. *A,* Excretory urogram. *B,* Cystogram. Reflux into both ureters.

sphincter mechanism or result in damage to the vagina, with the possible development of a vesicovaginal fistula. Although some experienced surgeons have reported good success with this approach and believe that ureterocele excision is an essential aspect of management (Brock and Kaplan; Hendren and Mitchell; Hendren and Monfort; Scherz et al; Williams and Woodard), it is my feeling, as discussed below, that an intravesical procedure is not necessary in each case.

Another approach for total reconstruction of ureteroceles with duplex ureters is to perform either a lower ureteroureterostomy or a common sheath reimplantation along with ureterocele excision (Amar). Although this approach allows the entire surgical procedure to be done through a single lower abdominal incision, these procedures have not gained general favor among urologists interested in ureteroceles. One of the drawbacks of this approach is that the upper segment is not visualized directly and thus very dysplastic tissue might be preserved. In addition, with lower ureteroureterostomy one might theoret-

ically be concerned that such an anastomosis would result in a situation in which yo-yo reflux could promote continued urinary stasis and urinary infection.

Because of these concerns, some surgeons have looked for less extensive means of managing these defects, especially in the very young infant. At diagnosis, ureteroceles may be very large and undermine and distort the trigone and bladder neck. They may prolapse into the bladder neck and cause bladder neck obstruction. However, once the upper segment of the kidney is detached from the ureterocele, the ureterocele collapses and becomes no more than a bit of redundant mucosa on the bladder floor (Fig. 15-92). After upper pole heminephrectomy, obstruction is generally relieved and the child should be able to void normally. In addition, any obstruction to ipsilateral or contralateral ureters will abate (Figs. 15-93 and 15-94). In some cases, mild reflux into the other ureters resolves, although new reflux can also be demonstrated on postoperative cystography (Figs. 15-95 and 15-96) (Uehling and Bruskewitz).

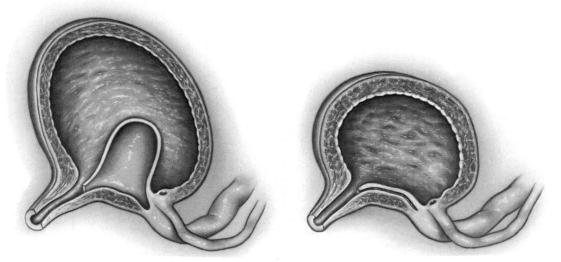

Figure 15–92 □ Schematic drawing of ectopic ureterocele before and after heminephrectomy and subtotal ureterectomy, showing collapse of ureterocele.

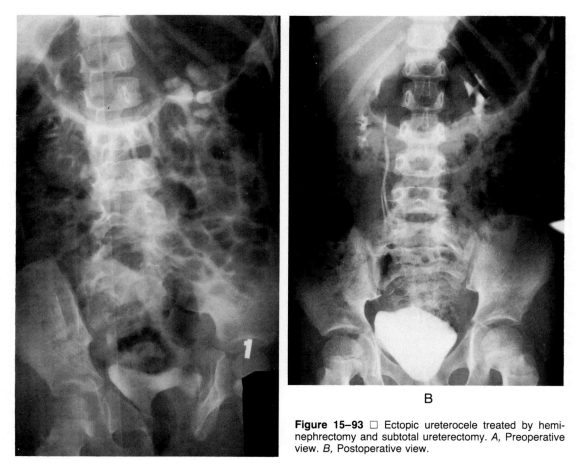

A

B

Figure 15–93 □ Ectopic ureterocele treated by heminephrectomy and subtotal ureterectomy. *A,* Preoperative view. *B,* Postoperative view.

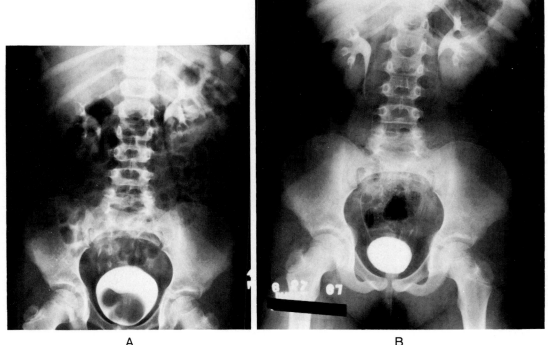

A   B

Figure 15–94 □ Ectopic ureterocele treated by heminephrectomy and subtotal ureterectomy. *A,* Preoperative view. *B,* Postoperative view.

Some pitfalls do remain, however. Sometimes the muscle behind the ureterocele is thinned and weakened and without repair forms a bladder diverticulum during voiding (Fig. 15–97). In addition, one must be aware of the possibility of a cecoureterocele (Balchick and Nasrallah) (Fig. 15–98). These unique ureteroceles have a ureteral meatus that is often patulous and within the bladder, but with a long, blind suburethral extension. During voiding, the ureterocele may fill by reflux, distending the suburethral extension and obstructing the bladder neck (Fig. 15–99). The degree of obstruction to the bladder neck at times seems to get worse in some cases after the distensible upper ureter and renal pelvis are excised. Despite these occasional drawbacks, excision of an infected, nonfunctioning, upper segment and relief of stasis by removal of the dilated ureter and decompression of the ureterocele generally results in a healthy child who can undergo a second-stage bladder level reconstruction electively when necessary. Two variations on this theme are now practiced.

Belman and colleagues originally proposed that upper segment heminephrectomy and subtotal ureterectomy through a subcostal or flank incision only was satisfactory (curative) for a majority of patients with ureteroceles and sev-

eral authors have adopted this approach (Hanson et al; King et al, 1983; Sen, 1987). In an infant, nearly all of the ureter can be excised in this fashion. In an older child, the dissection usually stops at about the level of the iliac vessels. If there is reflux into the ureter, it is simply tied off. If there is no reflux, the ureter is left open and a drain is left at the ureteral stump. The ureterocele then decompresses out the ureteral stump until this seals. With this approach, somewhere between 10 and 50 per cent of children require a second procedure to correct reflux and to complete ureterocele excision and reconstruction of the bladder neck (Barrett et al; Caldamone et al). Several factors are predictive of the possibility of requiring further surgical intervention:

1. Persistence of significant vesicoureteral reflux.
2. A remaining distal piece of upper segment ureter that is long and dilated.
3. Poor detrusor backing behind the ureterocele.

Although some may argue that this high percentage of patients requiring a second operation justifies a planned one-stage repair, the second-stage reconstruction is often much easier technically than if the bladder recon-

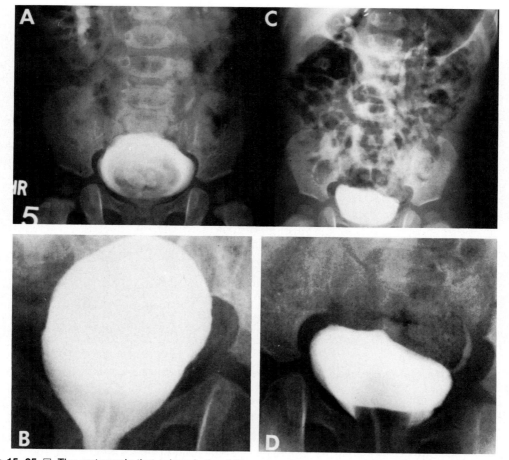

Figure 15–95 □ The ureterocele that subtends the right upper pole segment is clearly seen in *(A)*. Cystogram of the same patient *(B)* shows no preoperative reflux. Postoperatively, after upper pole heminephrectomy on the right and partial ureterectomy, there is good function of the right lower pole *(C)*. The ureterocele has collapsed. The interesting finding *(D)* is the appearance of low-grade contralateral reflux after the ureterocele has collapsed. (From King LR: Urologic Surgery in Neonates and Young Infants. Philadelphia, WB Saunders Co, 1989.)

struction is done at the time of the hemine-phrectomy. Hydroureters generally decompress after the first operation, a thickened bladder wall should decrease, and, in my experience, the limits of the collapsed uretero-cele are more easily defined than when it is tense and distended.

Kroovand and Perlmutter have proposed a somewhat more aggressive, although still limited, approach to reconstruction of uretero-celes (Kroovand; Kroovand and Perlmutter). After appropriate management of the parenchymal anomaly, the ureter is excised in total, usually through two separate incisions (flank and transverse suprapubic). Dissection must be carefully performed and must stay right on the adventitia of the upper segment ureter lest the common vascular tissue between the two ureters be damaged and the remaining lower

pole ureter be rendered ischemic. In addition, if the ureterocele extends beyond the bladder neck, there is a risk of damaging the urethra or vagina. But with care and experience, one can identify the ureteral wall and excise some of the ureterocele extravesically without opening the bladder mucosa (Fig. 15–100). To date, no second-stage procedures were required in the nine children reported in this study. I have found the above-mentioned procedure technically difficult in the very small infant and have violated the bladder mucosa during dissection of the ureterocele extravesically. If this occurs, it is important to be sure that a blind-ending suburethral extension, which could obstruct voiding, is not left behind, and I have then opened the bladder and converted these procedures to total excision of the ureterocele transvesically.

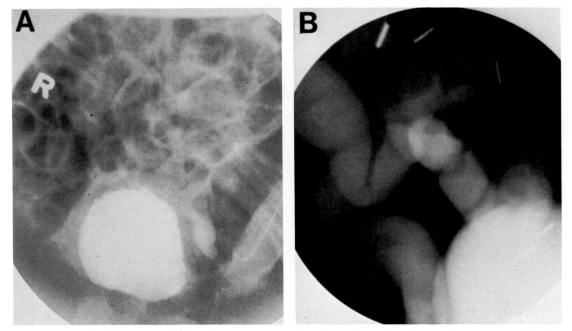

Figure 15–96 □ Ureterocele subtending left upper segment in a 2-month-old girl. Preoperative cystogram *(A)* shows some filling of the distal left lower pole ureter. After left upper pole heminephrectomy and partial ureterectomy, cystogram *(B)* demonstrates massive bilateral vesicoureteral reflux. (From King LR: Urologic Surgery in Neonates and Young Infants. Philadelphia, WB Saunders Co, 1989.)

Summary of Ureterocele Repair

When the surgeon is challenged with managing a ureterocele in a newborn or very young infant, I believe the primary principle should be to do only as much surgery as is necessary to relieve outflow obstruction, improve urinary stasis, and maintain an uninfected, healthy, growing child. In my opinion, an elective staged reconstruction is preferred over primary, total reconstruction in nearly all cases in this age group (Decter et al). With this philosophy in mind, I have adhered to the

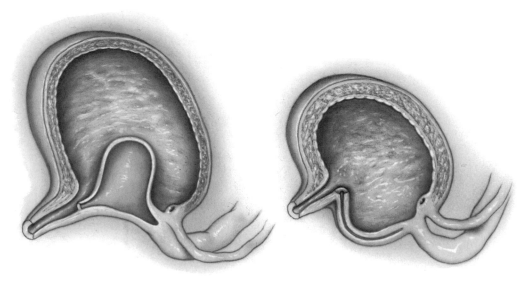

Figure 15–97 □ Schematic drawing of ureterocele with poor backing and conversion to diverticulum.

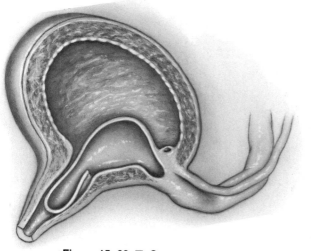

Figure 15–98 □ Cecoureterocele.

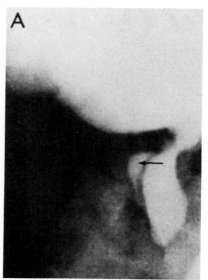

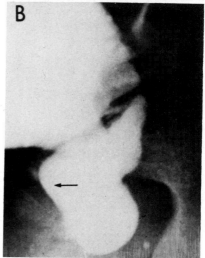

Figure 15–99 □ Cecoureterocele. Micturition cystoure-throgram of a child aged 3 years, showing opaque medium filling the tongue of the cecoureterocele and compressing the urethra *(arrows)* early *(A)* and late *(B)* during efforts to void. (Courtesy of Dr. F.D. Stephens.)

following guidelines for managing the child with ureteral duplication with a ureterocele:

1. Endoscopic incision of the ureterocele is considered as primary treatment for infants with:
   a. Urinary infection not responding to appropriate chemotherapy.
   b. Prolapsing ureteroceles.
   c. Severe vesicoureteral reflux into other ureteral segments.
   d. Small ureteroceles with salvageable upper segments where endoscopic incision might be definitive therapy if reflux does not result.

In my experience, children with prolapse or massive reflux have always required a definitive bladder reconstruction ultimately anyway.

2. For those ureteroceles with only mild associated reflux or with obstruction alone to other segments, I prefer upper pole heminephrectomy and partial ureterectomy through a single flank incision. In about half of the children, an upper procedure alone is all that appears necessary. In the other half, a ureterocelectomy and bladder reconstruction is ultimately required, but in my experience it has been elective and with less need for extensive lower ureteral remodeling.

Clearly, no single approach is appropriate for all children with ureteroceles. Each case must be individualized. These principles, though, have been successful in my hands when dealing with this complex anomaly in the infant.

TRIPLICATION OF THE URETER

Complete triplication of the ureter is one of the rarest anomalies in the upper urinary tract. Most cases are trifid ureters. The condition occurs more often on the left side and in females. It may be asymptomatic, being detected only during investigation of the other abnormalities that frequently are present. Triplicate ureters also may be responsible for infection, incontinence, or pain. Surgical treatment, when necessary, depends on the specific

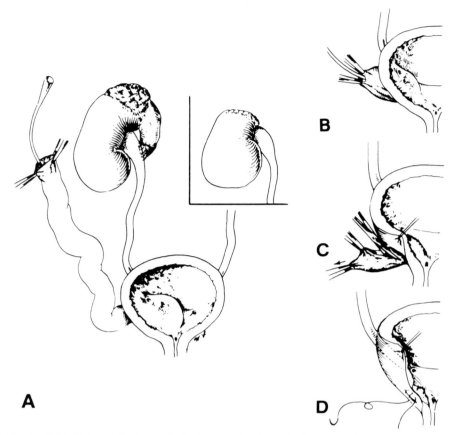

A

B

C

D

Figure 15–100 □ Kroovand and Perlmutter's technique of extravesical ureterocele excision. *A,* Inset shows the situation after either upper pole heminephrectomy or ureteroureterostomy. The lower portion of the upper pole ureter is cannulated with a straight catheter and subsequently excised completely through a second incision. The extravesical dissection of the ureterocele is demonstrated (*B* and *C*), and after its complete removal the detrusor muscle is coapted (*D*). This is another alternative to the management of the ureterocele. (Reprinted with permission from Kroovand RL, Perlmutter AD: A one-stage surgical approach to ectopic ureterocele. J Urol 122:367, 1979. © by Williams & Wilkins, 1979.)

problems in individual cases. Parvinen found a total of 23 cases of complete triplication. Ureteral quadruplication is exceedingly rare but has been reported (Soderdahl et al).

Bibliography

Ahmed S, Pope R: Uncrossed complete ureteral duplication with upper system reflux. J Urol 135:128, 1986.

Amar AD: Ipsilateral ureteroureterostomy for single ureteral disease in patients with ureteral duplication: a review of eight years of experience with sixteen patients. J Urol 119:472, 1978.

Amis ES, Cronan JJ, Pfister RD: Lower moiety hydronephrosis in duplicated kidneys. Urology 26:82, 1985.

Arey LB: Developmental Anatomy: A Textbook and Laboratory Manual of Embryology, 7th ed. Philadelphia, WB Saunders Co, 1974.

Ashcraft KW, Hendren WH: Bladder outlet obstruction after operation for ureterocele. J Pediatr Surg 14:819, 1979.

Assadi F, Caldamone A, Cornfield D, et al: Ureteroceles in children: clinical study and report of 58 cases. Clin Nephrol 21:275, 1984.

Babcock JR Jr, Belman AB, Shkolnik A, et al: Familial ureteral duplication and ureterocele. Urology 9:345, 1977.

Balchick RJ, Nasrallah PF: Cecoureterocele. J Urol 137:100, 1987.

Barrett DM, Malek RS, Kelalis PP: Problems and solutions in surgical treatment of 100 consecutive ureteral duplications in children. J Urol 114:126, 1975.

Belman AB, Filmer RB, King LR: Surgical management of duplication of the collecting system. J Urol 112:316, 1974.

Bisset GS, Strife JL: The duplex collecting system in girls with urinary tract infection: prevalence and significance. AJR Am J Roentgenol 148:497, 1987.

Brock WA, Kaplan GW: Ectopic ureteroceles in children. J Urol 119:800, 1978.

Caione P, Zaccara A, Capozza N, De-Gennaro M: How prenatal ultrasound can affect the treatment of ureterocele in neonates and children. Eur Urol 16:195, 1989.

Caldamone AA, Snyder HM, Duckett JW: Ureteroceles in children: follow-up of management with upper tract approach. J Urol 131:1130, 1984.

Campbell JE: Ureteral peristalsis in duplex renal collecting systems. Am J Roentgenol Radium Ther Nucl Med 99:577, 1967.

Campbell MF: Clinical Pediatric Urology. Philadelphia, WB Saunders Co, 1951.

Cendron J, Melin Y, Valayer J: Simplified treatment of ectopic ureterocele in 35 children. Eur Urol 7:321, 1981.

Chwalla R: The process of formation of cystic dilation of the vesical end of the ureter and of diverticula at the ureteral ostium. Urol Cutan Ren 31:499, 1927.

Cobb LM, Desai PG, Price SE: Surgical management of infantile (ectopic) ureteroceles: report of a modified approach. J Pediatr Surg 17:745, 1982.

Coughlan JD: Blind ending branch of a trifid ureter. Urol Radiol 7:172, 1985.

Cox CE, Hutch JA: Bilateral single ectopic ureter: a report of 2 cases and review of the literature. J Urol 95:493, 1966.

Culp OS: Ureteral diverticulum, classification of the literature and report of an authentic case. J Urol 58:308, 1947.

Decter RM, Roth DR, Gonzales ET: Individualized treatment of ureterocele. J Urol 142:535, 1989.

Diamond T, Boston VE: Reflux following endoscopic treatment of ureteroceles: a new approach using endoscopic subureteric Teflon injection. Br J Urol 60:279, 1987.

Ericsson NO: Ectopic ureterocele in infants and children: a clinical study. Acta Chir Scand 197 (Suppl):1, 1954.

Fehrenbaker LG, Kelalis PP, Stickler GB: Vesicoureteral reflux and ureteral duplication in children. J Urol 107:862, 1972.

Geringer AM, Berdon WE, Seldin DW, Hensle TW: The diagnostic approach to ectopic ureterocele and the renal duplication complex. J Urol 129:539, 1983.

Gerridzen R, Schillinger JF: Transurethral puncture in management of ectopic ureteroceles. Urology 23:43, 1984.

Glassberg KI, Braren V, Duckett JW, et al: Suggested terminology for duplex systems, ectopic ureters, and ureteroceles. J Urol 132:1153, 1984.

Gross RD, Clatworthy WH: Ureterocele in infancy and childhood. Pediatrics 5:58, 1950.

Hanson E, Enger EA, Hjalmas K: Heminephrectomy-ureterectomy as the sole procedure in ectopic uretero-cele in children. Z Kinderchir 39:355, 1984.

Hartman GW, Hodson CJ: The duplex kidney and related abnormalities. Clin Radiol 20:387, 1969.

Hendren WH, Monfort FJ: Surgical correction of ureteroceles in childhood. J Pediatr Surg 6:235, 1971.

Hendren WH, Mitchell ME: Surgical correction of ureteroceles. J Urol 121:590, 1979.

Jona JZ, Glicklich M, Cohen RD: Ectopic single ureter and severe renal dysplasia: an unusual presentation. Urology 121:369, 1979.

Kaplan N, Elkin M: Bifid renal pelves and ureters: radiographic and cinefluorographic observations. Br J Urol 40:235, 1968.

Keane TE, Fitzgerald RJ: Blind-ending duplex ureter. Br J Urol 60:275, 1987.

Kesavan P, Ramakrishnan MS, Fowler R: Ectopia in unduplicated ureters in children. Br J Urol 49:481, 1977.

King LR, Koglowski JM, Schacht MJ: Ureteroceles in children: a simplified and successful approach to management. JAMA 249:1461, 1983.

Kroovand RL: Ureterocele. Urol Clin North Am 10:445, 1983.

Kroovand RL, Perlmutter AD: A one-stage approach to ectopic ureterocele. J Urol 122:367, 1979.

Lenaghan D: Bifid ureters in children: an anatomical, physiological and clinical study. J Urol 87:808, 1962.

Lund AJ: Uncrossed double ureter with rare intravesical orifice relationship: case report with review of literature. J Urol 62:22, 1949.

Macki GG, Stephens FD: Duplex kidneys: a correlation of renal dysplasia with position of ureteral orifice. J Urol 114:274, 1975.

Malek RS, Kelalis PP, Stickler GB, et al: Observations on ureteral ectopy in children. J Urol 107:308, 1972.

Mandell J, Colodny AH, Lebowitz R, et al: Ureteroceles in infants and children. J Urol 123:921, 1980.

Marshall FF, McLoughlin MG: Long blind-ending ureteral duplications. J Urol 120:626, 1978.

Meyer R: Zur Anatomie und Entwicklungsgeschichte der Ureterverdoppelung. Virchow's Arch (Pathol Anat) 87:408, 1907.

Monfort G, Morrisson-Lacombe G, Coquet M: Endoscopic treatment of ureteroceles revisited. J Urol 133:1031, 1985.

Muller SC, Riedmiller H, Walz PH, Hohenfellner R: Blind-ending bifid ureter with an intravesical ectopic orifice. Eur Urol 10:416, 1984.

Musselman BC, Barry JJ: Varying degrees of ureteral ectopia and duplication in 5 siblings. J Urol 110:476, 1973.

Nation EF: Duplication of the kidney and ureter: a statistical study of 230 new cases. J Urol 51:456, 1944.

Nordmark B: Double formations of the pelves of the kidneys and the ureters: embryology, occurrence and clinical significance. Acta Radiol 30:267, 1948.

Nussbaum AR, Dorst JP, Jeffs RD, et al: Ectopic ureter and ureteroceles: their varied sonographic manifestations. Radiology 159:227, 1986.

O'Reilly PH, Shields RA, Testa HJ, et al: Ureteroureteric reflux. Pathological entity or physiological phenomenon? Br J Urol 56:159, 1984.

Parvinen T: Complete ureteral triplication. J Pediatr Surg 11:1039, 1976.

Passerini GG, Calabro A, Aragona F, et al: Blind ureterocele. Eur Urol 12:331, 1986.

Peppos DS, Skoog SJ, Canning DA, Belman AB: Non-surgical management of primary vesicoureteral reflux in complete ureteral duplication: is it justified? Submitted.

Rich MA, Keating MA, Snyder HM, Duckett JW: Low transurethral incision of single system intravesical ureteroceles in children. J Urol 144:120, 1990.

Scherz HC, Kaplan GW, Packer MG, Brock WA: Ectopic ureteroceles: surgical management with preservation of continence—review of 60 cases. J Urol 142:538, 1989.

Scholtmeijer RJ: Surgical treatment of ureteroceles in childhood—a reappraisal. Z Kinderchir 42:103, 1987.

Schulman CC: The single ectopic ureter. Eur Urol 2:64, 1976.

Seeds JW, Mittelstaedt CA, Mandell J: Pre- and postnatal ultrasonographic diagnosis of congenital obstructive uropathies. Urol Clin North Am 13:131, 1986.

Sen S, Ahmed S: Management of double system uretero-cele. Aust NZ J Surg 57:655, 1987.

Sen S, Ahmed S: Single system ureteroceles in childhood. Aust NZ J Surg 58:903, 1988.

Snyder HM, Johnson JH: Orthotopic ureteroceles in children. J Urol 119:543, 1978.

Soderdahl DW, Shiraki IW, Schamber DT: Bilateral ureteral quadruplication. J Urol 116:255, 1976.

Sole GM, Randall J, Arkell DG: Ureteropyelostomy: a simple and effective treatment for symptomatic ureter-oureteric reflux. Br J Urol 60:325, 1987.

Stephens FD: Anatomical vagaries of double ureters. Aust NZ J Surg 28:27, 1958.

Stephens FD: Caecoureterocele and concepts on the embryology and aetiology of ureteroceles. Aust NZ J Surg 40:239, 1971.

Stephens FD: Congenital Malformations of the Rectum, Anus, and Genitourinary Tracts. London and Edinburgh, Livingstone, 1963, p. 187.

Stephens FD: Congenital Malformations of the Urinary Tract. New York, Praeger, 1983, p 320–322, 329.

Tanagho EA: Embryogenic basis for lower ureteral anomalies: a hypothesis. Urology 7:451, 1976.

Tank ES: Experience with endoscopic incision and open unroofing of ureteroceles. J Urol 136:241, 1986.

Timothy RP, Decter A, Perlmutter AD: Ureteral duplication: clinical findings and therapy in 46 children. J Urol 105:445, 1971.

Tokunaka S, Gotoh T, Koyanagi T, Tsuji I: The morphological study of ureterocele: a possible clue to its embryogenesis as evidenced by a locally arrested myogenesis. J Urol 126:726, 1981.

Uehling DT, Bruskewitz RC: Initiation of vesicoureteral reflux after heminephrectomy for ureterocele. Urology 33:302, 1989.

Uson AC: A classification of ureteroceles in children. J Urol 85:732, 1961.

Uson AC, Schulman CC: Ectopic ureter emptying into the rectum: report of a case. J Urol 108:156, 1972.

Weigert C: Uber einige Bildungsfehler der Ureteren. Virchow's Arch (Pathol Anat) 70:490, 1877.

Weiss JP: Embryogenesis of ureteral anomalies: a unifying theory. Aust NZ J Surg 58:631, 1988.

Weiss JP, Duckett JW, Snyder HM: Single unilateral vaginal ectopic ureter: is it really a rarity? J Urol 132:1177, 1984.

Whitaker J, Danks DM: A study of the inheritance of duplication of the kidneys and ureters. J Urol 95:176, 1966.

Williams DI, Lightwood RG: Bilateral single ectopic ureters. Br J Urol 44:267, 1972.

Williams DI, Woodard JR: Problems in the management of ectopic ureteroceles. J Urol 92:635, 1964.

Young HH, Frentz WA: Congenital obstruction of the posterior urethra. J Urol 3:289, 1919.

BLADDER AND URACHAL ABNORMALITIES: THE EXSTROPHY-EPISPADIAS COMPLEX

John P. Gearhart

The variants of the exstrophy-epispadias complex of genitourinary malformations can be as simple as glandular epispadias or an overwhelming multisystem defect such as cloacal exstrophy. This subchapter deals mainly with the surgical management of bladder exstrophy, cloacal exstrophy, and epispadias. Other conditions involving the bladder are also discussed, but a detailed approach to the management of the exstrophy-epispadias complex and the results of such therapy are emphasized.

The primary objectives in the surgical management of bladder exstrophy are to obtain (1) secure abdominal wall closure, (2) urinary continence with the preservation of renal function, and (3) reconstruction of a functional and cosmetically acceptable penis in the male. These objectives can be achieved with primary bladder closure, bladder neck reconstruction, and epispadias repair. Although many reconstructive techniques have been described, a unified approach to the surgical management of this disorder has only recently evolved because all modalities formerly were associated with a substantial failure rate and, at times, unacceptable operative morbidity.

Formerly, surgical reconstruction of cloacal exstrophy, the most severe variant of the exstrophy-epispadias complex, was considered futile. However, advances in anesthesia, neonatal care, and nutrition, along with the application of principles that have evolved in the treatment of classic bladder exstrophy, have improved the outcome in this unfortunate group of patients. The surgical management of epispadias, the least extensive anomaly in this group, is fairly straightforward and involves reconstruction of the genitalia and restoration of continence in complete epispadias. In this text, the techniques for managing the various epispadias-exstrophy variants are discussed, a detailed description of the author's surgical approach to these anomalies is presented, and the results of surgical intervention are summarized.

BLADDER EXSTROPHY

Incidence and Inheritance

The incidence of bladder exstrophy has been estimated at between 1 in 10,000 (Rickham) and 1 in 50,000 (Lattimer and Smith) live births. However, new data from the International Clearinghouse for Birth Defects monitoring system estimated the incidence to be 3.3 in 100,000 live births (Lancaster). Two series have reported a 5:1 to 6:1 ratio of male to female exstrophy births (Ives et al; Lancaster). The risk of recurrence of bladder exstrophy in a given family is approximately 1 in 100 (Ives et al). Shapiro et al (1984) conducted a questionnaire of pediatric urologists and surgeons in North America and Europe and identified the occurrence of exstrophy and epispadias in only nine of approximately 2500 index cases. Shapiro's series identified five sets of male and female non-identical twins in which only one twin was affected with exstrophy; five sets of male identical twins in which both twins were affected; one set of identical male twins in which only one twin was affected; and three sets of female identical twins in which only one twin had the exstrophy anomaly (Shapiro et al, 1985).

In a literature review by Clemetson, the inheritance pattern of bladder exstrophy was studied in 45 females with bladder exstrophy who produced 49 offspring; none of their offspring demonstrated features of the exstrophy-epispadias complex. Until recently, bladder exstrophy or epispadias had not been reported in offspring of parents with the exstrophy-epispadias complex. Shapiro (1984) determined that the risk of bladder exstrophy in the offspring of individuals with bladder exstrophy and epispadias is 1 in 70 live births, a 500-fold greater incidence than in the general population. In a multinational review of exstrophy patients (Lancaster) two interesting trends were found: (1) bladder exstrophy tended to occur in infants of younger mothers, and (2) an increased risk at higher parity was seen for bladder exstrophy but not for epispadias.

Embryology

Bladder exstrophy, cloacal exstrophy, and epispadias are variants of the exstrophy-epispa-

dias complex. The etiology of this complex has been attributed to the failure of the cloacal membrane to be reinforced by ingrowth of mesoderm (Muecke). The cloacal membrane is a bilaminar layer situated at the caudal end of the germinal disc, which occupies the infraumbilical abdominal wall (Fig. 15–101). Mesenchymal ingrowth between the ectodermal and endodermal layers of the cloacal membrane results in formation of the lower abdominal muscles and the pelvic bones. After mesenchymal ingrowth occurs, downgrowth of the urorectal septum divides the cloaca into a bladder anteriorly and a rectum posteriorly (Fig. 15–101). The paired genital tubercles migrate medially and fuse in the midline cephalad to the dorsal membrane before perforation. The cloacal membrane is subject to premature rupture; depending upon the extent of the infraumbilical defect and the stage of development when rupture occurs, bladder exstrophy, cloacal exstrophy, or epispadias results (Ambrose and O'Brien).

The present theory of embryonic maldevelopment in exstrophy, held by Marshall and Muecke, is that the basic defect is an abnormal overdevelopment of the cloacal membrane,

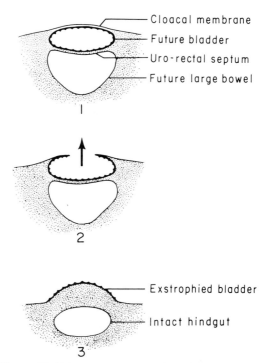

Figure 15–101 ☐ Diagram of events leading to classic exstrophy. (From Muecke EC: Exstrophy, epispadias, and other anomalies of the bladder. *In* Campbell's Urology, 4th ed. Edited by JH Harrison, RF Gittes, AD Perlmutter, et al. Philadelphia, WB Saunders Co, 1978.)

preventing medial migration of the mesenchymal tissue and proper lower abdominal wall development. The timing of the rupture of this cloacal defect determines the variant of the exstrophy-epispadias complex that results. The high incidence of central perforations results in a preponderance of classic exstrophy variants. Classic exstrophy accounts for 60 per cent of the patients born with this complex (Marshall and Muecke; Muecke). Thirty per cent are epispadias variants, and 10 per cent are cloacal exstrophies or minor variants, such as superior vesical fissure, duplicate exstrophy, and pseudoexstrophy.

Other plausible theories concerning the cause of the exstrophy-epispadias complex have been formulated. One group has postulated an abnormal caudal development of the genital hillocks with fusion in the midline below rather than above the cloacal membrane, a view that has been accepted by other authors (Ambrose and O'Brien; Patton and Barry). Another interesting hypothesis is that there is an abnormal caudal insertion of the body stalk (Mildenberger et al). This results in failure of interposition of the mesenchymal tissue in the midline. As a consequence of this failure, the translocation of the cloaca into the depths of the abdominal cavity does not occur. A cloacal membrane that remains in a superficial infraumbilical position represents an unstable embyonic state with a strong tendency to disintegrate (Johnston, 1974). However, the theory of an abnormal caudal insertion of the body stalk remains controversial, as the embryogenesis of the rat in this area differs in many ways from that of the human.

Anatomic Considerations

Exstrophy of the bladder is part of a spectrum of anomalies involving the urinary and genital tracts, the musculoskeletal system, and sometimes the intestinal tract. In bladder exstrophy, most anomalies are related to defects of the abdominal wall, bladder, genitalia, pelvic bones, rectum, and anus (Fig. 15–102). Because of the involved nature of this defect, the deficits will be described as they affect each organ system.

Musculoskeletal Defects

All cases of exstrophy show the characteristic widening of the symphysis pubis caused

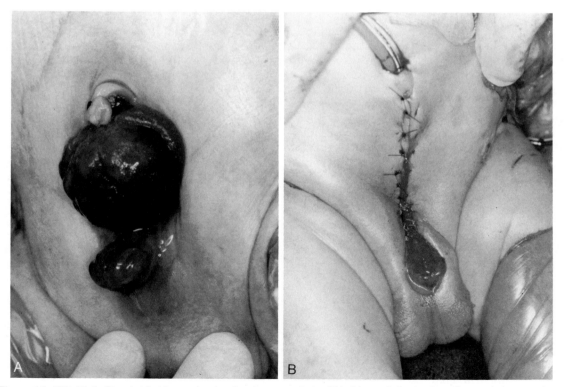

Figure 15–102 □ *A*, Classic bladder exstrophy showing a good-sized bladder and short epispadiac penis in a newborn male. *B*, Closure of classic bladder exstrophy plus anterior innominate osteotomy in the same patient.

by the outward rotation of the innominate bones, in relation to the sagittal plane of the body, along both sacroiliac joints. In addition, there is an outward rotation or eversion of the pubic rami at their junction with the ischial and iliac bones. These rotational deformities of the pelvic skeletal structures contribute to the short pendular penis seen in exstrophy. The outward rotation and lateral displacement of the innominate bones also account for the increased distance between the hips, the waddling gait, and the outward rotation of the lower limbs in these children, which in itself causes little disability.

The triangular defect caused by the premature rupture of the abnormal cloacal membrane is occupied by the open bladder. The fascial defect is limited inferiorly by the intersymphyseal band, which represents the divergent urogenital diaphragm. The anterior sheath of the rectus muscles has a fan-like extension behind the urethra and bladder neck that inserts into the intersymphyseal band.

At the upper end of the triangular defect and bladder is the umbilicus. In bladder exstrophy, the distance between the umbilicus and the anus is always foreshortened. Because the umbilicus is situated well below the horizontal line of the iliac crest, there is an unusual expanse of uninterrupted abdominal skin. Although an umbilical hernia is always present, it is usually of insignificant size. The umbilical hernia should be repaired at the time of the abdominal wall closure. Omphaloceles are rarely seen in conjunction with bladder exstrophy; however, they are frequently associated with cloacal exstrophy. The omphaloceles associated with exstrophy-epispadias complex are usually small and can be closed at the time of bladder closure. A large omphalocele in a cloacal exstrophy patient may necessitate repair before the exstrophy itself can be closed. The frequent occurrence of indirect inguinal hernias is attributed to a persistent processus vaginalis, large internal and external inguinal rings, and lack of obliquity of the inguinal canal. An inguinal hernia should be treated at the time of presentation by both excision of the hernial sac and repair of the transversalis fascia and muscle defect to prevent recurrence or direct hernia.

Anorectal Defects

The perineum is short and broad, with the anus situated directly behind the urogenital diaphragm, displaced anteriorly, and corresponding to the posterior limit of the triangular fascial defect. The anal sphincter mechanism is also anteriorly displaced, and it should be preserved intact in case internal urinary diversion is required in future patient management.

The divergent levator ani and puborectalis muscles and the distorted anatomy of the external sphincter contribute to varying degrees of anal incontinence and rectal prolapse. Anal continence is usually imperfect at an early age. In some patients, the rectal sphincter mechanism may never be adequate to control liquid content of the bowel. Rectal prolapse frequently occurs in untreated exstrophy patients with a widely separated symphysis. It is usually transient and easily reduced. Prolapse virtually always disappears after bladder closure or cystectomy and urinary diversion. The appearance of prolapse is an indication to proceed with definitive management of the exstrophied bladder.

Male Genital Defects

The male genital defect is severe and may be the most troublesome aspect of the surgical reconstruction, independent of the decision to treat by staged closure or by urinary diversion. The individual corpus cavernosum in bladder exstrophy is usually of normal caliber; however, the penis appears foreshortened because of the wide separation of the crural attachments, the prominent dorsal chordee, and the shortened urethral groove. A functional and cosmetically acceptable penis can be achieved when the dorsal chordee is released, the urethral groove lengthened, and the penis lengthened by mobilizing the crura in the midline. Duplication of the penis and unilateral hypoplasia of the glans and corpus are rare variants that further complicate surgical management. Patients with a very small or dystrophic penis should be considered for sex reassignment.

The vas deferens and ejaculatory ducts are normal, provided that they are not injured iatrogenically (Hanna and Williams). Testicular function has not yet been comprehensively studied in a large series of postpubertal exstrophy patients, but it is generally believed that fertility is not impaired. The autonomic innervation of the corpus cavernosum is provided by the cavernous nerves. These autonomic nerves are displaced laterally in patients with exstrophy (Schlegel and Gearhart). Potency is preserved following functional bladder closure, penile lengthening, and dorsal chordee release. Retrograde ejaculation may occur following bladder closure, since the internal sphincter sometimes remains dilated. The testes frequently appear undescended in their course from the widely separated pubic tubercles to the flat, wide scrotum. Most testes are retractile and have an adequate length of spermatic cord to reach the scrotum without the need for orchiopexy.

Female Genital Defects

Reconstruction of the female genitalia presents a less complex problem than do such procedures in the male (Fig. 15–103). The urethra and vagina are short; the vaginal orifice is frequently stenotic and displaced anteriorly; the clitoris is bifid; and the labia, mons pubis, and clitoris are divergent. The uterus, fallopian tubes, and ovaries are normal except for occasional uterine duplication. Approximation of the clitoral halves in the hair-bearing skin of the mons pubis provides satisfactory cosmetic restoration of the external genitalia (Dees). Vaginal dilatation or episiotomy may be required to allow satisfactory intercourse in the mature female. The defective pelvic floor may predispose mature females to uterine prolapse development, making uterine suspension necessary. Uterine prolapse does not appear to

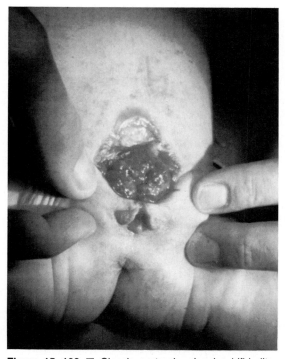

Figure 15–103 □ Classic exstrophy showing bifid clitoris, separated labia, and open urethra in a newborn girl.

occur when osteotomy and closure of the anterior defect are performed early in life.

Urinary Defects

At birth the bladder mucosa may appear normal; however, ectopic bowel mucosa or an isolated bowel loop may present on the bladder surface. Abnormal histology was observed in each of 23 bladder specimens obtained from individuals between the ages of 1 month and 52 years with bladder exstrophy. Squamous metaplasia, cystitis cystica, cystitis glandularis, and acute and chronic inflammation were commonly identified in these exstrophied bladder specimens (Culp). Abnormal histologic features demonstrated by both light and electron-microscopy may represent chronic mucosal change secondary to persistent infection.

The size, distensibility, and neuromuscular function of the exstrophied bladder as well as the size of the triangular fascial defect to which the bladder muscles attach affect the decision to attempt functional closure. When the bladder is small, fibrosed, and inelastic, functional closure may be impossible. The more normal bladder may be invaginated or may bulge through a small fascial defect, indicating the potential for satisfactory capacity.

Ultimate bladder function has been assessed in a group of continent closed exstrophy patients and normal reflexive bladders. Normal electromyograms were obtained in 70 and 90 per cent of cases, respectively (Toguri et al). In addition, Shapiro et al (1985), using radioligand receptor-binding techniques, demonstrated that exstrophied and control bladders contained similar levels of muscarinic cholinergic receptors.

The upper urinary tract is usually normal, but anomalous development does occur. Horseshoe kidney, pelvic kidney, hypoplastic kidney, solitary kidney, and dysplasia with megaureter are all encountered in these patients. The ureters have an abnormal course and termination. The peritoneal pouch of Douglas between the bladder and rectum is enlarged and unusually deep, forcing the ureter down and laterally in its course across the true pelvis. The distal segment of the ureter approaches the bladder from a point inferior and lateral to the orifice, and it enters the bladder with little or no obliquity. Therefore, reflux in the closed exstrophied bladder occurs in nearly 100 per cent of cases and subsequent surgery is required. Terminal ureteral dilatation frequently appears on pyelograms and is usually the result of edema, infection, and fibrosis of the terminal ureter acquired after birth.

Prenatal Diagnosis and Management

Sonographic evaluation of the fetus, especially by means of high-resolution, real-time units, allows a thorough survey of fetal anatomy, even during routine obstetric sonograms. Most studies, however, have dealt with the prenatal evaluation of hydronephrosis. However, reports have indicated that it is indeed possible to diagnose classic bladder exstrophy prenatally (Mirk; Verco). In the quoted reviews, the absence of a normal fluid-filled bladder on repeated examinations suggested the diagnosis, as did a mass of echogenic tissue lying on the lower abdominal wall (Verco). In a review of prenatal ultrasound examinations, the absence of bladder filling, along with a low-set umbilicus, was the key factor of note in eight exstrophy pregnancies summarized in retrospect (Gearhart et al, 1988). Prenatal diagnosis of exstrophy allows for optimal perinatal management, including delivery near a pediatric center prepared to handle this complex malformation.

Exstrophy Complex and Variants

Because the entire exstrophy group represents a spectrum of anomalies, it is not surprising that transitions between the bladder exstrophy–epispadias–cloacal exstrophy have been reported. There is a close relationship among all forms of the exstrophy-epispadias complex, for the fault in its embryogenesis is common to all; therefore, all clinical manifestations are merely variations on a theme.

The presence of the characteristic musculoskeletal defect of the exstrophy anomaly with no major defect in the urinary tract has been named "pseudoexstrophy" (Marshall and Muecke). Predominant characteristics include an elongated, low-set umbilicus and divergent rectus muscles that attach to the separated pubic bones. In this variant, the mesodermal migration has been interrupted in its superior aspect only, thus wedging apart the musculoskeletal elements of the lower abdominal wall without obstructing the formation of the genital tubercle (Marshall and Muecke).

In the superior vesical fissure variant of the exstrophy complex, the musculature and skeletal defects are exactly as those in classic exstrophy; however, the persistent cloacal membrane opens only at the uppermost portion and a superior vesical fissure thus results. Bladder extrusion is minimal and is present only over the abnormal umbilicus.

Duplicate exstrophy occurs when a superior vesical fissure opens, but there is later fusion of the abdominal wall and a portion of the bladder elements (mucosa) remains outside. In a case report by Muecke, the patient had exstrophy of the mucosa but a normal bladder inside. The patient also had a very widened symphysis and a stubby, upward-pointing penis. Three additional cases have been reported by Arap and Giron in which the patients had classic musculoskeletal defects and two of the three were continent. In the two males, one had an associated complete epispadias whereas the other had a completely normal penis. Thus, the external genital manifestations of duplicate exstrophy can be quite variable.

Besides pseudoexstrophy, superior vesical fissure, and duplicate exstrophy, isolated occurrences of a fourth entity—*covered exstrophy*—have been reported (Cerniglia et al; Narasimharao). These have also been referred to as *split symphysis variants*. A common factor present in these patients is the musculoskeletal defect associated with classic exstrophy with no significant defect of the urinary tract. However, in most cases reported as covered exstrophy (Cerniglia et al; Narasimharao et al), there has been an isolated ectopic bowel segment present on the inferior abdominal wall near the genital area, which can be either colon or ileum with no connection with the underlying gastrointestinal tract and only epispadias in the male (Fig. 15–104).

Staged Surgical Reconstruction

Sweetser et al (1952) initially described a staged surgical approach for bladder exstrophy. Four to 6 days prior to bladder closure, bilateral iliac osteotomies were performed. Epispadias repair was also performed as a separate procedure. The continence procedure was limited to freeing the fibrous intersymphyseal band and wrapping this band around the urethra at the time of closure. A staged approach to functional bladder closure that in-

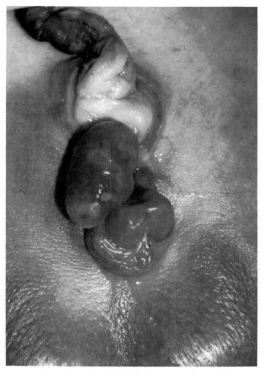

Figure 15–104 □ Covered exstrophy with isolated ectopic bowel segment on the inferior abdominal wall just above the penis. (Courtesy of Dr. Frank Cerniglia.)

cludes three separate stages (bladder closure, bladder neck reconstruction with an antireflux procedure, and epispadias repair) have been recommended for most cases of exstrophy reconstruction beginning in the early 1970s (Cendron; Gearhart and Jeffs, 1989a; Jeffs et al, 1972; Williams and Keaton).

Patient Selection

Successful treatment of exstrophy by functional closure demands that the potential for success in each child be considered at birth. Size and functional capacity of the detrusor muscle are important considerations in the eventual success of functional closure. The correlation between apparent bladder size and potential bladder capacity must not be confused. In minor grades of exstrophy that approach the condition of complete epispadias with incontinence, the bladder may be small yet may demonstrate acceptable capacity, either by bulging when the baby cries or by indenting easily when touched by a gloved finger (Chisholm, 1962). Once removed from surface irritation and repeated trauma, the small bladder enlarges and gradually increases

its capacity, even in the absence of continence or outlet resistance. The exstrophied bladder that is estimated at birth to have a capacity of 3 ml or more and demonstrates elasticity and contractility may be expected to develop useful size and capacity following successful closure.

Delivery Room and Nursery

At birth the bladder mucosa is usually smooth, thin, and intact; it is also sensitive and easily denuded. In the delivery room, the umbilical cord should be tied relatively close to the abdominal wall so that the umbilical clamp or long cord does not traumatize the bladder mucosa and cause excoriation of the bladder surface. The bladder may be covered with a nonadherent film of plastic wrap (e.g., Saran Wrap) to prevent the mucosa from sticking to clothing or diapers.

The distraught parents at this stage need reassurance. The counseling of the parents and decisions regarding eventual therapy should be made by surgeons with special interest and experience in managing cases of bladder exstrophy. This is especially true regarding the sex of rearing of males with bladder exstrophy. The author has seen several families who were made even more distraught by being told that the child also needed a change of gender. The need for changing the sex of rearing is extremely rare in the male child born with bladder exstrophy.

Early Management

Cardiopulmonary and general physical assessment can be carried out in the first few hours of life. Immediate intravenous pyelographic assessment of the kidneys in the newborn may lack clarity and detail. Radionuclide scans and ultrasound studies can provide evidence of renal function and drainage even in the first few hours of life.

Circumstances may be less than ideal at birth. A thorough neonatal assessment may have to be deferred until transportation to a children's medical center can be arranged. In these days of modern transportation, no child should be more than few hours away from a neonatal center with full diagnostic and consultative services. During travel the bladder should be protected by a plastic membrane (not petroleum jelly gauze) to prevent contact of dressing or clothing with the delicate newborn bladder mucosa.

The Small Bladder Unsuitable for Closure

A small fibrotic bladder patch that is stretched between the edges of a small triangular fascial defect without either elasticity or contractility cannot be selected for the usual closure procedure. Examination with the patient under anesthesia may at times be required to assess the bladder adequately, particularly if considerable edema, excoriation, and polyp formation have developed between birth and the time of assessment. The elasticity of the bladder can be demonstrated in this way, and the size of the triangular fascial defect can be appreciated by simultaneous abdominal and rectal examination. A neonatal closure, even when the bladder is small, allows for later assessment of bladder potential and provides an initial step in genital reconstruction that is helpful in reassuring the family. Other conditions that preclude primary closure include penile-scrotal duplication, ectopic bowel within the exstrophied bladder, a hypoplastic bladder, and significant hydronephrosis.

A review by Oesterling and Jeffs showed that of 51 patients treated solely at one institution, only one required initial diversion instead of primary closure. However, in some patients, for reasons mentioned above, primary closure cannot be used. In most cases, there is no need at birth for alternative management of these cases. Later, options include excision of the bladder and a nonrefluxing colon conduit or ileocecal ureterosigmoidostomy. Another appealing alternative involves urinary diversion and placing the small bladder inside to be used later for a posterior urethra in an Arap type procedure. Additionally, one could wait for several months to see whether the bladder plate increases in size. This has been seen in one patient in whom after 6 to 12 months the bladder did increase in size and primary closure was effected. Lastly, augmentation cystoplasty at the time of initial closure is not recommended.

Operative Procedure

Over the past two decades, modifications in the management of functional bladder closure have contributed to a dramatic increase in the success of the procedure. The most significant changes in management of bladder exstrophy have been (1) staging the reconstructive procedures, (2) performing bilateral osteotomies, (3) reconstructing a competent bladder neck, and (4) defining strict criteria for the selection of patients suitable for this approach.

The primary objective in functional closure of classic bladder exstrophy is to convert the exstrophy to a complete epispadias with incontinence while preserving renal function. The best management for the incontinence and epispadias is determined secondarily in a later stage or stages.

Osteotomy

Schultz combined primary bladder closure with bilateral iliac osteotomies. The efficacy of iliac osteotomies is still somewhat controversial. The primary arguments against osteotomy are that (1) the pubic bones retract eventually, (2) the penis retracts farther, and (3) continence can be achieved without osteotomies (Marshall and Muecke, 1968). The advantages of bilateral iliac osteotomies are that (1) reapproximation of the symphysis diminishes the tension on the abdominal closure and eliminates the need for fascial flaps, (2) placement of the urethra within the pelvic ring reduces the excessive urethrovesical angle and permits urethral suspension after bladder neck plasty, and (3) reapproximation of the urogenital diaphragm and approximation of the levator ani may aid in eventual urinary control. After pubic approximation with osteotomy, some patients show the ability to stop and start the urinary stream (Gearhart and Jeffs, 1989a; Jeffs et al, 1982). Ezwell and Carlson (1970) observed that urinary diversion was subsequently performed in 20 per cent of functional closures in patients who had undergone osteotomies whereas 75 per cent of individuals who had not undergone prior osteotomies during bladder closure eventually required urinary diversion. The majority of patients referred to our institution following partial or complete dehiscence have not undergone a prior osteotomy (Gearhart and Jeffs, 1990).

The author's recommendation is to perform bilateral iliac osteotomy when primary bladder closure is performed after 72 hours of life. In addition, if the pelvis is not malleable or if the pubic bones are unduly wide at the time of the examination with the patient under anesthesia, osteotomy should be performed even if the closure is performed before 72 hours of age. Osteotomy should be carried out at the same time as bladder closure. A well-coordinated surgical and anesthesia team can perform osteotomy and proceed to bladder closure without undue loss of blood or risk of prolonged anesthesia to the child. However, one must realize that osteotomy and bladder closure is a 5- to 7-hour procedure in these patients.

Two separate approaches are currently being used for osteotomy in the exstrophy group: posterior bilateral iliac osteotomy and anterior bilateral transverse innominate osteotomy. Both of these approaches can improve the ease of symphyseal approximation in the exstrophy patient. With appropriate approximation, tension on the midline abdominal closure is lessened. Also, in my experience, the dehiscence rate is lower if osteotomies are performed (Gearhart and Jeffs, 1990; Oesterling and Jeffs). In addition, pubic closure allows approximation of the levator and puborectile sling, inclusion of the bladder neck and urethra within the pelvic ring, and eventually, an improved continence rate (Gearhart and Jeffs, 1989a; Oesterling and Jeffs).

Several reports have demonstrated experience with an anterior approach through the innominate bone just above the acetabulum (Gokcora et al; Montagnani; Sponseller et al). Although my experience with posterior iliac osteotomy was not associated with any failure of the initial closures, I was disappointed with the poor mobility of the pubis, the occasional delayed or malunion of the ilium, and, most importantly, the need to turn the patient intraoperatively from the prone to the supine position. Initially, my experience in anterior osteotomy was in those patients who had failed to benefit from an initial exstrophy closure with or without prior posterior iliac osteotomy (Sponseller et al). The results with the new approach were so satisfactory that anterior innominate osteotomy is now being used also for primary closure of bladder exstrophy (Fig. 15–105). The anterior iliofemoral approach to the pelvis is similar to that used for a Salter osteotomy. Both sides may be exposed simultaneously, and a horizontal innominate anterior osteotomy performed using a Gigli saw. If the patient is younger than 6 months of age, an oscillating saw instead of a Gigli saw can be used (Sponseller et al). In order to leave a sizable inferior bone segment for fixation, the level of the osteotomy is from 5 mm above the anterior-inferior iliac spine to the most cranial part of the sciatic notch. An external fixator is commonly used and the pins are inserted before wound closure (Fig. 15–106). A horizontal mattress suture of No. 2 nylon is placed between the fibrous cartilage of the pubic rami

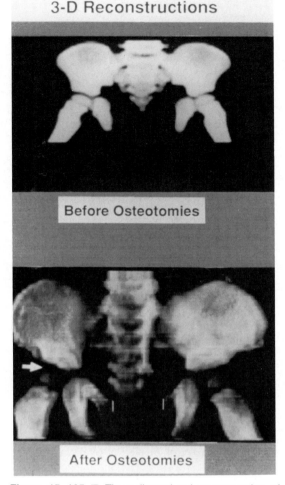

Figure 15–105 □ Three-dimensional reconstruction of pelvic CT scan before and after anterior innominate osteotomy. Arrow shows site of transverse osteotomy. (Courtesy Dr. Paul D. Sponseller.)

and tied anterior to the pubic closure at the time of bladder closure. Should this suture work loose or cut through the tissues during subsequent healing, the anterior placement of the knot in the horizontal mattress suture ensures that it will not erode into the urethra and interfere with the bladder or urethral lumen.

Whether posterior or anterior osteotomy is performed, the pelvic ring closure not only allows midline approximation of the abdominal wall structures but also permits the levator ani and puborectalis muscles to lend potential support to the bladder outlet, thereby adding resistance to urinary outflow. Furthermore, the incontinence procedure can be performed on the bladder neck and urethra within the closed

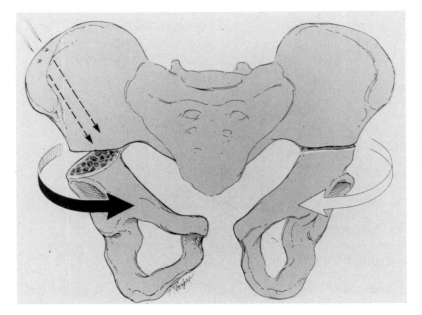

Figure 15–106 □ The sites of both the transverse innominate osteotomy and fixator pin placement are depicted. (Courtesy of Dr. Paul D. Sponseller.)

pelvic ring at a distance from the surface and without independent movement of the two halves of the pubis. When the urethra and bladder neck are set more deeply in the true pelvis, they are in a more normal relationship with the vertical axis of the bladder rather than being acutely angulated.

Postoperatively, both the bladder exstrophy patient who undergoes closure without osteotomies in the first 48 hours of life and the patient undergoing posterior osteotomies are immobilized in modified Bryant's traction with adhesive skin traction in a position in which the hips have 90 degrees of flexion and the knees are somewhat bent to protect the arterial tree. When modified Bryant's traction is used, the traction is employed for 3 to 4 weeks (Fig. 15–107). If anterior osteotomy has been performed, an external fixator is employed. Light Buck's traction is also used for 2 weeks to maintain comfort and bed rest. External fixation is continued for 6 weeks.

Bladder and Prostatic Urethra Closure

The various steps in primary bladder closure are illustrated in Figure 15–108. A strip of mucosa 2 cm wide, extending from the distal trigone to below the verumontanum in the male and to the vaginal orifice in the female, is outlined for prostatic and posterior urethral reconstruction. The male urethral groove length may be adequate, and no transverse incision of the urethral plate need then be made for urethral lengthening. However, when the length of the urethral groove from the verumontanum to the glans is so short that it interferes with eventual penile length or produces dorsal angulation, the urethral groove is lengthened after the manner of Johnston (1974) or Duckett. The diagrams in Figure 15–108C, D indicate that an incision is made outlining the bladder mucosa and the prostatic plate. The urethral groove is transected distal to the verumontanum, but continuity is maintained between the thin, mucosa-like, non–hair-bearing skin adjacent to the posterior urethra and bladder neck and the skin and mucosa of the penile shaft and glans. Flaps from the area of thin skin are subsequently

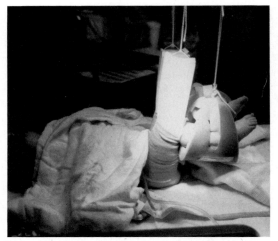

Figure 15–107 □ Modified Bryant's traction after posterior iliac osteotomy and exstrophy reclosure.

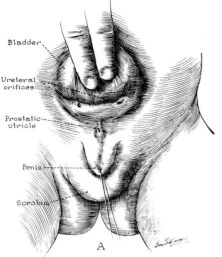

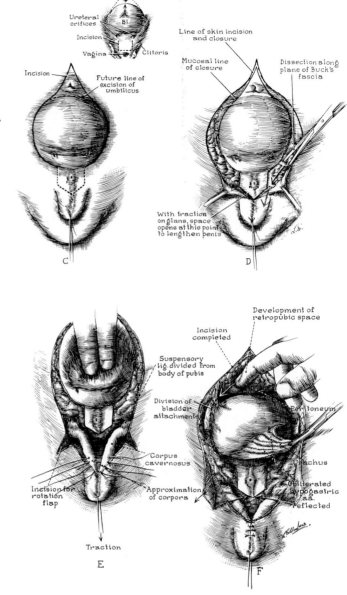

Figure 15–108 □ Steps in primary bladder closure following osteotomy or without osteotomy in the newborn younger than 72 hours of age.

A–D, Incision line around the umbilicus and bladder down to the urethral plate. If the male urethral groove is adequate, incision is made in the urethral plate for initial urethral lengthening.

E, Lateral skin incisions allow rotation of paraexstrophy skin to cover the elongated penis if the urethral groove has been transected.

F, Development of the retropubic space from below the area of umbilical dissection to facilitate separation of the bladder from the rectus sheath and muscle.

*Illustration continued
on following page*

moved distally and rotated to reconstitute the urethral groove, resurfacing the penis dorsally; the groove may be lengthened by 2 to 4 cm. Further urethral lengthening can then be performed at the time of epispadias repair by the method of Cantwell and Ransley et al.

Penile lengthening is achieved by exposing the corpora cavernosum bilaterally and freeing the corpora from their attachments to the suspensory ligaments and anterior part of the inferior pubic rami. If the mucosal plate has been transected, the partially freed corpora

are joined in the midline and the bare corpora are then covered with flaps of the thin paraexstrophy skin, which are rotated medially to be attached to the distal mucosa of the posterior urethral plate (Fig. 15–108E to I). These are inward rotation flaps and not long paraexstrophy skin flaps running up the lateral aspect of the exstrophied bladder. Lengthening at the time of closure is not usually required in the female urethra.

Bladder closure then proceeds by excision of the umbilical area, the redundant skin ad-

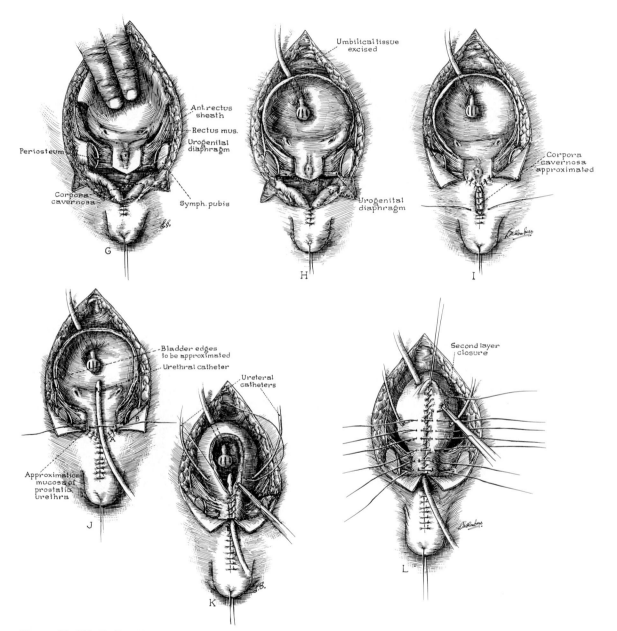

Figure 15–108 □ *Continued*

G, Fibers of rectus muscle attaching behind the prostate to urogenital diaphragm. The urogenital diaphragm and anterior corpus are freed from the pubis in a subperiosteal plane.

H, I, Anastomosis of the paraexstrophy skin to the prostatic plate.

J–L, Closure of bladder in two layers with placement of supraperiosteal tube and ureteral stents.

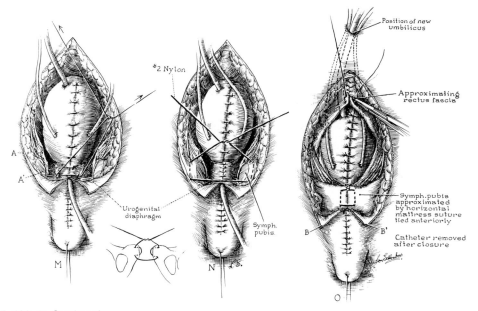

Figure 15–108 □ *Continued*

M, Urogenital diaphragm is closed with a separate layer of sutures if possible. Oftentimes, this is not possible.

N, Horizontal mattress suture is tied on the external symphysis while assistant applies medial rotation of greater trochanters.

O, Catheter is removed from closed bladder neck and urethra. Approximation of skin point B to B′ provides an anterior step from penile closure to abdominal wall closure.

(Drawings by Leon Schlossberg.)

jacent to the superior aspect of the bladder mucosa being discarded and the bladder muscle being freed from the fused rectus sheaths on each side. This dissection is facilitated by exposing the peritoneum above the umbilicus and then carefully dissecting extraperitoneally to enter the retropubic space on each side from above. The wide band of fibers and muscular tissue representing the urogenital diaphragm is detached subperiostally from the pubis bilaterally. The dissection must be extended onto the inferior ramus of the pubis to allow the bladder neck and posterior urethra to fall back and achieve a position deep within the pelvic ring. Reluctance to free the bladder neck and urethra well from the inferior ramus of the pubis certainly moves the neobladder opening cephalad if any separation of the pubis occur during healing. The mucosa and muscle of the bladder and posterior urethra are then closed in the midline anteriorly. This orifice should accommodate a 14 French (Fr.) sound comfortably. The size of the opening should allow enough resistance to aid in bladder adaptation and to prevent prolapse but not enough outlet resistance to cause upper tract changes. The posterior urethra and bladder neck are but-tressed with a second layer of local tissue if possible (Fig. 15–108 *J* to *M*).

The bladder is drained by a suprapubic Malecot catheter for a period of 3 to 4 weeks. The urethra is *not* stented in order to avoid pressure necrosis or the accumulation of infected secretions in the neourethra. Ureteral stents provide drainage during the first 7 to 10 days, when swelling or the pressure of closure of a small bladder may obstruct the ureters and give rise to obstruction and transient hypertension. If there are no problems with the stents during healing, the author sometimes leaves the stents in place for up to 2 weeks. When the bladder and urethra have been closed and the drainage tubes placed, pressure over the greater trocanters bilaterally allows the pubic bones to be approximated in the midline. Horizontal mattress sutures are placed in the pubis and tied with the knot away from the neourethra (Fig. 15–108*N*, *O*). Oftentimes, the author is able to use another stitch or two of No. 2 nylon as the most caudal stitches in the rectus fascia; these may help add to the security of the pubic closure. A V-shaped flap of abdominal skin at a point corresponding to the normal position of the umbilicus is tacked down to the abdominal fascia, and the drainage tubes exit this orifice.

Before and during this procedure, the patient is given broad-spectrum antibiotics in an attempt to convert a contaminated field into a clean surgical wound. Nonreactive sutures of polyglycolic acid (Dexon) and nylon are used to avoid undesirable stitch reaction or stitch abscesses.

Management after Primary Closure

The procedure just described converts a patient with exstrophy into one with complete epispadias and incontinence. Prior to removal of the suprapubic tube, 4 weeks postoperatively the bladder outlet is calibrated by a urethral catheter, urethral sound, or cystoscope to ensure free outlet drainage. An excretory urogram (IVP) is obtained to ascertain the status of the renal pelvis and ureters, and appropriate urinary antibiotics are administered to treat any bladder contamination that may be present after removal of this suprapubic tube. Residual urine is estimated by clamping the suprapubic tube, and specimens for culture are obtained before the patient leaves the hospital and at subsequent intervals to detect infection and to ensure that the bladder is emptying. If the initial IVP shows good drainage, upper tract imaging by ultrasonography is repeated 3 months after discharge from the hospital and at intervals of 6 months to 1 year during the next 2 to 3 years to detect any upper tract changes caused by reflux or infection. Prophylactic antibacterials should be continued at least through the first 6 months and then as necessary thereafter. Should bladder outlet resistance be such that urine is retained within the bladder and reflux and ureteral dilatation develop with infected urine, it may be necessary to dilate the urethra or, occasionally, to begin intermittent catheterization. If bladder outlet resistance persists, an antireflux procedure may be required as early as 6 months to 1 year after the initial bladder closure. If a useful continent interval has resulted unexpectantly from the initial closure, no further operation for incontinence may be required; however, this is a situation that is quite unusual.

In conversion from exstrophy to complete epispadias with incontinence, the bladder gradually increases in capacity and inflammatory changes in the mucosa resolve. Cystograms with the patient *under anesthesia* at 2 to 3 years of age detect bilateral reflux in nearly 100 per cent of patients and provide an estimate of bladder capacity. Even in the completely incontinent patient, bladder capacity gradually increases to the point at which the bladder can be distended at cystography to a capacity of 50 to 60 ml. In some patients with very small bladders, 4 to 5 years may be necessary to achieve this capacity.

A tight bladder closure, uncontrolled urinary tract infection, and reflux may cause uncontrollable ureteral dilatation. If severe upper tract changes occur, surgical revision of the bladder outlet by advancing skin flaps into the orifice may be necessary to prevent scarring and further obstruction. Judgment is required to know when to abort attempts at functional closure and when to turn to urinary diversion as a means of preserving renal function. This change of plan is seldom necessary if an adequate outlet has been constructed at initial closure and if careful attention has been paid to details of follow-up.

Penile and Urethral Reconstruction in Exstrophy

Formerly, the author performed bladder neck reconstruction prior to urethral and penile reconstruction. However, the significant increase in bladder capacity after epispadias repair in those patients with extremely small bladder capacities prompted a change in the management program (Gearhart and Jeffs, 1989). In this group of patients with small bladders, after initial closure there was a mean increase in capacity to 55 ml in only 22 months after epispadias repair. Construction of the neourethra and further penile lengthening and dorsal chordee release are usually performed between 2 and 3 years of age. Because the majority of boys with exstrophy have a somewhat small penis and a shortage of available penile skin on the dorsum, most patients undergo testosterone stimulation prior to urethroplasty and penile reconstruction (Gearhart and Jeffs, 1987).

Many surgical techniques have been described for reconstruction of the penis and urethra in patients with classic bladder exstrophy. Four key concerns must be addressed to ensure a functional and cosmetically acceptable penis:

- Dorsal chordee
- Urethral reconstruction
- Penile skin closure
- Glandular reconstruction

Although it is possible to achieve some penile lengthening with release of chordee at the time of initial bladder closure, it is often necessary to perform formal penile elongation with release of chordee at the time of urethroplasty in exstrophy patients. Certainly, all remnants of the suspensory ligaments and old scar tissue from the initial bladder closure must be excised. Also, further dissection of the corpora cavernosa from the inferior pubic ramus can be achieved. It is often surprising how little was accomplished at the time of initial exstrophy closure (Gearhart and Jeffs, 1989a). Lengthening of the urethral groove is also essential. Whether or not paraexstrophy skin flaps were used at the time of bladder closure, further lengthening will be needed. This can be as simple as Cantwell's original principle to transection of the urethral plate and replacement with other genital tissue (Hendren, 1979; Monfort et al; Thommala and Mitchell; Vyas et al).

Chordee

Besides lengthening, dorsal chordee must be addressed. To release dorsal chordee, one may lengthen the dorsomedial aspect of the corpora by incision and anastomosis of the corpora themselves (Ransley et al) or place a dermal graft to allow lengthening of the distal aspect of the corpora (Brzezinski et al; Woodhouse and Kellett, 1984). Another technique to improve dorsal chordee prior to urethroplasty is shortening or medial rotation of the ventral corpora (Koff and Eakins). Lastly, osteotomy initially or repeated with approximation of the inferior pubis ramus may correct lateral drift of the pubis with subsequent shortening and curvature of the phallus (Schillinger and Wiley).

Urethral Reconstruction

Urethral reconstruction is an important aspect of external genitalia reconstruction in exstrophy. This can be accomplished by many previously reported methods. Tubularization of the dorsal urethral groove as a modified Young urethroplasty is currently the author's preference when there is sufficient penile skin for both construction and coverage of the neourethra. Nonetheless, interposition of a free graft of genital or extragenital skin or even bladder mucosa can be used (Hendren, 1979; Vyas et al). In addition, ventral transverse island flaps and double-faced ventral island flaps have been used with some success for urethral reconstruction in exstrophy patients (Monfort et al; Thommala and Mitchell). After construction, the urethra can be mobilized almost completely and transferred to the ventrum of the penis under the separated corpora. Ransley et al have modified and refined this concept in exstrophy and epispadias patients with good success.

Penile Skin Closure

Skin closure remains a problem in genital reconstruction because of the paucity of skin in this condition. A Z-plasty incision and closure at the base of the penis prevents skin contraction and upward tethering of the penis. The ventral foreskin can be split in the midline and brought to the dorsum as lateral preputial flaps for coverage of the penile shaft. If the flaps are made a bit assymetric, a staggered dorsal suture line results with less upward tethering. Alternately, a buttonhole can be made and the ventral foreskin simply transposed to the dorsum for additional skin coverage.

Technique of Epispadias Repair

As stated, the author's preference for urethroplasty in the exstrophy patient when the urethral groove has adequate length is the modified Young procedure. The Young urethroplasty (Fig. 15–109A to K) is begun by placing a nylon suture through the glans; this provides midline traction on the penis. Incisions are made in two parallel lines, previously marked on the dorsum of the penis, that outline an 18-mm strip of penile skin extending from the prostatic urethral meatus to the tip of the glans. Triangular areas of the dorsal glans are excised adjacent to the urethral strip, and glanular flaps are constructed. The lateral skin flaps are mobilized, and a Z incision over the suprapubic area permits exposure and division of remaining suspensory ligaments and old scar tissue. The urethral strip is outlined, and the edges are mobilized for closure if no further lengthening is required. The urethral strip is then closed in a linear manner from the prostatic opening to the glans over a No. 10 synthetic rubber (Silastic) stent with 6-0 polyglycolic acid sutures.

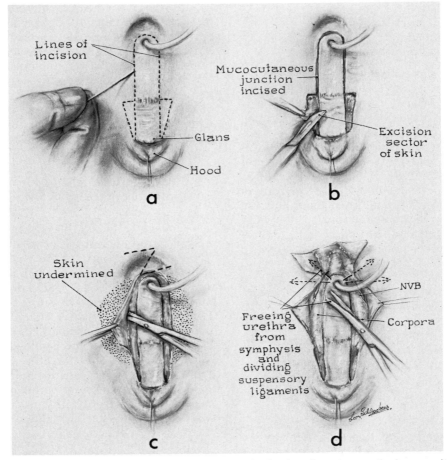

Figure 15–109 □ *a–k*, Modified Young urethroplasty for repair of epispadias when urethral groove is of sufficient length naturally or following prior lengthening procedure. (Drawings by Leon Schlossberg.)

A ventral meatotomy has already been made in the glans to move the urethral meatus to a more ventral position at the tip. Several sutures of 5-0 polyglycolic acid are used to approximate the glans over the neourethra. The skin of the glans is then closed with vertical mattress sutures of 4-0 Prolene. These sutures are removed in 10 days. Small pieces of a soft plastic vessel loop are used under both the knot and the loop of these sutures to prevent pressure necrosis of the glandular tissue and scarring secondary to edema. The Z-plasty is closed with interrupted 6-0 polyglycolic acid sutures. Several 6-0 polyglycolic acid sutures are inserted between the polypropylene (Prolene) sutures in the glans for proper skin approximation. A No. 10 Silastic stent is left indwelling in the neourethra as a drip tube and sewn to the glans with 5-0 Prolene. Drainage occurs through this catheter at low pressure and may be further ensured by a percuta-

neously placed suprapubic tube. If there is abundant subcutaneous tissue and the urethra is not to be transferred below the corporal bodies, the subcutaneous tissue is simply closed with two separate continuous layers of 6-0 polyglycolic acid suture. Occasionally, when there is an excess of ventral foreskin, part of this can be denuded and used as an extra layer over the urethra suture line. The skin is then reapproximated with interrupted 5-0 polyglycolic acid sutures.

Management of Postoperative Problems

One problem with the Young procedure is that it may not give adequate support to the reconstructed neourethra. At this stage, however, if further lengthening or correction of dorsal

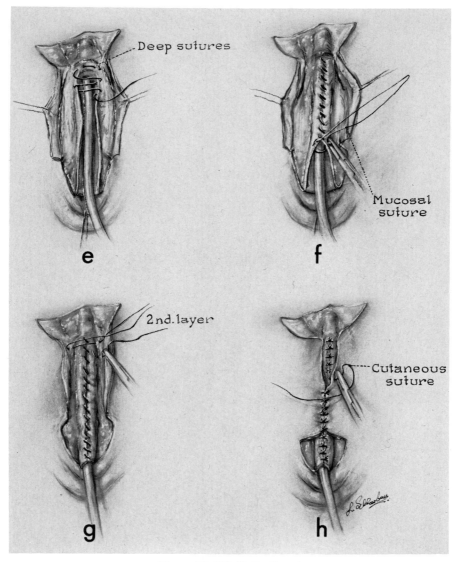

Figure 15–109 □ *Continued*

Illustration continued on following page

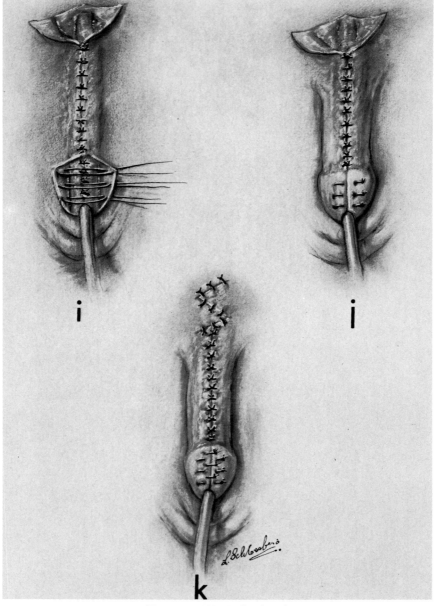

Figure 15–109 □ *Continued*

chordee is required, the Cantwell-Ransley method can be employed (Fig. 15–110A to J). The urethral strip is approached from below when one is seeking additional urethral lengthening (Fig. 15–110E). The urethral strip is mobilized, and the neurovascular bundles are freed bilaterally (Fig. 15–110F). Vessel loops are then used to retract these structures laterally (Fig. 15–110C to G). The urethra is then closed and transferred below the corporal bodies. Matching incisions are made in the medial aspect of the corporal bodies, and these are sewn together with 5-0 polydioxanone (PDS) suture (Fig. 15–110H). This not only causes a downward deflection of the penis but also helps to bury the urethra under the corporal bodies (Fig. 15–110I). After transferring the urethra to the ventrum and closing the corpora above, one proceeds with the rest of the procedure as described in performing the Young procedure (Fig. 15–110J).

Female Genitalia

After these reconstructive efforts, in the mons area there may remain shiny hairless skin, which becomes more apparent as puberty ap-

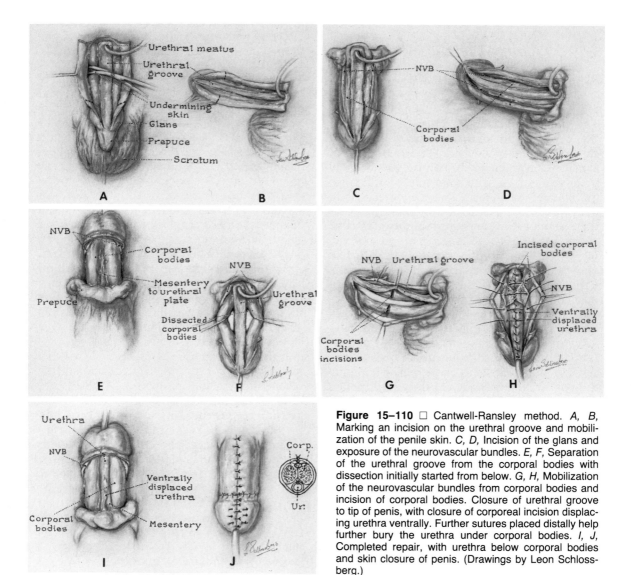

Figure 15–110 □ Cantwell-Ransley method. *A, B,* Marking an incision on the urethral groove and mobilization of the penile skin. *C, D,* Incision of the glans and exposure of the neurovascular bundles. *E, F,* Separation of the urethral groove from the corporal bodies with dissection initially started from below. *G, H,* Mobilization of the neurovascular bundles from corporal bodies and incision of corporal bodies. Closure of urethral groove to tip of penis, with closure of corporeal incision displacing urethra ventrally. Further sutures placed distally help further bury the urethra under corporal bodies. *I, J,* Completed repair, with urethra below corporal bodies and skin closure of penis. (Drawings by Leon Schlossberg.)

proaches. This can be obviated by lateral mobilization of the mons at the time of initial closure and by bringing this area to the midline. Also, this can be accomplished by Z-plasty or laterally based inguinal flaps rotated medially. The author prefers to wait until puberty and uses rhomboid skin flaps to rotate hair-bearing skin into the mons area if this was not done at the initial closure (Kramer and Jackson).

Also, the bifid clitoris can be denuded medially and brought together in the midline at the time of exstrophy closure or later if needed. However, a good closure with an attractive mons area is more important to the cosmetic appearance of the female genital area than is clitoral approximation.

Obstetric Implications

Clemetson's review of the literature identified 45 women with bladder exstrophy who were successfully delivered of 49 normal offspring. The main complication following pregnancy was cervical and uterine prolapse, which occurred frequently (Krisiloff et al). Burbige et al (1986) reviewed 40 women ranging from 19 to 36 years of age who were treated in infancy for bladder exstrophy. Fourteen pregnancies in 11 women resulted in nine normal deliveries, three spontaneous abortions, and two elective abortions. Uterine prolapse occurred in seven of 11 patients during pregnancy. All had undergone prior permanent urinary diversions. Patients must be informed of the likelihood of uterine prolapse following pregnancy. Spontaneous vaginal deliveries were performed in women who had undergone prior urinary diversions, and cesarean sections were performed in women with functional bladder closures to eliminate stress on the pelvic floor and to avoid traumatic injury to the reconstructed urinary sphincter mechanism (Krisiloff et al; Lattimer et al).

Incontinence and Antireflux Procedures

Bladder capacity is measured with the child under anesthesia after the third year of life. If the bladder capacity is 60 ml or higher, bladder neck reconstruction can be planned. The incontinence and antireflux procedures are illustrated in Figure 15–111A to I. The bladder is opened through a transverse incision at the bladder neck, but a vertical extension is also employed (Fig. 15–111A). The later midline closure of this incision narrows the width of the bladder neck area and enlarges the vertical dimension of the bladder, which in exstrophy is often short. The illustration depicts a Leadbetter or transtrigonal advancement procedure for correcting reflux in which a new hiatus lateral to the original orifice is selected prior to advancing the ureter across the bladder above the trigone. Also, the ureter can be taken in a more cephalic direction, as in the cephalotrigonal reimplant (Fig. 15–111B, C) (Canning et al, 1990). In addition, if the ureters are low on the trigone and there is a need to move the ureteral hiatus higher on the trigone, the hiatus is simply cut in a cephalic direction and cross trigonal reimplants are performed on the upper aspect of the trigone (Fig. 15–111C).

The incontinence procedure is begun by selecting a posterior strip of mucosa 15 to 18 mm wide and 30 mm long that extends distally from the midtrigone to the prostate or posterior urethra (Fig. 15–111D, E). The bladder muscle lateral to this mucosal strip is denuded of mucosa. It is often helpful at this juncture to use 1:200,000 epinephrine-soaked sponges to aid in the control of bleeding and in visualization of the denuded area. Tailoring of the denuded lateral triangles of bladder muscle is aided by multiple small incisions in the free edges bilaterally that allow the area of reconstruction to assume a more cephalic position. The edges of the mucosa and underlying muscle are formed into a tube by interrupted sutures of 4-0 polyglycolic acid (Fig. 15–111F). The adjacent denuded muscle flaps are overlapped and sutured firmly in place with 3-0 polyglycolic acid sutures in order to provide reinforcement of the bladder neck and urethral reconstruction (Fig. 15–110G). An 8 Fr. urethral stent may be used as a guide during urethral reconstruction, but it is removed after the bladder neck reconstruction is complete.

Somewhat radical dissection of the bladder, bladder neck, and posterior urethra is required within the pelvis and from the posterior aspect of the pubic bar to provide enough mobility for the bladder neck reconstruction. This maneuver allows for subsequent anterior suspension of the newly created posterior urethra and bladder neck. If visualization of this area is problematic, the intersymphyseal bar can simply be cut, thus providing a widened field of

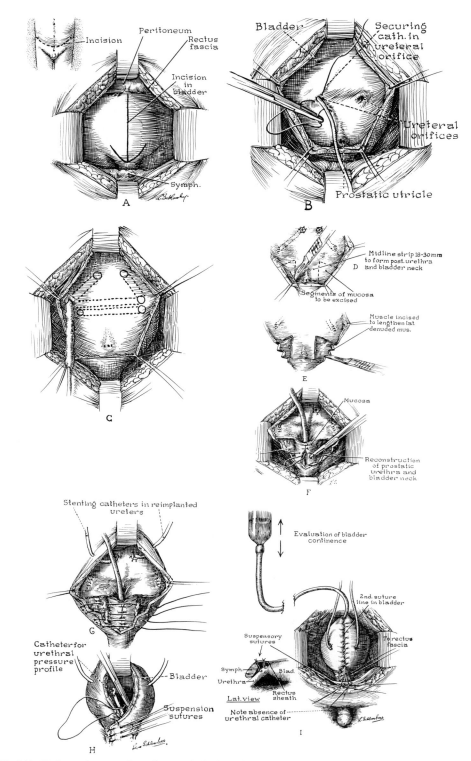

Figure 15–111 □ Steps in transtrigonal or cephalotrigonal reimplantation of ureters and bladder neck reconstruction for continence. *A,* Transverse bladder incision with vertical extensions subsequently closed in midline to narrow bladder near bladder neck. *B–F,* Ureteral mobilization with either transtrigonal or cephalotrigonal course for reimplantation. Mucosal strip of trigone to form bladder neck and prostatic urethra. Lateral denuded muscle triangles are lengthened by several small incisions to allow easy tailoring of the bladder neck reconstruction. *G–H,* The double-breasted nature and exact suture placement of the bladder neck reconstruction are depicted. A pressure profile catheter can be left and a urethral pressure profile obtained prior to closure of the bladder dome. Suspension sutures are elevated manually to estimate the final urethral pressure profile. *I,* Bladder neck and urethra are left *unstented.* Drainage is by urethral catheters and suprapubic tube. Bladder outlet resistance is estimated by water manometer. (Drawings by Leon Schlossberg.)

exposure (Peters and Hendren). This tissue is simply reapproximated with heavy sutures of PDS. Patient mobility should be restricted postoperatively to allow proper healing of the intersymphyseal bar.

Intraoperative Manometrics

Experience with intraoperative urodynamics shows that an intraoperative continence length of 2.5 to 3.5 cm is desirable (Gearhart et al, 1986). Also, intraoperative closure pressures ranging between 70 and 100 ml of water are required to prevent leakage when the bladder pressure is raised to 50 cm of water intraoperatively (Gearhart et al, 1986). At the end of the procedure, the bladder neck reconstruction is further enhanced by suspending the urethra and bladder neck to the structures of the pubis and anterior rectus sheath in the manner of Marshall, Marchetti, and Krantz. The continence length increases by at least 1 cm, and the closure pressure is at least doubled in all patients (Gearhart et al, 1986).

Ureteral stents are placed in the reimplanted ureters, and the bladder is drained by a suprapubic catheter, which is left indwelling for a 3-week period. Suprapubic catheter drainage prevents stretching or pressure on the reconstructed bladder neck. No *urethral* stent is used, and catheterization or instrumentation through the urethra is strictly avoided for a minimum of 3 weeks. The adequacy of bladder neck reconstruction is tested by water manometer at the end of the procedure. The bladder neck should support 50 cm of water pressure without leakage if the bladder neck plasty and suspension are adequate. Immediate revision is advisable when this degree of resistance is not obtained. Attempts are made to reduce postoperative frequency and severity of bladder spasms by the use of propantheline bromide (Pro-Banthine), oxybutynin HCl (Ditropan), diazepam (Valium), or imipramine HCl (Tofranil).

Patients are given intravenous antibiotics for 7 days to prevent infection. Prophylactic antibacterials are then begun and continued for the foreseeable future. Little or no leakage of urine should occur through the urethra during the 3 weeks of suprapubic drainage. Prior to removal of the suprapubic catheter, a clamp is applied to initiate voiding and the urethra is calibrated with a soft 8 Fr. catheter. Specimens for culture are obtained so that specific medi-

cation may be given to clear any bacteria. In some patients, immediate voiding after suprapubic clamping will not occur. Occasionally, a gentle cystoscopy using the infant cystoscope to help "find the way" will be needed. Oftentimes at this juncture a soft 8 Fr. Foley catheter is left in place for 24 to 48 hours to help dilate the passage. It is mandatory that there be catheterizable access through the urethra and bladder neck before the suprapubic tube is removed. In some patients, a period of intermittent catheterization may be required if reasonable bladder emptying does not occur. When the catheter is removed, a short dry interval is expected to occur but bladder size and operative reaction may result in a capacity no more than a few milliliters initially. Patients must learn to recognize bladder filling and to initiate a detrusor contraction, which they may not have experienced previously. A readjustment period occurs that may extend for many months before a useful bladder volume and long dry interval develop. Initially, the absence of stress incontinence and continuous urethral dribbling suggests that urethral resistance has been produced and that an increasing dry interval will occur. The patient should learn to use this interval profitably for daytime and later for nighttime continence.

Results

Staged Functional Closure

Reviews of functional bladder closure in bladder exstrophy have demonstrated dramatic improvements in the frequency of successful reconstructions. Several series (Ansell; Chisholm, 1979; Gearhart and Jeffs, 1989a; Mollard) have shown the success and applicability of the staged functional closure approach to bladder exstrophy. Series by Conner et al, Hussman et al (1988), and Canning et al (1989) have documented acceptable continence rates with the preservation of renal function in the vast majority of patients (Table 15–2).

Primary Bladder Closure

Sixty-seven of 68 consecutive patients with bladder exstrophy referred to our pediatric urology service between 1972 and 1989 underwent bladder closure (Canning et al, 1989). One patient had only a small bladder patch unsuitable for bladder closure and was treated

Table 15–2 □ Urinary Continence Following Functional Bladder Closure

Series*	No. of Closures Evaluated	Patients Who Remained Continent	
		No.	*%*
Chisholm (1979)	95	43	45
Mollard (1980)	16	11	69
Jeffs et al (1982)	55	33	60
Ansell (1983)	23	10	43
Husmann et al (1989)	80	60	75
Connor et al (1988)	40	35	82
Canning et al (1989)	67	51	76

From Gearhart JP, Jeffs RD: Exstrophy of the bladder, epispadias, and other bladder anomalies. *In* Campbell's Urology, 6th ed. Edited by PC Walsh, AB Retik, TA Stamey, ED Vaughn Jr., Philadelphia, WB Saunders Co, 1992.

by primary urinary diversion. The complications following primary bladder closure and the additional surgical procedures required to correct these complications are presented in Table 15–3. The importance of a successful initial closure has been emphasized by Oesterling and Jeffs and Hussman et al (1989), who found that the onset of eventual continence was quicker and the continence rate higher in those who underwent a successful initial closure with or without osteotomy. Also, the importance of an early initial bladder closure is emphasized by the data of Hussman et al (1989) showing that only 10 per cent of those patients who had bladder closure prior to 1 year of age needed eventual augmentation whereas 40 per cent of those who underwent bladder closure after 1 year of age required eventual bladder augmentation.

Table 15–3 □ Complications in 75 Primary Bladder Closures

	No.
Complication	
Bladder prolapse	11
Outlet obstruction (hydronephrosis)	2
Bladder calculi	2
Renal calculi	1
Wound dehiscence	3
Stitch granuloma	2
Corrective Surgical Procedure	
Repair of bladder prolapse/ dehiscence	14
Cystolithopexy	2
Urethrotomy	1
Augmentation cystoplasty	2

From Gearhart JP, Jeffs RD: Exstrophy of the bladder, epispadias, and other bladder anomalies. *In* Campbell's Urology, 6th ed. Edited by PC Walsh, AB Retik, TA Stamey, ED Vaughn Jr., Philadelphia, WB Saunders Co, 1992.

Bladder Neck Reconstruction

Seventy-five patients, some of whom underwent initial closure elsewhere, underwent initial bladder neck reconstruction at our institution between 1975 and 1989 (Canning et al, 1989). Current voiding status of each patient was obtained based on parental or patient interview or by direct observation by the nursing and physician staff. The patients were categorized as spontaneously voiding or on intermittent catheterization and were assigned a "continence number" as follows:

1. Dry
2. Dry during the day with occasional nighttime wetting
3. Dry for greater than 3 hours during the day with occasional nighttime wetting
4. Dry for more than 3 hours during the day but wet at nighttime
5. Wet

Patients in groups 1, 2, and 3 were considered continent; patients in groups 4 and 5 were defined as intermediately continent and incontinent, respectively. Fifty-five patients (74 per cent) were continent following bladder neck reconstruction; 12 (16 per cent) were dry for 1 to 2 hours during the day and wet at nighttime; and eight (10 per cent) remained totally wet. The vast majority (84 per cent) were voiding, and 12 (16 per cent) were on intermittent catheterization (Table 15–4).

Renal units from 75 patients have been evaluated by IVP or ultrasound between 6 months and 10 years following bladder neck reconstruction to assess the preservation of renal function following the continence procedure. Only two patients have shown significant hydronephrosis and deterioration of renal

Table 15–4 □ Urinary Continence Following 75 Initial Bladder Neck Reconstructions*

Result	Average Daytime Dry Interval (hr)	Patients	
		No.	*Per Cent*
Continent	3	55	74
Intermediate	1–3	12	16
Wet	1	8	10

From Gearhart JP, Jeffs RD: Exstrophy of the bladder, epispadias, and other bladder anomalies. *In* Campbell's Urology, 6th ed. Edited by PC Walsh, AB Retik, TA Stamey, ED Vaughn Jr., Philadelphia, WB Saunders Co., 1992.

function. There were 23 complications in 20 patients. Major complications included ureteral obstruction in three patients and bladder outlet obstruction requiring intermittent catheterization or prolonged suprapubic drainage that occurred in 14 patients.

There were several additional interesting findings in the bladder neck reconstruction group. Eventual continence was more likely in those patients who underwent initial bladder closure before 72 hours of age or after 72 hours of age with an osteotomy, whereas those who underwent closure after 72 hours of age without osteotomy had a very low continence rate (25 per cent). These patients were often referred to us because of a dehiscence. These findings agree with Hussman et al (1989), who found that patients who underwent delayed closure without osteotomy showed a significantly lower rate of eventual continence (10 per cent). Another important factor is bladder capacity at the time of bladder neck reconstruction. In this series and others, the continence rate is certainly higher in those patients who have a good bladder capacity at the time of bladder neck reconstruction (Hussman et al, 1989). Thus, the bladder capacity under anesthesia prior to bladder neck reconstruction is an important predictor of eventual urinary continence. The incontinence procedure should often be deferred until the bladder reaches a capacity of 60 to 75 ml.

Half of our patients underwent epispadias repair prior to bladder neck reconstruction. The mean increase in bladder volume was 49.7 ml over a 2-year period. The onset of continence was an interesting time period in this group of exstrophy patients. All but four patients achieved continence within the first 2 years following bladder neck reconstruction. Of a select group of 34 patients included in the above group of 75, 23 actually became continent in the first year after bladder neck reconstruction.

Urethroplasty

Fifty-five patients with bladder exstrophy underwent initial urethral reconstruction at Johns Hopkins between 1975 and 1989. A modified Young urethroplasty was performed in 51 patients, a distal urethral free graft in two, a bladder mucosal graft in one, and a ventral preputial pedicle flap in one. The average age at the time of urethral reconstruction was 3.5 years.

Fistulas developed in 21 patients following epispadias repair. One of the fistulas closed spontaneously, and 20 patients required surgical closure. The majority of these fistulas occurred at the junction of the corona and glans. This area is not only where a paucity of skin occurs but also where the most tension lies in the skin closure. Fistulas were closed by excising a small rim of penile skin and separating the fistulous tract from the adjacent penile skin. The urethra is then closed with 6-0 Vicryl suture. Multiple layers of soft tissue are brought together over the urethra to further bolster the repair. Again, most of these patients have had preoperative testosterone to increase the availability of local penile skin (Gearhart and Jeffs, 1987). All of the fistulas were repaired in a separate procedure.

In a prior review by Lepor and Jeffs, five parameters were evaluated as to their effect on subsequent fistula formation: (1) osteotomy, (2) sequence of bladder neck reconstruction and epispadias repair, (3) hospital of initial treatment, (4) number of prior bladder closures performed, and (5) preoperative hormonal administration. Of 55 patients (89 per cent), 49 underwent bilateral osteotomy prior to epispadias repair. As reported in Lepor and Jeffs' original series, a prior osteotomy appeared to decrease the number of fistulas requiring surgical closure. In our expanded series, more than one half of the fistulas occurred in patients without prior osteotomy. Again, the fistula rate was found to be independent of the sequence of bladder neck reconstruction and epispadias repair, the number of prior bladder closures, or the use of hormonal stimulation of the genitalia.

In the Lepor and Jeffs original report, an attempt was made to evaluate the current status of the genital reconstruction from parental interviews. Forty-nine parents were interviewed. The angulation of the flaccid penis when standing was directed downward in 83 per cent of boys. This finding compares favorably with the series of Mesrobian et al of 18 patients who had undergone primary closure with a straight penis and downward angulation in 55 per cent of cases. Erections were witnessed in 83 per cent of the youngsters in the Lepor and Jeffs series. In these individuals, the erect penis was directed upward in 47 per cent, horizontally in 47 per cent, and downward in 6 per cent. Every parent was extremely satisfied with the appearance of the penis, although some expressed concern about whether the penis would attain adequate size for sexual intercourse after puberty. In follow-up of a group of postpubertal patients, Mesrobian et al found that of those postpubertal patients with a straight penis, 86 per cent could achieve satisfactory intercourse whereas when the penis was angulated upward, one in two could also have what they reported as satisfactory sexual intercourse.

Fertility and Pregnancy

Reconstruction of the male genitalia and preservation of fertility were not primary objectives of the early surgical management of bladder exstrophy. Sporadic accounts of pregnancy or the initiation of pregnancy by males with bladder exstrophy had been reported. In two large exstrophy series, male fertility was rarely documented. Only three of 68 men (Bennett) and four of 72 men (Woodhouse et al) had successfully fathered children. Six of 26 and seven of 27 women with bladder exstrophy in these respective series successfully bore offspring. A survey of 2500 exstrophy and epispadias patients identified 38 males who had fathered children and 131 female patients who had borne offspring (Shapiro et al, 1985).

Hanna and Williams compared semen analyses of men who had undergone primary bladder closure and ureterosigmoidostomy. A normal sperm count was found in only one of eight men following functional bladder closure

and in four of eight men with urinary diversions. The difference in observed fertility potential was probably attributable to iatrogenic injury of the verumontanum during functional closure. Retrograde ejaculation may also account for the low sperm counts observed following functional bladder closure.

Preservation of libido in exstrophy patients is normal (Woodhouse et al). The erectile mechanism in patients who had undergone epispadias repair appears intact, since 87 per cent of boys and young men in our series had experienced erections following epispadias repair (Lepor et al).

Other Techniques

Unfortunately, not all children born with bladder exstrophy are candidates for staged functional closure, usually because of a small bladder plate or significant hydronephrosis. Additional reasons for seeking other methods of treatment include failure of initial closure with a small remaining bladder and failure of incontinence surgery. Therefore, in excluding those patients with a failure in initial treatment, this discussion deals with options available if staged functional closure is not suitable or for other reasons has not been chosen by the surgeon.

Ureterosigmoidostomy

Whichever diversion option is chosen, the upper tracts and renal function initially are usually normal. This allows the reimplantation of normal-sized ureters in a reliable nonrefluxing manner into the colon or other suitable urinary reservoir. Historically, *ureterosigmoidostomy* was the first form of diversion to be popularized in the exstrophy patient group. Although the initial series was associated with multiple metabolic problems, when newer techniques of reimplantation of the ureter into the colon were developed, results improved markedly (Leadbetter; Zarbo and Kay). Ureterosigmoidostomy is favored by some because of the lack of an abdominal stoma. However, this form of diversion should not be offered until one is certain that anal continence is normal and after the family has been made aware of the potential for serious complications, including pyelonephritis, hyperchloremic acidosis, rectal incontinence, ureteral obstruction, and the late development of malignancy (Duckett and Gazak; Spence et al). More recently, ureterosigmoidostomy has been proposed again as the initial treatment for bladder exstrophy with acceptable continence and renal preservation in a 10-year follow-up period (Stoeckel et al). However, data from Woodhouse and Strachan (1990) showed that of 34 patients followed carefully for more than 20 years, a colonic tumor developed in 22 per cent. Thus, the long-term cancer risk of ureterosigmoidostomy must be carefully considered in the young child. This is especially true in regard to today's very mobile society, in which careful, long-term follow-up may be difficult to guarantee. Ileocecal ureterosigmoidostomy appears to offer the advantages of intact ureterosigmoidostomy without the increased risk of cancer.

Trigonosigmoidostomy

Owing to the many complications associated with ureterosigmoidostomy, several alternative techniques of urinary diversion for bladder exstrophy have been described. Madyl described a method of trigonosigmoidostomy. Boyce and Vest reviewed 23 trigonosigmoidostomies followed for a mean interval of 10 years. Renal function, assessed by excretory urography, was normal in 21 cases (91 per cent); stones formed in two patients (9 per cent), and hypokalemic acidosis developed in approximately 50 per cent. Only a few individuals required chronic alkalinization, however, and reoperation was performed in only two cases (9 per cent). All of the children achieved daytime continence, and, overall, results were considered to be excellent in 18 cases (78 per cent). Kroovand's update of Boyce's 37-year experience with this procedure found that the majority of patients showed stable upper urinary tracts, minimal leakage, and no electrolyte imbalances or malignant change in the vesicorectal reservoir.

The Heitz-Boyer–Hovelacque procedure includes diverting the ureters into an isolated rectal segment and pulling the sigmoid colon through the anal sphincter muscle just posterior to the rectum. Taccinoli et al reviewed 21 staged Heitz-Boyer–Hovelacque procedures for bladder exstrophy that were followed for between 1 and 16 years. They reported 95 per cent fecal and urinary continence; no cases of urinary calculi, electrolyte abnormalities, or postoperative mortality; and the development of ureterorectal strictures requiring surgical revision in three patients (14 per cent).

Urinary Diversion

The early results following ileal conduit urinary diversions suggested that this technique might be useful for urinary drainage in bladder exstrophy patients, since fecal contamination and acidosis due to reabsorption were avoided. Unfortunately, significant long-term complications developed in children, especially 10 to 15 years following ileal conduit diversion (Jeffs and Schwarz, 1975; Shapiro et al, 1975). Ileal conduit diversion is not generally acceptable for exstrophy patients who otherwise have a normal life expectancy (MacFarland et al).

As an alternative method of treatment, Hendren (1976) first established an antirefluxing colonic conduit and later, after reflux was demonstrably absent, anastomosed the distal end to sigmoid colon. The nonrefluxing ureterointestinal anastomosis represents the primary advantage of colon conduits. The colon conduit is constructed when the child is 1 year of age. When anal continence is achieved, if the ureterocolonic anastomosis is indeed nonrefluxing, and if there is no upper tract deterioration, the colon conduit is undiverted into the colon when the child is age 4 to 6. Sixteen colon conduits and 11 subsequent colocoloplasties were reported by Hendren. The postoperative complications were intestinal obstruction in three cases (19 per cent) and ureteral obstruction in one case (6 per cent). There have been no instances of stomal complications, persistent reflux, pyelonephritis, or upper tract deterioration in the Hendren series. The long-term assessment of renal function and continence following colon conduit diversion and subsequent colocoloplasty requires further investigation. Despite the author's preference for primary functional bladder closure in bladder exstrophy, colon conduit urinary diversion represents the most attractive alternative, since a nonrefluxing anastomosis is achieved, which protects the kidney to a significant degree, and undiversion can be performed when clinically indicated.

An additional innovative approach by Retik and Rink was the creation of a nonrefluxing ileocecal segment that can be rejoined to the sigmoid colon. In this procedure, the terminal ileum is intussuscepted through the ileocecal valve and stabilized against the cecal wall to prevent dissusception. The nipple then serves as the antireflux mechanism. The cecum is anastomosed to the lower sigmoid colon, and the ureters to the ileal "tail" proximal to the intussusception. The result, from the patient's point of view, is the same as after intact ureterosigmoidostomy. Urine is passed mixed with feces. Control is dependent upon an intact anal sphincter. However, since the transitional epithelium of the ureters is in a sterile environment above the antireflux nipple, the increased risk of later malignancy is avoided, at least on theoretical grounds.

Leonard reported on the series of Gearhart and Jeffs (1990) in which good success was obtained in difficult failed exstrophy reconstructions by the use of multiple reconstructive techniques, including the Mitrofanoff and Benchekroun principles, which facilitate a continent urinary diversion.

Arap et al (1976) managed bladder exstrophy by initially constructing a colon urinary conduit. The entire bladder is then tubularized into a 5- to 6-cm neourethra, and the colon conduit is then later anastomosed to the urethrovesical tube. This technique may be useful for the patient with a failed Young-Dees-Leadbetter bladder neck procedure with a small contracted bladder or for the initial treatment of a bladder exstrophy when the bladder capacity is less than 3 ml.

The most reliable method for permanent urinary diversion currently in children is the nonrefluxing colon conduit, for which an external stoma and appliance are required. However, techniques of continent urinary diversion are rapidly improving, as are the results in the treatment of the bladder exstrophy patient, especially those with an initial failure. The author feels strongly that the optimal method of treating bladder exstrophy today is the staged functional reconstructive approach. Those patients with small bladders that are unsuitable for closure, late closure, or multiple closures who do not achieve an adequate bladder capacity after the first stage of reconstruction are the problematic patients. These patients are reasonably treated with any of the multiple reconstructive procedures mentioned above (Leonard et al).

EPISPADIAS

Epispadias varies from a glanular defect in a stubby covered penis to the complete variety associated with exstrophy of the bladder.

Classification

Epispadias in males is classified according to the position of the dorsally displaced urethral meatus. The degree of penile deformity and the occurrence of urinary incontinence are usually related to the extent of displacement of the urethral meatus. The displaced meatus may be found on the glans, penile shaft, or penopubic region. All types of epispadias are associated with varying degrees of dorsal chordee. In penopubic or subsymphyseal epispadias, the entire penile urethra is open and the bladder outlet may be large enough to admit the examining finger, indicating obvious gross incontinence. The pubic symphysis is divergent and contributes to the deficiency of the external urinary sphincter mechanism. The divergence of the pubis symphysis and the shortened urethral plate result in prominent dorsal chordee and a penis that appears short. The penile deformity is virtually identical to that seen in bladder exstrophy.

Kramer and Kelalis reviewed their surgical experience in 82 males with epispadias. Penopubic epispadias occurred in 49 cases, penile epispadias in 21 and glanular epispadias in 12. Urinary incontinence was observed in 46 of 49 patients with penopubic epispadias, and 15 of 21 patients with penile epispadias, but in none with glanular epispadias.

In a combined study, Dees reported the incidence of complete epispadias to be 1 in 117,000 males and 1 in 484,000 females. The reported male-to-female ratio of epispadias varies between 3:1 (Dees, 1949) and 5:1 (Kramer and Kelalis, 1982). Epispadias is apparently becoming more common.

Epispadias in the female is characterized by a bifid clitoris, flattening of the mons, and separation of the labia. There are three types of epispadias in females: In the least degree, the urethral orifice merely appears patulous; in intermediate epispadias, the urethra is dorsally split along most of the urethra; and in the most severe degree, the urethral cleft involves the entire length of the urethra and the sphincter mechanisms are then completely absent.

Associated Anomalies

The anomalies associated with complete epispadias are usually confined to deformities of the external genitalia, diastasis of the pubic symphysis, and deficiency of the urinary continence mechanism. The only renal anomaly observed in 11 cases of complete epispadias was agenesis of the left kidney (Campbell). In a review by Arap et al (1988), in 38 patients there was one case of unilateral renal agenesis and one ectopic pelvic kidney. The uretero-vesical junction is often also abnormal in complete epispadias, and reflux has been reported in a number of series to be around 30 to 40 per cent (Arap et al, 1988; Kramer and Kelalis).

Surgical Management

The objectives for the repair of penopubic epispadias include achievement of urinary continence with preservation of the upper urinary tract and reconstruction of functional and cosmetically acceptable and attractive genitalia. The surgical management of incontinence in penopubic epispadias is virtually identical to that of a closed bladder exstrophy.

Young reported the first cure of incontinence in a male with complete epispadias. Since Young described his approach, published results have been good. The operation has been progressively refined and standardized (Arap et al, 1988; Burkholder and Williams; Kramer and Kelalis; Peters et al, 1988). In patients with complete epispadias and good bladder capacity, epispadias and bladder neck reconstruction can be performed in a single operation. Urethroplasty formerly was performed after the bladder neck reconstruction in most cases (Arap et al; Kramer and Kelalis). However, results with both the small bladder associated with exstrophy (Gearhart and Jeffs, 1989b) or epispadias alone (Peters et al) have led us to perform urethroplasty and penile elongation prior to bladder neck reconstruction. A small incontinent bladder with reflux is hardly an ideal situation for bladder neck reconstruction and ureteral reimplantation. With urethroplasty prior to bladder neck reconstruction, there was an average increase in bladder capacity of 95 ml within 18 months in those patients with an initial small bladder capacity associated with epispadias and a continence rate overall of 87 per cent after the continence procedure (Peters et al, 1988).

In epispadias, much as in the exstrophy group, bladder capacity is the most accurate prognostic indicator of eventual continence (Ritchey et al). In one series Arap et al (1988) noted a much higher continence rate in those with adequate bladder capacity (71 per cent) prior to bladder neck reconstruction than in those with a smaller capacity (20 per cent). In addition, in Arap's group of complete epispadias patients, most attained continence within

2 years, much like patients with classic bladder exstrophy (Canning et al, 1989).

A firm intersymphyseal band bridges the divergent symphysis, and an osteotomy is not usually performed. The Young-Dees-Leadbetter bladder neck plasty, Marshall-Marchetti-Krantz bladder neck suspension, and ureteral reimplantation are performed when the bladder capacity reaches approximately 60 ml, which usually occurs when the child is between 3 and 4 years of age.

The genital reconstruction and urethroplasty in epispadias and exstrophy are quite similar. There must be a release of dorsal chordee and division of suspensory ligaments, dissection of the corpora from their attachment to the inferior pubic ramus, lengthening of the urethral groove, and lengthening of the corpora, if needed, by incision and anastomosis or grafting, or by medial rotation of the ventral corpora in a more downward direction.

Urethral reconstruction in complete epispadias can be as simple as a modified Young urethroplasty (Gearhart and Jeffs, 1989a) to even a two-stage repair (Kramer and Kelalis). All modern techniques of hypospadias repair have been used to aid in the repair of epispadias from the utilization of the prepuce to bladder mucosa and full-thickness skin grafts. The use of a transverse ventral island flap has been popularized by Monfort. The urethra, once reconstructed, can be positioned between and below the corpora (Cantwell; Ransley et al). A planned two-stage repair has been used with success in these reconstructions (Kramer and Kelalis). The glanular and skin closure is performed as in reconstruction of the penis in patients with bladder exstrophy.

The achievement of urinary continence following bladder neck reconstruction in patients with epispadias is summarized in Table 15–5 (Arap et al, 1988; Burkholder and Williams; Dees; Kramer and Kelalis; Peters et al). The majority of these patients underwent reconstruction by means of a Young-Dees-Leadbetter bladder neck plasty. Urinary continence was achieved in 74 per cent of males and 85 per cent of females following bladder neck reconstruction. Urinary diversion should therefore seldom be considered in the initial management of complete epispadias. Delayed development of urinary continence occurred in more than half the males with complete epispadias who eventually became continent following the continence operations (Kramer and Kelalis). The effect that urethral lengthening and prostatic enlargement may have on

Table 15–5 □ Urinary Continence Following Bladder Neck Reconstruction (BNR) in Patients with Complete Epispadias

	Kramer and Kelalis (1982)	Canning et al (1989)	Arap et al (1988)	Burkholder and Williams (1965)	Dees (1949)	Total
Total patients with complete epispadias	53	17	38	27	6	141
Number of males with complete epispadias treated with BNR*	32*	11	21	17	5	86
Number of males with surgically corrected incontinence	22	11	15	8	5	61
Percentage of males with surgically corrected incontinence	69	83	71	47	100	74
Number of females with complete epispadias treated with BNR	8	6	9	10	1	34
Number of females with surgically corrected incontinence	8	6	7	7	1	29
Percentage of females with surgically corrected incontinence	88	90	77	70	100	85

From Gearhart JP, Jeffs RD: Exstrophy of the bladder, epispadias, and other bladder anomalies. *In* Campbell's Urology. 6th ed. Edited by PC Walsh, AB Retik, TA Stamey, ED Vaughn Jr. Philadelphia, WB Saunders Co, 1992.
*Male patients with penopubic epispadias and total incontinence included.

increasing bladder outlet resistance is emphasized by these observations in the epispadias group. However, in a series by Arap et al (1988), continence had no relationship to puberty and usually occurred within 2 years; in the majority of patients, continence preceded puberty by several years.

The results of urethroplasty for epispadias have been reviewed by Kramer and Kelalis (1988). A Thiersch-Duplay procedure (modified Young urethroplasty) was selected in 49 of 67 cases (73 per cent), and several other reconstructive techniques were used in the remaining 18 cases. Urethral fistulas necessitating surgical repair occurred in 21 per cent of these urethroplasties.

Kramer et al (1986) reported the success of genital reconstruction in epispadias with a straight penis angled downward in almost 70 per cent of patients in whom erectile function was normal. Of this group, 80 per cent have experienced satisfactory sexual intercourse, and of 29 married patients, 19 have fathered children. This carefully constructed and well-planned approach to the management of urinary incontinence and genital deformities associated with complete epispadias should provide a gratifying cosmetic appearance, normal genital function, and preservation of fertility potential in most patients.

CLOACAL EXSTROPHY

Cloacal exstrophy represents one of the most severe congenital anomalies that is compatible with intrauterine viability. Fortunately, this entity is exceedingly rare, occurring in approximately 1 in 200,000 to 400,000 live births (Gravier). More recent reports indicate a sex ratio of approximately two males to one female patient (Gearhart and Jeffs, 1990; Hurwitz et al). Also, reports have shown that this condition can be diagnosed reliably antenatally (Meizner and Bar-Ziv). The inheritance pattern of cloacal exstrophy is unknown, since offspring have never been produced by individuals with this disorder.

Anatomy and Embryology

Anatomically, there is exstrophy of the foreshortened hindgut or cecum, which displays its bulging mucosa between the two exstrophied hemibladders (Fig. 15–112). The orifices of the terminal ileum, rudimentary tailgut, and a single (or paired) appendix are apparent on the surface of the everted cecum. The tailgut is blind-ending, and the ileum may be prolapsed. The pubic symphysis is widely separated, the hips are externally rotated and abducted, and the phallus is separated into right and left halves with adjacent labium or scrotal half (Fig. 15–113).

Schlegel and Gearhart have defined the neuroanatomy of the pelvis in the child with cloacal exstrophy. The autonomic innervation to the hemibladders and corporal bodies arise from a pelvic plexus on the anterior surface of the rectum. The nerves to the hemibladders travel in the midline along the posterior-infe-

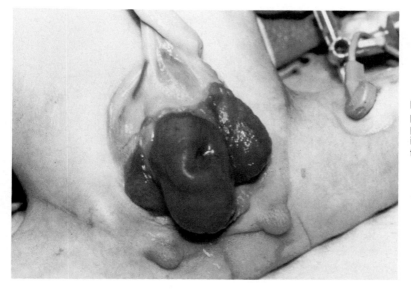

Figure 15–112 ☐ Cloacal exstrophy in a newborn male. Small omphalocele shows prolapse of the ileum through ileocecal area between exstrophied hemibladders.

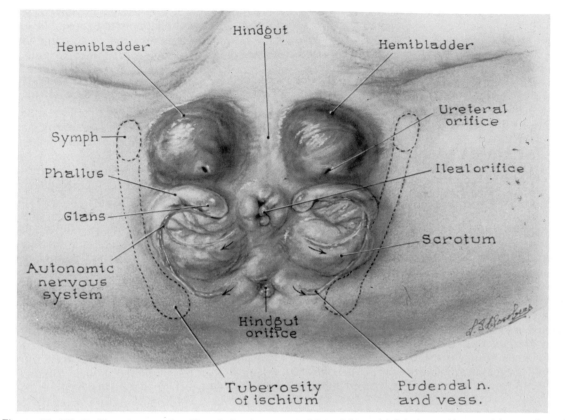

Figure 15–113 □ Cloacal exstrophy. The phallus is separated into right and left halves with neural innervation of corporal bodies and marked separation of pubic symphysis. (Drawing by Leon Schlossberg.)

rior surface of the rectum and extend laterally to the hemibladders. The autonomic innervation to the duplicated corporal bodies arises from the sacral pelvic plexus, travels in the midline, perforates the inferior portion of the pelvic floor, and courses medially to the hemibladder (Schlegel and Gearhart).

During normal embryogenesis, after 4 weeks of life the urorectal septum divides the cloaca into an anterior urogenital sinus and a posterior anorectal canal. Simultaneously, the infraumbilical abdominal wall is formed by primitive mesoderm, which migrates around the cloacal membrane. The cloacal membrane reaches its greatest dimension at 5 weeks of gestation and then regresses in size. Normally, the membrane ruptures after 6 weeks, when the urorectal septum has been formed, and the urethral, vaginal, and anal orifices then open onto the perineum. According to Marshall and Muecke, an abnormally extensive cloacal membrane produces a wedge effect by serving as a mechanical barrier to mesodermal migra-

tion, which results in impaired development of the abdominal wall, failure of fusion of the paired genital tubercles, and diastasis pubis. Exstrophy of the cloaca results when the wedge effect occurs before formation of the urorectal septum at 6 weeks.

Associated Conditions

A review of a large series of cloacal exstrophy patients by Hurwitz et al found associated anomalies in 85 per cent of cases. The most common genitourinary anomalies were pelvic kidneys, unilateral renal agenesis, multicystic kidneys, and ureteral duplication, in that order. Forty-eight per cent of patients had vertebral anomalies, and 46 per cent had associated gastrointestinal anomalies. Twenty-nine per cent had central nervous system anomalies (myelomeningocele, meningocele, or lipomeningocele) and 26 per cent had severe deformities of the lower extremities.

Surgical Management

Until recently, surgical reconstruction of cloacal exstrophy was considered futile and untreated neonates usually died from prematurity, sepsis, short bowel syndrome, or renal and central nervous system deficits. Rickham reported the first patient with cloacal exstrophy to survive surgical reconstruction. The omphalocele was repaired, the intestinal strip was separated from the hemibladders, and the blind-ending colon was externalized through the perineum. The hemibladders were then reapproximated. A ureteroileal conduit was constructed when the child was 18 months old, and a cystectomy was subsequently performed.

The only practical approach to reconstruction of cloacal exstrophy is by staged surgical reconstructive procedures (Table 15–6). The child's condition at birth may be critical, and attempts to reconstruct and repair may be futile or morally or ethically unwise. The more robust infant will survive and reparative surgery is then initiated in early infancy. Most individuals with cloacal exstrophy should be reared as females owing to the severe deformity and deficiency of the paired phallus

Table 15–6 ☐ Staged Functional Closure of Cloacal Exstrophy

Immediate Neonatal Assessment
 Evaluate associated anomalies
 Decide whether to proceed with reparative surgery

Functional Bladder Closure *(Immediately After Neonatal Assessment)*
 Bilateral iliac or innominate osteotomies
 Gonadectomy in males with a very small or absent penis
 Terminal ileostomy
 Closure of hemibladders

Anti-incontinence and Antireflux Procedure *(Age 3–5 Years)*
 Bladder capacity > 60 ml: Young-Dees-Leadbetter bladder neck plasty with Cohen ureteral reimplantations and Marshall-Marchetti-Krantz bladder neck suspension
 Bladder capacity < 60 ml: tubularized bladder into a urethrovesical tube. Ureters are reimplanted into a bladder or a bowel segment used to augment bladder capacity or continent diversion with/without abdominal stoma; Arap procedure as for bladder exstrophy
 Anti-incontinence devices: used for refractory incontinence; artificial sphincter

Vaginal Reconstruction *(Age 14–18 Years)*
 Vagina constructed or augmented using rudimentary colon

From Gearhart JP, Jeffs RD: Exstrophy of the bladder, epispadias, and other bladder anomalies. *In* Campbell's Urology, 6th ed. Edited by PC Walsh, AB Retik, TA Stamey, ED Vaughn Jr. Philadelphia, WB Saunders Co, 1992.

(Hussman et al, 1989). A gonadectomy is done when sex reassignment is indicated. At birth the omphalocele is repaired. A terminal ileostomy or a colostomy is performed to preserve as much of the hindgut as possible, including the rudimentary terminal colon (Howell et al). A very short terminal colonic segment can be used as the vagina. The exstrophied bladder is closed, and the bifid phallus is reapproximated in the midline. Both anterior innominate osteotomy and posterior iliac osteotomy have been used in the closure of cloacal exstrophy. With a large omphalocele defect, bladder closure and osteotomy must be delayed until respiratory and gastrointestinal stability is achieved. Anterior osteotomy allows placement of pins for external fixation and is preferred when severe lumbosacral dysraphism is present.

An additional operation may be required to join the terminal ileum to the colon segment to form a colostomy. Usually, intestinal absorption problems are resolved at approximately 3 to 4 years of age, and the most advantageous type of urinary tract reconstruction can then be considered. Urinary continence can be achieved in these individuals in many ways. An orthotopic urethra can be constructed from local tissue, vagina, ileum, or even ureter. A catheterizable stoma can be constructed from ileum when enough bowel is present and fluid loss by the intestine is not a problem. The bladder may be augmented with unused hindgut, ileum, or stomach (Gearhart and Jeffs, 1990; Mitchell and Peiser). However, surgery to produce a continent reservoir should be delayed until a method of evacuation can be taught and the child is old enough to participate in self-care. The choice between a catheterizable urethra and an abdominal stoma depends on the adequacy of the urethra and bladder outlet, interest and dexterity of the child, and orthopedic status regarding the spine, hip joints, braces and ambulation.

In one series, Gearhart and Jeffs (1990) used multiple techniques to produce continence in a selected group of ten cloacal exstrophy patients who underwent staged functional closure, including Young-Dees-Leadbetter bladder neck and urethral reconstruction in three, intermittent catheterization in one, ileal nipple plus augmentation in four, Kropp procedure plus bladder augmentation in one, and Benchekroun procedure plus augmentation in one. Staged reconstruction can therefore produce urinary continence in this complex anomaly. An innovative approach is required to find the most suitable solution for each individual patient concerning bladder size and function and mental, neurologic, and orthopedic status. With the advent of modern pediatric anesthesia and intensive care, the newborn survival rate is high. Improving survivorship makes reconstructive techniques applicable in a large percentage of infants born with this condition.

ANOMALIES OF BLADDER FORMATION

Agenesis and Hypoplasia

Agenesis of the bladder is an extremely rare congenital anomaly, with only 44 cases reported in the English literature up to 1988. Campbell reported seven cases in 19,046 autopsies (two were anencephalic monsters and in all seven, other severe anomalies coexisted). Glenn found only one case in 600,000 patients seen at Duke University Hospital in 28 years. Agenesis of the bladder is seldom compatible with life, and only 15 live births have been reported, all except one being female subjects (Akdas et al; Aragona et al; Krull et al).

The cause of agenesis of the bladder is uncertain. Because the hindgut is normal in these infants, it may be assumed that embryologic division of the cloaca into the urogenital sinus and anorectum had proceeded normally. Bladder agenesis may be the result of secondary loss of the anterior division of the cloaca, perhaps owing to a lack of distention with urine caused by failure of incorporation of the mesonephric ducts and ureters into the trigone, thus preventing urine from accumulating in the bladder (Krull et al, 1988).

The results of this anomaly depend on the sex of the fetus. In the female with normally developed müllerian structures, the ureteral orifice may end in the uterus, anterior vaginal wall, or vestibule. In these cases with ectopic ureteral openings, there is usually some preservation of renal function (Krull et al, 1988). In the male, the only means of achieving adequate outlet drainage would be cloacal persistence, with the ureters draining into the rectum, or a patent urachus. With the severity of this defect, it is not surprising that other urologic anomalies, including solitary kidney, renal agenesis, dysplasia, and the absence of prostate and seminal vesicles, coexist (Aragona et al). Treatment in most reported cases of surviving infants has included urinary diver-

sion either by ureterosigmoidostomy or by an external stoma (Glenn).

The small bladder may be dysplastic or hypoplastic. Dysplasia is seen in conditions such as duplicate exstrophy or hemibladder exstrophy, in which the rudiment is small, fibrotic, and nondistensible. Hypoplastic bladders have the potential to enlarge and are similar to those seen in conditions of severe incontinence, such as complete epispadias and bilateral ectopic ureters.

Bladder Duplication

Complete duplication of the bladder and urethra is rare, with only 45 cases reported in the literature (Kapoor and Saha). Duplications of the bladder comprise two bladder halves, each with a full-thickness muscular wall and each with its own ipsilateral ureter and urethra (Fig. 15–114). This anomaly is seen more commonly in males than in females. Associated congenital anomalies of other organ systems are present in the majority of cases of complete duplication of the bladder and urethra. In 40 cases reviewed by Kossow and Morales, 90 per cent had some type of duplication of the external

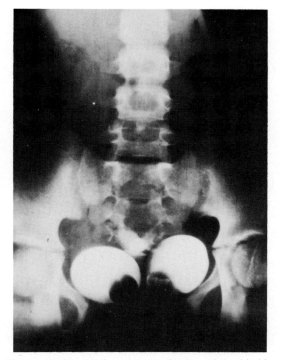

Figure 15–114 □ Complete duplication of the bladder and urethra.

genitalia and 42 per cent had duplication of the lower gastrointestinal tract. Spinal duplication and fistulas between the rectum, vagina, and urethra were other associated abnormalities.

Incomplete bladder duplication has been reported (Abramson). This entity involves two full-thickness bladders, each with its own ureter; unlike with complete bladder duplication, however, the two communicate and drain into a common urethra.

Diverticula

Congenital bladder diverticula unassociated with posterior urethral valves or neurogenic bladder are unusual but not rare (Barrett et al; Johnston, 1960). This entity is more common in male patients. Congenital diverticula usually occur in a smooth-walled, unobstructed bladder and are most often solitary and occur without evidence of outflow obstruction. The cause of these diverticula is an inherent weakness in the bladder musculature. The diverticula probably start near the ureteral orifice but not in the hiatal area. As the diverticulum enlarges, it may incorporate the ureteral tunnel and the ureter may drain into the diverticulum with resulting reflux. These congenital diverticula are often larger than those associated with neurogenic bladder or lower tract obstructive anomalies. Huge diverticula may cause outlet obstruction of the bladder neck or urethral (Taylor et al) or ureteral obstruction (Lione and Gonzalez). Diverticula are easy to diagnose on a voiding cystourethrogram, especially with post-voiding images (Fig. 15–115). Upper tract imaging, although important, is not the best method to diagnose a bladder diverticulum. Only two of 24 diverticula in Atwell's series were seen on IVP.

Recently, 11 cases of congenital bladder diverticula have been described in children with Ehlers-Danlos syndrome. This is a congenital connective tissue disorder characterized by abnormalities of collagen structure and function. However, the link between the connective tissue disorder and the occurrence of these bladder diverticula has yet to be proven. All of the reported cases of congenital bladder diverticula associated with Ehlers-Danlos syndrome have been males (Levard et al).

Megaureter (Megacystis)

Historically, "congenital megacystis" is a descriptive entity describing the bladder associated with massively refluxing megaureters. This term was first employed by Williams. The physiologic result of severe reflux is constant cycling of urine between the massively dilated refluxing megaureters and the bladder. Bladder contractibility is normal, although most of the urine at each vesicle contraction empties into the upper tracts. The effect of this constant recycling of urine is a progressive increase in residual urine and bladder capacity. The trigone is wide and poorly developed, with lateral gaping incompetent orifices. Correction

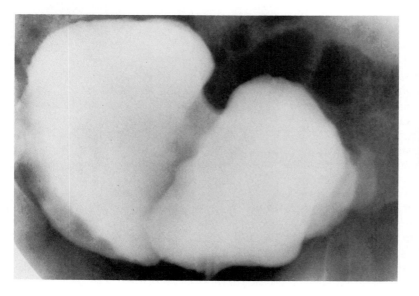

Figure 15–115 □ Congenital bladder diverticulum in an 8-year-old male. (Courtesy of Dr. George Taylor.)

of the reflux should lead to a resumption of normal voiding dynamics. The rarity of this condition in present urologic practice suggests an acquired causation as in the "neurogenic non-neurogenic bladder" syndrome. *E. coli* infection and reflux in a normal system may cause bladder and ureteral atony with subsequent dilatation. The cause of the dilated bladder in neonates may be difficult to determine when reflux, obstruction, and neurogenic abnormalities are excluded. There remains a group of patients with large bladders of unknown etiology. Prenatal temporary obstruction, metabolic abnormality, and cerebral anoxia have been implicated.

URACHAL ABNORMALITIES

Anatomy and Histology

The urachus lies between the peritoneum and transversalis fascia and extends from the anterior dome of the bladder toward the umbilicus. The urachus varies from 3 to 10 cm in length and 8 to 10 mm in diameter. The urachus is encased between two layers of umbilicovesical fascia, which tend to contain the spread of urachal disease. The urachus is adjacent to the umbilical ligaments, the remnants of the umbilical arteries. When the urachus is present as a muscular tube, three distinct tissue layers are recognized: (1) an epithelial canal of cuboidal or, more typically, transitional epithelium; (2) a submucosal connective tissue layer; and (3) an outer layer of smooth muscle that is thickest near the bladder. The central lumen is irregular and beaded and is filled with desquamated epithelial debris and epithelial islands. When the upper urachus becomes a fibrous cord, there are generally no recognizable urachal elements (Begg; Hammond et al; Hector; Steck and Helwig).

Embryology

The allantois is an extraembryonic cavity located within the body stalk that projects onto the anterior surface of the cloaca, the future bladder. The descent of the bladder into the pelvis is associated with elongation of the urachus, a tubular structure that extends from the fibrotic allantoic duct to the anterior bladder. During the 4th and 5th months of gestation, the urachus narrows to a small caliber epithelial tube (Nix et al). As the bladder descends into the pelvis during fetal development, its apical portion narrows progressively into a fibromuscular strand of urachus that maintains continuity with the allantoic duct. As the fetus develops, the urachus loses its attachment to the umbilicus. Hammond et al observed that continuity of the urachus with the posterior surface of the umbilicus and the apex of the bladder persisted in only 50 per cent of fetal specimens. Shortly after the embryonic stage of development, the tract obliterates because patency was observed in only 2 per cent of adult specimens. The obliteration of the urachus results in different patterns of urachal termination: (1) A well-defined urachal remnant may maintain an identifiable attachment to the umbilicus; (2) at a variable distance above the bladder the urachal cord may merge with one or both of the obliterated umbilical arteries, resulting in a single common ligament to the umbilicus—the medial vesicular ligament; or (3) an atrophic extension from a short tubular urachus may terminate within the fascia or blend into a plexus of fibrous tissue, the plexus of Luschka, formed by the urachus and the umbilical arteries (Blichert-Toft et al, 1971a; Hammond et al).

Congenital patent urachus is a lesion that is usually recognized in the neonate (Fig. 15–116*A*). It is a rare anomaly occurring in only three of more than 1 million admissions to a large pediatric center (Nix et al). The two forms of congenital patent urachus are persistence of the patent urachus with a partially distended bladder, and a vesicoumbilical fistula, representing failure of the bladder to descend at all (Fig. 15–116*B*). When the bladder forms, the bladder apex then never forms a true urachal tract. The more common form of a patent urachus results when there is failure of obliteration of a urachal remnant. Persistence of the urachus has been attributed to intrauterine urinary obstruction; however, only 14 per cent of neonates born with a patent urachus demonstrate evidence of urinary obstruction (Herbst). It is unlikely that urinary obstruction is directly related to the development of a patent urachus because even the most severe cases of posterior urethral valves are not associated with this anomaly. Furthermore, urethral tubularization occurs after obliteration of the urachal remnant, suggesting that urinary obstruction is not the major factor producing a patent urachus in humans (Schreck and Campbell).

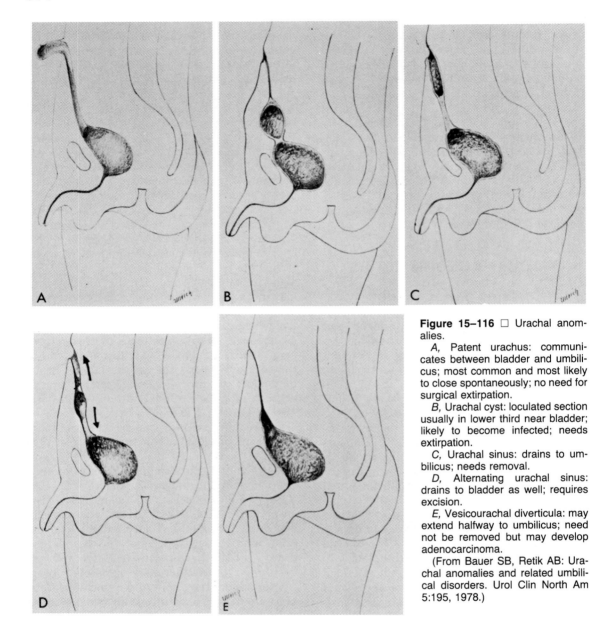

Figure 15–116 □ Urachal anomalies.

A, Patent urachus: communicates between bladder and umbilicus; most common and most likely to close spontaneously; no need for surgical extirpation.

B, Urachal cyst: loculated section usually in lower third near bladder; likely to become infected; needs extirpation.

C, Urachal sinus: drains to umbilicus; needs removal.

D, Alternating urachal sinus: drains to bladder as well; requires excision.

E, Vesicourachal diverticula: may extend halfway to umbilicus; need not be removed but may develop adenocarcinoma.

(From Bauer SB, Retik AB: Urachal anomalies and related umbilical disorders. Urol Clin North Am 5:195, 1978.)

Acquired patent urachus in the adult is usually a urinary umbilical fistula that results from bladder outflow obstruction. In these cases, extravasation of infected urine into the periurachal space ultimately may result in erosion through the umbilical region, a relatively weak segment of the abdominal wall. Since the urachus can remain attached to the umbilicus in a minority of normal adults, at least some acquired umbilical urinary fistulas may drain through the existing urachal canal. A patent urachus is diagnosed when there is free discharge of urine through the umbilicus. Patent urachus should be suspected when the umbilical cord is enlarged and edematous or when its normal slough is delayed. On occasion, the fistula is tiny and the discharge of urine may be minimal or intermittent.

The diagnosis of a patent urachus is confirmed by catheterization or probing of the urachal tract, intravesical instillation of colored dye, and analysis of the discharge fluid for blood urea nitrogen (BUN) and creatinine. Voiding cystourethrography is helpful in fully evaluating the lesion and any associated bladder outlet obstruction. Fistulography distinguishes the condition from a patent omphalomesenteric duct. Although cystoscopy is helpful in an older patient, it is not necessary in the neonate if the urethra appeas radiologically normal. Differential diagnosis of a wet umbilicus in the infant includes patent urachus, omphalitis (an infection of the umbilical stump), simple granulation of the healing stump, a patent vitelline or omphalomesenteric duct (enteroumbilical fistula), an infected umbilical vessel, and external urachal sinus. The presence of both urinary and enteric fistulas at the umbilicus is exceedingly rare (Davis and Nikhaus; Herbst; Kenigsberg; Mendoza et al; Steck and Helwig). Antenatal diagnosis of patent urachus was reported by Persutte et al. Not only is prenatal diagnosis helpful but postnatal confirmation of these omphalovesical anomalies can be readily accomplished with high-resolution ultrasound imaging (Avni et al).

A cyst may form within the isolated urachal canal if the lumen is enlarged by epithelial desquamation and degeneration. A persistent connection between a urachal sinus and the bladder may permit bacterial infection, which becomes loculated (Fig. 15–116*B*). Infected cysts occur most commonly in adults (Blichert-Toft and Neilson, 1971b; Sterling and Goldsmith); however, they have been reported in infants (Geist; Hinman). The cyst manifests itself because infection occurs. The most common organism cultured in the cyst fluid is *Staphylococcus aureus* (MacMillan et al). Untreated, the infected cyst may drain into the bladder or through the umbilicus, or it may drain intermittently internally and externally, resulting in an alternating sinus (Blichert-Toft and Neilson, 1971b; Hinman; Neidhart et al; Sterling and Goldsmith).

Serious complications of infected umbilical cysts include rupture into the preperitoneal tissues, rupture into the peritoneal cavity with significant peritonitis, and, rarely, inflammatory involvement of the adjacent bowel with the formation of enteric fistulas (Berman et al; Nunn). The symptoms and signs of a loculated, infected urachal cyst are lower abdominal pain, fever, voiding symptoms, midline hypogastric tenderness, often a palpable mass, and evidence of urinary infection. The urachal cyst should be suspected whenever localized suprapubic pain and tenderness are present with disturbed micturition, even when the urine remains clear. Useful diagnostic studies include excretory urography, cystography, cystoscopy, and high-resolution ultrasonography (Avni). Computed tomography (CT) of the abdomen may be helpful in determining the extent of the disease and the possibility of involvement of other organ systems (Berman et al).

External Urachal Sinus

Persistence of the urachal apex alone results in a blind external sinus that opens at the umbilicus (Fig. 15–116*C, D*). This may become symptomatic at any age with an infected discharge. In the adult, umbilical pilonidal disease can mimic an external sinus (Helwig). Because the differential diagnosis also includes lesions listed in the previous section, probing and radiographic evaluation should be undertaken before surgery. A urachal sinus extends inferiorly, unlike an omphalomesenteric duct remnant, which extends inward toward the peritoneal cavity.

Urachal Diverticulum

A diverticulum of the bladder apex (Fig. 15–116*E*), or "blind internal sinus," may be an incidental finding on radiographic studies not requiring treatment when it is small and minimally contractile. However, these lesions have been reported to attain massive proportions in adults, with cutaneous drainage. Surgical excision is then required (Berman et al). The large urachal diverticula, frequently seen in prune-belly syndrome (Lattimer) and occasionally associated with severe urethral obstruction, may necessitate resection. These may be poorly contractile or may expand paradoxically during voiding. Urachal diverticula occasionally contain calculi (Bandler et al; Ney and Friedenberg).

Treatment

Adequate therapy for a patent urachus involves excision of all anomalous tissue with a cuff of bladder. Some authors advocate nonoperative treatment initially while reserving radical surgical excision of the urachus for persisting cases or recurrences. Similarly, simple drainage of urachal cysts is associated with recurrent infections in 30 per cent of cases, and late occurrence of adenocarcinoma has been reported (Blichert-Toft and Neilson, 1971b; Nix et al).

In the treatment of benign urachal lesions in children, it is rarely necessary to remove the umbilicus; whenever possible, cosmetic considerations should prevail. In infants, a small curved, subumbilical incision is usually ample, for at this age the bladder dome is still high and readily accessible through this exposure.

A transverse midhypogastric incision permits adequate exposure in older children and adults and allows for both superior and inferior dissection. The urachal stalk or fibrous urachal remnant should be detached from the dermis posterior to the umbilicus. A "buttonhole" in the umbilical area is of no consequence. Application of a small gauze pledget under the dressing obliterates dead space, maintains umbilical configuration, and allows the skin to close secondarily.

When peritoneum and the umbilical ligaments are adherent to the inflammatory mass, these structures should be excised in continuity with the lesion. A vertical midline incision is the best approach for removal of an extensive inflammatory mass. Elliptical excision of the umbilicus may be necessary if it is involved in the inflammatory process, especially with an external urachal sinus or alternating sinus. A suppurating infection within a cyst or external sinus may require initial incision and drainage, and treatment as for an abscess. After healing is complete, a complete excision of the urachal tissue should be performed.

Bibliography

Abramson J: Double bladder and related anomalies: clinical and embryological aspects in a case report. Br J Urol 33:195, 1965.

Akdas A, Iseri C, Ozgur S, Kirkali Z: Bladder agenesis. Int Urol Nephrol 20:261, 1988.

Allen NH, Atwell JD: The paraureteral diverticulum in children. Br J Urol 52:264, 1980.

Ambrose SS, O'Brien DP: Surgical embryology of the exstrophy-epispadias complex. Surg Clin North Am 54:1379, 1974.

Ansell JE: Exstrophy and epispadias. In Urologic Surgery. Edited by JF Glenn. Philadelphia, JB Lippincott Co, 1983, p 647.

Aragona F, Passerini G, Zarembella P, Zorzi C, Talenti E, Perali R, Marigio A: Agenesis of the bladder: a case report and review of the literature. Urol Radiol 10:207, 1988.

Arap S, Giron A, Degoes GM: Complete reconstruction of bladder exstrophy. Urology 7:413, 1976.

Arap S, Giron AN: Duplicated exstrophy: report of three cases. Eur Urol 12:451, 1986.

Arap S, Nahas WC, Giron AM, Bruschini H, Mitra I: Incontinent epispadias: surgical treatment of 38 cases. J Urol 140:577, 1988.

Avni F, Matos C, Diard F, Schulman C: Midline omphalovesical anomalies in children: contribution of ultrasound imaging. Urol Radiol 48:189, 1988.

Bandler CG, Milbed AH, Alley JL: Urachal calculus. NY State J Med 42:2203, 1942.

Barrett DM, Malek RS, Kelalis PP: Observations of vesical diverticulum in children. J Urol 116:234, 1976.

Begg RC: The urachus and umbilical fistulae. J Anat 64:170, 1927.

Bennett AH: Exstrophy of the bladder treated by ureterosigmoidostomies. Urology 2:165, 1973.

Berman SM, Tolia BM, Laor E, Reid RE, Schweizerhof SP, Freed SZ: Urachal remnants in adults. Urology 31:17, 1988.

Blichert-Toft M, Nielson OV: Congenital patent urachus and acquired variants. Acta Chir Scand 137:807, 1971b.

Blichert-Toft M, Nielson OV: Diseases of the urachus simulating intra-abdominal disorders. Am J Surg 112:123, 1971a.

Boyce WH, Vest SA: A new concept concerning treatment of exstrophy of the bladder. J Urol 677:503, 1952.

Brezinski AE, Homsy YL, Leberg I: Orthoplasty in epispadias. J Urol 136:259, 1986.

Burbige KA, Hensle TW, Chambers WJ, Leb R, Jeter KF: Pregnancy and sexual function in women with bladder exstrophy. Urology 28:12, 1986.

Burkholder GV, Williams DI: Epispadias and incontinence: surgical treatment of 27 children. J Urol 94:674, 1965.

Campbell M: Epispadias: a report of fifteen cases. J Urol 67:988, 1952.

Canning DA, Gearhart JP, Oesterling JE, Jeffs RD: A computerized review of exstrophy patients managed during the past thirteen years (abstract 219). American Urological Association Annual Meeting, Dallas, May 7, 1989.

Canning DA, Gearhart JP, Jeffs RD: Cephalotrigonal reimplant as an adjunct to bladder neck reconstruction (abstract 219). American Urological Association Annual Meeting, New Orleans, May 1990.

Cantwell FV: Operative technique of epispadias by transplantation of the urethra. Ann Surg 22:689, 1895.

Cendron J: La reconstruction vesicale. Ann Chir Infant 12:371, 1971.

Cerniglia FR, Roth DA, Gonzalez ET: Covered exstrophy and visceral sequestration in a male newborn: case report. J Urol 141:903, 1989.

Chisholm TC: Exstrophy of the urinary bladder. In Long-Term Follow-up in Congenital Anomalies. Pediatric Surgical Symposium, Vol 6, p 31. Edited by WB Kiesewetter. Pittsburgh, Pittsburgh Children's Hospital, 1979.

Chisholm TC: Pediatric Surgery, Vol 2. Chicago, Year Book Medical Publishers, 1962, p 933.

Clemetson CAB: Ectopia vesicae and split pelvis. J Obstet Gynaecol Br Commonw 65:973, 1958.

Coffey RC: Transplantation of the ureter into the large intestine in the absence of a functioning bladder. Surg Gynecol Obstet 32:383, 1921.

Conner JP, Lattimer JK, Hensle TW, Burbige KA: Primary bladder closure of bladder exstrophy: long-term functional results in 137 patients. J Pediatr Surg 23:1102, 1988.

Culp DA: The histology of the exstrophied bladder. J Urol 91:538, 1964.

Davis HH, Nikhaus FW: Persistent omphalomesenteric duct and urachus in the same case. JAMA 86:685, 1926.

Dees JE: Congenital epispadias with incontinence. J Urol 62:513, 1949.

Devine CJ Jr, Horton CE, Scarff JE Jr: Epispadias: symposium on pediatric urology. Urol Clin North Am 7:465, 1980.

Duckett JW: Use of paraexstrophy skin pedicle grafts for correction of exstrophy and epispadias repair. Birth Defects 13:171, 1977.

Duckett JW, Gazak JM: Complications of ureterosigmoidostomy. Urol Clin North Am 10:473, 1983.

Engel RM, Wilkinson HA: Bladder exstrophy. J Urol 104:699, 1970.

Ezwell WW, Carlson HE: A realistic look at exstrophy of the bladder. Br J Urol 42:197, 1970.

Gearhart JP, Jeffs RD: Augmentation cystoplasty in the failed exstrophy reconstruction. J Urol 139:790, 1988.

Gearhart JP, Jeffs RD: Bladder exstrophy: increase in capacity following epispadias repair. J Urol 142:525, 1989b.

Gearhart JP, Jeffs RD: Complications of exstrophy and epispadias repair. In Complications of Urologic Surgery, 2nd ed. Edited by Smith RB, Ehrlich RM. Philadelphia, WB Saunders Co, 1990, p 569.

Gearhart JP, Jeffs RD: State of the art reconstructive surgery for bladder exstrophy at the Johns Hopkins Hospital. Am J Dis Child 143:1475, 1989a.

Gearhart JP, Jeffs RD: Techniques for continence in the cloacal exstrophy patient. J Urol 146:616, 1991.

Gearhart JP, Jeffs RD: The use of parenteral testosterone therapy in genital reconstructive surgery. J Urol 138:1077, 1987.

Gearhart JP, Jeffs RD, Saunders R: Prenatal diagnosis of congenital bladder exstrophy—a retrospective review for diagnostic clues. Unpublished data.

Gearhart JP, Williams KA, Jeffs RD: Intraoperative urethral pressure profilometry as an adjunct to bladder neck reconstruction. J Urol 136:1055, 1986.

Geist D: Patent urachus. Am J Surg 84:118, 1952.

Glenn JF: Agenesis of the bladder. JAMA 169:2016, 1959.

Gokcora IH, Yazar T: Bilateral transverse iliac osteotomy in the correction of neonatal bladder exstrophy. Int Surg 74:123, 1989.

Gravier L: Exstrophy of the cloaca. Am Surg 34:387, 1968.

Hammond G, Yglesias L, David JE: The urachus, its anatomy and associated fasciae. Anat Rec 80:271, 1941.

Hanna MK, Williams DJ: Genital function in males with vesical exstrophy and epispadias. Br J Urol 44:1969, 1972.

Hector A: Les vestiges de l'ouraque et leur pathologie. J Chir (Paris) 81:449, 1961.

Heitz-Boyer M, Hovelaque A: Creation d'une nouvelle vessie et d'une nouvelle uretre. J Urol 1:237, 1912.

Hendren WH: Exstrophy of the bladder: an alternative method of management. J Urol 115:195, 1976.

Hendren WH: Penile lengthening after previous repair of epispadias. J Urol 12:527, 1979.

Herbst WP: Patent urachus. South Med J 30:711, 1937.

Hinman F Jr: Surgical disorders of the bladder and umbilicus of urachal origin. Surg Gynecol Obstet 113:605, 1961.

Hurwitz RS, Manzoni GA, Ransley PG, Stephens FD: Cloacal exstrophy: a report of 34 cases. J Urol 138:1060, 1987.

Husmann DA, McLorie GA, Churchill BM: A comparison of renal function in the exstrophy patient treated with staged reconstruction vs. urinary diversion. J Urol 140:1204, 1988.

Husmann DA, McLorie GA, Churchill BM: Closure of the exstrophic bladder: an evaluation of the factors leading to its success and its importance on urinary continence. J Urol 142:522, 1989a.

Husmann DA, McLorie GA, Churchill BM: Phallic reconstruction in cloacal exstrophy. J Urol 142:563, 1989b.

Ives E, Coffey R, Carter CO: A family study of bladder exstrophy. J Med Genet 17:139, 1980.

Jeffs RD, Charrios R, Many M, Juransz AR: Primary closure of the exstrophied bladder. In Current Controversies in Urologic Management. Edited by R. Scott. Philadelphia, WB Saunders Co, 1972, p 235.

Jeffs RD, Guice SL, Oesch I: The factors in successful exstrophy closure. J Urol 127:974, 1982.

Jeffs RD, Schwarz GR: Ileal conduit urinary diversion in children: computer analysis follow-up from 2 to 16 years. J Urol 114:285, 1975.

Johnston JH: Lengthening of the congenital or acquired short penis. Br J Urol 46:685, 1974.

Johnston JH: Vesical diverticula without urinary obstruction in childhood. J Urol 84:535, 1960.

Johnston JH, Kogan SJ: The exstrophic anomalies and their surgical reconstruction. Curr Probl Surg August 1974, pp 1–39.

Kapoor R, Saha MM: Complete duplication of the bladder, common urethra and external genitalia in the neonate: a case report. J Urol 137:1243, 1987.

Kenigsberg K: Infection of umbilical artery simulating patent urachus. J Pediatr 86:151, 1975.

Koff SA, Eakins M: The treatment of penile chordee using corporeal rotation. J Urol 131:931, 1984.

Kossow JH, Morales PA: Duplication of bladder and urethra and associated anomalies. Urology 1:71, 1973.

Kramer SA, Jackson IT: Bilateral rhomboid flaps for reconstruction of the external genitalia in epispadias-exstrophy. Plast Reconstr Surg 77:621, 1986.

Kramer SA, Kelalis P: Assessment of urinary continence in epispadias: review of 94 patients. J Urol 128:290, 1982.

Kramer SA, Mesrobian HJ, Kelalis PP: Long-term follow-up of cosmetic appearance and genital function in male epispadias: review of 70 cases. J Urol 135:543, 1986.

Krisiloff M, Puchner PJ, Tretter W, MacFarlane MT, Lattimer JK: Pregnancy in women with bladder exstrophy. J Urol 119:478, 1978.

Kroovand RL, Boyce WH: Isolated vesicorectal internal urinary diversion: a 37-year review of the Boyce-Vest procedure. J Urol 140:572, 1988.

Krull CL, Hanes CF, DeKlerk DP: Agenesis of the bladder and urethra: a case report. J Urol 140:793, 1988.

Lancaster PAL: Epidemiology of bladder exstrophy: a communication from the International Clearinghouse for Birth Defects monitoring systems. Teratology 36:221, 1987.

Lattimer JK: Congenital deficiency of the abdominal musculature and associated genitourinary anomalies: a report of 22 cases. J Urol 79:343, 1958.

Lattimer JK, Beck L, Yeaw S, Puchner PJ, MacFarlane MT, Krisiloff M: Long-term follow-up after exstrophy closure: late improvement and good quality of life. J Urol 119:664, 1978.

Lattimer JK, Smith MJK: Exstrophy closure: a follow-up on 70 cases. J Urol 95:356, 1966.

Leadbetter WF: Consideration of problems incident to performance of ureteroenterostomy: report of a technique. J Urol 73:67, 1955.

Leonard MP, Gearhart JP, Jeffs RD: Continent urinary diversion in childhood. J Urol 144:330, 1990.

Lepor H, Jeffs RD: Primary bladder closure and bladder neck reconstruction in classical bladder exstrophy. J Urol 130:1142, 1983.

Lepor H, Shapiro E, Jeffs RD: Urethral reconstruction in males with classical bladder exstrophy. J Urol 131:512, 1984.

Levard G, Aigrain Y, Ferkadji L, Elghoneimi A, Pichon J, Boureau M: Urinary bladder diverticula and the Ehlers-Danlos syndrome in children. J Pediatr Surg 24:1184, 1989.

Lione PM, Gonzalez ET: Congenital bladder diverticula causing ureteral obstruction. Urology 25:273, 1985.

Lowe FC, Jeffs RD: Wound dehiscence in bladder exstrophy: an examination of the etiologies and factors for initial failure and subsequent closure. J Urol 130:312, 1983.

MacMillan RW, Schulinger JN, Santulli VT: Pyourachus: an unusual surgical problem. J Pediatr Surg 8:87, 1973.

Marshall VF, Marchetti AA, Krantz KE: The correction of stress incontinence by simple vesicourethral suspension. Surg Gynecol Obstet 88:509, 1949.

Marshall VF, Muecke EC: Congenital abnormalities of the bladder. In Handbuch de Urologie. New York, Springer-Verlag, 1968, p 165.

Maydl K: Uber die Radicaltherapie der ectopia vesical urinarie. Wien Med Wochenschr 25:1113, 1894.

Meizner I, Bar-Ziv J: In utero prenatal ultrasonic diagnosis of a rare case of cloacal exstrophy. J Clin Ultrasound 13:500, 1985.

Mendoza CB, Jr, Cueto J, Payan H, Gerwig WH, Jr: Complete urachal tract associated with Meckel's diverticulum. Arch Surg 96:438, 1968.

Mesrobian HJ, Kelalis PP, Kramer SA: Long-term follow-up of cosmetic appearance and genital function in boys with exstrophy: review of 53 patients. J Urol 136:256, 1986.

Mildenberger H, Kluth D, Dziuba M: Embryology of bladder exstrophy. J Pediatr Surg 23:116, 1988.

Mirk M, Calisti A, Feleni A: Prenatal sonographic diagnosis of bladder exstrophy. J Ultrasound Med 5:291, 1986.

Mitchell ME, Peiser JA: Intestinocystoplasty and total bladder replacement in children and young adults: follow-up in 129 cases. J Urol 138:579, 1987.

Mollard P: Bladder reconstruction in exstrophy. J Urol 124:523, 1980.

Monfort G, Morisson-Lacombe GM, Guys JM, Coquet M: Transverse island flap and double flap procedure in the treatment of congenital epispadias in 32 patients. J Urol 138:1069, 1987.

Montagni CA: Functional reconstruction of exstrophied bladder: timing and technique. Follow-up of 39 cases. Kinderchirurgie 43:322, 1988.

Muecke EC: The role of the cloacal membrane in exstrophy: the first successful experimental study. J Urol 92:659, 1964.

Narasimharao KI, Chana RS, Mitra SR, Pathak IC: Covered exstrophy and visceral sequestration: a rare exstrophy variant. J Urol 133:274, 1985.

Neidhardt JH, Morin A, Spay G, Guelpa G, Chavvier J: Mise au oint sur les kystes suppures de l'ouraque. J Urol Nephrol (Paris) 74:793, 1968.

Ney C, Friedenberg RM: Radiographic findings in the anomalies of the urachus. J Urol 99:288, 1968.

Nix JT, Menville JG, Albert M, Wendt DL: Congenital patent urachus. J Urol 79:264, 1958.

Nunn LL: Urachal cysts and their complications. Am J Surg 84:252, 1952.

Oesterling JE, Jeffs RD: The importance of a successful initial bladder closure in the surgical management of classical bladder exstrophy: analysis of 144 patients treated at the Johns Hopkins Hospital between 1975 and 1985. J Urol 137:258, 1987.

Patton BM, Barry A: The genesis of exstrophy of the bladder and epispadias. Am J Anat 90:35, 1952.

Persutte WH, Lenke RR, Kropp K, Ghareb C: Antenatal diagnosis of fetal patent urachus. J Ultrasound Med 7:399, 1988.

Peters CA, Gearhart JP, Jeffs RD: Epispadias and incontinence: the challenge of the small bladder. J Urol 140:1199, 1988.

Peters CA, Hendren WH: Splitting the pubis for exposure in difficult reconstruction for incontinence (Abstract 23). American Academy of Pediatrics Urology Section, San Francisco, October 15, 1988.

Ransley PG, Duffy PG, Wollin M: Bladder exstrophy closure and epispadias repair. In Operative Surgery: Paediatric Surgery, 4th ed. Edinburgh, Butterworths, 1989, p 620.

Rickham PP: Vesicointestinal fissure. Arch Dis Child 35:967, 1960.

Rink RC, Retik AB: Ureteroileocecalsigmoidostomy and avoidance of carcinoma of the colon. In Bladder Reconstruction and Continent Urinary Diversion. Edited by LR King, AS Stone. Chicago, Year Book Medical Publishers, 1987, p 172.

Ritchey ML, Kramer SA, Kelalis PP: Vesical neck reconstruction in patients with epispadias-exstrophy. J Urol 139:1278, 1988.

Schillinger JF, Wiley MJ: Bladder exstrophy: penile lengthening procedure. Urology 24:434, 1984.

Schlegel PN, Gearhart JP: Neuroanatomy of the pelvis in an infant with cloacal exstrophy: a detailed microdissection with histology. J Urol 141:583, 1989.

Schreck WR, Campbell WA: The relationship of bladder outlet obstruction to urinary umbilical fistula. J Urol 108:641, 1972.

Schultz WG: Plastic repair of exstrophy of the bladder combined with bilateral osteotomy of the ilia. J Urol 92:659, 1964.

Shapiro E, Jeffs RD, Gearhart JP, Lepor H: Muscarinic cholinergic receptors in bladder exstrophy: insights into surgical management. J Urol 134:309, 1985.

Shapiro E, Lepor H, Jeffs RD: The inheritance of classical bladder exstrophy. J Urol 132:308, 1984.

Shapiro SR, Lebowitz R, Colodny AH: Fate of 90 children with ileal conduit urinary diversion a decade later. Part 3. J Urol 114:133, 1975.

Soper RT, Kilger K: Vesico-intestinal fissure. J Urol 92:490, 1965.

Spence HM, Hoffman WW, Fosmire PP: Tumors of the colon as a later complication of ureterosigmoidostomy of exstrophy of the bladder. Br J Urol 51:466, 1979.

Spence HM, Hoffman WN, Pate VA: Exstrophy of the bladder: long-term results in a series of 37 cases treated by uretersigmoidostomy. J Urol 114:133, 1975.

Sponseller PD, Gearhart JP, Jeffs RD: Iliac osteotomies

for revision of bladder exstrophy failures. J Urol 146:137, 1991.

Steck WD, Helwig EB: Umbilical granuloams, pilonidal disease, and the urachus. Surg Gynecol Obstet 120:1043, 1965.

Sterling JA, Goldsmith R: Lesions of urachus which appear in the adult. Ann Surg 137:120, 1953.

Stoeckel M, Becht E, Voges G, Riedmiller H, Hohenfellner R: Ureterosigmoidostomy: an outdated approach to bladder exstrophy. J Urol 143:770, 1990.

Sweetser TH, Chisholm TC, Thompson WH: Exstrophy of the urinary bladder: discussion of anatomic principles applicable to its repair with a preliminary report of a case. Minn Med 35:654, 1952.

Taccinoli M, Laurenti C, Racheli T: Sixteen years experience with the Heitz-Boyer Hovelacque procedure for exstrophy of the bladder. Br J Urol 49:385, 1977.

Tauber J, Bloom B: Infected urachal cyst. J Urol 66:692, 1951.

Taylor WN, Alton D, Toguri A, et al: Bladder diverticulum causing posterior urethral obstruction in children. J Urol 122:415, 1979.

Thomalla J, Mitchell ME: Ventral preputial island flap technique for the repair of epispadias with or without exstrophy. J Urol 132:985, 1984.

Toguri AG, Churchill BM, Schillinger JF, Jeffs RD: Continence in cases of bladder exstrophy. J Urol 119:538, 1987.

Verco PW, Khor BH, Barbary J, Enthoven C: Ectopic vesicae in utero. Australas Radiol 30:117, 1986.

Vyas PR, Roth DPR, Perlmutter AB: Experience with free grafts in urethral reconstruction. J Urol 137:471, 1987.

Williams DI: Congenital bladder neck obstruction and megaureter. Br J Urol 29:389, 1957.

Williams DI, Keaton J: Vesical exstrophy: twenty years' experience. Br J Surg 60:203, 1973.

Woodhouse CRJ, Kellett MJ: Anatomy of the penis and its deformities in exstrophy and epispadias. J Urol 132:1122, 1984.

Woodhouse CRJ, Ransley PC, Williams DI: The exstrophy patient in adult life. Br J Urol 55:632, 1983.

Woodhouse CRJ, Strachan JR: Malignancy in exstrophy patients. (Abstract 61). The British Association of Urological Surgeons, Scarborough, England, July 11, 1990.

Young HH: An operation for the cure of incontinence associated with exstrophy. J Urol 7:1, 1922.

Zarbo A, Kay R: Uterosigmoidostomy in bladder exstrophy: a long-term follow-up. J Urol 136:396, 1986.

☐ HYPOSPADIAS AND OTHER URETHRAL ABNORMALITIES

A. Barry Belman

In the past editions of this text, an attempt was made to cover both historical and current aspects of hypospadias. Rather than present a rehash of those chapters, the current edition emphasizes up-to-date trends and approaches, although of necessity some of the basic aspects are repeated. I therefore refer the interested reader to the previous editions or to one of the other many excellent treatises that review that portion of the subject in depth.

HYPOSPADIAS

Although the term hypospadias is applied to females and may fulfill its Greek derivation (*hypo,* meaning "below" or "under," and *spadon,* meaning "rent" or "opening"), female hypospadias does not truly fit into this category. Rather, this abnormality is likely a failure of complete development of the urogenital sinus and is commonly seen in girls with urogenital sinus and cloacal abnormalities. Surgical correction of the cloacal deformity as

performed by the posterior midsagittal approach allows ready access to the anterior wall of the urogenital sinus. Urethral lengthening can then be achieved relatively simply to allow both better direction of the urinary stream as well as access for clean catheterization, should that be required (see Chapter 19). Hendren (1980) reported success in resolving urinary incontinence in a group of girls with short urethras, the majority representing the result of previous manipulation. He employed both anterior vaginal mucosa and an associated perineal pedicle flap to create a longer urethra, thus bringing the meatus to the more normal position.

In males nonglanular hypospadias is the result of failure of the urethral fold to unite over and cover the urethral groove (Fig. 15–117); thus, the urethral meatus exits proximal to the glans. The glanular urethra forms from the urethral or glanular plate, an outgrowth of the early urogenital sinus, which divides the glans ventrally. An ingrowth of ectoderm at the tip of the glans joins the tubularizing urethral

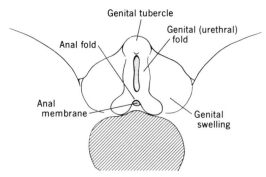

Figure 15–117 □ Sexually indifferent fetal genitalia. (From Bellinger MF: Embryology of the male external genitalia. Urol Clin North Am 8:375, 1981.)

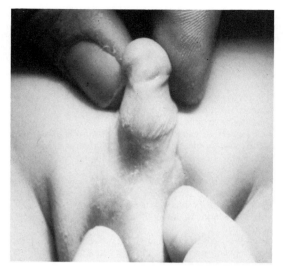

Figure 15–119 □ Megameatal hypospadias variant. Typical of this group, hypospadias was unrecognized and the child was circumcised at birth.

plate to finalize distal urethral development (Fig. 15–118) (Arey). Evidence of unsuccessful efforts to form the distal urethra persist in the pits seen in the distal urethral plate very often present in boys with hypospadias. The foreskin forms late in the first trimester as an overgrowth from the base of the glans. Thus, it is not surprising that the ventral prepuce is incomplete in boys with hypospadias. Nevertheless, a megameatal variant of hypospadias (Fig. 15–119) has been described in which the foreskin is complete and the abnormality goes unrecognized at birth unless the child is circumcised (Hatch et al).

Etiology

There is no single known cause of hypospadias. Unquestionably, a genetic factor exists, most

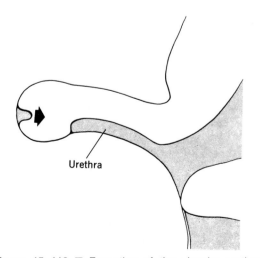

Figure 15–118 □ Formation of the glanular urethra. (From Bellinger MF: Embryology of the male external genitalia. Urol Clin North Am 8:375, 1981.)

Urethra

likely based on a multifactorial mode of inheritance. Bauer et al reviewed the family histories of 307 children with hypospadias (Fig. 15–120). In 21 per cent, a second family member was affected; in 14 per cent, there were brothers with hypospadias; and in 7 per cent, the father of the affected child also had hypospadias. The risk that a family without a previous positive history will have a second child with hypospadias is 12 per cent. If another family member (cousin or uncle) has hypospadias, the chances of another child with hypospadias rises to 19 per cent. If the father has hypospadias, the risk of having a second son with hypospadias becomes 26 per cent.

Androgen stimulates penile growth and development. It is therefore evident that whatever factors cause hypospadias, genetic or otherwise, act endocrinologically. Two possible mechanisms then exist. Either the stimulating factors are inadequate to force penile development, or the tissue is incapable of responding to the stimulant. Disregarding those severe cases with complete or partial failure to masculinize as a result of the inability to incorporate testosterone into the cell (Reifenstein's syndrome, testicular feminization), efforts have been made to determine whether a more mild failure of testosterone utilization is responsible for hypospadias. Schweikert et al noted a reduction in penile intracellular and nuclear testosterone binding capacity in six of 11 boys with hypospadias and concluded that this may play a role in some with severe hypospadias. Svensson and Snochowski iden-

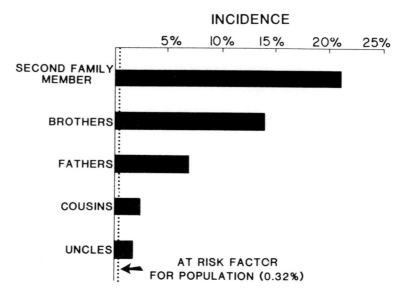

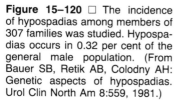

Figure 15–120 □ The incidence of hypospadias among members of 307 families was studied. Hypospadias occurs in 0.32 per cent of the general male population. (From Bauer SB, Retik AB, Colodny AH: Genetic aspects of hypospadias. Urol Clin North Am 8:559, 1981.)

tified a partial deficiency in androgen receptors at the cytoplasmic level. However, Coulam et al found no difference in concentrations of androgen receptors in boys with hypospadias compared with normal controls. And Gearhart et al, looking at both androgen receptor–binding activity and 5α-reductase activity (which converts testosterone to the more active dihydrotestosterone) in preputial and chordee tissues of boys with hypospadias found no difference in contrast to controls.

On the other hand, accumulating evidence suggests that endocrine responsiveness to stimulation may be abnormal in some of these children. Allen and Griffin, Knorr et al, Nonomura et al, and Shima et al all found a diminished testosterone response to human chorionic gonadotropin (HCG) stimulation in boys with hypospadias. Walsh et al, on the other hand, found no difference in testosterone response to hCG in 11 boys with hypospadias. Of interest is information regarding certain maternal factors in boys with hypospadias. For example, Polednak and Janerich reported the mean age of menarche in mothers of boys with hypospadias was significantly later than controls and the first pregnancy of these women produced fewer male fetuses than controls. Källén et al reported an increased risk of hypospadias both with increasing maternal age as well as in male-male twins, even when dizygotic, and a decreased risk for the male in male-female twins. Maternal ingestion of progestational hormones has variously been reported as correlating with hypospadias (Aar-

skog, 1979; Allen and Griffin; Nonomura et al) and bearing no relationship to hypospadias (Czeizel and Tóth). All of this suggests that there may be a failure of appropriate hCG stimulation of the fetal testes in some boys with hypospadias, resulting in delayed or inadequate testosterone production. This may then impact on the timing of development of the urethra and cause its incomplete formation. This hormonal effect appears to be more generalized than just in its effect on urethral formation. Bracka noted a correlation between the erect penile length and severity of hypospadias in a group of adults (Table 15–7).

Incidence and Classification

There may be a true geographic difference in the incidence of hypospadias independent of underascertainment. Källén et al reported a prevalence ranging from 0.26 per 1000 births (both sexes) in Mexico to 2.11 in Hungary.

Table 15–7 □ Penile Length Versus Severity of Hypospadias

Meatal Location	Erect Penile Length
Glanular	15.0 cm
Coronal	14.5 cm
Distal shaft	13.5 cm
Mid shaft	13.0 cm
Proximal shaft	11.0 cm

Modified from Bracka A: A long term view of hypospadias. Br J Plast Surg 42:250, 1989.

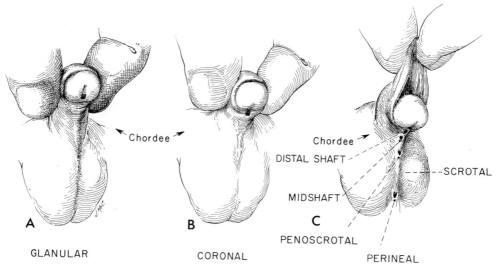

Figure 15–121 □ *A–C*, Classification of hypospadias based on anatomic location of urethral meatus. Associated chordee is best described in terms of severity: mild, moderate, or severe.

These same authors concluded that the true prevalence in Scandinavia is 2.6 per 1000 live births (approximately 5.2 per 1000 male births). Sweet et al reported 8.2 per 1000 male births in Minnesota.

Historically, classification of hypospadias has been based on meatal position. Communication can be improved by describing the position anatomically instead of using some arbitrary system of "degrees" of hypospadias. The types referred to in this chapter are (1) glanular; (2) coronal; (3) distal, mid, and proximal shaft; (4) penoscrotal; (5) scrotal; and (6) perineal (Fig. 15–121). Localization of meatal position can best be achieved by pulling outward on the ventral skin (Fig. 15–122). This maneuver serves to differentiate the functioning, more ventral meatus from the blind-ending pits often seen more distally. The meatus, which is attached to the skin, then opens when traction is applied, and its position becomes obvious. Because chordee is usually associated with hypospadias, including a description of its severity assists in mentally visualizing a given case. An example would be midshaft hypospadias with moderate chordee or penoscrotal hypospadias with severe chordee.

As is true in the spectrum of most diseases, the milder forms of hypospadias occur more frequently. It appears that about 80 to 85 per cent of these boys have coronal to glanular hypospadias whereas 10 to 15 per cent have a penile form. Only 3 to 6 per cent present with penoscrotal-perineal varieties (Table 15–8).

Presentation of the Child with Hypospadias

The surgical subspecialist rarely has the opportunity to be the first physician dealing with this problem, as these children are almost

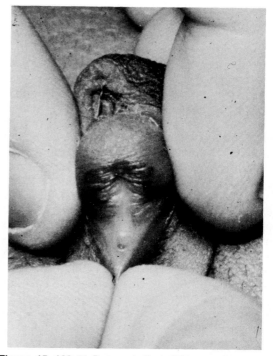

Figure 15–122 □ Demonstration of hypospadiac meatus by pulling outward on ventral shaft skin.

Table 15–8 □ Incidence (%) of Meatal Location

	Coronoglanular	Distal Shaft	Penile	Penoscrotal-Perineal
Sweet et al	87%		10%	3%
Kallen et al	81%		19%	
Standoh	45%	35%	14%	6%

always referred by others. Therefore, oftentimes a certain amount of "undoing" is required when the child is initially seen. There are advantages to seeing the child in the first weeks of life—misconceptions can be corrected and a plan outlined, thereby alleviating much familial anxiety. Additionally, if the penis is small, earlier return may be arranged to plan a course of hormonal stimulation prior to definitive surgical repair.

As previously mentioned, historical information should include that of the family and any previous members with hypospadias. Additionally, knowledge of maternal ingestion of hormonal medication during pregnancy may be of interest and helpful to future pregnancies. Other physical abnormalities that may require evaluation preoperatively should be noted and, if applicable, corrected at the same time.

Physical examination is almost always straightforward, as most of these children are otherwise healthy. Foreskin formation, meatal position, the presence or absence of chordee, and the amount of ventral skin present should all be carefully noted in anticipation of the upcoming repair. Chordee may be difficult to fully evaluate, and final disposition as to extent of repair may have to await an intraoperative artificial erection test.

Sexual Ambiguity

Buccal smears and karyotype are not necessary as a routine in all, but in the newborn with hypospadias and nonpalpable testes they become essential to rule out masculinization of a girl with adrenogenital syndrome. Gender identification may be a problem in children with ambiguous genitalia, and rapid resolution becomes paramount in the first days of life. In general, the presence of palpable scrotal testes can be taken as evidence of the patient's being a genetic male. Unsuspected chromosomal abnormalities are rare in this group (Aarskog, 1970; Chen and Wooley). Chromosomal abnormalities should be suspected, however, in those with only one palpable testis and are, of

course, to be considered in boys with dysmorphic features suggesting other syndromes (see Chapter 8).

There is no question that further evaluation is in order in patients with truly ambiguous genitalia or nonpalpable testes. Cystography (genitography) may be particularly helpful in determining the state of the internal genitourinary structures in such cases (Fig. 15–123).

Microphallus

The ability of the abnormally small phallus to respond to testosterone stimulation should be established in the newborn period. The parenteral administration of testosterone cypionate, 25 mg every 3 weeks, or testosterone enanthate in oil, 25 mg monthly (Guthrie et al), can determine within several weeks whether there is hope for a reasonably functional phallus. Alternatively, one may administer a course of exogenous gonadotropin, which will determine whether the testes are capable of producing testosterone as well as phallic responsiveness. This can then be followed by two doses of testosterone enanthate (25 mg) a few months apart to further stimulate phallic growth.

The normal penile stretched length in the newborn is 3.5 cm (Feldman and Smith), with a range of 2.8 cm to 4.2 cm for the 3rd and 97th percentile. If no significant growth response is noted by 8 to 12 weeks, serious consideration should be given to raising the child in question as a girl.

Associated Anomalies

A correlation is thought to exist between hypospadias, undescended testes, and inguinal hernia. This is probably a reflection of a common endocrinologic etiology. The incidence of undescended testes in boys with hypospadias has been reported by Khuri et al to be as high as 10 per cent (that has not been my experience).

Although one would not expect an increase in urinary abnormalities, considering the dif-

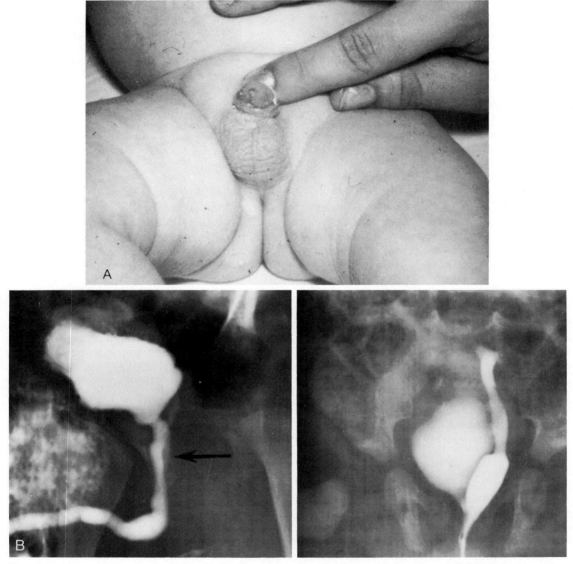

Figure 15–123 □ *A,* Totally masculinized circumcised female with adrenogenital syndrome. *B,* Voiding cystourethrogram in same patient with verumontanum clearly evident *(arrow).* Endoscopic retrograde vaginohysterogram demonstrates normal female internal genitalia.

ferent fetal developmental timing and stimulus for formation of these two systems, some authors report more urinary abnormalities than normal in boys with hypospadias (Fallon et al; H.S. Ikoma et al). Nevertheless, most agree that routine excretory urography does not appear to be justifiable (Kelly et al; Rozenman et al). Sonographic screening of the kidneys may be considered (Lutzker et al) but, again, does not appear to be justified by the low incidence of upper urinary tract abnormalities found (Davenport and MacKinnon).

A surprising finding reported by Shafir et al was increased vesicoureteral reflux in a group of 305 boys with hypospadias. Reflux was found in 37 (17 per cent). The majority were of low grade and were unassociated with renal damage. The four with radiographic evidence of reflux nephropathy appear to have had a history of urinary infections. Shelton and Noe found reflux in 10 per cent of a group with hypospadias, most of low grade and, again, of no consequence. I would continue to recommend cystography *only* in that subgroup with a history of urinary tract infection (UTI) and in evaluation of the child with truly ambiguous genitalia.

Cystoscopy adds nothing to our understanding of the child with hypospadias (Fallon et al), although in more severe forms one might note utricular enlargement (Fig. 15–124). Devine et al (1980) reported enlargement of the utriculus masculinus in 57 per cent of boys with perineal and 10 per cent with penoscrotal hypospadias. F. Ikoma et al (1985) found an enlarged utricle in 84 of 280 (27.5 per cent) boys with hypospadias evaluated with voiding or retrograde urethrograms. The incidence and severity correlated directly with the degree of hypospadias. It was suggested that the enlarged utricle is a result of failure of complete production of müllerian-inhibiting substance (MIS).

The early clinical significance of the enlarged utricle rests primarily with difficulty in inserting a urethral catheter. Although potentially a source of urinary stasis with inherent risks for infection and stone formation, in actuality indications for surgical intervention appear to be quite limited. F. Ikoma et al (1986) reported excision in 14 of 85 utricles for UTI, urinary dribbling, and stone formation. In eight, an actual uterus and tubes were present, suggesting a greater degree of intersex involvement than is being addressed in this chapter. Ritchey et al reported on 36 cases, 13 with hypospadias, advising a suprapubic or transvesical approach for symptoms of urinary dribbling or UTI. Donahoe recommends excision, although the indications are unclear, and suggests preserving and tubularizing the lateral walls of the utricle, over which the vasa run, to try to maintain fertility. Surgical excision of an enlarged utricle should be recommended only after direct correlation with a specific symptom or illness and not simply because of their presence.

Timing of Surgical Repair

Most now agree that surgical correction is best carried out as early as possible but certainly prior to the second birthday. Aside from ancillary support in relation to proper anesthesia and nursing and the general health of the child, the only limiting factor is penile size. In most instances, technical considerations do not limit planning correction at 6 months for the full-term infant. Correction can be performed even earlier if timed with another, more pressing problem (hernia). Occasionally, hormonal stimulation may be necessary in those with a small glans or limited preputial skin in whom that skin may be necessary to complete the repair. Testosterone enanthate, 25 mg given intramuscularly 6 weeks and 3 weeks preoperatively, is generally effective in achieving adequate growth. Testosterone cream (10 per

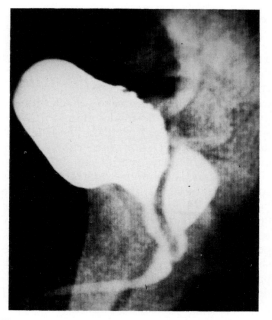

Figure 15–124 □ Voiding cystourethrogram in a boy with hypospadias and significant utricular enlargement.

cent testosterone propionate) applied locally has also been used (Tsur et al).

In 1975 a committee of the Section on Urology of the Academy of Pediatrics stated that "psychological considerations suggest that the optimal time for elective surgery on the genitalia is either the first six months of life or sometime during the fourth year." Separation anxiety begins at about 6 months of age, peaking at 18 months. Genital awareness begins at about the time that separation anxiety begins to wane and becomes significant by age 3 to 5 years (Table 15–9). Schultz et al, in a review of the psychologic ramifications of surgery in childhood, concluded that the ideal age for genital surgery is between 6 weeks and 12 months of age. Manley and Epstein reported a series of repairs in 17 children between 10 and 18 months of age who clearly showed less anxiety than did older children. Belman and Kass noted the same experience in 37 children ranging in age from 2 to 11 months (average 6 months) with no evidence of increased technical problems in this group. With application of modern techniques, there should be no increased incidence of complications based on the child's age.

Although there are no studies comparing groups of patients undergoing surgery at different ages to support the thesis that early surgery is psychologically advantageous, there is evidence that those who had repairs at an older age in the past are at risk emotionally. The literature documents the relationship between genital surgery and aberrant behavior (Sandberg et al). Berg and Berg published two studies in adults who had undergone hypospadias repairs in earlier years. In comparison with age-matched controls, 33 men evaluated by the Rorschach test were noted to be deficient in ego strength, self-esteem, and interpersonal relations. Anxiety and hostility levels were both also notably increased. Thirty-four men with repaired hypospadias demonstrated uncertainty regarding gender identity when compared with age-matched controls, with the probands taking more feminine sex roles. Nevertheless, the sexual orientation of the test group was similar to that of the controls. The

mean age at surgery for the patient study was 5.6 years. The control group was made up of patients who had undergone appendectomy at about the same age (mean 5.7 years). It must be recognized that the earliest age at which hypospadias repair had been carried out in this group was 3 years.

Further information exists regarding a large degree of dissatisfaction in some adults who had previously undergone repair. Of 213 patients interviewed in a report by Bracka published in 1989, 38 per cent expressed feelings of being deformed whereas about 75 per cent thought that the ultimate cosmetic result was important. In my own experience of obtaining the family history of an infant with glanular hypospadias, occasionally the father will admit to a similar deformity. When told that the degree of hypospadias is mild and will not interfere with function, the father usually agrees and responds that it did not, of course, bother him. However, he quickly adds that he would, nevertheless, like to have his son's penis repaired, if that is possible. Nevertheless, there are those with mild hypospadias who are truly unaware of their difference or unaffected by it. Our problem is an inability to select those who will not be affected by the abnormality and in whom, therefore, surgical correction is not necessary. This author's recommendation is to repair all but the most minimal glanular variants.

Chordee

The severity of chordee is generally proportional to the degree of hypospadias. Overall, chordee is present in only about 35 per cent (Sweet et al). This statistic correlates with the preponderance of the milder forms of hypospadias and may even overstate the true incidence by including some with "chordee" secondary to inadequate ventral skin.

Kaplan and Lamm, in studies of abortus specimens, found that ventral penile curvature persisted in 44 per cent of fetuses through the 6th gestational month (Fig. 15–125). They concluded that chordee is a normal phase of penile development and that one therefore should not expect to find ventral fibrosis in all patients operated upon for hypospadias. Chordee is best demonstrated by direct injection of normal saline into the corpora after applying a tourniquet at the penile base as introduced by Gittes and McLaughlin. True chordee is

Table 15–9 ☐ Timing of Surgical Correction

Age	Psychological Considerations
0–6 months	Minimal separation anxiety
6–12 months	Anxious with separation
1–3 years	Trauma with separation
4 and up	Genital anxiety

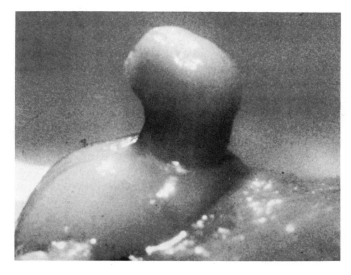

Figure 15–125 □ Fetal penis demonstrating chordee as part of phallic development. (Courtesy of Dr. George W. Kaplan.)

infrequent in boys with distal hypospadias (Fig. 15–126).

There have been reports of dorsal chordee both independent of and associated with hypospadias (Redman, 1983). Its cause is likely the result of disproportionate corporal growth and its association with hypospadias probably coincidental. One must wonder how often it has clinical significance, other than in its most severe form. Surgical correction should probably be delayed to the onset of sexual activity to ensure that treatment is warranted.

Chordee without Hypospadias

A small number of patients present with chordee despite a more or less normally placed urethral meatus. A clue to this defect lies in recognizing that most patients with this problem do not have a completely formed ventral foreskin.

Devine and Horton (1973) described three distinct pathologic classes of chordee without hypospadias. In the first, spongiosum is absent from the point of origin of the chordee to the glans. The urethra itself is often paper-thin, and the meatus is less than perfect (Fig. 15–127). Dorsal to the thin urethra lies a thick fibrous layer similar to that present in chordee seen with the more severe forms of hypospadias. It is to this group of patients that the confusing term *hypospadism without hypospadias* has been applied. Cendron and Melin call this a "concealed hypospadias." In all likelihood, this form of chordee without hypospadias and the obviously hypospadiac penis are

similar abnormalities except for the presence of a thinned urethra. One might attempt surgical correction by elevating the urethra and excising or resecting the underlying fibrous bands without urethral transection. However, considering the wispy nature of the urethra in this condition that may be inadvisable or even impossible. Apparent initial success may result

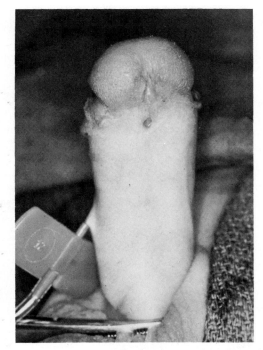

Figure 15–126 □ Artificial erection test in a boy with subcoronal hypospadias demonstrating absence of chordee.

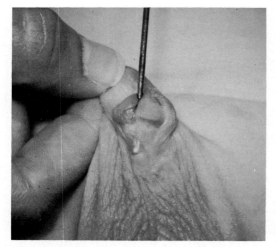

Figure 15–127 □ Probe in glanular meatus demonstrating area of absence of spongiosum. Urethra is extremely superficial at this juncture.

in increased postoperative complications (Hurwitz et al).

Type I chordee, in which the actual urethra is abnormal, in almost every instance should be dealt with as one would treat true hypospadias. That is, the entire urethra is freed up proximally until chordee is released and nor-

mal urethra exposed. In some instances in this group of patients, the meatus may be fairly normal and the distal urethra less pathologic, justifying its use. After it becomes evident that dissection of the urethra from the corpora (allowing the meatus to remain attached) results in a "bowstring" effect (causing chordee), an option is to transect the mid urethra rather than perform dorsal tucks to achieve a straight penis. By leaving the original meatus in the glans, one can create an interpositional pedicle tube to bridge this gap, performing well-spatulated anastomoses both proximally and distally.

In Devine and Horton's second class, the urethra is more completely developed; the Buck's and dartos layers are thought to be abnormal. The urethra itself must be mobilized from the corpus followed by extension dissection of the deep tunic to straighten the penis (Fig. 15–128). Mobilization of the urethra proximal to the penoscrotal junction may then be necessary to achieve adequate urethral length in these instances (Persky et al). Transection may also be necessary in this group if tethering by the urethra is noted (Kramer et al).

The third class is described as caused by an

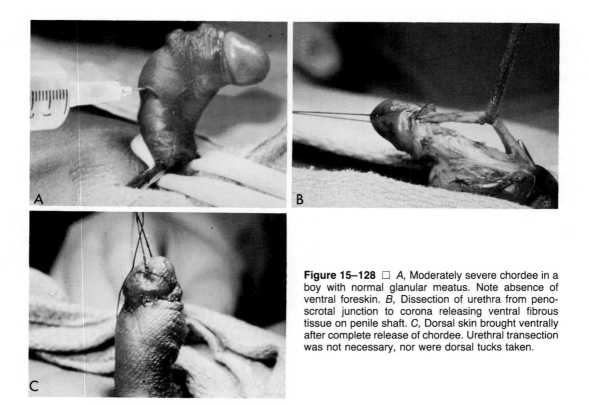

Figure 15–128 □ *A,* Moderately severe chordee in a boy with normal glanular meatus. Note absence of ventral foreskin. *B,* Dissection of urethra from penoscrotal junction to corona releasing ventral fibrous tissue on penile shaft. *C,* Dorsal skin brought ventrally after complete release of chordee. Urethral transection was not necessary, nor were dorsal tucks taken.

abnormality of the superficial fascia (dartos) and has been described as skin chordee (Allen and Spence). Dissection of the ventral skin superficial to the urethra entirely frees the penis, resulting in retraction of the scrotum from its base. These are often recognizable as "high-riding" scrota, release of which may result in a significant ventral defect requiring extensive skin transfer from the dorsum for coverage.

A fourth class (Kramer et al) has been attributed to a disproportion in length between dorsal and ventral corpora, similar to lateral penile bend. This may not much differ from type II described above; however, it has been recommended that since the urethra is normal, correction can be achieved by excising dorsal fascial wedges, as proposed by Nesbit (Kramer et al; Livne et al). One must be extremely cautious of injury to the dorsal neurovascular bundle, a task that may be difficult in the very small child, particularly when dealing with more distal chordee or glanular tilt. Some have advised this approach when faced with more severe forms of hypospadias with chordee when preserving the urethral plate for onlay pedicle repairs (Hollowell et al). However, there remains a question as to whether chordee recurs with penile growth during adolescence when this approach is employed and the primary, ventral process is not resolved (Bennett and Gittes).

Chordee with Hypospadias

In those with actual hypospadias, chordee is thought to be caused by thickened bands formed by the rudimentary spongiosum of the uncanalized urethral groove that are splayed distal to the hypospadiac meatus, by the thickening of the deep penile fascia, or by both (Creevy; Jones and Scott). To correct the chordee, it is necessary to excise or transect these bands, which may extend proximal to what appears to be normal urethra. In fact, dissection of the more proximal urethra off the corpora should be a fairly routine part of release of chordee and can be achieved with only slight bleeding in many instances if the dissection, using a fine pointed scissors (tenotomy), is kept along the fascia. Nevertheless, fulguration of venous bleeders or injection of epinephrine is often required in this area. After release of chordee, the meatus may retract substantially. It might be more reasonable, then, to relabel the degree of pathology in these patients based on the position of the

meatus following penile straightening. Culp and McRoberts, in their classic chapter published in 1968, defined the meatus in 28 per cent as penile, 45 per cent as penoscrotal, 16 per cent as scrotal, and 10 per cent as perineal after dissection compared with that stated in Table 15–8. Obviously, they were dealing with a highly selected group of patients; nevertheless, one should be aware that the problem may be more severe than suggested by original meatal position alone.

With more severe forms of hypospadias, chordee may persist even following extensive ventral dissection as well as mobilization of the urethra proximal to the hypospadiac meatus. Devine (1983) recommended the use of fine, superficial, transverse incisions through the remaining fascia just down to the deepest layers of the corporal tunica albuginea. These have been affectionately termed "fairy cuts"; the name implies how delicately these incisions must be made. If chordee still remains, Devine suggests cutting through the midline longitudinally for the extent of the exposed corpora in the avascular septum between the corporal bodies. This is often definitive in releasing chordee. The neourethra then overlies this defect, serving as its covering. Should chordee persist even after the above tricks have been applied, it may be necessary to deeply incise ventral fascia, transversely exposing erectile tissue. The resulting defect can be covered with a free dermal (Devine and Horton, 1975; Kogan et al) or tunica vaginalis graft (Perlmutter et al). Most suggest that this be carried out as the first stage of a planned two-stage repair. However, one could proceed in a single-stage procedure if the urethra is then formed from a well-vascularized pedicle flap. Hendren and Keating reported success using a dermal graft as the corporal patch in conjunction with a free, full-thickness skin graft for urethral construction. However, they reserve the single-stage approach for those in whom the penis can be "degloved" for access to the pathology, thereby reducing risks related to skin coverage. An alternative to applying a free patch to the ventral corpora is to attack the problem by excising diamond-shaped divots from the fascia dorsally (Nesbit).

Repair of Hypospadias

Technical Considerations

A marked reduction in complications joined with better cosmetic and functional results makes the repair of hypospadias considerably more gratifying and less burdensome than in the past. The use of fine, nonreactive suture material made possible by routine optimal magnification has probably played the major role. However, the maturation of our subspecialty allowing a greater number of repairs to be done by fewer individuals has also contributed tremendously to our experience and, secondarily, to our success.

Most "hypospadiologists" are satisfied with 2.5 to 3.5 *optical magnification*. However, there are those who prefer using the operating microscope, although it is not clear whether results are improved with that adjunct (Shapiro, 1989; Wacksman, 1984, 1987; Wesson and Mandell).

Bartone et al attempted to objectively determine which *suture material* is most appropriate by comparing reaction and granuloma formation as well as abscess formation and resorption using baboon foreskin as a laboratory model. They concluded that catgut is the most appropriate suture, causing the least reaction and resorbing the quickest. They recommended against both polyglycolic acid (Dexon) and polydioxanone (PDS). This does not conform to this author's experience, and since using coated polyglactin (Vicryl) exclusively (in conjunction with other modifications), complications have fallen to a minimum. Admittedly, the suture material lasts for several weeks and in some children can result in troublesome "suture tracks" (epithelial subcutaneous bridges). To avoid cutaneous problems, many surgeons use newer synthetic monofilament sutures to form the urethra but continue to prefer catgut on the skin.

Tissue viability plays an important role in the success of the procedure. Fine, noncrushing instruments and the liberal use of stay sutures are used to limit tissue trauma. Scheuer and Hanna recommended the application of nitroglycerine ointment as a means of increasing flap viability. However, Duckett (1981b) reported excellent viability of the island pedicle without the use of any adjuvant as evaluated by fluoroscein. Walker and Graham substantiated this observation. In general, it can be assumed that if flaps are visibly cyanotic, one can anticipate problems. Clinical experience suggests that the viability of penile skin flaps is dependent upon the amount of subcutaneous tissue attached. On the other hand, it is always surprising how well vascularized an island flap appears even when based on an extremely thin pedicle.

Hemostasis can be achieved by intermittent application of a tourniquet to the base of the penis. A rubber band held in position by a mosquito clamp is very effective for penile hypospadias; however, it can get in the way for more proximal repairs. Release of the tourniquet every 10 minutes to allow circulation is advisable, although no problems were reported by Redman (1986), who maintained continuous application for 12 to 50 minutes with a mean of 28 minutes. On the other hand, many experts inject a 1:100,000 dilution of epinephrine as a means of limiting intraoperative bleeding without any reported negative sequelae (Duckett, 1987). Finally, the judicious use of pinpoint electrocautery is an invaluable aid. Electrocautery can also be used to fulgurate erectile tissue both in the shaft and glans; however, it is most effective for individual bleeders.

Avoiding crossing suture lines is the single most essential step in *preventing urethrocutaneous fistulas*. Smith, in applying a de-epithelialized flap to a planned two-stage repair, lowered the fistula rate to less than 5 per cent at a time when others were pleased to have 50 per cent complication-free repairs. Of course, his patients had at least two operations, since all were staged. The application of his approach was successfully applied to repair of fistulas (Geltzeiler and Belman; Walker, 1981) and, finally, to single-stage repairs (Belman, 1988), with a marked reduction in complications.

Assuming that adequate tissue remains following creation of the urethra, cutis is removed from the residual preputial skin (Fig. 15–129). This subcutaneous tissue is brought over the neourethra to apply a barrier between it and the final penile cover. This barrier not only covers suture lines but also brings a layer of well-vascularized tissue over the repair, ideally to the meatus. Retik et al recommended a similar type of covering. If inadequate skin exists, a pedicle of tunica vaginalis based on the spermatic cord is swung from the scrotum to achieve the same result (Snow). Shapiro (1986) recommended the use of scrotal fat, advanced distally, to cover a free skin graft.

Cosmesis

One of the major changes in the last decade has been the unwillingness to accept repairs that result in an abnormally appearing penis. The question as to why the meatus should be normally placed in the glans rather than ac-

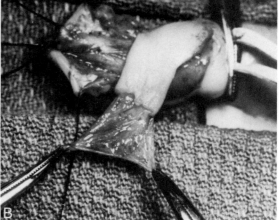

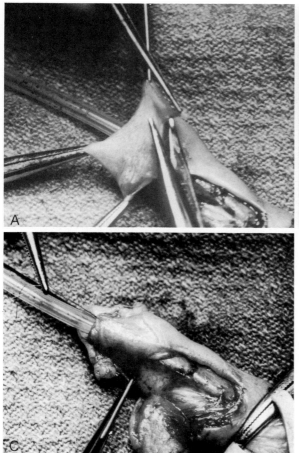

Figure 15–129 □ *A,* Left one half of hooded prepuce de-epithelialized using tenotomy scissors. *B,* Flap completely de-epithelialized. *C,* De-epithelialized segment placed into glans covering urethroplasty.

cepting it at the coronal sulcus is no longer asked. The confident hypospadiologist does not feel the need to leave unsightly residual skin "just in case"—which may later require trimming. Transferring dorsal skin by the buttonhole technique with its resultant "dog ears" is rarely applied. If possible, the skin is closed in the midline, having fashioned a collar proximal to the corona (Firlit). This is achieved by designing the initial lateral skin incisions 0.5 cm proximal to the glans, particularly ventrolaterally (Fig. 15–130). The result is a penis that is not dissimilar from that of other circumcised boys. In those with more mild forms of hypospadias, European efforts have been made to preserve foreskin and bring it ventral (VanDorpe). However, a high complication rate (26 per cent) has been reported when foreskin preservation was applied to the meatal advancement–glanuloplasty (MAGPI) procedure by Frey and Cohen.

Urinary Diversion

Postoperative urinary diversion has also undergone a remarkable transformation in recent years. In a survey of 86 American and Canadian pediatric urologists (with a 98 per cent response rate) the most remarkable finding was the limited use of suprapubic (SP) diversion (Oesterling et al). For distal shaft repairs, only 7 per cent used SP drainage, 26 per cent for mid-shaft and 81 per cent for penoscrotal-perineal hypospadias. Perineal urethrostomy is rarely employed. The second remarkable finding is the move to nondiversion for more distal repairs. In the report by Oesterling et al, 85 per cent of those undergoing glanular repairs (MAGPI) have no period of urinary diversion. Rabinowitz found no increase in complications in boys having outpatient, catheterless meatal-based flap repairs.

The move to more simple forms of urinary

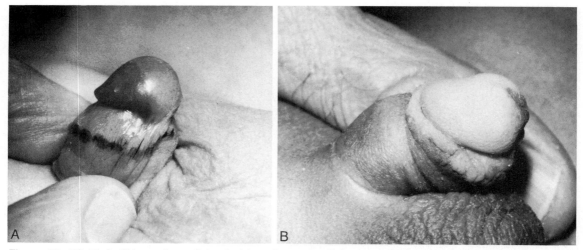

Figure 15–130 □ *A,* Skin marks outlining incision allow preservation of a subcoronal (Firlit's) collar. *B,* Healing hypospadias repair (2 weeks) demonstrates subcoronal collar.

diversion and outpatient postoperative care has led to the use of stents through which the patient voids directly (extravesical) or through which the urine continuously drains (intravesical). *Extravesical stents* are generally of silicone and extend from the bulbous urethra to just beyond the neomeatus. They may be intact or split on one side (pleated stent or splent) (Mitchell and Kulb) and are held by a suture to the glans for security. Boys beyond 18 months of age may find voiding through the stent painful. However, because there is no intravesical portion of the tube, bladder spasms are not a problem. Alternately, one may use silicone tubing or a small feeding tube that extends into the bladder through which urine drips constantly. This may also end just beyond the meatus (Gonzalez and Vivas), or it can be left long, and is either attached to a drainage bag or allowed to drain into a second diaper applied directly over the first diaper. When plastic disposable diapers are used, the inner diaper, and thus the healing penis, can be kept dry without the necessity of a drainage bag with the double-diaper technique. Low-dose antibacterial prophylaxis postoperatively appears to obviate infection with closed urinary diversion (Sugar and Firlit) and in our clinical experience is also effective with the open, double-diaper drainage system.

Postoperative Dressings

A variety of postoperative dressings have been employed through the years, some of which have required extensive nursing care (Devine, 1983). At the time of this writing, a popular dressing is application of a simple transparent dressing (Tegaderm) applied directly to the penis (Gilbert et al; Retik et al). In infants, a small sheet of Tegaderm is cut in half, each applied separately (Fig. 15–131). Therefore, a double layer results, the initial layer started on the ventral surface, the second from the dorsal. No adhesive spray is required, nor is any other method used to make the dressing adhere, although some apply adhesive strips (Steri-Strips) at the base to prevent rolling. To obtain best results, the surface should be dry at the time of application. This author removes the dressing in an outpatient setting on the 3rd to 4th postoperative day. In small chubby boys whose penises tend to retract into the fat pad, the dressing generally spontaneously falls off in 48 hours. In older boys, it may remain securely in place for several days and is ideal for the postpubertal male. For those with severe hypospadias in whom scrotal or perineal dissection is required, a short interval using a bulky compression dressing is added (Fig. 15–132) (Falkowski and Firlit). The other method that remains popular is the use of silicone foam applied within a mold surrounding the penis (DeSy and Oosterlinck). After the foam "sets," a rigid cast supports the penis as well as the catheter. It has been suggested that this type of dressing actually protects the glanuloplasty (Gaylis et al).

Pain Management

Postoperative pain relief for up to 6 hours can be achieved with long-acting local anesthetic (0.25 to 0.5 per cent bupivacaine) injected either at the penile base (Lau) or as a caudal block (Fig. 15–133) (Broadman). Post-

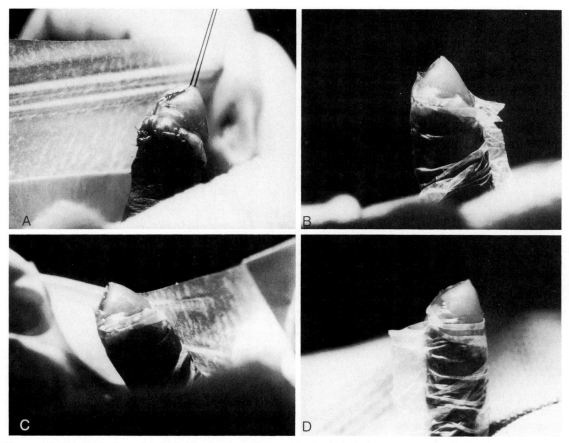

Figure 15–131 □ *A,* Completed Mathieu hypospadias repair. Penis is held up by traction suture, and one half of Tegaderm strip is held taut (background). *B,* First one half of Tegaderm is applied from ventral to dorsal. *C,* Second one half of Tegaderm strip is applied to dorsal aspect of penis. *D,* Completed Tegaderm application. *Note:* Meatus is exposed to allow unimpeded urination.

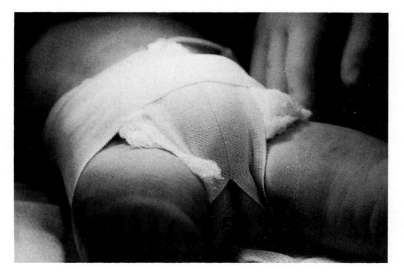

Figure 15–132 □ Modification of the Falkowski-Firlit compression dressing.

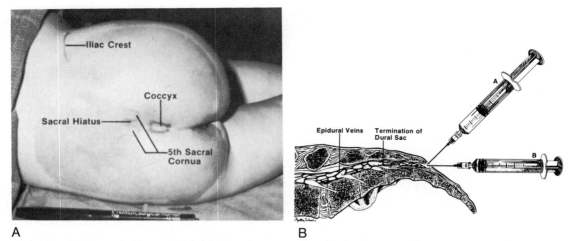

A   B

Figure 15–133 □ *A,* Patient positioning and external landmarks for the performance of a pediatric caudal block. The coccyx, sacral cornua, and sacral hiatus have been outlined with a surgical marker.

B, A 23-gauge × 1.0-inch needle attached to a 6-ml syringe is about to penetrate the sacrococcygeal ligament (A). Note that the bevel of the needle has been positioned in a ventral direction in order to minimize the likelihood of inadvertent injections into the periosteum lining the ventral side of the caudal canal. Following puncture of the sacrococcygeal ligament, the needle and syringe are lowered into a plane that parallels the spinal axis (B). The needle is advanced 2 mm, and following aspiration the local anesthetic is introduced into the caudal epidural space.

(From Broadman LM. Regional anesthesia for the pediatric outpatient. Anesth Clin North Am 5:59, 60, 1987.)

operative local anesthesia is particularly advantageous by preventing excessive crying and thrashing about, which can lead to bleeding or disruption of the dressing as the child awakens. Caudal block rather than penile injection is our preference because the latter may lead to more penile swelling and, theoretically, risk flap viability.

Surgical Procedures

An enormous number of procedures and their variations exist for the repair of hypospa-dias. As previously stated, this chapter confines itself to a relatively few that have proved highly effective (Table 15–10). These include methods for dealing with simple glanular hypospadias as well as meatal based flap techniques, which can be applied to coronal or distal shaft hypospadias with or without chordee.

Flap repairs are best for more severe hypospadias: an onlay for those without chordee and a pedicle tube when chordee is released. When the meatus is proximal to the penoscrotal junction, a midline tube (Thiersch-type)

Table 15–10 □ Procedures of Choice

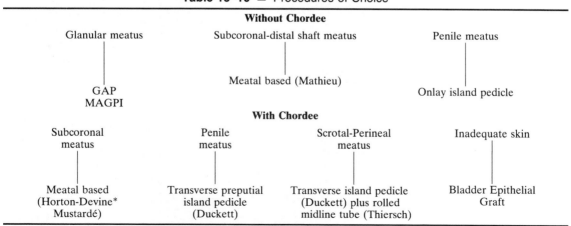

Without Chordee		
Glanular meatus	Subcoronal-distal shaft meatus	Penile meatus
	Meatal based (Mathieu)	
GAP MAGPI		Onlay island pedicle

With Chordee			
Subcoronal meatus	Penile meatus	Scrotal-Perineal meatus	Inadequate skin
Meatal based (Horton-Devine* Mustardé)	Transverse preputial island pedicle (Duckett)	Transverse island pedicle (Duckett) plus rolled midline tube (Thiersch)	Bladder Epithelial Graft

*Flip flap.
Abbreviations: GAP, glans approximation procedure; MAGPI, meatal advancement–glanuloplasty.

brings the meatus to the penoscrotal junction. This is then attached to a tubularized pedicle (Duckett type) that allows even those with the most proximally placed meatus to undergo reconstruction in a single stage.

Finally, for the true challenges in which adequate skin does not exist to both form a pedicle flap and cover the repair, an ability to harvest viable tissue for a successful free graft repair becomes a necessity. Bladder epithelium has become the most favored tissue for this situation at present.

Prior to performing the following procedures for glanular and distal hypospadias, one must be convinced that no true chordee exists. Should the question arise, skin dissection, with preservation of the prepuce in the event that a urethroplasty becomes necessary, followed by an artificial erection test (Gittes and McLaughlin) is the first step.

Glanular Hypospadias

MAGPI. Introduced by Duckett (1981), MAGPI changed the scope of hypospadias repairs by offering a simple approach to glanular hypospadias. Prior to its introduction, patients with coronoglanular meatuses were often advised that they were functionally normal and that creation of a more distal meatus

was not possible. Unfortunately, attempts to apply the MAGPI to those who have a more proximal meatus or a patulous, fibrotic, or hypoplastic meatus (Gibbons and Gonzales) have resulted in some degree of dissatisfaction with its results. Reports of a degree of meatal regression ranged from 26 of 28 (Hastie et al) to eight of 142 (Issa and Gearhart). Therefore, based on the excellent success of the meatal-based flap procedures, which can also be performed in catheter-free outpatients (Rabinowitz), attempts to extend the usefulness of the MAGPI and similar procedures should be abandoned and its application reserved only for those with glanular defects alone.

A dorsal meatotomy is performed well into the glans incising the bridge of tissue commonly existing between the meatus and the glanular groove (Fig. 15–134). A wide V configuration results. Two or three 7-0 Vicryl sutures are used to extend the dorsal urethral epithelium to the end of the incision created in the glans. Although it appears that a glanular tilt should result from this maneuver, that is not the case. A circumscribing incision is made, carefully preserving ventrolateral skin to create Firlit's collar. Great care is taken on the ventral surface not to enter the distal urethra, which is oftentimes extremely superficial and thin. By performing the initial sub-

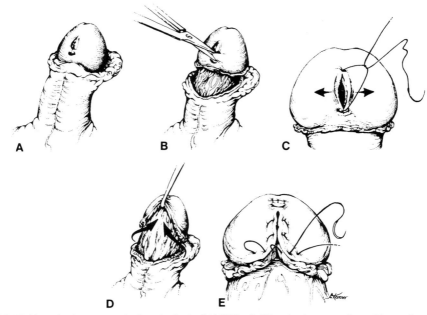

Figure 15–134 □ Meatal advancement–glanuloplasty (MAGPI). *A,* Glanular hypospadias without chordee. *B,* Division of septum distal to meatus. *C,* Advancement of dorsal epithelium distally. *D, E,* Advancement of ventral glans and approximation in midline.

cutaneous dissection lateral to the urethra, urethral damage can be avoided. Then, with double skin hooks used, the ventral skin is held away from the shaft on either side of the urethra and the blades of a fine scissors are gently spread subcutaneously between urethra and skin. Ventral skin can be safely dissected proximally following this maneuver. Using a single hook, one draws the ventral subglanular skin distally, effectively converting the skin line from its original transverse axis to vertical. This then brings ventral glanular and subglanular tissue into the midline overlying the advanced meatus. These edges are sutured in the midline. Therefore, although the meatal position itself has not moved, glanular tissue is placed proximal to it, making the meatus appear relatively more distal. Redundant skin is excised, and skin edges are approximated with 6-0 suture.

Arap Procedure. A direct modification of the MAGPI, the Arap repair advances two flaps of lateral coronal tissue distally (instead of one), approximating them in the midline, effectively lengthening the urethra. The glans is then closed over this tissue, normalizing its ventral appearance. In the original published description, a 90 per cent success rate was reported in ten patients (Arap et al). Subsequently, Scherz et al (1989) published excellent cosmesis in 93 per cent of 31 patients.

Glans Approximation Procedure (GAP). Similar modifications reported by Dimler et al and Zaontz apply de-epithelialization of skin lateral to the glanular groove (Fig. 15–135). This then results in two raw edges, the medial aspect of which can be brought together in the midline to actually lengthen the urethra distally. The lateral margins are then brought into the midline, over the first layer, to approximate the glans. This procedure is best applied when a moderately deep glanular groove exists distal to the glanular hypospadiac meatus. Its application to a flattened ventral glans may well result in disruption. Because there is actual lengthening of the urethra, fistulas may be a complication. Since little or no tissue then exists in the region of the repair to support closure of such a fistula, cutting back on the new urethra may be required to resolve this problem should it occur.

Urethral Advancement. Mobilization and advancement of the anterior urethra as a means of advancing the meatus to the glans dates back to the earlier part of the century (Beck; Duval). More recently, interest in this

approach was reintroduced by Belman (1977b) and a satisfactory experience has been reported by Waterhouse and Glassberg. Nasrallah and Minott combined this with a vigorous glanuloplasty to normalize the penile appearance. This is a more aggressive modification of the classic flip-flap procedure of Devine and Horton (1961). Chang reports ability to advance the urethra 1.8 cm in a 2-year-old boy after mobilizing 5 cm of proximal urethra and 5.0 cm in a 20-year-old following 14.0 cm of mobilization.

The procedure involves significant urethral dissection to gain the necessary length to bring the meatus to the glans and may result in brisk bleeding because spongiosum may be dissected. It therefore has all the risks inherent to any formal repair and consequently requires the same postoperative care. It is this author's opinion that a meatal-based flap achieves comparable or better cosmetic and functional results with less morbidity.

Distal Hypospadias Without Chordee

Procedure for the Megameatus Variant of Distal Hypospadias. Hatch et al reported a hypospadias variant with an intact foreskin. The patient is often circumcised prior to recognition of the abnormal meatus. However, because the glans in such a boy is broad and the meatus excessively wide and floppy, repair is generally not compromised by circumcision. Duckett and Keating describe the "pyramid procedure" for repair of this problem. Because the glans is so wide in this group, the urethra can be lengthened by rolling a tube distally using glanular tissue (King procedure). The wide meatus is tailored, and excessive ventral skin is de-epithelialized and brought to the distal glans to prevent crossing suture lines. The glans is brought together in the midline using 6-0 mattress sutures. One or two deep horizontal stitches in the glans may be helpful if undue tension appears to exist when the glans is closed (Fig. 15–136).

Mathieu Procedure. The various meatal-based flaps are applicable only to the more distal varieties of hypospadias and then only when sufficient ventral skin is present. Longer flaps are at risk not only for devascularization with the inherent complication of distal stenosis and stricture but also may incorporate hair-bearing skin. This procedure, popularized by Wacksman (1981), is particularly applicable when the hypospadiac meatus is at the corona

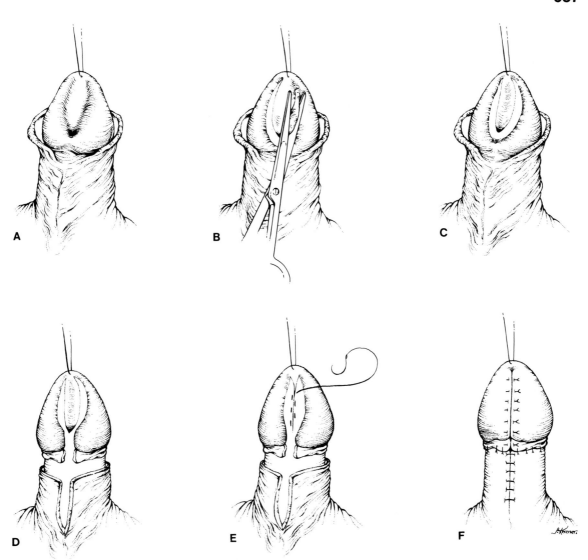

Figure 15–135 □ Glans approximation (GAP). *A,* Glanular hypospadias with wide glanular groove. *B, C,* De-epithelialization of glans lateral to groove. *D,* Extension of glanular de-epithelialization ventrally as well as circumcision. Redundant skin excised. *E,* Urethral lengthening—inner aspect of de-epithelialized glans closed in midline. *F,* Glans closure completed over lengthened urethra and skin edges approximated.

or in the distal shaft. When chordee is secondary to skin alone or in the absence of chordee, it is not necessary to divide the skin distal to the meatus. The Mathieu procedure (an updated application of the Ombredanne approach) is an excellent choice in this situation. It has the capability of producing a normal glanular meatus and is applicable to those with either a rounded or deeply grooved ventral glans.

A skin flap is outlined proximal to the meatus measurably long enough to reach the tip of the glans (Fig. 15–137). This flap is freed up with as much subcutaneous tissue attached

to the undersurface as possible. Skin incisions are then carried distally into the glans, penetrating to Buck's fascia. Dissection can also be carried laterally to create glans wings, should that be necessary, to allow closure of the glans over the new urethra in the midline without tension. The neourethra is formed by flipping the meatal-based flap distally into the glans. Running 7-0 Vicryl subcuticular sutures are used to close the lateral walls and have the advantage of inverting the skin edges, thereby reducing the risk of fistulas. Additionally, interrupted 7-0 Vicryl sutures can be used to bring flap subcutaneous tissue over the original

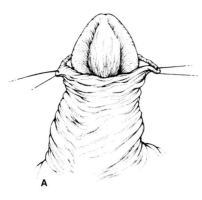

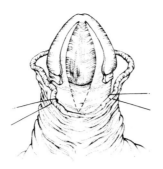

A

B

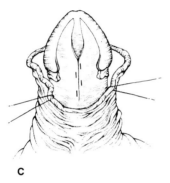

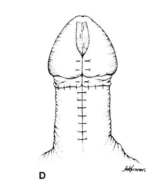

C

D

Figure 15–136 ☐ Megameatal variant repair. *A,* Meatus concealed by redundant ventral foreskin. *B,* De-epithelialization of glans lateral to urethral groove plus narrowing of patulous distal urethra (dotted line). *C,* Urethral lengthening in midline. *D,* Completion of repair after excision of redundant skin.

suture line, further reinforcing it. Finally, to reduce the risk of fistula to its absolute minimum, one half of the split prepuce can be de-epithelialized and brought over the entire distal urethra to be sutured to the depths of the glanular incisions using 7-0 Vicryl. The glans is approximated in the midline with mattressed 6-0 Vicryl suture, redundant tissue is excised, and skin edges are approximated with 6-0 Vicryl. A double layer of Tegaderm is applied, and the patient is discharged the same day, voiding directly through the repair. The Tegaderm is removed 3 days later.

Onlay Island Flap Repair. When *inadequate* ventral skin exists for a meatal-based flap repair for distal hypospadias or for those patients with mid to distal shaft hypospadias without chordee, the urethral plate may serve as the base for an onlay pedicle (Elder et al; Hodgson; Hollowell et al). Hodgson may have been the first to apply this principle, using a longitudinal double-faced dorsal flap flipped ventrally to create the floor of the urethra (Fig. 15–138). However, use of the undersurface of

the foreskin as a transverse island ensures that non–hair-bearing skin will be employed to create the urethra and a more cosmetic result can be achieved (Fig. 15–139). Parallel incisions are brought distally along the lateral border of the urethral plate to the corona and into the glans. These incisions join proximal to the hypospadiac meatus. Ventral skin is dissected to free the scrotum, if it is high-riding. The length of the onlay flap is determined by measuring the distance from the meatus to the tip of the glans. This length is then marked on the undersurface of the foreskin, and the foreskin is split appropriately. The portion of the prepuce to be used to create the floor of the urethra is swung ventrally as a double-faced pedicle, and an island is created by removing cutis from the outer surface of the flap, leaving the undersurface isolated as an island. Alternately, the undersurface of the foreskin can be freed on a vascular pedicle, as illustrated in Figure 15–139. The width of this island is tailored, and the anastomosis to the urethral plate is made with running 7-0 Vicryl.

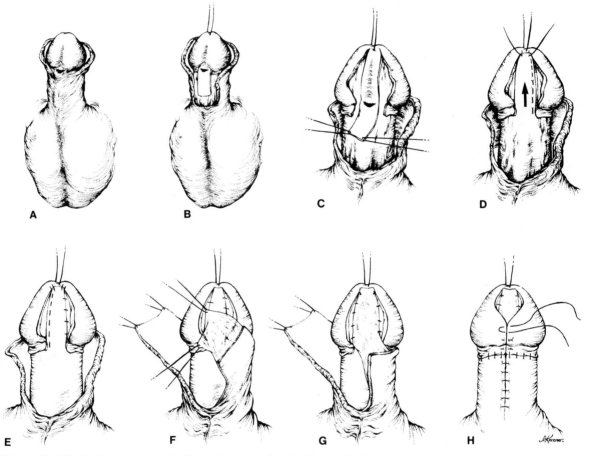

Figure 15–137 □ Mathieu repair. *A,* Coronal hypospadias. *B,* Flap outlined proximal to meatus. *C,* Deep incisions in glans to form urethral roof (dorsal aspect). *D,* Left side of anastomosis completed with running subcuticular suture. *E,* Second layer bringing subcutaneous tissue of flap over first suture line on left and completion of right sided anastomosis. *F, G,* De-epithelialized dorsal skin flap brought into glans covering neourethra. *H,* Completion of repair.

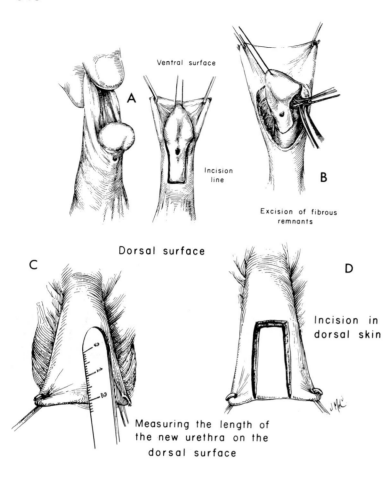

Figure 15–138 □ *A–J,* Hodgson II repair for mid to distal hypospadias without chordee. An island flap using the undersurface of the hooded prepuce is brought ventral and used as an onlay to complete the floor of the urethra. This island uses sagittal rather than transverse tissue. (From Hodgson NB: Hypospadias and urethral duplications. *In* Campbell's Urology. Fourth ed. Edited by JH Harrison, RF Gittes, AD Perlmutter, et al. Philadelphia, WB Saunders Co, 1978.)

The edge on the pedicle side is run first with a simple suture on the inner aspect of the proposed urethra, thus inverting its edges. The opposite edge is run on its outer aspect using a subcuticular stitch to achieve the same result. The remaining portion of the previously split preputial flap is de-epithelialized and brought ventrally to completely cover the newly constructed urethra, carrying it into the glans to offer a complete covering protecting the suture lines. Excessive skin is excised, and skin edges are tailored with 6-0 Vicryl suture.

Distal Hypospadias with True Chordee

In those situations in which chordee persists following release of the ventral skin, transection of the skin distal to the hypospadiac meatus becomes necessary to achieve penile straightening. Shapiro (1986) recommended a free graft as a means of dealing with the problem. This author's current choice would be an island pedicle tube utilizing foreskin.

However, meatal-based flap techniques can also be applied.

Flip-Flap Procedure. Horton and Devine (1973) introduced a meatal-based flap procedure combining contributions by Bevin and Mustardé that allows release of distal chordee as well as creation of a glanular meatus in a single stage (Fig. 15–140). The distal urethra is freed to release chordee, resulting in its retraction proximally. Assuming adequate, potentially hairless skin exists proximal to that recessed meatus, that skin is flapped distally. The glans is triangularized to accept the flap, thereby diminishing the risk of meatal stenosis but creating a glans with a characteristic snub-nosed appearance. Transposed prepuce is used to cover the resultant ventral skin defect.

Mustardé Procedure. The meatal-based flap in this urethroplasty is wider and is itself completely tubularized to form the neourethra. Therefore, because no tissue distal to the hypospadiac meatus is utilized in formation of the urethra, dissection to release chordee at that juncture is possible. One disadvantage is

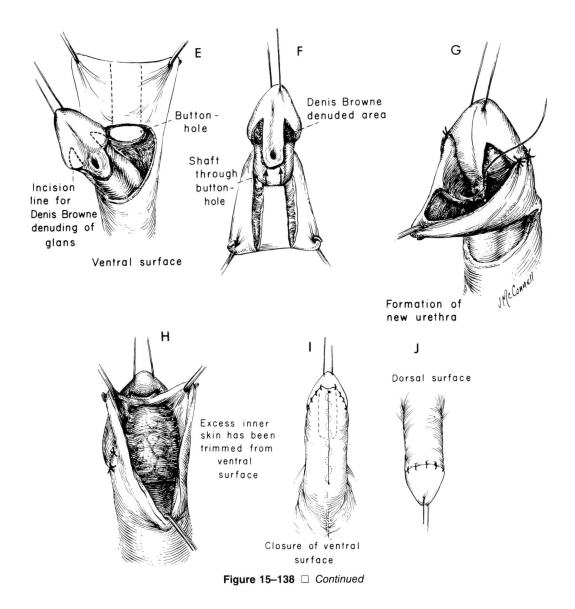

E

Button-hole

Incision line for Denis Browne denuding of glans

Ventral surface

F

Denis Browne denuded area

Shaft through button-hole

G

Formation of new urethra

H

Excess inner skin has been trimmed from ventral surface

I

Closure of ventral surface

J

Dorsal surface

Figure 15–138 □ *Continued*

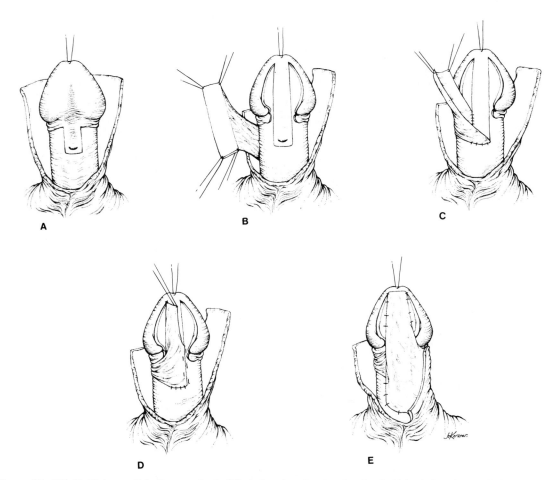

A

B

C

D

E

Figure 15–139 □ Onlay pedicle flap repair. *A,* Skin is freed up leaving the distal urethral plate intact. *B,* Incisions are carried distally into the glans incising to Buck's fascia and a segment of the hooded prepuce is freed on its pedicle and swung ventral. *C, D,* The anastomosis to the urethral plate is made. *E,* The remaining segment of prepuce unused for formation of the neourethra is de-epithelialized and used to cover the repair. Closure is completed as in the Mathieu repair.

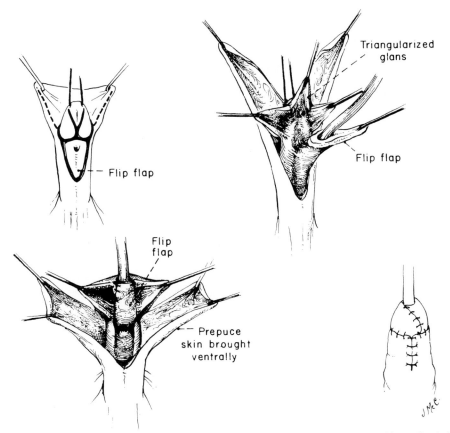

Figure 15–140 ☐ Horton and Devine's flip-flap repair for distal shaft hypospadias with or without distal chordee. (From Hodgson NB: Hypospadias and urethral duplications. *In* Campbell's Urology, 4th ed. Edited by JH Harrison, RF Gittes, AD Perlmutter, et al. Philadelphia, WB Saunders Co, 1978.)

that the flap must be considerably wider than that used in the Mathieu procedure with the potential risk for distal devascularization and meatal stenosis. Obtaining a wider meatal based flap also leaves a larger ventral defect which oftentimes makes closing the ventral skin in the midline difficult. On the other hand, a single dorsal suture line that is abutted against the ventral corpora and glans may serve to reduce the risk for a fistula. This procedure is particularly well suited to the glans channel technique for glansplasty, and success has been reported by both Belman (1982) and Klimberg and Walker.

Penile Hypospadias with Chordee

Asopa et al, Hodgson, Standoli, Duckett (1981a), and Harris and Jeffrey have contributed variations on an isolated pedicle flap using transposed dorsal skin to create the urethra. Each has its advocates, advantages, and dis-

advantages. The most recent procedure offered by Asopa and Asopa and by Hodgson (Wacksman) utilized a double-faced preputial island. The advantage of this technique is reduction of crossing suture lines, thereby theoretically decreasing the likelihood of fistula. A disadvantage is reduced ability to tailor skin ventrally and the transposition of dorsal skin of different pigmentation, possibly resulting in a patchwork appearance on the ventral aspect of the penis. It has been suggested that this appearance is not long-lasting. Duckett's variation, using an isolated island on its own pedicle, allows complete separation of the flap from its surrounding skin, creating the opportunity to cover the ventrum of the penis in the midline with split transposed prepuce. This offers ultimate cosmesis with a midline raphe. By combining Duckett's approach with a second layer of de-epithelialized skin or tunica vaginalis, as described previously, one can keep complications to a minimum (Belman, 1988).

Finally, in plastic surgery literature, use of a midline scrotal septal "neurovascular" island pedicle has been advocated (S. Y. Li). The theory is based on the prediction of a hairless midline scrotal raphe 1 cm wide that can be widely swung to form the urethra. Yachia, on the other hand, suggests that this repair might necessitate low-dose irradiation or depilation to achieve a hairless tube. It is this author's belief that long-term success with scrotal skin does not equal that of prepuce and one should probably consider reserving this approach for those circumstances in which alternatives do not exist.

Transverse Island Flap Urethroplasty (Fig. 15–141). Chordee is completely released by

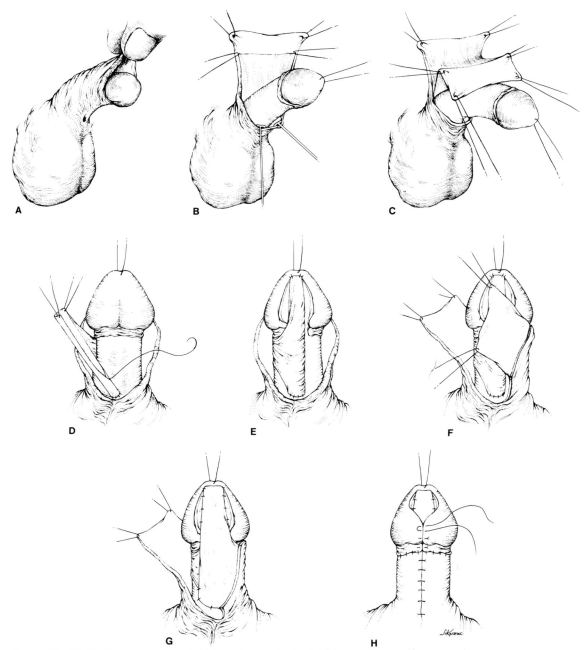

Figure 15–141 ☐ Transverse preputial island flap repair. *A–C*, Release of chordee and dissection of undersurface of dorsal prepuce. *D*, Anastomosis and tubularization of island flap. *E*, Creation of meatus (glans split). *F*, De-epithelialization of one half of remaining hooded prepuce used to cover neourethra *(G)*. *H*, Completion of ventral skin closure using midline technique for better cosmesis.

the usual techniques. The dorsal skin is dissected from the shaft between the superficial and deep fascial layers to the penile base. The four corners of the under surface of the prepuce are held with fine sutures, and a transverse incision is made at the junction between the inner and outer preputial layers.

Generally, the length of the undersurface of the prepuce is equal to the length of the penile shaft plus glans, thereby being adequate to form the entire neourethra. For a small child, a width of 1 cm forms about a 10 Fr. urethra. Superficial subcutaneous tissue is incised between the two preputial layers until a plane is established, preserving a thin vascular pedicle to its undersurface (Fig. 15–142). These layers are gently teased apart for a distance approximately equal to two-thirds the length of the shaft. Further dissection may be necessary if transposition of the pedicle flap results in penile torque. The resultant flap is then swung ventrally and laid parallel to the penis. The spatulated hypospadiac meatus is fixed to the ventral penile fascia with fine absorbable suture to prevent its retraction, and an anastomosis made between it and the proximal end of the pedicle flap with interrupted 7-0 Vicryl suture over a No. 8 feeding tube. The knots are placed on the outside of the urethra. The flap is then tubularized over the feeding tube using running subcuticular inverting 7-0 Vicryl suture. Any redundant tissue is carefully trimmed to prevent formation of an overly wide urethra. Some prefer forming the neourethra initially (Duckett, 1981), carrying out the proximal anastomosis secondarily. Either way, the suture line should be placed to allow abutment against Buck's fascia.

The meatus is created by splitting the glans and developing lateral wings to allow the urethra to be brought to its tip. Alternately, a wide glans channel can be created if the glans is more of the rounded variety and is not deeply grooved. The meatus is constructed using 7-0 Vicryl, carefully avoiding outpouching or gathering of the neourethra, which could end up in a roughened, asymmetric opening. There is usually adequate dorsal skin remaining to de-epithelialize and bring into the glans to completely cover the new urethra. If a glans channel is created, the de-epithelialized tissue can also be brought through the channel into the glans to achieve the same results (Fig. 15–143). If inadequate skin exists, tunica vaginalis is swung on a pedicle to cover the new urethra entirely, as suggested by Snow.

The glans is closed with mattressed 6-0 Vicryl suture and excess penile skin excised to obtain optimum cosmesis. The 3-0 silk suture that had been placed *longitudinally* in the distal glans at the start of the procedure as a traction suture (vertically placed traction sutures leave a telltale glanular scar) is used to secure the No. 8 feeding tube, which serves as an intravesical drip stent.

A double layer of Tegaderm is used for the dressing, and a double diaper is applied. The child goes home the same day, and a regimen

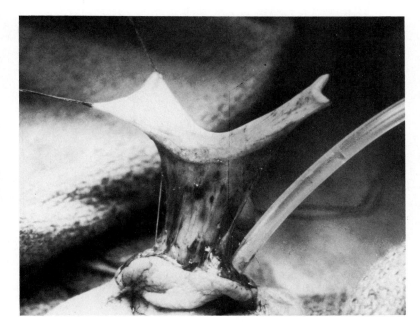

Figure 15–142 □ Transverse island pedicle flap as seen from the patient's head. Silk sutures used as traction. Redundant dorsal penile skin bunched up at base of pedicle. Silicone stent (right) exits meatus (not visible).

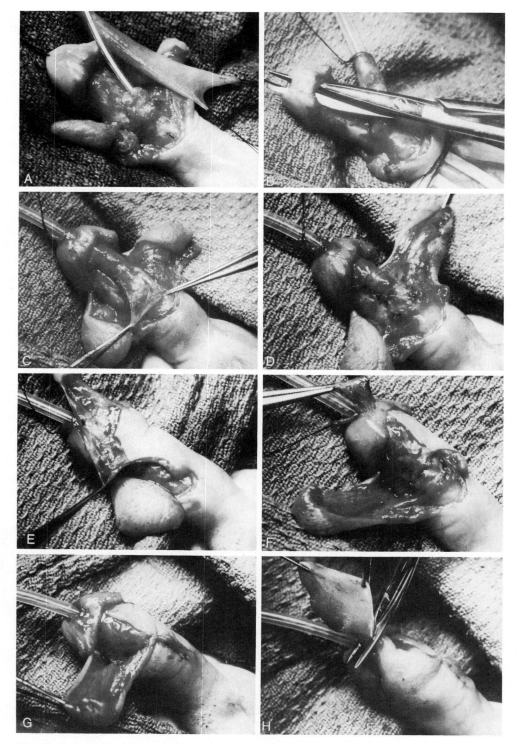

Figure 15–143 □ *A,* Midshaft hypospadias, chordee released, and island flap transferred ventral paralleling penile shaft. *B,* Neourethra formed and glans channel created. Note tourniquet at base for hemostasis. *C,* Redundant pedicle tissue brought over proximal anastomosis to cover suture line. *D,* Redundant split-hooded prepuce abundant. *E,* Prepuce de-epithelialized to provide additional coverage between neourethra and skin. *F,* De-epithelialized tissue brought with urethra through glans channel and tacked laterally to cover urethra. *G,* Skin tailored for midline closure. *H,* Redundant contralateral preputial tissue excised.

of oxybutinin chloride (Ditropan) and prophylactic trimethoprim-sulfamethoxazole is prescribed. The dressing is removed at 3 days and the intravesical stent at 7 to 10 days.

Scrotal or Perineal Hypospadias

Combined or Augmented Repair (Fig. 15–144). Rarely is the prepuce adequate to create a urethra that can extend from the perineal-scrotal area distally, even following administration of exogenous testosterone. The trick, then, is to create a tube from the hypospadiac meatus to the penoscrotal junction using other tissue. Devine (1983) recommended rolling midline, shiny, presumably hairless skin from the perineal meatus distally in a Thiersch-type fashion in combination with a free graft as the distal urethra. Glassberg (1987) applied the same principle using a transverse island pedicle distally. Alternately, if insufficient non–hair-bearing tissue exists from the hypospadiac meatus to the penoscrotal junction, a narrow

tail of the island flap, which might otherwise be discarded, may be used as an onlay. The remainder of the transverse island is then rolled in continuity to produce the distal urethra. In these complicated cases, it is rare for sufficient dorsal skin to remain after dissection of the island flap for creation of an additional de-epithelialized covering. It is in this circumstance that tunica vaginalis, easily accessible because of the previous scrotal dissection necessary to create the proximal portion of the urethra, is most applicable and advantageous.

Postoperatively, these patients require more conservative management. In a survey by Oesterling et al, 81 per cent of those pediatric urologists who responded used temporary suprapubic diversion, with two thirds also applying some form of urethral stent for penoscrotal hypospadias. Intraurethral drainage alone was used by only 13 per cent for penoscrotal repairs and 6 per cent for perineal repairs. Additionally, a short interval of scrotoperineal compression may be advisable, particularly when

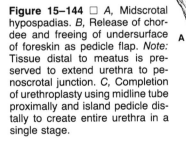

Figure 15–144 □ *A,* Midscrotal hypospadias. *B,* Release of chordee and freeing of undersurface of foreskin as pedicle flap. *Note:* Tissue distal to meatus is preserved to extend urethra to penoscrotal junction. *C,* Completion of urethroplasty using midline tube proximally and island pedicle distally to create entire urethra in a single stage.

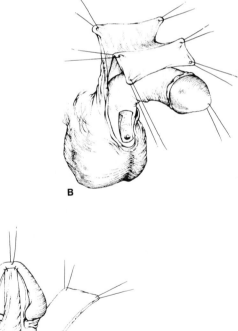

A

B

C

tunica vaginalis is used as an adjunct to prevent hematoma. The dressing, introduced by Falkowski and Firlit and applied for 48 to 72 hours, remains this author's choice in that circumstance, particularly since it compresses the perineum (see Figure 15–132).

Free Grafts. There have been many attempts to find the ideal nonpenile tissue for free graft repairs. Vessels, appendix, and skin from various sites have all been utilized. Split-thickness grafts tend to contract and therefore are not recommended. Full-thickness skin taken from "non–hair-bearing" areas other than the penis had transient popularity (Devine and Horton, 1961) but, again, are also not ideal. They may not keep up with penile growth and still have the potential to bear hair, regardless of harvest site. When skin is harvested from the undersurface of the prepuce, the majority of problems involving the use of free grafts may be obviated (Hendren and Horton; Kaplan), however, if that source is to be used, it seems more logical to swing the same skin on a well-vascularized pedicle, avoiding inherent risks related to use of a free graft.

Nevertheless, there are situations in which adequate skin does not exist to both construct urethra from a pedicle flap and cover the penis. One alternative (not recommended) is to form the urethra from penile skin and cover the shaft itself with a split-thickness graft. The cosmetic result, both visually and functionally, is never ideal, and split-thickness coverage of the penis itself should be reserved for those circumstances when no alternative exists (burns or skin avulsion).

Free bladder epithelium (popularly referred to as bladder mucosa) to form the urethra was originally described by Memmelaar in 1947. Three of four patients reported showed good results; however, the fourth died of sepsis. Subsequently, in 1981 Coleman et al and Z. Li et al reintroduced the use of bladder epithelium. Subsequently, there have been many reports of its utility (Decter et al; Ehrlich et al; Hendren and Reda; Ransley et al).

Often the bladder epithelial graft is reserved for those at greatest risk, such as "redo" hypospadias repair. Therefore, the complication rates reported tend to be high (Decter et al; Vyas et al). One predictable problem that occurs with bladder epithelium is proliferation at the site of the meatus. The epithelium at this point tends to "pout" and appear sticky (Ransley et al, 1986). It has been suggested that this can be prevented by avoiding redundancy of the distal urethra at the meatus (Ehr-

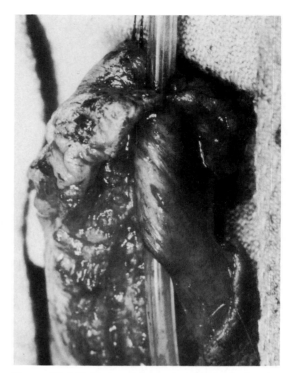

Figure 15–145 □ An adolescent male who had undergone four previous procedures had a scarred hair-bearing urethra with persistent chordee. Urethra was completely excised and chordee released. The proximal urethra from penoscrotal junction to corona was replaced with a bladder epithelial free graft. Glanular portion, formed from island pedicle taken from distal lateral penile skin shown here, tubularized around silicone stent.

lich et al). Other options include the application of a free penile skin graft (Ransley et al, 1987) distally. This author prefers to use a short offset pedicle skin flap for the glanular urethra (Fig. 15–145).

Technique. The penis is prepared with complete release of chordee as in other procedures. To best accommodate a free graft, a well-vascularized bed, free of scar, must exist. If a cavernosus patch is required to complete release of chordee, it is probably advisable to delay construction of the urethra to another stage. Nevertheless, success has been reported with a single-stage approach in this circumstance by Hendren and Keating. A few centimeters of distal penile shaft skin are advanced as an island pedicle into the glans, tubularized, and attached to the meatus with 6-0 or 7-0 Vicryl sutures. If insufficient shaft skin exists to create this pedicle flap, a free graft, preferably of penile skin, may be substituted. (However, if adequate penile skin exists to form a free graft, a pedicle can be created.)

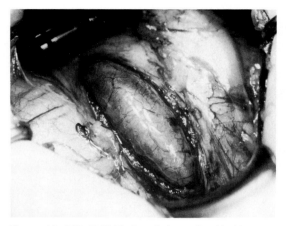

Figure 15–146 □ Epithelium bulges after bladder muscular layer is split and mobilized laterally.

After preparation of the penis, the bladder epithelium is harvested through a lower abdominal incision, the bladder having been partially filled in advance. The bladder may either be opened and the epithelium dissected directly from the inside or muscle split to the level of bulging epithelium, then peeled off as widely as necessary before harvesting epithelium (Fig. 15–146) (Hendren and Keating). In either case, more epithelium should be taken than would initially appear necessary. One should plan to use about 20 to 25 per cent greater width than measured (1.5 cm for a 12 Fr. urethra) because contraction, as may occur with all free grafts, should be anticipated. The graft is wrapped in a saline-soaked sponge while the bladder is closed. The graft is kept continuously moist during tubularization and anastomosis by means of a cool, normal saline drip. A suprapubic tube is left in the bladder.

Tubularization is accomplished over an appropriate-sized silicone tube that is left as an extravesical, intraurethral stent. A locked 7-0 running Vicryl suture is used to tubularize the urethra to prevent gathering. A widely spatulated anastomosis is created both proximally and distally to the glanular urethra, which had been previously constructed from an offset pedicle flap. If insufficient skin exists to create the glanular urethra from a pedicle flap, bladder epithelium can be employed directly; however, special care must be taken not to allow any distal redundancy. Two 7-0 sutures tacking the graft to the proximal glans may be helpful to achieve this.

Postoperatively, a compression dressing is applied for 3 days and the patient kept at bed rest for 5 days. Neovascularization (inoscula-tion) and establishment of lymphatic drainage require 4 to 5 days (Jordan et al). The patient is discharged, with both suprapubic drainage and the urethral stent intact. The stent is removed at 10 days and the suprapubic tube clamped for an additional 48 hours to test voiding prior to its removal.

Multistage Repairs

Applying the principles previously detailed, few situations exist that lead to use of a planned, multistage repair. These exceptions include the most bizarre forms of perineal hypospadias, wherein skin paucity persists in spite of pretreatment with testosterone; some instances of prescrotal transposition; and chordee, requiring corporal patch grafting.

Hypospadias in Association with Penoscrotal Transposition. Penoscrotal transposition is likely the result of failure of caudal migration of the labioscrotal folds. In its most extreme form, the penis itself may barely be visible until the scrotum is retracted laterally (Fig. 15–147). When unassociated with hypospadias, repair simply requires mobilization of the upper aspects of the scrotum and transfer below the penoscrotal junction (Fig. 15–148). However, moderate to severe chordee generally coexists and a long length of urethra may be necessary for its correction. This may be complicated by a paucity of foreskin. Staged

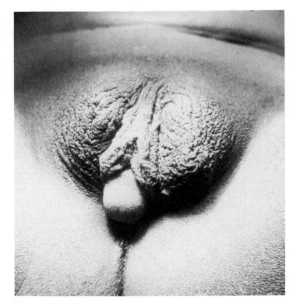

Figure 15–147 □ Severe penoscrotal transposition requiring multistage repair.

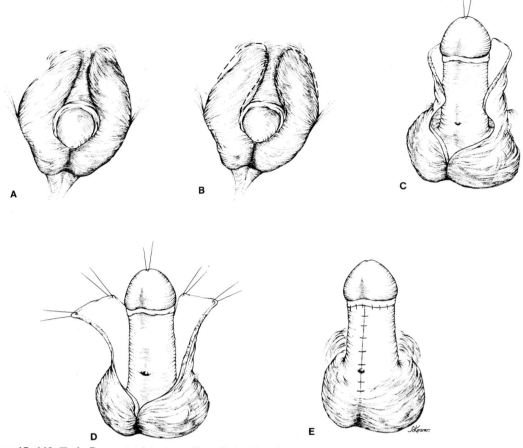

Figure 15–148 □ *A,* Penoscrotal transposition. *B,* Incision *(dotted line)* circumscribes scrotal folds leaving dorsal penile skin intact. *C–E,* Release of chordee and transposition of skin ventrally. Urethroplasty was to be completed at a later date.

repair in that circumstance may be advisable (Ehrlich and Scardino; Glenn and Anderson; Mori and Ikoma). Assuming, however, that the penile skin has remained well vascularized (a bridge of dorsal skin should be left intact) and is adequate to offer ventral skin coverage, a free bladder epithelial graft may be applied using tunica vaginalis as the additional covering layer. The postoperative care would be similar to that for a perineal hypospadias.

Redo Hypospadias Repairs

For those patients who have had multiple repairs complicated by strictures, fistulas, or persistent chordee, all one's ingenuity may be taxed to achieve a satisfactory result. These cases are not for the faint of heart, and often a very aggressive approach is necessary for success. Preoperative cystourethrography may help define urethral pathology. Additionally,

urethroscopy at the time of the planned repair is advisable, particularly when an attempt is made to evaluate the length of urethra bearing hair. Urine specimens for culture should be obtained preoperatively and specific antibiotics based on organism sensitivity initiated. Broad-spectrum (two-drug) therapy started at the onset of anesthesia is given even to those whose urine culture is negative because bacteria reside in skin crevices, suture tracts, and hair follicles. In fact, one should probably use parenteral antibiotics perioperatively in all postpubertal males undergoing urethroplasty, regardless of history of previous procedures.

All the basic steps of hypospadiology apply to this group; however, because of scarring, limited skin, and a generally older age, the application is much more difficult. Chordee must be released, and in this situation excision of dorsal fascia in the manner of Nesbit to achieve this result may be the only alternative.

As a general rule, all hair-bearing and circumferentially contracted segments of previously constructed urethra should be excised. Occasionally, however, portions may be utilized as part of the repair. If an extremely dilated portion exists, oftentimes part of its wall can be swung as a pedicle to widen strictured areas. If adequate tissue is unavailable for a pedicle flap repair, bladder epithelium may be the only reasonable tissue available for additional urethral construction. As anticipated, the complication rate in this group may be quite high in contrast to those with primary repairs (Burbige et al; Vyas et al). A more involved dressing and a greater period of bed rest and urinary diversion lead to a longer hospitalization in almost all cases. This can be justified, of course, if the problem is resolved definitively.

Complications After Repair

Chordee

Persistent chordee that interferes with function is a grievous complication that may necessitate sacrificing a functional urethra to achieve a straight penis. In that event, extensive dissection may be necessary to relieve the chordee. If the meatus has been successfully formed to the tip of the glans, then midurethral transection and simultaneous add-on urethroplasty using a pedicle flap or free graft should be considered. To avoid this complication, complete release of the penis should be verified by an artificial erection test prior to initial urethroplasty.

Meatal Stenosis

It is interesting to observe that meatal stenosis is a far less common complication than had been previously reported in spite of consistent efforts to bring the urethral meatus to the glans tip. The conclusion is that stenosis was probably the result of devascularization of the distal neourethra rather than secondary to manipulation of the glans. The use of a well-vascularized covering, such as de-epithelialized skin or tunica vaginalis, may have the value of making additional blood supply available to the distal urethra. Needless to add, however, is the importance of creating a loose tunnel in the glans through which the new urethra passes. This occurs as a natural consequence of the Mathieu procedure but must be carefully attended to with the glans channel technique.

The caliber of the post-hypospadias-repair meatus cannot be determined simply by visualization. Observing the urinary stream, or, ideally, measuring the flow rate, is the first step in evaluation for potential stenosis. Actual calibration of the urethra may be necessary in the small child in whom it is impossible to observe voiding should a question arise. It is not this author's habit to routinely calibrate or catheterize the urethra following repair or to have the family or patient dilate the meatus. If a period of meatal dilation becomes necessary, the tip of a tube of ophthalmic ointment is useful both as a dilator and simultaneous lubricant.

Post-hypospadias meatoplasty can be relatively simple when adequate, healthy distal tissue exists. Cutting back on the urethra ventrally with reapproximation of the ventral glans in a MAGPI or GAP type manner often cures the problem. Unfortunately, in most instances of significant stenosis, a portion of the distal urethra is stenotic and a more aggressive approach to its cure is required. This is discussed in the next section.

Urethral Stricture and Stenosis

Stenosis and stricture are most likely the results of poor vascularity of a flap or graft or contraction at a suture line. Symptoms in the very young child include a dribbling stream and straining to void. Often UTI is the first sign of a problem. Evaluation by urethrography is advisable prior to surgical correction, but the appearance of areas of dilatation and folds can be very misleading, since many well-functioning neourethras have a terrible appearance on urography (Figure 15–149). After determination, by observation of the stream, that there is a problem, endoscopic evaluation is the next step. A thin, iris-type stricture may respond to a single dilation or incision by urethrotomy. Scherz et al (1988) reported successful manipulative therapy (dilation or visual urethrotomy) in 55 per cent of early strictures. These were defined as presenting within 3 months of surgery. Only 16 per cent of late strictures responded to such manipulation. Barraza et al found that two thirds of strictures, most frequently occurring at the proximal anastomosis, were responsive to dilation. Generally, however, incision and reconstruction using a pedicle flap to widen the urethra is required. Should a dilated portion of the urethra lie proximal to the stenosis, part of its wall may be swung distally to serve as an onlay

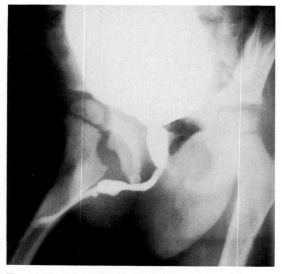

Figure 15–149 □ Post-hypospadias repair voiding cystourethrogram with relative narrowing and diverticula formation at site of proximal anastomosis. Patient asymptomatic with excellent flow.

flap. For longer areas, a pedicle of hairless penile skin can almost always be mobilized and inverted to serve as a new floor of the urethra. Scherz et al (1988) reported 79 per cent success in those who had undergone an open procedure.

Distal stenoses that extend into the glans require splitting of the glans in the midline, cutting proximal to healthy tissue. Again, an onlay similar to that described in the section on distal hypospadias without chordee (see p. 636) is best applied (Palmer and Bishai). It has been suggested that a meatal-based flap can also be useful in this situation, but its application is inadvisable if an incision has been placed proximal to the site of the current problem because vascularity to the flap would be in question (Duckett).

Urethocutaneous Fistula

Fistula remains the most common complication following hypospadias repair and serves as a bellwether regarding success of technique. Since the publication of the last edition of this book, remarkable reduction in such complications with primary repairs has been reported. With the application of a de-epithelialized or tunica vaginalis flap, this author reported a 3 per cent fistula rate in 131 consecutive cases, excluding those who had undergone MAGPI (Belman, 1988). Kass and Boling noted only one fistula in 181 such repairs. Hendren and Horton, using a free graft of prepuce to form

the urethra, reported only six fistulas in 103 cases (5.8 per cent).

To prevent fistulas, Horton and Horton suggest retrograde injection of methylene blue on completion of formation of the urethra at the time of the primary repair to ensure a watertight closure. Should a fistula occur, reoperation should be delayed for approximately 6 months to allow complete healing and resolution of tissue reaction. At that time, a retrograde injection of a dilute povidone-iodine (Betadine) solution may be used both for antisepsis and to localize all possible leaks. After approximating the edges of the defect with fine interrupted or running 7-0 vicryl, one can best achieve success by completely covering the defect with a de-epithelialized flap (Fig. 15–150) (Geltzeiler and Belman; Walker). The skin over this de-epithelialized flap acts as a second, complete covering to avoid crossing suture lines. Finally, a layer of collodian is applied as a dressing. In most instances, these problems can be resolved on an outpatient basis without the necessity for post-repair urethral stenting (Geltzeiler and Belman).

Urethral Diverticula

Urethral diverticula are usually a complication of postoperative infection or early stenosis of the distal urethra. Prevention of infection, particularly in those patients undergoing reoperation or who are beyond puberty, can be achieved by the use of parenteral bactericidal antibiotics given immediately preoperatively. Occasionally, even in the absence of infection or stenosis, the entire neourethra becomes saccular. This has been termed "acquired megalourethra" (Aigen et al) and usually presents when the family observes ballooning of the penis with voiding followed by post-micturition dribbling. It may be the result of tubularizing an excessively wide flap; if so, it can be prevented by tailoring the skin flap to form a tube of appropriate circumference at the time of the initial operation. However, it may also be the result of inadequate support of the urethra by overlying tissue.

The treatment of diverticula is generally straightforward, as more than enough tissue is present for urethroplasty. For small, less adherent diverticula, degloving of the penis to allow skin coverage without crossing suture lines after closure of the fistula has been advocated by Zaontz et al (1989). Aigen et al recommended treating the acquired megalourethra in a fashion similar to that of primary megalourethra with a de-epithelialized layer to

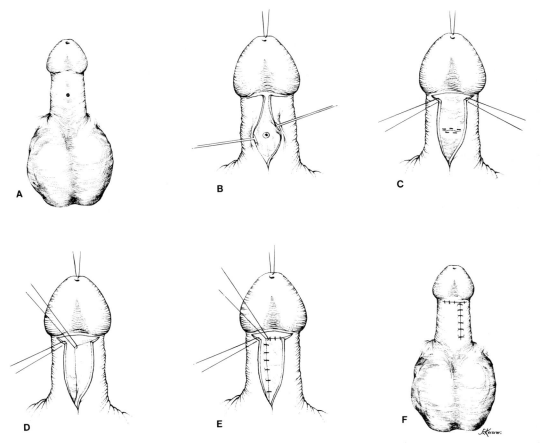

Figure 15–150 □ *A,* Repair of urethrocutaneous fistula. *B,* Fistula circumscribed and skin flaps freed laterally. *C,* Fistula closed with inverting suture. *D,* Left flap de-epithelialized. *E,* Left flap closed over fistula site. *F,* Skin closure completes two-layered covering.

both prevent fistula and to add reinforcement to prevent recurrence.

CONGENITAL URETHRAL FISTULA

Congenital fistulas of the urethra are rare. This author has seen one instance of mid-shaft fistula with an otherwise normal distal urethra in a boy who had an imperforate anus and sacral abnormality (Fig. 15–151). Goldstein, presenting a case and reviewing the literature, suggested that this is an anomaly of urethral plate development. Repair can be carried out as one would perform a second-stage Johanson urethroplasty, if adequate lateral skin is present, or by using an onlay pedicle flap.

URETHRAL PROLAPSE

Prolapse of urethral epithelium occurs most commonly in black girls under 10 years of age.

White girls represent fewer than 10 per cent of reported cases (Jerkins et al; Lowe et al). Mitie et al reported congenital prolapsed urethras in a pair of identical twins.

Patients generally present with blood spotting on their underwear and mild dysuria. Hematuria is not a frequent complaint. On physical examination, a rather typical-appearing everted, hemorrhagic, donut-shaped mass is seen superior to, but often hiding, the hymenal ring. Its size may be quite impressive (Fig. 15–152). It has been suggested that these children be evaluated to exclude bladder or vaginal sarcoma or a prolapsed ureterocele. Neither of these more serious diagnoses has the classic appearance of urethral prolapse. Therefore, should the appearance be atypical, pelvic sonography is in order.

Etiology

Lowe et al noted a cleavage plane between the two urethral muscle layers on an autopsy spec-

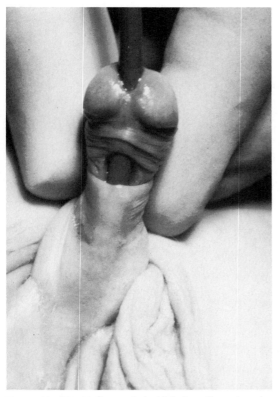

Figure 15–151 □ Congenital midshaft urethrocutaneous fistula.

imen and proposed that prolapse is the result of poor attachments between the longitudinal and circular-oblique smooth muscle of the urethra. Given the factor of race, the cause of urethral prolapse appears to be hereditary.

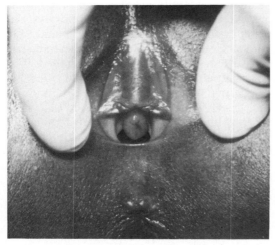

Figure 15–152 □ Urethral prolapse, which presented as "vaginal" bleeding.

Treatment

Most authors have advocated surgical excision, which can be performed rather simply as an outpatient procedure by incising the prolapsed epithelium at the 12 o'clock position and securing these edges with a holding suture. Each quadrant is then excised in turn, again approximating the edges as they are cut to avoid their retraction with potential bleeding. Use of a catheter postoperatively is not necessary. Devine and Kessel, on the other hand, advocated suprapubic vesicourethral suspension. In a child, this technique is probably overkill. Nonsurgical measures have also been advocated (Richardson et al), including application of an antimicrobial ointment only (Redman, 1982). In most instances, sitz baths appear as adequate initial treatment for girls with primary urethral prolapse. Generally, prolapse disappears within weeks, and excision should be reserved for those that either do not resolve or recur.

MEGALOURETHRA

Megalourethra is a rare congenital abnormality characterized by severe dilatation of the penile urethra. In its mildest forms, it differs little from a large congenital urethral diverticulum. In fact, it may be difficult to differentiate a urethral diverticulum secondary to an anterior epithelial flap (valve?) from an isolated area of sacular dilatation. Stephens defined the two classic types of megalourethra. The more mild form involves the urethra and spongiosum

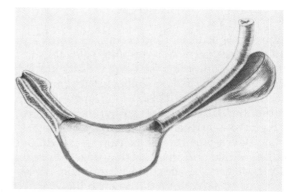

Figure 15–153 □ Scaphoid megalourethra. The corpus spongiosum is presumed to be deficient at the site of urethral expansion. (From Stephens FD: Congenital Malformations of the Rectum, Anus and Genitourinary Tracts. Edinburgh, Churchill Livingstone Ltd, 1963.)

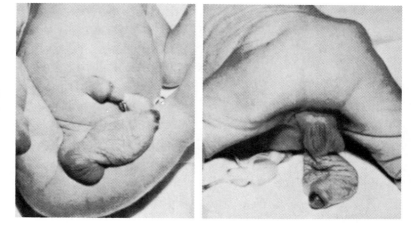

Figure 15–154 □ Fusiform megalourethra. Three-day-old infant with complete absence of corpora spongiosum and cavernosa and many other congenital anomalies, including imperforate anus.

alone. During urination the urethra dilates in a scaphoid (boat-shaped) fashion because the dorsal aspect is supported by the intact corpora (Fig. 15–153). A similar abnormality may be seen after hypospadias repair (Aigen et al). When the pathology involves all the erectile tissue with both spongiosum and cavernosum deficient, the entire phallus dilates in a fusiform (spindle) fashion with voiding (Fig. 15–154).

The etiology of the problem is unknown. It is presumed that this represents an embryologic arrest at an early phase in the development of the corpus spongiosum and corpora cavernosa, resulting in their absence or atresia. No true anatomic obstruction has been identified in either form. Neither appears to be an isolated abnormality. In boys with the scaphoid variety, often there is both associated dilatation of the prostatic urethra and vesicoureteral reflux (Fig. 15–155). This would suggest a possible relationship to the prune-belly syndrome. Fusiform megalourethra is known to be most frequently associated with prune-belly syndrome, and the majority of patients have other serious problems often incompatible with survival. All these patients require complete urologic evaluation.

Scaphoid megalourethra may first become apparent when an infant is observed voiding, although excessive, floppy penile skin is obvious even when the child is not urinating. Post-voiding dribbling is common, a result of gradual drainage of urine from the diverticular

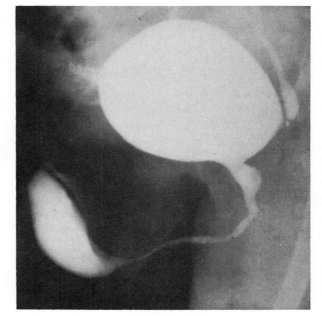

Figure 15–155 □ Voiding cystourethrogram demonstrating scaphoid expansion of the penile urethra in a 3-year-old male with reflux. (From Firlit CF: Urethral abnormalities. Urol Clin North Am 5:1, 1978.)

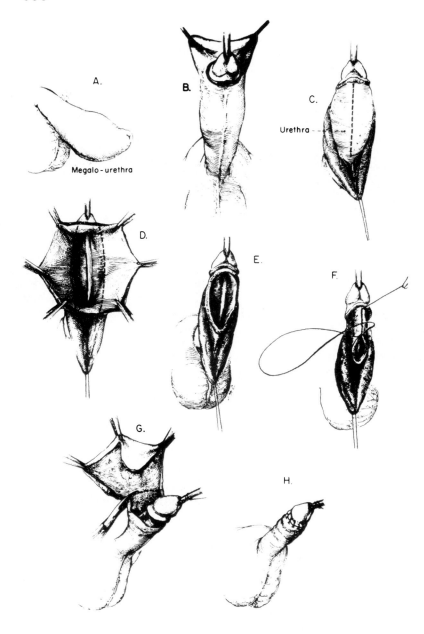

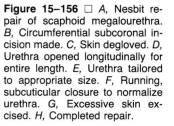

Figure 15–156 □ *A*, Nesbit repair of scaphoid megalourethra. *B*, Circumferential subcoronal incision made. *C*, Skin degloved. *D*, Urethra opened longitudinally for entire length. *E*, Urethra tailored to appropriate size. *F*, Running, subcuticular closure to normalize urethra. *G*, Excessive skin excised. *H*, Completed repair.

defect. T. Nesbit described the classic approach to its resolution (Fig. 15–156). A circumferential incision is used subcoronally, and the skin is "degloved" to the base of the penis. The urethra is tailored over an appropriate-sized catheter, reinforcing the closure with multiple layers to prevent recurrence. Excessive skin is excised and the edges reapproximated. The only area at risk for fistula is at the corona, where suture lines may cross. The catheter remains in place for 1 week.

Unless fusiform megalourethra presents as an incomplete variant, hopes for creation of a functional phallus appear nil. Should the child survive, gender reassignment is recommended at the earliest date.

URETHRAL DUPLICATION

Accessory urethra, or duplication of the urethra, is a rare anomaly. The vast majority occur in the sagittal plane; however, collateral, or side-by-side duplication in the absence of bladder duplication also exists (Kennedy et al). These lateral urethral anomalies, in the absence of an associated bladder deformity, occur almost exclusively in males and are often seen with other pelvic pathology, such as imperforate anus or partial penile duplication.

Embryology

The embryology of urethral duplication is vague because there are probably different provocations for the various types of anomalies. It is difficult to consider the cause of a Y type accessory perineal urethra as related to that causing an incomplete distal epispadiac duplication. There appears to be a misalignment of sorts between the termination of the cloacal membrane and its relationship with formation of the genital tubercle and urogenital sinus. It appears that in almost every instance, however, the ventral urethra is the normal variant.

Classification

A variety of classifications differentiate between complete and incomplete duplication. Das and Brosman applied the following simplified classification:

1. *Type I.* Complete duplication in which the accessory urethra is always more dorsally situated. Urine flows from both urethras, since they originate from the bladder.
2. *Type II.* A bifid urethra that may or may not have two external openings.
3. *Type III.* The ventral meatus is in a perineal location. This has been called an H or Y fistula.

Woodhouse and Williams divided the anomaly into four groups (Table 15–11) based primarily

Table 15–11 □ Classification of Male Urethral Duplications

Sagittal Duplication
Y-duplication: pre-anal or perineal accessory channel
Spindle urethra: urethra splits into two and then reunites
Epispadiac: dorsal penile accessory urethra
Hypospadiac: both urethrae ventral to corpora
Complete: 2 channels leave the bladder separately
Incomplete: urethra divides below the bladder
Abortive: accessory urethra is a blind sinus
Collateral Duplication
Complete with diphallus
Abortive: one urethra being a blind sinus

From Woodhouse CRJ, Williams DI: Duplications of the lower urinary tract in children. Br J Urol 51:481, 1979.

on the position of the ectopic urethral meatus. Both hypospadiac and epispadiac forms can be either complete (from the bladder), incomplete, or abortive (blind-ending sinus) (Figs. 15–157 and 15–158). A urethra that splits part way along its course and then reunites without an additional ectopic meatus is defined as a spindle duplication (Fig. 15–159), whereas one that ends ectopically in the perineum or anus is called a Y duplication (Figure 15–160).

The most complete classification has been offered by Effmann et al:

1. *Type I.* Incomplete urethral duplication.
2. *Type II.* Complete urethral duplication
   a. Two meatuses
      (1) Noncommunicating urethras arising independently from the bladder
      (2) A second channel arising from the first and exiting independently
   b. Complete duplication joining at one meatus
3. *Type III.* Duplication as a component of caudal duplication.

This classification can apply to either dorsal or ventral duplication. The Y type perineal or rectal fistula associated with a stenotic, normally located penile urethra, is placed in the IIa category.

Few cases of urethral triplication have been reported, including one in which all three channels extended from the bulbous urethra to the glans penis (Wirtshafter et al). One child had been noted to have combinations of hypospadiac and epispadiac accessory urethras (Forgaard and Ansell), and another had a hypospadiac accessory urethra extending from the prostatic urethra as well as a Y-type anomaly (Toguri et al). Zimmermann and Mildenberger reported a patient with a double Y fistula—two urethras extending to the perineum. This child also exhibited partial stenosis of the normally located urethra with a megalourethra distal to that stenosis.

The Y type fistula usually takes its origin from the prostatic urethra and is commonly associated with stenosis of the anterior portion of the normally situated urethra (Stephens and Donnellan). Rice et al reported a case without urethral stenosis, and Glassberg et al reported two children with vesicoperineal accessory urethras. Woodhouse and Williams noted a high incidence of associated urinary abnormalities in this group.

Urethral duplication in females in the absence of duplication of the bladder is extremely rare. However, a form of apparent urogenital

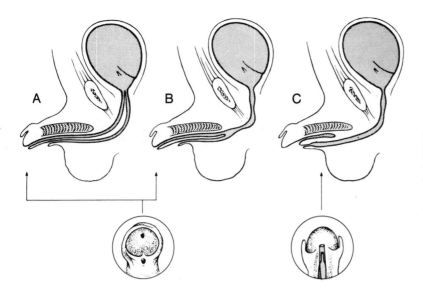

Figure 15–157 □ Hypospadiac duplication. *A,* Complete. *B,* Incomplete. *C,* Abortive. (From Woodhouse CRJ, Williams DI: Duplication of the lower urinary tract in children. Br J Urol 51:481, 1979.)

sinus abnormality exists in which an often stenotic hypospadiac ventral urethra opens into the anterior vaginal wall while a second urethra is found in the clitoris (Thiry et al). Bellinger and Duckett reviewed the subject in 1982. The external genitalia are typically flattened and posteriorly displaced, and the perineal body is deficient in this rare group of girls.

Presenting Symptoms

Children with complete and incomplete forms of accessory urethras usually present when they are observed to have two urinary streams. Occasionally, infection in a partially stenotic accessory urethra is the presenting complaint. Those with blind-ending (abortive) types rarely have symptoms. Children with Y-type abnormalities and stenosis of the normally situated urethra may void only from the perineal or anal component. Those with the ectopic orifice proximal to the anal sphincter behave similarly to the patient with a uretosigmoidostomy, voiding from the anus. Since the bladder neck is generally intact, children in this group have two levels of continence—both bladder and rectal.

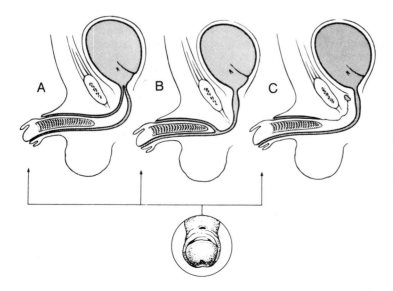

Figure 15–158 □ Epispadiac urethral duplication. *A,* Complete. *B,* Incomplete. *C,* Abortive. (From Woodhouse CRJ, Williams DI: Duplications of the lower urinary tract in children. Br J Urol 51:481, 1979.)

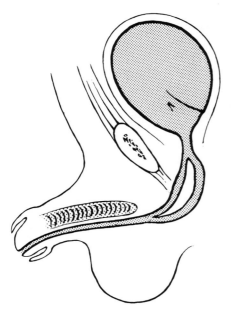

Figure 15–159 □ Spindle duplication of the urethra. (From Woodhouse CRJ, Williams DI: Duplication of the lower urinary tract in children. Br J Urol 51:481, 1979.)

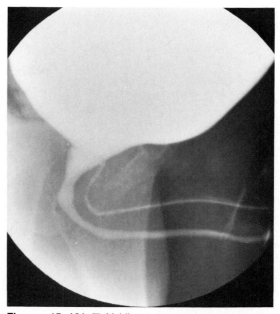

Figure 15–161 □ Voiding cystourethrogam demonstrates complete epispadiac duplication. Ventral urethra is normal.

Evaluation

An effort to determine the length of the defect should be made by retrograde urethrography. For urethras that are complete, a standard voiding cystourethrogram (VCUG) may be diagnostic (Fig. 15–161).

Treatment

Blind-ending accessory urethras generally do not cause symptoms and therefore do not

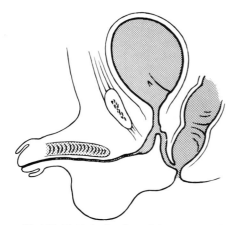

Figure 15–160 □ Y-duplication of the urethra. The accessory track may open just inside or just outside the anus. (From Woodhouse CRJ, Williams DI: Duplication of the lower urinary tract in children. Br J Urol 51:481, 1979.)

require excision. When indicated, those urethras that bifurcate distally and have closely adjacent meatuses may be joined by simply crushing and dividing the common septum. For larger septa, visual urethrotomy is a consideration (Goldstein and Hensle). Epispadiac duplications may be associated with dorsal chordee and also tend to cause irritative symptoms at the meatus. Excision with the release of the dorsal chordee is generally quite simple (Fig. 15–162).

In children with complete forms of duplication, other than joining the two tubes distally to allow a single stream, treatment is generally not necessary. Patients with a Y fistula obviously require intervention. Mobilization of the perineal limb with distal urethroplasty has been advocated (Belman, 1977b; Williams), although use of scrotal tissue to create the proximal urethra may lead to problems in the future. Alternately, one could consider a free bladder epithelial graft. Stephens and Donnellan recommended marsupialization of the atretic urethra with a secondary urethroplasty at a later date. Again, one could consider application of more updated repairs, such as an onlay pedicle or free bladder graft, in an effort to achieve this in one stage. Passerini had success with progressive dilation of an atretic penile urethra associated with the prune belly syndrome. Holst and Peterson reported fulguration of the perineal portion of a Y

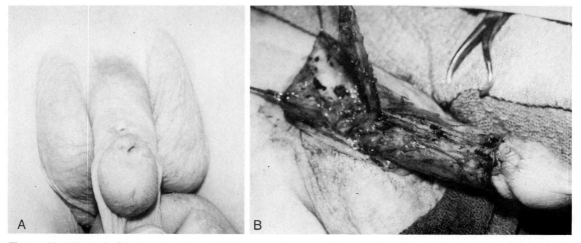

Figure 15–162 □ *A,* Blind ending (incomplete) epispadiac duplication. *B,* Dissection of duplicated urethra to penile base.

fistula in a patient in whom the dorsal urethra was the more normal of the two.

URETHRAL AGENESIS AND ATRESIA

Complete absence or stenosis of the urethra is incompatible with normal renal development. Therefore, surviving newborns must have an ancillary means for the egress of urine. Either a patent urachus or a urethrorectal communication must exist. Specific management of such a patient depends upon the underlying cause and is dealt with in the chapters pertaining to those anomalies.

URETHRAL DIVERTICULA

Primary congenital urethral diverticula are uncommon. Most are associated with some underlying cause, such as utricular enlargement occurring in intersex states, megalourethra, or as a consequence of an anterior urethral valve or deficiency of the corpus spongiosum. Most of this has been addressed previously.

Bibliography

Aarskog D: Clinical and cytogenetic studies in hypospadias. Acta Pediatr Scand (Suppl) 203:1, 1970.

Aarskog D: Maternal progestins as a possible cause of hypospadias. N Engl J Med 300:75, 1979.

Aigen AB, Khawand N, Skoog SJ, et al: Acquired megalourethra: an uncommon complication of the trans-verse preputial island flap urethroplasty. J Urol 137:712, 1987.

Allen TD, Griffin JE: Endocrine studies in patients with advanced hypospadias. J Urol 131:310, 1984.

Allen TD, Spence HM: The surgical treatment of coronal hypospadias and related problems. J Urol 100:504, 1968.

Arap S, Mitre AI, DeGoes GM: Modified meatal advancement and glanuloplasty repair of distal hypospadias. J Urol 131:1140, 1984.

Arey LB: The external genitalia. *In* Developmental Anatomy, 7th ed. Philadelphia, WB Saunders Co, 1974, p 337.

Asopa R, Asopa HS: One stage repair of hypospadias using double island preputial skin tube. Indian J Urol 1:41, 1984.

Asopa HS, Elhence EP, Atria SP, et al: One stage correction of penile hypospadias using a foreskin tube: a preliminary report. Int Surg 55:435, 1971.

Bartone F, Shore N, Newland J, et al: The best suture for hypospadias? Urology 29:517, 1987.

Bauer SB, Retik AB, Colodny AH: Genetic aspects of hypospadias. Urol Clin North Am 8:559, 1981.

Beck C: A new operation for balanic hypospadias. NY Med J 67:147, 1898.

Bellinger MF, Duckett JW: Assessory phallic urethra in the female patient. J Urol 127:1159, 1982.

Belman AB: De-epithelialized skin flap coverage in hypospadias repair. J Urol 140:1273, 1988.

Belman AB: The modified Mustarde hypospadias repair. J Urol 127:88, 1982.

Belman AB: The repair of a congenital H-type urethrorectal fistula using a scrotal flap urethroplasty. J Urol 118:659, 1977a.

Belman AB: The urethral advancement procedure. Society for Pediatric Urology Newsletter, December 28, 1977b.

Belman AB, Kass EJ: Hypospadias repair in children under one year of age. J Urol 128:1273, 1982.

Bennett AH, Gittes RF: Congenital penile curvature without hypospadias. Urology 16:364, 1980.

Berg G, Berg R: Castration complex: evidence from men operated for hypospadias. Acta Psychiatr Scand 68:143, 1983.

Berg R, Berg G: Penile malformation, gender identity

and sexual orientation. Acta Psychiatr Scand 68:154, 1983.

Bracka A: A long term view of hypospadias. Br J Plast Surg 42:250, 1989.

Broadman LM: Regional anesthesia for the pediatric outpatient. Urol Clin North Am 5:53, 1987.

Burbige KA, Hensle TW, Edgerton P: Extragenital split thickness skin graft for urethral reconstruction. J Urol 131:1137, 1984.

Cendron J, Melin Y: Congenital curvature of the penis without hypospadias. Urol Clin North Am 8:389, 1981.

Chang TS: Anterior urethral advancement: a one stage technique for hypospadias repair. Br J Plast Surg 37:530, 1984.

Chen YC, Wooley PV Jr: Genetic studies on hypospadias in males. J Med Genet 8:153, 1971.

Coleman JW, McGovern JH, Marshall VF: The bladder mucosal graft technique for hypospadias repair. Urol Clin North Am 8:457, 1981.

Creevy CD: The correction of hypospadias: a review. Urol Surg 8:2, 1958.

Coulam CB, Razel AJ, Kelalis PP, et al: Androgen receptor in human foreskin: II. Characterization of the receptor from hypospadiac tissue. Am J Obstet Gynecol 147:513, 1983.

Culp OS, McRoberts JW: Hypospadias. *In* Encyclopedia of Urology, Vol II/1. Edited by CE Alken, VW Dix, WE Goodwin, et al. New York, Springer-Verlag, 1968.

Czeizel A, Tóth J: Correlation between the birth prevalence of isolated hypospadias and parental subfertility. Teratology 41:167, 1990.

Das S, Brosman SA: Duplication of male urethra. J Urol 117:452, 1977.

Davenport M, MacKinnon AE: The value of ultrasound screening of the upper urinary tract in hypospadias. Br J Urol 62:595, 1988.

Decter RM, Roth DR, Gonzales ET Jr: Hypospadias repair by bladder mucosal graft: an initial report. J Urol 140:1256, 1988.

DeSy WA, Oosterlinck WIM: Silicone foam elastomer: a significant improvement in postoperative penile dressing. J Urol 128:39, 1982.

Devine CJ Jr: Chordee in hypospadias. *In* Urologic Surgery, 3rd ed. Edited by James F. Glenn. Philadelphia, JB Lippincott Co., 1983.

Devine CJ Jr, Gonzales-Serva L, Stecker JF Jr, et al: Utricular configuration in hypospadias and intersex. J Urol 123:407, 1980.

Devine CJ, Horton CE: A one stage hypospadias repair. J Urol 85:166, 1961.

Devine CJ Jr, Horton CE: Chordee without hypospadias. J Urol 110:264, 1973.

Devine CJ Jr, Horton CE: Use of dermal graft to correct chordee. J Urol 113:56, 1975.

Devine PC, Kessel HC: Surgical correction of urethral prolapse. J Urol 123:856, 1980.

Dimler M, Gibbons MD, Haley A: A modification of the MAGPI procedure. J Pediatr Surg 19:627, 1984.

Donahoe PK: Neoseminal vesicle created from retained mülerian duct to preserve the vas in male infants. J Pediatr Surg 23:272, 1988.

Duckett JW: Hypospadias. *In* Adult and Pediatric Urology. Edited by JY Gillenwater, JT Grayhack, SS Howards, JW Duckett. Chicago, Year Book Medical Publishers, 1987.

Duckett JW: MAGPI (meatoplasty and glanuloplasty): a procedure for subcoronal hypospadias. Urol Clin North Am 8:513, 1981b.

Duckett JW: The island flap technique for hypospadias repair. Urol Clin North Am 8:503, 1981a.

Duckett JW, Keating MA: Technical challenge of the megameatus intact prepuce hypospadias variant: the pyramid procedure. J Urol 141:1407, 1989.

Duval P: Chirugie del appareil genital de l'homme. *In* Precise de Technique Operatoir. Paris, Maisson et Cie, 1920, pp 170–172.

Effman EL, Lebowitz RL, Colodny AH: Duplication of the urethra. Radiology 119:179, 1976.

Ehrlich RM, Reda EF, Koyle MA, et al: Complications of bladder mucosal graft. J Urol 142:626, 1989.

Ehrlich RM, Scardino PT: Surgical correction of scrotal transposition and perineal hypospadias. J Pediatr Surg 17:175, 1982.

Elder JS, Duckett JW, Snyder HM: Onlay island flap in the repair of mid and distal penile hypospadias without chordee. J Urol 138:376, 1987.

Falkowski WS, Firlit CF: Hypospadias surgery: the X-shaped elastic dressing. J Urol 123:904, 1980.

Fallon B, Devine CJ Jr, Horton CE: Congenital anomalies associated with hypospadias. J Urol 116:585, 1976.

Feldman KW, Smith DW: Fetal phallic growth and penile standards for newborn male infants. J Pediatr 86:395, 1975.

Firlit CF: The mucosal collar in hypospadias surgery. J Urol 137:80, 1987.

Forgaard DM, Ansell JS: Trifurcation of the anterior urethra. J Urol 95:785, 1966.

Frey P, Cohen SJ: Reconstruction of foreskin in distal hypospadias repair. Prog Pediatr Surg 23:192, 1989.

Gaylis FD, Zaontz MR, Dalton D, Sugar EC, Maizels M: Silicone foam dressing for penis after reconstructive pediatric surgery. Urology 33:296, 1989.

Gearhart JP, Linhard HR, Berkovitz GD, et al: Androgen receptor levels and 5 alpha-reductase activities in preputial skin and chordee tissue of boys with isolated hypospadias. J Urol 140:1243, 1988.

Geltzeiler J, Belman AB: Results of closure of urethrocutaneous fistulas in children. J Urol 132:734, 1984.

Gibbons MD, Gonzales ET Jr: The subcoronal meatus. J Urol 130:739, 1983.

Gilbert DA, Devine CJ Jr, Winslow BH, et al: Microsurgical hypospadias repair. Plast Reconstr Surg 77:460, 1986.

Gittes RF, McLaughlin AP III: Injection technique to induce penile erection. Urology 4:473, 1974.

Glassberg KI: Augmented Duckett repair for severe hypospadias. J Urol 138:380, 1987.

Glassberg KI, Schwarz R, Haller JO: Vesicoperineal accessory urethra. J Urol 120:255, 1978.

Glenn JF, Anderson EE: Surgical correction of incomplete penoscrotal transposition. J Urol 110:603, 1973.

Goldstein HR, Hensle TW: Visual urethrotomy in management of male urethral duplication. Urology 18:374, 1981.

Goldstein M: Congenital urethrofistula with chordee. J Urol 113:138, 1975.

Gonzalez R, Vivas C: Pediatric urethral reconstruction without proximal diversion. J Urol 136:264, 1986.

Guthrie RD, Smith DW, Graham CB: Testosterone treatment for micropenis during early childhood. J Pediatr 83:247, 1973.

Harris DL, Jeffrey RS: One stage repair of hypospadias using split preputial flaps (Harris): the first 100 patients treated. Br J Urol 63:401, 1989.

Hastie KJ, Deshpande SS, Moisey CU: Long-term follow-up of the MAGPI operation for distal hypospadias. Br J Urol 63:320, 1989.

Hatch DA, Maizels M, Zaontz MR, et al: Hypospadias hidden by a complete prepuce. Surg Gynecol Obstet 169:233, 1989.

Hendren WH: Construction of female urethra from vaginal wall and perineal flap. J Urol 123:657, 1980.

Hendren WH, Horton CE Jr: Experience with one-stage repair of hypospadias and chordee using free graft of prepuce. J Urol 140:1259, 1988.

Hendren WH, Keating MA: Use of dermal graft and free urethral graft in penile reconstruction. J Urol 140:1265, 1988.

Hendren WH, Reda EF: Bladder mucosa graft for construction of male urethra. J Pediatr Surg 21:189, 1986.

Hodgson NB: Use of vascularized flaps in hypospadias repairs. Urol Clin North Am 8:471, 1981.

Hollowell JG, Keating MA, Snyder HM, et al: Preservation of the urethral plate in hypospadias repair: extended applications and further experience with the onlay island flap urethroplasty. J Urol 143:98, 1990.

Holst S, Peterson NE: Fulguration-ablation of atypical accessory urethra. J Urol 140:347, 1988.

Horton CE, Devine CJ Jr: One stage repair-III. In Plastic and Reconstructive Surgery for the Genital Area. Edited by CE Horton. Boston, Little, Brown & Co, 1973, p 278.

Horton CE Jr, Horton CE: Complications of hypospadias surgery. Clin Plast Surg 15:371, 1988.

Hurwitz RS, Ozersky D, Kaplan HJ: Chordee without hypospadias: Complications and management of hypoplastic urethra. J Urol 138:372, 1987.

Ikoma F, Shima H, Yabumoto H: Classification of enlarged prostatic utricle in patients with hypospadias. Br J Urol 57:334, 1985.

Ikoma F, Shima H, Yabumoto H, et al: Surgical treatment for enlarged prostatic utricle and vagina masculina in patients with hypospadias. Br J Urol 58:423, 1986.

Ikoma HS, Terakawa T, Satoh Y, et al: Developmental anomalies associated with hypospadias. J Urol 122:619, 1979.

Issa MM, Gearhart JP: The failed MAGPI: management and prevention. Br J Urol 64:169, 1989.

Jerkins GR, Verheeck K, Noe HN: Treatment of girls with urethral prolapse. J Urol 132:732, 1984.

Jones HW Jr, Scott WW: Hermaphroditism, Genital Anomalies and Related Endocrine Disorders, 2nd ed. Baltimore, William & Wilkins, 1971.

Jordan GH, Schlossberg SM, McGraw JB: Tissue transfer techniques for genitourinary reconstructive surgery: Part I. Principles, Definitions, Basic Techniques and Graft Techniques. AUA Update Series 7 (9:68), 1988.

Källen B: Case control study of hypospadias, based on registry information. Teratology 38:45, 1988.

Källen B, Bertollini R, Castilla E, et al: A joint international study on the epidemiology of hypospadias. Acta Paediatr Scand Suppl 324:1, 1986.

Kaplan GW: Repair of proximal hypospadias using a preputial free graft for neourethral construction and a preputial pedicle flap for ventral skin coverage. J Urol 140:1270, 1988.

Kaplan GW, Lamm DL: Embryogenesis of chordee. J Urol 114:769, 1975.

Kass EJ, Boling D: Single stage hypospadias reconstruction without fistula. J Urol 144:520, 1990.

Kelly D, Harte FB, Roe P: Urinary tract anomalies in patients with hypospadias. Br J Urol 56:316, 1984.

Kennedy HA, Steidle CP, Mitchell ME, et al: Collateral urethral duplication in the frontal plane: a spectrum of cases. J Urol 139:332, 1988.

Khuri FJ, Hardy BE, Churchill BM: Urologic anomalies associated with hypospadias. Urol Clin North Am 8:565, 1981.

King LR: Hypospadias—a one stage repair without skin graft based on a new principle: chordee is sometimes produced by the skin alone. J Urol 103:660, 1970.

Klimberg I, Walker RD: A comparison of the Mustarde and Horton Devine flip-flap techniques of hypospadias repair. J Urol 134:103, 1985.

Knorr D, Beckmann D, Bidlingmaier F, et al: Plasma testosterone in male puberty: II. HCG stimulation test in boys with hypospadias. Acta Endocrinol (Copenh) 90:365, 1979.

Kogan SJ, Reda EF, Smey PL, et al: Dermal graft correction of extraordinary chordee. J Urol 130:952, 1983.

Kramer SA, Aydin G, Kelalis PP: Chordee without hypospadias in children. J Urol 128:539, 1982.

Lau JTK: Penile block for pain relief after circumcision in children. Am J Surg 147:797, 1984.

Li SY, Li SK, Zhuang HX: Use of scrotal septal neurovascular pedicle island skin flap in one stage repair of hypospadias. Ann Plast Surg 15:529, 1985.

Li Z, Zheng Y, Sheh Y, et al: One stage urethroplasty for hypospadias using a tube constructed with bladder mucosa—a new procedure. Urol Clin North Am 8:463, 1981.

Livne PM, Gibbons MD, Gonzales ET Jr: Correction of disproportion of corpora cavernosa as cause of chordee in hypospadias. Urology 22:608, 1983.

Lowe FC, Hill GS, Jeffs RD, et al: Urethral prolapse in children: Insight into etiology and management. J Urol 135:100, 1986.

Lutzker LG, Kogan SJ, Levitt SS: Is routine intravenous urography indicated in patients with hypospadias? Pediatrics 59:630, 1977.

Manley CB, Epstein ES: Early hypospadias repair. J Urol 125:698, 1981.

Memmelaar J: Use of bladder mucosa in a one-stage repair of hypospadias. J Urol 58:66, 1947.

Mitchell ME, Kulb TB: Hypospadias repair without a bladder drainage catheter. J Urol 135:321, 1986.

Mitie A, Nahas W, Gilbert A, et al: Urethral prolapse in girls: familial case. J Urol 137:115, 1987.

Mori Y, Ikoma F: Surgical correction of incomplete penoscrotal transposition associated with hypospadias. J Pediatr Surg 21:46, 1986.

Nasrallah PF, Minott HB: Distal hypospadias repair. J Urol 131:928, 1984.

Nesbit RM: Congenital curvature of the phallus: report of three cases with description of corrective operation. J Urol 93:230, 1965.

Nesbit TE: Congenital megalourethra. J Urol 73:839, 1955.

Nonomura K, Fujieda K, Sakakibara N, et al: Pituitary and gonadal function in prepubertal boys with hypospadias. J Urol 132:595, 1984.

Oesterling JE, Gearhart JP, Jeffs RD: Urinary diversion in hypospadias surgery 1987. Urology 29:513, 1987.

Palmer JM, Bishai MB: Island pedicle graft in the correction of urethral meatal stenosis following hypospadias repair. J Urol 135:1227, 1986.

Passerini G: Severe urethral hypoplasia: new concepts in treatment. Presented at the annual meeting of the Section on Urology, American Academy of Pediatrics. New Orleans, November 2, 1987.

Perlmutter AD, Montgomery BT, Steinhardt GF: Tunica vaginalis free graft for the correction of chordee. J Urol 134:311, 1985.

Persky L, Hoffman A, DesPrez J: The repair of chordee without hypospadias. J Urol 98:216, 1967.

Polednak AP, Janerich DT: Maternal characteristics and hypospadias: a case control study. Teratology 28:67, 1983.

Rabinowitz R: Outpatient catheterless modified Mattieu hypospadias repair. J Urol 138:1074, 1987.

Ransley PG, Duffy PG, Oesch IL, et al: Autologous

bladder mucosa graft for urethral substitution. Br J Urol 58:331, 1986.

Ransley PG, Duffy PG, Oesch IL, et al: The use of bladder mucosa and combined bladder mucosal preputial skin grafts for urethral substitution. J Urol 138:1096, 1987.

Redman JF: Conservative management of urethral prolapse in female children. Urology 19:505, 1982.

Redman JF: Dorsal curvature of penis. Urology 21:479, 1983.

Redman JF: Tourniquet as hemostatic aid in repair of hypospadias. Urology 28:241, 1986.

Richardson DA, Hajj SN, Herbst AL: Medical treatment of urethral prolapse in children. Obst Gynec 59:69, 1982.

Ritchey ML, Benson RC Jr, Kramer SA, et al: Management of müllerian duct remnants in the male patient. J Urol 140:795, 1988.

Retik AB, Keating M, Mandell J: Complications of hypospadias repair. Urol Clin North Am 15:223, 1988.

Rozenman J, Hertz M, Boichis H: Radiological findings of the urinary tract in hypospadias: a report of 110 cases. Clin Radiol 30:471, 1979.

Sandberg DE, Meyer-Bahlburg HFL, Aranoff GS, et al: Boys with hypospadias: A survey of behavioral difficulties. J Pediatr Psychology 14:491, 1989.

Scherz HC, Kaplan GW, Packer MG: Modified meatal advancement and glanuloplasty (Arap hypospadias): experience of 31 patients. J Urol 142:620, 1989.

Scherz HC, Kaplan GW, Packer MG, et al: Posthypospadias repair urethral strictures: a review of 30 cases. J Urol 140:1253, 1988.

Scheuer S, Hanna MK: Effective nitroglycerine ointment on penile skin flap survival in hypospadias repair: experimental and clinical studies. Urology 27:438, 1986.

Schultz JR, Klykylo WM, Wacksman J: Timing of elective hypospadias repair in children. Pediatrics 71:349, 1983.

Schweikert HU, Schluter M, Romalo G: Intracellular and nuclear binding of (3H) dihydrotestosterone in cultured genital skin fibroblasts of patients with severe hypospadias. J Clin Invest 83:662, 1989.

Section on Urology, American Academy of Pediatrics: The Timing of Elective Surgery on the Genitalia of Male Children with Particular Reference to Undescended Testes in Hypospadias. Pediatrics 56:479, 1975.

Shafir R, Hertz M, Boichis H: Vesicoureteral reflux in boys with hypospadias. Urology 20:29, 1982.

Shapiro SR: Free graft patch one-stage procedure to repair penile hypospadias unsuitable for the flip-flap procedure: indications and experience. J Urol 136:433, 1986.

Shapiro SR: Hypospadias repair: optical magnification versus zeiss reconstruction microscope. Urology 33:43, 1989.

Shelton TB, Noe HN: The role of excretory urography in patients with hypospadias. J Urol 134:97, 1985.

Shima H, Ikoma F, Yabumoto H, et al: Gonadotropin and testosterone response in prepubertal boys with hypospadias. J Urol 135:539, 1986.

Smith ED: Malformations of the bladder and urethra, and hypospadias. In Pediatric Surgery. Edited by TM Holder, KW Ashcraft. Philadelphia, WB Saunders Co., 1980, page 785.

Snow BW: Use of tunica vaginalis to prevent fistulas in hypospadias surgery. J Urol 136:861, 1986.

Standoli L: One stage repair of hypospadias: preputial island flap technique. Ann Plast Surg 9:81, 1982.

Stephens FD: Congenital intrinsic lesions of the anterior urethra. In Congenital Malformations of the Urinary Tract. New York, Praeger, 1983, pp 128–130.

Stephens FD, Donnellan WL: "H-type" urethroanal fistula. J Pediatr Surg 12:95, 1977.

Sugar EC, Firlit CF: Urinary prophylaxis and postoperative care of children at home with an indwelling catheter after hypospadias repair. Urology 32:48, 1988.

Svensson J, Snochowski M: Androgen receptor levels in preputial skin from boys with hypospadias. J Clin Endocrinol Metab 49:340, 1979.

Sweet RA, Schrott HG, Kurland R, et al: Study of the incidence of hypospadias in Rochester, Minnesota, 1940–1970, and a case-controlled comparison of possible etiologic factors. Mayo Clin Proc 49:52, 1974.

Thiry AJ, Wincqz PJ, Schulman CC: Female pseudohermaphroditism with supplementary plastic urethra. Urol 5:285, 1979.

Toguri AG, Churchill BM, Rabinowitz R: Y-type urethral triplication. J Urol 118:684, 1977.

Tsur H, Shafir R, Shachar J, et al: Microphallic hypospadias: Testosterone therapy prior to surgical repair. Br J Plast Surg 36:398, 1983.

VanDorpe EJ: Correction of distal hypospadias with reconstruction of the preputium. Plast Reconstr Surg 80:290, 1987.

Vyas PR, Roth DR, Perlmutter AD: Experience with free grafts in urethral reconstruction. J Urol 137:471, 1987.

Wacksman J: Modification of the one stage flip flap procedure to repair distal penile hypospadias. Urol Clin North Am 8:527, 1981.

Wacksman J: Repair of hypospadias using new mouth-controlled microscope. Urology 29:276, 1987.

Wacksman J: Results of early hypospadias surgery using optical magnification. J Urol 131:516, 1984.

Wacksman J: Use of the Hodgson XX (modified Asopa) procedure to correct hypospadias with chordee: surgical technique and results. J Urol 136:1264, 1986.

Walker RD: Outpatient repair of urethral fistulae. Urol Clin North Am 8:582, 1981.

Walker RD, Graham B: Measurement of blood flow in hypospadias flaps with subvisual doses of fluorescein. J Urol 136:266, 1986.

Walsh PC, Curry N, Mills RC, et al: Plasma androgen response to HCG stimulation in prepubertal boys with hypospadias and cryptorchidism. J Clin Endocrinol Metab 42:52, 1976.

Waterhouse K, Glassberg KI: Mobilization of the anterior urethra as an aid in the one stage repair of hypospadias. Urol Clin North Am 8:521, 1981.

Wesson L, Mandell J: Single stage hypospadias repair using the operating microscope. Microsurgery 6:182, 1985.

Williams DI: Male urethral anomalies. In Pediatric Urology, 2nd ed. Edited by DI Williams, JH Johnston. London, Butterworth Scientific, 1982.

Wirtschafter A, Carrion HM, Morillo G, et al: Complete trifurcation of urethra. J Urol 123:431, 1980.

Woodhouse CRJ, Williams DI: Duplications of the lower urinary tract in children. Br J Urol 51:481, 1979.

Yachia D: Correction of penile curvatures caused by unsuccessful hypospadias repair using the scrotal septum pedicled skin tube principle combined with corporoplasty and a modified meatoglanuloplasty. Ann Plast Surg 23:269, 1989.

Zaontz MR: The GAP (glans approximation procedure) for glanular/coronal hypospadias. J Urol 141:359, 1989.

Zaontz MR, Kaplan WE, Maizels M: Surgical correction of anterior urethral diverticula after hypospadias repair in children. Urology 33:40, 1989.

Zimmermann H, Mildenberger H: Posterior urethral duplication and triplication in the male. J Pediatr Surg 15:212, 1980.

☐ Index

Note: Page numbers in *italics* indicate illustrations; page numbers followed by t indicate tables.

i